ECHOCARDIOGRAPHIC DIAGNOSIS OF CONGENITAL HEART DISEASE

An Embryologic and Anatomic Approach

ECHOCARDIOGRAPHIC DIAGNOSIS OF CONGENITAL HEART DISEASE

An Embryologic and Anatomic Approach

Edited by

Lilliam M. Valdes-Cruz, M.D.
Professor of Pediatrics
Director, Cardiac Imaging Laboratory
Associate Chief, Division of Cardiology
The Children's Hospital
University of Colorado Health Sciences Center
Denver, Colorado

Raul O. Cayre, M.D.
Former Assistant Professor of Pediatrics
Division of Cardiology
The Children's Hospital
University of Colorado Health Sciences Center
Denver, Colorado
and
Professor
Facultad de Medicina
Universidad Nacional del Nordeste
Corrientes, Argentina

with the technical assistance of Ole A. Knudson, Jr.

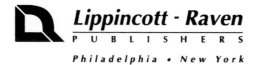

Lippincott - Raven
P U B L I S H E R S
Philadelphia • New York

Acquisitions Editor: Ruth W. Weinberg
Developmental Editor: Ellen DiFrancesco
Manufacturing Manager: Tim Reynolds
Production Manager: Jodi Borgenicht
Production Editor: Deirdre Marino-Vasquez
Cover Designer: Levavi & Levavi
Indexer: Frances Lennie
Compositor: CJS Tapsco
Printer: Courier Westford

Printed and bound in the United States of America

9 8 7 6 5 4 3 2 1

Library of Congress Cataloging-in-Publication Data

Echocardiographic diagnosis of congenital heart disease: an embryologic and
    anatomic approach/edited by Lilliam M. Valdes-Cruz, Raul O. Cayre.
        p.   cm.
    Includes index.
    ISBN 0-7817-1433-8
    1. Ultrasonic cardiography.   2. Congenital heart disease—Diagnosis.
3. Echocardiography.   4. Embryology, Human.   5. Anatomy, Pathological.
I. Valdes-Cruz, Lilliam M.   II. Cayre, Raul O.
    [DNLM: 1. Heart Defects, Congenital—diagnosis.   2. Echocardiography—
methods.   3. Heart Defects, Congenital—embryology.   WG 220E18 1998]
RC683.5.U5E23   1998
616. 1'207543—dc21
DCLM/DLC
for library of Congress   98-26987
                                                                        CIP

To my brothers, for their unconditional support; my daughters Ana
and Lorena, for accepting my absence; and my wife Diana, whose support,
understanding, and love enabled me to participate in the completion of this book.

R.O.C.

To my parents Dr. Oscar and Mrs. Clara Valdes-Cruz, who always served as
examples of academic excellence and honesty;
and Alina U. Borges, for her trust in us and her support of this book.

L.V-C.

Contents

Contributors

Raul O. Cayre, M.D.   *Former Assistant Professor of Pediatrics, Division of Cardiology, The Children's Hospital, University of Colorado Health Sciences Center, Denver, Colorado 80218; and Professor, Facultad de Medicina, Universidad Nacional del Nordeste, Corrientes, Argentina*

Kevin Y. Chung, R.D.M.S.   *President, Cardiovascular Imaging Consultants, 344 DeClaire Way, Marietta, Georgia 30067*

Curt G. DeGroff, M.D.   *Assistant Professor of Pediatrics, Division of Cardiology, The Children's Hospital, University of Colorado Health Sciences Center, 1056 East 19th Avenue, Denver, Colorado 80218*

D. Dunbar Ivy, M.D.   *Assistant Professor of Pediatrics, Division of Cardiology, The Children's Hospital, University of Colorado Health Sciences Center, 1056 East 19th Avenue, Denver, Colorado 80218*

Ole A. Knudson, Jr.   *Senior Professional Research Assistant, Department of Pediatrics, Division of Cardiology, The Children's Hospital, University of Colorado Health Sciences Center, 1056 East 19th Avenue, Denver, Colorado 80218*

Elizabeth M. Shaffer, M.D.   *Associate Professor of Pediatrics, Division of Cardiology, The Children's Hospital, University of Colorado Health Sciences Center, 1056 East 19th Avenue, Denver, Colorado 80218*

Robin S. Shandas, Ph.D.   *Adjunct Assistant Professor, Department of Mechanical Engineering, University of Colorado, Boulder, Colorado; Assistant Professor of Pediatrics, Cardiovascular Flow Dynamics Laboratory, Division of Cardiology, The Children's Hospital, University of Colorado Health Sciences Center, 1056 East 19th Avenue, Denver, Colorado 80218*

Lilliam M. Valdes-Cruz, M.D.   *Professor of Pediatrics, Director, Cardiac Imaging Laboratory, Associate Chief, Division of Cardiology, The Children's Hospital, University of Colorado Health Sciences Center, 1056 East 19th Street, Denver, Colorado 80218*

Foreword

I am delighted to write the foreword to *Echocardiographic Diagnosis of Congenital Heart Disease: An Embryologic and Anatomic Approach,* edited and primarily written by Drs. Raul O. Cayre and Lilliam Valdes-Cruz, both at the time of this writing at the University of Colorado, Department of Pediatrics, Division of Pediatric Cardiology.

This is a very comprehensive and contemporary textbook devoted to the echocardiographic diagnosis of congenital heart disease. Very complete and beautifully illustrated, it is divided into 13 parts and is organized in a thoughtful and indeed logical and comprehensive manner. Part I focuses on general considerations and appropriately begins with the embryological development of the heart and great vessels, and then moves on to the nomenclature and segmental analysis of congenital cardiac malformations. It is important to understand the physics and instrumentation of diagnosis, and in the remainder of Part I, the co-authors examine the techniques of the echocardiographic examination of the heart and great vessels, the aspects of quantitative and Doppler echocardiography, and the more novel applications of three-dimensional echocardiography.

Part II focuses on anomalies of visceroatrial situs. There is considerable discussion of the concepts of bilateral right-sidedness and left-sidedness syndromes, placing these into important clinical perspectives. The following parts discuss anomalies of cardiac septation, anomalies of the atrioventricular valves, and anomalies of ventricular looping. Part VI provides a very important discussion of anomalies of the ventricles. In this section the authors focus on various descriptive terms of the atrioventricular univentricular connection, including double-inlet ventricle, classic tricuspid atresia, and mitral atresia. Part VII focuses on anomalies of the ventricular outflow tracts and Parts VIII and IX move on to hypoplastic left-heart syndrome and conotruncal abnormalities. In Part X there is considerable discussion on the anomalies of the aortic arches, including coarctation of the aorta, interruption of the aortic arch, patent arterial duct, and vascular rings. The final three parts of this very thorough book detail anomalies of systemic and pulmonary venous connections; abnormal origins of the coronary arteries, including fistulas and aneurysms; and give an echocardiographic evaluation of patients with pulmonary hypertension.

Among the many attractive features of this wonderful book are the historical aspects, the beautiful line drawings that are carefully and constructively labeled, and the "art quality" of the echocardiographic imaging. Almost all of the common forms of congenital heart disease are well-represented and many very rare anomalies are well-documented, including isolated ventricular inversion, which perhaps should be termed "isolated atrioventricular discordance"; heart with superior-inferior ventricles and crossed atrioventricular connections; and other forms of complex double-inlet ventricles. From simple to very complex, the authors provide in a logical and stepwise fashion the approach to diagnostic echocardiographic imaging, providing insights from their vast clinical experiences, including the potential pitfalls, hazards, and errors that we have all encountered.

I am very pleased to write this Foreword because this book illustrates so clearly the reality that the student soon becomes the teacher, which is the important aspect of academic medicine. I have known

Dr. Valdes-Cruz since she was a resident at Johns Hopkins and I am very proud of her signal accomplishments in pediatric cardiovascular medicine and in the development and application of echocardiographic imaging and diagnosis of congenital heart disease.

Robert M. Freedom, M.D., F.R.C.P. (C), F.A.C.C.
Head, Division of Cardiology
The Hospital for Sick Children
Professor of Pediatrics (Cardiology) & Pathology
The University of Toronto
Faculty of Medicine
Toronto, Canada

Preface

Those who have dissected or inspected many bodies, have at least learned to doubt; when others, who are ignorant of anatomy and do not take the trouble to attend to it, are in no doubt at all.

De Sedibus et Causis Morborum per Anatomen Indagatis
J. B. Morgagni, 1760

Echocardiographic Diagnosis of Congenital Heart Disease: An Embryologic and Anatomic Approach is based on the fundamental consideration that the objective of echocardiography is to define the form and determine the function of the heart. Defining the form is the first step in the echocardiographic study of congenital cardiac malformations. The normal anatomic characteristics of a form, in this case of the heart and great vessels, are the consequence of normal embryologic development, while an abnormal developmental process is expressed anatomically as a malformation. In this context, it becomes self-evident that if the normal morphogenetic processes are not comprehended thoroughly, malformations cannot be understood. Further, specifically as applied to any imaging modality and to echocardiography in particular, the observer cannot appreciate structures in the images that he or she does not recognize. In this book, we have attempted to address these needs by amalgamating three basic concepts: embryologic development, anatomic expression, and functional assessment. We appreciate the suggestion of Dr. Maria Victoria de la Cruz, Director of the Laboratory of Experimental Embryology and Teratology at the Hospital Infantil de Mexico "Federico Gomez," who first proposed the need for this approach.

In order to analyze the probable morphogenesis of the various congenital cardiac malformations, it is of absolute importance to understand the normal development of the heart and great vessels. As such, the first chapter discusses the normal embryologic development of the heart and great vessels, including information provided by descriptive embryology as well as that contributed by experimental embryologic techniques. It is possible that there may be some contention regarding certain theories as addressed in that chapter. Nonetheless, we feel that it provides a solid foundation for the understanding of normal and abnormal cardiac morphogenesis.

Each of the subsequent chapters on the various congenital cardiac anomalies includes a brief historical perspective on the first publication of each particular case. This is followed by a section on embryologic considerations, which includes the various theories that attempt to explain the probable morphogenesis of each lesion. The anatomic characteristics and echocardiographic study of the specific malformation, in the classic anatomic expression, their anatomic variants, and the associated anomalies, are discussed in detail. Finally, issues pertinent to the intraoperative and postoperative studies, including early and late follow-up, are specifically defined for the various surgical procedures currently utilized.

In all chapters, the sections on the echocardiographic study include the use of M-mode, two-dimensional imaging, and spectral and color Doppler techniques. In addition, the intraoperative evaluation describes the transesophageal approach to imaging congenital cardiac anomalies. The chapter on echocardiographic evaluation of pulmonary hypertension includes recent findings on intravascular imaging of small pulmonary arteries.

In this book we aim to provide the reader with the information necessary to approach the difficult art of imaging congenital cardiac malformations in a sequential and scientific manner. Therefore, we have addressed the book to cardiologists and cardiology fellows, in both pediatric and medical training programs, who are faced with the care of children and adults with congenital heart disease; to cardiovascular surgeons who operate on patients with congenital cardiac malformations; and to sonographers who most directly have the responsibility of obtaining images that will lead to correct diagnoses.

If, as a result of our efforts, we contribute, even in a small way, to a better life for these patients and their families, we will have accomplished our most desired goal.

Lilliam M. Valdes-Cruz
Raul O. Cayre

Acknowledgments

A book devoted to the echocardiographic diagnosis of congenital cardiac malformations must stand as a tribute to the support and collaboration of innumerable individuals. We would like to acknowledge the unwavering support offered us by all the members of the Division of Pediatric Cardiology at The Children's Hospital, University of Colorado Health Sciences Center, Denver. Specifically we would like to thank Mark M. Boucek, Chief of the Division of Cardiology, for offering an environment where academic productivity and scientific excellence is fostered; Henry M. Sondheimer, who patiently and caringly edited the manuscript; and Michael S. Schaffer, who revised parts of the text and is consistently willing to contribute his knowledge in our daily reading sessions. We would like to thank The Children's Hospital Foundation and Demosthenes A. Argys, Administrator, Department of Pediatrics, for the financial support offered us, without which this project would not have been accomplished.

The physicians and sonographers in our Cardiac Imaging Laboratory at The Children's Hospital provided us with the moral, professional, and skilled support needed to complete this seemingly impossible task. We thank Elizabeth M. Shaffer, our closest colleague, for her willingness to "cover" for us during innumerable hours of writing, editing, drawing, photographing, and so on. Curt DeGroff, the newest member of our echo lab team, was always ready to help us in the service duties and in obtaining beautiful transesophageal intraoperative images. His contribution, most evident in his excellent chapter on Doppler echocardiography, is deeply appreciated. Without the consistent production of high-quality echocardiograms by our skilled sonographers we would not have had the clinical material to present in this book. We specially thank K. Scott Kirby, RDCS, Supervisor of the Cardiac Imaging Laboratory, for his meticulous attention to detail.

Ole A. Knudson, Jr. has been our colleague for a number of years. His level of knowledge, expertise of ultrasound technology, and understanding of congenital heart disease have made him an invaluable contributor and collaborator in our clinical and research laboratories. He single-handedly completed all the schematic drawings and helped select all clinical echocardiograms used in this book. He edited the manuscript for technical accuracy and participated in all levels of its preparation. We deeply thank him for his consistent commitment to excellence.

We thank our colleagues in the Cardiovascular Flow Dynamics Laboratory, Robin S. Shandas, PH.D., and Jeffrey Kwon, MSEE, for their dedication to the study of flow phenomena that so deepens our understanding of clinical echocardiography.

A meticulous research of the literature serves as the backbone for this type of book. We began each chapter by acquiring a thorough list of pertinent references and obtaining copies of all available publications in order to confirm their content and the accuracy of the citations. All references that were not readily found were then procured for us by Becky Berg, Cathy LeGrand, and Carol Freimark, the untiring personnel of the Forbes Medical Library at The Children's Hospital. We also thank the librarians at the Dennison Library, University of Colorado Health Sciences Center, for allowing us to enter the Waring Room, where old medical books are kept.

Most of the echocardiographic material in the book is from the Cardiac Imaging Laboratory at The Children's Hospital. Nonetheless, we have also utilized material made available to us by echocardiographers from other institutions. Although we have acknowledged their contributions and, when previously published, that of the publishers, we would like to thank them for their generosity.

We must acknowledge the support, motivation, humor, and wise perspective offered by Alina U. Borges, who for the last three years has lived through the journals, references, illustrations, manuscripts, and endless hours at the computer, while always providing an environment where we could work quietly and carefully. We thank you.

We would like to extend our appreciation to Ruth Weinberg, our editor at Lippincott-Raven Publishers. She provided us with guidance and support through difficult times during the preparation of the illustrative material. Her trust in the project gave us the stimulus to continue working until its completion.

Finally, we must recognize the role of Shari Borcherding, Administrative Assistant of the Cardiac Imaging Laboratory and the Cardiovascular Flow Dynamics Laboratory at The Children's Hospital. She carefully typed the multiple drafts and maintained order throughout chaotic times. She managed to keep the laboratories at full functioning capacity, untiringly staying ahead of deadlines for grants, abstracts, and scientific meetings, and sustaining the flow of manuscripts while at the same time seeing the book to its completion. We deeply acknowledge her contribution to the clinical and scientific productivity of our laboratories.

Lilliam M. Valdes-Cruz
Raul O. Cayre

This book represents a multitude of important moments in my life. In addition to the scientific and technical information, it is filled with different times and places, colleagues and moments, embryos and specimens, a search for knowledge, and a living next to children and their parents involved in the reality of suffering a congenital cardiac malformation. It is also filled with moments of solitude, absence, and loss.

The arrival at a specific moment in one's life is not an isolated event. There are innumerable individuals who contributed to this accomplishment. I would like to express my gratitude to all who were important at one point or another in my life. I would first like to thank God for allowing me to arrive at what I am today. Secondly, I would like to thank all my professors in the Escuela Normal, Quitilipi, Argentina, my birthplace, for fostering in me the desire to learn. I would especially like to thank my professor of Botany and Zoology, Mrs. Maria L. Carrio de Rodriguez, for putting a microscope in my hands and creating a love for research in me. To Dr. Abel Bengolea, former Chief of Cardiology of the Hospital Instituto de Cardiologia "Fundacion H. Pombo de Rodriguez," Buenos Aires, Argentina, for encouraging my love of cardiology. To Dr. Eliseo Segura, former Associate Chief of Cardiac Surgery of the Hospital Instituto de Cardiologia "Fundacion H. Pombo de Rodriguez," for putting in my hands for the first time a heart with a congenital malformation and awakening my interest in this condition. To Dr. Manuel Quero Jimenez, Chief of Pediatric Cardiology, and to my friends and members of the staff at the Centro Especial Ramon y Cajal, Madrid, Spain, for contributing to my education as a pediatric cardiologist. To my colleagues during residency, Drs. Carlos Alvarez, Alfonso Robles, Mario Cazzaniga, and Oscar Saravalli, for their thoughts and discussions that helped to cement my knowledge of cardiology and pediatrics, and for the friendship that has united us for so many years. To my former colleagues in the Laboratory of Cardiovascular Embryology at the Centro Especial Ramon y Cajal, Madrid, and in the Laboratory of Experimental Embryology and Teratology at the Hospital Infantil de Mexico "Federico Gomez" for sharing their interest in cardiovascular embryology. To Dr. Hector Bidogia, Emeritus Professor of the Faculty of Medicine, Universidad del Salvador, Buenos Aires, Argentina, for being an example of a physician and teacher, for his wise advice, and for the honor of his friendship. To Prof. Dr. Samuel Bluvstein, Dean, and Dr. Julio D. Civetta, Vice-Dean, Faculty of Medicine, Universidad Nacional del Nordeste, Corrientes, Argentina, and to Professors Edgardo Marecos, Juan F. Gomez Rinesi, and Miguel Ramos of the VI Clinical Medicine Department, Faculty of Medicine of the Universidad del Nordeste, for offering me the opportunity to continue my academic activities in my country and for honoring me with their friendship.

I would like to thank my friends Drs. Pedro Gimenez, Diego Micheli, Alicia Marquez, and Mario Cazzaniga for offering their suggestions during revisions of several chapters in the initial manuscript.

To my father Luis and my mother Rosa, who passed away before the completion of this book. To my aunt Elisa, my gratitude for teaching me honesty and decency as a way of life. To my brothers for offering me unconditional love and the privilege of a family. To my daughters Ana and Lorena who, beyond their desire to have me at their side, accepted my absence and encouraged my participation in this book.

Finally and most especially to my wife Diana, to whom I dedicate this book, as evidence of my gratitude for understanding love as respect and freedom. I thank her for allowing me to use that freedom without which I could not have participated in the writing of this book.

R.O.C.

Nearly 38 years ago my family left Cuba for the United States following the realization that they were ideologically in disagreement with the Communist policies that were being implanted there. As a physician, my father had to validate his credentials in Florida and I, as a 12-year-old continued my studies in the United States. As I reflect back on those years, a number of individuals stand out for the encouragement and inspiration they provided me both professionally and personally. Dr. Emilio Soto Pradera, former Professor of Pediatrics at Georgetown University School of Medicine, served as an example of the ultimate pediatrician for his wisdom, compassion, and breadth of knowledge of childhood diseases. He was a personal friend of my family and had been my pediatrician when I was a child in Cuba. As a medical student at Georgetown he provided me with my first experience in clinical pediatrics in the summer between my second and third years and inspired me to dedicate my career to the care of children. As a third-year medical student rotating through the Neonatal Service at Georgetown University Hospital, I met Dr. Joseph K. Perloff, who was offering a consult on a neonate with truncus arteriosus. His lucid explanation of the physiology of this complex malformation caught my imagination and I immediately decided to pursue a career in pediatric cardiology, with the purpose of investigating the morphogenetic processes and hopefully preventing these lesions. Joe has remained a mentor and has offered me his friendship throughout these years; I thank him for both. I had the privilege of meeting Dr. Richard D. Rowe while I was in training at The Johns Hopkins Hospital. He was present also when, as a fellow, I presented my first paper at a Scientific Sessions of the American Heart Association. His integrity, honesty, gentleness, and ability to always encourage the best in people have continued to be a source of inspiration in my career. Dr. Daniel R. Pieroni taught me all the echocardiography I know and, while I was still a fellow at Johns Hopkins, patiently encouraged and helped me through my first experiences in research and my first scientific publications. He is still a close friend and colleague. Dr. Robert M. Freedom saw me through my first cardiac catheterization as a first-year fellow at Johns Hopkins. I thank him for writing the Foreword to this book and for his interest in my career. I would also like to acknowledge the support and motivation I received from the pediatric cardiology faculty at Johns Hopkins, all of whom were pioneers in the field: Helen B. Taussig, Catherine Neill, Glenn Rosenquist, P. Jacob Varghese, Jerry Krovetz, and Lulu Haroutunian.

About 20 years ago I met Drs. Stanley J. Goldberg, Hugh D. Allen, and David J. Sahn, who approached me with the proposal that I join their group at the University of Arizona Health Sciences Center as an Assistant Professor. At that time they were the premier group in pediatric ultrasound and were responsible for many of the technical advances in the field. With them I had the opportunity to be involved in the advancement of two-dimensional imaging and in the first developments and validations of spectral and, later, color Doppler techniques.

In 1983 David and I moved to the University of California at San Diego and continued to pursue research in the field of ultrasound together. Eventually this led to a mutual interest in analyzing flow phenomena in the heart from a fundamental approach using Doppler techniques. Our dialogue with engineers led us to utilize *in vitro* models and flow visualization methods and, in collaboration with an old friend and colleague from Johns Hopkins, Dr. Michael Jones of the National Heart, Lung and Blood Institute, Bethesda, to apply our insights in complex animal models. I will always be indebted to David for offering me the opportunity and for providing an environment where I could develop intellectually and professionally, and where my interests in research were appreciated and encouraged. He remains a dear friend and close collaborator, despite our presently working at different institutions.

I thank my parents, to whom I personally dedicate this book, for their encouragement and their effort in always providing me with the means to pursue my academic interests, despite the hardships of a political exile. They were a source of inspiration for their dedication to intellectual honesty and scholarly pursuits. I am sorry my father died before I completed my medical studies. Finally, I would like to thank Alina U. Borges for her support and trust in us and in this book.

L.V-C.

PART I

General Considerations

CHAPTER 1

Embryologic Development of the Heart and Great Vessels

Lilliam M. Valdes-Cruz and Raul O. Cayre

To understand the probable morphogenesis of the various congenital cardiac malformations, it is essential to know the changes that occur at the different stages of normal cardiac development. Knowledge to date is based on descriptive embryologic studies of human embryos and on the contributions of experimental embryologic techniques applied to biologic models whose cardiac development is considered to be similar to that of humans. Results from descriptive embryology are somewhat questionable (1,2), however, as are those from experimental embryology (3), because no confirmation has been obtained in the human embryo. Nonetheless, much information is available on normal human cardiac development, which is summarized in this chapter.

The processes of cardiac development have been grouped into two stages. The first stage, early cardiogenesis, or the premorphologic stage, starts at the fertilization process and ends at the formation of the two lateral endothelial heart tubes. The second stage, the morphologic stage, starts at the straight or primitive heart tube and ends at the mature heart stage.

EARLY CARDIOGENESIS, OR PREMORPHOLOGIC STAGE

Embryologic development begins with the fertilization process (4)—that is, the fusion of the male and female gametes. In the human species, this usually takes place in the ampullary region of the uterine tube (5), giving rise to the fertilized ovum or zygote.

Initially, the zygote is unicellular, but then it undergoes a series of cleavages that results in an increase in the number of cells, or blastomeres, without an increase in overall size. This dense, multicellular structure is the morula (Fig. 1-1A). As the process of segmentation continues, the morula is transformed into a blastocyst, which consists

of an outer cell mass, or trophoblast, an eccentrically located inner cell mass, the embryoblast, and a central cavity, the blastocyst cavity (Fig. 1-1B). The embryoblast has two cell layers, an external layer, or epiblast, and an internal layer, or hypoblast; these form a flat disc, known as the bilaminar germ disc or embryonic disc (Fig. 1-1C).

In the blastocyst stage, the cell groups that will give rise to the different organs are already present and occupy precise topographic locations (2,6). The precardiac cells are located in the epiblast at each side of the primitive streak along its middle third (6,7) (Fig. 1-1D).

At the end of the blastocyst stage, a series of cellular movements, the morphogenetic movements, begins; these give origin to the gastrula (Fig. 1-1E–G). The epiblast cells migrate through the primitive streak to a position between the epiblast and the hypoblast, giving rise to an intermediate cell layer, the intraembryonic mesoderm (Fig. 1-1E). The gastrula is composed of three layers of cells: an external one, the ectoderm, originating from the epiblast; a middle one, the mesoderm; and an internal one, the endoderm, formed primarily of cells derived from the epiblast and probably from a portion of the hypoblast (Fig. 1-1F).

The precardiac or prospective heart cells also migrate through the primitive streak and come to be located in the mesoderm on both sides of the Hense node in the anterior half of the primitive streak; these constitute the cardiogenic areas. They are joined at the midline in the prechordal region, forming the cardiogenic plate (6–8) (Fig. 1-1F–G).

The rapid development of the cephalic process and neural tube as well as the formation of the foregut bring about an anterior folding of the cardiogenic plate (Fig. 1-2). Simultaneously, the rapid development of the somite areas results in a ventral folding of the lateral portions of the embryo. This folding process also occurs in the region

A   **MORULA**

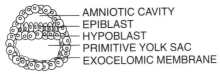

INNER CELL MASS
BLASTOCYST CAVITY
TROPHOBLAST

B   **EARLY BLASTOCYST**

AMNIOTIC CAVITY
EPIBLAST
HYPOBLAST
PRIMITIVE YOLK SAC
EXOCELOMIC MEMBRANE

C   **LATE BLASTOCYST**

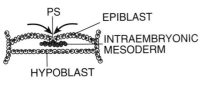

AMNIOS CUT EDGE

EPIBLAST
PN
PS

PRECARDIAC CELLS

D   **LATE BLASTOCYST**

PS
EPIBLAST
INTRAEMBRYONIC MESODERM
HYPOBLAST

E

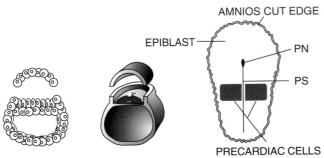

ECTODERM   MESODERM
ECTODERM
PN
ENDODERM   CARDIOGENIC AREAS
PS
MESODERM

F

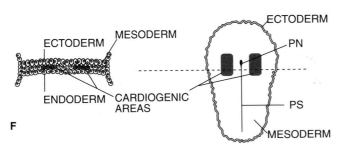

ECTODERM
ECTODERM   MESODERM
PN
ENDODERM   CARDIOGENIC PLATE
PS
MESODERM

G

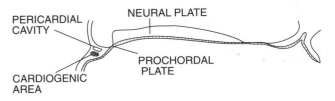

PERICARDIAL CAVITY   NEURAL PLATE
PROCHORDAL PLATE
CARDIOGENIC AREA

A

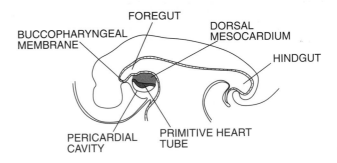

FOREGUT
BUCCOPHARYNGEAL MEMBRANE   DORSAL MESOCARDIUM
HINDGUT
PERICARDIAL CAVITY   PRIMITIVE HEART TUBE

B

FIG. 1-2. Schematic drawing of a right lateral view of a sagittal cut of an embryo, showing the location of the cardiogenic areas and the rotation over its transverse axis. See text for details. **A:** Presomite embryo. **B:** Embryo of 14 paired somites.

of the cardiogenic plate, resulting in the formation of two lateral endothelial heart tubes, right and left, located between the endoderm and the embryonic splachnopleura, which thickens in the region next to the endothelial heart tube to form the myocardial plate (9) (Fig. 1-3A). The two endothelial heart tubes migrate toward the midline, through a process of ventralization, and fuse (10). The fusion of the medial walls of both tubes occurs in a cephalocaudal direction (5) and gives origin to the straight-tube heart or primitive heart tube (Fig. 1-3B).

It is important to point out that initially, in the presomite embryo, the location of the cardiogenic area is anterior to the prechordal plate in a ventral position relative

FIG. 1-1. Schematic drawing of the various stages of early cardiogenesis. **A:** Morula. **B:** Early blastocyst. **C:** Frontal section of embryo in the late blastocyst stage. **D:** Resection of the amniotic sac during late blastocyst stage, showing the location of the precardiac cells in the epiblast on both sides of the primitive streak. **E:** Frontal section of the late blastocyst, showing the migration of the cells of the epiblast, which will give origin to the intraembryonic mesoderm. **F:** Frontal section of the gastrula after resection of the amniotic sac and the ectoderm, showing the three layers that compose it and the cardiogenic areas of the mesoderm. **G:** Frontal section of the gastrula after resection of the amniotic sac and ectoderm, showing the location of the cardiogenic plate within the mesoderm. *PS*, primitive streak; *PN*, primitive node.

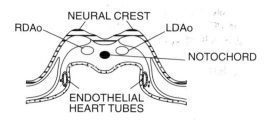

A

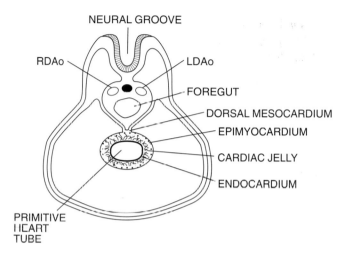

B

FIG. 1-3. Schematic drawing of a frontal cut of an embryo, showing the location of the endothelial heart tubes and the formation of the primitive heart tube. See text for details. **A:** Embryo of two paired somites. **B:** Embryo of 12 paired somites. *RDAo*, right dorsal aorta; *LDAo*, left dorsal aorta.

to the pericardial cavity, which originates in the intraembryonic coelom (Fig. 1-2A). With the rapid development of the central nervous system, the cardiac primordium rotates 180 degrees over its transverse axis and comes to lie caudally, behind the buccopharyngeal membrane and below the anterior wall of the foregut (11) (Fig. 1-2B). The pericardial cavity now has a ventral position with respect to the straight-tube heart (compare Fig. 1-2A and Fig. 1-2B).

LATE CARDIOGENESIS, OR MORPHOLOGIC STAGE

The fusion of the endothelial heart tubes gives rise to the primitive heart tube, which is a medial structure joined to the ventral wall of the foregut by the dorsal mesocardium (Fig. 1-3B). The straight-tube heart has an inner layer, the endocardium, and an outer layer, the epimyocardium, which will give rise to the myocardium and epicardium. Between these two layers is a substance

composed of hyaluronic acid and sulfated glycosaminoglycans (12); it contains few cells and has been called cardiac jelly by Davis (13) (Fig. 1-3B). This cardiac jelly plays an important role in the fusion of the endothelial heart tubes (14), in the process of looping, and in cardiac septation (15).

The morphologic stage of cardiac morphogenesis is divided into three periods or stages: the preloop stage, corresponding to the straight-tube heart; the loop stage, during which the process of looping occurs; and the postloop stage, which starts at the beginning of cardiac septation (early postloop stage) and ends with the incorporation of the posteromedial conus into the left ventricle (late postloop stage) (2). This marks the end of the embryologic development of the heart.

Preloop Stage

Classically, it has been thought that in the preloop stage, which corresponds to the straight-tube heart, all primitive cardiac cavities that will give rise to the definitive cardiac cavities are already present (Fig. 1-4). In 1927, Davis (1) pointed out that the straight-tube heart has four regions, called primitive cardiac cavities, separated by three pairs of ectodermal grooves and their corresponding endodermal crests. It was proposed that these primitive cavities give rise to the definitive cardiac cavities. Following a cephalocaudal sequence, Davis (1) described the aortic bulb, the right and left interbulbar grooves, the bulbus cordis, the right and left bulboventricular grooves, the primitive ventricle, the right and left atrioventricular grooves, and the right and left atria (Fig. 1-4)

Recently, however, De la Cruz and others (16–20), using *in vivo* labeling techniques in the chick embryo,

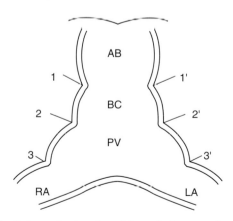

FIG. 1-4. Schematic drawing of the primitive cardiac cavities in the preloop stage, according to Davis (1). See text for details. *AB*, aortic bulb; *BC*, bulbus cordis; *PV*, primitive ventricle; *RA*, right atrium; *LA*, left atrium; *1*, right interbulbar groove; *1'*, left interbulbar groove; *2*, right bulboventricular groove; *2'*, left bulboventricular groove; *3*, right atrioventricular groove; *3'*, left atrioventricular groove.

demonstrated that only the primordia of the trabeculated portions of the ventricles are present in the straight-tube heart: that of the right ventricle, located cephalically, and that of the left ventricle, located caudally (18) (Fig. 1-5A). Neither the conus nor primordium of the ventricular infundibula (17) nor the atria (16) are present at this stage of development. Rather, the primitive cardiac cavities arise sequentially during development of the heart (19–21) (Fig. 1-5B).

Loop Stage

The primitive heart tube, which is initially straight, develops rapidly and acquires the form of a loop that is convex to the right and concave to the left (Fig. 1-5B). This defines the dextro (or D) loop (22), which determines that the primordium of the trabecular portion of the anatomic right ventricle is located to the right and that the primordium of the trabecular portion of the anatomic left

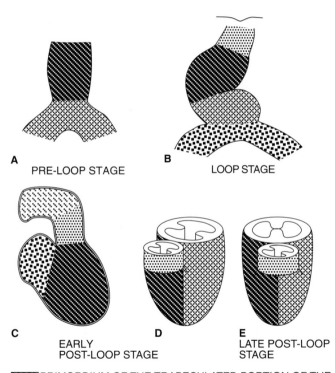

A PRE-LOOP STAGE
B LOOP STAGE
C EARLY POST-LOOP STAGE
D
E LATE POST-LOOP STAGE

▨ PRIMORDIUM OF THE TRABECULATED PORTION OF THE RIGHT VENTRICLE

▨ PRIMORDIUM OF THE TRABECULATED PORTION OF THE LEFT VENTRICLE

▨ CONUS

▨ ATRIA

▨ TRUNCUS

FIG. 1-5. Schematic drawing of the various stages during late morphogenesis. See text for details. **A:** Preloop stage. **B:** Loop stage. **C:** Early postloop stage, showing the appearance of the truncus. **D:** Early postloop stage, showing the start of cardiac septation. **E:** Late postloop stage.

ventricle is located to the left. This is the normal spatial position of the ventricles (Fig. 1-5B). If the looping is to the left—that is, a levo (or L) loop (22)—the primordium of the trabecular portion of the anatomic right ventricle will be on the left and the primordium of the trabecular portion of the anatomic left ventricle will be on the right.

Simultaneously, during the loop stage, the conus or primordium of the infundibula of both ventricles appears as a new segment at the extreme cephalic end of the heart (17), and the primordium of the right and left atria (primitive atrium) appears at the caudal end (16) (Fig. 1-5B). The aortic bulb, or truncus, which will give rise to the aortic and pulmonary semilunar valves, the ascending aorta, and the pulmonary trunk, is not yet present at this stage (17).

In the loop stage, the sinus venosus is included in the transverse septum and communicates with the primitive atrium through the sinoatrial orifice, which is guarded by the right and left sinus valves. At this point, the primitive atrium occupies the caudal segment of the heart (Figs. 1-5B, 1-6A); however, as the loop develops, the dorsal mesocardium disappears and the atria move cephalad, acquiring a dorsal position with respect to the ventricles.

Postloop Stage

In the early postloop stage, cardiac septation begins (2) and the aortic bulb, or truncus, appears at the extreme cephalic end of the heart (17) (Fig. 1-5C). At this stage in the embryologic development of the heart, all primitive cardiac cavities are present (2,19–21): the truncus, which is continuous distally with the aortic sac and proximally with the conus, the conus, the primordium of the trabeculated portion of the right ventricle, the primordium of the trabeculated portion of the left ventricle, the atrioventricular canal, the right and left primitive atria, and the sinus venosus (Figs. 1-5C, 1-6A). In the late postloop stage, the left ventricle acquires its outflow tract by incorporating the posteromedial conus (Figs. 1-5D–E).

Atrial Septation

Atrial septation starts with the appearance of the septum primum in the inside of the middorsal wall of the primitive atrium (Fig. 1-7A–B). It is sickle-shaped and has two limbs that are directed toward the atrioventricular canal, where they become continuous with the endocardial cushions, which appear simultaneously in the atrioventricular canal (23) (Fig. 1-7A). The free border of the septum primum and the free border of the endocardial cushions delineate an orifice, the ostium primum, or foramen primum, which allows the passage of blood from the right to the left atrium (Fig. 1-7A,B). The foramen primum closes with tissue originating from the septum primum and from the endocardial cushions (23,24), particularly the inferior one (23). Before the foramen primum closes,

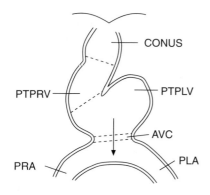

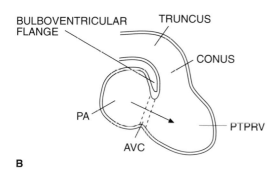

FIG. 1-6. Schematic drawing demonstrating the spatial location of the atrioventricular canal in the loop and early post-loop stages. **A:** Loop stage. **B:** Early postloop stage. *PRA,* primitive right atrium; *PLA,* primitive left atrium; *PA,* primitive atrium; *AVC,* atrioventricular canal; *PTPRV,* primordium of the trabeculated portion of the right ventricle; *PTPLV,* primordium of the trabeculated portion of the left ventricle. *Arrows* indicate the spatial orientation of the atrioventricular canal.

however, small orifices form in its dorsocephalic portion through a process of cellular death; these rapidly coalesce to form a new foramen, the ostium secundum, or foramen secundum, which stays open until birth (Fig. 1-8).

Within the right atrium, in the space between the right surface of the primum septum and the left surface of the left sinus venous valve, called the interseptovalvular space (23), a new septum appears, the septum secundum (23,25) (Fig. 1-8). It is also sickle-shaped; its limbs are directed toward the orifice of the inferior vena cava, outlining an incomplete oval ring called the limbus of the foramen ovale; its floor is constituted by the septum primum (Fig. 1-8). Between the free border of the septum secundum on the right and the free border of the septum primum at the level of the foramen secundum on the left side, a communication is established that is called the foramen ovale. During fetal life, the septum secundum and the septum primum form a valvular system allowing the passage of blood from the inferior vena cava to the left atrium (Fig. 1-8). After birth, the septum primum and septum secundum fuse, the foramen ovale disappears, and the limbus of the foramen ovale transforms itself into the

fossa ovalis, clearly visible from the right surface of the interatrial septum (Fig. 1-8D).

Development and Incorporation of the Sinus Venosus

The sinus venosus is a structure that is originally paired and related to the septum transversum. Caudally, each sinus venosus receives two extraembryonic veins, a vitelline vein medially and an umbilical vein laterally. In addition, each also receives one intraembryonic vein—a com-

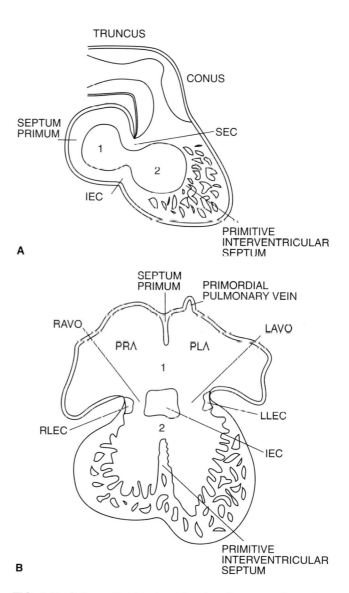

FIG. 1-7. Schematic drawing showing the start of cardiac septation in the early postloop stage. **A:** View from the right side of a sagittal cut of the heart. **B:** Transverse cut of the heart. *PRA,* primitive right atrium; *PLA,* primitive left atrium; *IEC,* inferior endocardial cushion; *SEC,* superior endocardial cushion; *LLEC,* left lateral endocardial cushion; *RLEC,* right lateral endocardial cushion; *LAVO,* left atrioventricular orifice; *RAVO,* right atrioventricular orifice; *1,* foramen primum; *2,* primary interventricular foramen.

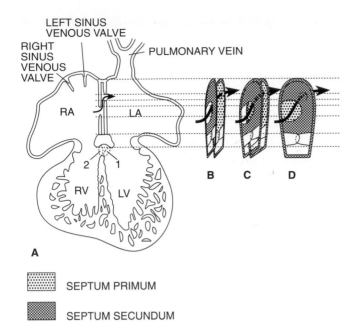

SEPTUM PRIMUM

SEPTUM SECUNDUM

FIG. 1-8. Schematic drawing of the formation of the interatrial and interventricular septa. See text for details. **A:** Transverse cut of the heart. **B–D:** The right and left atrial septal surfaces. The *arrow* indicates the direction of blood flow across the foramen ovale. *RA*, right atrium; *LA*, left atrium; *RV*, right ventricle; *LV*, left ventricle; *1*, orifice of the proximal portion of the left ventricular outflow tract (primary interventricular foramen); *2*, secondary interventricular foramen.

mon cardinal vein, or duct of Cuvier—laterally and cephalically (Fig. 1-9). Both sinus venosi fuse and, while maintaining their paired condition (24), form a cavity that is flattened dorsoventrally (2), located behind the primitive atrium, and made up of a small transverse portion and right and left sinus horns (Fig. 1-9A,B). The sinus venosus communicates with the primitive atrium through the sinoatrial orifice (Figs. 1-8A, 1-9B), which is guarded by the right and left sinus valves (25,26); these prevent backward flow during atrial contraction (27). Initially, this communication between the sinus venosus and the primitive atrium is wide and centrally located (5,23); however, the profound changes occurring in the venous circulation of the embryo during the fourth and fifth weeks of gestation, particularly the shunting of blood from left to right, cause the sinoatrial orifice to shift to the right.

The obliteration first of the left umbilical vein and later of the left vitelline vein bring about the progressive diminution in size of the transverse portion and the left horn of the sinus venosus (Fig. 1-9C), which are now separated from the left dorsal wall of the primitive atrium by a deep fold called the sinoatrial fold (5,24). The right horn increases in size, acquires a more vertical orientation, and becomes progressively incorporated into the right atrium, so that the sinoatrial orifice is now totally related to the right horn (24) (Fig. 1-9C). As the sinus venosus separates

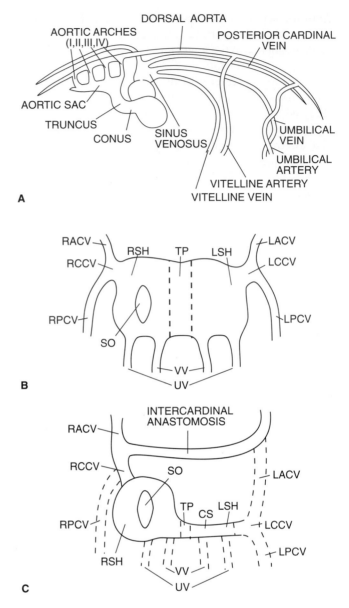

FIG. 1-9. Schematic drawing showing the intraembryonic and extraembryonic blood vessels as well as the development and incorporation of the sinus venosus. See text for details. **A:** View from the right side of a sagittal cut of the embryo. **B:** Schema of the sinus venosus, showing its various components. The *thick dotted lines* indicate the borders of the transverse portion of the sinus venosus. **C:** Schema demonstrating incorporation of the sinus venosus and development of the cardinal veins and coronary sinus. The *thin dotted lines* indicate the portions of the sinus venosus and of the systemic veins that disappear. *RSH*, right sinus horn; *LSH*, left sinus horn; *TP*, transverse portion of the sinus venosus; *RCCV*, right common cardinal vein; *RACV*, right anterior cardinal vein; *RPCV*, right posterior cardinal vein; *LCCV*, left common cardinal vein; *LACV*, left anterior cardinal vein; *LPCV*, left posterior cardinal vein; *VV*, vitelline veins; *UV*, umbilical veins; *SO*, sinoatrial orifice; *CS*, coronary sinus.

from the septum transversum, the left common cardinal vein and the distal portion of the left horn become obliterated, giving rise to the ligament of Marshall. The proximal portion of the left horn and the transverse portion of the sinus venosus give rise to the coronary sinus while the right horn is progressively absorbed into the right atrium (Fig. 1-9C).

The right and left sinus valves fuse at their cephalic end to form the septum spurium. As the right horn is absorbed into the right atrium, the sinus venous valves progressively diminish in size, the septum spurium and the left sinus venous valve become attached to the right surface of the atrial septum, the superior portion of the right sinus venous valve disappears, and the inferior portion divides in two parts: one forms the eustachian valve of the inferior vena cava, and the other one forms the thebesian valve of the coronary sinus.

The incorporation of the sinus venosus into the right atrium gives rise to the smooth or sinus portion of this atrium, where the superior and inferior venae cavae enter. The primordium of the right atrium forms only the right atrial appendage in the definitive atrium (24).

Development of the Systemic Veins

As previously stated, the sinus venosus receives three venous systems. Two of these systems, the vitelline, or omphalomesenteric, veins and the umbilical veins, are extraembryonic, and the other, the cardinal veins, is intraembryonic (24,27) (Fig. 1-9A,B).

The vitelline, or omphalomesenteric, veins transport the blood from the yolk sac to the sinus venosus. Before emptying into the caudal medial portion of the sinus veno-

sus, they form a vascular network at the level of the transverse septum where the liver develops and around the duodenum (Fig. 1-10A). This vascular anastomotic network is called the hepatic sinusoids (28). Those proximal portions of the vitelline veins that connect the hepatic sinusoids with the sinus venosus are called the hepatocardiac channels (24,28) (Fig. 1-10A). The vascular network around the developing duodenum undergoes a series of transformations and gives rise to only one vessel, the portal vein (Fig. 1-10B). The distal portion of the left vitelline vein disappears, and the distal portion of the right vitelline vein becomes the superior mesenteric vein (Fig. 1-10B,C). As the right side of the sinus venosus increases in size, the blood is rerouted to the proximal right vitelline vein (the right hepatocardiac channel), which progressively enlarges to become the suprahepatic portion of the inferior vena cava (Fig. 1-10B,C). The proximal portion of the left vitelline vein disappears.

The umbilical veins, which initially empty caudally and laterally into the sinus venosus, also establish connections with the hepatic sinusoids. The proximal portion of the right and left umbilical veins and the distal portion of the right umbilical vein progressively diminish in size and disappear. The distal portion of the left umbilical vein persists, establishing connections with the right hepatocardiac channel and becoming the ductus venosus (Fig. 1-10B,C). The ductus venosus allows blood to pass directly into the heart, bypassing the hepatic sinusoids. The ductus venosus and the left umbilical vein become obliterated after birth.

The system of cardinal veins also undergoes profound transformations during development. The right and left common cardinal veins enter the sinus venosus laterally and

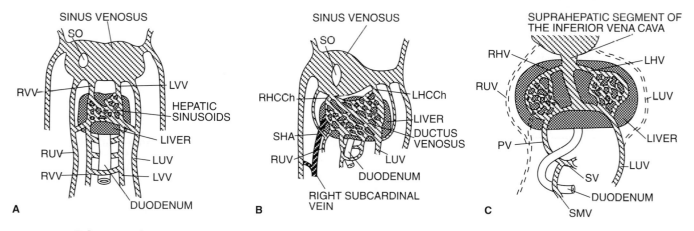

FIG. 1-10. Schematic drawing of the development of the vitelline and umbilical veins. See text for details. **A:** Development of the hepatic sinusoids. **B:** Development of the hepatocardiac channels. **C:** Development of the suprahepatic portion of the inferior vena cava, the ductus venosus, the hepatic veins, and the portal veins. The *dotted lines* indicate the portions of the umbilical veins that disappear. *SO,* sinoatrial orifice; *LUV,* left umbilical vein; *LVV,* left vitelline vein; *RUV,* right umbilical vein; *RVV,* right vitelline vein; *RHCCh,* right hepatocardiac channel; *LHCCh,* left hepatocardiac channel; *SHA,* subcardiac hepatic anatomosis; *SV,* splenic vein; *SMV,* superior mesenteric vein; *PV,* portal vein; *RHV,* right hepatic vein; *LHV,* left hepatic vein.

cephalically (Figs. 1-9; 1-10A,B; 1-11). The common cardinal veins receive the anterior and posterior cardinal veins, which drain the cephalic and caudal portions of the embryo, respectively (29) (Figs. 1-9A,B; 1-10A,B; 1-11).

The right and left anterior cardinal veins, also called precardinal veins (27), are related to the development of the head and neck. Their distal portions participate in the formation of the cerebral veins (27), the intracranial or dural venous plexus, and the internal jugular vein (27). Their proximal portions undergo transformation when an anastomosis, the intercardinal anastomosis, forms between them during the eighth week of development (Fig. 1-9C). This anastomosis permits the flow of blood between the left and right anterior cardinal veins. The right common cardinal vein and the adjacent caudal end of the proximal portion of the right anterior cardinal vein will become the superior vena cava (Fig. 1-9C). The cephalic end of the same proximal portion of the right cardinal vein will develop into the right brachiocephalic vein. The intercardinal anastomosis persists as the innominate and

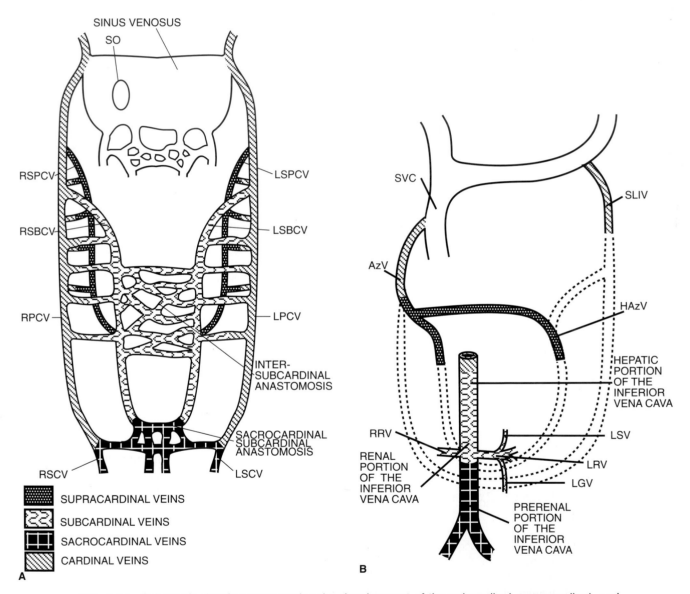

FIG. 1-11. Schematic drawing representing the development of the subcardinal, supracardinal, and sacrocardinal venous systems and of the inferior vena cava. See text for details. **A:** Development of the subcardinal, supracardinal, and sacrocardinal venous systems. **B:** Development of the azygous venous system and of the different portions of the inferior vena cava. The *dotted lines* indicate the portions of the posterior cardinal, subcardinal, and supracardinal veins that disappear. *SO,* sinoatrial orifice; *RSPCV,* right supracardinal vein; *LSPCV,* left supracardinal vein; *RSBCV,* right subcardinal vein; *LSBCV,* left subcardinal vein; *RPCV,* right posterior cardinal vein; *LPCV,* left posterior cardinal vein; *RSCV,* right sacrocardinal vein; *LSCV,* left sacrocardinal vein; *SVC,* superior vena cava; *AzV,* azygous vein; *HAzV,* hemiazygous vein; *SLIV,* superior left intercostal vein; *RRV,* right renal vein; *LRV,* left renal vein; *LGV,* left gonadal vein; *LSV,* left suprarenal vein.

left brachiocephalic veins. The portion of the left cardinal vein located between the intercardinal anastomosis and the left common cardinal vein also undergoes transformation; the caudal portion adjacent to the common left cardinal vein will become the oblique vein, and the cephalic portion persists as the highest intercostal vein (27).

Important transformations occur in the caudal portions of the intraembryonic venous system between the sixth and eighth weeks of development (Fig. 1-11). The right and left posterior cardinal veins are the first to appear; their location is dorsal to the mesonephron, and they are closely related to the development of this structure. The right and left subcardinal veins appear later and are ventral and medial to the mesonephron; they establish connections with both the mesonephric sinusoids and the posterior cardinal veins (Fig. 1-11A). Simultaneously, a network of anastomotic vessels, called the subcardinal anastomosis, develops between both subcardinal veins. Later, the right and left supracardinal veins appear in a position dorsal and medial to the posterior cardinal veins. They establish connections with the posterior cardinal and the subcardinal veins (Fig. 1-11A). Simultaneously, in the caudal region of the embryo, the right and left sacrocardinal veins emerge in a dorsal and lateral position, and the right and left caudal veins appear in a more ventral and medial location (24). A number of anastomotic connections develop between the sacrocardinal and caudal veins and between the sacrocardinal and subcardinal systems; these are called sacrocardinosubcardinal anastomoses (24) (Fig. 1-11A).

The posterior cardinal veins, which were the first to appear, along with the mesonephron, progressively diminish in size and disappear simultaneously with the mesonephron. Only a small portion of the proximal end of the right posterior cardinal vein persists, giving rise, along with the proximal end of the right supracardinal vein, to the azygous vein (Fig. 1-11B). A small portion of the proximal end of the left posterior cardinal vein also persists as the superior left intercostal vein (28) (Fig. 1-11B).

The anastomotic connections that develop between the proximal segments of right and left supracardinal veins, along with the proximal segment of the left supracardinal vein itself, give rise to the hemiazygous vein (Fig. 1-11B).

The intersubcardinal anastomosis will become the left renal vein. The proximal portion of the left subcardinal vein adjacent to the left renal vein gives rise to the left suprarenal vein; the remainder of the proximal segment disappears. The distal portion persists as the left gonadal vein (24) (Fig. 1-11B). The proximal end of the right subcardinal vein connects with the right hepatocardiac channel to form the subcardinohepatic anastomosis, which will become the hepatic portion of the inferior vena cava (24) (Fig. 1-10). The remainder of the proximal segment of the right subcardinal vein will become the renal portion of the inferior vena cava (Fig. 1-11B).

The origin of the prerenal portion of the inferior vena cava is controversial. McClure and Butler (29) as well as Arey (27) state that the distal segment of the right supracardinal vein and a distal remnant of the right posterior cardinal vein participate in its formation. Van Mierop (24), on the other hand, maintains that this portion of the inferior vena cava originates from the distal segment of the right subcardinal vein, from the sacrocardinosubcardinal anastomoses, and from the right sacrocardinal vein.

The left common iliac vein is formed by the sacrocardinal anastomosis (28).

Development of the Pulmonary Veins

The respiratory system originates from an outgrowth of the ventral wall of the foregut, called the respiratory diverticulum. The diverticulum grows caudally and at its most caudal end divides into two lung buds; these are surrounded by a capillary plexus called the splanchnic plexus.

When pulmonary differentiation occurs, part of the splanchnic plexus forms the pulmonary venous plexus, where the pulmonary veins develop (30). The pulmonary venous plexus shares the drainage sites of the splanchnic plexus with the cardinal venous system and the umbilical-vitelline venous system (31), so that these are the initial drainage sites of the pulmonary venous flow (30). Simultaneously, an endothelial sprout grows from the superior wall of the left atrium toward the pulmonary venous plexus, forming the primordial pulmonary vein (32), or common pulmonary vein (30,31) (Fig. 1-7B). Eventually, a lumen forms and connects with the pulmonary venous plexus (32); this structure bifurcates into right and left pulmonary veins, which in turn divide into two further branches (27) (Fig. 1-8A).

Once the left atrium and the pulmonary venous plexus are joined, the latter loses its connection with the splanchnic plexus and the cardinal and umbilical-vitelline venous systems (30,31). The common pulmonary vein is absorbed into the wall of the left atrium and later the branches are also absorbed, so that eventually the four pulmonary veins drain separately into the left atrium (32). The absorbed portions of the pulmonary venous plexus give origin to the smooth portion of the left atrium. The primordium of the left atrium is represented in the definitive left atrium only by the left atrial appendage (24).

Septation of the Atrioventricular Canal and Development of the Atrioventricular Valves

During the loop stage, a new cardiac segment, called the conus, appears in the cephalic end of the heart (17) while the primordia of the right and left atria appear in the caudal end (16) (Fig. 1-5B). At the atrioventricular junction, between the atrial primordia and the primordium of the trabecular portion of the left ventricle, is a tunnel-like stricture, the atrioventricular canal, with a cephalo-caudal longitudinal axis (Figs. 1-5B, 1-6A). It has a cephalic ventricular orifice and a caudal atrial orifice (1,2) (Fig. 1-6A). In the early postloop stage, when the primitive atria acquire a posterior position with respect to the primordia of the trabecular portions of the ventricles, the longitudinal axis of the atrioventricular canal changes to a dorsoventral orientation, with the atrial orifice in a dorsal position and the ventricular orifice in a ventral one (2) (Figs. 1-5C, 1-6B).

During the early postloop stage, two mesenchymal tissue masses appear inside the atrioventricular canal (2,11,23,33,34). The one on the superior, or ventral, surface is called the ventral or superior cushion of the atrioventricular canal; the second one, on the inferior, or dorsal, surface, is the dorsal or inferior cushion of the atrioventricular canal (Figs. 1-7A, 1-12A–B). Before fusing, these cushions perform a valvelike action (2,11,22,33) conjointly with the lateral cushions that simultaneously appear on the right and left walls of the atrioventricular canal. They occlude the canal in systole and divide the atrioventricular blood flow into two separate streams (23,34) (Fig. 1-12B).

From the time of their appearance, the inferior and superior cushions of the atrioventricular canal are in continuity with the interatrial and interventricular septa without any boundary (19,23) (Fig. 1-7A) and divide the orifice of the atrioventricular canal into a right orifice and a left orifice; these connect each atrium with its corresponding ventricle (Figs. 1-7B, 1-12B). Between the free border of the septum primum and the free atrial border of the

atrioventricular canal is the foramen primum (Fig. 1-7). Likewise, between the free ventricular border of the cushions and the free border of the primitive interventricular septum is the primary interventricular foramen, or bulbo-ventricular foramen (Fig. 1-7). The inferior cushion undergoes a rapid growth and becomes superimposed on the superior cushion on the right side (23); at the same time, the superior cushion thins and acquires the shape of an arc, with its concave surface toward the right ventricle and its convex surface toward the left ventricle (23,35).

Simultaneously, two crests appear in the conus: a dextrodorsal crest and a sinistroventral crest (Fig. 1-12). A new orifice is then configured, which is limited posteroinferiorly by the free border of the inferior cushion, anteriorly by the free border of the primitive interventricular septum, and superiorly by the conal crests. This new orifice, called the secondary interventricular foramen, is located to the right of the primary interventricular foramen and connects the right ventricle with the left ventricle, while the primary interventricular foramen, which in reality is a tunnel (23), becomes the proximal portion of the outflow tract of the left ventricle (9) (Fig. 1-8A).

The inferior cushion of the atrioventricular canal gives rise to the septum that separates both ventricular inflow tracts (20,23)—that is, the portion of septum that separates the right atrium from the left ventricle, called the atrioventricular septum. It is located between the septal insertion of the anterior mitral leaflet dorsally and the insertion of the septal tricuspid leaflet ventrally. The inferior cushion also gives rise to the portion of the interventricular septum adjacent to the atrioventricular septum

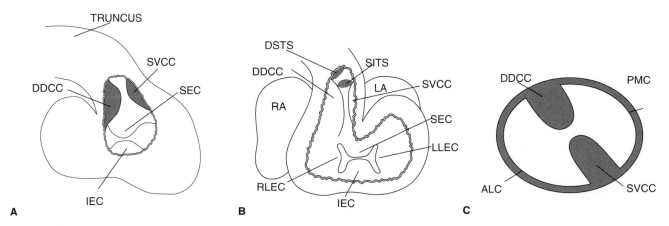

FIG. 1-12. Schematic drawing showing septation of the atrioventricular canal and conus. **A:** View from the right side of the heart, showing the cushions of the atrioventricular canal and the conal crests. The superior portion of the right wall of the atrioventricular canal and the right wall of the conus have been resected. **B:** Frontal view of the atrioventricular canal and conus. The apical portion of the ventricular chambers and the anterior wall of the conus have been resected. **C:** Transverse cut of the conus demonstrating conal septation. *DDCC,* dextrodorsal conal crest; *SVCC,* sinistroventral conal crest; *SEC,* superior endocardial cushion; *IEC,* inferior endocardial cushion; *RLEC,* right lateral endocardial cushion; *LLEC,* left lateral endocardial cushion; *DSTS,* dextrosuperior truncal swelling; *SITS,* sinistroinferior truncal swelling; *ALC,* anterolateral conus; *PMC,* posteromedial conus; *RA,* right atrium; *LA,* left atrium.

that constitutes the inlet of both ventricles (20,23). The inferior cushion probably also gives rise to the atrioventricular and interventricular portions of the membranous septum (23,36). The membranous septum is the closure point of the secondary interventricular foramen by tissue from the conal crests, the endocardial cushions, and the primitive interventricular septum (9,24). However, for some authors this is a point of contention (37).

The atrioventricular valves develop from the cushions of the atrioventricular canal, the dextrodorsal conal crest, and the ventricular walls (9,23,24,38) (Fig. 1-13). The posterior mitral leaflet originates from the left lateral cushion of the atrioventricular canal (23,24). The anterior mitral leaflet has two embryologic origins: The septal portion originates from the inferior cushion of the atrioventricular canal (23,24), and the free portion, which also constitutes the external wall of the left ventricular infundibulum, originates from the superior cushion (23,24,35,36). The right lateral cushion gives rise to the posterior tricuspid leaflet (23,24,34), and the inferior cushion contributes to the septal tricuspid leaflet (23).

The anterolateral tricuspid leaflet has dual embryologic origins (23,24): The medial portion adjacent to the septal leaflet originates from the dextrodorsal conal crest (23,24) and the lateral portion from the right lateral cushion (23,24). Leaflet tissue initially is muscular, and later, by a process of cellular differentiation, it transforms into connective tissue, thins, and becomes membranous (35). The tendinous chords and papillary muscles of both atrioventricular valves arise through a process of diverticulation and undermining of the ventricular walls (35).

Development of the Trabecular Portion of the Ventricles

The primordia of the trabecular portion of the ventricles appear in the straight-tube heart stage, the right one located cephalically and the left one caudally (16,20) (Fig. 1-5A). As looping occurs, the trabecular portion of the right ventricle shifts to the right, and the trabecular portion of the left ventricle shifts to the left (D loop) (Fig. 1-5B). Both primordia undergo a rapid development that results from centrifugal growth of the myocardium followed closely by a process of diverticulation and trabecular formation (24). In the wall of the developing ventricles, a septum, called the primitive interventricular septum, emerges; this corresponds externally to the interventricular sulcus (Fig. 1-7). From its appearance, it is aligned with the endocardial cushions and along with them delineates the primary interventricular foramen (Fig. 1-7). According to Van Mierop (24), this septum is formed by apposition and fusion of the medial walls of the growing and expanding ventricles and separates the trabecular portions of both ventricles. However, other authors mention that this septum is formed by cellular migration of the ventricular walls and not through a process of apposition (39,40).

The ventricles constitute an anatomic unit but not an embryologic one (20). The tripartite concept that divides the ventricle into inlet, trabecular, and outlet portions (41) and serves as the basis for the segmental analysis of congenital cardiac anomalies in fact corresponds to the different embryologic origins of the ventricles. The inlet portion is derived from the cushions of the atrioventricular canal, the trabecular portion from the primordia of the trabecular portion of the ventricles, and the outlet portion from the conus, which gives rise to the infundibula of both ventricles.

Septation of the Conus and Truncus

The conus, or primordium of the ventricular infundibula, appears during the loop stage (17) and forms the cephalic end of the heart (2) (Fig. 1-5B). Caudally, it is continuous with the primordium of the trabecular portion of the right ventricle; it is separated from the primordium of the trabecular portion of the left ventricle laterally and

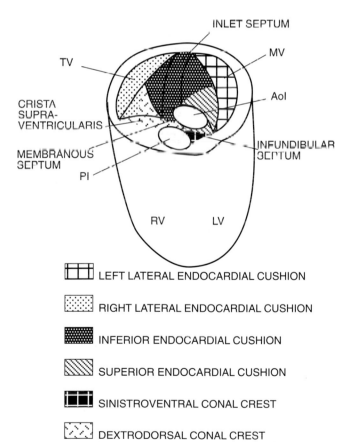

FIG. 1-13. Schematic drawing of the base of the heart, demonstrating the embryologic origin of the atrioventricular valves, the crista supraventricularis, and the inlet, membranous, and outlet portions of the interventricular septum. *TV*, tricuspid valve; *MV*, mitral valve; *RV*, right ventricle; *LV*, left ventricle; *PI*, pulmonary infundibulum; *AoI*, aortic infundibulum.

from the atrial wall posteriorly by the bulboventricular (conoventricular) flange (Fig. 1-5C). Cephalically, it is continuous with the truncus, which appears during the early postloop stage (Fig. 1-5C).

Three morphogenetic processes contribute to the embryologic development of the conus: septation (9,42), migration, and absorption (9,42-44). Initially, neither the conus nor the truncus is septated. During the early postloop stage, two mesenchymal masses appear along the inside wall of the conus; these are the dextrodorsal and sinistroventral conal crests (42) (Figs. 1-12, 1-14A1). Simultaneously, two opposing masses appear within the truncus, the dextrosuperior and sinistroinferior truncal swellings (24) (Figs. 1-12B, 1-14B1) The conal crests divide the conus into an anterolateral and a posteromedial conus (Figs. 1-12C, 1-14A1). At their caudal, or proximal, end, the conal crests form the superior border of the secondary interventricular foramen. The sinistroventral conal crest is continuous with the primitive interventricular septum. The dextrodorsal conal crest forms a unit with the superior cushion of the atrioventricular canal and the conoventricular flange and becomes continuous with the right lateral cushion of the atrioventricular canal. The dextrodorsal conal crest also contributes to the development of the medial portion of the anterolateral tricuspid leaflet (Fig. 1-13) and, along with the right lateral cushion

of the atrioventricular canal, participates in the formation of the crista supraventricularis (36). The crista supraventricularis is a muscular or fibrous structure that in the normal, mature heart separates the tricuspid and pulmonic valves (Fig. 1-13). At the cephalic, or distal, end, the sinistroventral conal crest becomes continuous with the sinistroinferior truncal swelling, while the dextrodorsal conal crest is continuous with the dextrosuperior truncal swelling (24) (Fig. 1-14).

When the conal crests fuse, they give rise to the right surface of the conal or outlet septum (36,38); the left surface of the conal septum is formed by the superior cushion (36,38) (Fig. 1-13). As the bulboventricular (conoventricular) flange diminishes in size, the conus migrates (43), shifting from a rightward position in the bulboventricular loop to an anteromedial position. The anterolateral conus then connects with the anatomic right ventricle and the posteromedial conus with the anatomic left ventricle (Fig. 1-5D–E).

Truncal septation is accomplished through growth of the truncal swellings and the aorticopulmonary septum (Figs. 1-12B, 1-14). The latter originates as an extracardiac septum in the aortic sac between the fourth and sixth aortic arches. Recently, Kirby et al. (45) found that cells from the neural crest participate in its formation. The aorticopulmonary septum is spiral, grows in a cephalocau-

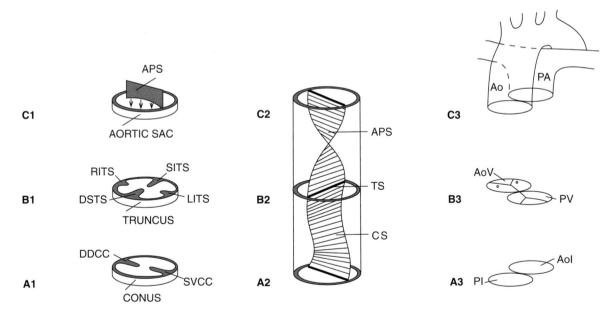

FIG. 1-14. Schematic drawing of the aorticopulmonary, truncal, and conal septation. **A1:** Location of the conal crests. **A2:** Spatial orientation and shape of the conal septum. **A3:** Normal spatial relationship of the infundibula. **B1:** Location of the truncal swellings. **B2:** Spatial orientation of the truncal septum. **B3:** Normal spatial relationship of the semilunar valves. **C1:** Septation of the aortic sac. **C2:** Spatial orientation and shape of the aorticopulmonary septum. **C3:** Normal spatial relationship of the great arteries at their cephalic end. *DDCC,* dextrodorsal conal crest; *SVCC,* sinistroventral conal crest; *DSTS,* dextrosuperior truncal swelling; *SITS,* sinistroinferior truncal swelling; *RITS,* right intercalated truncal swelling; *LITS,* left intercalated truncal swelling; *PI,* pulmonary infundibulum; *AoI,* aortic infundibulum; *AoV,* aortic valve; *PV,* pulmonic valve; *Ao,* aorta; *PA,* pulmonary artery; *CS,* conal septum; *TS,* truncal septum; *APS,* aorticopulmonary septum.

dal direction, and, conjointly with the truncal septum formed by fusion of the truncal swellings, separates the aortic and pulmonary trunks (Fig. 1-14). Its spiral shape determines the normal spatial relationship of the great arteries. The aorta, which cephalically is anterior and to the right, becomes continuous with the posteromedial conus, which forms the infundibulum of the left ventricle. The pulmonary artery, which cephalically is posterior and leftward, becomes in turn connected with the anterolateral conus, which is the infundibulum of the right ventricle (Fig. 1-14).

The sigmoid aortic and pulmonary valves develop at the boundary between the conus and truncus. As the sinistroinferior and dextrosuperior truncal swellings fuse to form the truncal septum, they also give rise to the posterior right and left pulmonary cusps and the anterior right and left aortic cusps. The dorsal, or right, intercalated truncal swelling gives origin to the posterior or noncoronary aortic cusp, and the ventral, or left, intercalated truncal swelling gives rise to the anterior pulmonary cusp (26) (Fig. 1-14).

Development of the Coronary Arteries

The coronary arteries appear late in development (44) at the time the myocardium begins its transformation from spongy to compact tissue (46,47). The cardiac walls receive nutrients during the initial stages of development by imbibition of circulating blood (48), and later through the intramyocardial sinusoids, which begin to form from the intertrabecular spaces (46,49–51).

During the fifth week of development, an endothelial vascular network appears in the subepicardial space of the atrioventricular and interventricular sulci (52–54); some of its branches penetrate the myocardium and establish contact with the intramyocardial sinusoids (Fig. 1-15). Conte and Pellegrini (54) describe the existence of two endothelial subepicardial networks: a right posterior one and a left anterior one (Fig. 1-15A). The right posterior subepicardial vascular network is distributed along the right atrioventricular sulcus, the posterior interventricular sulcus, the diaphragmatic surface of both ventricles, and the anterior wall of the right ventricle. The left anterior subepicardial vascular network develops in the region of the left atrioventricular sulcus, the anterior interventricular sulcus, and the adjacent walls of both ventricles.

There are two schools of thought regarding the origin of the proximal portions of the coronary arteries: One invokes the existence of coronary buds around the arterial trunk, and another states that the subepicardial vascular networks penetrate the aortic wall to reach the sinuses of Valsalva.

According to the first school of thought, a series of coronary buds appears in the proximal portions of the walls of the unseptated truncus arteriosus, in the region

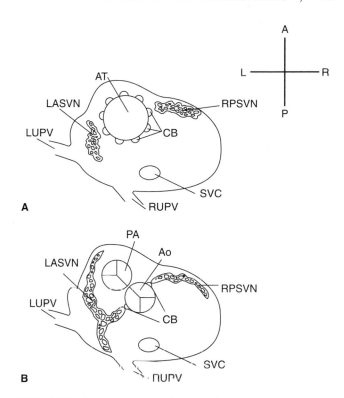

FIG. 1-15. Schematic drawing of the heart viewed from above, showing the embryologic development of the coronary arteries. A: Schema demonstrating the development of the coronary buds along the walls of the arterial trunk and the development of the subepicardial vascular network. B: Schema demonstrating the disappearance of most of the coronary buds, with persistence of only those related to the aortic sinuses, which will establish connection with the subepicardial vascular network. CB, coronary buds; AT, arterial trunk; RPSVN, right posterior subepicardial vascular network; LASVN, left anterior subepicardial vascular network; SVC, superior vena cava; RUPV, right upper pulmonary vein; LUPV, left upper pulmonary vein; Ao, aorta; PA, pulmonary artery. A, anterior; P, posterior; L, left; R, right.

where both the aortic and pulmonary semilunar valves are developing (52–55). The coronary buds are initially solid, and their growth starts from the endothelium of the truncal walls. The yolks related to the right and left anterior sinuses of Valsalva become hollow and grow outward from the walls of the aorta. The remaining coronary buds disappear (Fig. 1-15B). After septation of the truncus arteriosus and formation of the sigmoid valves have been completed, the coronary buds establish a connection with the subepicardial endothelial vascular networks. The coronary bud related to the right anterior sinus of Valsalva connects with the right posterior vascular network; the coronary bud becomes the right main coronary artery, and the vascular network becomes its branches. The coronary bud of the left anterior sinus of Valsalva connects with the left anterior subepicardial vascular network, giving rise to the main and branch left coronary arteries (54). The vascular networks lose contact with the intramyocardial sinusoids when they connect with the coronary buds.

The ideas of the second school of thought have recently been proposed by Bogers et al. (56) and Gittenberger-de Groot et al. (57) utilizing monoclonal antiendothelial antibodies in quail embryos, and by Waldo and Kirby (58) using India ink injections in chick embryos. According to these investigators, no evidence can be found for the existence of coronary buds at any stage of development. They postulate that the subepicardial vascular networks penetrate the wall of the aorta and establish small channels; only the channels related to the aortic sinuses that face the pulmonary sinuses persist to give rise to the right and left coronary arteries (56,58).

Development of the Aortic Arches

The embryologic development of the aortic arches is intimately related to the development of the head and neck. During the fourth week of development, the pharyngeal arches appear in a cephalocaudal sequence along the ventral and lateral walls of the pharyngeal gut, which is the most anterior portion of the foregut.

The pharyngeal arches are bars of mesenchymal tissue separated by deep grooves, the pharyngeal clefts. Likewise, the pharyngeal pouches, which also appear on the lateral walls of the pharyngeal gut, separate the individual pharyngeal arches from each other. Along the dorsal wall of the embryo on both sides of the pharyngeal gut are two arteries, named the right and left dorsal aortas, and in front of the ventral wall of the foregut is the aortic sac, which is continuous with the truncus. As each pharyngeal arch appears, the aortic sac contributes right and left arterial branches; these connect with the right and left dorsal aortas, respectively, to form six pairs of arteries, called the aortic arches (Fig. 1-16A). The aortic arches appear in the same cephalocaudal sequence as the pharyngeal arches, and the first ones to appear are also the first ones to undergo the transformations resulting from the cephalization process.

The *first aortic arch* is the earliest one to disappear (Fig. 1-16B); only one portion persists to give rise to the maxillary arteries (24,27,28). It can also contribute to the development of the external carotid arteries (4).

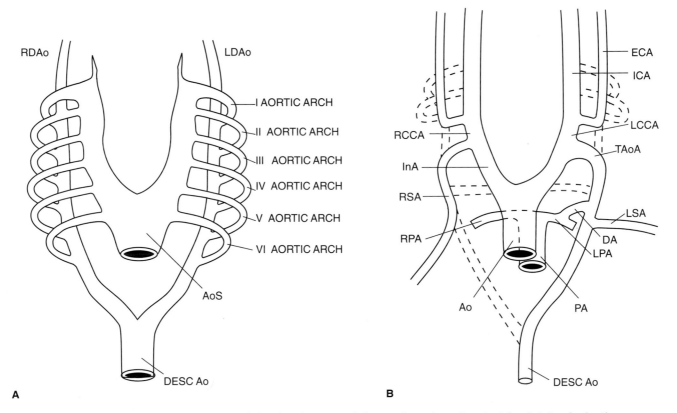

FIG. 1-16. Schematic drawing of the development of the aortic arches. See text for details. **A:** Aortic arches. **B:** Development of the innominate, carotid, and subclavian arteries as well as the branches of the pulmonary artery and the ductus arteriosus. The *dotted lines* indicate the aortic arches and the portions of the right dorsal aorta that disappear. *RDAo*, right dorsal aorta; *LDAo*, left dorsal aorta; *AoS*, aortic sac; *Desc Ao*, descending aorta; *InA*, innominate artery; *RCCA*, right common carotid artery; *LCCA*, left common carotid artery; *ECA*, external carotid artery; *ICA*, internal carotid artery; *TAoA*, transverse aortic arch; *RSA*, right subclavian artery; *LSA*, left subclavian artery; *DA*, ductus arteriosus; *RPA*, right pulmonary artery; *LPA*, left pulmonary artery; *Ao*, aorta; *PA*, pulmonary artery.

The *second aortic arch* also disappears (Fig. 1-16B); only its dorsal portion persists, giving origin to the stapedial arteries.

The *third aortic arch* contributes to the development of the carotid arteries (Fig. 1-16B). Its proximal portion gives rise to the common carotid arteries. Its distal portion, along with the segments of the right and left dorsal aortas located between the first and second aortic arches, gives rise to the internal carotid arteries. The portions of the right and left dorsal aortas located between the third and fourth aortic arches disappear (Fig. 1-16B).

The *fourth aortic arch* undergoes different transformations on each side. On the right side, the proximal end of the fourth aortic arch and an elongation of the right portion of the aortic sac give rise to the right brachiocephalic, or innominate, artery (27) (Fig. 1-16B). The distal right fourth arch gives rise to the proximal right subclavian artery. The distal right subclavian artery originates from the proximal segment of the caudal portion of the right dorsal aorta and from the right seventh intersegmental artery. The distal segment of the caudal portion of the right dorsal aorta disappears. On the left side, the fourth arch gives rise to the transverse aortic arch. The ascending aorta comes from the aortic sac, and the descending aorta from the left dorsal aorta.

The *fifth aortic arch* is never well developed and is transitory (Fig. 1-16B). It does not give rise to any definitive arterial structure (24,27,28).

The *sixth aortic arch*, in addition to connecting with the right and left dorsal aortas, also connects with the primitive right and left pulmonary arteries, which originate from the pulmonary capillary plexus of the developing lungs. The proximal portion of the right sixth arch gives rise to the proximal right pulmonary artery; the distal right arch disappears (Fig. 1-16B). The proximal portion of the left sixth arch gives rise to the proximal left pulmonary artery, and the distal left arch becomes the ductus arteriosus (Fig. 1-16B). The main pulmonary trunk stems from the aortic sac.

The left subclavian artery originates from the left seventh intersegmental artery (Fig. 1-16B).

REFERENCES

1. Davis CL. Development of the human heart from its first appearance to the stage found in embryos of twenty paired somites. *Contrib Embryol* 1927;19:245–284.
2. De la Cruz MV, Cayre R. Desarrollo embriologico del corazon y las grandes arterias. In: Sanchez PA, ed. *Cardiologia pediatrica, clinica y cirugia*, Vol 1. Barcelona: Editorial Salvat, 1986:10–18.
3. Anderson RH. The present-day place of correlations between embryology and anatomy in the understanding of congenitally malformed hearts. In: Aranega A, Pexieder T, eds. *Correlations between experimental clinic embryology and teratology and congenital cardiac defects*. Granada: Universidad de Granada, 1989:265–295.
4. Moore KL. *The developing human. Clinically oriented embryology*, 4th ed. Philadelphia: WB Saunders, 1988.
5. Sadler TW. Ovulation to implantation. In: Tracy TM, ed. *Langman's medical embryology*, 5th ed. Baltimore: Williams & Wilkins, 1985:19–38.
6. Rosenquist GC, DeHaan RL. Migration of precardiac cells in the chick embryo: a radioautographic study. *Contrib Embryol* 1966;38:111–121.
7. DeHaan RL. Migration patterns of the precardiac mesoderm in the early chick embryo. *Exp Cell Res* 1963;29:544–560.
8. Rawles ME. The heart-forming areas of the early chick blastoderm. *Physiol Zool* 1943;16:22–42.
9. Domenech Mateu JM. Desarrollo del corazon. In: Soler J, Bayes de Luna A, eds. *Cardiologia*. Barcelona: Editorial Doyma, 1986:3–13.
10. Domenech Mateu JM, Reig Vilallonga J. Embriologia experimental cardiaca. In: Sanchez PA, ed. *Cardiologia pediatrica, clinica y cirugia*, Vol 1. Barcelona: Editorial Salvat, 1986:19–31.
11. Colvin EV. Cardiac embryology. In: Garson JR, Bricker JT, McNamara DG, eds. *The science and practice of pediatric cardiology*, Vol 1. Philadelphia: Lea & Febiger, 1990:71–108.
12. Nakamura A, Manasek FJ. An experimental study of the relation of cardiac jelly to the shape of the early chick embryonic heart. *J Embryol Exp Morphol* 1981;65:235–256.
13. Davis CL. The cardiac jelly of the chick embryo. *Anat Rec* 1924;27:201–202.
14. Ojeda JL, Hurle JM. Cell death during the formation of the tubular heart of the chick embryo. *J Embryol Exp Morph* 1975;33:523–534.
15. Nakamura A, Kulikowski RR, Lacktis JW, Manasek FJ. Heart looping: a regulated response to deforming forces. In: Van Praagh R, Takao A, eds. *Etiology and morphogenesis of congenital heart disease*. Armonk, NY: Futura Publishing, 1980:81–98.
16. Castro-Quesada A, Nadal-Ginard B, De la Cruz MV. Experimental study of the formation of the bulboventricular loop in the chick. *J Embryol Exp Morphol* 1972;27:623–637.
17. De la Cruz MV, Sanchez Gomez C, Arteaga MM, Arguello C. Experimental study of the development of the truncus and the conus in the chick embryo. *J Anat* 1977;123:661–686.
18. De la Cruz MV, Sanchez Gomez C, Palomino MA. The primitive cardiac regions in the straight tube heart (stage 9−) and their anatomical expression in the mature heart: an experimental study in the chick embryo. *J Anat* 1989;165:121–131.
19. Arteaga M, Garcia Pelaez I. Nomenclature in the embryonic heart. In: Aranega A, Pexieder T, eds. *Correlations between experimental cardiac embryology and teratology and congenital cardiac defects*. Granada: Universidad de Granada, 1989:17–35.
20. De la Cruz MV, Sanchez Gomez C, Cayre R. The developmental components of the ventricles: their significance in congenital cardiac malformations. *Cardiol Young* 1991;1:123–128.
21. Markwald RR. Overview: formation and early morphogenesis of the primary heart tube. In Clark EB, Markwald RR, Takao A, eds. *Developmental mechanisms of heart disease*. Armonk, NY: Futura Publishing, 1995:149–155.
22. Van Praagh R, Dehaan RL. *Morphogenesis of the heart: mechanism of curvature*. Annual report of the Director, Department of Embryology. Washington: Yearbook Carnegie Institute of Washington, DC, 1967:536.
23. De la Cruz MV, Gimenez-Ribotta M, Saravalli O, Cayre R. The contribution of the inferior endocardial cushion of the atrioventricular canal to cardiac septation and to the development of the atrioventricular valves: study in the chick embryo. *Am J Anat* 1983;166:63–72.
24. Netter FH, Van Mierop LHS. Embryology. In: Netter FH, Yonkman FF, eds. *Heart*. Summit, NJ: Ciba Publications Department, 1969:112–130 (*The Ciba collection of medical illustrations*, Vol 5).
25. Odgers PNB. The formation of the venous valves, the foramen secundum and the septum secundum in the human heart. *J Anat* 1935;69:412–422.
26. Kramer TC. The partitioning of the truncus and the formation of the membranous portion of the interventricular septum in the human heart. *Am J Anat* 1942;71:343–370.
27. Arey LB. *Developmental anatomy. A textbook and laboratory manual of embryology*, 7th ed. Philadelphia: WB Saunders, 1966.
28. Sadler TW. Cardiovascular system. In: Tracy TM, ed. *Langman's medical embryology*, 5th ed. Baltimore: Williams & Wilkins, 1985:168–214.
29. McClure CFW, Butler EG. The development of the vena cava inferior in man. *Am J Anat* 1925;35:331–383.

30. Lucas RV Jr, Anderson RC, Amplatz K, Adams P Jr, Edwards JE. Congenital causes of pulmonary venous obstruction. *Pediatr Clin North Am* 1963;10:781–836.
31. Edwards JE. Pathologic and developmental considerations in anomalous pulmonary venous connection. *Proc Staff Meet Mayo Clin* 1953;28:441–452.
32. Neill CA. Development of pulmonary veins with reference to embryology and anomalies of pulmonary venous return. *Pediatrics* 1956;18:880–887.
33. Icardo JM. Heart anatomy and developmental biology. *Experientia* 1988;44:910–919.
34. Thompson RP, Losada Cabrera MA, Fitzharris TP. Embryology of cardiac cushion tissue. In: Aranega A, Pexieder T, eds. *Correlations between experimental cardiac embryology and teratology and congenital cardiac defects.* Granada: Universidad de Granada, 1989: 147–169.
35. Van Mierop LHS, Alley RD, Kausel HW, Stranahan A. The anatomy and embryology of endocardial cushion defects. *J Thorac Cardiovasc Surg* 1962;43:71–83.
36. De la Cruz MV, Quero-Jimenez M, Arteaga Martinez M, Cayre R. Morphogenèse du septum interventriculaire. *Coeur* 1982;13:443–448.
37. Allwork SP, Anderson RH. Developmental anatomy of the membranous part of the ventricular septum in the human heart. *Br Heart J* 1979;41:275–280.
38. Garcia-Pelaez I, Diaz-Gongora G, Arteaga Martinez M. Contribution of the superior atrioventricular cushion to the left ventricular infundibulum. Experimental study on the chick embryo. *Acta Anat* 1984;118:224–230.
39. Harth JY, Paul MH. Experimental cardiomorphogenesis. I. Development of the ventricular septum in the chick. *J Embryol Exp Morphol* 1975;33:1–28.
40. De la Cruz MV. Different concepts of univentricular heart. Experimental embryological approach. *Herz* 1979;4:67–72.
41. Goor DA, Lillehei CW. *Congenital malformations of the heart. Embryology, anatomy, and operative considerations.* New York: Grune & Stratton, 1975.
42. De la Cruz MV, Munoz Armas S, Castellanos L. *Development of the chick heart.* Baltimore: The Johns Hopkins Press, 1971.
43. Goor DA, Dische R, Lillehei CW. The conotruncus. I. Its normal inversion and conus absorption. *Circulation* 1972;46:375–384.
44. Anderson RH, Wilkinson RA, Lubkiewicz K. Morphogenesis of bulboventricular malformations. I: Consideration of embryogenesis in the normal heart. *Br Heart J* 1974;36:242–255.
45. Kirby ML, Gale TF, Stewart DE. Neural crest cells contribute to normal aorticopulmonary septation. *Science* 1983;220:1059–1061.
46. Rychter Z, Rychterova V. Angio- and myoarchitecture of the heart wall under normal and experimentally changed morphogenesis. In: Pexieder T, ed. *Mechanisms of cardiac morphogenesis and teratogenesis. Perspectives in cardiovascular research.* New York: Raven Press, 1981:431–452.
47. De la Cruz MV, Noriega Ramos N, Sanchez Gomez C, Martinez Sanchez A. Embriologia normal de las arterias coronarias, malformaciones congenitas de las coronarias. Embriopatologia y clasificacion. In: Bezerra de Carvalho V, Macruz R, eds. *Cardiopatia isquemica. Aspectos de importancia clinica.* Sao Paulo, Brazil: Editorial Sarvier, 1989:13–38.
48. Dbaly J, Ostadal B, Rychter Z. Development of the coronary arteries in rat embryos. *Acta Anat* 1968;71:209–222.
49. Licata RH. A continuation study of the development of the blood supply of the human heart. Part II: The deep or intramural circulation. *Anat Rec* 1956;124:326(abst).
50. Manasek FJ. The ultrastructure of embryonic myocardial blood vessels. *Dev Biol* 1971;26:42–54.
51. Rychter Z, Ostadal B. Fate of "sinusoidal" intertrabecular spaces of the cardiac wall after development of the coronary vascular bed in the chick embryo. *Folia Morphol (Warsz)* 1971;19:31–44.
52. Ogden J. The origin of the coronary arteries. *Circulation* 1968; 38[Suppl VI]:150.
53. Hirakow R. Development of the cardiac blood vessels in staged human embryos. *Acta Anat* 1983;115:220–230.
54. Conte G, Pellegrini A. On the development of the coronary arteries in human embryos, stages 14–19. *Anat Embryol* 1984;169:209–218.
55. Sissman NJ. Developmental landmarks in cardiac morphogenesis: comparative chronology. *Am J Cardiol* 1970;25:141–148.
56. Bogers AJJC, Gittenberger-deGroot AC, Dubbeldam JA, Huysmans HA. The inadequacy of existing theories on development of the proximal coronary arteries and their connexions with the arterial trunks. *Int J Cardiol* 1988;20:117–123.
57. Gittenberger-de Groot AC, Bogers AJJC, Poelmann RE, Peault BM, Huysmans HA. Development of the coronary arterial orifices. *Ann N Y Acad Sci* 1990;588:377–379.
58. Waldo K, Kirby ML. A new perspective on the development of the coronary arteries in the chick embryo. *Ann N Y Acad Sci* 1990;588: 459–460.

CHAPTER 2

Nomenclature and Segmental Analysis of Congenital Cardiac Malformations

Lilliam M. Valdes-Cruz and Raul O. Cayre

The terminology that has been used in the literature to define the various positions of the heart in the chest, and the nomenclature used to denote the different types of congenital cardiac malformations have created great confusion. Applying different names to the same anomaly and the same name to different anomalies has added to this confusion. Therefore, the terms should first be defined and then applied in a segmental sequence, allowing congenital cardiac malformations to be classified according to their different anatomic types and labeled using the most appropriate terminology.

DEFINITION OF TERMS

Levocardia. Classically, this term is used when the heart is located in the left side of the thorax or when its base-to-apex axis is directed downward and to the left. It can occur in the presence of situs solitus, situs inversus, or situs ambiguus. In situs solitus, it is considered the normal cardiac position (Fig. 2-1A) and has also been called pure levocardia (1). We will use the term levocardia when the heart is located on the left side of the thorax, irrespective of visceroatrial situs (Fig. 2-1).

Cardiac Malposition. This term is used to indicate any position of the heart that is not levocardia with situs solitus (2). Shaher et al. (3) define cardiac malposition as those situations in which the cardiac apex is not on the same side as the morphologic left atrium. We will not use malposition in this sense. We will use the term cardiac malposition to indicate any cardiac position other than levocardia in situs solitus.

Isolated Levocardia. This term has been used to indicate that the heart is on the left side of the chest in the presence of visceroatrial situs inversus (4,5). This has also been called levoversion (3,6–11) or true levocardia (12). We will not use any of these terms. Rather, we will use

the terms levocardia in situs inversus or levocardia by levoversion (Fig. 2-1B).

Levocardia and Ventricular Inversion. A heart in levocardia with situs solitus or situs inversus can present with or without ventricular inversion. This type of association has been called mixed levocardia with ventricular inversion in cases with situs solitus and mixed levocardia with atrial inversion in situs inversus (1,13,14). This is simply atrioventricular discordance (Fig. 2-1C,D). The situs must be defined independently.

Levoposition. Location of the heart in the left side of the chest resulting from displacement from an extracardiac cause has been called levoposition in the literature (7,8,14,15). We agree with this terminology and will use the term levocardia resulting from extracardiac displacement synonymously with levoposition.

The terms pure levocardia, isolated levocardia, levoversion without further qualification, true levocardia, levocardia and ventricular inversion, mixed levocardia with ventricular inversion, and mixed levocardia with atrial inversion should be abandoned to avoid confusion.

Dextrocardia. This term has been used to indicate that the heart is located in the right side of the thorax (2,16–21) or that the base-to-apex axis is directed downward and to the right (1,14,22–24). This can present in situs solitus, situs inversus, or situs ambiguus. In the presence of situs inversus, it is classically called mirror-image dextrocardia. It has also been called pure dextrocardia or complete dextrocardia (25). Dextrocardia is the normal situation in the presence of total situs inversus (Fig. 2-2A). We will use the term dextrocardia when the heart is located on the right side of the thorax irrespective of situs, which needs to be defined separately (Fig. 2-2). The Kartagener triad or syndrome (26) describes situs inversus, bronchiectasis, and sinusitis and typically includes dextrocardia.

19

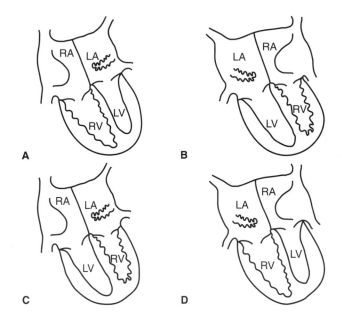

FIG. 2-1. Schematic drawings showing hearts in levocardia with situs solitus and situs inversus, with atrioventricular concordance and atrioventricular discordance. **A:** Situs solitus and atrioventricular concordance. **B:** Situs inversus and atrioventricular concordance (levocardia by levoversion). **C:** Situs solitus and atrioventricular discordance. **D:** Situs inversus and atrioventricular discordance. *RA*, right atrium; *LA*, left atrium; *RV*, right ventricle; *LV*, left ventricle.

Isolated Dextrocardia. This term indicates that the heart is located in the right thorax in the presence of visceroatrial situs solitus (1,17,23,27–29). This type of cardiac malposition has also been called dextroversion (7–10,18,29–31), incomplete dextrocardia (25), pivotal dextrocardia (1), and pure dextrocardia (32). We will not use any of these terms. Rather, we will use the term dextrocardia in situs solitus or dextrocardia by dextroversion (Fig. 2-2B). The Cantrell syndrome includes dextrocardia; situs solitus; a defect in the medial abdominal wall, such as umbilical hernia or omphalocele; a defect in the lower portion of the sternum; deficiency in the anterior diaphragm; defect in the diaphragmatic portion of the parietal pericardium; and left ventricular diverticulum (33).

Dextrocardia with Ventricular Inversion. A heart in dextrocardia can present with or without ventricular inversion independently of situs. This type of cardiac malposition in the presence of situs solitus has been called mixed dextrocardia with ventricular inversion (34) and mixed dextrocardia with atria in pivotal position and ventricles in mirror image (14,35). Cases with situs inversus have been termed mixed dextrocardia with atrial inversion (34) and mixed dextrocardia with mirror-image atria and ventricles in pivotal position (14,35). This is dextrocardia with atrioventricular discordance (Fig. 2-2C,D). The situs must be defined separately.

Dextroposition. This term has been used to indicate location of the heart in the right chest resulting from

displacement from extracardiac causes (7,8,14,19,22,31). To define this type of dextrocardia, various terms have been used, such as acquired dextrocardia (16,17,30,36), secondary dextrocardia (30), and extrinsic dextrocardia (37). The terms congenital dextrocardia (16,17,36–38) and primary dextrocardia (30) have been reserved to indicate an anomaly intrinsic to the development of the heart. Jones (16) has used the term dextroversion to indicate hearts displaced to the right but without cavity inversion. We will use the terms dextrocardia resulting from extracardiac displacement and dextroposition synonymously.

The terms pure dextrocardia, complete dextrocardia, isolated dextrocardia, incomplete dextrocardia, dextroversion without further qualification, pivotal dextrocardia, pure dextrocardia, dextrocardia with ventricular inversion, mixed dextrocardia with ventricular inversion, mixed dextrocardia with atria in pivotal position and ventricles in mirror image, mixed dextrocardia with atrial inversion, mixed dextrocardia with mirror-image atria and ventricles in pivotal position, congenital dextrocardia, acquired dextrocardia, primary dextrocardia, secondary dextrocardia, and extrinsic dextrocardia should be abandoned to avoid confusion.

Mesocardia. There are several definitions of the term mesocardia: (a) heart located in midthorax (20,21,39) or in the midline (2,8,20,21,39); (b) long axis of the heart found in the midsagittal plane with no apex (35,40); and

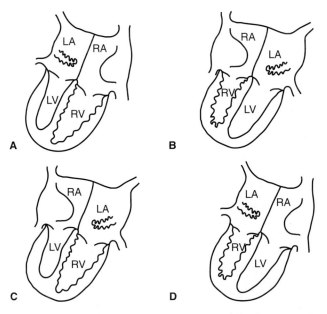

FIG. 2-2. Schematic drawings showing hearts in dextrocardia with situs solitus and situs inversus, with atrioventricular concordance and atrioventricular discordance. **A:** Situs inversus and atrioventricular concordance (mirror-image dextrocardia). **B:** Situs solitus and atrioventricular concordance (dextrocardia by dextroversion). **C:** Situs solitus and atrioventricular discordance. **D:** Situs inversus and atrioventricular discordance. *RA*, right atrium; *LA*, left atrium; *RV*, right ventricle; *LV*, left ventricle.

(c) base-to-apex axis pointing ventrally (14). A heart in mesocardia can present in situs solitus, situs inversus, or situs ambiguus. Mesocardia in situs solitus (Fig. 2-3A) has been given various denominations, such as mesoversion, incomplete dextroversion, pivotal mesocardia, and mesoversion type I (14,35,40). Mesocardia in situs inversus (Fig. 2-3B) has been called mesoversion type II (14,35). Mesocardia in the presence of situs ambiguus has been termed presumptive mesoversion or indeterminate type of mesocardia (14,40). We will use the term mesocardia to denote a heart located in the middle of the thorax, irrespective of situs (Fig. 2-3).

Mesocardia and Ventricular Inversion. Mesocardia in situs solitus or inversus can present with or without ventricular inversion. Cases in situs solitus have been called mixed mesocardia with ventricular inversion or mixed mesocardia with pivotal atria and inverted ventricles. Those with situs inversus have been called mixed mesocardia with atrial inversion (14,35). We will use the term mesocardia with atrioventricular discordance (Fig. 2-3C,D). The situs must be defined independently.

Mesoposition. This term has been used to characterize a heart in mesocardia resulting from displacement from an extracardiac cause (14).

The terms mesoversion, incomplete dextroversion, pivotal mesocardia, type I and type II mesoversion, presumptive mesoversion, indeterminate type of mesocardia, mixed mesocardia with ventricular inversion, mixed mesocardia with pivotal atria and inverted ventricles, and mixed mesocardia with atrial inversion should be abandoned to avoid confusion.

SEGMENTAL ANALYSIS OF CONGENITAL CARDIAC MALFORMATIONS

The sequential segmental analysis of congenital heart defects was originally proposed by Van Praagh (41) and later by De la Cruz and Nadal-Ginard (42), Kirklin et al. (43), Shinebourne et al. (44), Tynan et al. (45), and Anderson et al. (46). The successive contributions by these authors have resulted in a current methodology for the sequential segmental analysis of cardiac malformations that has clarified most of the confusion regarding the nomenclature used to classify congenital heart disease, although the methodology continues to be somewhat controversial among some cardiac embryologists, anatomists, clinicians, and surgeons (9,10,18–21,47–52). This approach is based on the sequential study of the different segments into which the heart has been divided—the atrial, ventricular, and arterial segments—and on the manner in which they are connected and related.

Atrial Segment

Analysis of the atrial segment considers the atrial arrangement or atrial situs. The situs is the location or position that an organ occupies in the bilateral system of symmetry. There are three types of situs: (a) solitus, (b) inversus, and (c) ambiguus, incertus, or indeterminate (Fig. 2-4).

Situs Solitus. Situs solitus (Fig. 2-4A) is the position that an organ normally occupies in the plane of bilateral symmetry. As the atrial situs usually corresponds to the visceral situs, the term visceroatrial situs can be used. In situs solitus, the liver is to the right, the trilobed right lung is to the right, and the bilobed left lung is to the left. The morphologic right main bronchus (eparterial), which is shorter and more vertically oriented, is located on the right, and the morphologic left main bronchus (hyparterial), which is longer and more horizontally oriented, is located to the left. The anatomic right atrium is on the right and the anatomic left atrium is on the left.

To establish atrial situs, it is necessary to recognize the morphologic characteristics of the right and left atria. The morphologic right atrium has a smooth or sinusal portion, which is found between the interatrial septum and the crista terminalis. It receives the drainage of the superior and inferior venae cavae and the coronary sinus. The trabecular portion is characterized by the presence of pectinate muscles, which are directed from the crista terminalis to the base of the right atrial appendage. The appendage is wide and its edge is blunt. The anatomic left atrium is totally smooth and lacks pectinate muscles. It receives

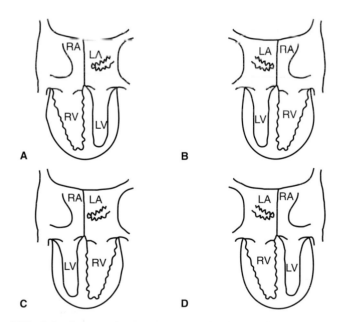

FIG. 2-3. Schematic drawings showing hearts in mesocardia with situs solitus and situs inversus, with atrioventricular concordance and atrioventricular discordance. **A:** Situs solitus and atrioventricular concordance. **B:** Situs inversus and atrioventricular concordance. **C:** Situs solitus and atrioventricular discordance. **D:** Situs inversus and atrioventricular discordance. *RA*, right atrium; *LA*, left atrium; *RV*, right ventricle; *LV*, left ventricle.

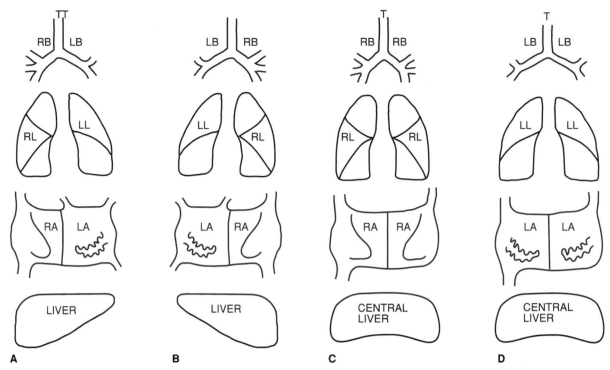

FIG. 2-4 Schematic drawings of the various types of visceroatrial situs. **A:** Situs solitus. **B:** Situs inversus. **C:** Situs ambiguus, bilateral right-sidedness syndrome. **D:** Situs ambiguus, bilateral left-sidedness syndrome. *T*, trachea; *RB*, right bronchus; *LB*, left bronchus; *RL*, right lung; *LL*, left lung; *RA*, right atrium; *LA*, left atrium.

the drainage of the pulmonary veins, and its appendage has a narrow base and fingerlike appearance.

The drainage of the systemic and pulmonary veins does not permit the conclusive identification of the atria, as drainage sites are sometimes anomalous. The atrial septum cannot always be used either, because it can have defects or be absent. The only structures that are constant and allow differentiation between the right and left atria are the appendages (53,54).

Situs Inversus. In situs inversus (Fig. 2-4B), the atria and viscera are in a position that is opposite the normal. The anatomic right atrium is located on the left and the anatomic left atrium is on the right. The major lobe of the liver is located to the left, the right lung and the right main bronchus are on the left, and the left lung and left main bronchus are on the right. The location of the atria and viscera are such that they form a mirror image of what is found in situs solitus.

Situs Ambiguus. Situs ambiguus (55) (Fig. 2-4C,D), also called uncertain or indeterminate situs (20,56), is characterized by a tendency toward bilateral visceroatrial symmetry. Generally, it is associated with bilateral right-sidedness (also called right isomerism or asplenia syndromes) (57) (Fig. 2-4C) or with bilateral left-sidedness (also denominated left isomerism or polysplenia syndromes) (58) (Fig. 2-4D). Rarely, it can present with a

normal spleen (20,56). The liver in the majority of cases occupies a central position.

In bilateral right-sidedness, both atria, lungs, and main bronchi are morphologically of the right type, whereas in bilateral left-sidedness, the atria, lungs, and main bronchi are morphologically of the left type. It is important to note that each organ has its own situs or location; therefore, discordance in the situs of the different organs can exist.

Ventricular Segment

Analysis of the ventricular segment includes the spatial position of the ventricles (i.e., the relationship between the two ventricles) and the manner in which they connect with the atrial segment (i.e., the atrioventricular connection).

Spatial Position of the Ventricles. A rightward (or "D") bulboventricular loop (59) determines embryologically that the anatomic right ventricle will be located on the right and that the anatomic left ventricle will be on the left; this is the normal spatial relationship of the ventricles (Fig. 2-5A). In leftward (or "L") bulboventricular looping (59), the morphologic right ventricle will be on the left and the morphologic left ventricle on the right, resulting in ventricular inversion (Fig. 2-5B).

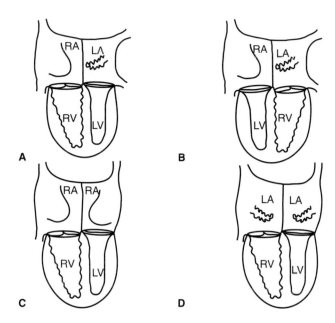

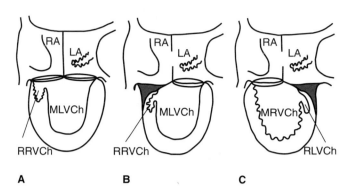

FIG. 2-5. Schematic drawings showing the different types of atrioventricular connection in the presence of two ventricles in the ventricular mass and two perforated atrioventricular valves. A: Concordant. B: Discordant. C: Ambiguous in bilateral right-sidedness syndrome. D: Ambiguous in bilateral left-sidedness syndrome. *RA*, right atrium. *LA*, left atrium; *RV*, right ventricle; *LV*, left ventricle.

FIG. 2-6. Schematic drawings demonstrating the various types of atrioventricular connection in the presence of one ventricle in the ventricular mass, or univentricular atrioventricular connection. A: Double-inlet ventricle. B: Atretic (absent) right atrioventricular connection. The shading indicates the fibrofatty tissue in the right atrioventricular sulcus. C: Atretic (absent) left atrioventricular connection. The *tone* shows the fibrofatty tissue in the left atrioventricular sulcus. *RA*, right atrium; *LA*, left atrium; *MLVCh*, main left ventricular chamber; *MRVCh*, main right ventricular chamber; *RRVCh*, rudimentary right ventricular chamber; *RLVCh*, rudimentary left ventricular chamber.

The anatomic right ventricle has the following characteristics: It has a trileaflet (tricuspid) atrioventricular valve comprising a septal, an anterosuperior, and a posterior leaflet. The ventricular cavity has thick trabcculations, and a medial papillary muscle can be recognized among them. This medial papillary muscle, also called the conal papillary muscle or muscle of Lancici, is located on the right ventricular surface adjacent to the posterior limb of the septomarginal trabecula and receives insertions from the septal and anterosuperior leaflets. The anterolateral papillary muscle is located in the anterior free wall of the right ventricle and receives insertions of the anterosuperior and posterior tricuspid leaflets. The posterior papillary muscle(s) can be single or multiple and receives tendinous chordal attachments of the posterior and septal leaflets. The septomarginal trabecula is prominently located on the right ventricular surface and has an apical and a basal end. The apical end is continuous with the moderator band, which is a band of muscular tissue extending from the interventricular septum to the base of the anterolateral papillary muscle. The basal end of the septomarginal trabecula bifurcates into an anterior and a posterior limb; between these limbs is found the septal portion of the crista supraventricularis (the outlet or infundibular septum). The crista supraventricularis is a fibrous or muscular structure; in hearts with normal outflow tracts, it separates the tricuspid and pulmonic valves. It has two portions—a septal portion that inserts between

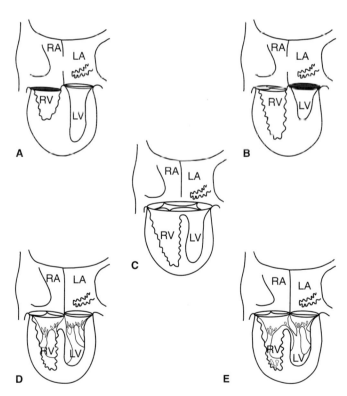

FIG. 2-7. Schematic drawings showing the various modes of atrioventricular connection. A: One perforated left and one atretic (imperforate) right atrioventricular valve. B: One perforated right and one atretic (imperforate) left atrioventricular valve. C: Common atrioventricular valve. D: Overriding tricuspid valve. E: Straddling tricuspid valve. *RA*, right atrium; *LA*, left atrium; *RV*, right ventricle; *LV*, left ventricle.

the limbs of the septomarginal trabecula and constitutes the infundibular or outlet septum and a parietal portion that extends from the interventricular septum to the free wall of the right ventricle. The infundibulum of the right ventricle is completely muscular and supports the pulmonic valve.

The anatomic left ventricle has a bileaflet (mitral) atrioventricular valve comprising an anterior and a posterior leaflet. The ventricular cavity is characterized by smooth walls and has fine trabeculations in its apical end. Within these are an anterolateral papillary muscle located in the free wall of the left ventricle and a posteromedial papillary muscle located in the posterior portion of the interventricular septum. Both papillary muscles receive tendinous insertions from the anterior and posterior mitral leaflets. The left ventricular infundibulum is fibromuscular and supports the aortic valve. Its muscular component is the outlet portion of the interventricular septum, and its fibrous component is the free portion of the anterior mitral leaflet.

Atrioventricular Connection. The different types and modes of connection between the atria and ventricles should be considered separately in this analysis (44–46,52,53).

The type of connection refers to the junction between the atrial and ventricular segments; therefore, it is important to note whether two separate or only one single ventricle is present in the ventricular mass. If there are two separate ventricles, then the connection is biventricular and can be one of three types (45,53,60) (Fig. 2-5). If the right atrium is connected with the morphologic right ventricle and the left atrium with the morphologic left ventricle, then the connection is said to be *concordant* (Fig. 2-5A). If the anatomic right atrium is connected with the morphologic left ventricle and the left atrium with the morphologic right ventricle, then the connection is said to be *discordant* (Fig. 2-5B). In situs ambiguus, the atrioventricular connection is said to be *ambiguous* because both atria are of the same anatomic type, either two morphologic right (Fig. 2-5C) or two morphologic left atria (Fig. 2-5D).

If there is only one ventricular chamber in the ventricular mass, the connection is a univentricular atrioventricular connection (61-63). There are also three types (Fig. 2-6). If both atria are connected to one ventricle, then a double-inlet ventricle is present (Fig. 2-6A). If the right atrioventricular valve is absent and no potential connection can be identified between the blind-ending right

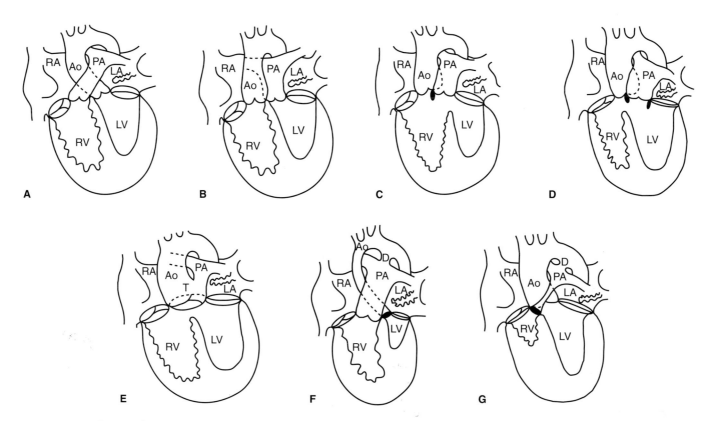

FIG. 2-8. Schematic drawings showing the different types of ventriculoarterial connection. **A:** Concordant. **B:** Discordant. **C:** Double-outlet right ventricle. **D:** Double-outlet left ventricle. **E:** Single-outlet truncus arteriosus type. **F:** Single-outlet aortic atresia type. **G:** Single-outlet pulmonary atresia type. *RA*, right atrium; *LA*, left atrium; *RV*, right ventricle; *LV*, left ventricle; *Ao*, aorta; *PA*, pulmonary artery; *D*, ductus arteriosus; *T*, truncus arteriosus.

atrium and the rudimentary ventricle but a potential connection is present to the main ventricular chamber, then this is called an absent right atrioventricular connection (64) (Fig. 2-6B). If the left atrioventricular valve is absent and no potential connection is identified between the blind-ending left atrium and the rudimentary ventricular chamber but a potential connection exists to the main ventricular chamber, then this is called an absent left atrioventricular connection (61–63) (Fig. 2-6C). (See chapter 17.)

The mode of connection refers to the morphologic characteristics of the atrioventricular valves and their subvalvular apparatus. There are five modes of connection (44–46,52,53): (a) through *two perforated atrioventricular valves* (Figs. 2-5A, 2-6A), (b) through *one perforated and one atretic atrioventricular valve* (Figs. 2-6B,C; 2-7A,B) (c) through a *common atrioventricular valve* (Fig. 2-7C), (d) through an *overriding atrioventricular valve* (Fig. 2-7D), and (e) through a *straddling atrioventricular valve* (Fig. 2-7E). The term overriding refers to the relation of the valvular ring to the interventricular septum and is used when the valve ring is above both surfaces of the ventricular septum in the presence of two ventricles or above the ventricular or the intercameral septum when a main ventricular and an accessory ventricular chamber are present (Fig. 2-7D). Straddling refers to an atrioventricular valve whose subvalvular apparatus has insertions on both sides of the ventricular septal surface (Fig. 2-7E).

Arterial Segment

Analysis of the arterial segment considers the ventriculoarterial connection and the spatial relationship of the great vessels. The arterial segment is composed of the aorta and pulmonary arteries. The location of the aorta is posterior and to the right of the pulmonary artery at the level of the valves. From its proximal end, the origin of the coronary arteries can be seen; distally, it is directed to the front, rightward, and superiorly and gives rise to the head and neck vessels. The location of the pulmonary artery, at the valvular level, is anterior and to the left of the aorta. It is directed leftward and superiorly and divides into two branches, a right pulmonary artery and a left pulmonary artery.

Ventriculoarterial Connection. The ventriculoarterial connection can be of a concordant, discordant, double-outlet, or single-outlet type (44–46,52,53,65,66) (Fig. 2-8). When the pulmonary artery emerges from the morphologic right ventricle and the aorta from the morphologic left ventricle, the connection is said to be *concordant* irrespective of the spatial position of the ventricles (Fig. 2-8A). If the aorta emerges from the morphologic right ventricle and the pulmonary artery from the morphologic left ventricle, the connection is said to be *discordant* (Fig. 2-8B). A *double-outlet* ventriculoarterial connection is

said to exist when both great arteries emerge completely or almost completely from the same ventricle, when one artery emerges completely from one ventricle and the other overrides the ventricular septum by more than 50% over the same ventricle, or when more than half of the circumference of each semilunar valve is connected with the same ventricle (43,65,67–71) (Fig. 2-8C,D). A *single-outlet* ventriculoarterial connection is present when only one artery emerges from the heart; this can be from a morphologic right or left ventricle, overriding the interventricular septum, from an outlet chamber of the right or left type, or from a double-inlet ventricle of the right, left, or indeterminate type. In this type of ventriculoarterial connection, three subtypes are seen: single-outlet truncus arteriosus type (Fig. 2-8E), single-outlet aortic atresia type (Fig. 2-8F), and single-outlet pulmonary atresia type (Fig. 2-8G).

Spatial Relation of the Great Arteries. The spatial relation can be analyzed by determining the position of the aorta with respect to the pulmonary artery (Fig. 2-9). When the great arteries are normally related, the location of the aorta is posterior and to the right of the pulmonary artery, which is anterior and to the left (Fig. 2-9A). In a side-by-side relationship of the great arteries, the aorta can be located to the right of the pulmonary artery (*side-by-side great arteries with aorta to the right*; Fig. 2-9B)

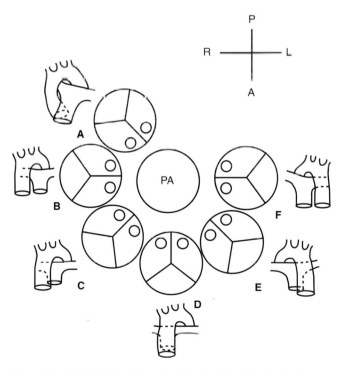

FIG. 2-9. Schematic drawing showing the different types of spatial relationship of the great arteries. **A:** Normally related great arteries. **B:** Side-by-side great arteries with aorta to the right. **C:** Aorta anterior and to the right. **D:** Aorta strictly anterior. **E:** Aorta anterior and to the left. **F:** Side-by-side great arteries with aorta to the left. *PA*, pulmonary artery. *R*, right; *L*, left; *A*, anterior; *P*, posterior.

or to the left of the pulmonary artery (*side-by-side great arteries with aorta to the left*; Fig. 2-9F). When the aorta is anterior with respect to the pulmonary artery, it can be either *anterior and to the right* (Fig. 2-9C), *strictly anterior* (Fig. 2-9D), or *anterior and to the left* (Fig. 2-9E).

REFERENCES

1. Lev M. Pathologic diagnosis of positional variations in cardiac chambers in congenital heart disease. *Lab Invest* 1954;3:71–82.
2. Stanger P, Rudolph AM, Edwards JE. Cardiac malpositions. An overview based on study of sixty-five necropsy specimens. *Circulation* 1977;56:159–172.
3. Shaher RM, Duckworth JW, Khoury GH, Moes CAF. The significance of the atrial situs in the diagnosis of positional anomalies of the heart. I. Anatomic and embryologic considerations. *Am Heart J* 1967;73:32–40.
4. Campbell M, Deuchar DC. Dextrocardia and isolated laevocardia. I: Isolated laevocardia. *Br Heart J* 1965;27:69–82.
5. Liberthson RR, Hastreiter AR, Sinha SN, Bharati S, Novak GM, Lev M. Levocardia with visceral heterotaxy—isolated levocardia: pathologic anatomy and its clinical implications. *Am Heart J* 1973;85:40–54.
6. Taussig HB. Situs inversus with levocardia. In: Taussig HB, ed. *Specific malformations.* Cambridge, MA: Harvard University Press, 1960:984–995 (*Congenital malformations of the heart*, Vol 2).
7. Elliot LP, Jue KL, Amplatz K. A roentgen classification of cardiac malpositions. *Invest Radiol* 1966;1:17–28.
8. Daves ML, Pryor R. Cardiac positions. A primer. *Am Heart J* 1970;79:408–421.
9. De la Cruz MV, Anselmi G, Munos-Castellanos L, Nadal-Ginard B, Munoz-Armas S. Systematization and embryological and anatomical study of mirror-image dextrocardias, dextroversions, and laevoversions. *Br Heart J* 1971;33:841–853.
10. Anselmi G, Munoz S, Blanco P, Machado I, De la Cruz MV. Systematization and clinical study of dextroversion, mirror-image dextrocardia, and laevoversion. *Br Heart J* 1972;34:1085–1098.
11. Attie F, Malpartida F, Poveda JJ, Testelli MR, Espino Vela J. Acyanotic levoversion in situs inversus. *Chest* 1973;64:668–670.
12. Moscovitz HL, Gordon AJ, Scherlis L. Levocardia. *Am Heart J* 1952;44:184–195.
13. Lev M, Rowlatt UF. The pathologic anatomy of mixed levocardia. A review of thirteen cases of atrial or ventricular inversion with or without corrected transposition. *Am J Cardiol* 1961;8:216–263.
14. Bharati S, Lev M. Positional variations of the heart and its component chambers [Editorial]. *Circulation* 1979;59:886–887.
15. Rowe GG, Paul LW. A case of abnormal cardiac position (levoposition). *Circulation* 1959;19:750–752.
16. Jones HW. Types of dextrocardia. *Br Med J* 1924;1:147–148.
17. Reinberg SA, Mandelstam ME. On the various types of dextrocardia and their diagnostics. *Radiology* 1928;11:240–249.
18. Van Praagh R, Van Praagh S, Vlad P, Keith JD. Anatomic types of congenital dextrocardia. Diagnostic and embryologic implications. *Am J Cardiol* 1964;13:510–531.
19. Wilkinson JL, Acerete F. Terminological pitfalls in congenital heart disease. Reappraisal of some confusing terms, with an account of a simplified system of basic nomenclature. *Br Heart J* 1973;35:1166–1177.
20. Van Praagh R. Terminology of congenital heart disease. Glossary and commentary [Editorial]. *Circulation* 1977;56:139–143.
21. Van Praagh R, Vlad P. Dextrocardia, mesocardia, and levocardia: the segmental approach to diagnosis in congenital heart disease. In: Keith JD, Rowe RD, Vlad P, eds. *Heart disease in infancy and childhood*, 3rd ed. New York: Macmillan, 1978:638–695.
22. Lev M, Liberthson RR, Eckner FAO, Arcilla RA. Pathologic anatomy of dextrocardia and its clinical implications. *Circulation* 1968;37:979–999.
23. Squarcia U, Ritter DG, Kincaid OW. Dextrocardia: angiocardiographic study and classification. *Am J Cardiol* 1973;32:965–977.
24. Huhta JC, Hagler DJ, Seward JB, Tajik AJ, Julsrud PR, Ritter DG. Two-dimensional echocardiographic assessment of dextrocardia: a segmental approach. *Am J Cardiol* 1982;50:1351–1360.
25. Parsons-Smith B. Dextrocardia, complete and incomplete, with four illustrative cases. *Lancet* 1919;2:1076–1078.
26. Kartagener M. Zur pathogenese der Bronchiektasien. I. Mitteilung: Bronchiektasien bei situs viscerum inversus. *Beitr Klin Tuberk* 1933;83:489–501.
27. Burchell HB, Pugh DG. Uncomplicated isolated dextrocardia (dextroversio cordis type). *Am Heart J* 1952;44:196–206.
28. Gubbay ER. Isolated congenital dextrocardia. *Am Heart J* 1955;50:356–365.
29. Campbell M, Deuchar DC. Dextrocardia and isolated laevocardia. II. Situs inversus and isolated dextrocardia. *Br Heart J* 1966;28:472–487.
30. Welsh RA, Felson B. Uncomplicated dextroversion of the heart. *Radiology* 1956;66:24–32.
31. Grant RP. The syndrome of dextroversion of the heart. *Circulation* 1958;18:25–36.
32. Capon NB, Chamberlain EN. A case of true dextrocardia. *Lancet* 1925;1:918–919.
33. Cantrell JR, Haller JA, Ravitch MM. A syndrome of congenital defects involving the abdominal wall, sternum, diaphragm, pericardium, and heart. *Surg Gynecol Obstet* 1958;107:602–614.
34. Gasul BM, Arcilla RA, Lev M. Dextrocardia and levocardia with situs inversus. In: Gasul BM, Arcilla RA, Lev M, eds. *Heart disease in children. Diagnosis and treatment.* Philadelphia: JB Lippincott Co, 1966:1050–1085.
35. Lev M, Bharati S. Abnormal position of the heart and its chambers. In: Edwards JE, Lev M, Abell MR, eds. *The heart.* Baltimore: Williams & Wilkins, 1974:327–331.
36. Senac M de (Jean-Baptiste). Traité de la structure du coeur, de son action, et de ses maladies. Paris 1749. Cited by Manchester B, White PD. Dextrocardia with situs inversus complicated by hypertensive and coronary heart disease. *Am Heart J* 1938;15:493–497.
37. Arcilla RA, Gasul BM. Congenital dextrocardia. Clinical, angiocardiographic, and autopsy studies on 50 patients. *J Pediatr* 1961;58:39–58.
38. Willius FA. Congenital dextrocardia with situs transversus complicated by hypertensive heart disease: electrocardiographic changes. *Am Heart J* 1931;7:110–113.
39. Van Praagh R, Weinberg PM, Matsuoka R, Van Praagh S. Malpositions of the heart. In: Adams FH, Emmanouilides GC, eds. *Moss' heart disease in infants, children, and adolescents*, 3rd ed. Baltimore: Williams & Wilkins, 1983:422–458.
40. Lev M, Liberthson RR, Golden JG, Eckner FAO, Arcilla RA. The pathologic anatomy of mesocardia. *Am J Cardiol* 1971;28:428–435.
41. Van Praagh R. The segmental approach to diagnosis in congenital heart disease. In: Bergsma D, ed. *Birth defects: original article series*, Vol 8. Baltimore: Williams & Wilkins, 1972:4–23.
42. De la Cruz MV, Nadal-Ginard B. Rules for the diagnosis of visceral situs, truncoconal morphologies, and ventricular inversions. *Am Heart J* 1972;84:19–32.
43. Kirklin JW, Pacifico AD, Bargeron LM Jr, Soto B. Cardiac repair in anatomically corrected malposition of the great arteries. *Circulation* 1973;48:153–159.
44. Shinebourne EA, Macartney FJ, Anderson RH. Sequential chamber localization—logical approach to diagnosis in congenital heart disease. *Br Heart J* 1976;38:327–340.
45. Tynan MJ, Becker AE, Macartney FJ, Quero-Jimenez M, Shinebourne EA, Anderson RH. Nomenclature and classification of congenital heart disease. *Br Heart J* 1979;41:544–553.
46. Anderson RH, Becker AE, Freedom RM, et al. Sequential segmental analysis of congenital heart disease. *Pediatr Cardiol* 1984;5:281–288.
47. Macartney FJ, Shinebourne EA, Anderson RH. Connexions, relations, discordance, and distortions. *Br Heart J* 1976;38:323–326.
48. De la Cruz MV, Berrazueta JR, Arteaga M, Attie F, Soni J. Rules for diagnosis of arterioventricular discordances and spatial identification of ventricles. Crossed great arteries and transposition of the great arteries. *Br Heart J* 1976;38:341–354.
49. Shinebourne EA. Introduction—terminology and nomenclature. In: Anderson RH, Shinebourne EA, eds. *Paediatric cardiology 1977.* Edinburgh: Churchill Livingstone, 1978:3–4.

50. Van Praagh R. Diagnosis of complex congenital heart disease: morphologic-anatomic method and terminology. *Cardiovasc Intervent Radiol* 1984;7:115–120.

51. Freedom RM. The anthropology of the segmental approach to the diagnosis of complex congenital heart disease. *Cardiovasc Intervent Radiol* 1984;7:121–123.

52. Anderson RH, Ho SY. The diagnosis and naming of congenital malformed hearts. In: Macartney FJ, ed. *Congenital heart disease.* Lancaster, England: MTP Press Limited, 1986:1–34.

53. Anderson RH, Macartney FJ, Shinebourne EA, Tynan M. Terminology. In: Anderson RH, Macartney FJ, Shinebourne EA, Tynan M, eds. *Paediatric cardiology*, Vol 1. Edinburgh: Churchill Livingstone, 1987:65–82.

54. Sharma S, Devine W, Anderson RH, Zuberbuhler JR. The determination of atrial arrangement by examination of appendage morphology in 1842 heart specimens. *Br Heart J* 1988;60:227–231.

55. Van Mierop LHS, Gessner IH, Schiebler GL. Asplenia and polysplenia syndromes. In: Bergsma D, ed. *Birth defects: original article series*, Vol 8. Baltimore: Williams & Wilkins, 1972:36–44.

56. Macartney FJ, Partridge JB, Shinebourne EA, Tynan M, Anderson RH. Identification of atrial situs. In: Anderson RH, Shinebourne EA, eds. *Paediatric cardiology 1977*. Edinburgh: Churchill Livingstone, 1978:16–26.

57. Ivemark BI. Implications of agenesis of the spleen on the pathogenesis of cono-truncus anomalies in childhood. An analysis of the heart malformations in the splenic agenesis syndrome, with fourteen new cases. *Acta Paediatr* 1955;44[Suppl 104]:1–110.

58. Moller JH, Nakib A, Anderson RC, Edwards JE. Congenital cardiac disease associated with polysplenia. A developmental complex of bilateral left-sidedness. *Circulation* 1967;36:780–799.

59. Van Praagh R, Ongley PA, Swan HJC. Anatomic types of single or common ventricle in man. Morphologic and geometric aspects of 60 necropsied cases. *Am J Cardiol* 1964;13:367–386.

60. Macartney FJ. Classification and nomenclature of congenital heart disease. In: Stark J, De Leval M, eds. *Surgery for congenital heart defects*, 2nd ed. Philadelphia: WB Saunders, 1994:3–12.

61. Anderson RH, Macartney FJ, Tynan M, et al. Univentricular atrioventricular connection: the single ventricle trap unsprung. *Pediatr Cardiol* 1983;4:273–280.

62. Anderson RH, Becker AE, Tynan M, Macartney FJ, Rigby ML, Wilkinson JL. The univentricular atrioventricular connection: getting to the root of a thorny problem. *Am J Cardiol* 1984;54:822–828.

63. Freedom RM, Smallhorn JF. Hearts with a univentricular atrioventricular connection. In: Freedom RM, Benson LN, Smallhorn JF, eds. *Neonatal heart disease*. London: Springer-Verlag, 1992:497–521.

64. Anderson RH, Wilkinson JL, Gerlis LM, Smith A, Becker AE. Atresia of the right atrioventricular orifice. *Br Heart J* 1977;39:414–428.

65. Tynan MJ, Anderson RH, Macartney FJ, Shinebourne EA. The ventricular origin of the great arteries. In: Anderson RH, Shinebourne EA, eds. *Paediatric cardiology 1977*. Edinburgh: Churchill Livingstone, 1978:36–42.

66. Quero-Jimenez M, Anderson RH, Tynan M, et al. Summation of anatomic patterns of atrioventricular and ventriculo-arterial connexions. In: Godman MJ, ed. *Pediatric cardiology*, Vol 4. Edinburgh: Churchill Livingstone, 1981:211–226.

67. Lev M, Bharati S, Meng CCL, Liberthson RR, Paul MH, Idriss F. A concept of double-outlet right ventricle. *J Thorac Cardiovasc Surg* 1972;64:271–281.

68. Wilcox BR, Ho SY, Macartney FJ, Becker AE, Gerlis LM, Anderson RH. Surgical anatomy of double-outlet right ventricle with situs solitus and atrioventricular concordance. *J Thorac Cardiovasc Surg* 1981;82:405–417.

69. Anderson RH, Becker AE, Wilcox BR, Macartney FJ, Wilkinson JL. Surgical anatomy of double-outlet right ventricle—a reappraisal. *Am J Cardiol* 1983;52:555–559.

70. Wilkinson JL. Double outlet ventricle. In: Anderson RH, Macartney FJ, Shinebourne EA, Tynan M, eds. *Paediatric cardiology*, Vol 2. Edinburgh: Churchill Livingstone, 1987:889–911.

71. Musumeci F, Shumway S, Lincoln C, Anderson RH. Surgical treatment for double-outlet right ventricle at the Brompton Hospital, 1973 to 1986. *J Thorac Cardiovasc Surg* 1988;96:278–287.

CHAPTER 3

Physics and Instrumentation of Ultrasound and Doppler Imaging

Robin S. Shandas

ULTRASOUND WAVES

Ultrasound waves are pressure waves similar to acoustic waves. Just as one hears differences in pitch and loudness among sounds in different environments, ultrasound signals are also modified depending on the characteristics of the environment through which they are traveling— in this case, the body. Ultrasound signals in the body can be classified as longitudinal compression waves, and by the definition of ultrasound, they contain frequencies above the audible human range (higher than 20 kHz). However, most medical ultrasound imaging systems utilize much higher frequencies (1 to 20 MHz) to provide adequate resolution of small structures within the body. It is important to consider some general properties of ultrasound signals to gain insight into some of the limitations and advantages of this noninvasive technique in imaging structure and flow within the body.

Four main factors should be kept in mind as the utility of ultrasound for medical imaging is examined: (a) the relationship between frequency and wavelength; (b) the diffraction of the ultrasound beam; (c) the effect of various media on the speed of signal transmission; and (d) the properties of wave transmission, reflection, and absorption. All these have fundamental effects on the quality of the image ultimately presented by the ultrasound scanner.

Frequency and Wavelength

The frequency and wavelength of an ultrasound signal are inversely related via the speed of the signal in the media, and can be represented by the following equation:

$$\lambda = \frac{c}{f} \qquad [1]$$

where λ is wavelength, c is the speed of the ultrasound signal in the tissue, and f is frequency.

Understanding the components and relationships within the above equation is essential to understanding the fundamental theoretical spatial resolution limitations in ultrasound imaging. As shown in Fig. 3-1, λ determines how close two targets can be and still be imaged as separate objects. Thus, Eq. 1 also explains the relationship between resolution and frequency, indicating that high frequencies are needed to image small structures, such as those within fetuses or children, adequately.

Ultrasound Beam Diffraction

Diffraction of an ultrasound signal is caused by multiple waves interacting with each other, canceling the signal at some spatial locations (destructive interference) and enhancing the signal in others (constructive interference). Because ultrasound transducers consist of a number of ultrasound signal generators (piezoelectric crystals), the beam that is eventually formed when all these elements are activated is shaped by diffraction processes. Thus, although each element can be thought of as producing a spherically growing ultrasound signal that expands equally in all directions, the interaction of signals from multiple elements produces a more focused and directed beam whose direction is determined by the spatial configuration of all the elements (Fig. 3-2). For optimal ultrasound imaging, it is important to direct the ultrasound beam precisely in the desired direction. This requires straight beam paths where diffraction processes are accurately controlled. Diffraction is related to the number of wavelengths that can be generated by the ultrasound transducer; the greater the number of wavelengths, the straighter the resulting ultrasound beam. The aperture of a transducer defines the number of wavelengths it can

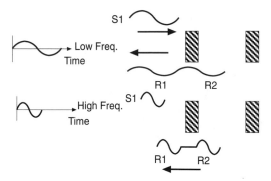

FIG. 3-1. The theoretical relationship between imaging resolution in the axial direction and transducer frequency can be understood by examining the differences in reflected waves from two closely spaced scatterers when signals of low and high frequencies are transmitted. The top illustrates one cycle of a low-frequency signal (S_1) transmitted toward two scatterers. Part of the transmitted wave is reflected from the first scatterer (R_1) while part of the signal moves through and is reflected by the second scatterer (R_2). Because of the closeness of the two scatterers, the two reflected signals R_1 and R_2 merge. The receiver cannot distinguish between R_1 and R_2 and thus cannot identify that the received signal is a result of two scatterers. On the ultrasound image, only a single scatterer would be displayed. By contrast, the reflections from a transmitted signal of a higher frequency (*bottom*) can be resolved because of the signal's shorter cycle length. Although in practice axial resolution is not purely dependent on frequency, such an illustration is useful to determine the theoretical maximum axial resolution for a particular transducer frequency.

produce for a particular frequency. Thus, a 15-mm-wide transducer has apertures of 20 λ at 2 MHz and 48 λ at 5 MHz.

Various Speeds in Various Media

The compression wave characteristic of ultrasound signals implies that the signal speed can be affected by the density of the media through which it propagates. Thus, the speed of an ultrasound signal in a dense structure such as bone is much faster (4,000 m/s) than the speed in blood (1,570 m/s), muscle (1,580 m/s), or fat (1,440 m/s). In Eq. 1, we saw that frequency and wavelength were inversely related via the speed of the signal *c*. This indicates that the wavelength of a constant-frequency signal generated at the transducer can change by the time the signal has traveled into the body.

Wave Transmission, Reflection, and Absorption

The effect of the properties of ultrasound wave transmission, reflection, and absorption can be illustrated with the analogy of headlights in fog. The fact that the headlights can be seen through the fog illustrates the *transmis-*

sion of the signal through the fog. Seeing the fog shows that the signal has been *reflected off* the particles within the fog. When water droplets are present, certain wavelengths are *absorbed* by the moisture, leaving the remaining colors to be seen.

Ultrasound wave transmission and reflection within the body depend on the small differences in tissue structures. Although the body appears as an extremely homogeneous material to the ultrasound signal, there are enough small differences to produce reflections of the ultrasound signal. Detection and processing of these extremely small reflections underlie the science of ultrasound imaging. For example, only 0.04% of the incident ultrasound energy is reflected from the interface between muscle and blood, whereas 46% of the incident energy is reflected from the interface between muscle and bone (1). Such reflection characteristics explain many of the problems that arise during imaging of areas where both soft and hard structures are found. The interface between soft and hard structures produces strong reflections that may overwhelm reflections from less distinct interfaces.

Absorption of ultrasound energy by the cells in the body is the primary mechanism by which the ultrasound signal is attenuated as it passes through the tissue. Absorption losses are energy transformations in which ultrasound energy is converted into heat. In general, absorption losses can be modeled as increasing with frequency. Thus, higher frequencies are associated with greater absorption of the signal and so cannot penetrate more deeply into the tissue, explaining the application differences between low- and high-frequency transducers. Low frequencies penetrate more deeply into the tissue and are therefore required to study structures relatively farther away, such as those in adults. In pediatric imaging, the structures to be studied are relatively closer, and a higher-frequency transducer with its advantage of better spatial resolution can be used.

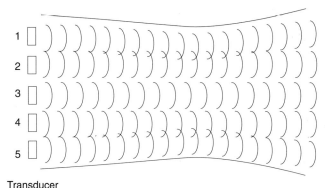

Transducer elements

FIG. 3-2. Illustration of the natural focusing of an ultrasound beam as a result of constructive and destructive interference from multiple signals. Diffractive focusing depends on the aperture of the ultrasound transducer. *1–5*, transducer elements.

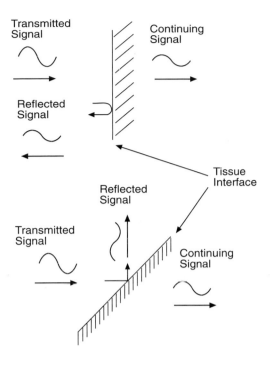

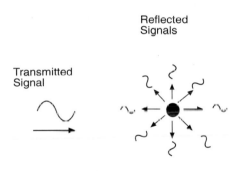

FIG. 3-3. Two major types of ultrasound reflections off tissue. **A:** Specular reflections. These are caused by differences in the density of the acoustic mass at the interface between two tissues. Specular backscatter is maximized when the tissue interface is at right angles to the transducer. **B:** Single scatterer. Single-scatterer reflections are caused by small, dense objects that are of the order of 1 λ in dimension. Single-scatterer reflections are strong and scatter in all directions. Ultrasound imaging of the body usually consists of a combination of specular and single-scatterer reflections, so that it is necessary for the transducer to be perpendicular to the tissue interface to maximize returning echoes.

Single-scatterer versus Specular Reflections. Ultrasound signal reflections off tissue interfaces are received by the ultrasound transducer and generated into an image by the scanner processing system. As shown in Fig. 3-3, two main types of reflections occur in the body: single-scatterer reflections and specular reflections. Single-

scatterer reflections are produced by dense objects that are about 1 λ in size. Single scatterers reflect ultrasound energy strongly in all directions regardless of the incident angle of the transmitted wave. Specular reflections occur off tissue interfaces and depend on the angle of the incoming wave. As stated above, these reflections are a product of the mismatch in density between two tissue structures. The strongest specular reflections occur when the incoming wave is perpendicular to the tissue interface—that is, the transducer is at an angle of 90 degrees to the tissue. Such a position also allows most of the reflected energy to be received by the transducer. Any deviation from perpendicular causes the reflected wave to bounce off toward another direction, as shown in Fig. 3-3, thereby preventing the signal from being received at the transducer. Most interfaces in the body consist of a combination of specular and single-scatterer reflectors. Thus, a perpendicular transducer position is needed to maximize returning echo signals.

ULTRASOUND SIGNAL GENERATION

Ultrasound waves are generated by transducers composed of numerous elements. Each element is composed of a piezoelectric crystal independently connected to the transmission waveform generator, which determines the shape, direction, and strength of the transmitted beam. Piezoelectric materials have the property that any applied deformation produces an electric field across the material. Likewise, a voltage difference applied to opposite sides of the material produces a deformation. When a rapidly changing sinusoidal voltage waveform is applied, the piezoelectric material elongates and compresses at the frequency of the applied signal. This high-frequency vibration can be transferred into various structures with the use of appropriate connecting material, thereby allowing ultrasound energy to be transmitted into the body. Returning echo signals are received in the opposite fashion, wherein the piezoelectric crystal transforms the returning vibrations into an electric signal, which is then processed to produce the ultrasound image.

The transducers that transmit and receive ultrasound signals are composed of multiple piezoelectric crystals, shaped to form rectangular or concentric arrays depending on the type of transducer. Figure 3-4 illustrates transducer shapes for linear and annular types of configurations. As stated above, each crystal is independently controlled and can be excited at different times and to different amplitudes. Varying the time at which each crystal fires the ultrasound signal in linear fashion allows the resulting ultrasound beam to be steered in different directions. Varying the crystal timing in nonlinear fashion permits both steering and focusing of the beam, which occur as a result of constructive and destructive interference

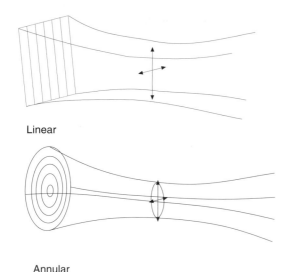

Linear

Annular

FIG. 3-4. Examples of two different types of transducer array configurations. Linear arrays (*top*) are usually found in electronically steered transducers. These have good focusing in one direction but not in the orthogonal direction. Annular arrays (*bottom*) are found in mechanically steered transducers and are composed of concentric circles. These arrays have symmetric focusing in lateral and azimuthal directions. *Arrows* indicate the focusing directions.

among all the signals. The various methods of producing timing delays and array configurations allow for a wide variety of transducer types. In linearly phased arrays, a rectangular piezoelectric crystal configuration is used, along with electronic beam steering and focusing accomplished by delaying crystal activation in a nonlinear manner. In annular arrays, the crystals are configured as concentric circles, which allows for accurate focusing of the beam in two planes but does not allow for electronic beam steering. Thus, annular arrays must be mechanically rotated for two-dimensional ultrasound imaging.

ULTRASOUND IMAGING (PULSED-ECHO AMPLITUDE IMAGING)

Ultrasound imaging consists of detecting and processing minute reflections from various parts of the imaged structure. Accordingly, the ultrasound scanner must distinguish signals reflected from various depths to reconstruct returning signal information into an accurate image of the heart or other organ of interest. To facilitate recognition of signals from different depths, ultrasound energy is transmitted into the body in short pulses. The frequency of these pulses, the pulse-repetition frequency, is carefully controlled, and so the time between each pulse, the pulse-repetition interval, is known and constant. Both transmission and reception of the signal occur at these known time intervals. Because the velocity of sound in tissue (blood, muscle) can be considered relatively constant

(1,580 m/s), the time needed for one ultrasound pulse to travel a certain distance and back can be calculated. The time interval between successive pulses, therefore, can be thought of as a depth interval. Once an ultrasound pulse is transmitted, the receiver picks up the returning echoes at successive pulse-repetition intervals, which in effect is the equivalent of picking up echoes from ever-increasing depths. Practical constraints related to signal absorption and dispersion create the need to transmit several pulses to receive signals from various depths. Other practical limits, such as transducer frequency and element configuration, create further trade-offs among spatial resolution, depth of imaging, temporal resolution, and suppression of artifactual noise.

Amplitude Mode

Amplitude mode (A mode) was the earliest and simplest ultrasound imaging modality. It consists of transmitting a single ultrasound pulse into the body, waiting for a specified period of time, and examining the returning echo signal on an oscilloscope. The echo from the distance corresponding to the time delay between transmission and reception will be seen as a low-amplitude, high-frequency burst with roughly the same frequency as the transmitted signal. The development of more advanced signal-processing techniques has made this imaging modality obsolete.

Motion Mode

Motion mode (M mode), an advancement over A-mode imaging, allowed appreciation of tissue motion along one ultrasound beam line by successively processing returning echoes from different depths, as explained above. The ability to process signals continuously over time allowed M-mode imaging to produce good images of fast-moving structures, such as cardiac walls and valve leaflets. M-mode imaging is still used today because its temporal and spatial resolution are better than those of two-dimensional imaging modalities.

Brightness Mode

The ultrasound imaging modality most commonly used today is brightness mode (B mode). B mode is a two-dimensional technique that displays a cross-section of the imaged structure on a conventional monitor. B mode is more advanced than M-mode imaging because it processes echoes from multiple depths along multiple, radially oriented scan lines. All these reflected echoes are processed by means of highly sophisticated digital signal-processing techniques, so that scanning and display of even rapidly moving structures, such as the heart, become possible. It is useful to examine some fundamental relationships between ultrasound pulse transmission, reflection, and reception. Figure 3-5 illustrates how an ultrasound pulse is reflected from two targets placed a distance D apart. The first target is placed at a distance R_1 from the transducer and the second at a distance R_2. The ultrasound pulse is generated into the medium and travels at a velocity c. The pulse reaches the first target in time R_1/c; it reflects part of the pulse, absorbs some of the pulse, and refracts the rest through toward the second target, which does the same. When the ultrasound transducer is turned to receive mode, it receives the first reflection at a time $t_1 = 2R_1/c$ after it sent out the pulse. Likewise, the second reflection occurs at a time $t_2 = 2R_2/c$. The difference in time between receiving these two reflections can be calculated using the distance between the targets ($\Delta t = 2D/c$). Therefore, to distinguish these two targets, the ultrasound pulse length T must be of sufficiently short duration that there is no overlap between the first and second reflected pulses. T must therefore be smaller than Δt for the two targets to be distinguished by the ultrasound scanner. Thus, it is the ultrasound pulse length T that truly determines the axial resolution of an ultrasound system. However, frequency plays an important role in increasing or reducing T because higher frequencies

shorten the total pulse length required and thereby increase resolution.

Another important point regarding two-dimensional echo imaging concerns the relationships among frame rate, lateral resolution, imaging depth, and transducer frequency. All these variables are interconnected; changing one causes a corresponding change in the other, and all must be kept in mind when two-dimensional echo scans are optimized. Two-dimensional echo imaging sequentially builds the received echoes from multiple points along one beam line before radially shifting the beam line and starting the process again. The time required to process one beam line is related to the maximum depth R at which the imaging scanner is set and is $2R/c$. The scanner also has to wait an additional time t_o to allow all the reverberations to die down before moving to the next beam line. Thus, the total time required for one beam line t_b is as follows:

$$t_b = \frac{2R}{c + t_o} \qquad [2]$$

If there are N number of beams within a two-dimensional sector, the frame rate FR can be calculated as the inverse of the total time required to process one frame:

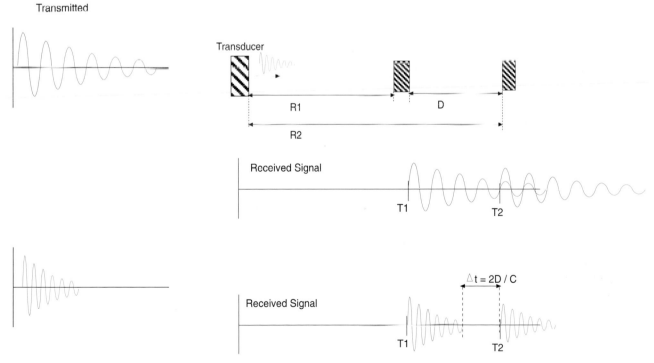

FIG. 3-5. The limitation of maximum axial resolution is not related purely to frequency but actually to transmitted ultrasound pulse length. Smaller pulse lengths (*bottom*) allow targets that are closer together to be detected. For two targets placed at distances R_1 and R_2 from the ultrasound transducer and a distance D apart, the pulse length required to resolve them would have to be less than $2D/c$, where c is the speed of the ultrasound signal in this tissue. The receiver would pick up the reflections from the first scatterer at time t_1 and from the second at time t_2.

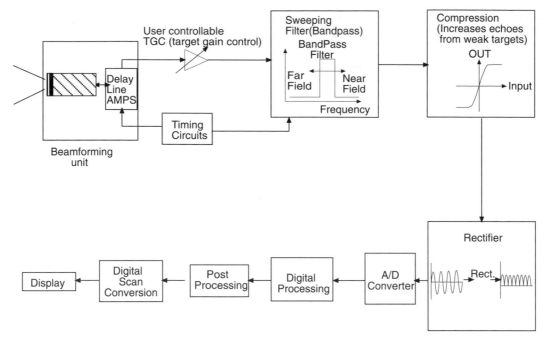

FIG. 3-6. Block diagram of a typical ultrasound imaging system. *AMPS*, amplifiers; *TGC*, time gain compensation; *A/D*, analog to digital. See text for details.

$$FR = \frac{1}{Nt_b} = \frac{1}{N[(2R/c) + t_o]} \qquad [3]$$

The frame rate for a depth of 16 cm at 128 lines per sector is computed as 30 frames per second. The above equation has important implications regarding the relationship between lateral resolution and transducer frequency. Higher-frequency transducers have a narrower ultrasound beam width, which means that a larger number of beam lines is required to fill up one two-dimensional sector. Therefore, to maintain high lateral resolution while keeping adequate frame rates, the overall sector size must be reduced, which will reduce N but maintain good continuity between adjacent structures. Low-frequency transducers have a larger beam width and thus lower inherent lateral resolution. This implies that a larger sector size can still be used without any significant loss of lateral image quality.

A schematic illustrating some of the main components of a B-mode scanner is shown in Fig. 3-6. The scanner can be divided into four units: beam former; analog signal-processing unit, which includes gain compensation, filtering, and rectification; digital conversion and processing; and lastly, analog reconversion and display. The beam-forming unit consists of an oscillator, delay lines, and amplifiers connected to the main transducer unit. The delay lines and amplifiers shape the ultrasound beam as it is transmitted and selectively "focuses" on particular areas for optimal reception. Once the ultrasound signal is reflected and received by the beam-forming unit, selective time or depth gain compensation is performed based on settings selected by the user, and the resulting signal is fed into the analog signal-processing unit to be prepared for digital sampling and processing. Analog filters enhance near and far field signals and compression-transforms work to enhance weak signals to a level comparable with the stronger signals. A rectifier cancels the negative portion of the signal for easier digital processing, and the rectified signal is then input into the digital processing unit. The digital processing unit consists of a sampler that produces a digital version of the analog signal; the sampled signal is then used by various digital signal-processing algorithms to extract intensity information, couple it to spatial coordinates, perform postprocessing "cleanup" of the image, and present it to the digital scan converter. The digital scan converter transforms the presented digital information into analog signals recognizable to a conventional video monitor. The monitor displays all the ultrasound information along with any additional overlays of text and graphics to produce the ultimate echocardiographic image.

ULTRASOUND DOPPLER VELOCITY MEASUREMENT

In addition to imaging structures such as cardiac walls, ultrasound imaging can be used to measure blood velocity via the use of the Doppler-shift principle. Before we examine some of the principles of the Doppler shift, it is useful to look at how blood interacts with the ultrasound beam.

Scattering of Ultrasound from Blood

The red blood cell is shaped like a biconcave disk. Its long-axis diameter is approximately 7 to 8 μ, and its volume is approximately 80 μ^3. Because the typical wavelength λ for ultrasound signals is on the order of 150 μ (10 MHz) or higher, the red blood cell is much too small to scatter an ultrasound signal by itself; scattering occurs from a group of red blood cells clustered together within the sample volume of the ultrasound signal. The typical volume element for an ultrasound signal contains hundreds of red blood cells, and the total integrated scatter from all these cells makes up the reflection signal from that particular sample volume. The concentration of the red blood cells within the ultrasound sample volume is crucial in determining how well the signal will be reflected; in fact, the backscatter intensity BI is proportional to the size of the volume element ΔV and the mean square of the red blood cell concentration fluctuation [σ_n^2] (2):

$$BI \propto \Delta V \cdot [\sigma_n^2] \qquad [4]$$

This has profound implications; how well blood reflects ultrasound depends on the hematocrit. Although backscatter intensity increases with increasing hematocrit for low and medium levels of red blood cell concentration, it actually decreases once the hematocrit increases past a certain point (Fig. 3-7). This decrease is a consequence of the fact that at high packing concentrations of red blood cells, there is more destructive interference than constructive interference of the reflected signals because the probability is significantly larger that a red blood cell is present at a distance of $\lambda/4$ from another red blood cell.

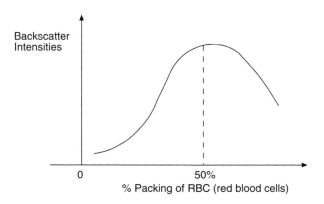

FIG. 3-7. The backscatter from red blood cells depends on the hematocrit. As the hematocrit increases from very low values, backscatter also increases. However, after a certain level (usually 40% to 50%), backscatter power begins decreasing owing to the increased effects of destructive interference from the large number of red blood cells present in the sample volume. Large values of hematocrit increase the possibility that red blood cells are present at distances of one fourth of a wavelength from the scatterer, thereby increasing the amount of destructive interference within the reflected ultrasound signals.

Such a configuration causes the maximum destructive interference between reflected ultrasound signals.

The fact that backscatter intensity depends on red blood cell concentration has several implications for optimal ultrasound Doppler blood velocity measurement. Primary among these is that the underlying flow character significantly affects the returning ultrasound signal because local red blood cell concentration may change significantly depending on the hydrodynamics of blood flow. There are four primary mechanisms that can change the dynamics of blood flow and so also alter backscatter intensity:

Convection. This is the main mechanism by which blood is transported, and it produces movement of blood down a pressure gradient. Convective blood flow produces small changes in red blood cell concentration, although high velocities can produce strong backscatter at locations where a significant velocity gradient can exist, such as near walls or at the boundaries of a regurgitant or stenotic jet.

Diffusion. This produces movement of red blood cells down a concentration gradient. However, the process of diffusion is too slow to affect red blood cell concentration to the degree at which backscatter intensity is affected.

Rouleaux Formation. In certain hemodynamic and disease states, red blood cells clump together in tight formations, producing extremely large local variations in red blood cell concentration. These rouleaux usually form in regions of lower convective pressures, such as venous beds, and produce bursts of high-amplitude backscatter. They are not generally present in arteries or cardiac chambers.

Turbulence. Turbulence within blood flow causes small- and large-scale disturbances in velocities and prevents the smooth lamination of flow layers. Turbulence usually results in the formation of small vortex structures within the flow; these vortices can exert significant centrifugal forces because of their rotation and thereby separate red blood cells from plasma. Such separations can cause dramatic changes in red blood cell concentration levels, leading to greater ultrasound backscatter intensity. Thus, turbulence within blood flow produces the strongest backscatter of ultrasound signals, leading to strong Doppler signals wherever it is present.

Principles of Doppler Shift

Ultrasound blood flow imaging is possible because a frequency shift occurs in the reflected signal when moving blood flow is encountered by the transmitted ultrasound signal. The frequency shift is caused by the Doppler effect, named after the person who first described the shift in the spectral content of certain stars toward the red or blue end of the frequency spectrum depending on whether the relative motion of the star was away from or toward the earth (3). Further research showed that the shift in

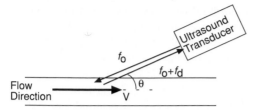

FIG. 3-8. The various parameters that influence the returning Doppler-shifted signal (f_d). The mean Doppler shift is related to transmitted ultrasound frequency (f_o), the angle between the transducer beam and flow direction (q), and the flow velocity (V).

frequency of the returning signal from the transmitted frequency is proportional to the speed of the reflecting object. This principle is used extensively for Doppler blood flow measurement and imaging to determine local flow velocities within the cardiovascular system. As illustrated by Fig. 3-8, the Doppler shift f_d is related to the frequency of the transmitted signal f_o, the speed of sound within the media c, and the relative angle Θ between the direction of flow and the direction of the transmitted ultrasound signal. This relationship can be expressed in the following equation:

$$f_d = \frac{2V\cos\Theta\, f_o}{c} \quad\quad [5]$$

One of the most important points to keep in mind when analyzing Doppler waveforms of blood flow is the cos Θ relationship inherent in the above equation. Essentially, this means that one must know the exact flow direction and the ultrasound beam direction at the point of velocity measurement to determine whether the given Doppler-measured velocity is true. If the ultrasound transducer is not held parallel to the direction of flow upstream or downstream to the velocity measurement site—that is, if Θ is not 0 degrees or 180 degrees—there will always be some error in the velocity measurement. Some ultrasound scanners offer the option of correcting this error automatically by having the user provide the system with the blood flow direction. The above Doppler shift equation is used to measure velocity in continuous-wave and pulsed-wave Doppler modes by extracting the shifted Doppler frequency in the reflected ultrasound signal, assuming that c is 1,580 m/s, and calculating $V\cos\Theta$. For color Doppler imaging, the necessity for real-time imaging prevents a direct calculation of the Doppler-shifted frequency at each sample point as is done for continuous and pulsed-wave Doppler. Instead, color Doppler imaging uses an estimate of the frequency content of the returning ultrasound signal to calculate mean frequency shift and thereby local velocity. The techniques of continuous-wave, pulsed-wave, and color Doppler are explained in further detail below.

Continuous-wave and Pulsed-wave Doppler

Continuous-wave and pulsed-wave Doppler measure velocity at a particular site by direct extraction of the Doppler-shifted frequency via a signal-processing routine called the fast Fourier transform (FFT). An in-depth explanation of FFT techniques is beyond the scope of this chapter; suffice to say that the FFT is a gateway between looking at a signal as a function of time and looking at the same signal as a function of frequency. Thus, FFT operation on a reflected Doppler-shifted ultrasound signal will reveal the dominant frequencies within the signal and will look something like Fig. 3-9, with a range of frequencies spread in a bell-shaped curve around the Doppler-shifted frequency f_d. Extraction of the mean frequency shift f_d after the FFT transformation becomes trivial, involving only a measurement of the statistical mean.

Continuous-wave Doppler measures velocity by continuously transmitting and receiving ultrasound signals into the body (4). The main advantage of continuous-wave Doppler is that it can measure velocities within a large range of values and so is used to measure high-velocity jets and peak flows. The disadvantage is that there is no information as to the exact location where the velocities are being measured along the ultrasound beam. Therefore, continuous-wave Doppler cannot be used to measure local velocities. Because transmission and reception are occurring simultaneously, two sets of ultrasound crystals are required, one for transmission and the other for reception. The transmitter emits the ultrasound signal at a predefined frequency set by the transducer specifications. Usually, the Doppler frequency differs slightly from the imaging frequency so that reflections from tissue versus flow signals can be separated more easily. Early implementations of continuous-wave Doppler velocity measurement allowed for velocity measurements along one ultrasound beam line only; recent advances in ultrasound transducer technology now allow the continuous-wave

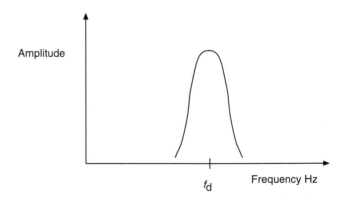

FIG. 3-9. The typical frequency spectrum of the returning Doppler-shifted signal is a Gaussian curve centered around the mean Doppler-shift frequency f_d. The mean Doppler shift is converted from frequency units (hertz) to velocity with the Doppler equation.

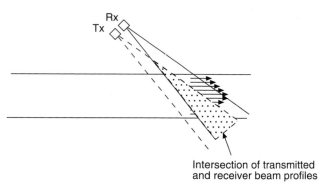

Intersection of transmitted
and receiver beam profiles

FIG. 3-10. Continuous-wave (*CW*) Doppler interrogation of flow. Continuous-wave Doppler detects all velocities located within the flow region consisting of the intersection between the transmitter (*Tx*) and receiver (*Rx*) beam profiles. Thus, continuous-wave Doppler cannot be used to obtain localized velocity information and is instead used to measure peak velocities within a flow region.

beam direction to be steered within the two-dimensional echo sector. As shown in Fig. 3-10, the measurement site for continuous wave Doppler lies on the intersection region between transmitting and receiving beam profiles. Thus, velocities recorded from continuous-wave Doppler are composed of multiple individual velocities all integrated into the overall continuous-wave Doppler waveform. Because of this integration, continuous-wave Doppler is used only for peak velocity detection and measurement, as these velocities stand out from the others within the Doppler velocity envelope.

As stated above, the transmitter and receiver elements for the continuous-wave processing system are located within the same transducer, and much of the front-end processing is the same for transmission and reception. The reflected ultrasound Doppler signal is first demodulated after reception to scale its frequency content downward for easier filtering and digital processing. The signal is then prepared for digital sampling by the use of various filters, amplifiers, and rectifiers; the resulting signal is then digitally sampled by passing it through an analog-to-digital converter, after which digital signal processing is performed to extract the mean frequency by use of the FFT. The digital signal processor usually outputs both velocity and signal power, both of which are used by the digital scan converter, which turns digital values into an analog signal to display the Doppler waveform on the monitor. The Doppler signal is displayed using a monochromatic color scheme, usually in varying shades of gray, with intensity of gray level corresponding to signal power and height of the signal corresponding to velocity.

Pulsed-wave Doppler velocity measurement is very similar to continuous-wave Doppler processing in regard to the manner in which velocities are extracted and displayed. Pulsed-wave Doppler also uses a FFT processor to extract Doppler shifts from the returning ultrasound signals and displays velocities according to returning sig-

nal power and mean frequency. The difference is that pulsed-wave Doppler is a spatial sampling technique in that it uses pulsed ultrasound with predefined intervals between successive pulses. The use of pulses at regular intervals allows for the recognition of depth information in the returning ultrasound Doppler signals, and this in turn allows the sample volume used for velocity measurement to be user-controlled and set anywhere within the two-dimensional sector. The ability to recognize depth information is the main advantage of pulsed-wave Doppler over continuous-wave Doppler. However, this ability also produces a drawback. Pulsed-wave Doppler is limited in the range of velocities it can measure accurately.

Causes of Spectral Variance in Continuous-wave and Pulsed-wave Doppler Signals

In general, an increase in the variance in the Doppler signal is attributed to blood flow disturbances. Although this is true for the most part, there can be circumstances in which the returning Doppler signal can contain large amounts of variance although the underlying flow pattern is relatively undisturbed. The reasons for this can be understood by examining the main cause of ultrasound backscatter, red blood cell concentration. Any process that changes red blood cell concentration will also cause variations in the reflected Doppler signal. As stated above, convection and turbulence can cause significant changes in red blood cell concentration. Variance in returning Doppler signal, however, can be ascribed to three dominant causes: velocity variance, transit time effect, and turbulence (1,5).

Velocity Variance. The effect of velocity variance on the Doppler signal can be seen when one examines a typical sample volume that is located close to a wall or other structure. As shown in Fig. 3-11, a sample volume close to a structure will contain a range of velocities.

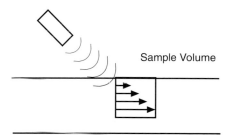

Sample Volume

FIG. 3-11. Velocities within a Doppler sample volume may not be uniform or equal. At locations where flow shear is high, such as near walls or adjacent to other flows, a gradient of velocities can exist within the sample volume. The returning Doppler signal will be influenced by all the variations in velocity that exist within the sample volume, resulting in a broadening of the Doppler frequency spectrum. Such increased spectral variance may be falsely interpreted as turbulence within the flow.

Velocities near the wall will be very low because of the frictional effects of the surface. At locations within the sample volume but away from the wall, flow will be at higher velocities. This range of velocities will produce a skewed red blood cell concentration profile within the sample volume, which will in turn cause an increase in backscatter intensity. The changes in backscatter intensity between locations close to the wall and farther away will produce a variation in the returning Doppler signal, although there are no inherent flow disturbances present at the measurement location.

Transit Time Effect. The transit time effect is a consequence of the inverse relationship between observation time t_1 and bandwidth *BW* of the returning Doppler signal, that is, $BW = 1/t_1$. The accuracy of the Doppler-shift calculation increases with the amount of time used for observing the blood flow because a better estimate of mean velocity can be obtained. Thus, a long observation time will result in a narrow band of frequencies detected because of the more accurate Doppler-shift estimate. By contrast, shorter observation times will result in a spreading of the Doppler frequency spectrum because of the relative ambiguity present in the measurement process. For a sample volume of length *L* with blood flowing at mean velocity *V*, the observation time t_1 is as follows:

$$t_1 = \frac{L}{V} \qquad [6]$$

The above equation shows that decreasing the sample volume size to obtain better spatial resolution will also have the effect of decreasing t_1 and increasing returning signal bandwidth. This will in turn increase the variance of the Doppler signal. However, increasing the sample volume size to obtain better velocity measurement may also increase signal variance because of an increase in the overall velocity variance within the sample volume by inclusion of other flow regions. Thus, changing sample size to optimize velocity measurement and spatial resolution requires careful consideration of the flow regime where velocity measurements are being made.

Turbulence. Turbulence, as stated previously, produces strong Doppler backscatter signals because of the variations in red blood cell concentration that can occur within the sample volume. Because turbulence by definition contains random velocities around the mean velocity, the returning Doppler frequency spectrum will also contain the various frequencies that correspond to this range of velocities. This results in an increase in the spectral variance of the Doppler signal.

Color Doppler Imaging

Color Doppler images can be thought of as echoes from multiple pulsed-wave Doppler sample volumes processed fast enough to provide a real-time image of the blood flow within the heart or vasculature. The requirement for real-time blood flow measurement over a two-dimensional ultrasound cross section, however, imposes strict time limitations on the mean frequency extraction capability of FFT processors. Usually, the number of calculations required for multiple velocity measurements cannot be performed in real time using FFT techniques. Current systems sample the Doppler signal for a short time period, usually between 4 and 10 ms, and estimate the actual energy or power spectrum of the returning signal from this sample using various algorithms. All of them calculate three main parameters that are then used to compose the color Doppler image: mean frequency f_d, which can be used to calculate mean velocity; total power

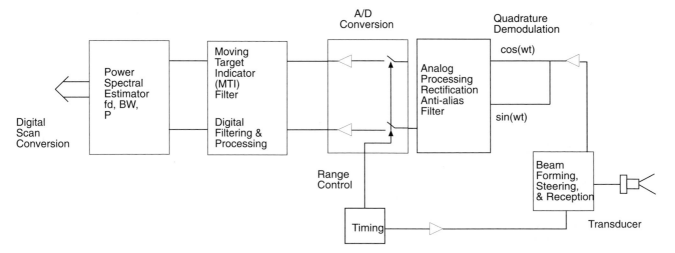

FIG. 3-12. Schematic of a typical color Doppler imaging system. f_d, Doppler-shifted frequency; *BW*, bandwidth; *P*, returning Doppler signal power; A/D, analog to digital; cos (*wt*), cosine of frequency-time; sin (*wt*), sine of frequency-time. See text for details.

of the Doppler-shifted signal *P*, which indicates the strength of the ultrasound Doppler backscatter signal; and bandwidth *BW* or variance of the Doppler-shifted signal, which reveals information about how much velocity variance is present in the underlying flow (6,7).

Figure 3-12 shows a schematic for a color Doppler system. Essentially the same processing as for the conventional pulsed-wave Doppler technique is performed on the received Doppler signal up to the point of digital conversion of the filtered analog signal. After digital conversion, a moving target indicator (MTI) filter is applied to separate the fast-moving components of the returning signal from the more slowly moving components (8). Moving structures such as cardiac walls are responsible for the more slowly moving components of the returning signal. The MTI filter essentially subtracts the signal sampled at one point from the signal sampled at the point immediately preceding it. This removes or severely attenuates nonmoving or slowly moving signals, leaving only those signals reflected from faster-moving blood. Digital signal processing to estimate the power spectrum of the remaining signal is then performed to produce estimates of f_d, *P*, and *BW*, which are then passed to the digital scan converter and displayed in various colors.

Flow information calculated by the color Doppler scanner is displayed on the monitor in a color scheme that identifies direction, velocity along the beam direction, and in some cases reflected signal bandwidth or signal power. The transformation from calculated values of f_d, *BW*, and *P* to a color scheme can be appreciated by examining the vector containing all three values plotted on a polar axis, as shown in Fig. 3-13. The length of the vector corresponds to the power of the signal, its angle offset from 0 degrees corresponds to the mean Doppler-shift frequency f_d, and the range of values it can take on is represented by the circle around the vector and corresponds to the bandwidth of the returning Doppler signal. This circular coordinate system can be divided into a number of bins representing discrete values of f_d and *P*. These circularly oriented bins can then be mapped onto a rectangular color scheme of various colors and intensities. This color bar is used by the color Doppler scanner to display the calculated values of mean frequency or velocity and bandwidth (variance) or power. Directional flow information—that is, whether the detected blood flow is moving away from or toward the transducer—is usually displayed in two primary colors, generally red and blue. Red indicates blood moving toward the transducer, and blue indicates blood moving away from the transducer. Additionally, intensities of green color are mixed in with the primary colors to provide a rough estimate of the amount of variance in the returning Doppler signal. However, the amount of green within a color Doppler map should be interpreted with caution because many color Doppler systems artificially enhance their color maps with additions of green for better visual appreciation of color Doppler flow images.

Some ultrasound systems offer a digital transfer of velocity information directly from the stage preceding digital scan conversion, and this represents the most accurate flow information available for off-line analysis. Digitization of the radio frequency data before signal demodulation and processing would be the ideal means of extracting truly raw data on the returning Doppler signal. However, apart from some experimental configurations, no commercially available system has this capability at present.

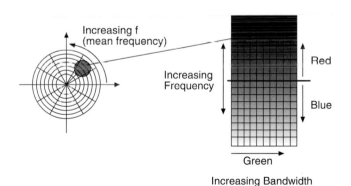

FIG. 3-13. One example of the conversion of flow information obtained from the power spectral estimator within the color Doppler system into a color scheme. The power spectral estimator produces an estimate of Doppler-shift frequency (*f*), reflected signal bandwidth, and signal power. These three parameters can be mapped onto a polar coordinate system as a vector with the angle of the vector representing Doppler-shift frequency, length of the vector representing power, and bandwidth represented as a range of radial locations around the mean. Such a circular representation can then be mapped onto a rectangular color bar as illustrated.

REFERENCES

1. Angelsen BAJ. Wave, signals and signal processing in medical ultrasound. 1997 (*in press*).
2. Angelsen BAJ. A theoretical study of the scattering of ultrasound from blood. *IEEE Trans Biomed Eng* 1980;BME-27:61–67.
3. White DN. Johann Christian Doppler and his effect—a brief history. *Ultrasound Med Biol* 1982;8:583–591.
4. Brody WR, Meindl JD. Theoretical analysis of the CW Doppler ultrasonic flowmeter. *IEEE Trans Biomed Eng* 1974;BME-21:183–192.
5. Cloutier G, Shung KK, Durand LG. Experimental evaluation of intrinsic and nonstationary ultrasonic Doppler spectral broadening in steady and pulsatile flow loop models. *IEEE Trans Ultrason Ferro Fre Control* 1993;40:786–795.
6. Kimme-Smith C, Tessler RN, Grant EG, Perella RR. Processing algorithms for color flow Doppler. *IEEE Ultrasonics Symposium*, 1989:887–879.
7. Angelsen BAJ, Kristoffersen K. Discrete time estimation of the mean Doppler frequency in ultrasonic blood velocity measurements. *IEEE Trans Biomed Eng* 1983;BME-30:207–214.
8. Angelsen BAJ, Kristoffersen K. On ultrasonic MTI measurement of velocity profiles in blood flow. *IEEE Trans Biomed Eng* 1979;BME-26:665–671.

CHAPTER 4

Echocardiographic Examination of the Heart and Great Vessels

Elizabeth M. Shaffer and Ole A. Knudson, Jr.

The echocardiographic examination of congenital heart disease differs from that of acquired heart disease in several important aspects. First, the diagnosis of the structural abnormalities found in congenital heart lesions requires a thorough knowledge of cardiac morphology. Secondly, dealing with children, especially sick children, presents unique challenges. The children are frequently frightened and need coaxing and distractions to cooperate with the study. In our laboratory, we distract the children with age-appropriate videotapes. This approach has significantly decreased, but not eliminated, the need for sedative medication (1). We use oral chloral hydrate (50 to 100 mg/kg, with a maximum dose of 1 g) as our primary sedative medication. The parents are instructed to have the children avoid food or drink for 2 to 4 hours before the scheduled echocardiogram. While sedated, the children are monitored continuously by pulse oximetry. The children are not allowed to leave the cardiac imaging laboratory until they can be aroused and the parents are comfortable. Using this approach, we have not had any major complications with patient sedation. With infants, maintaining appropriate body temperature can be difficult during the examination; to minimize heat loss, the infants are placed on a heating pad and the ultrasonic gel is warmed (2).

In our laboratory, we start the echocardiographic examination by obtaining the two-dimensional anatomic information from all transducer positions and recording the M-mode and spectral Doppler traces from the appropriate views. Color Doppler flow mapping is performed after all basic anatomic recording has been completed and in conjunction with the spectral Doppler.

VIEWS IN THE NORMAL HEART AND GREAT VESSELS

The segmental approach to congenital heart disease is used in our laboratory. The position of the heart mass and apex within the chest and the situs or laterality are determined. Each level of the heart is described: systemic and pulmonary venous return, atria, ventricles, and great vessels. The connections and spatial relations of the chambers and great vessels are also determined. When this approach is used, the most complex heart can be described with an understanding of the relationships between the cardiac structures and the physiology of the circulation (3–8).

Each cardiac structure has various morphologic features that aid in its identification. The septal surfaces of the heart hold many of the keys to chamber morphology (9). The atrial septum has a left and a right side. The thin flap valve of the foramen ovale is on the left side, and the eustachian and thebesian valves are positioned on the right side. The atrial appendages also guide in distinguishing the left atrium from the right atrium. The left atrial appendage is thin and fingerlike, whereas the right atrial appendage has a broad base and is triangular in shape (5). The atrioventricular valves are always associated with the appropriate ventricle—namely, the mitral valve with the morphologic left ventricle and the tricuspid valve with the morphologic right ventricle. The tricuspid valve has three leaflets and is positioned more toward the apex than is the mitral valve. The mitral valve is bileaflet and is attached to the ventricular wall by two papillary muscles (9). The tricuspid valve has attachments to the interventricular septum, whereas the mitral valve has no septal attachments. The surfaces of the interventricular septum are also helpful in defining the ventricular morphology. The left side of the interventricular septum is smooth, as opposed to its right side, which has the septal attachments of the tricuspid valve and is heavily trabeculated (5,6,9). The right ventricle has the septomarginal trabecula, or moderator band, whereas the left ventricle is smooth-

41

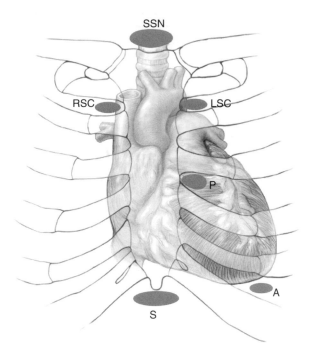

FIG. 4-1. Schematic drawing of the transthoracic echocardiographic windows. *P*, parasternal; *A*, apical; *S*, subcostal; *SSN*, suprasternal; *LSC*, left subclavicular; *RSC*, right subclavicular. (*Drawing by Richard Gersony*)

walled. The aorta is distinguished from the pulmonary artery by the head and neck vessels and the coronary arteries. The pulmonary artery normally bifurcates into branch pulmonary arteries.

The position of the heart in the chest along with the position of the ventricular apex should be described. The heart may be positioned in the left side of the chest (levocardia), the right side (dextrocardia), or in the middle of the chest (mesocardia) (see Figs. 2-1–2-3). Likewise, the apex may be oriented leftward, rightward, or straight down. If most of the heart is positioned in the right side of the chest, then dextrocardia is present (see Fig. 2-2). The heart may be in this position because a space-occupying lesion in the left side of the chest is pushing the heart into the right side, or the volume of the right side of the chest may be small, pulling the heart into the right side. In these circumstances, the cardiac apex is usually to the left despite the heart's being located in the right side of the chest; this is called dextroposition. The heart may be positioned in the right chest because of failure of the cardiac apex to pivot into the left chest but the visceroatrial situs is solitus. This is termed dextrocardia in situs solitus or dextrocardia by dextroversion (10–13). In situs inversus totalis, the abdominal and cardiac situs are both reversed and dextrocardia is normal; this is called mirror-image dextrocardia or dextrocardia with situs inversus. In this situation, the incidence of congenital

heart disease is low. In contrast, when the cardiac and abdominal situs are discordant (dextrocardia by dextroversion), the incidence of congenital heart disease is high (6).

Situs refers to laterality (see Fig. 2-4). Some organs in the body are symmetric, such as the kidneys, whereas other organs have a definite left and right side, such as the lungs. The heart also has a left and right side. Situs is generally described in three terms: solitus, inversus, and ambiguus. Situs solitus refers to the usual situation, in which the right-sided atrial structures are located to the right of the left-sided atrial structures (see Fig. 2-4A). In situs inversus, the morphologically right-sided atrial structures are located to the left and the morphologically left-sided atrial structures are located to the right (see Fig. 2-4B). In situs ambiguus, atrial laterality cannot be identified or does not exist. The heterotaxy syndromes are described as bilateral left-sidedness or bilateral right-sidedness (see Fig. 2-4C,D). These syndromes are associated with complex cardiac abnormalities. The spatial relationship between the descending aorta and the systemic venous return from the lower body (inferior vena cava, azygous and/or hemiazygous vein) provides valuable clues in defining situs. The spatial relationship of these structures can be assessed echocardiographically from the abdominal short- and long-axis views (see Figs. 4-12–4-15). In situs solitus, the inferior vena cava is usually positioned on the right side of the spine and is anterior to the left-sided descending aorta (see Figs.

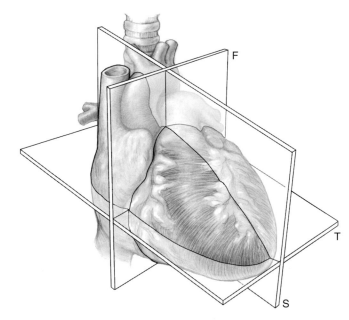

FIG. 4-2. Schematic rendition of the frontal, transverse, and sagittal axes of the heart. These correspond to the short, long, and sagittal echocardiographic planes, respectively. *F*, frontal axis; *T*, transverse axis; *S*, sagittal axis. (*Drawing by Richard Gersony*)

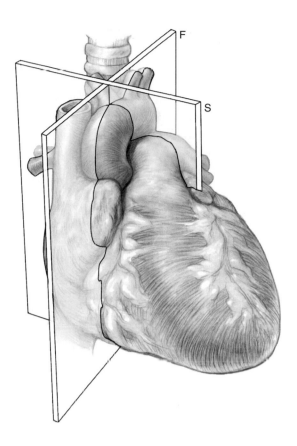

FIG. 4-3. Schematic rendition of the frontal and sagittal axes of the great vessels. These correspond to the long and short suprasternal echocardiographic planes, respectively. *F*, frontal axis; *S*, sagittal axis. (*Drawing by Richard Gersony*)

4-12, 4-13). In situs inversus, the inferior vena cava is usually located on the left and is anterior to the right-sided descending aorta (see Echo. 8-7). In situs ambiguus, several situations may be present. In bilateral left-sidedness, the aorta is anterior and to the left of the spine, the inferior vena cava is frequently interrupted, and an azygous and/or hemiazygous vein can be present posterior to the aorta. The azygous is to the right and the hemiazygous is to the left side of the aorta (see Echo. 8-10). In the situation of bilateral right-sidedness, the inferior vena cava is usually not interrupted and is anterior to the descending aorta. The vena cava and descending aorta are usually juxtaposed—that is, both are located either on the left or on the right side of the spine (14) (see Echo. 8-8).

The echocardiographic examination in congenital heart disease utilizes five standard echocardiographic windows: parasternal, apical, subcostal, suprasternal, and subclavicular. In addition, right and left subclavicular windows are commonly used (Fig. 4-1). At each window, multiple views are obtained in the long, short, and sagittal planes of the heart or great vessels by rotation of the transducer clockwise or counterclockwise and angulation superiorly

or inferiorly (Figs. 4-2, 4-3). In this way, a three-dimensional image of the heart is reconstructed through the use of multiple two-dimensional images. Our laboratory conforms to the standards of the American Society of Echocardiography for the display of images (15). The parasternal long-axis views have a cranial-caudal orientation (Fig. 4-4) with the cranial structures displayed on the right side of the screen and the caudal structures on the left side of the screen. For views that have a left-right orientation, such as the parasternal short-axis, apical, abdominal short-axis, and suprasternal views (see Figs. 4-6, 4-8, 4-12, 4-20, 4-22), the structures on the patient's left are displayed on the right side of the screen and the patient's right-sided structures on the left side of the screen. For views with a superior-inferior, anterior-posterior orientation (see Figs. 4-10, 4-14, 4-16, 4-18), the image is oriented in an anatomic position (i.e., up and down inverted on the screen). This orientation facilitates the understanding of complex cardiac anatomy (16).

Parasternal Long-axis Views

The family of parasternal long-axis views is usually obtained by positioning the patient in the left lateral de-

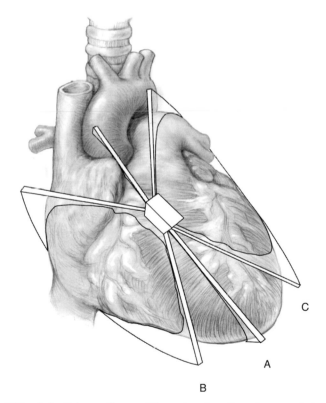

FIG. 4-4. Schematic rendition showing the planes of the ultrasound beam to obtain the family of parasternal long-axis views. **A:** Standard long axis. **B:** Long axis of the inflow of the right ventricle. **C:** Long axis of the outflow of the right ventricle. (*Drawing by Richard Gersony*)

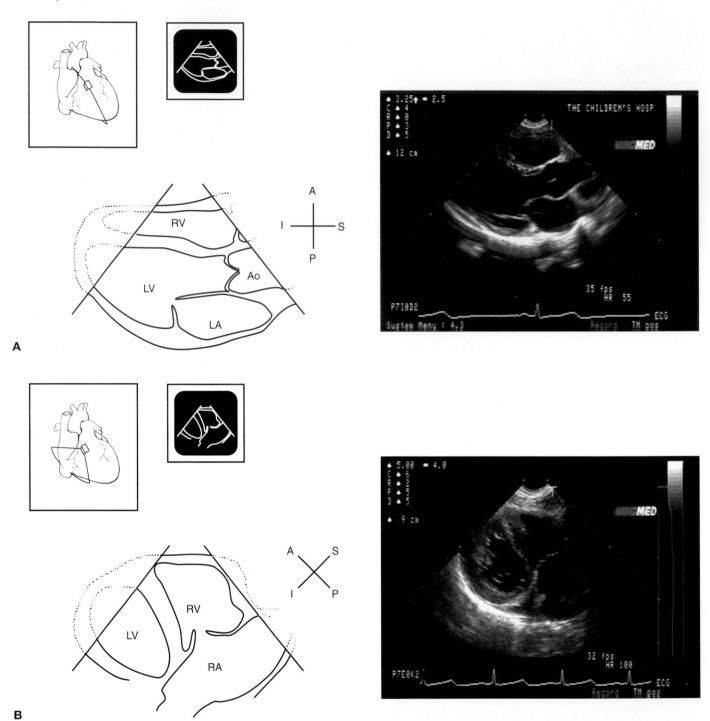

FIG. 4-5. Schematic drawings and echocardiograms demonstrating the family of parasternal long-axis views. **A:** Standard long axis. **B:** Long axis of the inflow of the right ventricle.

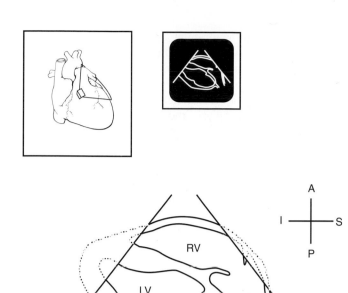

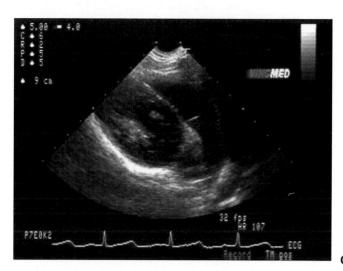

FIG. 4-5. (*Continued.*) **C:** Long axis of the outflow of the right ventricle. *RV*, right ventricle; *LV*, left ventricle; *RA*, right atrium; *LA*, left atrium; *I V*, tricuspid valve; *MV*, mitral valve; *AoV*, aortic valve; *PV*, pulmonic valve; *Ao*, aorta; *PA*, pulmonary artery. *A*, anterior; *P*, posterior; *S*, superior; *I*, inferior.

cubitus position. The transducer is placed in the second to fourth intercostal space to the left of the sternum roughly along a line oriented between the right shoulder and the left hip (17–20) (Fig. 4-4). The orientation of the heart in the chest changes early in life, from a nearly horizontal lie in the newborn to a more vertical orientation in the adult. In the standard parasternal long-axis view, the left atrium, mitral valve, left ventricle, left ventricular outflow tract, aortic valve, interventricular septum, and right ventricle are assessed (Figs. 4-4A, 4-5A). Note that the interventricular septum should be fairly horizontal in this view (2), with the mitral valve in the center of the image. The interventricular septum is a complex anatomic structure requiring examination from multiple views. From the parasternal long-axis view, portions of the trabecular and outlet septum are visualized. As stated previously, the smooth septal and free wall surfaces of the left ventricle serve to differentiate it from the anatomic right ventricle. The right and noncoronary cusps of the aortic valve are visualized, whereas the left coronary cusp is out of this plane. The anterior leaflet of the mitral valve is continuous with the posterior aortic wall, confirming the mitral aortic fibrous continuity. There is also continuity between the interventricular septum and the anterior aortic wall. The posterior leaflet of the mitral valve and the posteromedial papillary muscle are also visualized. Frequently, the coronary sinus can be appreciated as a small circle in the atrioventricular groove (21) (Fig. 4-5A). The coronary sinus may be enlarged if a left-sided

superior vena cava drains into it. A left-sided superior vena cava may be seen in 3% to 10% of patients with congenital heart disease but is also present in 0.5% of the general population (22,23). The descending aorta in cross section is posterior to the left atrium (24).

The transducer is then angled from the parasternal long axis view toward the right hip and rotated approximately 30 degrees counterclockwise to assess the inflow of the right ventricle (Figs. 4-4B, 4-5B). In this view, the inlet muscular septum is seen under the septal leaflet of the tricuspid valve, and the proximal portion of the trabecular septum is also visualized. In addition, the anterior leaflet of the tricuspid valve comes into view. The attachments of the tricuspid valve to the interventricular septum, when seen, may help define the morphologic right ventricle. The inferior vena cava and right atrial appendage can also be seen from this view.

The transducer is then angled toward the left shoulder to the outflow portion of the right ventricle (Figs. 4-4C, 4-5C). The infundibular septum, right ventricular outflow, pulmonary valve, and proximal pulmonary artery are visualized.

Parasternal Short-axis Views

From the parasternal long axis, the transducer is rotated 90 degrees clockwise to a parasternal short axis (25) (Fig. 4-6). A family of views is obtained by sweeping the trans-

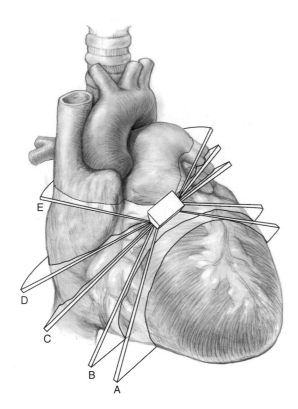

FIG. 4-6. Schematic rendition showing the planes of the ultrasound beam to obtain the family of parasternal short-axis views. **A:** Level of the left ventricular papillary muscles. **B:** Level of the mitral valve leaflets. **C:** Level of the base of the heart at the great vessels. **D:** Level of the pulmonary arterial trunk. **E:** Level of the main pulmonary artery and branches. (*Drawing by Richard Gersony, modified by the authors*)

ducer from the left ventricular apex to the base of the heart. Two papillary muscles, the anterolateral and the posteromedial, are normally positioned at 4 o'clock and 8 o'clock, respectively, at the middle left ventricular level (Figs. 4-6A, 4-7A). Occasionally, accessory papillary muscles or left ventricular strands can be visualized in the normal heart. A portion of the trabecular interventricular septum is seen at this level. The transducer is then slowly angled superiorly to the level of the anterior and posterior mitral valve leaflets (Figs. 4-6B, 4-7B). As the sweep to the base of the heart continues, the fibrous continuity between the anterior leaflet of the mitral valve and the aortic valve is confirmed. At the base of the heart, the aortic valve is in the center of the image with the right side of the heart anterior to it (Figs. 4-6C, 4-7C). The right, left, and noncoronary cusps of the aortic valve are best examined from this view. Posterior to the aortic valve is the left atrium. Clockwise from the left atrium is a portion of the interatrial septum and the right atrium. Further clockwise are the septal and anterior leaflets of the tricuspid valve, part of the right ventricular body and free wall, the right ventricular outflow tract, the pulmonary valve, and the proximal main pulmonary artery. The left atrial appendage can be seen with slight superior angulation (Figs. 4-6D, 4-7D). Its characteristically long, fingerlike appearance along with its narrow mouth where it joins the left atrium confirm the situs of the atrium. To visualize the distal main pulmonary artery and its bifurcation into the right and left pulmonary arteries, the transducer must be angled farther superiorly with slight clockwise rotation (Figs. 4-6E, 4-7E).

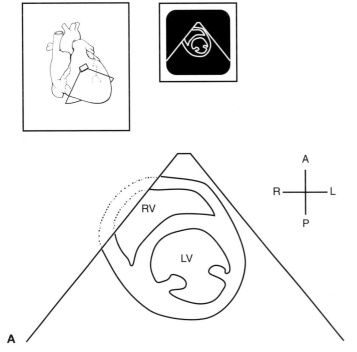

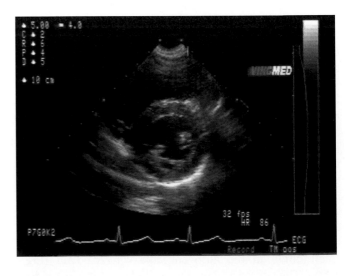

FIG. 4-7. Schematic drawings and echocardiograms demonstrating the family of parasternal short-axis views. **A:** Short axis at the level of the papillary muscles.

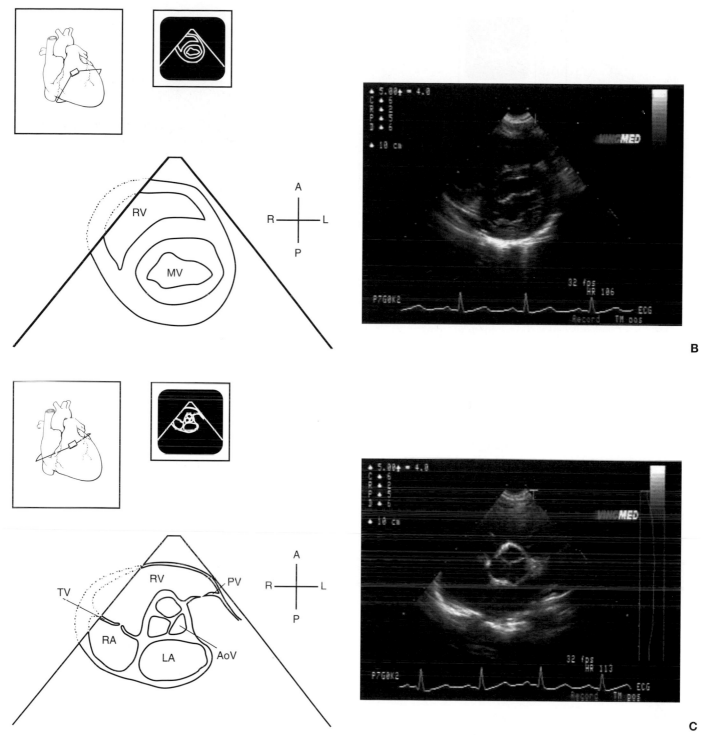

FIG. 4-7. (*Continued.*) **B:** Short axis at the level of the mitral valve leaflets. **C:** Short axis at the level of the great vessels.

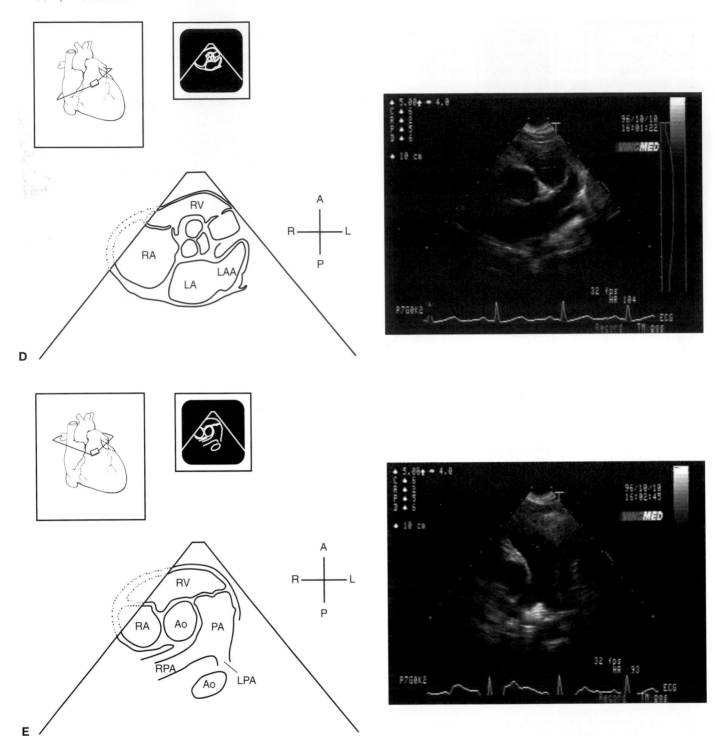

FIG. 4-7. (*Continued.*) **D:** Short axis at the level of the pulmonary trunk. **E:** Short axis at the level of the main pulmonary artery and branches. *RA*, right atrium; *LA*, left atrium; *LAA*, left atrial appendage; *RV*, right ventricle; *LV*, left ventricle; *TV*, tricuspid valve; *AoV*, aortic valve; *PV*, pulmonic valve; *Ao*, aorta; *PA*, pulmonary artery; *RPA*, right pulmonary artery; *LPA*, left pulmonary artery. *A*, anterior; *P*, posterior; *R*, right; *L*, left.

Several portions of the interventricular septum are visualized in the sweep of the parasternal short-axis views. At the level of the papillary muscles (Fig. 4-7A), the trabecular septum is seen extending to the level of the left ventricular outflow tract (Fig. 4-7B). At the base of the heart, the membranous septum is identified under the septal leaflet of the tricuspid valve and the noncoronary aortic cusp extending to the midportion of the right anterior coronary cusp (Fig. 4-7C). In this view, a portion of the outlet septum can be seen between the membranous septum and the pulmonic valve. Further anterior angulation demonstrates the full extension of the infundibular septum (Fig. 4-7D,E).

Apical Views

From the parasternal short axis views, the transducer is moved caudally and leftward and positioned over the cardiac apex without rotation (Fig. 4-8). The visual display of this family of views may be inverted and shown anatomically with the atria on the top of the screen and the ventricles on the bottom of the screen (18,19,26) (Figs. 4-9A–D, see 4-11A,B). The patient is usually best scanned from the left lateral decubitus position. In infants, true apical views may be difficult to obtain because of the horizontal lie of the heart. Nonetheless, it is important to try to obtain a true apical view because this is the best view for visualization of the left ventricular apex. If a true apical view is not obtained, abnormalities such as apical ventricular septal defects may be missed.

The four chambers of the heart, coronary sinus, mitral and tricuspid valves, portions of the ventricular septum, and ventricular outflows are assessed in the sweep of the apical four-chamber views (Fig. 4-9A–D). The scan starts posterior to the inlet of the heart to view the coronary sinus as it runs behind the left atrium; the mouth of the coronary sinus is in the right atrium (21) (Figs. 4-8A, 4-9A). From this position, the transducer is slowly angled anteriorly to visualize the four chambers of the heart at the level of the ventricular inlets and atrioventricular valves (Figs. 4-8B, 4-9B). In a true four-chamber view, the left ventricle should be positioned at the apex of the display and the atrial and ventricular septa should be visualized parallel to the ultrasound beam. From this view, the relative positions of the atrioventricular valves can be seen. The insertion of the tricuspid valve is closer to the apex than the insertion of the mitral valve, with a small portion of the septum, called the atrioventricular septum, separating the two atrioventricular valves (Fig. 4-9B). It is important to note that anteriorly the insertions of the atrioventricular valves approach each other (Fig. 4-9C). This area should be carefully imaged by slowly sweeping the transducer anteroposteriorly to demonstrate the apical displacement of the tricuspid valve. The septal

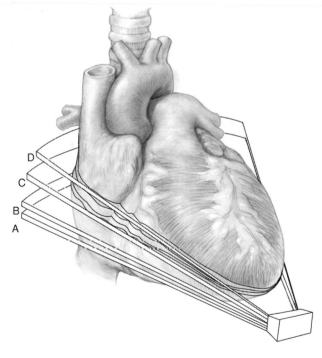

FIG. 4-8. Schematic rendition showing the plane of the ultrasound beam to obtain the family of apical four-chamber views. **A:** Level of the coronary sinus. **B:** Level of the ventricular inlets and atrioventricular septum. **C:** Level of the four chambers. **D:** Level of the left ventricular outflow tract. (*Drawing by Richard Gersony*)

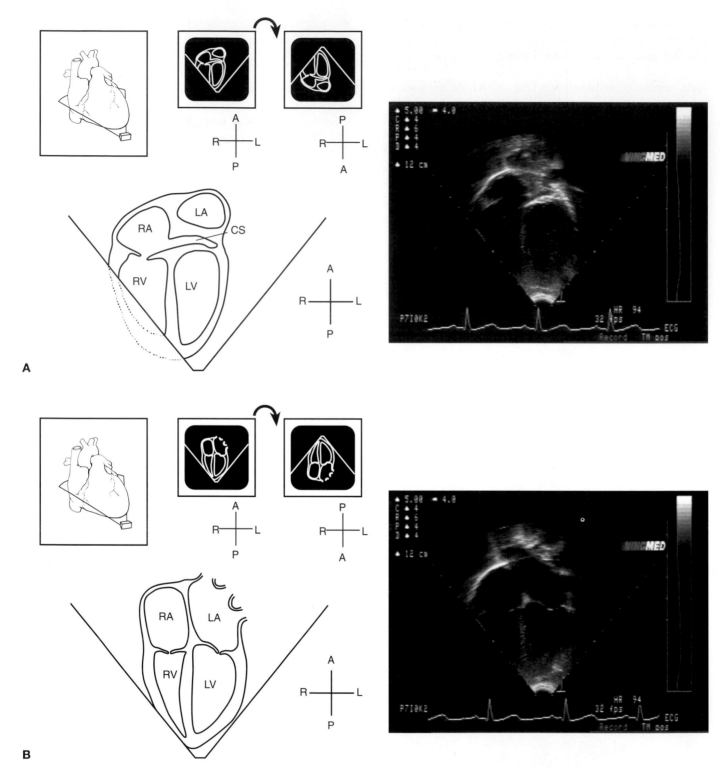

FIG. 4-9. Schematic drawings and echocardiograms demonstrating the family of apical four-chamber views. **A:** Level of the coronary sinus. **B:** Level of the inlet portion of the ventricles and atrioventricular septum.

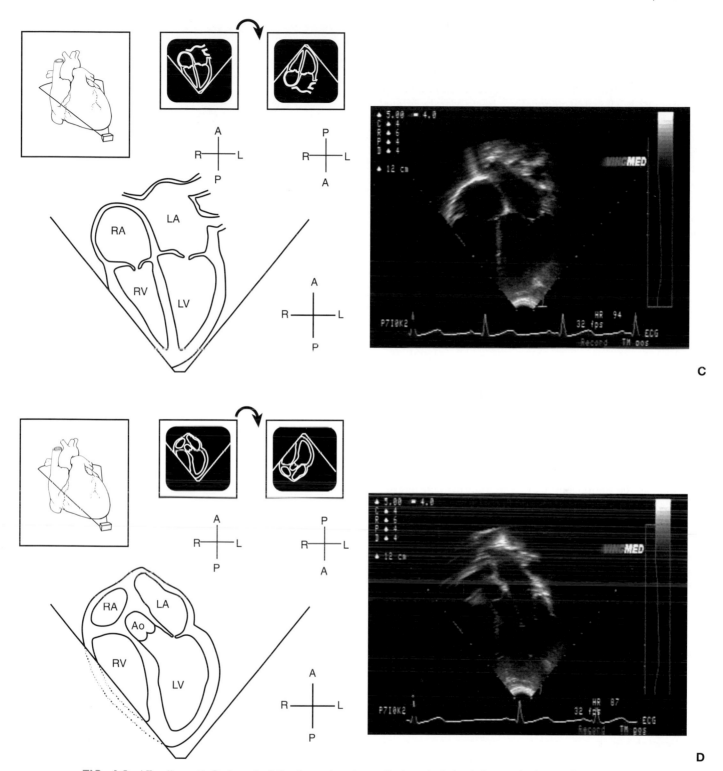

FIG. 4-9. (*Continued.*) **C:** Level of the four chambers. **D:** Level of the left ventricular outflow tract. *RA,* right atrium; *LA,* left atrium; *RV,* right ventricle; *LV,* left ventricle; *CS,* coronary sinus; *Ao,* aorta. *A,* anterior; *P,* posterior; *R,* right; *L,* left.

and anterior leaflets of the tricuspid valve and the anterior and posterior leaflets of the mitral valve, as well as their chordal attachments to the papillary muscles, are clearly seen from this view. The anatomic characteristics that differentiate the ventricular chambers are appreciated. The right ventricle is heavily trabeculated and the moderator band is present, whereas the left ventricle is smooth-walled without prominent muscle bundles. The left and right upper pulmonary veins and sometimes the left lower pulmonary vein can be seen entering the left atrium (Fig. 4-9B,C). The descending aorta in cross section can also be seen near the left atrium. Further anterior angulation demonstrates the left ventricular outflow tract, aortic valve, and ascending aorta (Figs. 4-8D, 4-9D). In infants and young children, the transducer can be angled even more anteriorly to visualize the body of the right ventricle, the right ventricular outflow tract, and the pulmonary valve.

From the apical four-chamber view, the transducer is rotated 90 degrees to obtain the apical long-axis or three-chamber view (15,18) (Figs. 4-10A, 4-11A). This view gives another perspective of the left ventricular outflow tract, proximal ascending aorta, mitral valve, and left atrium. The septal and posterior free wall of the left ventricle can be examined from this position. If the transducer is further rotated from the apical long-axis view, the apical two-chamber view is obtained (Figs. 4-10B, 4-11B). In this view, the left atrium and left ventricle are visualized as well as the entire lengths of the anterior and inferior left ventricular walls.

Like the parasternal views, the apical views permit examination of different anatomic portions of the ventricular septum. The inlet portions of the muscular interventricular septum are seen posteriorly (Fig. 4-9A,B). The atrioventricular septum is seen from the four-chamber plane separating the septal insertions of the tricuspid and mitral valves (Fig. 4-9B). Anteriorly, the membranous septum is visualized below the aortic valve (Fig. 4-9D). Almost the entire length of the trabecular septum can be examined from these views (Fig. 4-9A–D). Between the pulmonary and aortic outlets, portions of the infundibular septum are seen.

Subcostal Views

Following apical imaging, the subcostal views are usually obtained (Figs. 4-12–4-19). With complex congenital heart disease, sometimes the examination begins from the subcostal windows to gain an appreciation of the viscero-atrial situs, location of the heart in the chest, and overall cardiac anatomy.

The subcostal views start with the abdominal short axis (Fig. 4-12). The transducer is positioned in the midline

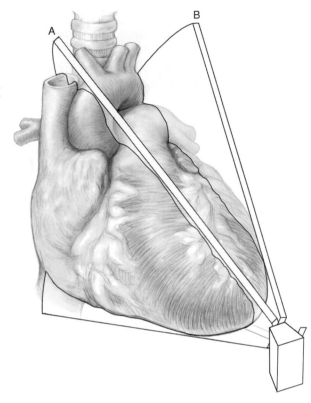

FIG. 4-10. Schematic rendition showing the plane of the ultrasound beam to obtain the apical long-axis and the apical two-chamber views. **A:** Level of the left ventricular outflow tract (long-axis view). **B:** Level of the inflow tract of the left ventricle (two-chamber view). (*Drawing by Richard Gersony*)

of the body caudal to the xiphoid process so that the left-sided structures are displayed to the right of the screen. In this view, the descending aorta and inferior vena cava should be identified. The aorta should be positioned on the left side of the spine, and the inferior vena cava should be to the right of the spine and slightly anterior to the aorta (Fig. 4-13). The left and right diaphragms are seen from this projection, and their movement with respiration can be assessed. The transducer is then rotated 90 degrees counterclockwise to assess the aorta and inferior vena cava in long axis (Fig. 4-14) and slowly swept toward the patient's left until the pulsatile descending aorta comes into view (Fig. 4-15A). The inferior vena cava is located by slowly sweeping the transducer to the patient's right until a parallel vascular structure is identified (Fig. 4-15B).

The transducer is returned to the abdominal short axis and angled cranially to visualize the heart (Fig. 4-16). As in the apical views, the subcostal images may be inverted and displayed in anatomic position (Figs. 4-17A–E, see 4-19A–D).

The family of subcostal coronal or long-axis views starts in the posterior portion of the heart (27–30). The

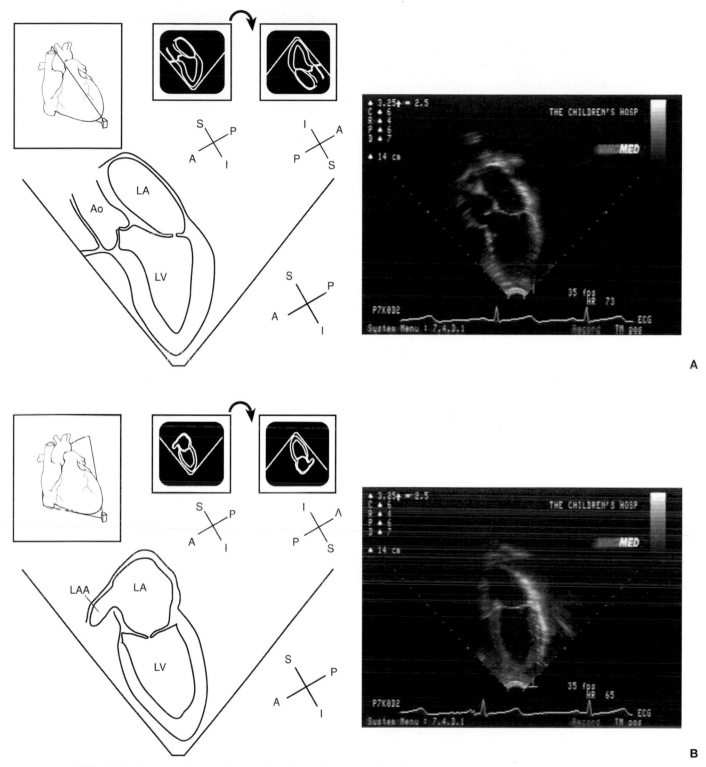

FIG. 4-11. Schematic drawings and echocardiograms demonstrating the apical long-axis and apical two-chamber views. **A:** Apical long-axis view. **B:** Apical two-chamber view. *LA,* left atrium; *LAA,* left atrial appendage; *LV,* left ventricle; *Ao,* aorta. *A,* anterior; *P,* posterior; *S,* superior; *I,* inferior.

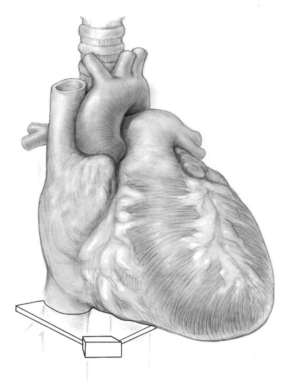

FIG. 4-12. Schematic rendition showing the plane of the ultrasound beam to obtain the abdominal short-axis view. (*Drawing by Richard Gersony*)

coronary sinus can be seen on the posterior surface of the left atrium with its mouth entering the right atrium (Figs. 4-16A, 4-17A). The transducer is slowly angled anteriorly to the inlet of the heart. The inferior vena cava, right atrium, tricuspid valve, atrial septum, left atrium, mitral valve, and inflow and bodies of the right and left ventricles are visualized (Figs. 4-16B, 4-17B). The atrioventricular septum and the inlet and trabecular portions of the muscular septum can also be seen. The eustachian valve appears as a thin membrane in this view, extending from the inferior vena cava along the posterior wall of the right atrium and approaching the inferior rim of the fossa ovalis. On the left side of the atrial septum, especially in the neonatal period, the portion of the primum septum constituting the valve of the foramen ovale or the floor of the fossa ovalis can be identified. The eustachian valve and the valve of the foramen ovale are identifying morphologic features of the right and left atria, respectively. Slight rotation of the transducer to the right of the patient emphasizes the atrial septum and its morphologic features (Figs. 4-16C, 4-17C). The transducer is then slowly angled anteriorly to visualize the left ventricular outflow tract and ascending aorta (Figs. 4-16D, 4-17D). The junction of the superior vena cava and right atrium is seen to the right of the ascending aorta. The parts of the ventricular septum visualized in this view include the trabecular

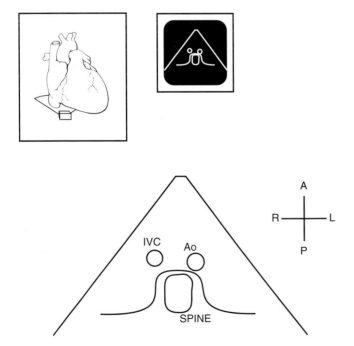

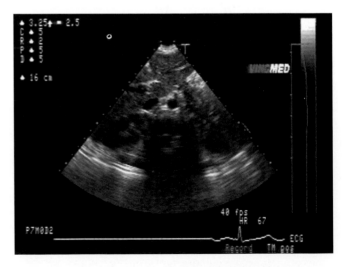

FIG. 4-13. Schematic drawing and echocardiogram demonstrating the abdominal short-axis view. *IVC*, inferior vena cava; *Ao*, aorta. *A*, anterior; *P*, posterior; *R*, right; *L*, left.

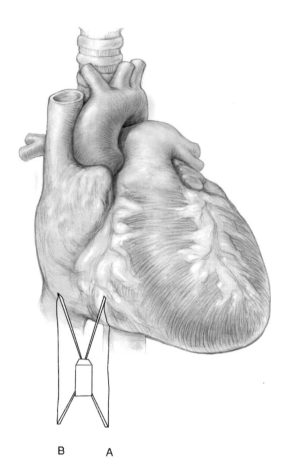

FIG. 4-14. Schematic rendition showing the planes of the ultrasound beam to obtain the subcostal long-axis views. **A:** Long axis of the aorta. **B:** Long axis of the inferior vena cava. (*Drawing by Richard Gersony*)

B   A

septum, portions of the membranous septum, and the subaortic outlet septum. Further anterior angulation demonstrates the right ventricular outflow tract crossing the left ventricular outflow tract (Figs. 4-16E, 4-17E).

The transducer is slowly returned to the inlet portion of the heart and rotated 90 degrees to obtain the subcostal sagittal or short-axis subcostal projections of the heart (Fig. 4-18). The family of subcostal short-axis views is obtained by angling the transducer from the patient's right to left. From the sagittal view positioned to the patient's right, the superior and inferior venae cavae are seen in their length as they enter the right atrium (Figs. 4-18A, 4-19A). The atrial septum is seen with the left atrium positioned posterior to the right atrium and receiving the pulmonary veins. The right pulmonary artery can be seen in cross section superior to the left atrium. The small azygous vein can occasionally be seen entering the superior vena cava superior to the right pulmonary artery. The transducer is then angled slowly to the patient's left, where the ascending aorta is imaged. In some patients, it is possible to visualize the entire aortic arch from this projection. The transducer is angled farther leftward to image the right ventricular outflow tract, pulmonary valve, and pulmonary artery (Figs. 4-18B, 4-19B). With

additional leftward angulation, the mitral valve and left ventricle are imaged in short axis (Figs. 4-18C,D; 4-19C,D). These views are very similar to the parasternal short-axis views and give another projection of the trabecular septum.

Suprasternal Views

The transducer is positioned in the suprasternal notch to obtain the suprasternal views (31–33). From the suprasternal notch, the long-axis (Fig. 4-20) and short-axis (see Fig. 4-22) views of the aorta are obtained. Imaging may be improved if the patient's neck is hyperextended and the head turned toward the left or right to facilitate placement of the transducer in the suprasternal notch. In infants, the transducer can sometimes be placed in a high right subclavicular position. The ascending, transverse, and descending thoracic aorta can be seen by orienting the transducer between the sagittal and coronal planes of the body, along the frontal axis of the aorta (Figs. 4-20A, 4-21A). The proximal head and neck vessels can be seen arising from the transverse aortic arch. The first large vessel is the in-

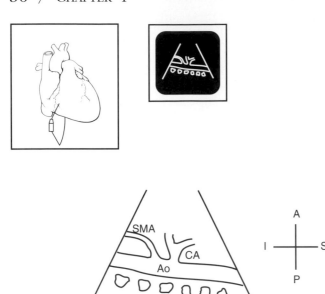

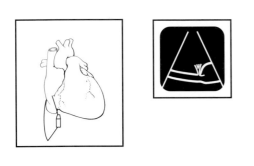

A

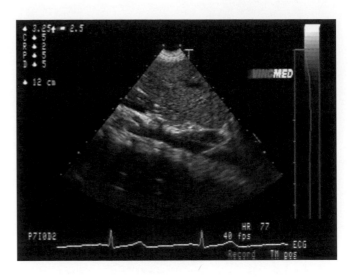

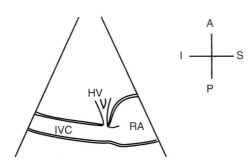

B

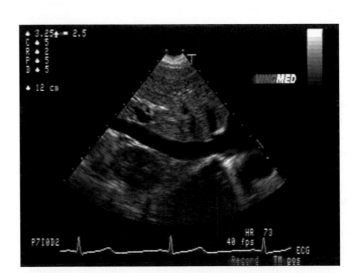

FIG. 4-15. Schematic drawings and echocardiograms demonstrating the abdominal long-axis views. **A:** Long-axis view of the descending aorta. **B:** Long-axis view of the inferior vena cava. *IVC*, inferior vena cava; *RA*, right atrium; *Ao*, aorta; *CA*, celiac artery; *SMA*, superior mesenteric artery; *HP*, hepatic vein. *A*, anterior; *P*, posterior; *S*, superior; *I*, inferior.

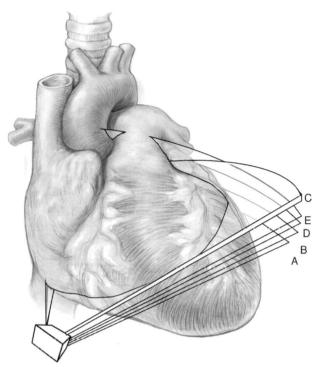

FIG. 4-16. Schematic rendition of the planes of the ultrasound beam to obtain the subcostal coronal or long-axis views. **A:** Level of the coronary sinus. **B:** Level of the inlet portion of both ventricles. **C:** Level of the atrial septum. **D:** Level of the left ventricular outflow tract. **E:** Level of the right ventricular outflow tract. (*Drawing by Richard Gersony*)

nominate artery; if one follows this vessel cranially and rightward, its bifurcation into the right subclavian artery and right carotid artery can be appreciated. The second brachiocephalic vessel is the left carotid, followed by the left subclavian artery. The location of the innominate vein is superior to the transverse arch. The right pulmonary artery is visualized in cross section below the ascending aorta. Manipulating the transducer farther posteriorly and leftward will emphasize the descending thoracic aorta (Figs. 4-20B, 4-21B). If the transducer is angled farther toward the patient's left, the proximal left pulmonary artery can be visualized (Figs. 4-20C, 4-21C).

The transducer is then rotated clockwise to obtain the short-axis view of the aorta (Fig. 4-22). The ultrasound plane should be parallel to the sternum. The suprasternal short-axis views are obtained by angling the transducer in an anterior-posterior direction (Fig. 4-23). The aorta is seen in cross section and appears circular. Superior to the aorta, the innominate vein is visualized as it joins the superior vena cava to the right of the aorta. The right pulmonary artery is visualized in its length under the aorta. From the suprasternal short-axis view, the left atrium is seen beneath the right pulmonary artery. The transducer may have to be angled slightly posteriorly to visualize all four pulmonary veins as they enter the left atrium. If the transducer is angled cranially, the first head and neck vessel and its branching can be assessed.

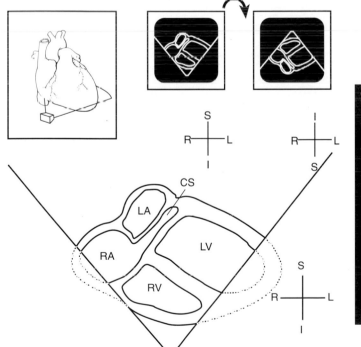

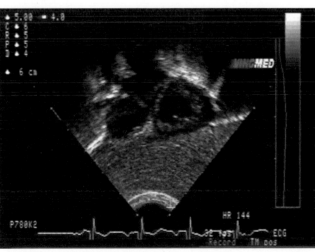

A

FIG. 4-17. Schematic drawings and echocardiograms demonstrating the subcostal coronal or long-axis views. **A:** Level of the coronary sinus.

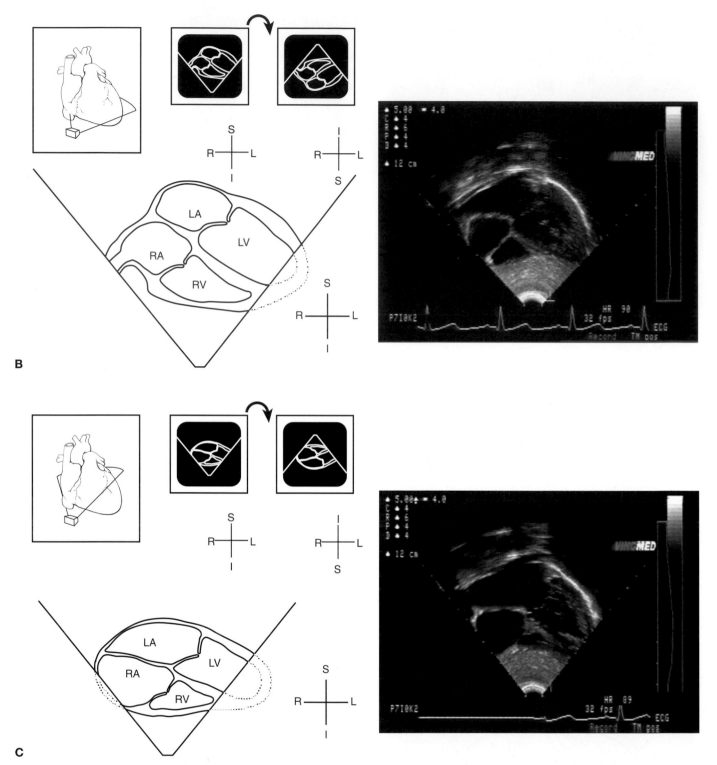

FIG. 4-17. (*Continued.*) **B:** Level of the inlet portion of both ventricles. **C:** Level of the atrial septum.

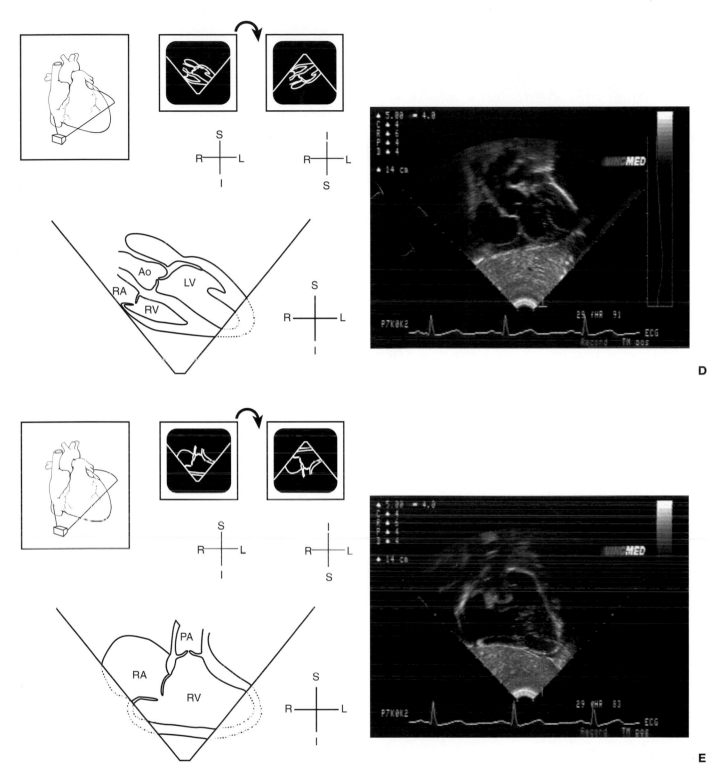

FIG. 4-17. (*Continued.*) **D:** Level of the left ventricular outflow tract. **E:** Level of the right ventricular outflow tract. *RA,* right atrium; *LA,* left atrium; *RV,* right ventricle; *LV,* left ventricle; *CS,* coronary sinus; *PA,* pulmonary artery. *S,* superior; *I,* inferior; *R,* right; *L,* left.

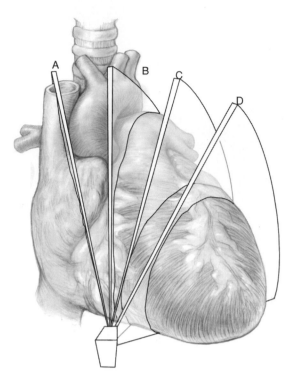

FIG. 4-18. Schematic rendition of the planes of the ultrasound beam to obtain the subcostal short-axis views. **A:** Level of the superior and inferior venae cavae. **B:** Level of the right ventricular outflow tract. **C:** Level of the mitral valve leaflets. **D:** Level of the left ventricular papillary muscles. (*Drawing by Richard Gersony*)

The normal aortic arch is left-sided, but occasionally a right-sided aortic arch will be present, even in an otherwise normal heart. The side of the aortic arch can be determined from the suprasternal views (34,35). When the transducer is placed in the suprasternal notch at the proper angle and the long axis of the aortic arch does not readily come into view, one should suspect a right aortic arch. In the presence of a right aortic arch, the long axis of the aorta is visualized by rotating the transducer counterclockwise from the standard long-axis position (Echo. 31-4). In the standard long-axis view of a left-sided aortic arch, the trachea is visualized by angling to the patient's right, demonstrating that the aortic arch is to the left of the trachea. On the other hand, with a right aortic arch, the aorta is to the right of the trachea. In a left-sided aortic arch, the first brachiocephalic vessel is directed to the patient's right side, whereas with a right aortic arch, it is directed to the patient's left side (compare Fig. 4-21A with Echo. 31-4).

Subclavicular Views

The left subclavicular view is useful for examining the branch pulmonary arteries (Figs. 4-24A, 4-25A). This becomes important in the assessment of conotruncal anomalies and pulmonary slings. The transducer is positioned in a transverse plane in the second left intercostal space (Fig. 4-24A). The main pulmonary artery is located to the left of the ascending aorta, which is seen on cross section. The proximal right and left pulmonary arterial branches are seen posteriorly (Fig. 4-25A).

The right subclavicular view is obtained from the second right intercostal space in a sagittal projection (Fig. 4-24B). This view is useful in the assessment of the superior vena cava and ascending aorta and the area of the superior vena caval-right atrial junction. The right upper pulmonary vein and the drainage of the azygous vein into the superior vena cava can also be examined in this view. With rightward angulation, the length of the superior vena cava and sometimes the inferior vena cava and their entry into the right atrium can be visualized (Fig. 4-25B). Sweeping leftward allows demonstration of the ascending aorta and aortic valve.

Coronary Arteries

It is important to elucidate the coronary artery anatomy in the study of congenital heart disease. The routine examination must include visualization of at least the origins of the left and right coronary arteries. If the coronary arteries are of particular interest, then a higher-frequency transducer must be used at a specific point during the examination. In the normal echocardiographic examination, slight modifications of the standard echocardiographic views can yield a full evaluation of the coronary arteries. Although every coronary artery segment may not be imaged in every patient in every view, enough of the coronary artery system should be imaged to provide adequate assessment (36,37).

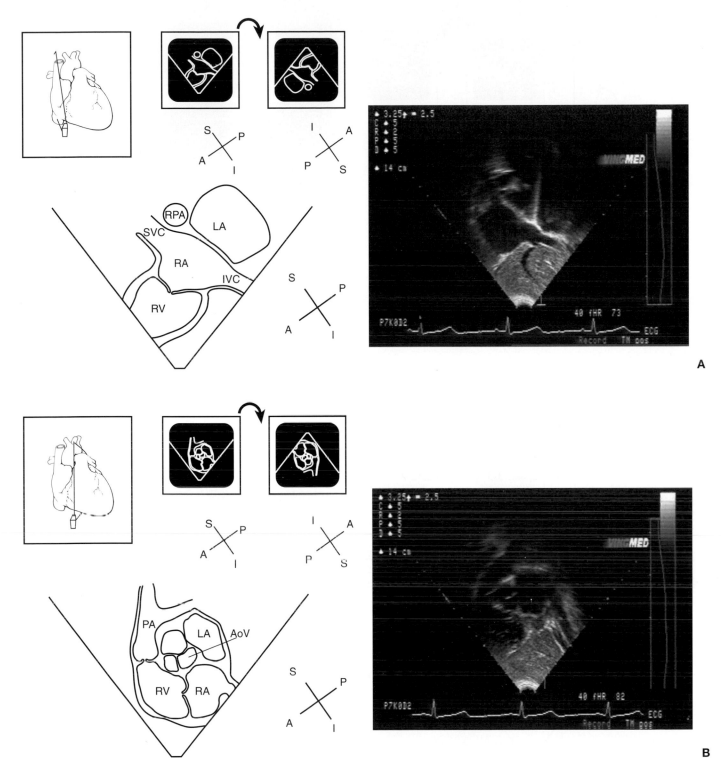

FIG. 4-19. Schematic drawings and echocardiograms demonstrating the subcostal short-axis views. **A:** Level of the venae cavae. **B:** Level of the right ventricular outflow tract.

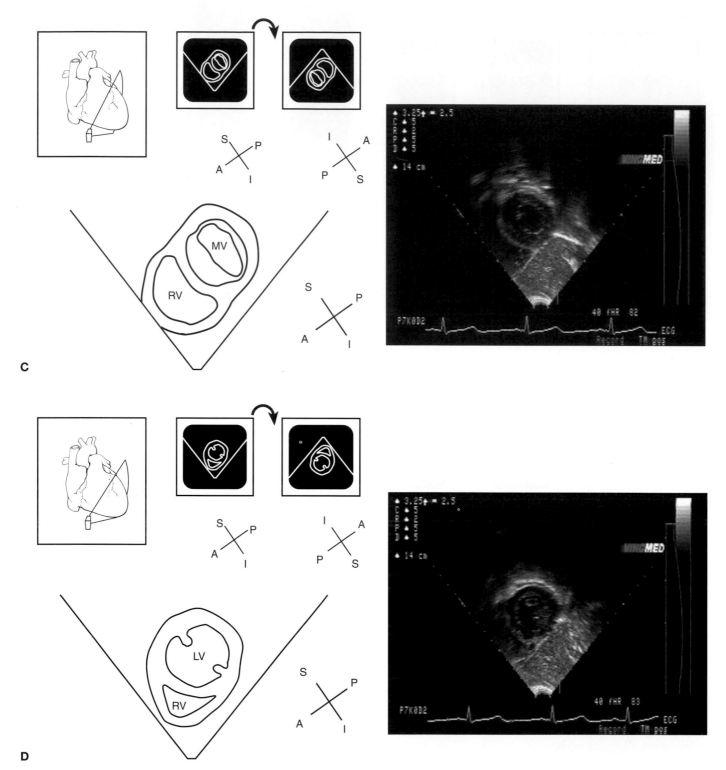

FIG. 4-19. (*Continued.*) **C:** Level of the mitral valve leaflets. **D:** Level of the left ventricular papillary muscles. *SVC*, superior vena cava; *IVC*, inferior vena cava; *RA*, right atrium; *RV*, right ventricle; *LA*, left atrium; *AoV*, aortic valve; *PA*, pulmonary artery. *S*, superior; *I*, inferior; *A*, anterior; *P*, posterior.

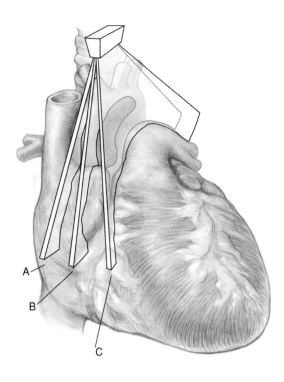

FIG. 4-20. Schematic rendition of the planes of the ultrasound beam to obtain the suprasternal long-axis views. **A:** Level of the transverse aortic arch. **B:** Level of the descending thoracic aorta. **C:** Level of the left pulmonary artery. (*Drawing by Richard Gersony*)

In the standard parasternal long-axis view, the ostium and proximal portion of the right coronary artery can sometimes be seen arising from the anterior aortic root (Fig. 4-5A). When the transducer is angled from the parasternal long-axis to the right ventricular inflow view, a portion of a right ventricular branch of the right coronary artery can usually be seen (Echo. 4-1). Imaging of this coronary artery can sometimes be maximized by dropping down one interspace on the chest from the standard parasternal long-axis position. In the routine echocardiographic examination, the transducer is then angled toward the left shoulder to image the right ventricular outflow tract. As the ultrasound plane is angled between the semilunar valves, a segment of the left anterior descending coronary artery is usually seen in the anterior portion of the ventricular septum (Echo. 4-2). Occasionally, a segment of the left main coronary artery can also be visualized in this view (38,39).

The parasternal short-axis view is very important in coronary artery imaging because this is the view in which the origins of the coronary arteries are best visualized (40,41). The transducer is positioned at the base of the heart with the aortic root in the center of the image. In this view, the three cusps of the aortic valve can be appreciated: the right coronary cusp near the tricuspid valve, the left coronary cusp near the pulmonary valve, and the noncoronary cusp immediately anterior to the left atrium. Usually, the origins of the left and right coronary arteries can be seen with little transducer manipulation (Echo. 4-3). Frequently, the left and right coronary artery origins

will be better imaged individually. From the standard parasternal short-axis view, the transducer is rotated slightly clockwise and angled slightly cranially to visualize the ostium and proximal right coronary artery. A major segment of the right coronary artery can be visualized coursing along the right atrioventricular sulcus by aiming the transducer toward the patient's right. Clockwise rotation of the transducer and cranial angulation are continued to visualize the ostium of the left coronary artery. The left main coronary artery and its bifurcation into the left anterior descending and circumflex coronary artery can usually be clearly seen (Echo. 4-4). The left anterior descending coronary artery can sometimes be followed as it traverses caudally in the ventricular septum.

Portions of the coronary arteries can be visualized from several of the apical planes. When the transducer is angled posteriorly, the right coronary artery can be visualized in the right atrioventricular groove (Echo. 4-5). The posterior descending coronary artery can also be seen in the interventricular sulcus (Echo. 4-6). If the transducer is angled anteriorly to visualize the left ventricular outflow tract, portions of the proximal left coronary artery and its branches can be seen (Echo. 4-7). The coronary arteries can also be imaged from the subcostal view. When the transducer is aimed posteriorly, the posterior descending artery is seen along the diaphragmatic surface of the heart. In the subcostal coronal view of the left ventricular outflow tract, the ostia and proximal portions of the left main and right coronary arteries can be seen. When the transducer is in the sagittal plane, angled to the left at the

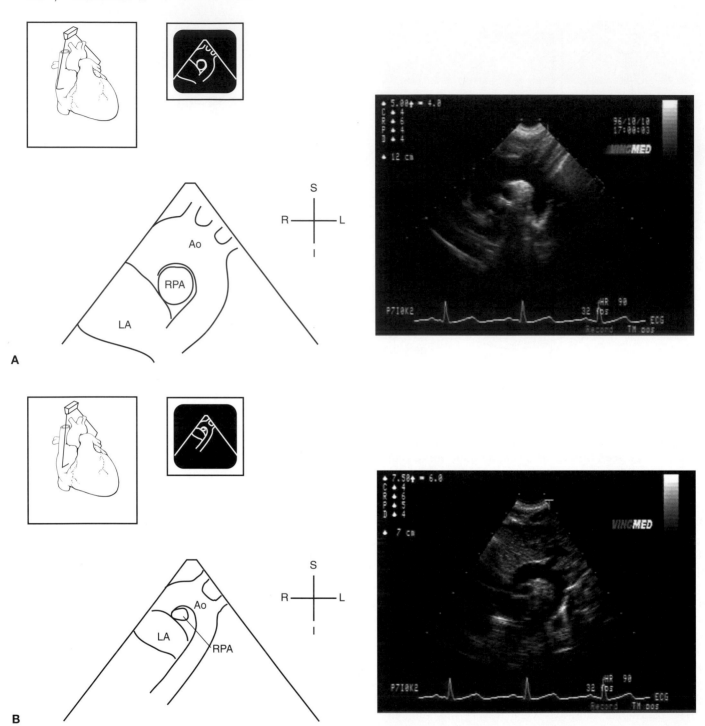

FIG. 4-21. Schematic drawings and echocardiograms demonstrating the suprasternal long-axis views. **A:** Level of the transverse aortic arch. **B:** Level of the descending thoracic aorta.

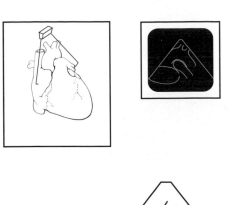

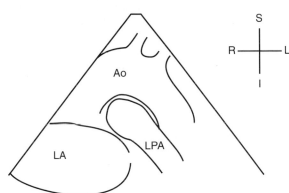

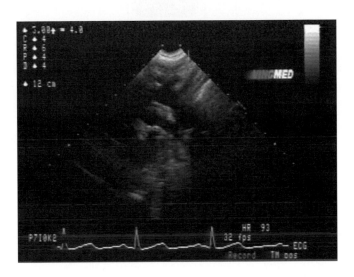

C

FIG. 4-21. (*Continued.*) **C:** Level of the left pulmonary artery. *Ao*, aorta; *RPA*, right pulmonary artery; *LPA*, left pulmonary artery; *LA*, left atrium. *S*, superior; *I*, inferior; *R*, right; *L*, left.

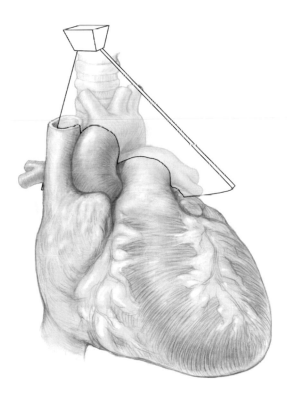

FIG. 4-22. Schematic rendition of the planes of the ultrasound beam to obtain the suprasternal short-axis view. (*Drawing by Richard Gersony*)

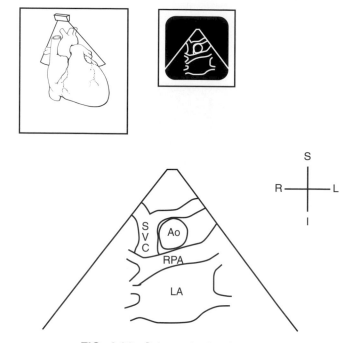

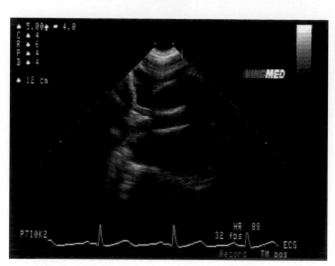

FIG. 4-23. Schematic drawing and echocardiogram demonstrating the suprasternal short-axis view. *Ao*, aorta; *RPA*, right pulmonary artery; *SVC*, superior vena cava; *LA*, left atrium. *S*, superior; *I*, inferior; *R*, right; *L*, left.

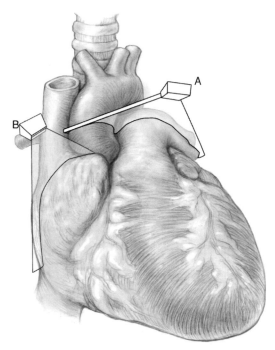

FIG. 4-24. Schematic rendition of the planes of the ultrasound beam to obtain the subclavicular views. **A:** Left subclavicular view. **B:** Right subclavicular view. (*Drawing by Richard Gersony, modified by the authors*)

level of the mitral valve, a long segment of the circumflex coronary artery can be imaged in the left atrioventricular groove (Echo. 4-7).

Positioning the transducer in the suprasternal notch allows another view of the origin and proximal course of the coronary arteries. From a classic long-axis view, the transducer is rotated counterclockwise and angled slightly anteriorly to achieve a suprasternal right anterior oblique cut from which the left coronary artery is seen (Echo. 4-8). Further counterclockwise rotation with rightward angulation brings the origin of the right coronary artery into view (Echo. 4-8). The left coronary artery can be examined in this fashion in most children; the right coronary artery may become more difficult to visualize in older children (42).

VIEWS IN THE MALPOSED HEART

It is usually easiest to start the echocardiographic examination with the subcostal views if cardiac malposition is suspected. From this approach, presence of dextrocardia or levocardia can quickly be determined, along with the position of the liver and the ventricular apex (see Echos. 8-1, 8-2). In addition, as stated previously, the situs can usually be determined from the subcostal abdominal

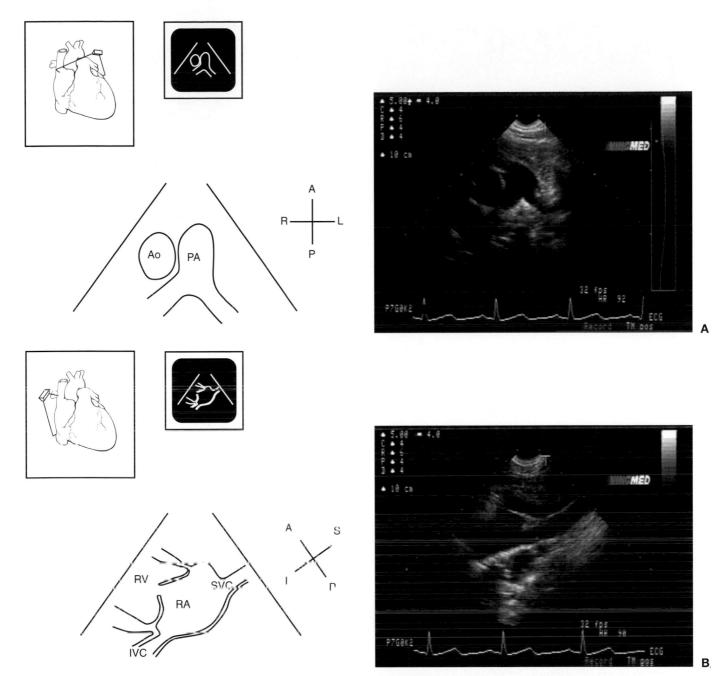

FIG. 4-25. Schematic drawings and echocardiograms demonstrating the subclavicular views. **A:** Left subclavicular view. **B:** Right subclavicular view. *Ao*, aorta; *PA*, pulmonary artery; *RA*, right atrium; *RV*, right ventricle; *SVC*, superior vena cava; *IVC*, inferior vena cava. *A*, anterior; *P*, posterior; *R*, right; *L*, left; *S*, superior; *I*, inferior.

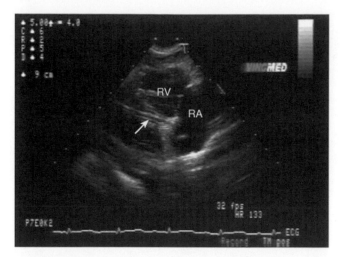

ECHO. 4-1. Parasternal long-axis view of the right ventricular inflow demonstrating a portion of a right ventricular branch of the right coronary artery (*arrow*). *RV*, right ventricle; *RA*, right atrium.

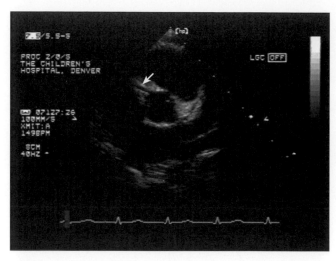

ECHO. 4-3. Parasternal short-axis view of the aorta demonstrating the ostia and proximal segments of the right (*arrow*) and left coronary arteries.

views by noting the relative positions of the aorta and the systemic venous return from the lower body (14) (see Echos. 8-7, 8-8, 8-10).

In situs inversus with mirror-image dextrocardia, the cardiac apex is positioned to the patient's right and all the cardiac chambers are in a mirror-image position: the morphologic left atrium is to the right of the morphologic right atrium, the morphologic left ventricle is to the right of the morphologic right ventricle, and the aorta is posterior and to the left of the pulmonary artery (see Echo. 8-2). It is important to note that all echocardiographic images are recorded in their anatomic positions and are not inverted from left to right to correct for dextrocardia. In the parasternal views, the transducer is positioned along

the long axis of the heart. With dextrocardia, the transducer is usually positioned to the right of the sternum. In mirror-image dextrocardia and dextrocardia by dextroversion, because the apex of the heart is oriented to the right of the patient, the line of ultrasound will be from the left shoulder to the right hip. In dextroposition when the cardiac apex is pointing toward the left of the patient, the ultrasound plane will be the same as in a normal subject—that is, from right shoulder to left hip. Because the standard parasternal long-axis view has anterior-posterior and cranial-caudal orientation, without right-left orientation, it will look the same in dextrocardia as in levocardia (Fig. 4-5A). On the other hand, the display of parasternal short-axis views, which have right-left orientation, will be the opposite of usual on the screen. The

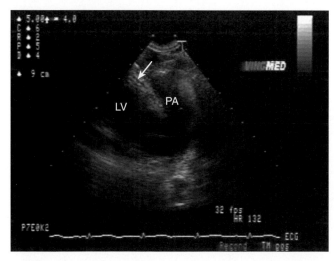

ECHO. 4-2. Parasternal long-axis view of the right ventricular outflow demonstrating a segment of the left anterior descending coronary artery (*arrow*). *LV*, left ventricle; *PA*, pulmonary artery.

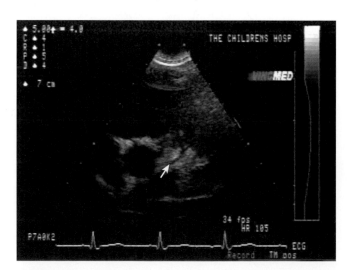

ECHO. 4-4. Parasternal short-axis view angled cranially to visualize the left main coronary artery and the bifurcation into left anterior descending and circumflex branches (*arrow*).

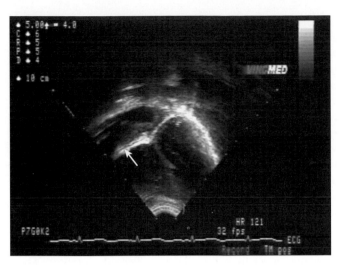

ECHO. 4-5. Apical view angled posteriorly to visualize the right coronary artery along the right atrioventricular groove (*arrow*).

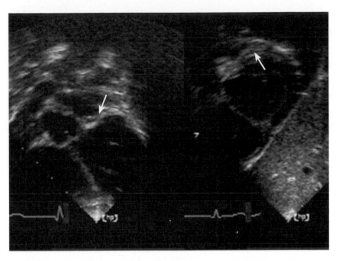

ECHO. 4-7. Left: Apical view aimed toward the left ventricular outflow demonstrating the course of the left circumflex coronary artery along the left atrioventricular groove. **Right:** Subcostal sagittal view at the level of the mitral valve leaflets demonstrating the course of the circumflex branch along the left ventricular groove (*arrow*).

right ventricular inflow will be positioned on the right side of the screen and the pulmonary artery will be on the left side of the screen.

The apical views are obtained by positioning the transducer over the apical impulse, be it on the left or right side of the chest. The apical and subcostal views have left-right orientation, so situs inversus will be the mirror image of situs solitus, with the morphologic left atrium and left ventricle positioned to the right of the morphologic right atrium and right ventricle, respectively.

M-MODE ECHOCARDIOGRAPHY

In our laboratory, the normal pediatric echocardiogram begins with two-dimensional imaging, followed by re-

cording of M-mode echocardiographic traces. These parts of the examination are considered complementary.

In the routine patient, M mode has a limited but important role. Although two-dimensional imaging has replaced M mode in the diagnosis of structural congenital heart disease, M-mode echocardiography has the advantage of high temporal resolution because of its rapid sampling rate (43). M mode is utilized to measure cardiac chamber size accurately and estimate systolic and diastolic function.

M-mode traces of the right and left ventricle are obtained from the parasternal long or short axis (44–51)

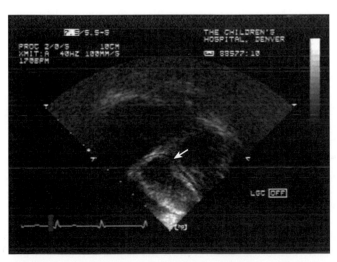

ECHO. 4-6. Apical view angled posteriorly to visualize the posterior descending coronary artery.

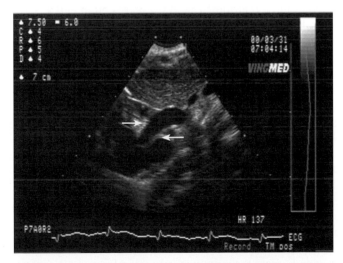

ECHO. 4-8. Suprasternal long-axis view rotated counterclockwise to visualize the origins of the left and right coronary arteries (*bottom* and *top arrows*, respectively).

(see Echo. 5-1). The M-mode cursor is positioned perpendicular to the interventricular septum and the M-mode line is swept from the apex to the base of the heart. The anterior surface of the right ventricle may be difficult to resolve from the surrounding structures because of its position in the near field of the image; however, the endocardial surface of the right ventricular wall can usually be visualized and its movement assessed. The left ventricular cavity is measured in diastole and systole and the measurements are compared with normal values adjusted for body surface area to evaluate overall cardiac size and systolic ventricular function (see Echo. 5-1). The interventricular septum and posterior wall are routinely measured in systole and diastole to establish the percentage of thickening during ventricular contraction. Diastolic values are compared with normal values to assess ventricular hypertrophy. The M-mode sweep is continued, with the motion of the mitral valve noted. At the base of the heart, the left atrium is visualized behind the aortic root and the measurements compared with normal values (40).

DOPPLER STUDY: SPECTRAL AND COLOR FLOW MAPPING

Spectral Doppler utilizing pulsed-wave, high pulsed repetition frequency (high PRF), and continuous-wave modes and color flow mapping are vital to the complete evaluation of the pediatric patient. Spectral Doppler traces are routinely recorded for the mitral, tricuspid, aortic, and pulmonary valves; the pulmonary veins, venae cavae, and hepatic veins; the main pulmonary artery and its branches; and the ascending and descending aorta.

From the parasternal long axis, color flow mapping is used to evaluate the left ventricular inflow and outflow tracts. Frequently, pulmonary venous flow can be seen entering the left atrium. The trabecular septum and a portion of the outlet ventricular septum are evaluated from this position with spectral and color Doppler to exclude the presence of any defects. As the transducer is angled to the right ventricular inflow tract, the membranous ventricular septum and the tricuspid valve inflow are evaluated. Velocities across the tricuspid valve can be sampled with pulsed-wave Doppler from this position and color flow mapping can reveal the presence of physiologic tricuspid regurgitation. The color image can help position the Doppler sample volume to measure the velocity of the regurgitant jet (see Echo. 6-12). The transducer is then angled toward the right ventricular outflow tract to assess the outlet portion of the interventricular septum and the pulmonary artery. Pulsed-wave Doppler is used to record velocities within the right ventricular outflow tract and across the pulmonic valve (see Echo. 6-9). Color flow imaging usually demonstrates the presence of physiologic pulmonic valve regurgitation and aids in positioning of the pulsed-wave sample volume for velocity recording (see Echo. 6-13).

From the parasternal short-axis views at the base of the heart, the right ventricular inflow can be evaluated with pulsed-wave and color flow Doppler. Like the long-axis view of the right ventricular inflow, this position allows complete spectral and color Doppler evaluation of the tricuspid valve flow, including the presence of tricuspid valve regurgitation. Physiologic tricuspid valve regurgitation has been seen in 83% of normal subjects (52). From a sweep into this position, the membranous septum is also seen under the septal leaflet of the tricuspid valve, which facilitates demonstration of any defects at this site with color Doppler mapping. Also in this position, the atrial septum can be evaluated by Doppler (spectral and color flow mapping) to reveal the presence of shunting. The aortic valve is seen on cross section in the center of the image, and color Doppler flow mapping can reveal even trivial amounts of aortic regurgitation. Although spectral sampling is not accurate for peak velocity determination because of the unfavorable interrogation angle, the spectral traces can be used to document the timing of the signals. The transducer is then aimed leftward toward the right ventricular outflow to reveal the outflow tract, pulmonic valve, and main and branch pulmonary arteries. The velocities in the right ventricular outflow tract and main pulmonary artery are recorded with pulsed-wave Doppler by placing the sample volume proximal to the pulmonary valve in the right ventricular outflow tract and slowly moving through the pulmonic valve into the main pulmonary artery (see Echo. 6-9). The peak velocity in the main pulmonary artery is approximately 0.9 m/s and is slightly higher than the peak velocity in the right ventricular outflow tract (50). In newborns, the peak velocity of flow in the pulmonary artery is less than that in older children (53). The velocity within the main pulmonary artery varies depending on the position of the sample volume, being slightly higher along the medial than the lateral arterial wall. This is also evident on color Doppler flow maps, where aliasing of velocities is commonly seen along the inner curvature of the main pulmonary artery. The pulsed-wave Doppler velocity trace should be obtained from the central main pulmonary artery between the pulmonic valve and the bifurcation. Physiologic pulmonary insufficiency has been detected with color flow mapping and confirmed with pulsed-wave Doppler in 93% of normal individuals (52) (see Echo. 6-13). The color Doppler signal in physiologic pulmonary regurgitation has the characteristic appearance of a small flame within the right ventricular outflow tract.

The transducer is then slowly angled inferiorly toward the cardiac apex. This scanning provides the best view of the entire trabecular ventricular septum. It should be undertaken carefully with color flow mapping because it can reveal the presence of tiny septal defects that would otherwise go undetected from other views. At the level of the mitral valve, color Doppler can reveal the presence of mitral regurgitation as well. Spectral Doppler is of limited use in these views because of the unfavorable angle of interrogation with most structures.

The transducer is then positioned over the cardiac apex. Pulsed-wave Doppler of the mitral and tricuspid valves is recorded from the apical four-chamber view. The sample volume is positioned on the atrial side of the respective valves and slowly advanced to the ventricular inflows. The maximal velocities of the tricuspid and mitral valves are obtained at the tips of the valve leaflets (see Echo. 6-7). The tricuspid and mitral valve Doppler patterns are qualitatively similar, but the peak velocity of the mitral valve is slightly higher than that of the tricuspid valve (54). Flow in early diastole, representing passive ventricular filling, is characterized by a peak called the E wave; it is followed by the A wave, which represents filling during atrial contraction (55) (see Echo. 6-7). In children, both the tricuspid and mitral valve Doppler velocity curves have a dominant E wave except for fetuses and neonates during the first few weeks of life, in whom the A wave is dominant (56,57). The tricuspid valve Doppler curves show more variation with respiration than those across the mitral valve (58–61). In children, the effect of heart rate must also be taken into account when the mitral and tricuspid inflow patterns are assessed (62,63).

The tricuspid and mitral valves should also be assessed with color flow mapping and spectral Doppler for the presence and severity of valvar insufficiency. As the Doppler sensitivity of echocardiographic instruments improves, trace amounts of valvar insufficiency are commonly detected (52,64–66). The significance of these findings must be evaluated within the context of the individual patient.

After tricuspid and mitral valve Doppler velocities have been recorded, the pulsed-wave sample volume is placed within a pulmonary vein with guidance by the color flow map (see Echo. 6-6). The flow in the normal pulmonary vein is continuous with peaks in diastole and systole. Often, flow reversal can be seen in the pulmonary vein during atrial contraction (pulmonary venous A wave). Although the peak velocity is higher during diastole than during systole, the velocity time integral is greater during systole than during diastole. The flow patterns do not vary with respiration (67).

The transducer is then tilted superiorly toward the left ventricular outflow tract, aortic valve, and proximal ascending aorta. The sample volume is initially positioned within the left ventricular outflow tract, where Doppler velocity is approximately 1 m/s in children (see Echo. 6-10). As the sample volume is advanced across the aortic valve annulus, the flow profile changes slightly, with a more rapid acceleration time and increased peak velocity

(53) (see Echo. 6-10). In contrast to the flow velocity in the pulmonary artery, the flow velocity in the ascending aorta is the same in newborns as in older children (53).

The subcostal views are particularly useful for assessment of the atrial septum with spectral and color Doppler in both the coronal and sagittal projections. The flow patterns in the venae cavae and hepatic veins are also assessed by pulsed-wave and color Doppler from the subcostal views. Normal flow in the superior vena cava is a continuous low-velocity flow, with both the peak velocity and velocity time integral greater in systole than in diastole (68) (see Echo. 6-5). This pattern is similar to that observed in adult patients; however, in most adults flow reversal is present with atrial systole (69), whereas flow reversal is present in only 17% of children. Respiratory variation is seen in vena caval flow, with an augmentation of the flow velocities on inspiration (55). Flow in the hepatic vein is also similar to that recorded in adult patients (69–71). The majority of children have a biphasic pattern, with the predominant flow in systole. Flow reversal is frequently seen at end-systole and with atrial contraction (68).

In the suprasternal long-axis view, the entire aortic arch can be interrogated with spectral Doppler and color flow mapping. The velocity should be approximately the same in the ascending and descending aorta (53) (see Echo. 6-11). In the descending aorta, a small amount of retrograde flow is normally seen during early diastole, which probably represents elastic recoil (2). In the short-axis suprasternal view and the left subclavicular view, a portion of the main pulmonary artery is visualized as well as the bifurcation and right and left branches. Pulsed-wave Doppler should be used to record velocities across the bifurcation and within both branches. Usually in newborns, particularly in premature infants, there is a slight increase in the velocity across the bifurcation because of mild peripheral pulmonary branch stenosis, which normally resolves with growth. Also from the short axis suprasternal view, the four pulmonary veins are seen entering the left atrium; thus, this is the best view to document the pulmonary venous return. Color Doppler flow mapping is particularly useful in demonstrating the inflows of the four veins and aids in the placement of the pulsed-wave Doppler sample volume to record and document the velocities.

TRANSESOPHAGEAL ECHOCARDIOGRAPHY

Transesophageal echocardiography has achieved an important role in pediatric echocardiography. Miniaturized single-plane (horizontal), biplane (horizontal and longitudinal), and more recently multiplane transesophageal probes are now available that allow patients as small as 3 kg to be imaged safely from a transesophageal approach. These probes utilize high-frequency ultrasound imaging crystals that provide excellent resolution of the septa, valves, left and right ventricular outflow tracts, pulmonary artery, aorta, venous return, and ventricular function in children (72–74). The probes are also equipped with full Doppler capabilities (pulsed-wave, continuous-wave, and color flow imaging), making hemodynamic assessment possible.

Transesophageal echocardiography is particularly useful in the operating room, where the patient can be evaluated intraoperatively both before and after cardiopulmonary bypass (75–79). In a study by O'Leary et al. (80), biplane intraoperative transesophageal echocardiography had a significant impact on intraoperative management in 16% of their patients despite routine preoperative assessment, including cardiac catheterization. In this same study, transesophageal echocardiography revealed residual abnormalities that resulted in immediate surgical revision in 8.7% of the patients (80). The transesophageal approach has also been used in difficult-to-image children (81,82) and in the cardiac catheterization laboratory to aid in the correct placement of intracardiac devices, balloon valvuloplasty catheters (79,83,84), and radiofrequency ablation catheters (85,86).

Complications of transesophageal echocardiography have been low (80,87–97) in children. Mechanical problems with the probe, such as buckling of the tip of the endoscope in the patient's esophagus, have been reported; these made probe removal difficult and necessitated advancement of the endoscope into the stomach, where the probe could be straightened, permitting safe removal (98). Compression of the airway or vascular structures by the endoscope has been observed, and these usually resolve with probe repositioning or removal. Supraventricular and ventricular arrhythmias have been reported in the adult literature (96–100) but have not been a problem in children.

Pediatric patients require heavy sedation or general anesthesia for this procedure. In our laboratory, transesophageal imaging is rarely required outside the operating room or cardiac catheterization laboratory. On these infrequent occasions, one physician is responsible for administering the sedation and maintaining the airway, leaving the echocardiographer free to focus on the echocardiographic study. A sonographer is responsible for adjusting the controls on the ultrasound machine. We have not had any significant complications related to sedation or airway compromise when following this protocol.

Images can be obtained from three general positions of the endoscope: transgastric, behind the left atrium, and at the level of the great vessels (see Figs. 4-27–4-31). For each position, imaging from the horizontal and longitudinal cardiac planes should be obtained with the biplane probe. If a multiplane probe is available, the entire range of images, from 0 degrees (horizontal plane of the chest) through 90 degrees (longitudinal plane of the chest) to 180 degrees (mirror image of the horizontal plane of the chest), is available (Fig. 4-26). The 45-degree plane corresponds to the short axis of the heart and the 135-degree plane to the long axis of the heart. The probe is manipulated by advancing and withdrawing, anteflexion and retroflexion, and clockwise and counterclockwise rotation of the endoscope. Many probes have a control that allows the probe to be moved laterally in the esophagus. This movement has limited applicability in children. Overall, manipulation of the endoscope is much reduced with the use of multiplane probes compared with the biplane probes. In our studies, we perform imaging and Doppler interrogation at each sequential site to minimize probe manipulation.

The probe is placed initially in the patient's stomach to obtain the transgastric views (Fig. 4-27). The probe is anteflexed and the transducer array is rotated through the horizontal and longitudinal planes. In the transgastric horizontal plane, a left ventricular short-axis view is obtained (Fig. 4-27A,B) (Echo. 4-9). These images are similar to the parasternal short-axis views of the left ventricle and allow an overall assessment of left ventricular function. Rotation of the ultrasound plane to the longitudinal axis of the heart with anteflexion of the endoscope provides images similar to the subcostal coronal views (Fig. 4-27C–E) (Echo. 4-10). These latter views allow for the best Doppler alignment of the left and right ventricular outflow tracts for recording

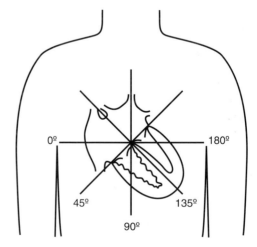

FIG. 4-26. Diagram of the planes of the chest and the heart with the degrees of rotation corresponding to the transesophageal multiplane probe positions. Note that the planes of the chest and the heart differ. The horizontal plane of the chest corresponds to 0 degrees and the longitudinal plane to 90 degrees. The short axis of the heart corresponds to 45 degrees and the long axis to 135 degrees.

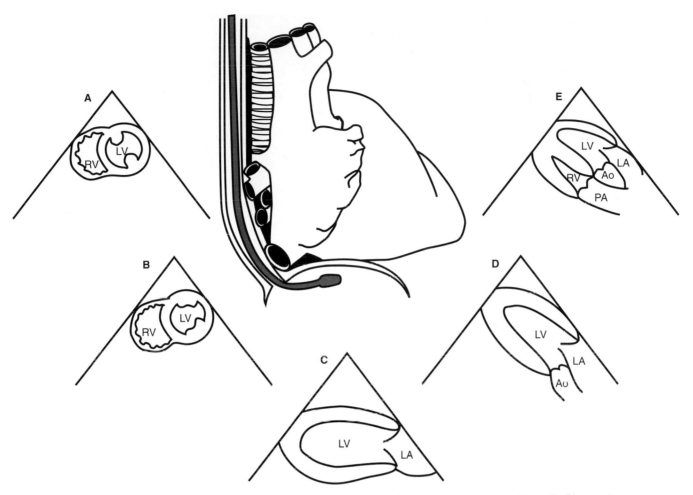

FIG. 4-27. Diagram of the transesophageal views obtained from a transgastric position. **A:** Short axis 0-degree view at the level of the papillary muscles. **B:** Short axis 45-degree view at the level of the mitral leaflets. **C:** Longitudinal 90-degree view of the left ventricle. **D:** Longitudinal 120-degree view of the left ventricular outflow tract. **E:** Longitudinal 120-degree view of the right ventricular outflow tract. *RV,* right ventricle; *LV,* left ventricle; *LA,* left atrium; *Ao,* aorta; *PA,* pulmonary artery. (*Drawing by Alina U. Borges*)

of velocities (Fig. 4-27D,E) (Echo. 4-11). The probe is then returned to a neutral plane and withdrawn to a retrocardiac position, behind the left atrium (Fig. 4-28). In the horizontal plane, the four chambers of the heart are viewed (Fig. 4-28A,B) (Echo. 4-12). The atrial septum can be seen almost in its entirety by counterclockwise rotation of the endoscope with the transducer at 0 degrees. This is equivalent to a subcostal coronal plane (Echo. 4-13). The coronary sinus can usually be imaged in its length behind the left atrium and its mouth visualized in the right atrium. As the probe is slightly withdrawn, the mitral and tricuspid valves are seen. The septal attachments of the tricuspid valve and its normal apical displacement relative to the point of insertion of the mitral valve are readily apparent. Inflow velocities of the tricuspid and mitral valves should be recorded with pulsed-wave and color Doppler flow imaging (Echo. 4-14). If tricuspid or mitral valve insuffi-

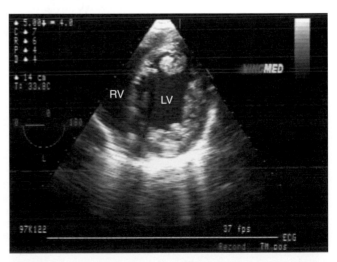

ECHO. 4-9. Transesophageal transgastric view of the short axis of the ventricles. *RV,* right ventricle; *LV,* left ventricle.

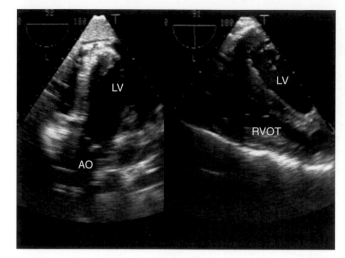

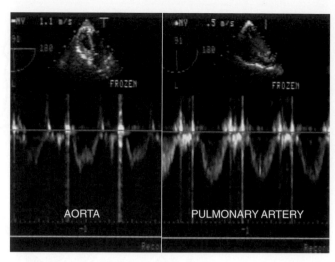

ECHO. 4-10. Transesophageal longitudinal views with extreme anteflexion of the transducer demonstrating the left ventricular outflow tract **(left)** and right ventricular outflow tract **(right)**. *LV*, left ventricle; *AO*, aorta; *RVOT*, right ventricular outflow tract.

ECHO. 4-11. Spectral Doppler recording of the velocities through the aorta **(left)** and pulmonary artery **(right)** obtained from transgastric longitudinal views.

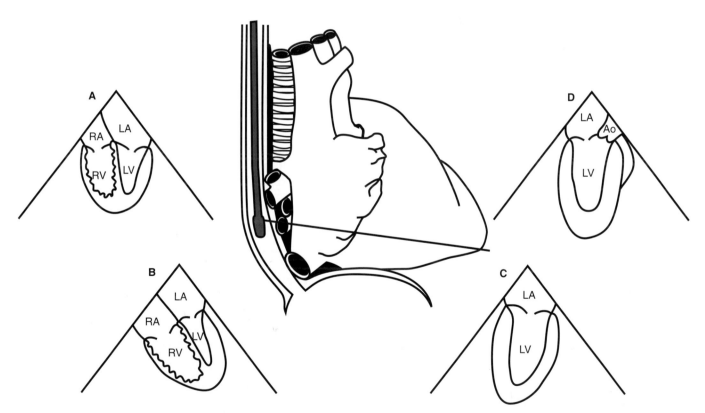

FIG. 4-28. Diagram of the transesophageal views obtained from a low retrocardiac position behind the left atrium. **A:** Four-chamber 0-degree view of the ventricular inlet. **B:** Four-chamber 45-degree view. **C:** Longitudinal 90-degree view of the left atrium and ventricle (two-chamber equivalent). **D:** Longitudinal 150-degree view of the left ventricular outflow (three-chamber equivalent). *RA*, right atrium; *LA*, left atrium; *RV*, right ventricle; *LV*, left ventricle; *Ao*, aorta. (*Drawing by Alina U. Borges*)

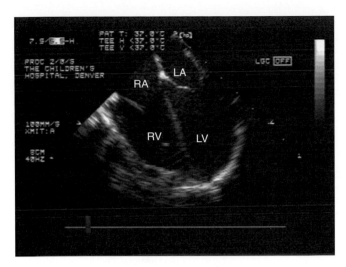

ECHO. 4-12. Transesophageal horizontal view obtained from a low retrocardiac position demonstrating the four cardiac chambers. *RA*, right atrium; *LA*, left atrium; *RV*, right ventricle; *LV*, left ventricle.

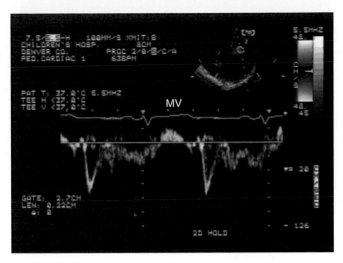

ECHO. 4-14. Spectral Doppler recording of the inflow velocities through the mitral valve obtained from the four-chamber transesophageal horizontal view. *MV*, mitral valve.

ciency is detected, spectral Doppler should be used to quantitate the amount of valvular insufficiency and the peak velocity of the insufficiency. The inlet and most of the trabecular portions of the interventricular septum are seen in these views, and they should be scanned with color Doppler for any defects. The probe can be withdrawn slightly to image the left ventricular outflow tract, the membranous septum, and the anterior right and posterior noncoronary aortic cusps (Echo. 4-15). With further rotation of the transducer array toward the

longitudinal plane of the heart (Fig. 4-28C), the mitral valve inflow is visualized in a view similar to an apical two-chamber view (Echo. 4-16). This allows imaging of the valve from a view orthogonal to the four-chamber orientation. With further rotation, the left ventricular outflow tract is seen, including the aortic root (Fig. 4-28D).

The transducer is then returned to 0 degrees and the endoscope withdrawn slightly to image the left ventricular outflow tract, with the aortic valve in the center of the image (Fig. 4-29). The right atrial appendage can be seen anterior to the aortic root (Fig. 4-29A) (Echo. 4-17). The

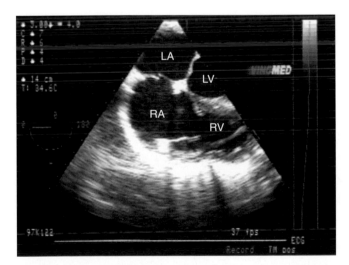

ECHO. 4-13. Transesophageal horizontal view obtained from a low retrocardiac position by counterclockwise rotation of the endoscope. The view displays the full length of the atrial septum. Note the flap of the foramen ovale with the primum septum on the left side. *LA*, left atrium; *RA*, right atrium; *RV*, right ventricle; *LV*, left ventricle.

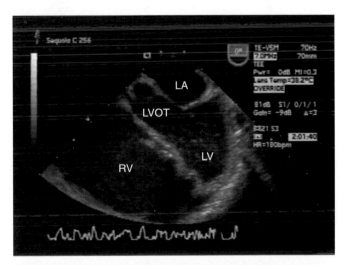

ECHO. 4-15. Transesophageal horizontal view obtained from a midretrocardiac position demonstrating the left ventricular outflow tract and aortic root. *RV*, right ventricle; *LA*, left atrium; *LV*, left ventricle; *LVOT*, left ventricular outflow tract.

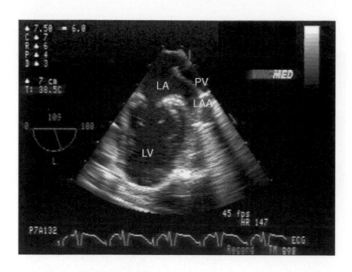

ECHO. 4-16. Transesophageal longitudinal view of the left atrium and ventricle (two-chamber equivalent) obtained from a low retrocardiac position. *LA*, left atrium; *LV*, left ventricle; *LAA*, left atrial appendage; *PV*, pulmonary vein.

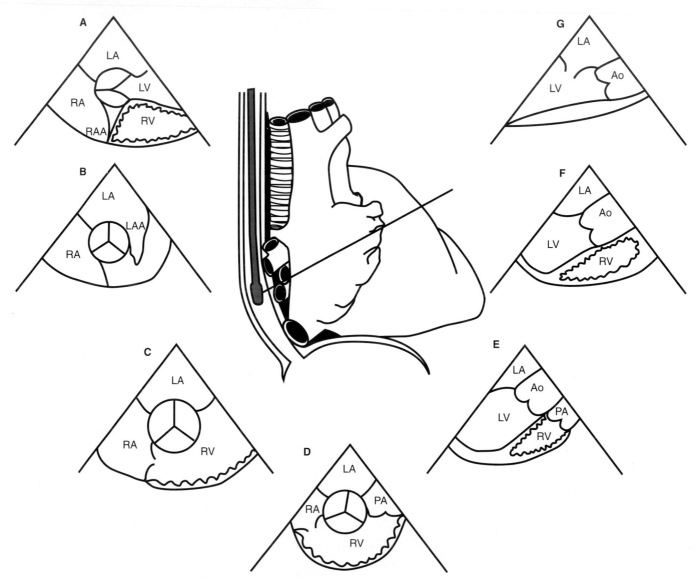

FIG. 4-29. Diagram of the transesophageal views obtained from a midretrocardiac position. **A:** Horizontal 0-degree view of the left ventricular outflow tract and aorta. **B:** Short-axis 45-degree view of the aorta. **C:** Longitudinal 60-degree view of the right ventricular inflow. **D:** Longitudinal 90-degree view of the right ventricular outflow. **E:** Longitudinal 100-degree view of the right and left ventricular outflows. **F:** Longitudinal 110-degree view of the left ventricular outflow. **G:** Longitudinal 140-degree view of the left ventricular outflow and ascending aorta. *LA*, left atrium; *RA*, right atrium; *LV*, left ventricle; *RV*, right ventricle; *RAA*, right arterial appendage; *LAA*, left atrial appendage; *Ao*, aorta; *PA*, pulmonary artery. (*Drawing by Alina U. Borges*)

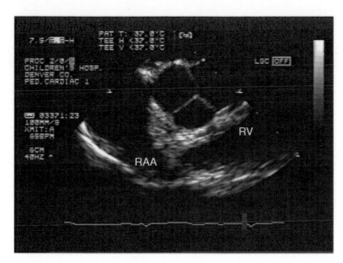

ECHO. 4-17. Transesophageal horizontal view of the aorta obtained from a midretrocardiac position. Note the right atrial appendage seen anterior to the aorta. *RAA*, right atrial appendage; *RV*, right ventricle.

array is then rotated until the aorta is seen in cross section in the middle of the image (Fig. 4-29B) (Echo. 4-18). These images are very similar to the parasternal short-axis view of the base of the heart, with the right side of the heart located anteriorly. The probe can be manipulated slightly to see the origins of the left and right coronary arteries in these positions (Echo. 4-19). Frequently, the bifurcation of the left main coronary artery into the left anterior descending and left circumflex coronary arteries can be imaged (Echo. 4-19A). The left and right upper pulmonary veins can also be seen as they enter the left atrium, and pulsed-wave and color Doppler can help iden-

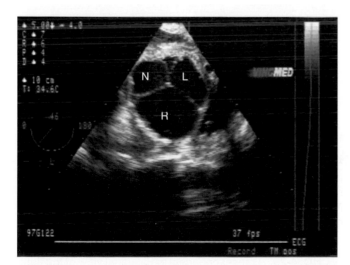

ECHO. 4-18. Transesophageal horizontal view of the aortic valve. *L*, left coronary cusp; *R*, right coronary cusp; *N*, noncoronary cusp.

tify and characterize their flows (Echo. 4-20). The left atrial appendage is also seen (Echos. 4-20, 4-21). Further steering toward the longitudinal plane of the heart allows imaging of the right ventricular inflow and outflow (Fig. 4-29C,D) (Echo. 4-22). Rotation to approximately 90 degrees will demonstrate the right and left ventricular outflow tracts, with the aortic and pulmonic valves parallel to each other in a longitudinal display (Fig. 4-29E) (Echo. 4-23). Further rotation will demonstrate the left ventricular outflow tract and ascending aorta (Fig. 4-29F,G). These views are important to identify defects of the infun-

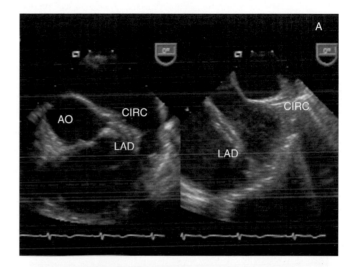

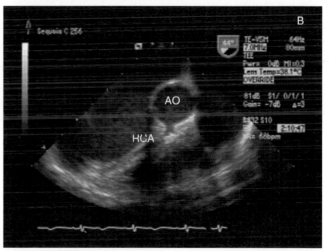

ECHO. 4-19. A: Left: Transesophageal horizontal view of the aortic valve adjusted to image the origin and bifurcation of the left main coronary artery. **Right:** Transesophageal horizontal view of the left ventricular outflow tract adjusted to image the distal courses of the left anterior descending and circumflex branches of the left coronary artery. **B:** Transesophageal horizontal view of the aorta adjusted to image the origin and distal course of the right coronary artery. *AO*, aorta; *CIRC*, circumflex branch; *LAD*, left anterior descending branch; *RCA*, right coronary artery.

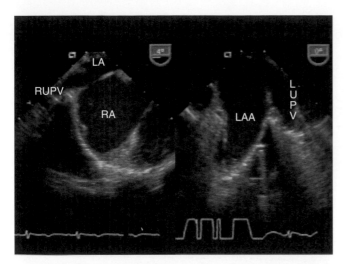 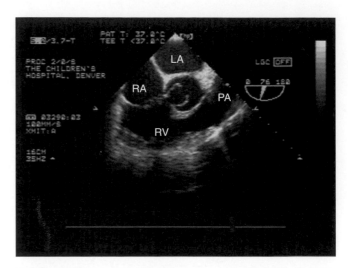

ECHO. 4-20. Left: Transesophageal horizontal view of the left ventricular outflow tract with counterclockwise rotation of the endoscope to image the atrial septum and right upper pulmonary vein. **Right:** Transesophageal horizontal view of the aortic valve rotated to image the left atrial appendage and left upper pulmonary vein. *LA*, left atrium; *RUPV*, right upper pulmonary vein; *RA*, right atrium; *LAA*, left atrial appendage; *LUPV*, left upper pulmonary vein.

ECHO. 4-22. Transesophageal view obtained from a mid-retrocardiac position at 76 degrees demonstrating the right ventricular inflow and outflow. *LA*, left atrium; *RA*, right atrium; *RV*, right ventricle; *PA*, pulmonary artery.

dibular or outlet septum, the presence of aortic valve override, displacement of the outlet septum leftward or rightward, and presence of doubly committed ventricular septal defects.

Detailed examination of the interatrial septum is particularly important in children because atrial defects can be present anywhere within the septum (Fig. 4-30) (Echo. 4-13). With the endoscope behind the left atrial cavity,

the atrial septum can be visualized from a horizontal position (Fig. 4-30A). Rotation of the transducer array to approximately 100 to 120 degrees provides the longitudinal view of the atrial cavities with the superior and inferior venae cavae as they enter the right atrium (Fig. 4-30D). The interatrial septum is perpendicular to the ultrasound beam, so that this structure is particularly well visualized (Echo. 4-24). This is an excellent view to assess shunting at the atrial level.

The endoscope is now withdrawn to the level of the great vessels (Fig. 4-31). The horizontal plane provides

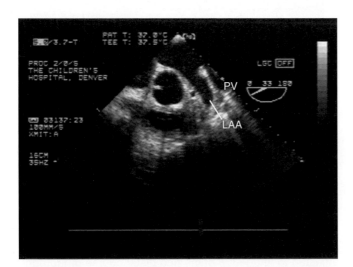 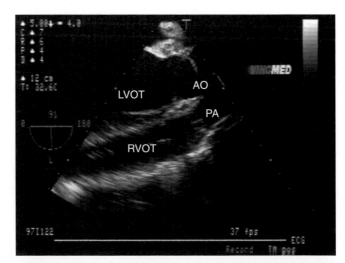

ECHO. 4-21. Transesophageal horizontal view of the aortic valve and left atrial appendage. *LAA*, left atrial appendage; *PV*, pulmonary vein.

ECHO. 4-23. Transesophageal longitudinal view of the right and left ventricular outflow tracts. *LVOT*, left ventricular outflow tract; *AO*, aorta; *RVOT*, right ventricular outflow tract; *PA*, pulmonary artery.

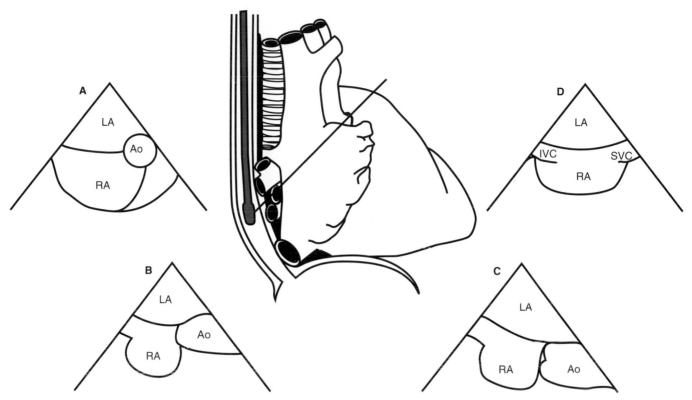

FIG. 4-30. Diagram of the transesophageal images obtained from a high retrocardiac position. **A:** Horizontal 0-degree view of the atrial septum. **B:** Horizontal 30-degree view of the atrial septum and superior vena cava. **C:** Longitudinal 90-degree view of the atrial septum. **D:** Longitudinal 120-degree view of the atrial septum and venae cavae. *LA*, left atrium; *RA*, right atrium; *Ao*, aorta; *IVC*, inferior vena cava; *SVC*, superior vena cava. (*Drawing by Alina U. Borges*)

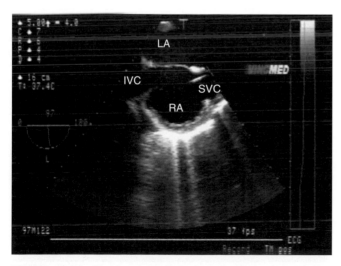

ECHO. 4-24. Transesophageal longitudinal view of the atrial septum and venae cavae. *LA*, left atrium; *RA*, right atrium; *IVC*, inferior vena cava; *SVC*, superior vena cava.

an excellent view of the main and branch pulmonary arteries, particularly the right (Fig. 4-31A,B) (Echo. 4-25). In addition to providing an anatomic image equivalent to that obtained from a left subclavicular position, this view also allows direct alignment of the Doppler beam along the direction of pulmonary flow for spectral and color Doppler sampling of velocities (Echo. 4-26). Although most intracardiac anatomy in children can be well defined with transesophageal echocardiography, there are some notable exceptions. The apical and outlet portions of the interventricular septum can be difficult to assess, and the left pulmonary artery can very seldom be adequately visualized because of its angulation (79). Occasionally, true peak velocities of intracardiac jets cannot be accurately defined with Doppler because of difficulty in correct alignment of the Doppler beam parallel to flow. With the advent of pediatric multiplane transesophgeal endoscopes, many of these difficulties are being resolved.

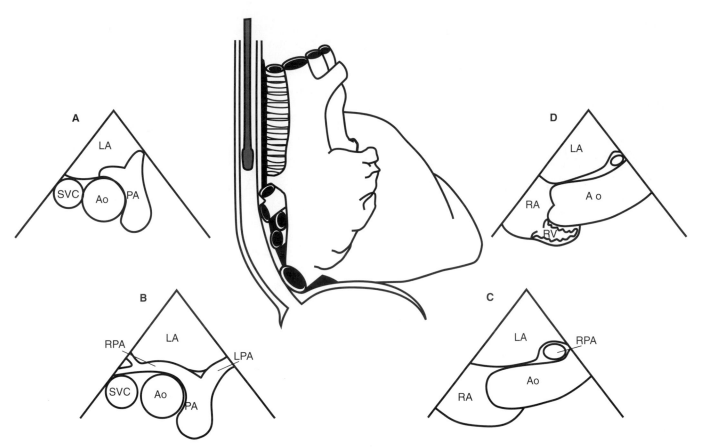

FIG. 4-31. Diagram of the transesophageal images obtained behind the great vessels. **A:** Horizontal 0-degree view of the main pulmonary artery and its bifurcation. **B:** Horizontal 40-degree view of the branch pulmonary arteries. **C:** Longitudinal 90-degree view of the ascending aorta. **D:** Longitudinal 120-degree view of the aortic root and ascending aorta. *LA,* left atrium; *RA,* right atrium; *Ao,* aorta; *SVC,* superior vena cava; *PA,* pulmonary artery; *RPA,* right pulmonary artery; *LPA,* left pulmonary artery. (*Drawing by Alina U. Borges*)

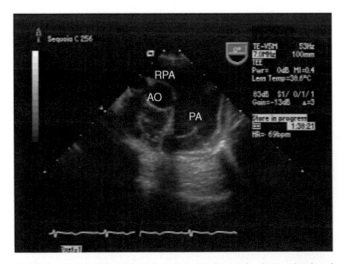

ECHO. 4-25. Transesophageal horizontal view obtained behind the great vessels demonstrating the main pulmonary artery, bifurcation, and proximal right pulmonary branch. *AO,* aorta; *PA,* main pulmonary artery; *RPA,* right pulmonary artery.

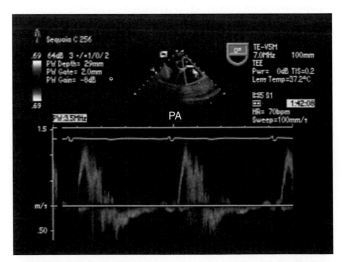

ECHO. 4-26. Spectral Doppler recording of velocities across the pulmonic valve obtained from the transesophageal horizontal view of the pulmonary artery. *PA,* pulmonary artery.

REFERENCES

1. Stevenson JG, French JW, Tenckhoff L, Maeda H, Wright S, Zamberlin K. Video viewing as an alternative to sedation for young subjects who have cardiac ultrasound examinations. *J Am Soc Echocardiogr* 1990;3:488–490.

2. Snider RA, Serwer GA. *Echocardiography in pediatric heart disease*. Chicago: Year Book, 1993.

3. Van Praagh R, Ongley PA, Swan HJC. Anatomic types of single or common ventricle in man: morphologic and geometric aspects of 60 necropsied cases. *Am J Cardiol* 1964;13:367–386.

4. Van Praagh R. The segmental approach to diagnosis in congenital heart disease. In: Bergsma D, ed. *Birth defects: original article series*. Baltimore: Williams & Wilkins, 1972:4–23.

5. Shinebourne EA, Macartney FJ, Anderson RH. Sequential chamber localization—logical approach to diagnosis in congenital heart disease. *Br Heart J* 1976;38:327–340.

6. Stanger P, Rudolph AM, Edwards JE. Cardiac malpositions. An overview based on study of sixty-five necropsy specimens. *Circulation* 1977;56:159–172.

7. Van Praagh R. Terminology of congenital heart disease. Glossary and commentary [Editorial]. *Circulation* 1977;56:139–143.

8. Tynan MG, Becker AE, Macartney FJ, Jimenez MQ, Shinebourne EA, Anderson RH. Nomenclature and classification of congenital heart disease. *Br Heart J* 1979;41:544–553.

9. Goor DA, Lillehie CW. *Congenital malformations of the heart*. New York: Grune & Stratton, 1975.

10. Silverman NH. *Pediatric echocardiography*. Baltimore: Williams & Wilkins, 1993.

11. Van Praagh R, Van Praagh S, Vlad P, Keith JD. Anatomic types of congenital dextrocardia: diagnostic and embryologic implications. *Am J Cardiol* 1964;13:510–531.

12. Calcaterra G, Anderson RH, Lau KC, Shinebourne EA. Dextrocardia—value of segmental analysis in its categorisation. *Br Heart J* 1979;42:497–507.

13. Anderson RH, Becker AE, Freedom RM, et al. Sequential segmental analysis of congenital heart disease. *Pediatr Cardiol* 1984;5:281–287.

14. Van Mierop LH, Gessner IH, Schiebler GL. Asplenia and polysplenia syndromes. In: Bergsma D, ed. *Birth defects: original article series*. Baltimore: Williams & Wilkins, 1972.

15. Henry WL, DeMaria A, Gramiak R, et al. Report of the American Society of Echocardiography Committee on Nomenclature and Standards in Two-dimensional Echocardiography. *Circulation* 1980;62:212–217.

16. Van Mill GJ, Moulaert AJ, Harinck E. *Atlas of two-dimensional echocardiography in congenital cardiac defects*. Boston: Martinus-Nijhoff Publishers, 1985.

17. Tanaka M, Neyazaki T, Kosaka S, et al. Ultrasonic evaluation of anatomical abnormalities of heart in congenital and acquired heart diseases. *Br Heart J* 1971;33:686–698.

18. Tajik AJ, Seward JB, Hagler DJ, et al. Two-dimensional real-time ultrasonic imaging of the heart and great vessels: technique, image orientation, structure identification and validation. *Mayo Clin Proc* 1978;53:271–303.

19. Seward JB, Tajik AJ. Two-dimensional echocardiography. *Med Clin North Am* 1980;64:177–203.

20. Sahn DJ. Real-time two-dimensional echocardiography. *J Pediatr* 1981;99:175–185.

21. Snider AR, Ports TA, Silverman NH. Venous anomalies of the coronary sinus: detection by M-mode, two-dimensional and contrast echocardiography. *Circulation* 1979;60:721–727.

22. Cha EM, Khoury GH. Persistent left superior vena cava. *Radiology* 1972;103:375–381.

23. Winter FS. Persistent left superior vena cava. Survey of world literature and report of thirty additional cases. *Angiology* 1954;5:90–132.

24. Mintz GS, Kotler MN, Segal BL, Parry WR. Two-dimensional echocardiographic recognition of the descending thoracic aorta. *Am J Cardiol* 1979;44:232–238.

25. Henry WL, Maron BJ, Griffith JM. Cross-sectional echocardiography in the diagnosis of congenital heart disease. *Circulation* 1977;56:267–273.

26. Silverman NH, Schiller NB. Apex echocardiography. A two-dimensional technique for evaluation of congenital heart disease. *Circulation* 1978;57:503–511.

27. Bierman FZ, Williams RG. Subxyphoid two-dimensional imaging of the interatrial septum in infants and neonates with congenital heart disease. *Circulation* 1979;60:80–90.

28. Lange LW, Sahn DJ, Allen HD, Goldberg SJ. Subxyphoid cross-sectional echocardiography in infants and children with congenital heart disease. *Circulation* 1979;59:513–524.

29. Marino B, Ballerini L, Marcelletti C, et al. Right oblique subxiphoid view for two-dimensional echocardiographic visualization of the right ventricle in congenital heart disease. *Am J Cardiol* 1984;54:1064–1068.

30. Isaaz K, Cloez JL, Danchin N, Marcon F, Worms AM, Pernot C. Assessment of right ventricular outflow tract in children by two-dimensional echocardiography using a new subcostal view. Angiocardiographic and morphologic correlative study. *Am J Cardiol* 1985;56:539–545.

31. Allen HD, Goldberg SJ, Sahn DJ, Ovitt TW, Goldberg SJ. Suprasternal notch echocardiography. Assessment of its clinical utility in pediatric cardiology. *Circulation* 1977;55:605–612.

32. Sahn DJ, Allen HD, McDonald G, Goldberg SJ. Real-time cross-sectional echocardiographic diagnosis of coarctation of the aorta: a prospective study of echocardiographic-angiographic correlations. *Circulation* 1977;56:762–769.

33. Snider AR, Silverman NH. Suprasternal notch echocardiography: a two-dimensional technique for evaluating congenital heart disease. *Circulation* 1981;63:165–173.

34. Huhta JC, Gutgesell HP, Latson LA, Huffines FD. Two-dimensional echocardiographic assessment of the aorta in infants and children with congenital heart disease. *Circulation* 1984;70:417–424.

35. Shrivastava S, Berry JM, Einzig S, Bass JL. Parasternal cross-sectional echocardiographic determination of aortic arch situs: a new approach. *Am J Cardiol* 1985;55:1236–1238.

36. Arjunan K, Daniels SR, Meyer RA, Schwartz DC, Barron H, Kaplan S. Coronary artery caliber in normal children and patients with Kawasaki disease but without aneurysms: an echocardiographic and angiographic study. *J Am Coll Cardiol* 1986;8:1119–1124.

37. Oberhoffer R, Lan D, Feilen K. The diameter of coronary arteries in infants and children without heart disease. *Eur J Pediatr* 1989;148:389–392.

38. Silverman NH, Schmidt KG. Echocardiographic demonstration of the coronary arteries in children. In: Anderson RH, Neches WH, Park SC, Zuberbuhler JR, eds. *Perspectives in paediatric cardiology*, Vol 1. Mount Kisco, NY: Futura Publishing, 1988:379–404.

39. Satomi G, Natamura K, Narai S, Takao A. Systematic visualization of coronary arteries by two-dimensional echocardiography in children and infants: evaluation in Kawasaki's disease and coronary arteriovenous fistulas. *Am Heart J* 1984;107:497–505.

40. Weyman AE, Feigenbaum H, Dillon JC, Johnston KW, Eggleton RC. Noninvasive visualization of the left main coronary artery by cross-sectional echocardiography. *Circulation* 1976;54:169–174.

41. Fisher EA, Sepehri B, Lendrum B, Luken J, Levitsky S. Two-dimensional echocardiographic visualization of the left coronary artery in anomalous origin of the left coronary artery from the pulmonary artery: Pre- and postoperative studies. *Circulation* 1981;63:698–704.

42. Feigenbaum H. *Echocardiography*. Philadelphia: Lea & Febiger, 1972.

43. Lundstron NR, Edler I. Ultrasound cardiography in infants and children. *Acta Paediatr Scand* 1971;60:117–128.

44. Gramiak R, Shah PM. Cardiac ultrasonography: a review of current applications. *Radiol Clin North Am* 1971;9:469–490.

45. Solinger R, Elbl F, Minhas K. Echocardiography in the normal neonate. *Circulation* 1973;47:108–118.

46. Meyer RA, Kaplan S. Noninvasive techniques in pediatric cardiovascular disease. *Prog Cardiovasc Dis* 1973;15:341–367.

47. Solinger R, Elbl F, Minhas K. Deductive echocardiographic analy-

sis in infants with congenital heart disease. *Circulation* 1974;50: 1072–1096.

48. Sahn DJ, Allen HD, Goldberg SJ, Solinger R, Meyer RA. Pediatric echocardiography: a review of its clinical utility. *J Pediatr* 1975; 87:335–352.

49. Meyer RA. Echocardiography in congenital heart disease. *Semin Roentgenol* 1975;10:277–290.

50. Popp RL. Echocardiographic assessment of cardiac disease. *Circulation* 1976;54:538–552.

51. Stevenson JG, Kawabori I, French JW. Critical importance of sedation when measuring pressure gradients by Doppler. *Circulation* 1984;70[Suppl 2]:II-363(abst).

52. Hatle L, Angelsen B. *Doppler ultrasound in cardiology. Physical principles and clinical applications*, 2nd ed. Philadelphia: Lea & Febiger, 1985:74–96.

53. Grenadier E, Oliveira Lima C, Allen HD, et al. Normal intracardiac and great vessel Doppler flow velocities in infants and children. *J Am Coll Cardiol* 1984;4:343–350.

54. Cohen GI, Pietrolungo JF, Thomas JD, Klein AL. A practical guide to assessment of ventricular diastolic function using Doppler echocardiography. *J Am Coll Cardiol* 1996;27:1753–1760.

55. Riggs TW, Snider AR. Respiratory influence on RV and LV diastolic filling in normal children. *J Am Coll Cardiol* 1989;13:205A.

56. Riggs TW, Rodriguez R, Snider AR, Batton D, Polluck JC, Sharp EJ. Doppler echocardiographic evaluation of right and left ventricular diastolic function in normal neonates. *J Am Coll Cardiol* 1989; 13:700–705.

57. Appleton CP, Hatle LK, Popp RL. Cardiac tamponade and pericardial effusion: respiratory variation in transvalvular flow velocities studied by Doppler echocardiography [Review]. *J Am Coll Cardiol* 1988;11:1020–1030.

58. Dabestani A, Takenaka K, Allen B, et al. Effects of spontaneous respiration on diastolic left ventricular filling assessed by pulsed Doppler echocardiography. *Am J Cardiol* 1988;61:1356–1359.

59. Harada K, Takahashi Y, Shiota T, et al. Effect of heart rate on left ventricular diastolic filling patterns assessed by Doppler echocardiography in normal infants. *Am J Cardiol* 1995;76:634–636.

60. Iliceto S, D Ambrosio G, Marangelli V, Amico A, Di Biase M, Rizzon P. Echo-Doppler evaluation of effects of heart rate increments on left atrial pump function in normal human subjects. *Eur Heart J* 1991;12:345–351.

61. Areias JC, Meyer R, Scott WA, Goldberg SJ. Serial echocardiographic and Doppler evaluation of left ventricular diastolic filling in full-term neonates. *Am J Cardiol* 1990;66:108–111.

62. Harada K, Suzuki T, Tamura M, et al. Role of age on transmitral flow velocity patterns in assessing left ventricular diastolic function in normal infants and children. *Am J Cardiol* 1995;76:530–532.

63. Maciel BC, Simpson IA, Valdes-Cruz LM, et al. Color flow mapping studies of physiologic pulmonary and tricuspid regurgitation: evidence for true regurgitation as opposed to a valve closing volume. *J Am Soc Echocardiogr* 1991;4:589–597.

64. Kostucki W, Vanderbossche JL, Friart A, Englert M. Pulsed Doppler regurgitant flow patterns of normal valves. *Am J Cardiol* 1986; 58:309–313.

65. Yoshida K, Yoshikawa J, Shakudo M, et al. Color Doppler evaluation of valvular regurgitation in normal subjects. *Circulation* 1988; 78:840–847.

66. Sahn DJ, Maciel BC. Physiological valvular regurgitation. Doppler echocardiography and the potential for iatrogenic heart disease. *Circulation* 1988;78:1075–1077.

67. Minich LL, Lloyd LY, Hawkins JA, McGough EC, Shaddy RE. Abnormal Doppler pulmonary venous flow patterns in children after repaired totol anomalous pulmonary venous connection. *Am J Cardiol* 1995;75:606–610.

68. Meyer RJ, Goldberg SJ, Donnerstein RL. Superior vena cava and hepatic vein velocity patterns in normal children. *Am J Cardiol* 1993;72:238–240.

69. Appleton CP, Hatle LK, Popp RL. Superior vena cava and hepatic vein Doppler echocardiography in healthy adults. *J Am Coll Cardiol* 1987;10:1032–1039.

70. Pennestri F, Loperfido F, Salvatori MP, et al. Assessment of tricuspid regurgitation by pulsed Doppler ultrasonography of the hepatic veins. *Am J Cardiol* 1984;54:363–368.

71. Sakai K, Nakamura K, Satomi G, Kondo M, Hirosawa K. Evaluation of tricuspid regurgitation by blood flow pattern in the hepatic vein using pulsed Doppler technique. *Am Heart J* 1984;108:516–523.

72. Weintraub R, Shiota T, Elkadi T, et al. Transesophageal echocardiography in infants and children with congenital heart disease [Review]. *Circulation* 1992;86:711–722.

73. Ritter SB. Transesophageal real-time echocardiography in infants and children with congenital heart disease. *J Am Coll Cardiol* 1991;18:569–580.

74. Wolfe LT, Rossi A, Ritter SB. Transesophageal echocardiography in infants and children: use and importance in the intensive care unit. *J Am Soc Echocardiogr* 1993;6:286–289.

75. Cyran SE, Kimball TR, Meyer RA, et al. Efficacy of intraoperative transesophageal echocardiography in children with congenital heart disease. *Am J Cardiol* 1989;63:594–598.

76. Kyo S, Koike K, Takanawa E, et al. Impact of transesophageal Doppler echocardiography on pediatric cardiac surgery. *Int J Card Imaging* 1989;4:41–42.

77. Sutherland GR, van Dael MERM, Stumper OFW, Hess J, Quaegebeur J. Epicardial and transesophageal echocardiography during surgery for congenital heart disease. *Int J Card Imaging* 1989;4: 37–40.

78. Dan M, Bonato R, Mazzucco A, et al. Value of transesophageal echocardiography during repair of congenital heart defects. *Ann Thorac Surg* 1990;50:637–643.

79. Lam J, Neirotti RA, Lubbers WJ, et al. Usefulness of biplane transesophageal echocardiography in neonates, infants and children with congenital heart disease. *Am J Cardiol* 1993;72:699–706.

80. O'Leary PW, Hagler DJ, Seward JB, et al. Biplane intraoperative transesophageal echocardiography in congenital heart disease. *Mayo Clin Proc* 1995;70:317–326.

81. Marcus B, Seward DJ, Khan NR, et al. Outpatient transesophageal echocardiography with intravenous propofol anesthesia in children and adolescents. *J Am Soc Echocardiogr* 1993;6:205–209.

82. Marcus B, Wong PC, Wells WJ, Lindesmith GG, Starnes VA. Transesophageal echocardiography in the postoperative child with an open sternum. *Ann Thorac Surg* 1994;58:235–236.

83. Stumper O, Witsenburg M, Sutherland GR, Cromme-Dijkhuis A, Godman MJ, Hess J. Transesophageal echocardiographic monitoring of interventional cardiac catheterization in children. *J Am Coll Cardiol* 1991;18:1506–1514.

84. Tumbarello R, Sanna A, Cardu G, Bande A, Napoleone A, Bini R. Usefulness of transesophageal echocardiography in the pediatric catheterization laboratory. *Am J Cardiol* 1993;71:1321–1325.

85. Lai WW, Al-Khatib Y, Klitzner TS, et al. Biplanar transesophageal echocardiographic direction of radiofrequency ablation in children and adolescents with the Wolff-Parkinson-White syndrome. *Am J Cardiol* 1993;71:872–874.

86. Drant SE, Klitzner TS, Shannon KM, Wetzel GT, Williams RG. Guidance of radiofrequency catheter ablation by transesophageal echocardiography in children with palliated single ventricle. *Am J Cardiol* 1995;76:1311–1312.

87. Stumper OF, Elzenga NJ, Hess J, Sutherland GR. Transesophageal echocardiography in children with congenital heart disease: an initial experience. *J Am Coll Cardiol* 1990;16:433–441.

88. Cyran SE, Myers JL, Gleason MM, Weber HS, Baylen BG, Waldhausen JA. Application of intraoperative transesophageal echocardiography in infants and small children. *J Cardiovasc Surg* 1991; 32:318–321.

89. Lam J, Neirotti RA, Nijveld A, Schuller JL, Blom-Muilwijk CM, Visser CA. Transesophageal echocardiography in pediatric patients: preliminary results. *J Am Soc Echocardiogr* 1991;4:43–50.

90. Roberson DA, Muhiudeen IA, Silverman NH, Turley K, Hass GS, Cahalan MK. Intraoperative transesophageal echocardiography of atrioventricular septal defect. *J Am Coll Cardiol* 1991;18:537–545.

91. Ritter SB. Transesophageal real-time echocardiography in infants and children with congenital heart disease. *J Am Coll Cardiol* 1991;18:569–580.

92. Stumper O, Kaulitz R, Elzenga NJ, et al. The value of transesophageal echocardiography in children with congenital heart disease. *J Am Soc Echocardiogr* 1991;4:164–176.

93. Wienecke M, Fyfe DA, Kline CH, et al. Comparison of intraoperative transesophageal echocardiography to epicardial imaging in children undergoing ventricular septal defect repair. *J Am Soc Echocardiogr* 1991;4:607–614.

94. Gilbert TB, Panico FG, McGill WA, Martin GR, Halley DG, Sell JE. Bronchial obstruction by transesophageal echocardiography probe in a pediatric cardiac patient. *Anesth Analg* 1992;74:156–168.

95. Lunn RJ, Oliver WC Jr, Hagler DJ, Danielson GK. Aortic compression by transesophageal echocardiographic probe in infants and children undergoing cardiac surgery. *Anesthesiology* 1992;77:587–590.

96. Klhandheria BK, Oh J. Transesophageal echocardiography: state-of-the art and future directions [Review]. *Am J Cardiol* 1992;69:61H–81H.

97. Daniel WG, Erbel R, Kasper W, et al. Safety of transesophageal echocardiography: a multicenter survey of 10,419 examinations. *Circulation* 1991;83:817–821.

98. Kronzo I, Cziner DG, Katz ES, et al. Buckling of the tip of the transesophageal echocardiography probe. A potentially dangerous technical malfunction. *J Am Soc Echocardiogr* 1992;5:176–177.

99. Seward JB, Khanderia BK, Oh JK, Freeman WK, Tajik AJ. Critical appraisal of transesophageal echocardiography: limitations, pitfalls, and complications [Review]. *J Am Soc Echocardiogr* 1992;5:288–305.

100. Chan KL, Cohen GI, Sochowski RA, Baird MG. Complications of transesophageal echocardiography in ambulatory adult patients: analysis of 1500 consecutive examinations. *J Am Soc Echocardiogr* 1991;4:577–582.

CHAPTER 5

Quantitative Echocardiography

Elizabeth M. Shaffer

Cardiac dimensions, systolic and diastolic ventricular function, cardiac output, pressures, and shunt flows can be measured using the various modalities of echocardiography. This chapter focuses on M-mode and two-dimensional echocardiographic quantitative techniques. Doppler methods are covered in detail in Chapter 6.

SYSTOLIC FUNCTION

Left ventricular systolic function is the result of a complex interrelationship of the myocardial contractile state, preload, afterload, and heart rate (1). Myocardial contractility is dependent on myocardial fiber shortening (2). Preload is the ventricular end-diastolic volume and relates to systolic performance through the Frank-Starling mechanism (3). Afterload is the resistance to myocardial fiber shortening during systole (4). Heart rate affects the systolic function of the heart through changes in diastolic filling time, as with increasing heart rates, the diastolic filling time decreases.

Ejection-phase Indices

Ejection-phase indices, despite being preload- and afterload-sensitive, are commonly used to assess left ventricular function (5).

M-mode Techniques

Measurements derived from left ventricular M-mode traces were the first used to assess ventricular function echocardiographically and remain useful today for evaluation of global function. The shortening fraction, fractional thickening of the left ventricular posterior wall and interventricular septum, mitral valve E-point septal separation, and mean velocity of circumferential fiber shortening are measurements of left ventricular ejection. Although ventricular volumes and ejection fraction can be calculated from the M mode, more accurate determinations of ventricular volumes can be made from two-dimensional imaging. Stroke volume and cardiac output can be derived from the ventricular volumes.

Left ventricular M-mode traces are obtained from the parasternal long- or short-axis views (Echo. 5-1). It is important to align the M-mode cursor so that it is perpendicular to the interventricular septum and the posterior wall of the left ventricle. For most measurements of left ventricular systolic function, the M mode should be recorded at the level of the posterior mitral valve leaflet. Standardizing the site of the M-mode recording is critical because the force of ventricular contraction is not uniform from cardiac base to apex. According to the recommendations of the American Society of Echocardiography, end-diastole should be measured at the beginning of the QRS complex (6). However, in children, this may lead to errors, and measuring at the largest and smallest ventricular dimension may be more appropriate than measuring at specific times on the electrocardiogram (7). Measuring from leading edge to leading edge of the M-mode trace is the preferred technique (6) (Echo. 5-1).

The *shortening fraction* (SF) is one of the measurements of left ventricular function most commonly used clinically. It is measured from M-mode traces derived from the short axis of the left ventricle. The equation for fractional shortening is

$$\text{SF}(\%) = \frac{\text{LVDD} - \text{LVSD}}{\text{LVDD}} \times 100 \qquad [1]$$

where LVDD is left ventricular diastolic dimension (cm) and LVSD is left ventricular systolic dimension (cm).

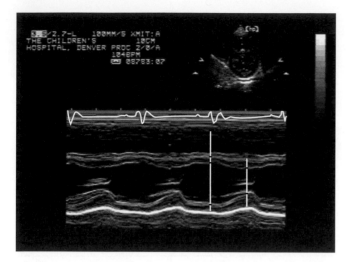

ECHO. 5-1. M-mode tracing of the right and left ventricle derived from a parasternal short-axis view.

The normal range for shortening fraction is 28% to 44% (8). The measurement is dependent on normal interventricular septal motion. If the interventricular septal motion is flat or paradoxical, the shortening fraction will not accurately reflect ventricular ejection. This measurement is independent of age and heart rate but is dependent on preload and afterload. The shortening fraction is increased in volume-overloaded ventricles (9) and with increased afterload, as in cases of aortic stenosis (10).

The *percentage of thickening of the interventricular septum and left ventricular posterior wall* is another measurement of systolic ejection (11–14). This measurement is also routinely made from the left ventricular M-mode recording by the following calculation:

$$\text{Thickening (\%)} = \frac{\text{STh} - \text{DTh}}{\text{STh}} \times 100 \qquad [2]$$

where STh is systolic thickness (cm) and DTh is diastolic thickness (cm).

The range of normal values for this measurement is wide, from 30% to 100%, making it difficult to interpret as an independent indicator of left ventricular systolic function (15–16).

E-point septal separation (*EPSS*) is another commonly used ejection-phase index (17–20). It is based on the observation that as the left ventricle dilates, the interventricular septum moves anteriorly, whereas mitral valve opening is dependent on the amount of flow through the valve. Thus, in the presence of a dilated left ventricle and low cardiac output, the EPSS will be increased. To measure the EPSS, a left ventricular M-mode recording is obtained at the level of the mitral valve, and the distance between the E point of the ante-

rior leaflet of the mitral valve and the most posterior portion of the interventricular septum is measured (Echo. 5-2). EPSS can be normalized to ventricular size by dividing it by the left ventricular end-diastolic dimension (LVEDD). In children with normal ventricular function, EPSS/LVEDD is 0.08 ± 0.06, compared with 0.39 ± 0.09 for children with congestive cardiomyopathy (21). If the ventricle is dilated but ventricular function is normal, there will be no significant EPSS. This measurement does not rely on normal septal motion, which is an advantage over measurement of the shortening fraction (20,22), but the mitral valve must be normal for it to be a reliable indicator of left ventricular function. EPSS will not accurately reflect the left ventricular function if significant aortic insufficiency is present because the aortic insufficiency jet may hit the anterior leaflet of the mitral valve, thus distorting its motion. Further, the regurgitant volume, which is included in left ventricular ejection, does not flow through the mitral valve.

The *rate of left ventricular fiber shortening* is another index of systolic function (23–25). The mean velocity of circumferential fiber shortening (mean V_{cf}), normalized for end-diastolic dimension, is calculated from the following formula:

$$\text{Mean } V_{cf} \text{ (cir/s)} = \frac{\text{LVDD} - \text{LVSD}}{\text{LVDD} \times \text{LVET}} \qquad [3]$$

where LVET is left ventricular ejection time.

Left ventricular systolic and diastolic dimensions are measured from M-mode traces of the left ventricle, and the ejection time is calculated from M-mode traces of the

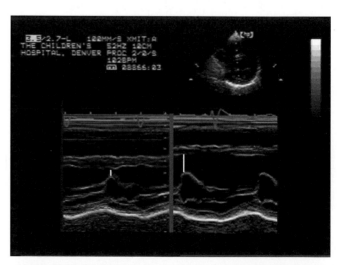

ECHO. 5-2. M-mode traces for measurement of the E-point septal separation (EPSS). **Left:** Normal EPSS. **Right:** An increased EPSS resulting from ventricular dilation.

aortic valve (Echo. 5-3). Ideally, the two M-mode traces should be obtained simultaneously, but as this is not possible with most ultrasound machines, at least the M-mode traces should be recorded at equal heart rates. This measurement of systolic function is heart rate- and afterload-dependent (26,27). It can be heart rate-corrected by dividing the left ventricular ejection time by the square root of the RR interval (28). The normal value for the heart rate-corrected mean V_{cf} is 0.98 ± 0.07 circ/s (25).

Two-dimensional Techniques

Several two-dimensional echocardiographic methods can be used to assess left ventricular function. These include measurement of the descent of the mitral annulus in systole, left ventricular volume at end-systole and end-diastole, left ventricular ejection fraction, stroke volume, and cardiac output.

Measurement of the descent of the mitral annulus in systole is a simple technique to assess global left ventricular function that uses two-dimensional imaging. With ventricular contraction, the base of the heart moves toward the apex. This technique has been used in adults and involves measuring the position of the mitral annulus in diastole and systole (29–32) (Echo. 5-4). The degree of annular descent has correlated well with radionuclide estimates of ejection fraction (30).

Left ventricular volumes at end-systole and end-diastole obtained by two-dimensional imaging are more accurate than measurements obtained by M-mode techniques (33,34). These have correlated well with left ven-

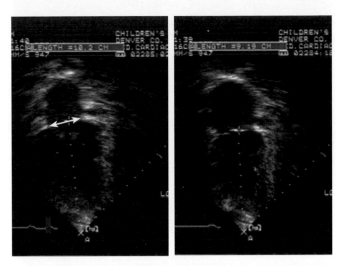

ECHO. 5-4. Measurement of mitral valve annular motion in diastole **(left)** and systole **(right)**. Determination of the degree of descent of the mitral valve annulus in systole is a technique to assess global left ventricular function. Arrow indicates mitral valve annulus.

tricular volumes and ejection fractions calculated from cineangiography (33–36), although ventricular volumes calculated from echocardiography are usually smaller than those derived from angiography (34). It is not clear whether this is a consequence of underestimation by echocardiography or overestimation by angiography. Echocardiography could easily underestimate the ventricular volume because of foreshortening of the left ventricle with two-dimensional imaging. With angiography, the ventricular volume may be overestimated when the volume of the papillary muscles or trabeculations is not taken into account.

Many geometric models and formulas have been used to calculate ventricular volumes (34–37). The most accurate estimates of ventricular volume are calculated from orthogonal apical views of the left ventricle by employing Simpson's rule. In this method, the ventricle is divided into equal slices; the volume of each slice is calculated and then summed to provide an estimate of the total ventricular volume. In children, the apical four-chamber and apical long-axis views are used (Echo. 5-5). This method requires that the endocardium be traced at end-diastole and end-systole; however, the endocardium may be difficult to define. A study by Bengur et al. (38) describes a promising technique in which color flow imaging is utilized to define the boundary between the ventricular cavity and endocardium. The color sector is placed over the left ventricle and the lowest possible Nyquist limit is used. The ventricular cavity is filled with mosaic color, but the motion of the walls gives rise to a nonaliased signal, allowing for easy measurement of left ventricular volume (38).

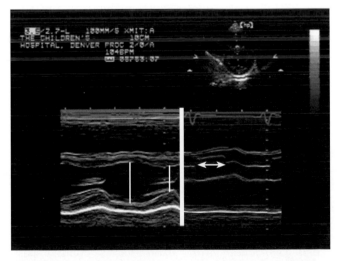

ECHO. 5-3. Measurement of the rate of left ventricular fiber shortening. **Left:** M-mode trace of the left ventricle derived from the parasternal short-axis view for measurement of the end-systolic and end-diastolic dimensions. **Right:** M-mode trace of the aortic valve for measurement of the left ventricular ejection time.

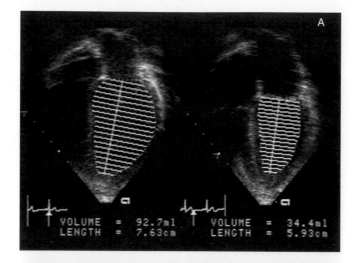

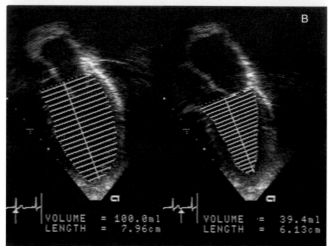

ECHO. 5-5. Measurement of left ventricular volumes with Simpson's rule. **A:** Apical four-chamber views of the left ventricle in diastole **(left)** and systole **(right)** traced to measure ventricular volumes. **B:** Apical long-axis views of the left ventricle in diastole **(left)** and systole **(right)** traced to measure ventricular volumes.

The *left ventricular ejection fraction* (EF) is derived from the end-systolic (LVESV) and end-diastolic (LVEDV) ventricular volumes by means of the following equation:

$$EF(\%) = \frac{LVEDV - LVESV}{LVEDV} \times 100 \qquad [4]$$

The normal range for ejection fraction at rest is 56% to 78%.

Ejection fractions measured by the technique proposed by Bengur et al. (38) correlate well with ejection fractions calculated from standard two-dimensional techniques and angiography.

Stroke volume (SV) is calculated as the difference between the end-diastolic and end-systolic volumes:

$$SV \ (cc) = LVEDV - LVESV \qquad [5]$$

Cardiac output is derived from the product of the stroke volume and the heart rate:

Cardiac Output (cc/s)

$$= Stroke \ Volume \times Heart \ Rate \qquad [6]$$

Afterload

Afterload is the wall stress or force per unit area encountered by the ventricle during ejection. The law of Laplace (39) states that

$$\frac{Chamber \ Wall}{Stress} = \frac{Pressure \times Cavity \ Diameter}{Wall \ Thickness} \qquad [7]$$

Ventricular ejection is a dynamic process; therefore, the determinants of wall stress—that is, ventricular pressure, wall thickness, and diameter—are constantly changing (40).

Meridional wall stress is defined as the force per unit area acting at the equatorial plane of the ventricle in the direction of the apex-to-base axis. Meridional wall stress is independent of the long-axis dimension of the left ventricle and can be calculated as follows (41):

$$\frac{Meridional \ Wall}{Stress \ (g/cm^2)} = \frac{0.334 \ P \times LVID}{LVPW \ (1 + LVPW/LVID)} \qquad [8]$$

where P is left ventricular pressure (mmHg), $LVID$ is dimension of the left ventricular minor axis (cm), and $LVPW$ is left ventricular posterior wall thickness (cm).

Circumferential wall stress is the force per unit area acting along the circumference of the left ventricle at its minor axis and is calculated by the following equation (41):

$$\frac{Circumferential \ Wall}{Stress \ (g/cm^2)} = \frac{1.35 \ Pr \ [1 - (2r^2/L^2)]}{LVPW} \qquad [9]$$

where P is left ventricular pressure (mmHg), r is the dimension of the left ventricular minor axis divided by 2 (cm), $LVPW$ is left ventricular posterior wall thickness, and L is the long axis of the left ventricle (cm).

Left ventricular wall stress varies continuously throughout systole (42). Wall stress can be calculated at different times during systole, and there is still controversy regarding which measurement of wall stress is the best index of left ventricular afterload (43–45). Peak systolic wall stress is the largest of all the values, mean systolic wall stress is the average of all wall stress values, and end-systolic wall stress is calculated at end-systole (46). Various techniques have been used to estimate left ventricular pressure. End-systolic wall stress can be determined from M-mode measurements taken when the ventricle is smallest; the systolic blood pressure determined from an arm cuff is used as the left ventricular pressure (42). In other approaches, a carotid pulse tracing is calibrated to the cuff arterial blood pressure and an estimate of the pressure at the dicrotic notch is made (47) to calculate end-systolic wall stress. In infants, an indirect axillary pulse tracing calibrated to an automated blood pressure monitoring device may be used (48).

Left ventricular mass is important in the evaluation of afterload and can be calculated using several formulas.

The Penn convention (49,50) assumes that the ventricle is a prolate ellipsoid with minor radii that are one-half the major radii. In this method, the endocardial echoes are included in the measurement of the left ventricular diastolic dimension. The formula is as follows:

Left Ventricular Mass (g)

$$= 1.04 \, [(LVID + PWT + IVST)^3 - LVID^3] - 13.6 \quad [10]$$

where *LVID* is left ventricular internal dimension, *PWT* is left ventricular posterior wall thickness, and *IVS* is thickness of the interventricular septum in diastole.

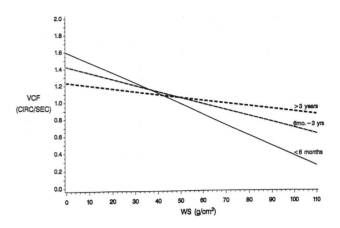

FIG. 5-2. The mean regression lines for the heart rate-corrected velocity of circumferential fiber shortening (V_{cf}) along the ordinate and left ventricular end-systolic meridional wall stress (WS) along the abscissa in infants less than 6 months of age (*solid line*), 6 months to 3 years of age (*dashed line*), and children over 3 years of age (*bold, dashed line*). With increasing age, the regression line has a shallower slope and a lower intercept. (From Kimball TR, Daniels SR, Khoury P. Age-related variation in contractility estimate in patients less than 20 years of age. *Am J Cardiol* 1991;68:1383–1387. Reprinted with permission.)

An alternative to the Penn convention is the American Society of Echocardiography convention (51). This method uses the leading edge-to-leading edge measuring technique. The formula is as follows:

$$(\text{Left Ventricular Mass})^3 = 1.04 \, [(LVID + PWT + IVST)^3 - LVID^3] \quad [11]$$

where *LVID* is left ventricular internal dimension, *PWT* is left ventricular posterior wall thickness, and *IVST* is thickness of the interventricular septum in diastole.

Left Ventricular Mass (g)

$$= 0.80 \, (\text{Left Ventricular Mass})^3 + 0.6 \quad [12]$$

Left ventricular mass should be indexed in children. In a study by Daniels et al. (52) using the Penn convention to calculate left ventricular mass in children, the left ventricular mass in grams per square meter of body surface area was 70.4 g/m² for male subjects and 60.7 g/m² for female subjects. In a more recent study from their group (53), indexing by the cube of the height appeared to be a better method for comparison with lean body mass. In this study, there was no difference between sexes when left ventricular mass was indexed to the cube of the height. The mean value for left ventricular mass in grams per cube of the height in meters was 25.8 g/m³.

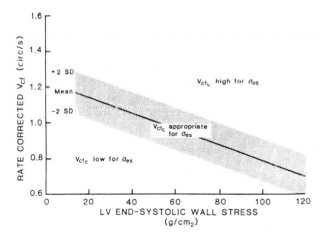

FIG. 5-1. Curve demonstrating the relationship between end-systolic wall stress and the rate-corrected velocity of fiber shortening (V_{cf}). A depressed contractile state (a low V_{cf} for the level of wall stress) may be distinguished from situations in which contractility is normal but afterload is increased. The *shaded area* represents 95% confidence intervals. (From Colan SD, Borow KM, Neumann A. Left ventricular end-systolic wall stress-velocity of fiber shortening relation: a load-independent index of myocardial contractility. *J Am Coll Cardiol* 1984;4:715–724. Reprinted with permission of the American College of Cardiology.)

Contractility

The ejection-phase indices that have been discussed are all load-dependent indices of ventricular function. Colan and colleagues (53) developed the *stress-velocity index*, which assesses contractility utilizing the relationship between end-systolic wall stress and the velocity of fiber shortening. This index is independent of preload and normalized for heart rate, and it incorporates afterload (53). The stress-velocity index assesses the relationship between left ventricular end-systolic meridional wall stress and the rate-corrected mean velocity of fiber shortening V_{cfc}. In their study of children ages 3 to 18 years, this relationship was constant over a wide variety of preload and afterload conditions; when contractility was augmented with dobutamine, an increase in the V_{cfc} was noted at all levels of end-systolic wall stress. An inverse linear relationship was demonstrated between the mean V_{cf} and left ventricular end-systolic wall stress (53) (Fig. 5-1). Another study, by Franklin et al., found similar results in children 2 to 13 years old (54). Studies by Kimball et al. (55) and Rowland and Gutgesell (56) in children under 3 years of age showed that the regression line had a steeper slope and a higher intercept than in older children; a family of curves was produced suggesting that age must be taken into account when contractility is assessed (Fig. 5-2). This technique has proved useful in a variety of disease states (7,57–63).

The measurement of the stress-velocity index requires simultaneous left ventricular M-mode recordings, phonocardiogram, indirect carotid or axillary pulse tracing, electrocardiogram, and determinations of systolic and diastolic blood pressure. Obtaining these measurements in infants and children can be technically difficult. Rowland and Gutgesel (64) observed in the catheterization laboratory that the mean arterial pressure approximated the end-systolic pressure in most patients, and they substituted the mean arterial pressure for the end-systolic pressure obtained by indirect carotid pulse tracing. They also simplified the method of Colan and colleagues by measuring the left ventricular ejection time from the aortic valve M-mode tracing instead of from the indirect carotid pulse tracing (64).

These modifications simplify the measurements involved in the stress-velocity index and may make this measurement of contractility easier for routine clinical use. Karr and Martin (65) used the simplified technique and were able to identify accurately patients with normal and abnormal contractility.

CARDIAC DIMENSIONS

Cardiac dimensions are important in evaluating patients with congenital heart disease. The size of chambers and vessels as well as the thickness of walls adds additional information to the anatomic and hemodynamic assessment. The cardiac chambers and great vessels grow in unison and at a predictable rate after birth, reaching 50% of their adult dimensions at birth, 75% by 5 years, and 90% by 12 years (66). Many studies have been performed using M-mode and two-dimensional imaging to obtain normal values for cardiac chambers (67–70). The dimensions can be indexed to the patient's height, weight, or body surface area.

M mode is well suited to the measurement of cardiac structures. Its inherently high temporal resolution allows for more accurate assessment of rapidly moving structures than does two-dimensional imaging. The M-mode measurements are performed using the leading edge-to-leading edge technique. Normal values indexed to body surface area were established by Roge et al. (69) (Fig. 5-3).

Two-dimensional imaging is commonly used in pediatric cardiology, and normal values for cardiac chambers, valves, and great vessels have been established. The measurements are performed from inner edge to inner edge. Imai et al. (71) have published normal values for 19 variables indexed to weight in preterm and term infants weighing between 0.5 and 4.0 kg (71) (Fig. 5-4). Normal values have also been established for children outside the newborn period. Measurements of the main and right pulmonary artery and aorta are available (72), as are left-sided dimensions indexed to body surface area (73,74) or height (66) (Fig. 5-5). Accurate normal values for the aortic root and ascending aorta are particularly useful in

(text continues on page 96)

FIG. 5-3. M-mode dimensions (mm) of cardiac structures and great vessels plotted against body surface area (m²). The 90% tolerance lines are shown by *heavy continuous lines*. *Curves* show the following dimensions: *RVAWD*, right ventricular anterior wall thickness in diastole; *RVDD*, right ventricular end-diastolic dimension; *SEPT D*, septal thickness at end-diastole; *LVESD*, left ventricular end-systolic dimension; *LVEDD*, left ventricular end-diastolic dimension; *LVPWD*, left ventricular posterior wall thickness at end-diastole; *AOS*, aortic diameter in systole; *AOD*, aortic diameter in diastole; *PAD*, pulmonary artery diameter; *LAS*, left atrial dimension in systole; *MVDE*, anterior mitral valve leaflet excursion; *TVDE*, anterior tricuspid valve leaflet excursion. (From Roge CL, Silverman NH, Hart PS, Ray RM. Cardiac structure growth pattern determined by echocardiography. *Circulation* 1978;57:285–290. Reprinted with permission of the American Heart Association.)

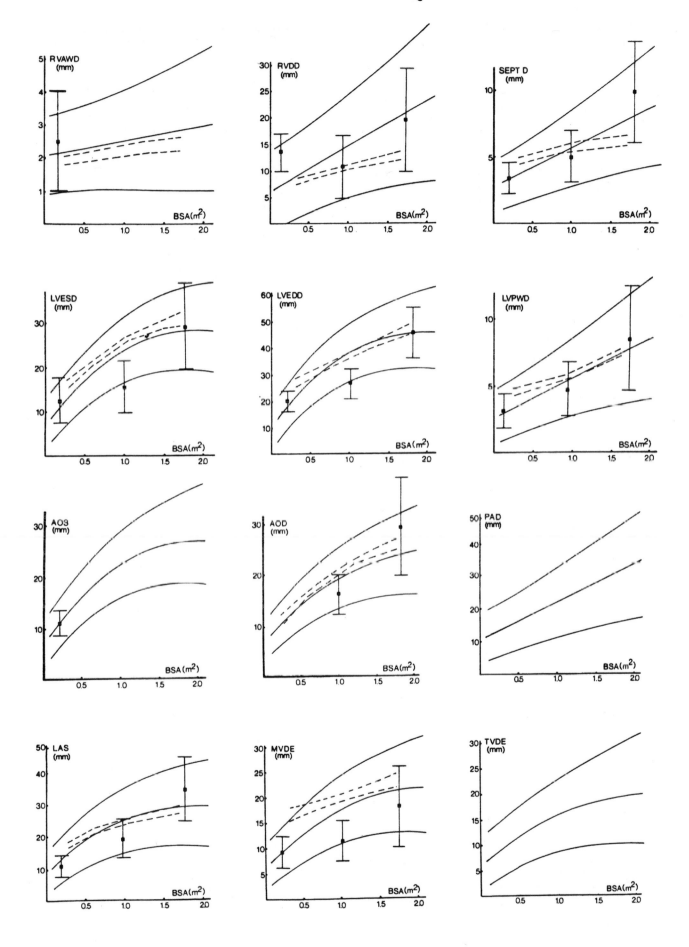

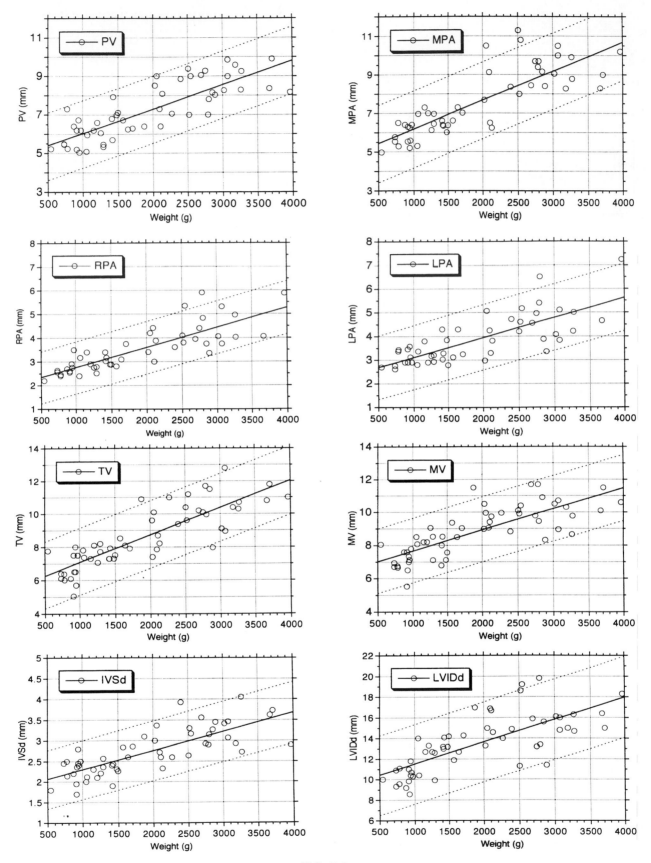

FIG. 5-4.

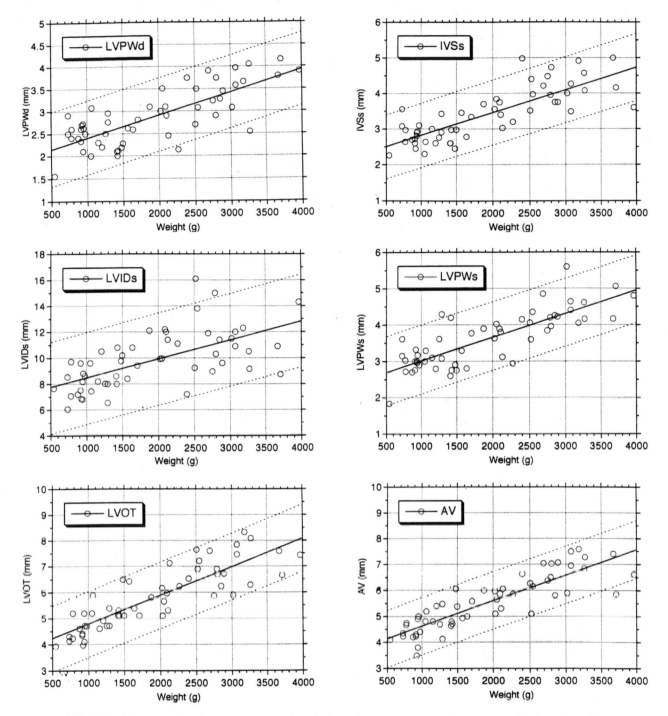

FIG. 5-4. Cross-sectional measurements (mm) of cardiac structures and great vessels plotted against body weight (g). The *solid line* represents the regression line. The 95% confidence intervals are shown as *dashed lines. Curves* show the dimensions. PV, end-systolic diameter of pulmonary valve measured from a parasternal long axis; *MPA*, end-systolic diameter of the main pulmonary artery measured from a parasternal short axis; RPA, right pulmonary artery measurement from a parasternal short axis; *LPA*, left pulmonary artery measurement from a parasternal short axis; *TV*, tricuspid valve annulus measurement from an apical four-chamber view; *MV*, mitral valve annulus measurement from an apical four-chamber view; *IVSd*, ventricular septal thickness at end-diastole measured from a parasternal short axis; *LVIDd*, left ventricular dimension in diastole measured from a parasternal short axis; LVPWd, left ventricular posterior wall in diastole measured from a parasternal short axis; *IVSs*, interventricular septum in systole measured from a parasternal short axis; *LVIDs*, left ventricular dimension in systole measured from a parasternal short axis; *LVPWs*, left ventricular posterior wall thickness in diastole measured from a parasternal short axis; *LVOT*, left ventricular outflow tract measured from a parasternal short axis; *AV*, systolic aortic valve measurement from a parasternal long axis.

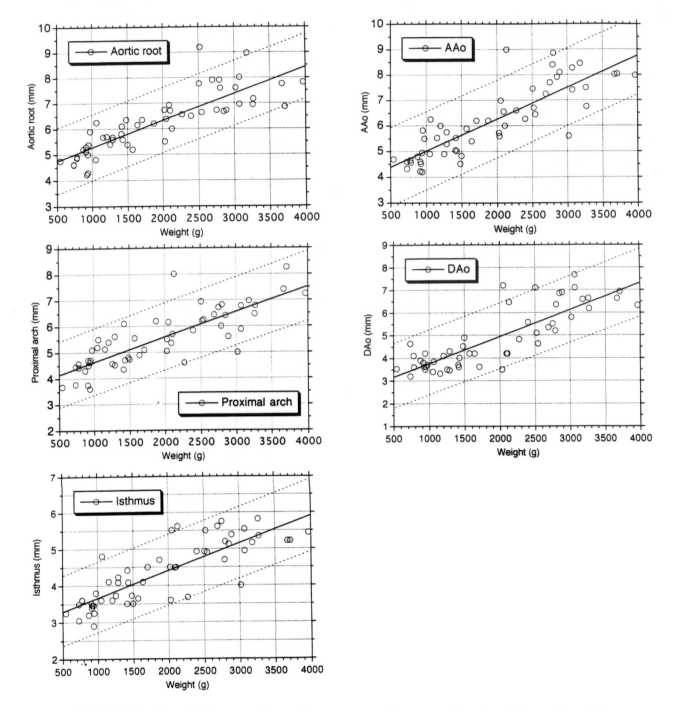

FIG. 5-4. (*Continued*) AAo, ascending aorta measurement from suprasternal or right parasternal view in systole; *DAo*, descending aorta measured at diaphragmatic level. (From Imai T, Satomi G, Yasukochi S, et al. Normal values for cardiac and great arterial dimensions in premature infants by cross-section echocardiography. *Cardiol Young* 1995;5:319–325. Reprinted with permission.)

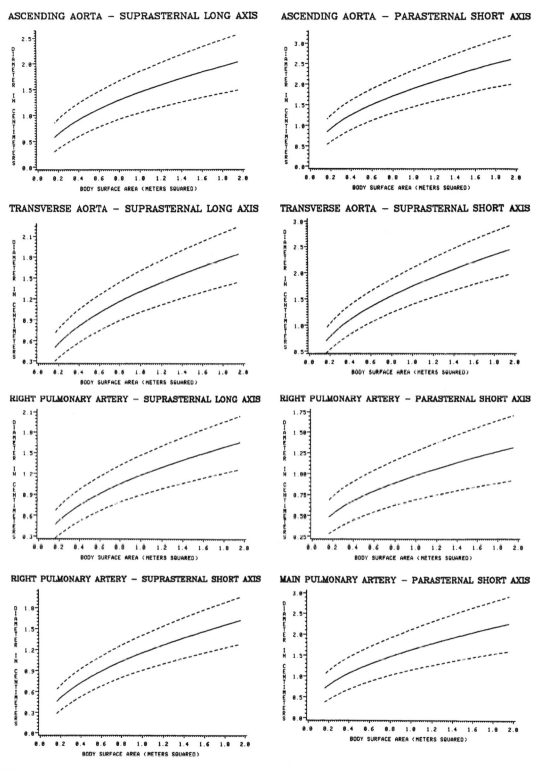

FIG. 5-5. Cross-sectional measurements (cm) of cardiac structures and great vessels in infants plotted against body surface area (m²). The measurements were made at end-diastole. The *dashed lines* are the tolerance limits weighted for body surface area, for prediction of normal values for 80% of the future population with 50% confidence. (From Snider AR, Enderlein M, Teitel S, Juster RP. Two-dimensional echocardiographic determination of aortic and pulmonary artery sizes from infancy to adulthood in normal subjects. *Am J Cardiol* 1984;53:218–224. Reprinted with permission.)

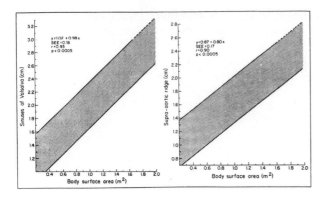

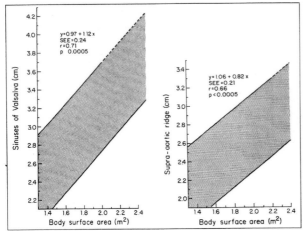

FIG. 5-6. Relation of body surface area to aortic root diameter at the sinuses of Valsalva and at the supraaortic ridge in normal infants and children (*top*) and in adults less than 40 years old (*bottom*). The *shaded areas* represent the 95% normal confidence limits. (From Roman MJ, Devereux RB, Kramer-Fox R, O'Loughlin J, Spitzer M, Robins J. Two-dimensional echocardiographic aortic root dimensions in normal children and adults. *Am J Cardiol* 1989;64:507–512. Reprinted with permission.)

the evaluation of children with connective tissue disorders, such as Marfan syndrome. M-mode measurements of the aortic valve opening may overestimate the true aortic size, leading to the false impression of aortic root dilatation. Roman et al. (75) have published normal values for the aorta measured at the annulus, sinuses of Valsalva, supraaortic ridge, and proximal ascending aorta (Fig. 5-6). A ratio of these aortic measurements, proposed by Sheil et al. (76), may obviate the need to index the measurements for growth.

REGIONAL WALL MOTION

Assessment of the regional wall motion of the left ventricle is important in the evaluation of patients with congenital heart disease, particularly when coronary arterial abnormalities are present and after surgical procedures, such as the arterial switch operation, that involve manipu-

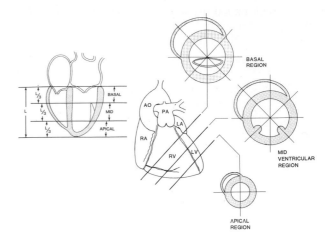

FIG. 5-7. Schematic representation of the ventricular segments used in evaluating regional wall motion according to the recommendations of the American Society of Echocardiography.

lation of the coronary arteries. Echocardiographic wall motion analysis is based on evaluation of the contractility of the various segments into which the left ventricle is divided, following a standardized system. According to the American Society of Echocardiography, the left ventricle is divided into three levels: basal, middle (papillary muscle), and apical. In addition, the basal and middle levels are further subdivided into six segments each and the apical level into four segments, making a total of 16 segments that are individually examined (Fig. 5-7). As illustrated in Fig. 5-7, these segments can be visualized from various two-dimensional transthoracic views that are easily obtained in most patients. These include the parasternal long-axis and short-axis views, with the transducer swept from the left ventricular apex to the level of the mitral valve, and the apical four- and two-chamber views. A score can be assigned to each segment based on the contractility, in which 1 is normal, 2 is hypokinetic, 3 is akinetic, 4 is dyskinetic, and 5 is aneurysmal. Further, a global wall motion score index can be calculated by summing all individual scores and dividing by the number of segments examined. We do not find this global calculation useful, as it fails to provide the cardiologist with the specific contractility of the individual wall segments.

DIASTOLIC FUNCTION

Echocardiography plays a major role in the assessment of diastole. Initially, digitized M mode was used to assess diastole (77–88). This method has largely been replaced by Doppler echocardiography (89–92). The mitral, tricuspid, pulmonary vein, and vena cava Doppler flow patterns are analyzed to evaluate diastole. In addition, other information, such as left atrial size and left ventricular mass, can be obtained from the echocardiogram to help in the interpretation of the Doppler flow patterns.

Diastole is divided into four phases (Fig. 5-8). The first phase of diastole is the isovolumic relaxation period. This is the time between aortic valve closure and mitral valve opening, when the left ventricular pressure falls. Following mitral valve opening, passive ventricular filling occurs, which is dependent on the pressure difference between the left atrium and left ventricle. After early filling, there is a period of diastasis, when relatively little ventricular filling occurs. The last phase of diastole is active, requiring atrial contraction.

Several distinct Doppler flow patterns are now recognized in adults with acquired heart disease (93). Patients with coronary artery disease (94–96), aortic stenosis (92), systemic hypertension (97), and various types of cardiomyopathy (92,98–104) have been studied. It has become apparent that the diastolic inflow patterns are not disease-specific but rather represent distinct hemodynamic states. Many factors, including age, preload, afterload, PR interval, and heart rate affect the Doppler diastolic flow curves (105–111).

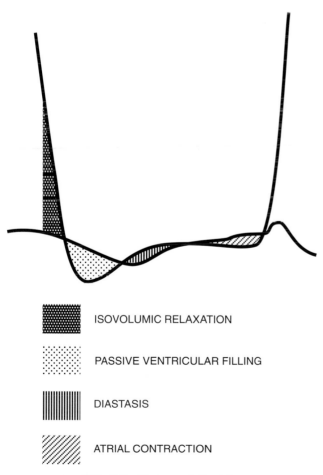

ISOVOLUMIC RELAXATION

PASSIVE VENTRICULAR FILLING

DIASTASIS

ATRIAL CONTRACTION

FIG. 5-8. Phases of diastole.

Diastolic function in children and adults with congenital cardiac malformation has been examined less frequently than in adults with acquired heart disease. The higher heart rates and frequent occurrence of postoperative rhythm disturbances result in Doppler curves that cannot be easily interpreted with the established criteria. Nonetheless, preliminary data suggest that Doppler assessment of diastolic function in this population is possible, despite the greater technical difficulties. These are covered in detail in Chapter 6.

REFERENCES

1. Braunwald E. Seminars in medicine of the Beth Israel Hospital, Boston. *N Engl J Med* 1974;290:1124–1129.
2. Weber KT, Janicki JS, Hunter WC, Shroff S, Pearlman ES, Fishman AP. The contractile behavior of the heart and its functional coupling to the circulation. *Prog Cardiovasc Dis* 1982;24:375–400.
3. Gordon AM, Huxley AF, Julian FJ. The variation in isometric tension with sarcomere length in vertebrate muscle fibres. *J Physiol* 1966;184:170–192.
4. St. John Sutton MG, Oldershaw PJ, Kotler MN. *Textbook of echocardiography and Doppler in adults and children*, 2nd ed. Oxford, England: Blackwell Science, 1996.
5. Branyas NA, Cassidy DM, Cain ME. Periodicity of global ventricular activation of sinus beats in patients with coronary artery disease and sustained ventricular tachycardia. *Am J Cardiol* 1991; 68:901–908.
6. Sahn DJ, DeMaria A, Kisslo J, Weyman A. Recommendations regarding quantitation in M-mode echocardiography: results of a survey of echocardiographic measurements. *Circulation* 1978;58: 1072–1083.
7. Silverman NH. *Pediatric echocardiography*. Baltimore: Williams & Wilkins, 1993.
8. Gutgesell HP, Paquet M, Duff DF, McNamara DG. Evaluation of left ventricular size and function by echocardiography. *Circulation* 1977;56:457–462.
9. Baylen B, Meyer RA, Korfhagen J, Benzing G, Bubb ME, Kaplan S. Left ventricular performance in the critically ill premature infant with patent ductus arteriosus and pulmonary disease. *Circulation* 1977;55:182–188.
10. McDonald IG. Echocardiographic assessment of left ventricular function in aortic valve disease. *Circulation* 1976;53:860–864.
11. Traill TA, Gibson DG, Brown DJ. Study of left ventricular wall thickness and dimension changes using echocardiography. *Br Heart J* 1978;40:162–169.
12. Corya BC, Rasmussen S, Feigenbaum H, Knoebel SB, Black MJ. Systolic thickening and thinning of the septum and posterior wall in patients with coronary artery disease, congestive cardiomyopathy, and atrial septal defect. *Circulation* 1977;55:109–114.
13. Sasayama S, Franklin D, Ross J Jr, Kemper WS, McKown D. Dynamic changes in left ventricular wall thickness and their use in analyzing cardiac function in the conscious dog. *Am J Cardiol* 1976;38:870–879.
14. Feneley MP, Hickie JB. Validity of echocardiographic determination of left ventricular systolic wall thickening. *Circulation* 1984; 70:226–232.
15. Mason SJ, Fortuin NJ. The use of echocardiography for quantitative evaluation of left ventricular function. *Prog Cardiovasc Dis* 1978;21:119–132.
16. Ghafour AS, Gutgesell HP. Echocardiographic evaluation of left ventricular function in children with congestive cardiomyopathy. *Am J Cardiol* 1979;44:1332–1338.
17. Massie BM, Schiller NB, Ratshin RA, Parmley WW. Mitral-septal separation: new echocardiographic index of left ventricular function. *Am J Cardiol* 1977;39:1008–1016.
18. Lew W, Henning H, Schelbert H, Karliner JS. Assessment of

mitral valve E point-septal separation as an index of left ventricular performance in patients with acute and previous myocardial infarction. *Am J Cardiol* 1978;41:836–845.

19. De Cruz IA, Lalmalani GG, Sambasivan V, Cohen HC, Glick G. The superiority of mitral E point-ventricular septum separation to other echocardiographic indicators of left ventricular performance. *Clin Cardiol* 1979;2:140–145.

20. Ahmadpour H, Shah AA, Allen JW, Edmiston WA, Kim SJ, Haywood LJ. Mitral E point septal separation: a reliable index of left ventricular performance in coronary artery disease. *Am Heart J* 1983;106:21–28.

21. Engle SJ, DiSessa TG, Perloff JK, et al. Mitral valve E point to ventricular septal separation in infants and children. *Am J Cardiol* 1983;52:1084–1087.

22. Ginzton LE, Kulick D. Mitral valve E-point septal separation as an indicator of ejection fraction in patients with reversed septal motion. *Chest* 1985;88:429–431.

23. Sahn DJ, Deely WJ, Hagan AD, Friedman WF. Echocardiographic assessment of left ventricular performance in normal newborns. *Circulation* 1974;49:232–236.

24. Sahn DJ, Vaucher Y, Williams DE, Allen HD, Goldberg SJ, Friedman WF. Echocardiographic detection of large left to right shunts and cardiomyopathies in infants and children. *Am J Cardiol* 1976;38:73–79.

25. Colan SD, Borow KM, Neumann A. Left ventricular end-systolic wall stress-velocity of fiber shortening relation: a load-independent index of myocardial contractility. *J Am Coll Cardiol* 1984;4:715–724.

26. Gutgesell HP, Paquet M. *Atlas of pediatric echocardiography.* Hagerstown, MD. Harper & Row, 1978.

27. Fisher EA, DuBrow IW, Hastreiter AR. Comparison of ejection phase indices of left ventricular performance in infants and children. *Circulation* 1975;52:916–925.

28. Bazett HC. An analysis of the time-relations of electrocardiograms. *Heart* 1920;7:353–370.

29. Simonson JS, Schiller NB. Descent of the base of the left ventricle: an echocardiographic index of left ventricular function. *J Am Soc Echocardiogr* 1989;2:25–35.

30. Pai RG, Bodenheimer MM, Pai SM, Koss JH, Adamick RD. Usefulness of systolic excursion of the mitral anulus as an index of left ventricular systolic function. *Am J Cardiol* 1991;67:222–224.

31. Jones CJH, Raposo L, Gibson DG. Functional importance of the long axis dynamics of the human left ventricle. *Br Heart J* 1990;63:215–220.

32. Keren G, Sonnenblick EH, LeJemtel TH. Mitral anulus motion. Relation to pulmonary venous and transmitral flows in normal subjects and in patients with dilated cardiomyopathy. *Circulation* 1988;78:621–629.

33. Folland ED, Parisi AF, Moynihan PF, Jones DR, Feldman CL, Tow DE. Assessment of left ventricular ejection fraction and volumes by real-time, two-dimensional echocardiography. A comparison of cineangiographic and radionuclide techniques. *Circulation* 1979;60:760–766.

34. Silverman NH, Ports TA, Snider AR, Schiller NB, Carlsson E, Heilbron DC. Determination of left ventricular volume in children: echocardiographic and angiographic comparisons. *Circulation* 1980;62:548–557.

35. Mercier JC, DiSessa TG, Jarmakani JM, et al. Two-dimensional echocardiographic assessment of left ventricular volumes and ejection fraction in children. *Circulation* 1982;65:962–969.

36. Schiller NB, Acquatella H, Ports TA, et al. Left ventricular volume from paired biplane two-dimensional echocardiography. *Circulation* 1979;60:547–555.

37. Wahr DW, Wang YS, Schiller NB. Left ventricular volumes determined by two-dimensional echocardiography in a normal adult population. *J Am Coll Cardiol* 1983;1:863–868.

38. Bengur AR, Snider AR, Vermilion RP, Freeland JC. Left ventricular ejection fraction measured with Doppler color flow mapping techniques. *Am J Cardiol* 1991;68:669–673.

39. Emmanouilides GC, Riemenschneider TA, Allen HD, Gutgesell HP. *Heart disease in infants, children, and adolescents including the fetus and young adult*, 5th ed. Baltimore: Williams & Wilkins, 1995.

40. Garson A Jr, Bricker JT, McNamara DG. *The science and practice of pediatric cardiology*, Vol 1. Philadelphia: Lea & Febiger, 1990.

41. Mehta N, Bennett D, Mannering D, Dawkins K, Ward DE. Usefulness of noninvasive Doppler measurement of ascending aortic blood velocity and acceleration in detecting impairment of the left ventricular functional response to exercise three weeks after acute myocardial infarction. *Am J Cardiol* 1986;58:879–884.

42. Reichek N, Wilson J, St. John Sutton M, Plappert TA, Goldberg S, Hirshfeld JW. Noninvasive determination of left ventricular end-systolic stress: validation of the method and initial application. *Circulation* 1982;65:99–108.

43. Grossman W, Jones D, McLaurin LP. Wall stress and patterns of hypertrophy in the human left ventricle. *J Clin Invest* 1975;56:56–64.

44. Borow KM, Neumann A, Lang RM. Milrinone versus dobutamine: contribution of altered myocardial mechanics and augmented inotropic state to improved left ventricular performance. *Circulation* 1986;73[Suppl III]:III-153–III-161.

45. Weber KT, Janicki JS. Myocardial oxygen consumption: the role of wall force and shortening. *Am J Physiol* 1977;233:H421–H430.

46. Carabello BA, Green LH, Grossman W, Cohn LH, Koster JK, Collins JJ Jr. Hemodynamic determinants of prognosis of aortic valve replacement in critical aortic stenosis and advanced congestive heart failure. *Circulation* 1980;62:42–48.

47. Marsh JD, Green LH, Wynne J, Cohn PF, Grossman W. Left ventricular end-systolic pressure-dimension and stress-length relations in normal human subjects. *Am J Cardiol* 1979;44:1311–1317.

48. Colan SD, Borow KM, MacPherson D, Sanders SP. Use of the indirect axillary pulse tracing for noninvasive determination of ejection time, upstroke time, and left ventricular wall stress throughout ejection in infants and young children. *Am J Cardiol* 1984;53:1154–1158.

49. Devereux RB, Reichek N. Echocardiographic determination of left ventricular mass in man. Anatomic validation of the method. *Circulation* 1977;55:613–618.

50. Devereux RB, Casale PN, Kligfield P, et al. Performance of primary and derived M-mode echocardiographic measurements for detection of left ventricular hypertrophy in necropsied subjects and in patients with systemic hypertension, mitral regurgitation and dilated cardiomyopathy. *Am J Cardiol* 1986;57:1388–1393.

51. Daniels SR, Meyer RA, Liang Y, Bove KE. Echocardiographically determined left ventricular mass index in normal children, adolescents and young adults. *J Am Coll Cardiol* 1988;12:703–708.

52. Daniels SR, Kimball TR, Morrison JA, Khoury P, Meyer RA. Indexing left ventricular mass to account for differences in body size in children and adolescents without cardiovascular disease. *Am J Cardiol* 1995;76:699–701.

53. Colan SD, Borow KM, Neumann A. Left ventricular end-systolic wall stress-velocity of fiber shortening relation: a load-independent index of myocardial contractility. *J Am Coll Cardiol* 1984;4:715–724.

54. Franklin RCG, Wyse RKH, Graham TP, Gooch VM, Deanfield JE. Normal values for noninvasive estimation of left ventricular contractile state and afterload in children. *Am J Cardiol* 1990;65:505–510.

55. Kimball TR, Daniels SR, Khoury P, Meyer RA. Age-related variation in contractility estimate in patients <20 years of age. *Am J Cardiol* 1991;68:1383–1387.

56. Rowland DG, Gutgesell HP. Noninvasive assessment of myocardial contractility, preload, and afterload in healthy newborn infants. *Am J Cardiol* 1995;75:818–821.

57. Kimball TR, Daniels SR, Weiss RG, et al. Changes in cardiac function during extracorporeal membrane oxygenation for persistent pulmonary hypertension in the newborn infant. *J Pediatr* 1991;118:431–436.

58. Newburger JW, Sanders SP, Burns JC, Parness IA, Beiser AS, Colan SD. Left ventricular contractility and function in Kawasaki syndrome. *Circulation* 1989;79:1237–1246.

59. Colan SD, Trowitzsch E, Wernovsky G, Sholler GF, Sanders SP, Castaneda AR. Myocardial performance after arterial switch operation for transposition of the great arteries with intact ventricular septum. *Circulation* 1988;78:123–141.

60. Kimball TR, Daniels SR, Meyer RA, Schwartz DC, Kaplan S. Left ventricular mass in childhood dilated cardiomyopathy: a possible predictor for selection of patients for cardiac transplantation. *Am Heart J* 1991;122:126–131.

61. Kimball TR, Daniels SR, Meyer RA, Hannon DW, Khoury P, Schwartz DC. Relation of symptoms to contractility and defect size in infants with ventricular septal defect. *Am J Cardiol* 1991;67:1097–1102.

62. Kimball TR, Daniels SR, Meyer RA, et al. Effect of digoxin on contractility and symptoms in infants with a large ventricular septal defect. *Am J Cardiol* 1991;68:1377–1382.

63. Kimball TR, Daniels SR, Loggie JMH, Khoury P, Meyer RA. Relation of left ventricular mass, preload, afterload and contractility in pediatric patients with essential hypertension. *J Am Coll Cardiol* 1993;21:997–1001.

64. Rowland DG, Gutgesell HP. Use of mean arterial pressure for noninvasive determination of left ventricular end-systolic wall stress in infants and children. *Am J Cardiol* 1994;74:98–99.

65. Karr SS, Martin GR. A simplified method for calculating wall stress in infants and children. *J Am Soc Echocardiogr* 1994;7:646–651.

66. Nidorf SM, Picard MH, Triulzi MO, et al. New perspectives in the assessment of cardiac chamber dimensions during development and adulthood. *J Am Coll Cardiol* 1992;19:983–988.

67. Epstein ML, Goldberg SJ, Allen HD, Konecke L, Wood J. Great vessel, cardiac chamber, and wall growth patterns in normal children. *Circulation* 1975;51:1124–1130.

68. Henry WL, Ware J, Gardin JM, Hepner SI, McKay J, Weiner M. Echocardiographic measurements in normal subjects. Growth-related changes that occur between infancy and early adulthood. *Circulation* 1978;57:278–285.

69. Roge CLL, Silverman NH, Hart PA, Ray RM. Cardiac structure growth pattern determined by echocardiography. *Circulation* 1978;57:285–290.

70. Henry WL, Gardin JM, Ware JH. Echocardiographic measurements in normal subjects from infancy to old age. *Circulation* 1980;62:1054–1061.

71. Imai T, Satomi G, Yasukochi S, et al. Normal values for cardiac and great arterial dimensions in premature infants by cross-sectional echocardiography. *Cardiol Young* 1995;5:319–325.

72. Snider AR, Enderlein MA, Teitel DF, Juster RP. Two-dimensional echocardiographic determination of aortic and pulmonary artery sizes from infancy to adulthood in normal subjects. *Am J Cardiol* 1984;53:218–224.

73. Pearlman JD, Triulzi MO, King ME, Newell J, Weyman AE. Limits of normal left ventricular dimensions in growth and development: analysis of dimensions and variance in the two-dimensional echocardiograms of 268 normal healthy subjects. *J Am Coll Cardiol* 1988;12:1432–1441.

74. Pearlman JD, Triulzi MO, King ME, Abascal VM, Newell J, Weyman AE. Left atrial dimensions in growth and development: normal limits for two-dimensional echocardiography. *J Am Coll Cardiol* 1990;16:1168–1174.

75. Roman MJ, Devereux RB, Kramer-Fox R, O'Loughlin J, Spitzer M, Robins J. Two-dimensional echocardiographic aortic dimensions in normal children and adults. *Am J Cardiol* 1989;64:507–512.

76. Sheil MLK, Jenkins O, Sholler GF. Echocardiographic assessment of aortic root dimension in normal children based on measurement of a new ratio of aortic size independent of growth. *Am J Cardiol* 1995;75:711–715.

77. Hanrath P, Mathey DG, Kremer P, Sonntag F, Bleifeld W. Effect of verapamil on left ventricular isovolumic relaxation time and regional left ventricular filling in hypertrophic cardiomyopathy. *Am J Cardiol* 1980;45:1258–1264.

78. Bahler RC, Vrobel TR, Martin P. The relation of heart rate and shortening fraction to echocardiographic indexes of left ventricular relaxation in normal subjects. *J Am Coll Cardiol* 1983;2:926–933.

79. Fifer MA, Borow KM, Colan SD, Lorell BH. Early diastolic left ventricular function in children and adults with aortic stenosis. *J Am Coll Cardiol* 1985;5:1147–1154.

80. St. John Sutton MG, Tajik AJ, Gibson DG, Brown DJ, Seward JB, Giuliani ER. Echocardiographic assessment of left ventricular filling and septal and posterior wall dynamics in idiopathic hypertrophic subaortic stenosis. *Circulation* 1978;57:512–520.

81. Hanrath P, Mathey DG, Siegert R, Bleifeld W. Left ventricular relaxation and filling pattern in different forms of left ventricular hypertrophy: an echocardiographic study. *Am J Cardiol* 1980;45:15–23.

82. Gibson DG, Brown D. Measurement of instantaneous left ventricular dimension and filling rate in man, using echocardiography. *Br Heart J* 1973;35:1141–1149.

83. Gibson DG, Brown DJ. Assessment of left ventricular systolic function in man from simultaneous echocardiographic and pressure measurements. *Br Heart J* 1976;38:8–17.

84. Kugler JD, Gutgesell HP, Nihill MR. Instantaneous rates of left ventricular wall motion in infants and children. Computer-assisted determination from single-cycle echocardiograms. *Pediatr Cardiol* 1979;1:15–21.

85. Upton MT, Gibson DG. The study of left ventricular function from digitized echocardiograms. *Prog Cardiovasc Dis* 1978;20:359–384.

86. St. John Sutton MG, Hagler DJ, Tajik AJ, et al. Cardiac function in the normal newborn. Additional information by computer analysis of the M-mode echocardiogram. *Circulation* 1978;57:1198–1204.

87. Friedman MJ, Sahn DJ. Computer-assisted analysis of M-mode echocardiogram: is it a gold mine? *Pediatr Cardiol* 1979;1:47–50.

88. Hofstetter R, Mayr A, Von Bernuth G. Computer analysis of cardiac contractility variables obtained by M-mode echocardiography in normal newborns. *Br Heart J* 1982;48:525–528.

89. Rokey R, Kuo LC, Zoghbi WA, Limacher MC, Quinones MA. Determination of parameters of left ventricular diastolic filling with pulsed Doppler echocardiography: comparison with cincangiography. *Circulation* 1985;71:543–550.

90. Friedman BJ, Drinkovic N, Miles H, Shih WJ, Mazzoleni A, DeMaria AN. Assessment of left ventricular diastolic function: comparison of Doppler echocardiography and gated blood pool scintigraphy. *J Am Coll Cardiol* 1986;8:1348–1354.

91. Spirito P, Maron BJ, Bonow RO. Noninvasive assessment of left ventricular diastolic function: comparative analysis of Doppler echocardiographic and radionuclide angiographic techniques. *J Am Coll Cardiol* 1986;7:518–526.

92. Pearson AC, Labovitz AJ, Mrosek D, Williams GA, Kennedy HL. Assessment of diastolic function in normal and hypertrophied hearts: comparison of Doppler echocardiography and M-mode echocardiography. *Am Heart J* 1987;113:1417–1425.

93. Nishimura RA, Abel MD, Hatle LK, Tajik AJ. Assessment of diastolic function of the heart: background and current applications of Doppler echocardiography. Part II. Clinical studies. *Mayo Clin Proc* 1989;64:181–204.

94. Labovitz AJ, Lewen MK, Kern M, et al. Evaluation of left ventricular systolic and diastolic dysfunction during transient myocardial ischemia produced by angioplasty. *J Am Coll Cardiol* 1987;10:748–755.

95. Koolen JJ, Visser CA, Wever E, Van Wezel H, Meyne NG, Dunning AJ. Transesophageal two-dimensional echocardiographic evaluation of biventricular dimension and function during positive end-expiratory pressure ventilation after coronary artery bypass grafting. *Am J Cardiol* 1987;59:1047–1051.

96. Fujii J, Yazaki Y, Sawada H, Aizawa T, Watanabe H, Kato K. Noninvasive assessment of left and right ventricular filling in myocardial infarction with a two-dimensional Doppler echocardiographic method. *J Am Coll Cardiol* 1985;5:1155–1160.

97. Phillips RA, Coplan NL, Krakoff LR, et al. Doppler echocardiographic analysis of left ventricular filling in treated hypertensive patients. *J Am Coll Cardiol* 1987;9:317–322.

98. Takenaka K, Dabestani A, Gardin JM, et al. Pulsed Doppler echocardiographic study of left ventricular filling in dilated cardiomyopathy. *Am J Cardiol* 1986;58:143–147.

99. Gidding SS, Snider AR, Rocchini AP, Peters J, Farnsworth R. Left ventricular diastolic filling in children with hypertrophic cardiomyopathy: assessment with pulsed Doppler echocardiography. *J Am Coll Cardiol* 1986;8:310–316.

100. Iwase M, Sotobata I, Takagi S, Miyaguchi K, Jing HX, Yokota M. Effects of diltiazem on left ventricular diastolic behavior in patients with hypertrophic cardiomypathy: evaluation with exercise pulsed Doppler echocardiography. *J Am Coll Cardiol* 1987; 9:1099–1105.

101. Maron BJ, Spirito P, Green KJ, Wesley YE, Bonow RO, Arce J. Noninvasive assessment of left ventricular diastolic function by pulsed Doppler echocardiography in patients with hypertrophic cardiomyopathy. *J Am Coll Cardiol* 1987;10:733–742.

102. Bryg RJ, Pearson AC, Williams GA, Labovitz AJ. Left ventricular systolic and diastolic flow abnormalities determined by Doppler echocardiography in obstructive hypertrophic cardiomyopathy. *Am J Cardiol* 1987;59:925–931.

103. Takenaka K, Dabestani A, Gardin JM, et al. Left ventricular filling in hypertrophic cardiomyopathy: a pulsed Doppler echocardiographic study. *J Am Coll Cardiol* 1986;7:1263–1271.

104. Agatston AS, Rao A, Price RJ, Kinney EL. Diagnosis of constrictive pericarditis by pulsed Doppler echocardiography. *Am J Cardiol* 1984;54:929–931.

105. Choong CY, Herrmann HC, Weyman AE, Fifer MA. Preload dependence of Doppler-derived indexes of left ventricular diastolic function in humans. *J Am Coll Cardiol* 1987;10:800–808.

106. Ishida Y, Meisner JS, Tsujioka K, et al. Left ventricular filling dynamics: influence of left ventricular relaxation and left atrial pressure. *Circulation* 1986;74:187–196.

107. Herzog CA, Elsperger KJ, Manoles M, Murakami M, Asinger R. Response of transmitral flow velocity to physiologic variables. *J Am Coll Cardiol* 1987;9:197A(abst).

108. Parker TG, Cameron D, Serra J, Morgan CD, Sasson Z. The effect of heart rate and A-V interval on Doppler ultrasound indices of left ventricular diastolic function. *Circulation* 1987;76[Suppl IV]: IV-124(abst).

109. Harrison TR, Dixon K, Russel RO, Bidwai PS, Coleman HN. The relation of age to the duration of contraction, ejection, and relaxation of the normal human heart. *Am Heart J* 1964;67: 189–199.

110. Valantine HA, Appleton CP, Hatle LK, Hunt SA, Stinson EB, Popp RL. Influence of recipient atrial contraction on left ventricular filling dynamics of the transplanted heart assessed by Doppler echocardiography. *Am J Cardiol* 1987;59:1159–1163.

111. Zile MR, Blaustein AS, Shimizu G, Gaasch WH. Right ventricular pacing reduces the rate of left ventricular relaxation and filling. *J Am Coll Cardiol* 1987;10:702–709.

CHAPTER 6

Doppler Echocardiography

Curt G. DeGroff

DOPPLER TECHNIQUES

Continuous wave (CW), pulsed wave (PW), and color Doppler flow mapping were introduced in Chapter 3. The following describes concepts important in the clinical application of these methods.

Spectral Doppler

In CW Doppler, the sampling rate is infinite, with no theoretic limit to display high velocities. CW Doppler imaging can be obtained using two different types of transducers, one with no imaging capabilities and one with simultaneous display of two-dimensional imaging. Simultaneous display leads to some loss in sensitivity of the signal (1).

In PW Doppler imaging, short bursts of ultrasound signals are transmitted at regular intervals (the pulse repetition frequency). PW Doppler's main advantage is range resolution in sampling blood flow velocities. The main disadvantage comes from sampling theory, which states the maximum detectable frequency shift (the Nyquist limit) is equal to half the sampling rate (the pulse repetition frequency). If the Nyquist limit is exceeded, then the velocities are recorded ambiguously; this is termed "aliasing," meaning an inability to obtain the maximum velocities accurately (Echo. 6-1). Images with shallow depth settings require less time for PW Doppler signals to return to the transducer, allowing for higher sampling rates, leading to higher maximal detectable velocities.

There are several methods that can be used to increase the maximum detectable velocity (2). The first method entails simply shifting the baseline (the zero velocity line) away from the direction of flow, allowing for the display of higher velocities in the direction of flow. One can also use the shallowest instrument depth setting to maximize pulse repetition frequency, as well as using the lowest frequency transducer applicable.

A relatively newer method used to increase the maximum detectable velocity relates to high pulse repetition frequency (HPRF) Doppler imaging (3). In HPRF, the pulse repetition rate is set so high that the signal from one pulse does not complete its return before the next pulse is transmitted. Thus, Doppler shifts are detected from more than one interrogation site. If all but one of these potential sites are positioned in areas where elevated flow velocities are unlikely (or not possible), then accurate high-velocity measurements can be obtained from the site of interest (Echo. 6-2).

In current echocardiography, there is a place for all of the Doppler methods described.

Color Doppler

Color Doppler imaging is a method where blood flow is displayed on the two-dimensional echocardiographic image by color-encoding the Doppler-generated flow signal. Flow toward the transducer is usually displayed in shades of red, and flow away from the transducer is usually displayed in shades of blue. Increasing velocities are displayed in varying hues of red and blue. For issues regarding variance mapping, see Chapter 3.

When simultaneously displaying a two-dimensional echocardiographic image and color flow information, compromises to overall image quality are usually unavoidable. In addition, balances between color, sector size, line density, and frame rate must be taken into account (4). Just as in PW Doppler imaging, aliasing can occur, depending on the pulse repetition frequency (PRF). As velocity increases, brighter and brighter colors are displayed until the aliasing point is reached, where there is reversal of color (bright blue to bright red or vice versa). The maximum PRF that can be utilized in most color flow imaging systems is relatively low, which leads to aliasing even in some normal flow situations (Echo. 6-3; see color plate 1 following p. 364) (5).

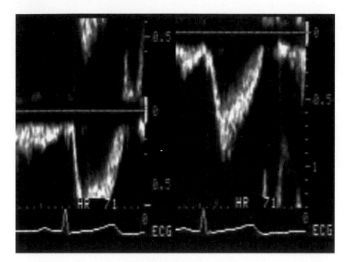

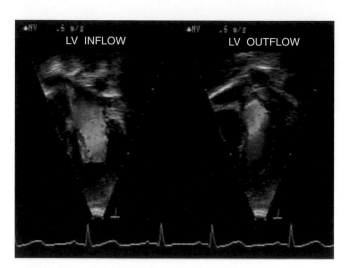

ECHO. 6-1. Example **(left)** of aliasing in a PW Doppler image where velocities in the Doppler signal exceed the Nyquist limit. The remainder of the signal is "wrapped around" and displayed as velocities in the opposite direction. Shifting the baseline (zero velocity line) away from the direction of flow **(right)** allows for display of higher velocities in the direction of flow.

ECHO. 6-3. Color Doppler aliasing can be seen in normal physiologic flow situations as shown here in the color Doppler flow images of the left ventricular inflow **(left)** and the left ventricular outflow **(right).** The maximum pulse repetition frequency (PRF), that can be utilized in most color flow imaging systems is relatively low which leads to such aliasing. *LV,* left ventricle.

Angle Dependence of Doppler: The Cosine Effect

The value of the recorded velocities when using spectral Doppler is dependent on the cosine of the angle between the ultrasound beam and the direction of flow in the region being interrogated. With angles between 0 and 20 degrees, the cosine of that angle will be 1 to 0.94, and, therefore, it can be disregarded (6). With larger angles, velocity magnitudes will be significantly underestimated.

Angle correction is available on many echocardiographic machines but is generally avoided.

The impact of angle dependence in color Doppler may be a more subtle concept than in spectral Doppler. In numeric simulations of regurgitant flow through a mitral valve, we have demonstrated how imaging such flow from various selected locations results in quite different color Doppler images (7). As we can see from Fig. 6-1 (see color plate 2 following p. 364), the appearance of the flow changes dramatically when imaging from various locations.

Velocity Time Integral

It is often important to measure the time-averaged velocity (TAV) of a Doppler velocity signal. The area under the spectral velocity-time curve is referred to as the velocity time integral (VTI). The TAV equals the area under the spectral velocity-time curve divided by the duration of the cardiac cycle (RR interval) (Echo. 6-4):

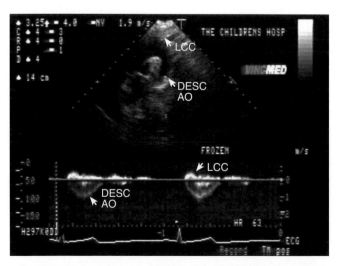

ECHO. 6-2. Example of HPRF where the pulse repetition rate is set such that the signal from one pulse does not complete its return before the next pulse is transmitted leading to detection of Doppler shifts from more than one interrogation site. Suprasternal notch view of descending aorta and left common carotid. *DESC AO,* descending aorta; *LCC,* left common carotid.

$$\text{TAV} = \frac{\text{VTI}}{\text{RR interval}} \qquad [1]$$

Most commercial echocardiographic equipment can automatically integrate the velocity-time curve and calculate TAV after the user traces the curve from the spectral signal. This is generally used in the calculation of volumetric flow rates, as discussed later in this chapter.

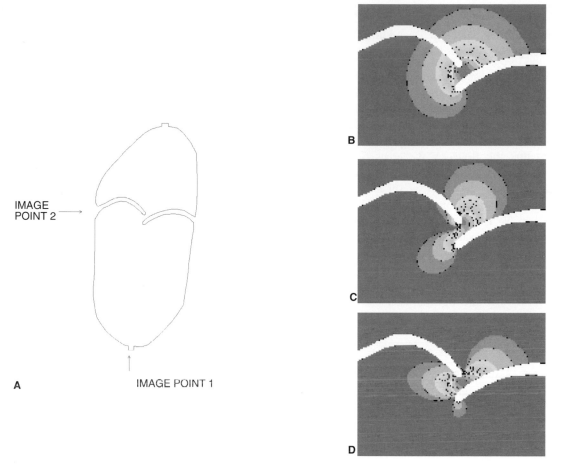

FIG. 6-1. Numerical simulation of regurgitant flow through a prolapsed mitral valve demonstrating the angle dependence of Doppler color imaging. "Echo" Doppler color images were simulated from two transducer sites in the numerical model (A). True isovelocity contours are shown (B), along with "echo" Doppler isovelocity contours imaging from point 1 (C) and point 2 (D). Note how the image changes depending on where the "transducer" is placed.

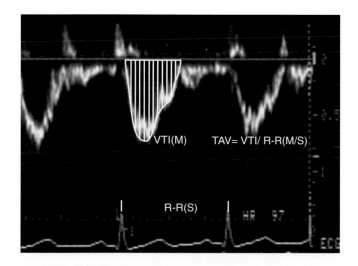

ECHO. 6-4. Doppler spectral velocity waveform is shown with an example of how the VTI and the TAV Doppler indices are measured. Note that the VTI is simply the area under the Doppler spectral velocity waveform with units equal to meters. TAV equals the area under the spectral velocity-time curve (i.e., VTI) divided by the duration of the cardiac cycle (RR interval), with units equal to meters/second.

NORMAL DOPPLER PATTERNS AND IMAGES

Normal Doppler Spectral Recordings and Optimal Echocardiographic Views

In order to detect abnormal Doppler velocity patterns, one has to have a sense of what can be seen in normal individuals. Normal ranges in velocity magnitude and pattern depend on the patient's age and size. As Doppler technology becomes more sophisticated, one needs to keep in mind that the flows in the areas of the heart under consideration may have complex structures, with nonuniform flow velocity profiles (8–10). Thus, samples of flow velocities at specific points (i.e., PW Doppler) or along lines (i.e., CW Doppler) may vary somewhat depending upon where one is sampling in the flow field (5).

We will now review Doppler velocity magnitudes and patterns seen in the normal pediatric and adult population in various locations within the cardiovascular system. We will also review the optimal echocardiographic planes used for this spectral interrogation.

Systemic Venous System

Blood flow in the superior vena cava (SVC) near its entrance into the right atrium can be best imaged and sampled from the suprasternal and subcostal planes. Flow in the inferior vena cava (IVC), where it enters the right atrium, can be best imaged and sampled from the subcostal, parasternal, and apical planes. The Doppler velocity signals for the vena caval inflows (5,11–13) are normally continuous, with two inflow phases in the velocity spectral display (Echo. 6-5). The first inflow phase has the

highest peak velocity and represents inflow during ventricular systole (S wave). The second inflow phase represents inflow during the rapid filling phase of ventricular diastole (D wave). Flow reversal can be seen between systolic and diastolic phases (H wave), as well as after atrial contraction (A wave).

Respiratory variation exists with increased forward velocity magnitudes and decreased reverse flow velocity magnitudes during inspiration. Therefore, it is often helpful to record a simultaneous respiratory tracing when interpreting these flows (14) (Echo. 6-5). Normal peak velocity values are well documented in adults (5,11,12); however, there are only a few reports of normal peak velocity values in children and especially in infants (5,13). Peak velocities range between 0.5 to 1.5 m/s in children and adults and can be higher in infants (5). Mean velocities in the superior vena cava in infants and children are 0.4 (±0.6) m/s (13). Higher heart rates often seen in infants and children may change the shape of the Doppler signal, leading to one peak in systole (5).

Pulmonary Venous System

Blood flow in the pulmonary veins near their entrance sites into the left atrium can be imaged from the suprasternal, parasternal, apical, and subcostal planes. The best alignment to sample flows is in the suprasternal, apical, and subcostal positions depending on which of the four veins is being interrogated. The Doppler velocity signal for pulmonary venous inflow (5,15–21) is typically continuous with two inflow phases in the velocity spectral display (Echo. 6-6). The first inflow phase (S or J wave) occurs during ventricular systole and represents reduction in left atrial pressure (LAP) secondary to left atrial relaxation, augmented by the descent of the base of the heart (15). This phase may consist of two distinct peaks (S1 and S2). The second inflow phase occurs during ventricular diastole (D or K wave). As in vena caval flow, there may be normal flow reversal between systolic and diastolic phases (H wave); reversal also occurs after atrial contraction (A wave) during the end of the diastolic phase.

The systolic phase of pulmonary venous flow depends on left atrial contraction, relaxation, compliance, and pressure, as well as left ventricular systolic function and cardiac output (17). The diastolic phase depends on left atrial pressure and left ventricular compliance and relaxation (17). The A wave of pulmonary venous flow depends on left atrial contraction, relaxation, and compliance, as well as left ventricular compliance (17).

There are documented variations in the significance of the diastolic phase with age that are felt to be secondary to age-related changes in left ventricular relaxation (22). Over the first 36 months of life, the peak diastolic velocity increases (22), which may reflect maturational improvement in left ventricular relaxation. In adults, as ventricular

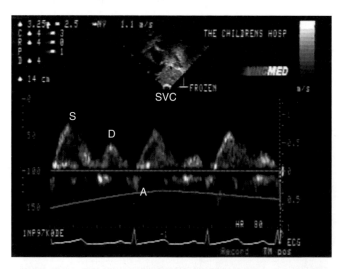

ECHO. 6-5. Example of a typical Doppler spectral velocity waveform of the superior vena cava (*SVC*). Note the two inflow phases. Inflow during ventricular systole is represented by the first inflow phase (*S*). The second inflow phase represents inflow during the rapid filling phase of ventricular diastole (*D*). Flow reversal may be seen between systolic and diastolic phases (not shown), as well as after atrial contraction (*A*).

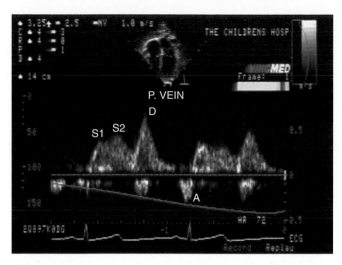

ECHO. 6-6. Example of a typical Doppler spectral velocity waveform of pulmonary vein inflow, which is continuous. During ventricular systole, the first inflow phase occurs with two peaks (*S1* and *S2*). During ventricular diastole, the second inflow phase occurs (*D*). Flow reversal may occur between systolic and diastolic phases (not shown) and in the diastolic phase after atrial contraction (*A*). *P*, pulmonary.

relaxation deteriorates in older age groups, there is a reduction in magnitude of the diastolic peak velocity (17,23). In contrast to vena cava flow, the diastolic phase in most age groups commonly has a higher peak velocity than the systolic phase (5).

Reported normal peak velocity values in adults range from 0.4 to 0.5 m/s (17) and 0.3 to 0.7 (24). In young adults, the reported peak velocity range is similar (0.38 to 0.68 m/s) (25). Reports of normal values in children and especially infants are sparse, though peak values under 2 m/s are felt to indicate lack of significant pulmonary venous pathology (26).

Adult studies have shown normal A wave reversal velocities up to 0.35 m/s (23). The duration of the pulmonary venous A wave should be less than that of the mitral A wave (16). The duration of the pulmonary venous A wave (T_{A-pulm}) can be compared to the duration of the mitral A wave ($T_{A-mitral}$) and a ratio ($T_{A-pulm}/T_{A-mitral}$) obtained. A preliminary study (27) of normal children (ages 5 to 12 years old) showed the mean value for this ratio was 0.5 (range 0 to 1.0).

In the early neonatal period the pulmonary venous waveform is felt to be strongly influenced by the increased pulmonary blood flow (secondary to the patent ductus arteriosus) and the rapid decline in pulmonary pressures that normally occurs at birth. Immediately after birth, the pulmonary venous waveform is quite different from that found later in life. The pattern in this early period shows a high flow phasic waveform without cessation of forward flow and without reverse flow during atrial contraction (28). The mean of the peak flow velocities is considerably higher than the normal range in adults (systolic 0.7 m/s and diastolic 0.81 m/s) (28).

Atrioventricular Valve Inflow

Mitral valve and tricuspid valve inflows are best sampled in the apical plane. One of the most important aspects of sampling atrioventricular valve inflow is beam alignment (29). Commonly the mitral valve is erroneously sampled with the transducer too close to the apex of the heart, which leads to a less than optimal nonparallel angle between the Doppler beam and inflow direction. Generally, for mitral valve inflow, the transducer should be positioned more laterally to obtain a sample beam directly parallel to mitral valve inflow. The most optimal location to place the PW Doppler sample volume for both the mitral and tricuspid valves is at the leaflet tips (29).

A typical atrioventricular valve Doppler velocity signal (5) consists of two inflow phases in the velocity spectral display (Echo. 6-7). The first inflow phase (E wave) has the highest peak velocity and represents early diastolic filling. The second inflow phase (A wave) corresponds to inflow during atrial contraction. Conceptually it may be more helpful to view the velocity curves as reflecting the time-dependent pressure gradient between the atrium and ventricle in diastole (14,30,31). After systole, the ventricular pressure decreases rapidly as a result of ventricular relaxation. The ventricular pressure eventually drops below atrial pressure and a driving pressure causes the atrioventricular valves to open and inflow to occur (early diastolic filling). As the ventricle fills, ventricular pressure rises, the pressure gradient lessens, and inflow velocities decrease (downslope of E wave). Eventually ventricular pressure exceeds or meets atrial pressure but inflow continues due to inertia (30). At this point there may be a short period of flow reversal (32) between the A and E waves. Lastly, atrial contraction occurs,

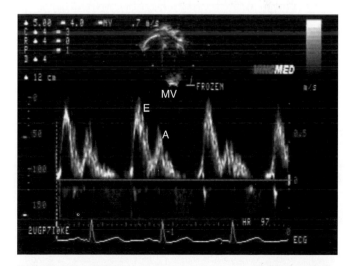

ECHO. 6-7. Example of a typical Doppler spectral velocity waveform of an atrioventricular valve inflow. Early diastolic filling is represented by the first inflow phase (*E*). The second inflow phase (*A*) corresponds to inflow during atrial contraction. There may be a short period of flow reversal between the A and E waves. *MV*, mitral valve.

causing an increase in atrial pressure and leading to an acceleration of inflow (A wave).

One may think of the inflow pattern somewhat simplistically as the E wave being related to ventricular relaxation and the A wave being related to active ventricular relaxation and passive ventricular compliance (33).

Normal mitral valve velocity indices have been reported in children (5,27,34–36). Normal peak velocities (5) range between 0.8 to 1.3 m/s. The normal E/A peak velocity ratio range is reported between 1.5 to 2.3 (37) and reported elsewhere between 0.8 to 2.8 with tighter ranges dependent on body surface area (35). Changes in the E wave peak velocity occur during respiration with 8% decrease during inspiration (34). There are essentially no changes in A wave peak velocity during respiration (34). The time duration of the downsloping portion (deceleration) of the E wave is called the deceleration time (DT) and ranges in normal children between 103 to 195 ms (27). The isovolumetric relaxation time (IVRT) will be discussed in detail later. Briefly, it is the time from the start of the aortic valve (AOV) closure signal to the start of the mitral valve opening signal but may be measured in a number of ways (Echo. 6-8). IVRT ranges in normal children are 30 to 70 m/s (35).

Many of these parameters change with age (35,38–41). Most notably E and A wave changes occur throughout life starting in the prenatal period. In early gestation (42), the A wave is dominant in peak magnitude compared to the E wave suggesting impaired ventricular relaxation and decreased compliance. Through gestation the E/A ratio increases suggesting improved relaxation and increased compliance. Neonates, infants, and young children have relative residual impaired ventricular relaxation compared to older children and young adults (38,43) with E waves that continue to increase through early childhood without

significant changes in A waves (38). In the normal adult aging process (27,44) the E/A ratio then gradually reverts back to an A wave dominant pattern with associated impaired ventricular relaxation and decreased compliance.

Normal tricuspid valve velocity indices have also been reported (5,34,36). Normal peak velocities range between 0.5 to 0.8 m/s. Normal E/A peak velocity ratios range between 0.6 to 2.6. Increases in both the E and A wave peak velocities occur during respiration with up to a 26% increase in the E wave during inspiration (34). Compared to mitral valve inflow there is much less reported in the literature regarding the normal changes in E and A waves of the tricuspid valve with aging; however, a similar increase in the E/A ratio has been reported to occur through gestation (42,45).

Right Ventricular Outflow Tract and Pulmonary Valve Outflow

Spectral Doppler sampling of the right ventricular outflow tract (RVOT) and pulmonary valve outflow is best obtained from the left parasternal short axis and the subcostal planes. In neonates and young children, one can also use the apical planes with steep angulation of the transducer anteriorly.

There is usually a slight increase in PW Doppler sampled velocity magnitude from the right ventricular outflow tract to the pulmonary valve outflow, with an earlier peak velocity at the pulmonary valve outflow (Echo. 6-9). Slight peaks in the velocity spectral signal can be seen in the right ventricular outflow tract during atrial contraction and early in ventricular diastole (5). A similar small peak can be seen in the pulmonary valve outflow velocity signal during atrial contraction. Hatle et al. (5) point out that the shape of the velocity signal may change depending on where the sample volume is located within the right ventricular outflow tract and the pulmonary artery with even reversal of flow velocity seen near the lateral or posterior wall in the right ventricular outflow tract during systole. There is spectral broadening on the downsloping side of the velocity signal, which is probably related to deceleration turbulence. There is normally a short period of reverse velocities at the end of systole, which is consistent with valve closure.

To obtain maximum Doppler velocity values in the pulmonary valve outflow, measurements from all of the above planes should be attempted and the highest velocity value used (10). When using CW Doppler sampling, one must be careful not to include increased velocities (if present) at the branches of the left and right pulmonary arteries when attempting to sample the pulmonary valve outflow area. Normal values for pulmonary valve outflow peak velocities range between 0.7 to 1.1 m/s (5). Samples of the left and right branch pulmonary arteries can be obtained in the left parasternal short axis and suprasternal planes. A general rule of thumb used by many pediatric

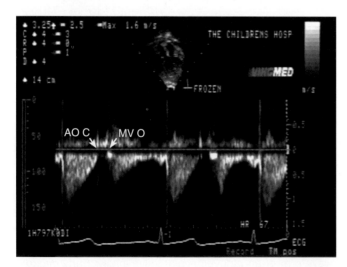

ECHO. 6-8. IVRT can be measured from the end of the aortic flow Doppler signal to the beginning of the mitral valve inflow Doppler signal as shown. *AOC*, aortic closure; *MVO*, mitral valve opening.

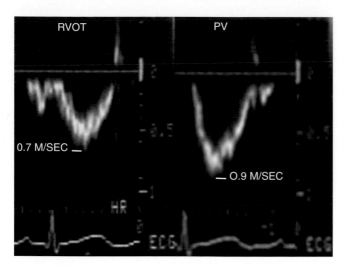

ECHO. 6-9. Differences in the PW Doppler sampled velocity signal from the right ventricular outflow tract **(left)** compared to the pulmonary valve outflow **(right)** with an earlier peak velocity at the pulmonary valve outflow. *PV*, pulmonary valve; *RVOT*, right ventricular outflow tract.

echocardiographers is that velocities below 2.0 m/s signify normal branch pulmonary artery velocities.

Left Ventricular Outflow Tract and Aortic Valve Outflow

Spectral Doppler sampling of the left ventricular outflow tract (LVOT) is best obtained in the apical plane. There is usually a slight increase in PW Doppler sampled velocity magnitude from the left ventricular outflow tract to the aortic valve outflow, with an earlier peak velocity at the aortic valve outflow (Echo. 6-10) (5). Normal val-

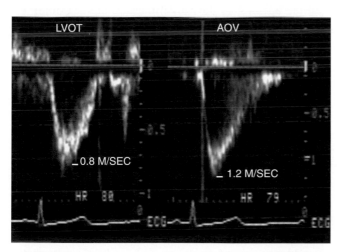

ECHO. 6-10. Differences in the PW Doppler sampled velocity signal from the left ventricular outflow tract **(left)** compared to the aortic valve outflow **(right)** with an earlier peak velocity at the aortic valve outflow. The *AOV* outflow signal has a sharp upstroke with a short acceleration time to peak velocity. Spectral broadening on the downsloping side of the velocity signal occurs. *AOV*, aortic valve; *LVOT*, left ventricular outflow tract.

ues for maximum velocity in the LVOT range between 0.7 to 1.2 m/s (5,36).

Spectral Doppler sampling of aortic valve outflow is best obtained in the apical, subcostal, and high right parasternal planes. The shape of the aortic valve outflow Doppler velocity signal is similar to that seen in the pulmonary valve outflow signal—with some important differences. The aortic valve outflow signal (5), measured just distal to the aortic valve leaflets, has a sharper upstroke with a shorter acceleration time (AT) to peak velocity and a higher peak velocity (Echos. 6-9 and 6-10). Similarities to the pulmonary valve outflow signal include spectral broadening on the downsloping side of the velocity signal, which is probably related to deceleration turbulence. The spectral signal may show a short period of reverse velocities at the end of systole, which is consistent with valve closure. Normal values for aortic valve outflow peak velocities range from 1.2 to 1.8 m/s (5).

Ascending and Descending Aorta

Flow velocities in the ascending and descending aorta are optimally recorded with a nonimaging Doppler transducer at the suprasternal notch (Echo. 6-11). In the pediatric patient a Doppler study is not complete until descending aortic velocities are measured past the takeoff of the last aortic arch branch vessel by PW and CW Doppler, if possible. There may be a short period of reverse velocities at the end of systole in the normal ascending and descending aorta Doppler spectral velocity display.

Normal Valvular Insufficiency

Prior to the development of color Doppler, studies using spectral Doppler demonstrated that valvular regurgita-

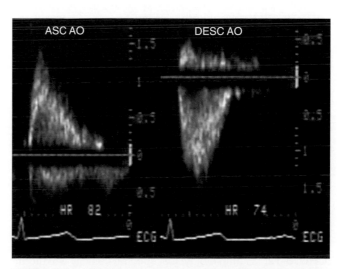

ECHO. 6-11. Typical CW Doppler sampled velocity signals of the ascending aorta **(left)** and descending aorta from the suprasternal notch approach **(right)**. *ASC AO*, ascending aorta; *DESC AO*, descending aorta.

tion (specifically pulmonary and tricuspid regurgitation) occurred in normal subjects and that Doppler methods were more sensitive than clinical examination (Echos. 6-12 and 6-13) (46). Once color Doppler was developed, it became obvious that silent Doppler-detected regurgitation exists in adults (47–49) and children (50,51) (Echos. 6-12 and 6-13). Fear of assigning iatrogenic heart disease to patients with normal hearts exists (47,48,52). The prevalence of valvular regurgitation from various studies listed herein should be viewed with some caution since various echocardiographic machines and machine settings can no doubt have dramatic influence on the ability to detect slight valvular regurgitation (53).

Tricuspid and Pulmonic Valves

Tricuspid regurgitation has been found in 6% to 75% of normal children, depending on the definition of tricuspid regurgitation (50,51). If tricuspid regurgitation flow of very short duration is excluded then regurgitation is present in only 6% to 8% of normal children (50,51). The short duration tricuspid regurgitation is attributed to the dynamics of valve closure. Short duration has been defined as duration of less than 0.5 systole (50) or less than 100 ms (51) on CW Doppler. Transient tricuspid regurgitation has been reported in the newborn (54,55).

The typical velocity curve in physiologic tricuspid regurgitation has a rapid upstroke that starts in early systole, immediately after closure of the tricuspid valve. Regurgitation is holosystolic; however, due to cardiac motion and the relatively weak Doppler signal intensity, frequently it is only recorded during early systole (Echo. 6-12).

Pulmonary insufficiency has been found in 22% to 84%

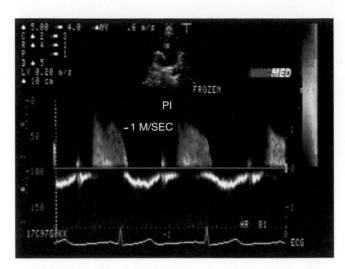

ECHO. 6-13. Example of a typical spectral velocity waveform of physiologic pulmonic valve regurgitation. There is a rapid early diastolic acceleration phase with a slower deceleration phase lasting throughout diastole. The velocity signal generally remains above the baseline until the opening of the valve marking the beginning of systole. The end diastolic velocity (1 m/s) can be used to estimate pressure gradient between the right ventricle and pulmonary artery. *PI*, pulmonary insufficiency.

of children with normal hearts (50,51). The prevalence of pulmonic regurgitation appears to increase with age in childhood (51). Interestingly, in adults the prevalence decreases with age (47).

The velocity curve of physiologic pulmonic valve regurgitation has a characteristic shape demonstrating rapid, early diastolic acceleration and a slower deceleration that lasts throughout diastole and remains above the baseline until the opening of the valve marking the beginning of systole (Echo. 6-13).

Mitral and Aortic Insufficiency

Mitral insufficiency has been found in 2% of children with normal hearts (51). Transient mitral regurgitation has also been reported in the newborn.

Aortic insufficiency has not been found in children (51) and adults (47) with normal hearts.

QUANTITATIVE DOPPLER TOOLS: GENERAL CONCEPTS

Flow Measurement

Fundamental Concepts

The fundamental concept in using Doppler to quantify blood flow is based on the principle of determining flow rate (FR) through a specified surface. Consider that any

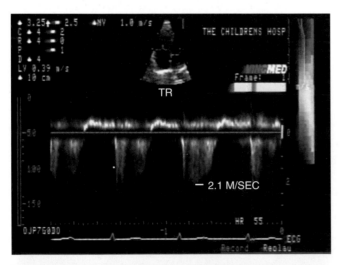

ECHO. 6-12. Example of typical spectral velocity waveform of physiologic tricuspid valve regurgitation. The regurgitation is holosystolic; however, frequently it is only recorded during early systole. The signal has a rapid upstroke in early systole. *TR*, tricuspid regurgitation.

surface can be divided into infinitesimally small surfaces, each called "dA." Fluid mechanics principles teach us that instantaneous flow rate (dIFR) through each incremental surface dA is equal to the normal velocity times its surface area (Fig. 6-2). The normal velocity is the magnitude of the velocity vector that is normal (or in two dimensions, perpendicular) to the incremental surface dA. The instantaneous flow rate through an entire surface is the sum (or more accurately integral) of all of the incremental instantaneous flow rates (dIFRs) through all infinitesimally small surface areas (dAs) making up the specified surface.

In many instances, overall (or average) flow rate over time (e.g., cardiac output) is more useful to clinicians than instantaneous flow rates. Therefore, the TAV (Eq. 1) is used in the equations to obtain overall flow rate (Echo. 6-4).

Traditional Flow Measurement Methods

Traditionally, flow rates have been calculated (5,56–91) taking a cross-section of a chamber/vessel as the measurement surface and assuming this cross-sectional surface is represented by a flat circular disk. In addition, this method assumes the velocity profile throughout this surface is uniform (i.e., velocities all along the cross-sectional surface are equal in magnitude and pointed uniformly directly downstream). With these assumptions calculating flow rate simplifies to cross-sectional area of a disk of radius r multiplied by the TAV (Eq. 1) measured in the chamber/vessel:

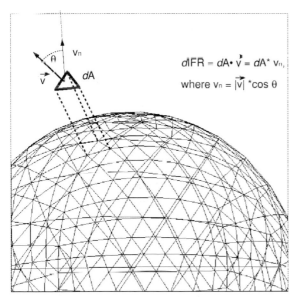

$$dIFR = dA \cdot \vec{v} = dA * v_n,$$
where $v_n = |\vec{v}| * \cos\theta$

FIG. 6-2. Demonstration of the concept of measuring flow rate through a surface by dividing that surface into infinitesimally small surfaces, each called "dA." dIFR through each incremental surface (dA) is equal to the component of the velocity (V) normal to that surface (V_n) times its surface area (dA).

$$FR = TAV * \pi r^2. \qquad [2]$$

The radius of the vessel r can be determined from either two-dimensional or M-mode images of the vessel itself, where r equals one half the measured diameter of the vessel. Stroke volume (SV) is easily determined using the VTI and cross-sectional area:

$$SV = VTI * \pi r^2. \qquad [3]$$

In clinical settings, this traditional method of measuring flow rate has proven to be useful but prone to errors (5,61,78–80,92). One source of error is that the chamber/vessel where flow is being measured may not be a cylinder. Another source of error is that velocities may not be uniform throughout the chosen cross-sectional surface of the chamber/vessel where flow is being measured (5,9,92–95). A third source of error is in measuring the chamber/vessel radius where this measurement on two-dimensional images is sometimes an approximation at best. Errors in this measurement are amplified in the flow rate equation since radius is squared (r^2). Also the vessel radius usually changes throughout the heart cycle (5,96). As an example the aortic diameter has been reported to change by as much as 10% (5).

A fourth source of error involves the fact that the spectral velocity signal may not represent a precise sample of backscattering particles (red blood cells) in the blood flow stream. This will be discussed in more detail in the section on power mode imaging methods.

Newer Flow Measurement Methods

Fundamental Concepts

It is impossible to accurately measure velocities throughout the surface of a flat circular disk using current Doppler technology since Doppler flow imaging only allows for the accurate measurement of velocity vectors parallel to the Doppler beam. Newer techniques using standard two-dimensional echocardiography do not use the assumed surface of a flat circular disk as the flow measurement surface to measure flow rate (97,98). In order to understand how these methods work, the concepts of a control volume and conservation of mass need to be introduced (99).

A control volume is an arbitrary volume in space through which fluid flows. The control surface is the geometric boundary of the control volume (Fig. 6-3). Assuming blood has constant density, conservation of mass dictates that the net rate of mass flow (mass flux) out of the control surface is zero (i.e., mass is neither created nor destroyed inside the control volume). Another way to put this is simply "what goes in must come out." If one assumes that all flow through the portion of the control surface we select as the flow measurement surface (inflow

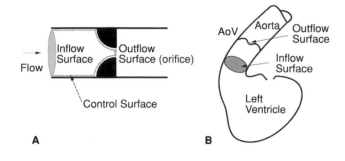

A

B

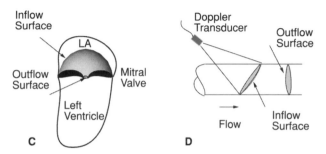

C

D

FIG. 6-3. Example of control volumes, control surfaces, and flow measurement surfaces. A control volume is any arbitrary volume drawn in space where the control surface is the geometric boundary of the control volume. **A:** An example of a control surface drawn around an orifice, where two parts of a control surface are shown (inflow surface and outflow surface). Examples of inflow and outflow surfaces are shown through the left ventricular outflow tract and the aortic valve **(B)**; through the mitral valve during ventricular filling **(C)**; and through a vessel with the inflow surface the "shape" of a Doppler signal fan **(D)**. LA, left atrium; *AoV,* aortic valve.

surface) is directed into the control volume and all flow out of the portion of the control surface we select as the outflow surface is directed outward, then the flow rate into the inflow surface must equal the flow rate out of the outflow surface (Fig. 6-3). Thus, flow rate can be derived from any arbitrarily drawn, irregularly shaped surface. Calculating flow rate through one of these surfaces is performed as described above, where the normal component of the velocity vector is multiplied by an incremental surface area and summed (or integrated) over the entire surface of interest.

Angle-Independent Two-Dimensional Flow Method

Due to the angle dependence of Doppler techniques it is virtually impossible to determine the normal component of the velocity vectors along most surfaces. However, this is possible if a flow measurement surface is chosen such that all points on the surface have equal distance from the Doppler transducer as in the example of where the surface becomes the surface of the ice cream in an ice cream cone (Fig. 6-3D). With this, Doppler measured velocity magnitudes along this surface are precisely the

magnitude of the component of the velocity vectors normal to its surface. Assuming that all flow through that surface is in the direction of the flow of interest (i.e., no recirculatory flow patterns), then one simply has to sum the incremental surface areas multiplied by their respective Doppler measured velocity to calculate flow rate (Fig. 6-4). These methods have shown promising initial results (97,98).

Automatic Cardiac Output Measurement

One recent attempt at improving the accuracy of flow rate measurements has been to sample velocities along an arc section (two-dimensional equivalent of a three-dimensional cone surface) of the chamber/vessel in space and time, giving space- and time-averaged velocities (STAVs) along discrete arc segments (Fig. 6-5). This method has been termed automatic cardiac output measurement (ACOM) (100–105). The discrete arc segments are then revolved 180 degrees in space (RS_{SAi} = surface area of 180-degree revolved arc segment) to make up an assumed three-dimensional STAV profile (Fig. 6-5). Flow rate is calculated as:

$$\text{Flow Rate} = \Sigma \ RS_{SAi} * STAV_i, \ i = 1, \ . \ . \ ., n \quad [4]$$

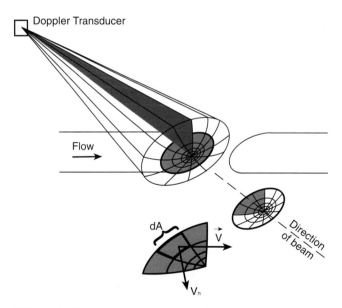

FIG. 6-4. Schematic diagram of a flow measurement surface created using a 180-degree rotation of equidistant scan planes giving a surface where all points on the surface have equal distance from the Doppler transducer. The Doppler measured velocity magnitudes along this surface are precisely the magnitude of the component of the velocity vector ($\vec{V}$) normal to its surface (V_n) as shown. Flow rate through the entire surface can be estimated by simply summing the incremental surface areas (dA) multiplied by their respective Doppler measured velocities (V_n).

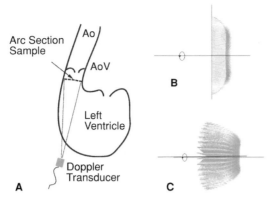

FIG. 6-5. ACOM method of estimating flow rate. **A:** Velocities are sampled along an arc section (two-dimensional equivalent of a three-dimensional cone surface) of the chamber/vessel in space and time giving STAVs along discrete arc segments. **B:** A discrete arc segment with velocity vectors shown. **C:** Arc segment is revolved 180 degrees in space to make up an assumed three-dimensional STAV profile. *Ao*, aorta; *AoV*, aortic valve.

where n = total number of discrete arc segments; RS_{SAi} = $\pi * radius_i * d$; and d = distance between segments.

Velocities measured along an arc section through the vessel are perpendicular to that arc section allowing for angle independence of velocity measurements normal to the flow surface as described above. Revolving the discrete arc segments to form the flow measurement surface is angle-dependent, however, and the flow rate equation above must be modified to account for this. This work is still in progress.

ACOM assumes the 180-degree revolution of discrete arc segments gives a close estimation of the three-dimensional flow velocity profile. Flows in most physiologic chambers/vessels do not generally have this level of symmetry (5,9,92–95) but this may well be a close approximation. ACOM has shown promising preliminary results (100–105).

Flow Convergence Method

Flow convergence methods (FCMs) were first introduced (106) after the observation was made that flow approaching a theoretic infinitesimally small orifice accelerates symmetrically, producing isovelocity surfaces that are hemispheric in shape. Isovelocity surfaces could be visualized in physiologic orifices as color Doppler aliasing hemicircular concentric rings (Echo. 6-14; see color plate 3 following p. 364). Since these color Doppler aliased hemicircular rings could be easily visualized and measured and the value of the velocity along the surface was known (i.e., the aliasing velocity or Nyquist limit) then one could use this as the inflow measurement surface described previously (Fig. 6-3C) to estimate flow rate

through an orifice. Assuming the isovelocity surface is a hemisphere and the magnitude of the isovelocity ($V_{isovelocity}$) along the inflow hemispheric surface measured by color Doppler is the magnitude of the velocity vector perpendicular to all portions of its entire surface, then IFR is simply:

$$IFR = 2\pi r^2 * V_{isovelocity},\qquad [5]$$

where r is the radius of the hemisphere and $2\pi r^2$ is the surface area of a hemisphere.

Unfortunately, the hemispheric flow convergence method is only an approximation to flow for several reasons (107). The first source of error occurs when dealing with physiologic finitely sized orifices rather than theoretic infinitesimally small orifices. The isovelocity surfaces near finitely sized orifices are nonhemispherical in shape (108–115), rather they are flattened hemispheres close to the orifice due to the effect of the finite size of the orifice. On the other hand, far from the orifice the isovelocity surfaces are elliptically shaped due to surrounding wall constraints. Assuming all isovelocity surfaces are hemispherical in shape leads to underestimation of flow rate too close to the orifice and overestimation of flow rate too far from the orifice.

Somewhere in the middle of this overestimation and underestimation, there is a "sweet spot" where the isovelocity contours are nearly hemispherical and the hemispherical flow convergence method are most accurate. Empirical studies have shown that this is somewhere between 1 to 2 orifice diameters distance from the orifice (114,116). However, one does not know the orifice diameter *a priori*; in fact, it is one of the indices of severity clinically sought. Thus, investigators have begun to de-

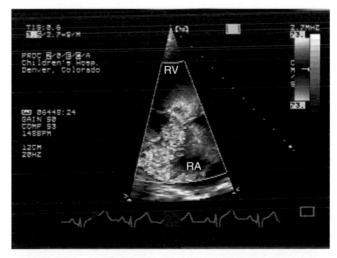

ECHO. 6-14. Color Doppler flow image of flow convergence region with isovelocity surfaces visualized as aliasing hemicircular concentric rings shown here on the right ventricular side of the tricuspid valve. *RV*, right ventricle; *RA*, right atrium.

velop methods to find the "sweet spot" based, among other things, on the spatial derivative of velocity in the flow convergence region and pressure gradients (109–111,117,118). Whether these refined methods will be useful clinically has not yet been determined.

In methods that attempt to measure the surface areas of the actual isovelocity contours using multiple two-dimensional planes (117) or three-dimensional color flow imaging (119), two additional errors are introduced. The angle dependence of color Doppler distorts the shape of the actual isovelocity surface (7) leading to measurement errors. Secondly, when dealing with finitely sized orifices and nonhemispherically shaped isovelocity contours, the magnitude of the isovelocity v is not equal to the magnitude of the component of the velocity vector normal (or perpendicular in two dimensions) to the isovelocity surface (Fig. 6-6; see color plate 4 following p. 364) (112,114,120). As we have discussed only the component of the velocity vector normal to the isovelocity surface should be used in the control volume calculation of flow rate (Fig. 6-2). This effect tends to cause overestimation of flow rates (114,120).

Modifications to the flow convergence method have been proposed when considering constrained orifices (109,113–115,121,122). Constrained orifices are those where the surrounding boundaries are at less than a 180-degree angle with the orifice (Fig. 6-7). Instead of a hemisphere, the isovelocity surface is the surface of a cone and IFR becomes:

$$\text{IFR}_\alpha = 2\pi r^2 \frac{\alpha}{180} * V_{\text{isovelocity}} \qquad [6]$$

where α = constraining angle.

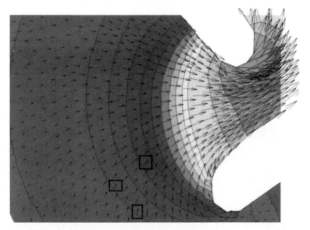

FIG. 6-6. Example of velocity vectors and an isovelocity surface in the flow convergence region of a finitely sized orifice. Note the velocity vectors are not normal **(boxes)** to the isovelocity surface. Only the component of the velocity vector normal to the isovelocity surface should be used in the control volume calculation of flow rate.

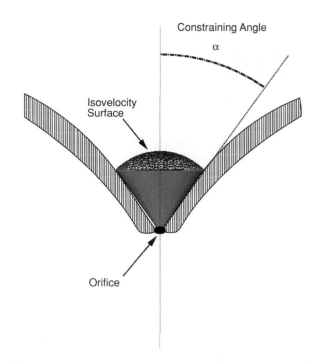

FIG. 6-7. Example of a constrained orifice and the modification of the hemispheric flow convergence method. The isovelocity surface becomes the surface of a cone instead of a hemisphere with constraining angle shown (α). See text for details.

Three-Dimensional Echocardiography

Three-dimensional echocardiography (123) color Doppler flow imaging (119,124,125) offers great potential in accurate volumetric flow quantitation. With this technique, true three-dimensional space and time velocity measurements can be implemented along with techniques that use the angle dependencies of Doppler sampling to their advantage (97,98) in defining specified surfaces where normal velocity vectors are accurately measured.

Power Mode Imaging

As discussed earlier, a source of error when using the spectral velocity signal for flow rates involves the fact that the spectral velocity signal may not represent a precise sample of backscattering particles (red blood cells) in the blood flow stream. Spectral velocity gives equal weight to velocity (frequency shift) signals coming from various volumes of red blood cells. Power-weighted and amplitude-weighted velocities (power mode) have been used with some success (126–128) to account for this phenomenon. In these methods, each velocity is weighted for the power or amplitude of that velocity, and thus weighted to the volume of red blood cells giving rise to that specific velocity (126). This method still depends on an accurate measurement of vessel radius. In addition,

Bascom et al. (129) have shown the backscatter power may not always be proportional to the actual volume of red blood cells.

Although this method has been used in the past (130,131), it is not currently used routinely in the clinical setting. Nonetheless, it may be incorporated into future algorithms.

Cardiac Output

Cardiac output can be measured by Doppler techniques at several locations in the heart. Traditionally the aorta has been used; however, flow rates through the pulmonary, tricuspid, and mitral valves have been measured using these Doppler techniques.

Left Ventricular Outflow Tract and Aorta

Cardiac output in adults has been traditionally measured using a cross-section of the aorta at various locations (5,59,64–83,132) including the left ventricular outflow tract, aortic annulus, and ascending aorta (Echo. 6-15). With the assumptions of this method, calculating cardiac output (CO) simplifies to surface area of a disk of radius r (cm) multiplied by the TAV (cm/s) measured in the left ventricular outflow tract or aorta:

$$CO\ (L/min) = TAV * \pi r^2 * \frac{60\ s/min}{1{,}000\ cm^3/L}. \quad [7]$$

The radius of the LVOT or aorta can be determined from either two-dimensional or M-mode images, where radius equals one half the measured diameter of the vessel (Echo. 6-15).

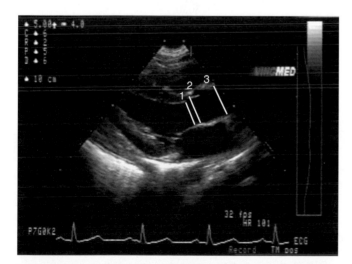

ECHO. 6-15. Locations traditionally used in the calculation of cardiac output, including the left ventricular outflow tract (1), aortic annulus (2), and ascending aorta (3).

Overall results from these studies show good correlations to the Fick and thermodilution methods for measuring cardiac output ($r = 0.83$ to 0.97). Studies in children (57,84–91,133) show similar results when compared to the Fick or thermodilution methods ($r = 0.86$ to 0.99).

We have already discussed sources of error using this method. Reviewing briefly: (a) the cross-section of the vessel where flow is being measured may not be represented well by the surface of a round flat disc; (b) velocities may not be uniform throughout the chosen cross-sectional surface of the chamber/vessel where flow is being measured (5,9,92–95); (c) the vessel radius is sometimes difficult to measure and changes throughout the heart cycle (5,96).

Variations in results in the clinical studies mentioned also depend on the varying reliability of different sites of measurements of aortic dimensions as well as different sites of Doppler velocity measurements. Some of these studies used CW Doppler of the ascending aorta and assumed the velocities obtained by CW Doppler are always from the narrowest portion of the aorta (at the aortic annulus) (65,68,69,84,88). Whether the highest velocities in the outflow tract and ascending aorta are always at the aortic annulus throughout the cardiac cycle may not always hold. Many of these studies measured the diameter of the aorta or outflow tract at one place and measured Doppler velocities at another. In addition, some of the early studies in adults and children, with technology available at that time, used blind PW Doppler (59,85,86,90,91).

For many of the reasons mentioned, this method of estimating cardiac output is not in favor universally (74,75). As Nanda (75) states, "The clinical utility for absolute measurements must be viewed with some reservation at present." Considering all of the above, this technique may not have received a fair assessment with the capabilities of current technology including HPRF Doppler and improved two-dimensional image quality. As Sahn (134) states, "If echocardiographers expect less than a 15% variability in a Doppler method for cardiac output applicable to a wide range of patients, . . ., they will need to give meticulous attention to detail, especially regarding the determination of flow area." Whether studies have been performed with today's technology and with that kind of attention is in question.

Mitral Valve

Calculating cardiac output through the mitral valve poses unique problems as studies have shown in adults (56,60–64,72,134–136) and children (137). The mitral valve is not circular and the shape of the valve changes throughout the flow period making it difficult to obtain an accurate cross-sectional area of flow.

Improved results have been shown experimentally assuming an elliptically shaped orifice (136). The mean mitral valve orifice area measured by planimetry of mitral valve M-mode images has been used (56,60). A more elaborate system has been proposed (62) that tracks the short axis dimensions of the mitral valve (assuming the long axis changes minimally) and integrates that with the instantaneous mitral valve velocities. Overall, these latter methods are not in routine clinical use, which may be partly due to how cumbersome they are.

Pulmonary Artery

Pulmonary blood flow can be measured using the same principles as the methods above (57,58,76,77,81,135, 138–142). In adults and some children it is sometimes difficult to visualize the walls of the pulmonary artery to measure its radius. Nonetheless, reported results have been fairly accurate when compared to invasive measures ($r = 0.72$ to 0.88) (57,139). With the capabilities of today's current echocardiographic technology including HPRF Doppler and improved two-dimensional image quality one would expect even better results than those published previously.

Tricuspid Valve

Blood flow through the tricuspid valve has been used to calculate cardiac output (63,135,142). Tricuspid diameter was measured as the distance from the anterior right ventricular endocardium to the septal endocardium at the level of insertion of the tricuspid valve leaflets. Excellent but limited clinical results have been reported in children ($r = 0.98$) (63) when compared to standard invasive measures.

Shunt Calculations and Regurgitant Volumes

The above flow rate methods allow for estimation of flow rates in more than one site of the heart allowing for calculations of cardiac shunt flow (138–147) and regurgitant flow rates.

Calculating Shunts

Once pulmonary blood flow rate (Qp) and a systemic blood flow rate (Qs) are determined, a shunt ratio can be calculated (Qp/Qs). One of the main drawbacks of this technique is that calculating flows by Doppler methods gives approximations and dividing one approximation by a second approximation tends to amplify errors introduced by the Doppler flow methods. However, the techniques have been shown to have acceptable results (139,140,142–144). The sites chosen to calculate flow volumes for a specific shunt flow calculation depend on the level of the shunt as described below.

Atrial Level Shunts

With atrial level shunts, the pulmonary or tricuspid valve flow is used to calculate pulmonary blood flow and the mitral or aortic flow is used to calculate systemic blood flow.

Ventricular Level Shunts

In ventricular level shunts various methods have been used including calculating the pulmonary blood flow from the pulmonary or mitral valves and the systemic blood flow from the aortic or tricuspid valves. A technique described by Teien (143) involves determining the volume flow through the ventricular septal defect by measuring the defect and the mean velocity determined from the CW Doppler trace of the ventricular septal defect (which assumes a round orifice with a uniform velocity profile through it). This volume flow was added to the aortic flow (systemic flow) to estimate the pulmonary blood flow. This approach had the best correlation with catheterization data of all methods mentioned (142).

Systemic to Pulmonary Artery Shunts

To calculate volume flows through a systemic to pulmonary artery shunt such as a patent ductus arteriosus, pulmonary blood flow can be calculated from the mitral or aortic valves and systemic blood flow can be calculated from the tricuspid valve.

Regurgitant Volumes and Regurgitant Fraction

To obtain regurgitant volume and regurgitant fraction (RF) (148–150), the stroke volume (Eq. 3) is measured at the regurgitant valve ($SV_{regurgitant\ valve}$) and at a valve where there is no regurgitation ($SV_{reference}$) (151). Regurgitant stroke volume (RSV) is given as:

$$RSV = SV_{regurgitant\ valve} - SV_{reference}. \qquad [8]$$

and RF can be calculated:

$$RF = \frac{RSV}{SV_{regurgitant\ valve}}. \qquad [9]$$

The methods described are derived from Doppler stroke volumes that have their own inherent inaccuracies. These methods then perform subtraction and division of stroke volumes, which in many cases can magnify such inaccuracies manyfold.

Pressure Gradients between Chambers: The Bernoulli Equation

Determining the pressure gradient between two chambers is an important tool in the echocardiographer's armamentarium. This tool allows for quantitating the severity of obstructive lesions (e.g., aortic stenosis) as well as determining pressures between various cardiac chambers (e.g., estimating right ventricular pressure using the tricuspid regurgitant jet or the ventricular septal defect jet velocity). Specific lesions will be discussed later. This discussion is of the general concepts involved in using the Bernoulli equation to estimate pressure gradients between chambers of the cardiovascular system.

Theoretic Considerations

A modification to the standard Bernoulli equation (99) is often used in the assessment of pressure gradient (5,152–160). In order to understand the limitations of what has been called the modified Bernoulli equation, which is used in clinical echocardiographic practice, one has to understand the assumptions made in its derivation. The standard Bernoulli equation applies to the situation of (a) steady flow; (b) incompressible flow; (c) frictionless flow; and (d) measuring pressure gradient along a streamline. Streamlines are lines drawn in a flow field such that they are always tangent (parallel) to the direction of flow at every point in the flow field (Fig. 6-8). The Bernoulli equation is as follows:

$$\Delta P = \frac{\rho}{2} \times (V_2^2 - V_1^2) \qquad [10]$$

where ΔP = pressure at point 2 − pressure at point 1; ρ = density of blood; V_2 = velocity at point 2; V_1 = velocity at point 1.

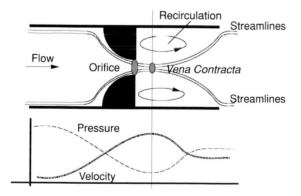

FIG. 6-8. Streamlines through an orifice. Streamlines are lines drawn in a flow field such that they are always tangent (parallel) to the direction of flow. The *vena contracta* represents a contraction in the edges of the flow streamlines as they move through an orifice. Graphs show the velocity and pressure magnitude along the centerline.

Normal blood flow is unsteady (i.e., pulsatile) and is viscous (i.e., not without friction); thus, the standard Bernoulli equation does not apply, and the "viscous unsteady" Bernoulli equation needs to be adopted. The "viscous unsteady" Bernoulli equation for flow along a streamline is (5):

$$\Delta P = \frac{\rho}{2} \times (V_2^2 - V_1^2) + \rho \int_1^2 \delta \, (V_s/(\delta t \, d_s + R\vec{V})) \qquad [11]$$

or

$$\Delta P = \text{convective acceleration} + \text{local acceleration}$$
$$+ \text{ viscous friction,} \qquad [12]$$

where V_s = velocity along streamline; d_s = incremental distance along streamline; $R(\vec{V})$ = viscous friction as a function of the vector velocity.

Convective acceleration refers to a particle being convected ("pushed") into a region of higher or lower velocity, which can occur in steady and unsteady flow (99). Local acceleration occurs because the velocity field is a function of time (99).

Local acceleration usually only becomes significant during the initial and final part of systole, where there is significant flow acceleration. If local acceleration is ignored, the pressure drop calculated using the Bernoulli equation is delayed in time during periods of significant acceleration (5). This delay is negligible in most clinical settings (5).

Viscous friction $R(\vec{V})$ forces, if neglected, cause underestimation of pressure drop (5) in (a) very small diameter orifices and/or in low-flow velocity states; and (b) long-segment and/or multiple obstructions where viscous forces become important.

What we call the simplified echo Bernoulli equation (5,30) used in clinical settings neglects local acceleration and viscous forces, leading to errors as described. As we will discuss subsequently for each specific lesion, errors within many clinical settings are quite acceptable.

The term "$\rho/2$" for blood is approximately equal to 4. The simplified echo Bernoulli equation thus becomes:

$$\Delta P = 4(V_2^2 - V_1^2). \qquad [13]$$

In many clinical settings, the velocity at point 1 (V_1) is much less (less than 1.5 m/s) (30) than at point 2 (V_2); thus, the simplified echo Bernoulli equation can be expressed as:

$$\Delta P = 4V_2^2. \qquad [14]$$

Peak Pressure Gradients

Often, the Doppler pressure gradient measured using the simplified echo Bernoulli equation is compared to the pressure gradient measured during cardiac catheterization. These two methods measure different pressure gradients (161–167) in space and time as we discuss later.

Measurement Differences in the Space Domain

In order to understand the measurement discrepancy in space one needs to understand the flow dynamics around a stenotic orifice (99). Figure 6-8 shows streamlines of flow through a stenotic orifice. As discussed, streamlines are lines drawn in a flow field such that they are always tangent (parallel) to the direction of flow. The *vena contracta* represents a contraction in the edges of the flow streamlines as they move through an orifice (99,160). For orifices without a smoothly tapering proximal geometry, inertia prevents proximal streamlines entering from the side from changing direction instantly; in this region, these streamlines are directed almost perpendicular to the general flow direction. As the flow passes through the orifice, the streamlines change direction to run parallel to the main flow direction but not before "squeezing" the main flow and causing a constriction in the cross-sectional area of flow immediately distal to the orifice. The mechanism that causes this reduction in distal flow area has been termed the *vena contracta* effect (99,160). Flow separation just distal to the orifice causes a recirculation zone to form. Through the middle of the recirculation zone the mainstream "fresh" flow continues to accelerate from the orifice to its highest magnitude presumably where the cross-sectional area of the mainstream flow is narrowest (i.e., at the *vena contracta*). Past the *vena contracta*, blood then decelerates again to fill the vessel.

The pressure along the centerline of blood flow is lowest at the *vena contracta* and then rises toward its original pressure (the pressure proximal to the orifice) further downstream. This is called pressure recovery (99,161,162,164–169). The amount of pressure recovery depends on the Reynolds number (161,164,165) and the shape of the orifice (99,161,162,170). The Reynolds number (RE_{number}) is a dimensionless quantity representing the ratio of inertial (momentum) forces to viscous (friction) forces:

$$RE_{number} = \frac{\rho V d}{\mu}, \qquad [15]$$

where ρ = density; V = velocity; d = diameter, and μ = viscosity.

At very low and very high Reynolds numbers (e.g., low and high velocities), the pressure recovery is not as significant (164,165) as at moderate Reynolds numbers (e.g., moderate velocities). At low Reynolds numbers this is due to the viscous (friction) forces being dominant and at high Reynolds numbers this is felt to be due to turbulence effects (164). Work is in progress (165) to define the "moderate" range of Reynolds numbers where pressure recovery is most significant in various clinical settings.

Since in most clinical settings the Reynolds number

may be in this "moderate" range, one can immediately see that the only way to measure maximum pressure drop across a stenotic orifice with a catheter is to have the catheter positioned exactly at the *vena contracta*, which is practically impossible. Thus, the catheter technique is measuring pressure gradients between two different points in space than the Doppler technique. When pressure recovery is prominent the catheter technique underestimates maximal pressure gradients.

The amount of pressure recovery not only depends on the Reynolds number, it also depends on the shape of the orifice (99,162). An orifice with a sharp edge will have flow in the turbulent range at much lower velocities than a same sized orifice with a smooth taper to it, thus causing pressure recovery differences between the two orifices. Quantitating just how much the shape of the orifice affects pressure recovery is beyond the scope of this text.

Measurement Differences in the Time Domain

Figure 6-9 depicts the difference in pressure gradients regarding timing for measurements made using Doppler and catheter techniques. Typical reported catheter pressure gradient measurements are the peak-to-peak pressure gradients ($\Delta P_{peak-to-peak}$); that is, the difference between the highest pressure in the proximal chamber subtracted from the highest pressure in the distal chamber, regardless of the timing of the two peaks. Doppler, on the other hand, measures the peak instantaneous pressure gradient ($\Delta P_{peak\ instantaneous}$) between the two chambers, which may not correlate with the peak-to-peak pressure gradient since the peak pressures in the two chambers may occur at different points in time. The peak instantaneous pressure gradient is in many instances higher than the peak-to-peak pressure gradient.

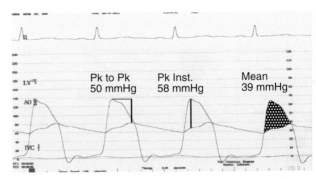

FIG. 6-9. Difference in various pressure gradients regarding timing for measurements using Doppler and catheterization techniques. Doppler measurements are typically recorded as peak instantaneous (Pk Inst) pressure gradients. Catheterization measurements are typically recorded as peak-to-peak (Pk to Pk) pressure gradients. Determination of mean pressure gradient (Mean) from catheterization pressure tracings is also shown. The catheter mean gradient is the area between the two pressure tracing curves divided by the ejection time.

It is possible to measure the peak instantaneous pressure gradient in the catheterization laboratory. It is important to remember, however, that this is different from the Doppler peak instantaneous pressure gradient since the catheter is usually distal to the *vena contracta* (see "Measurement Differences in the Space Domain"). For accuracy, measurement of the peak instantaneous pressure gradient in the catheterization laboratory usually requires simultaneous catheters in two chambers of the heart, which may not be appropriate or cost-effective in many clinical studies. Further, most protocols indicating the appropriate timing for intervention are based on the value of the peak-to-peak pressure gradient. As such, new studies would be required to adjust the protocols to peak instantaneous pressure gradient.

Total Measurement Differences

Thus, there is an overall "balance" of measurement differences when comparing the Doppler and the catheter pressure gradient measurement techniques. Timing (peak-to-peak versus instantaneous peak) and pressure recovery tend to cause the Doppler peak instantaneous pressure gradient to be higher than the catheter peak-to-peak pressure gradient. Viscous forces and local acceleration effects, on the other hand, tend to cause the Doppler peak instantaneous pressure gradient to be less than the catheter peak-to-peak pressure gradient. Different hemodynamic states (i.e., changes in cardiac output → changes in velocities → changes in Reynolds number) change the "balance" of these measurement differences (164), and work is in progress to define these changes (165) in various clinical settings.

Mean Pressure Gradient

In an attempt to find Doppler and catheterization methods that would more closely correlate, investigators have used mean pressure gradients. Theoretically, averaging over an entire ejection phase incorporates underestimation effects at the beginning and end of the ejection phase where the Reynolds number is low, therefore cancelling some of the overestimation effects of Doppler measured pressure gradients seen at high flow rates (midejection phase) when compared to catheter measured pressure gradients (164). Also, averaging over an entire ejection phase removes the issue of peak-to-peak versus peak instantaneous pressure gradient differences.

Figure 6-9 outlines how the mean gradient (ΔP_{mean}) is calculated using catheterization pressure measurements. The catheter mean pressure gradient is the area between the two pressure curves throughout the ejection phase

divided by the ejection time (ET). Figure 6-10 outlines how the mean pressure gradient is determined with the Doppler technique and the Bernoulli equation. The area under the velocity squared ($4V^2$) curve must be measured throughout the ejection phase and the average gradient obtained dividing this area by ET:

$$\text{Doppler } \Delta P_{mean} = \frac{\int_o^{ET} 4V^2 dt}{ET} \qquad [16]$$

where ET = duration of velocity envelope. Less precisely, one can sum individual incremental pressure gradients along the Doppler velocity curve and obtain an average:

$$\text{Doppler } \Delta P_{mean} \approx \Sigma \Delta P_i/n \qquad [17]$$

where i = 1, 2, 3, . . ., n (n = number of samples along velocity curve), and

$$\Delta P_i = 4(V_{2i}^2 - V_{1i}^2). \qquad [18]$$

Mean pressure gradients between the Doppler and catheterization methods have shown improved correlation in certain clinical situations (163,165,171).

Other Bernoulli-Like Equations

Investigators have introduced the concept of a "loss coefficient" *(K)* in another modification to the Bernoulli equation (172):

$$\Delta P = K(V_2^2 - V_1^2) \qquad [19]$$

The loss coefficient is determined empirically in *in vitro* experiments and applied to clinical situations (in this case, using magnetic resonance imaging) with similar relative dimensions and flow rates. The loss coefficient is set up to compensate for the errors introduced when disregarding local acceleration, viscous forces, and Reynolds number-

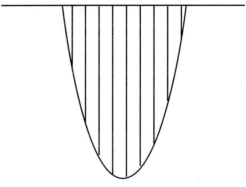

FIG. 6-10. Determination of mean pressure gradient (ΔP_{mean}) from Doppler spectral velocity waveforms. To determine the Doppler mean gradient, the area between the velocity curves is not used. Instead one has to measure the area between the two "velocity squared" ($4 * velocity^2$) curves. See text for details.

related pressure recovery. Though this method provides a practical way to compensate for these errors and may become quite useful clinically, there is a danger this could be misinterpreted as an analytical rather than an empirical method and lead one away from the basic fluid dynamic principles of the flow problem.

Statistical Comparison between Doppler and Catheter Pressure Gradients

Most of the studies that are quoted for various lesions use linear regression analysis to demonstrate agreement between Doppler and catheterization methods. Weiss (173) points out linear analysis gives little information about the agreement between two methods measuring the same variable. Use of linear analysis is quite valid in all of these studies since Doppler and catheterization pressure gradient measuring methods never really measure the same variable so all the authors are attempting to demonstrate with linear analysis is a consistent relationship between two variables. As we have discussed, Doppler and catheterization methods are measuring two inherently different variables, even, when measuring and comparing the Doppler and catheter mean pressure gradients or the Doppler peak instantaneous and the catheter peak-to-peak pressure gradient.

Valve Areas

The impetus for assessing valve areas arose from the fact that pressure gradients across valves are flow-dependent (77). It was initially felt that calculation of valve area with these methods would be a flow-independent parameter, thus not dependent on the patient's cardiovascular status at the time of the study. A major problem with all of these Doppler methods is that there is no real gold standard measurement of valve area available for comparison. Even the Gorlin and Gorlin formula used in the catheterization laboratory (174) to estimate valve area is itself flow-dependent (175–178).

Doppler Continuity Equation

Originally a modified form of the Gorlin and Gorlin formula was used in the Doppler quantification of valve areas (179). The continuity equation was introduced (180) as an alternative Doppler method to estimate valve areas and since then has become quite popular in use.

The continuity equation is derived from control volume theory (99). To reiterate, a control volume is an arbitrary volume in space through which fluid flows. The control surface is the geometric boundary of the control volume. Assuming blood has constant density, conservation of mass dictates that what goes in must come out. In calculating valve area, the following conditions are set: (a) a

control volume is drawn such that it contains only two portions where flow is crossing its surface; (b) one of those portions is an area where flow volume can be measured easily, and the other portion is the area where one is interested in measuring the valve area (Fig. 6-3B). Methods for calculating flow rate through a surface have been discussed earlier in this chapter (Fig. 6-2). The continuity equation is derived from the concept of conservation of mass and can be expressed as:

$$\text{Flow Rate}_{\text{inflow surface}} = \text{Flow Rate}_{\text{outflow surface}} . \quad [20]$$

As we have discussed, assuming a flat uniform velocity profile through the valve orifice and at the reference flow location, flow rate is given as shown in Eq. 2, where TAV is as in Eq. 1 and $\text{Area}_{\text{surface}} = \pi r^2$ (r is the radius of the cross-sectional area where flow is being measured).

Theoretically, since stroke volume is not exactly the same with each heartbeat, these two flow rates need to be measured simultaneously for the most accurate results. Since this is not clinically practical, attempts should be made to either use time-averaged velocities from Doppler velocity waveforms having similar RR intervals or obtain averages for both.

The Doppler continuity equation for valve area becomes:

$$\text{Area}_{\text{valve}} = \text{Area}_{\text{reference flow}} * \frac{\text{TAV}_{\text{reference flow}}}{\text{TAV}_{\text{valve}}} . \quad [21]$$

Similarly, substituting the VTI (Eq. 1), the Doppler continuity equation can be written as follows:

$$\text{Area}_{\text{valve}} = \text{Area}_{\text{reference flow}} * \frac{\text{VTI}_{\text{reference flow}}}{\text{VTI}_{\text{valve}}} . \quad [22]$$

It is likely for many stenotic valves that the valve area changes during the ejection period so the above equations give an average valve area. Peak velocities can be used in the equation to obtain a peak flow valve area. This assumes the peak velocities (V_{peak}) in the two areas of flow being measured occur simultaneously. The Doppler continuity equation then becomes:

Peak Area$_{\text{valve}}$

$$= \text{Area}_{\text{reference flow}} * \frac{V_{\text{peak − reference flow}}}{V_{\text{peak − valve}}} . \quad [23]$$

Generally, the CW Doppler sample through the valve is used to acquire the TAV, the VTI, and the peak velocity through the valve. CW Doppler measures the highest velocity, which is assumed to be at the *vena contracta* and not at the valve itself. Thus, the Doppler valve area calculated is not exactly the actual anatomic area, which is what the Gorlin and Gorlin formula attempts to measure. Rather, the Doppler method using the continuity equation calculates effective orifice area (177), which is the area of the *vena contracta*. As described above, the *vena con-*

tracta is the point distal to the orifice where the mainstream fresh flow continues to accelerate from the orifice through the middle of the recirculation zone to the point of highest velocity magnitude, corresponding to where the cross-sectional area of the mainstream flow is narrowest (Fig. 6-8).

Various investigators have found that estimation of the valve area using the Doppler continuity equation is flow-dependent in certain clinical settings (177,181–183). This may be due to the valve leaflets opening further with increased flow rate (177,183). It appears to be also related to the fact that the above formula assumes uniform flow velocities across the valve orifice (flat velocity profile). If the velocity profile changes at different flow rates, then the valve area equation above will be flow-dependent. Investigations in our laboratory have demonstrated in *in vitro* models (182) and numeric models (181) of discrete rigid orifices that the velocity profile varies with different flows. At low flow rates (i.e., low Reynolds number), viscous effects predominate and the velocity profile through an orifice acquires an elliptical shape, whereas at higher flow rates (high Reynolds numbers) inertial effects predominate and the velocity profile flattens out (Fig. 6-11). Thus, at low flow rates the time-averaged peak velocity measured with CW Doppler overestimates the

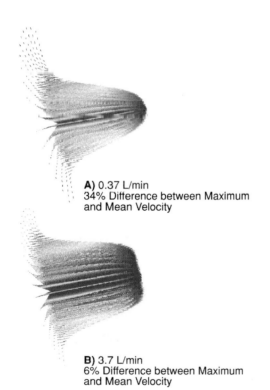

A) 0.37 L/min
34% Difference between Maximum and Mean Velocity

B) 3.7 L/min
6% Difference between Maximum and Mean Velocity

FIG. 6-11. Computer simulations of blood flow through a stenotic orifice showing velocity vector profiles at low flow rate **(A)** and high flow rate **(B)**. The length of individual vectors represent the magnitude of each velocity vector. Note the shape of the profile is parabolic at low flow rate **(A)** and flattened at high flow rate **(B)**.

time- and space-averaged velocity through the orifice, resulting in underestimation of valve areas with the continuity equation since this velocity is in the denominator (Eqs. 21 and 22).

Flow Convergence Method

A method has been proposed to estimate orifice areas using the flow convergence method (Eq. 5) in regurgitant orifices (184–187) and stenotic orifices (188–191). The FCM can measure the peak instantaneous flow rate (IFR_{peak}) through the valve in question:

$$IFR_{peak} = 2\pi r_{peak}^2 * V_{isovelocity\text{-}peak} \qquad [24]$$

where $V_{isovelocity\text{-}peak}$ and r_{peak} are the value of the velocity and radius of the isovelocity shell chosen at peak flow. This is easily determined by setting a particular Nyquist limit on the echocardiographic machine and tracking the first aliased boundary in the color flow image through the ejection cycle and recording the first aliased boundary with the largest radius (r_{max}) from the orifice. The peak orifice velocity (V_{peak}) can then be measured by CW Doppler and the flow convergence method orifice area ($Area_{orifice}$) can be computed:

$$Area_{orifice} = \frac{IFR_{peak}}{V_{peak}}. \qquad [25]$$

Stenotic and regurgitant orifices are sometimes found to have surrounding boundaries that form less than a 180-degree angle with the orifice (Fig. 6-7) (109,113–115,192). Instead of a hemisphere, the isovelocity surface is the surface of a cone and peak flow rate (Eq. 6) becomes:

$$IFR_{peak} = 2\pi r_{peak}^2 \frac{\alpha}{180} * V_{isovelocity\text{-}peak} \qquad [26]$$

where α = constraining angle. The flow convergence method orifice area equation remains the same.

Momentum Analysis

A method has been proposed for use in estimating regurgitant orifice areas (ROAs) (193) using the conservation of momentum principle, which implies that momentum calculated through planes orthogonal to a jet axis should be constant. This method neglects the effects of jet impingement. Thus, momentum (or more properly momentum flux) through the orifice equals momentum through a plane downstream to the orifice (Fig. 6-12). If one assumes a flat velocity profile at the orifice with velocity of $v_{orifice}$ (measured by CW Doppler), the momentum through the orifice ($M_{orifice}$) is simply:

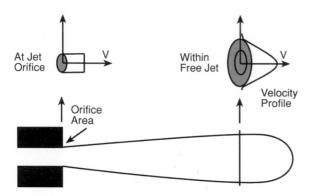

FIG. 6-12. Diagram of a jet leaving an orifice. The momentum flux crossing any given plane through the jet should be equal. Thus, momentum through the orifice equals momentum through a plane downstream to the orifice. See text for details. V, velocity.

$$M_{orifice} = V^2_{orifice} * Area_{orifice} \qquad [27]$$

Calculating the momentum through the plane downstream is what has made this technique impractical to date. Obviously the flow through the plane of the downstream jet will not have a flat velocity profile. Thus, theoretically one would have to break up this cut plane into small incremental areas (ΔA) and multiply each by the square of the measured velocity through that incremental area (V_i). The momentum through the cut plane (M_{plane}) would then be a summation:

$$M_{plane} = \Sigma \Delta A * v^2, i = 1, . . ., n \qquad [28]$$

where n = number of discrete area segments.

Then by conservation of momentum the orifice area is given by:

$$Area_{orifice} = \frac{M_{plane}}{V^2_{orifice}}. \qquad [29]$$

With current technology the angle dependency of Doppler velocity mapping comes into play when determining these incremental velocities through this flat cut plane. Assumptions of axisymmetric jet flow (which is physiologically probably a gross approximation) have been made to simplify the calculation of M_{plane} (193). Whether this method can be applied to turbulent jets has not been determined (74).

Taking into account these noninsurmountable problems, it will be interesting to see if newly developing Doppler technologies (i.e., three-dimensional color digital Doppler) breathe new life into this technique.

Valve Resistance

Valve resistance has been proposed as another attempt at finding an index that would be independent of flow (194–196). In this approach, resistance (R) is the pressure gradient (ΔP) divided by flow rate (FR): $R = \Delta P/FR$.

The pressure gradient can be obtained by catheterization or by Doppler through the Bernoulli equation (197,198). Unfortunately valve resistance using Doppler to measure pressure gradient was also found to be flow-dependent in at least one clinical setting (197). Normal and abnormal values have not yet been established in children for any heart valve.

Spectral Doppler Velocity Waveform Measurements

Many characteristics of spectral velocity waveforms can be used in the assessment of various hemodynamic parameters. Here, each velocity waveform index will be discussed. Below, the significance of each index according to where the velocity waveform was obtained are addressed.

Acceleration Time

The acceleration time in a Doppler velocity waveform (199,200) is the time from initial flow to peak flow (Echo. 6-16). Mean acceleration is the peak velocity divided by acceleration time. These measurements are performed on signals derived from ventricular ejection such as semilunar valve forward flows as well as atrioventricular valve regurgitant flows. They are often used in measures of systolic ventricular performance as well as measures of downstream impedance (e.g., pulmonary valve flow and assessment of pulmonary hypertension).

Deceleration Time

The deceleration time (DT) is the time period from the peak velocity to the time at which an extrapolated line,

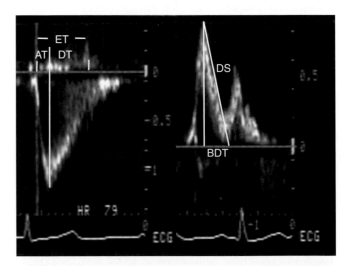

ECHO. 6-16. Doppler spectral velocity waveform with demonstration of how one measures specific indices. See text for details. These include *AT*, acceleration time; *BDT*, baseline deceleration time; *ET*, ejection time; and *DS*, deceleration slope.

following the downward slope of the Doppler velocity waveform, crosses the zero velocity axis (Echo. 6-16).

There are two different deceleration times reported in the literature regarding inflow of atrioventricular valves. There are usually two peaks in atrioventricular inflow signals where after the first peak (E wave) the velocity waveform may or may not reach the zero velocity axis prior to the start of the A wave. The deceleration time has been defined as the time of E wave velocity descent (200). The deceleration time has also been defined as the time from peak velocity on the E wave to the time at which an extrapolated line, following the downsloping E wave, crosses the zero velocity axis (30). To avoid confusion we will call the second definition the baseline deceleration time (BDT).

Ejection Time

The ejection time (ET) is the time from onset to cessation of flow (Echo. 6-16) (77,200).

Deceleration Slope

Many CW Doppler signals obtained from forward or regurgitant flows through valves have a linear slope in the deceleration phase of the Doppler signal (Echo. 6-16). The slope of this straight line drawn on the deceleration phase of the CW Doppler velocity waveform is called the deceleration slope (DS) (201).

Pressure Half-Time or Diastolic Half-Time

The measurement of pressure half-time (PHT), also called the diastolic half-time (DHT), by Doppler techniques (200–202) was an adaptation from the pressure half time measured at cardiac catheterization. This measurement was used in the catheterization laboratory as a measurement that was thought to be independent of heart rate or cardiac output (202). Pressure half-time is by definition the time it takes for the pressure drop across a valve to fall to one half its maximum value (202). It is used in the assessment of pressure gradients across valves during forward or regurgitant flow periods as well as in the assessment of the severity of valve regurgitation and stenosis.

Determining this time interval from the Doppler velocity waveform, the interval is sometimes erroneously measured as the time from peak velocity to one half the peak velocity. Thus, the term velocity half-time used synonymously for pressure half-time may be misleading and probably should be avoided.

Using the simplified echo Bernoulli equation (Eq. 14), it is evident that the measurement should be the time period from peak velocity (V_{peak}) to a velocity ($V_{pressure-half-time}$) where the pressure gradient is half the value of the peak gradient.

Using the echo simplified Bernoulli equation and solving for $V_{pressure-half-time}$ gives (202):

$$V_{pressure-half-time} = 2\tfrac{1}{2} * V_{peak} \cong 0.7 * V_{peak} . \quad [30]$$

To obtain the pressure half-time, the time between V_{peak} and $V_{pressure-half-time}$ (Echo. 6-17) can be measured directly; however, there are several simpler ways of measuring pressure half-time. Using simple algebra and the discussed previously, one can show (202):

$$PHT = DHT = 0.29 * \frac{V_{peak}}{DS} . \quad [31]$$

Using the baseline deceleration time as discussed previously, one can show that BDT = V_{peak}/DS; therefore:

$$PHT = DHT = 0.29 * BDT. \quad [32]$$

Isovolumetric Relaxation Time or Preejection Period

Isovolumetric relaxation time (IVRT), also called the "preejection period" (PEP), measured by Doppler is an adaptation from cardiac catheterization methods. By definition the IVRT for a right or left ventricle is the time from the respective semilunar valve closing to the onset of diastolic flow velocity through its respective atrioventricular valve. A method has been developed to measure this quantity by Doppler techniques for the left ventricle (203). A CW Doppler velocity waveform is obtained where the mitral valve inflow signal and the aortic outflow signal are recorded simultaneously (Echo. 6-8). The IVRT is ideally measured from the start of the aortic valve closure signal to the start

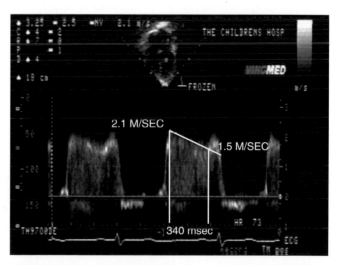

ECHO. 6-17. Demonstration of proper method to determine PHT from the Doppler spectral velocity waveform. The PHT equals the time from peak pressure gradient to a time when the pressure gradient equals half the peak pressure gradient. Using the echo simplified Bernoulli equation, this translates to the time period from peak velocity (V_{peak} = 2.1 m/s) to a velocity where the pressure gradient is half the value of the peak gradient ($V_{pressure-half-time}$ = 1.5 m/s).

of the mitral valve opening signal (203), which usually is visible on the CW signal obtained. Less accurately, the IVRT is measured from the end of the aortic flow signal to the beginning of the mitral valve inflow signal. Normal values in adults for the IVRT are 55 to 90 m/s (204).

Time Constant of Ventricular Relaxation

The time constant of ventricular relaxation (Γ) measured by Doppler is an adaptation from cardiac catheterization methods. It serves as an index for ventricular diastolic function (204–207). In this technique the downslope of a regurgitant atrioventricular valve Doppler velocity waveform is translated into a pressure-time waveform using the simplified echo Bernoulli equation (Eq. 14). The resultant curve is then numerically fit into the following exponential equation:

$$P(t) = P_o e^{-t/\Gamma} \qquad [33]$$

where $P_o = 4V_{peak}^2$.

Numerical curve fitting may not be practical; therefore, Scalia et al. (207) have used a simpler method to determine the time constant of ventricular relaxation using IVRT, peak systolic blood pressure (P_s), and left atrial pressure (P_{LA}):

$$\Gamma = \frac{\text{IVRT}}{\ln (P_s) - \ln (P_{LA})}. \qquad [34]$$

Rate of Pressure Rise (dP/dt)

The rate of pressure rise (RPR or dP/dt) measured by Doppler (208,209) is an adaptation from cardiac catheterization methods. It is used in the assessment of ventricular systolic function by examining an atrioventricular valve regurgitant CW Doppler velocity waveform.

The mean rate of pressure rise (mean dP/dt) is defined as the rate of pressure change on the velocity curve from a velocity of V_1 to V_2 m/s. By the simplified echo Bernoulli equation (Eq. 14), the pressure gradients at V_1 and V_2 m/s are 4 V_1^2 and 4 V_2^2 mmHg, respectively. To obtain the mean rate of pressure rise then:

$$\text{mean } dP/dt = \frac{4 V_2^2 - 4 V_1^2}{\Delta t} \qquad [35]$$

where Δt equals the time measured between these two points on the Doppler velocity waveform.

The peak rate of pressure rise was developed because the mean is an average slope and may underestimate true peak dP/dt (209). To determine the peak rate of pressure rise, the simplified echo Bernoulli equation is used on the entire Doppler velocity waveform and a complete pressure gradient curve is produced (209,210). From that curve the peak dP/dt can be determined as the point on the pressure gradient curve with the greatest slope. The peak rate of pressure rise is usually measured on off-line analysis systems.

Peak Acceleration Rate

The peak acceleration rate (PAR) of blood traveling out of a ventricle has been shown to be a measure of ventricular systolic performance (211,212). The peak acceleration rate is derived from the CW Doppler velocity waveform and is, by definition, the point on the velocity-time signal where there is maximum slope. Typically, this is measured on off-line analysis systems.

Jets: Regurgitant and Stenotic

There have been numerous methods proposed to quantitate the severity of a regurgitant or stenotic valve from the flow jets visualized on spectral and color Doppler flow mapping.

PW Velocity Mapping

Early in echocardiographic Doppler development, determination of the spatial distribution of flow jets was felt to be important for quantitating the severity of the lesion causing the flow disturbance. Prior to the development of color Doppler flow imaging the only way to map out the area occupied by a jet was to sample the entire receiving chamber of the flow jet stream with PW Doppler (213–215). A disturbed flow pattern was defined as a PW Doppler velocity signal with a wide bandwidth.

PW velocity mapping is mentioned here primarily for historic purposes. In general it is not in regular clinical use since most echocardiographic machines in use today display color Doppler velocity images.

CW Doppler Signal Strength

Qualitative methods of assessing the severity of valve regurgitation include CW Doppler signal strength. CW Doppler signal intensity relies on the observation that the larger the regurgitant volume, the stronger and harsher the CW signal since a greater number of backscattering particles (red blood cells) contribute to its formation (74). It is important to compare the forward flow signal to the regurgitant flow signal when making a judgment about regurgitant CW Doppler signal strength to avoid errors due to machine setting and imaging factors (74).

Spatial Distribution of Color Flow Jets

Once color Doppler velocity imaging was introduced (initially referred to as multigated pulsed Doppler), determining the distribution of a jet in its receiving chamber became much simpler compared to the same practice using PW velocity mapping (216). Despite a multitude of problems, it is still in use today in many clinical laboratories. Spatial distribution of jets produced by stenotic valves has generally not been used in the assessment of the severity of stenosis.

Jet length (Jet$_{Length}$) and jet area (Jet$_{area}$) are parameters that have been used in the quantitation of the spatial distribution of jets. In assessing jet area the absolute two-dimensional (217,218) or three-dimensional (119) area is determined or a ratio of the two-dimensional or three-dimensional jet area to receiving chamber area (Jet$_{ratio}$) is obtained. Doppler color flow jet areas change throughout the ejection cycle (219). When using two-dimensional measurements the maximal jet area from multiple two-dimensional echocardiographic planes should be used (74) as well as the maximum jet area throughout the ejection period. Of course, maximum jet area or length depends mostly on the peak regurgitant flow rate and not on total flow rate.

Regarding the assessment of lesions by the spatial distribution of the color Doppler image of the jet, as long as the clinician is aware that the Doppler velocity image displays blood velocities, not blood flow (200), and is aware of the consequent pitfalls associated with the method, then it can still be a useful tool. Factors that may or may not be associated with the severity of the lesion have been shown to affect the spatial distribution of the flow jet image. These include (a) pressure, volume, and compliance of the receiving chamber (128,220–223); (b) instrumentation factors (223–226); (c) the effects of solid boundaries into which the jet may impinge (113,227,228); and (d) interobserver variability (229).

The solid boundary effect on jets is quite interesting and highlights the fact that color Doppler velocity imaging only gives a two-dimensional view of the three-dimensional process of turbulent jets interacting with walls. Turbulent jets within the heart expand primarily by entrainment of adjacent fluid from the receiving chamber (160,227). If there is an adjacent wall in the receiving chamber near the orifice this can limit the amount of receiving chamber fluid locally available for entrainment. With that limitation the jet tends to be pulled towards the adjacent wall. This is called the Coanda effect (113,227,228). These wall jets tend to spread out significantly in a thin layer along the wall and may lose their momentum faster than free jets. A cross-section of this thin layer will lead to gross underestimation of the severity of the lesion, as shown in Echo. 6-18 (see color plate 5 following p. 364).

Width of Proximal Color Flow Jet

Measuring the width of the color Doppler velocity image of the proximal flow jet (also called the color Doppler imaged vena contracta) is another technique developed to qualitatively assess the severity of a lesion (Echo. 6-19; see color plate 6 following p. 364). When originally

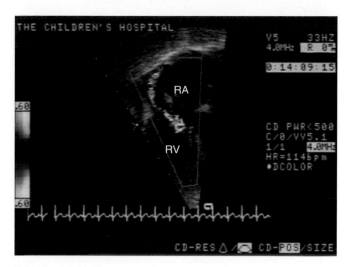

ECHO. 6-18. Example of a jet spreading out over a wall. Two-dimensional color Doppler flow images of such a jet may not show full extent of regurgitant flow area. *RA,* right atrium; *RV,* right ventricle.

proposed, the expectation was that many of the factors that affect the ability of jet area and jet length to predict lesion severity would not affect this method. It has been used primarily in the assessment of aortic regurgitation (230–233) and mitral regurgitation (234–238).

In preliminary numeric (239) and *in vitro* (240) studies in our laboratory, we have demonstrated the low-velocity cutoff setting on a Doppler device may affect the width of the visualized proximal flow jet. Also in our laboratory, we have demonstrated *in vitro* that the vena contracta area does not change to a measurable degree with flow rate (241), implying that two patients with the same sized regurgitant orifice but different flow rates will have the same proximal flow jet width. This leads to the fundamental question of what the best indicator of severity is in a stenotic or regurgitant lesion, the flow rate, the orifice size, or some combination of the two. With further advancements in color Doppler technology and three-dimensional flow visualization, this question may soon be answered.

Color Doppler M-Mode: Propagation Velocity

Current Doppler imaging does not allow tracking of particles traveling through the heart. However, it does allow the tracking of particle velocities. Color Doppler M-mode displays tracking of particle velocities or, in other words, displays propagation velocity. By tracking particle velocities with color M-mode, the speed at which a set of velocities moves through a one-dimensional sample volume is visualized.

Color Doppler M-mode propagation velocity imaging has been shown to be quite useful in assessing diastolic left ventricular dysfunction (24,242–245) as is discussed

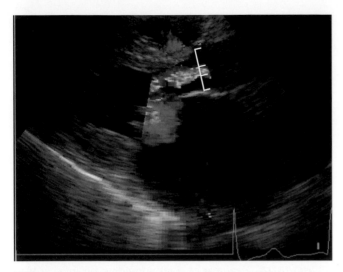

ECHO. 6-19. Example of proximal flow jet width measurement *(inner bars)* taken from the color Doppler velocity parasternal long-axis image of aortic regurgitation.

below. In this context, velocities are tracked as they propagate into the left ventricle during early diastolic filling, a function of how fast the ventricle is relaxing.

This technique may eventually show broader applicability to the assessment of pathophysiologic abnormalities in other parts of the cardiovascular system.

VENTRICULAR FUNCTION

Systolic Function: Left Ventricle

One of the most obvious ways to quantitate left ventricular systolic function is to measure cardiac output. We have previously discussed the Doppler techniques that are used to measure cardiac outputs in various locations of the left heart (see "Quantitative Doppler Tools"). Other Doppler tools for assessing left ventricular systolic function will be introduced here.

Peak Aortic Velocity

Doppler peak velocities of the ascending aorta have been used to separate adult patients with normal cardiac output from those with impaired function (246). Since the normal range for peak velocities is so wide this method has generally not been useful in the assessment of cardiac output in children except for separating out the extreme cases where cardiac output is significantly decreased.

Aortic Velocity Time Integral

The aortic VTI has been used in the assessment of cardiac output. As we have discussed, this, along with aortic diameter, is used in estimating cardiac output directly. Thus, simply using the aortic VTI is a less-than optimal index of cardiac output since VTI alone does not consider aortic diameters, which vary greatly in various age groups. VTI alone, however, can be used in the immediate serial evaluation of therapies and/or interventions where anatomic size can reasonably be assumed to not be substantially different.

Peak and Mean Acceleration Rate

The peak acceleration rate (PAR) and the mean acceleration rate (MAR) of blood traveling out of the left ventricle has been shown to be a measure of left ventricular systolic performance in adults (211,212,247–252) and children (253).

As we have discussed in "Quantitative Doppler Tools," the peak acceleration rate is derived from the CW Doppler velocity waveform and is, by definition, the point on the velocity-time signal where there is maximum slope. Typically, this is measured with off-line analysis systems. The mean acceleration is the average of acceleration rates from initial flow to peak flow, which is approximated by dividing the peak aortic velocity by the acceleration time (77).

The peak and mean acceleration rates for the aorta were found to be dependent on heart rate and left ventricular preload and afterload (211,212,247,248,250,254,255). Since the duration of maximum acceleration is short this index is quite sensitive to measurement errors (253). The reported average for mean acceleration rate varies widely in normal children: 9.55 m/s^2 (7.35 to 13.18 m/s^2) (256), 21.1 m/s^2 (17.5 to 24.7 m/s^2) (257), and 21.3 m/s^2 (15.5 to 27.1 m/s^2) (253). These indices are not commonly used in the evaluation of ventricular systolic function in pediatric patients.

Acceleration Time and Ejection Time

The acceleration time and ejection time as well as the acceleration/ejection time interval (AT/ET) have been investigated as measures of left ventricular function in adults (246,258) and normal children (253). The reported normal mean for AT/ET ratio in children older than 6 months of age is 0.23 (±0.05) (253). These indices are not routinely used in the evaluation of ventricular systolic function in pediatric patients.

Mitral Regurgitation: Rate of Pressure Rise (dP/dt)

The mean rate of pressure rise (mean *dP/dt*) was discussed previously (Eq. 35) and for the left ventricle is measured conventionally as the rate of pressure change on the acceleration phase of the mitral regurgitation Doppler velocity curve from velocities (V_1 and V_2) of 1 m/s to

3 m/s (208) (Echo. 6-20). The equation for mean rate of pressure rise becomes:

$$\text{mean } dP/dt = \frac{36 - 4}{\Delta t} \qquad [36]$$

where Δt equals the time measured between 1 m/s and 3 m/s on the Doppler velocity waveform. It has been suggested that this index is afterload-independent since the measurement is usually taken during the preejection phase of systole (259–261). The Doppler-derived mean rate of pressure rise has shown good correlation to catheter-derived values in adults (206,208,260–262). Similar extensive studies have not been performed in children. In adults the mean rate of pressure rise has shown good correlation to M-mode echocardiographic estimation of ejection fraction (259) as well.

Preload has been shown to affect these values of rate of pressure rise, and, therefore, a normalized dP/dt has been proposed as a more reliable assessment of the left ventricular contractile state (263). In this method, the ventricular dP/dt is divided by ventricular end diastolic volume as determined by M-mode echocardiography.

Systolic Function: Right Ventricle

Estimating ventricular systolic function by Doppler methods may be even more important for the right ventricle compared to the left ventricle for which there are a number of accurate non-Doppler methods available. Right ventricular systolic function based on volume analysis is difficult due to the complex geometry of the right ventricle. Similar to the assessment of left ventricular systolic function, one of the most obvious ways to quantitate right ventricular systolic function is to measure cardiac output. We have previously discussed the Doppler techniques that

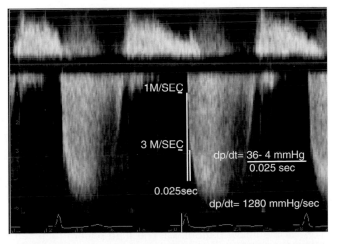

ECHO. 6-20. The mean rate of pressure rise (mean *dP/dt*) is defined as the rate of pressure change on the Doppler spectral velocity waveform. By convention this is measured from a velocity of 1 m/s to a velocity of 3 m/s.

are used to measure cardiac outputs in various locations of the right heart (see "Quantitative Doppler Tools"). Other Doppler tools for assessing right ventricular systolic function will be introduced here.

Acceleration Rate, Acceleration Time, and Ejection Time: Right Ventricle

The mean acceleration rate, acceleration time, and ejection time have been used in the assessment of systolic right ventricular function in children who have undergone intraatrial repair of aortopulmonary transposition in whom the right ventricle is the systemic ventricle (257). In these children, the mean acceleration rate was lower and the acceleration time and AT/ET were greater in patients who had their repair after three months of age (257). This suggested impaired systolic function in the group repaired after three months of age as opposed to the group repaired earlier in life.

In general, in patients where the right ventricle is the normal pulmonary ventricle, these indices are not used in the assessment of systolic function. However, AT and ET measured through the pulmonary artery are used in the detection of pulmonary hypertension, which will be covered in chapter 35.

Tricuspid Regurgitation: Rate of Pressure Rise (dP/dt)

The mean rate of pressure rise (mean *dP/dt*) has been discussed (Eq. 35) and is defined as the rate of pressure change on the acceleration phase of the tricuspid regurgitation Doppler velocity curve between two velocities (V_1 and V_2). Exactly which two velocities are chosen for the right ventricle has varied among investigators. V_1 and V_2 of 0 to 2 m/s (264), 0.5 to 2 m/s (264), and 0.5 to 1.5 m/s (265) have been used in adult studies, and all correlated well with catheter-derived *dP/dt* values. Similar studies in children have not been reported. Imanishi et al. (210) looked at the peak rate of pressure rise in adults. As discussed previously, the peak rate of pressure rise is determined from the reconstructed atrioventricular pressure curve where the peak *dP/dt* is the point on the pressure-time curve with the greatest slope. Doppler values correlated quite closely with catheter-derived peak *dP/dt* values.

One study examined the mean rate of pressure rise in the systemic right ventricle of children with hypoplastic left heart syndrome and sufficient tricuspid regurgitation. With systemic pressures in the right ventricle the standard left ventricular formula for mean rate of pressure rise was used (Eq. 36) and demonstrated a good correlation with catheter-derived *dP/dt* values (145).

Diastolic Function

The study of Doppler techniques and their application in the assessment of diastolic function can quite easily take an entire chapter or, for that matter, an entire book to explain fully. We will attempt a concise review here.

Atrioventricular Doppler Inflow Patterns

Effects From Changes in Preload and Afterload

In order to understand how atrioventricular inflow patterns are used in the assessment of diastolic function it will be helpful to understand how changes in afterload and preload affect these inflow patterns. With simple perturbations to a patient's hemodynamic status the subsequent changes to the inflow velocity waveform can be easily explained (30). The reader should review the physiology underlying normal inflow patterns (see ''Normal Doppler Patterns and Images'') before proceeding.

Regarding changes in preload, with an increase in preload the atrial pressure prior to atrioventricular valve opening is elevated, leading to a higher driving pressure with increased flow velocities when the atrioventricular valve opens (higher E wave). Since the diastolic pressure-volume curve is nearly linear (at least for the left ventricle) there is a faster and larger increase in ventricular pressure that rapidly decelerates inflow, leading to a decreased deceleration time. In the case of decreased preload, there is a lower pressure gradient just prior to atrioventricular valve opening leading to lower inflow velocities (lower E wave). Opposite to increased preload, there is a slower rate of rise of ventricular pressure leading to a prolongation of the deceleration time.

With changes in afterload, an increase in afterload prolongs ventricular relaxation. Thus, after systole, ventricular pressures drop more slowly and by the time the atrioventricular valve opens the initial driving pressure is decreased leading to decreased initial inflow velocities (smaller E wave). There is a continued delay in ventricular relaxation due to the increased afterload, which leads to a prolonged deceleration time. Overall, there is less filling in early diastole. To compensate for this decreased filling in early diastole, there is increased filling during atrial contraction leading to higher inflow velocities during atrial contraction (increased A wave).

Left Ventricular Diastolic Function

Inflow velocity waveforms appear to be most helpful in assessing patients with diastolic dysfunction. Most studies assessing diastolic function with atrioventricular valve Doppler inflow patterns have been performed in adults with the left ventricle in mind. We have previously dis-

cussed the relative diastolic left ventricular dysfunction found in the normal fetus and normal neonate.

In adults, three abnormal left ventricular Doppler inflow patterns have been recognized (14,30,31,204,266–269) (Fig. 6-13). The first pattern represents abnormal left ventricular relaxation. Similar to the case of increased afterload, when abnormal relaxation is present the normal drop in ventricular pressures is delayed, causing a reduction in initial driving pressure, leading to decreased early filling and decreased early filling velocities (decreased E wave). This delay in ventricular relaxation continues and leads to a prolonged deceleration time. To compensate, the filling that occurs with atrial contraction is increased (increased A wave); thus, the E/A ratio is decreased. This pattern of abnormal ventricular relaxation has been observed in children with systemic hypertension and hypertrophic cardiomyopathy (270). In addition to the reduced E/A ratio and longer deceleration time, as we will discuss, there is an increase in the IVRT. The increase in IVRT is due to the delay in relaxation of the ventricle. This delay maintains a high left ventricular pressure and results in late opening of the mitral valve.

The second inflow pattern occurs when there is abnormal ventricular relaxation and the left atrial pressure is increased. The increased filling pressure counteracts the abnormal ventricular relaxation, and the result is a ''pseudonormal'' inflow pattern. This pattern can be difficult to distinguish from the normal pattern, which emphasizes the importance of serial studies and evaluating the Doppler patterns in the context of the patient's overall clinical status. The IVRT can also normalize. In adults, pseudonormal filling is typically detected by the presence of atrial or ventricular dilation (271).

As the filling pressure continues to increase, a third characteristic Doppler pattern emerges that has been described as a restrictive filling pattern (272–274). Because of the very high filling pressures and abnormally rapid increase in diastolic left ventricular pressure, flow occurs

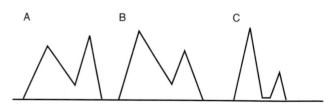

FIG. 6-13. Three classic mitral valve inflow patterns found with left ventricular diastolic dysfunction. **A:** The first pattern represents abnormal left ventricular relaxation with a delay in ventricular relaxation leading to a decreased E wave and a compensative increased A wave. **B:** The second pattern represents abnormal left ventricular relaxation with increased left atrial pressure leading to a ''pseudonormalization'' of the inflow pattern. **C:** The third pattern represents a restrictive filling pattern, whereas left ventricular diastolic pressure continues to increase, flow occurs mostly in early diastole, leading to a high peak E wave velocity with rapid deceleration time and a small A wave.

early in diastole with a rapid, short rush into the ventricle. This results in a high peak velocity and rapid DT of the E wave and a very small A wave. Also, the DT and IVRT are shortened.

Inflow velocity patterns not only depend on preload, afterload, and diastolic function but also depend on heart rate, systolic function, autonomic status (200). Thus, one must include all of these factors into the assessment of diastolic function. The mean for left ventricular DT in normal adults 21 to 49 years old is 179 m/s (139 to 219 m/s) (24).

Right Ventricular Diastolic Function

Unfortunately, most diastolic function studies using atrioventricular Doppler inflow patterns have been performed in adults regarding the left ventricle. We have previously discussed the relative diastolic right ventricular dysfunction found in the normal fetus and normal neonate. Diastolic Doppler inflow studies regarding the right ventricle in adults (275) and in children (276,277) have been limited.

In children with pulmonary stenosis a tricuspid valve inflow pattern reflecting diastolic dysfunction similar to that seen with increased afterload has been described (276,277). As we have discussed, an increase in afterload prolongs ventricular relaxation. Thus, after systole, right ventricular pressures drop slowly, and by the time the tricuspid valve opens the initial driving pressure is decreased, leading to decreased initial inflow velocities (smaller E wave). There is a prolonged deceleration time due to a continued delay in right ventricular relaxation from the increased afterload. Overall there is less filling in early diastole. There is increased filling during atrial contraction to compensate for this decreased filling in early diastole, leading to higher inflow velocities during atrial contraction (increased A wave). Interestingly this abnormal inflow pattern was felt not to be due solely to increased afterload since immediately after the obstruction was relieved the inflow pattern did not change significantly (276). However, upon long-term follow-up, inflow patterns in these patients did tend to normalize, indicating that the initial pattern was suggestive of diastolic dysfunction secondary to ventricular hypertrophy which subsequently resolved (277).

The mean for right ventricular deceleration time in normal adults 21 to 49 years old is 188 m/s (144 to 232 m/s) (24).

Isovolumetric Relaxation Time or Preejection Period: Left Ventricle

As we have discussed, the IVRT for the left ventricle is the time from the aortic valve closing to the onset of diastolic flow through the mitral valve. CW Doppler can be used to measure this quantity in the left ventricle (203).

A CW Doppler velocity waveform may be obtained where the mitral valve inflow signal and the aortic outflow signal are present simultaneously. The IVRT is ideally measured from the start of the aortic valve closure signal to the start of the mitral valve opening signal (203) which usually is visible on the CW signal obtained. Less accurately the IVRT is measured from the end of the aortic flow signal to the beginning of the mitral valve inflow signal (Echo. 6-8). Care must be taken when comparing studies using these differing definitions (278).

The IVRT is dependent not only on the rate of ventricular relaxation, but also on the left ventricular pressure at the time of aortic valve closure (afterload), the left atrial pressure at the time of mitral valve opening (preload) (14,75), and heart rate. Regarding preload, it has been shown that with elevated left atrial pressure the IVRT shortens (204).

As with most of the other measures of diastolic function there is only a limited number of studies in children using IVRT (279,280). The mean IVRT value for adults with normal hearts who are between 21 to 49 years old, is reported as 76 m/s (54 to 98 m/s) (24), with another source quoting the normal range in adults of all ages is between 70 m/s and 100 m/s (281).

Time Constant of Ventricular Relaxation: Left Ventricle

As discussed (Eqs. 33 and 34), the time constant of ventricular relaxation (Γ) serves as an index for left ventricular diastolic function. Here the downslope of a regurgitant mitral valve (24,205,206,282) or regurgitant AOV (283,284) Doppler velocity waveform is translated into a pressure-time waveform using the simplified echo Bernoulli equation (Eq. 14). The resultant curve is then numerically fitted into Eq. 33, where the value of Γ is determined. This method is felt by some to be a "semi-quantitative" method of assessing the rate of left ventricular relaxation in adults (205) with no adequate studies performed in infants or children to date.

Pulmonary Venous Inflow Patterns

Pulmonary venous velocity inflow patterns can be used in the assessment of diastolic function. The type of abnormal pattern depends on the type of diastolic dysfunction. With abnormal ventricular relaxation and increased left atrial pressure, the systolic to diastolic ratio (S/D) of the pulmonary venous flow pattern is decreased from normal and there is increased flow reversal (A wave greater than 35 cm/s) (16,24,30,271). One can measure the duration of the pulmonary venous A wave ($T_{A\text{-pulm}}$) and compare it to the duration of the mitral A wave ($T_{A\text{-mitral}}$). In abnormal relaxation, termination of transmitral flow prior to the ending of pulmonary venous reverse flow occurs

(16,24,30,271). Thus, with abnormal ventricular relaxation, the ratio of pulmonary venous A wave duration to mitral valve A wave duration ($T_{A\text{-pulm}}/T_{A\text{-mitral}}$) will be greater than normal. The mean $T_{A\text{-pulm}}/T_{A\text{-mitral}}$ ratio for children with normal hearts is 0.5 (range 0 to 1.0) (285).

With restrictive filling the pulmonary venous flow exhibits almost no systolic phase with tall diastolic and tall atrial reversal components (200).

Systemic Venous Inflow Patterns

It seems the same reasoning can be applied to the systemic venous inflow and its use in assessing diastolic right ventricular function. There does not appear to be much in the current literature regarding this, however.

Color Doppler M-Mode: Propagation Velocity

Color Doppler M-mode propagation velocity imaging has been shown to be quite useful when assessing diastolic dysfunction in adults (24,242–244,286). To date there are no published data on measuring propagation velocity in children.

Color Doppler M-mode displays trackings of particle velocities or in other words displays propagation velocity. By tracking particle velocities one is visualizing how fast a set of velocities moves through the one-dimensional sample volume (M-mode). Specifically, regarding mitral valve inflow, if velocities are tracked as they move into the left ventricle during early diastolic filling, then how fast these velocities propagate is a function of how fast the ventricle is relaxing.

A typical color Doppler M-mode display of flow through a mitral valve is shown in Echo. 6-21 (see color

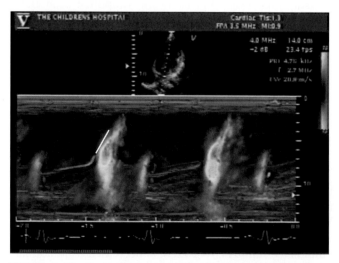

ECHO. 6-21. Color Doppler M-mode tracings of mitral valve inflow demonstrating how propagation velocity is measured. A line is drawn from the leading edge of the early diastolic inflow wave on the color Doppler M-mode signal, and the slope of this line represents the propagation velocity (a measure of diastolic function). A diminished propagation slope occurs with worsening ventricular diastolic function.

plate 7 following p. 364). One way to measure the propagation velocity is to determine the slope of the line drawn from the leading edge of the early diastolic inflow wave on the color Doppler M-mode signal. With worsening ventricular diastolic function (i.e., worsening relaxation) it will take longer for a velocity to travel a certain distance, leading to a diminished propagation slope. This technique may help in distinguishing pseudonormalization from normal filling (24).

OBSTRUCTIVE LESIONS

In the Doppler echocardiographic assessment of obstructive lesions we will be using several of the quantitative Doppler tools we introduced previously, most notably pressure gradients between chambers and valve areas.

Atrioventricular Valve Stenosis

Mitral Valve Stenosis

As the severity of mitral valve stenosis increases, changes to the mitral valve inflow velocity waveform include (a) increased flow acceleration (steeper acceleration slope); (b) increased peak velocity; and (c) decreased flow deceleration (lesser deceleration slope) (74).

Valve Area

Early on workers in the field developed empirical formulas using the Doppler mitral inflow signal to estimate valve area in the assessment of mitral valve stenosis. It was noted that the slope of the deceleration side of the mitral valve inflow velocity waveform was dependent on stenosis severity. Using this dependency mitral valve area ($\text{Area}_{\text{mitral valve}}$) has been estimated by the following two formulas:

$$\text{Area}_{\text{mitral valve}} = \frac{220}{\text{PHT}} \text{ (5)} \qquad [37]$$

and

$$\text{Area}_{\text{mitral valve}} = \frac{750}{\text{BDT}} \text{ (287)} \qquad [38]$$

where PHT and BDT are both measured as previously described. These methods not only depend on the valve area but also on the left atrial and left ventricular compliance and pressures (77,288,289). This dependence is evident after percutaneous mitral balloon valvuloplasty where this method remains inaccurate 24 to 48 hours post procedure (30,290).

This method has been shown to be clinically useful in adults (291), mostly for valve areas less than 2.0 cm^2 (292,293). The constants, 240 and 750, in these equations were derived from studies in adults and may not apply to children with faster heart rates (77,294). In at least one study in children this method has been shown to correlate poorly ($r = 0.57$) with catheterization methods (294); however, these were not simultaneous measurements.

Mitral valve area has also been estimated using the continuity equation discussed previously (Eq. 22). If there are no significant shunts or mitral or aortic regurgitation, the left ventricular outflow tract is used as the reference flow location (295) giving:

$$\text{Area}_{\text{mitral valve}} = \frac{A_{\text{LVOT}} * \text{VTI}_{\text{LVOT}}}{\text{VTI}_{\text{mitral valve}}}. \qquad [39]$$

This method has been shown to be superior to pressure half-time methods when compared to catheterization results in adults (295,296).

We have previously discussed the use of the flow convergence method in estimating stenotic valve areas, including constrained stenotic orifices. This method has been applied in the assessment of mitral valve stenosis in adults with encouraging results (121,188,189,191,297). Similar studies in children have not been performed.

In adults mitral valve areas have been categorized as mild stenosis (MV_{area} greater than 1.5 cm^2), moderate stenosis ($\text{MV}_{\text{area}} = 1.0$ to 1.5 cm^2), and severe stenosis (MV_{area} less than 1.0 cm^2) (30).

Pressure Gradient

Peak transmitral pressure gradient assessed by Doppler has been shown to be a useful index in assessing the severity of mitral stenosis in children (298). However, at least in adults, the mean transmitral pressure gradient (ΔP_{mean}) has been shown to have better correlation than the peak gradient when compared to the respective gradient measured at cardiac catheterization (30,291,292,299, 300). In adults, mean transmitral pressure gradients have been categorized as mild stenosis (ΔP_{mean} less than 5 mmHg), moderate stenosis ($\Delta P_{\text{mean}} = 5$ to 10 mmHg), and severe stenosis (ΔP_{mean} greater than 10 mmHg) (30). The mitral mean pressure gradient depends on the heart rate as well as on the severity of the obstruction (30); thus, corollaries in children need to be addressed. A fair correlation ($r = 0.73$) with catheterization mean gradients was found in one study in children (294); however, these were nonsimultaneously performed measurements.

Tricuspid Valve Stenosis

Similar to mitral stenosis, as the severity of tricuspid stenosis increases, changes to the inflow velocity waveform include (a) increased flow acceleration (steeper acceleration slope); (b) increased peak velocity; and (c) decreased flow deceleration (lesser deceleration slope) (74).

Valve Area

In contrast to the mitral valve, the tricuspid valve orifice area is large and the degree of obstruction needed to cause hemodynamic compromise may be different (301). Much less has been written on the Doppler evaluation of tricuspid stenosis (74,301–306) compared to mitral stenosis, especially regarding tricuspid stenosis in children. Again mean gradients tend to be the preferred severity assessment index, at least in adults (74,306).

It is rare to find patients where the continuity equation (Eq. 22) can be used to estimate tricuspid valve area ($\text{Area}_{\text{tricuspid valve}}$) since tricuspid regurgitation is often present (74,304). If there are no significant shunts, as well as no significant tricuspid or aortic regurgitation, the left ventricular outflow tract can be used as the reference flow location:

$$\text{Area}_{\text{tricuspid valve}} = \frac{A_{\text{LVOT}} * \text{VTI}_{\text{LVOT}}}{\text{VTI}_{\text{tricuspid valve}}}. \qquad [40]$$

In theory, the flow convergence method can be used to estimate tricuspid valve area, but this has not been tested clinically to date.

Lastly, use of the PHT method requires that empirical formulas be developed that are similar to those used in the pressure half-time method in mitral stenosis (Eqs. 37 and 38). One study (303) has shown that the formula

$$\text{Area}_{\text{tricuspid valve}} = \frac{190}{\text{PHT}} \qquad [41]$$

correlated well with catheterization data ($r = 0.74$), but more studies are required (74).

Semilunar Valve Stenosis

Aortic Valve Stenosis

Increased flow velocities in the ascending aorta may indicate aortic stenosis, left ventricular outflow tract obstruction, or increased overall flow secondary to aortic regurgitation (77,307). If the increased flow velocities are from left ventricular outflow tract obstruction or increased overall flow, the left ventricular outflow tract will have high flow velocities as well. It may be necessary to use HPRF Doppler to accurately measure left ventricular outflow tract flow velocities. In valvar aortic stenosis as the sample volume in PW Doppler is moved through the aortic annulus there will be a marked increase in flow velocities (5).

The Doppler velocity waveform pattern in aortic stenosis has a high peaking maximum velocity, with this peak occurring later in systole as the severity of the stenosis increases (74).

Pressure Gradients

Aortic value peak instantaneous pressure gradient ($\Delta P_{\text{peak instantaneous}}$) assessed by Doppler has been shown to be a useful index in assessing the severity of aortic stenosis (5) where the simplified echo Bernoulli equation is (Eq. 13):

$$\Delta P_{\text{peak instantaneous}} = 4 \ (V^2_{\text{max} - \text{aortic valve}} - V^2_{\text{max-LVOT}}). \quad [42]$$

In many clinical settings, the velocity in the left ventricular outflow tract is much less (less than 1.5 m/s) (30) than through the aortic valve; thus, the simplified echo Bernoulli equation (Eq. 14) then becomes:

$$\Delta P_{\text{peak instantaneous}} = 4 \ V^2_{\text{max} - \text{aortic valve}} \cdot \quad [43]$$

As we have discussed, the peak instantaneous pressure gradient measured by Doppler measures the pressure gradient at a different place in time and space when compared to the catheterization measurement of the peak-to-peak pressure gradient ($\Delta P_{\text{peak-to-peak}}$) (Fig. 6-9).

We discussed the "balance" of measurement differences when comparing the Doppler and the catheter pressure gradient measurement techniques. Spatial (pressure recovery) and timing ($\Delta P_{\text{peak-to-peak}}$ versus $\Delta P_{\text{peak instantaneous}}$) tend to cause the Doppler peak instantaneous gradient to be greater than the catheter peak-to-peak gradient. Viscous forces and local acceleration effects tend to cause the Doppler peak instantaneous gradient to be less than the catheter peak-to-peak gradient. Therefore, different hemodynamic states change the balance of these measurement differences (164) and work is in progress to define these changes (165) in aortic stenosis and other clinical settings.

Considering this, linear regression analysis in many studies has shown a surprising somewhat close correlation between these two measurements (catheter $\Delta P_{\text{peak-to-peak}}$ versus Doppler $\Delta P_{\text{peak instantaneous}}$) in adults ($r = 0.79$ to 0.94) (5,291,308–317) and children ($r = 0.68$ to 0.94) (179,310,318,319). However, there is generally an overestimation of the catheter peak-to-peak gradient by Doppler. The differences between catheter peak-to-peak gradient and Doppler peak instantaneous gradient are greater in mild to moderate stenosis (5,313,317) and less in patients with severe stenosis where pressure gradient is more evenly maintained during systole. The differences between these two methods is also worsened with aortic regurgitation (5,311,313) where it is felt the regurgitation affects the peak instantaneous gradient more than it does the peak-to-peak gradient.

Most of these studies were nonsimultaneous, which may account for some of the error. In fact, one study compared nonsimultaneous and simultaneous Doppler measurements to catheterization peak-to-peak pressure gradients and showed improved results ($r = 0.92$ to 0.98) with simultaneous measurements (320). Better correlation has been shown in studies that have compared simultaneous Doppler peak instantaneous gradient and catheter peak-to-peak gradient in adults (320) and children (179).

Catheter measured peak-to-peak pressure gradients ($\Delta P_{\text{peak-to-peak}}$) have been categorized for mild stenosis (25 to 50 mmHg), moderate stenosis (50 to 75 mmHg), and severe stenosis (greater than 75 mmHg) (321).

Studies that have compared Doppler peak instantaneous gradient and catheter peak instantaneous gradient in adults (157,163,308,322,323) and children (165) have generally shown improved correlation ($r = 0.79$ to 0.95) over the correlation between Doppler peak instantaneous gradient and catheter peak-to-peak gradient measurements, especially when measured simultaneously (163,165). In addition to the improved correlation the linear regression line more closely matches the line of identity with less overestimation by Doppler. Degrees of stenosis have not been defined for peak instantaneous gradients (Doppler or catheterization).

Those studies where the mean gradient (ΔP_{mean}) using the catheterization data was compared to the Doppler mean gradient (Eqs. 16 and 17) have found good correlation ($r = 0.82$ to 0.95) in adults (157,163,308,313,317, 323–330) and children (163), with generally little overestimation of the mean catheter gradient by the Doppler mean gradient method. However, in many studies, Doppler mean pressure gradient significantly overestimated the catheter mean pressure gradient (157,316,327). The best correlation between the two mean pressure measurement methods again was in those studies where the mean pressure gradients by the two methods were measured simultaneously (157,163).

Mean pressure gradients were introduced in an attempt to find Doppler and catheterization methods that would more closely correlate. Theoretically, averaging over an entire ejection phase incorporates underestimation effects at the beginning and end of the ejection phase where the Reynolds number is low, which cancels out some of the overestimation effects of Doppler measured pressure gradients seen at high flow rates when compared to catheter measured pressure gradients (164). Also, averaging over an entire ejection phase removes the issue of peak-to-peak versus peak instantaneous pressure gradient differences.

Values of the mean pressure gradient have been used to select those patients with critical aortic stenosis in adults (324,328). In the first of two studies (324,328) where critical aortic stenosis was defined as catheterization determined valve area less than 0.75 cm^2, the investigators concluded that patients with a Doppler mean pressure gradient greater than 50 mmHg likely have critical aortic stenosis (324). In those with intermediate mean gradients (30 to 50 mmHg) additional information is required (e.g., cardiac output) to assess if critical aortic stenosis exists. Those with a Doppler mean pressure gradient less than 30 mmHg are likely not to have critical aortic stenosis. However, there was much overlap between groups, with no sensitivity or specificity reported. In the other similar study of adult patients, a Doppler mean pressure gradient ≥50 mmHg had a 94% specificity but only a 48% sensitivity for severe aortic stenosis (328).

Similarly, Doppler mean gradients in children have been assessed to determine whether severe aortic stenosis is present (319,331,332). In the first two of these studies, severe aortic stenosis was defined as a patient having a catheter peak-to-peak gradient ≥75 mmHg (331). In the first study (331) a Doppler mean pressure gradient greater than 27 indicated a catheter peak-to-peak gradient ≥75 mmHg with 100% specificity, while a Doppler mean pressure gradient less than 17 mmHg predicted mild aortic stenosis. Patients with (a) Doppler ΔP_{mean} greater than 27 mmHg; or (b) Doppler ΔP_{mean} = 17 to 27 mmHg and with symptoms or abnormal exercise test indicated a catheter peak-to-peak gradient ≥75 mmHg with 80% specificity and 96% sensitivity. In the second study in children, the investigators demonstrate how aortic regurgitation reduces the predictive value of Doppler mean pressure gradient (319). In this study, 15 of 21 patients with a Doppler mean pressure gradient greater than 27 mmHg had a catheter peak-to-peak gradient less than 75 mmHg. Twelve of these 15 patients had aortic regurgitation and that was postulated as at least part of the reason for the poor predictive value of mean pressure gradients greater than 27 mmHg. In the third study, where Doppler valve area (see below) less than 0.7 cm²/m² defined patients with severe aortic stenosis, 10 of 33 patients with severe aortic stenosis had a Doppler mean pressure gradient ≤27 mmHg; however, many of these patients had low cardiac output (332).

Valve Area

In contrast to adults many children with aortic stenosis do not have diminished left ventricular stroke volume (331). However, some do (especially neonates), and pressure gradients overall are a flow-dependent index of aortic stenosis. The impetus for determining aortic valve area was to find a flow-independent index of stenosis severity.

A major problem with judging the Doppler assessment of valve area is that there is no real reference standard measurement of valve area to compare with since the catheterization method uses the Gorlin and Gorlin formula which is itself flow-dependent (175–177).

From our previous general discussion of valve area (Eqs. 21 and 22) calculations and using the left ventricular outflow tract as the reference flow location, the Doppler continuity equation becomes:

$$Area_{aortic\ valve} = Area_{LVOT} * \frac{TAV_{LVOT}}{TAV_{valve}}, \quad [44]$$

or

$$Area_{aortic\ valve} = Area_{LVOT} * \frac{VTI_{LVOT}}{VTI_{valve}}, \quad [45]$$

where TAV and VTI are as in Eq. 1.

As discussed (Eq. 23), valve area calculations can be simplified with an approximation to the Doppler continuity equation using peak velocities (V_{peak}) giving:

$$Peak\ Area_{aortic\ valve} = Area_{LVOT} * \frac{V_{peak-LVOT}}{V_{peak-aortic\ valve}}. \quad [46]$$

Comparisons between aortic valve areas estimated by the Doppler continuity equation using averaged velocities versus using peak velocities have shown excellent correlation in adults (333) and children (r = 0.95 to 0.97) (332).

Linear regression analysis comparing aortic valve area measured by the Gorlin and Gorlin formula at catheterization and the standard Doppler continuity equation (Eq. 45 or 46) (158,180,314,315,328,334,335), as well as the Doppler continuity equation using peak velocities (Eq. 47) (180,314,323,328–330,336,337) has shown close correlations (r = 0.80 to 0.99). Similar analysis in children has shown generally less desirable correlation (r = 0.73 to 0.81) (179,332). In patients with low cardiac output or relatively large valve areas, the discrepancy between the Doppler and catheterization methods worsens in children (332) and adults (175,178,323,325,328,336,338).

Most of these studies were done where the catheter and Doppler methods were performed nonsimultaneously, which could lead to some of the discrepancies noted. One should also keep in mind that these two methods are estimating two different entities, where the continuity equation reflects effective valve area (i.e., the area of the vena contracta) and the catheterization Gorlin and Gorlin formula reflects actual anatomic valve area. Another source of discrepancy may come from the errors introduced into the Doppler continuity equation when estimating the area, flow rate, stroke volume, or velocities through the reference flow location. Errors in estimating cross-sectional area are particularly a problem in children since a small error in measurement of the radius at the reference flow location may be relatively large compared to its overall small radius (332). The Doppler continuity equation and its approximations all assume the subaortic cross-sectional flow profiles at the reference location (usually the left ventricular outflow tract) and at the valve orifice (or actually the vena contracta) are flat. If this is not the case, errors will be introduced. Several studies have shown that the flow profile through the left ventricular outflow tract (339) and at the vena contracta of a stenotic orifice are, in fact, not flat (181,182). Specifically, the shape of the velocity profile at the vena contracta appears to depend on flow rate (181,182).

Some investigators have found the Doppler continuity equation to be flow-independent (178). Various other investigators have found estimation of valve area by the Doppler continuity equation to be flow-dependent (177,181–183,197), with generally ''underestimation'' at low flow rates and ''overestimation'' at high flow rates. This may be due to the valve actually ''stretching'' open with increased flow rates (177,183). On the other hand, it may be due to the fact that at low flow rates (as discussed in "Doppler Tools") the time-averaged peak velocity (which is that measured with CW Doppler) overestimates the space and TAV through the orifice (181,182), causing orifice valve areas to be underestimated.

In adults, aortic valve areas have been categorized as mild stenosis (greater than 1.0 cm^2), moderate stenosis (0.75 to 1.0 cm^2), and severe stenosis (less than 0.75 cm^2) (328,335). In children, aortic valve areas have been categorized as a function of body surface area as mild stenosis (0.8 to 2.0 cm^2/m^2), moderate stenosis (0.5 to 0.8 cm^2/m^2), and severe stenosis (less than 0.5 cm^2/m^2) (37). One study of children with normal hearts obtained a mean aortic valve area of 1.33 cm^2/m^2, implying the range for mild aortic stenosis just quoted may be too wide (340).

Pulmonary Valve Stenosis

As with aortic stenosis an increased flow velocity in the main pulmonary artery can be indicative of pulmonary stenosis or increased flow. Increased flow can be secondary to pulmonary insufficiency or a significant left to right shunt (e.g., ventricular septal defect). To distinguish between these the flow velocities in the right ventricular outflow tract should be measured and incorporated into the Bernoulli equation. As with all lesions, flow velocities across the pulmonary valve should be measured from all possible echocardiographic windows (341) to obtain the highest velocities and best Doppler velocity waveform signals.

Pulmonary valve peak instantaneous pressure gradient ($\Delta P_{peak\ instantaneous}$) assessed by Doppler has been shown to be a useful index in assessing the severity of pulmonary stenosis (5) where the simplified echo Bernoulli equation is (Eq. 13):

$\Delta P_{peak\ instantaneous}$

$$= 4\ (V^2_{max\ -\ pulmonic\ valve} - V^2_{max\ -\ RVOT}). \quad [47]$$

In many clinical settings, the velocity in the right ventricular outflow tract is much less (less than 1.5 m/s) than through the pulmonary valve; thus, the simplified echo Bernoulli equation (Eq. 14) then becomes:

$$\Delta P_{peak\ instantaneous} = 4\ V^2_{max\ -\ pulmonic\ valve}. \quad [48]$$

Studies comparing the peak instantaneous pressure gradient measured by Doppler compared to the catheter peak-to-peak pressure gradient in children (2,3,77,156,179, 341–343) and adults (344) have generally shown equal or better correlations than similar studies of patients with aortic stenosis. The regression line in many of these studies closely approximates the line of identity whereas in aortic stenosis the Doppler peak-to-peak instantaneous pressure gradients tend to overestimate catheter peak-to-peak gradients. There is at least one study that disagrees with this concept, in which investigators have found a consistent overestimation of catheter peak-to-peak gradient across the pulmonary valve using the simplified echo Bernoulli equation (345). Again the importance of whether the catheter and Doppler measurements have been performed simultaneously when comparing these two methods needs to be considered (346).

With the Doppler techniques already described, the mean gradient and pulmonary valve area can be obtained (179,340,345). However, in the clinical setting, these indices of the severity of pulmonary stenosis are seldom used probably because of the belief among many echocardiographers that the Doppler peak instantaneous gradient matches the catheter peak-to-peak gradient so well.

In the neonatal period it is important to assess if the patent ductus arteriosus (PDA) is open. In these instances the pressure gradient across the pulmonary valve may underestimate the degree of valvular stenosis severity due to high pressures transmitted through the PDA. Once the PDA closes the transvalvular pressure gradient could change dramatically.

Subvalvular Obstruction

This section will specifically cover the Doppler aspects of subvalvular obstruction of the semilunar valves. We will not specifically be covering the aspects of subvalvular obstruction for atrioventricular valves. There are several types of subvalvular obstructions in the ventricular outflow tracts, especially in congenital heart disease, which include (a) fixed discrete obstruction; (b) fixed tunnel obstruction; (c) dynamic obstruction. Any of these can coexist with semilunar valvar obstruction.

Considerations of Doppler Velocity Waveforms and the Simplified Echo Bernoulli Equation

With simple fixed discrete subvalvular obstructions the CW velocity curve in the respective great artery should be similar to that found in semilunar valvular stenosis (5) and the assumptions of the simplified echo Bernoulli equation (Eq. 14) should allow for an acceptable representation of peak instantaneous pressure gradient. The PW Doppler sample point can be "walked" through the ventricular outflow tract and the level of the discrete obstruction identified at the location of a significant increase in velocities (5). It may be difficult to determine whether valvular stenosis exists in addition to the subvalvular obstruction. HPRF Doppler can be used to help identify such multiple obstructions, by sampling at selective locations through the outflow tract and the semilunar valve area.

In fixed tunnel obstructions, the applicability of the Bernoulli equation comes into question (162,347) since viscous forces may become more prominent, causing the simplified echo Bernoulli equation to underestimate pressure gradients.

Dynamic obstruction in the ventricular outflow tract produces interesting Doppler signals (5). The obstruction increases with the emptying of the ventricle; thus, there is a late peaking of the velocity waveform with dynamic obstruction so the waveform takes on a characteristic "dagger" appearance (77) (Echo. 6-22). The obstruction is highly dependent on loading conditions and can change in the same patient from one point in time to another.

When subvalvular dynamic obstruction coexists with semilunar valve stenosis, CW Doppler through both areas may show the "dagger" waveform of the dynamic obstruction superimposed on the signal from the valvular stenosis (5). Whether this type of superimposition of waveforms occurs depends on the relative degree of the two obstructions. When it does occur, this phenomenon can be explained (5) by the fact that early in systole the main pressure drop is at the semilunar valve so that the early high velocities on the superimposed waveforms are from the semilunar valve stenosis. Later in systole, as the dynamic obstruction becomes more prominent, the main pressure drop is across the dynamic obstruction so that the high velocities on the superimposed waveform seen later in systole are from the dynamic obstruction.

These subvalvular and valvar obstructions in series also create interesting alterations to the assumptions that have been made regarding the simplified echo Bernoulli equation when dealing with discrete orifices. One of the terms left out in the simplified echo Bernoulli equation is viscous friction. This may or may not be a factor (depending on the Reynolds number) in causing errors when the simplified echo Bernoulli equation is used in subvalvular obstructions in series with valve obstructions, especially

long tunnel-type subvalvular obstructions (162,347). Also, the phenomenon of pressure recovery is quite different with obstructions in series. Yoganathan et al. (162) describe the fluid dynamics through such a series of obstructions (fixed subvalvular and valvar). They show that the vena contracta occurs between the subvalvular obstruction and the stenotic valve, where the velocity is maximum and the pressure is the lowest. Past the stenotic valve, there is a significant pressure recovery (which probably depends on the Reynolds number). The CW Doppler velocity through this series of obstructions records the highest velocity, which is at the vena contracta. Catheter pressures are generally measured at both ends of the entire series of obstructions (subvalvular and valvar). Thus, with pressure recovery the Doppler instantaneous pressure gradient will overestimate the catheter peak-to-peak gradient. This leads to a difference of measurement in space for these methods. Of course there is still the difference of measurement in time (peak instantaneous versus peak-to-peak gradients). In this study (in vitro and in vivo experiments) the Reynolds numbers for the flow rates and orifice sizes tested (RE_{number} greater than 15,000) allowed viscous effects to be neglected.

Left Ventricular Outflow Tract Obstruction

Doppler studies of left ventricular outflow tract obstruction have mostly focused on the dynamic obstruction found in hypertrophic cardiomyopathy (5,348–362), though some studies have included fixed discrete and tunnel subaortic stenoses (162,347,363–367). The signal from mitral regurgitation has to be excluded when measuring the left ventricular outflow tract obstruction (349,351). In hypertrophic cardiomyopathy the mitral valve apparatus as well as the ventricular walls probably in combination cause the overall obstruction (348,353,362).

The Doppler peak instantaneous gradient using the simplified Bernoulli equation is (Eq. 14):

$$\Delta P_{\text{peak instantaneous}} = 4\,(V^2_{\text{max} - \text{LVOT}}).\qquad [49]$$

Suggesting that viscous effects can be neglected, surprisingly good correlations have been shown between Doppler peak instantaneous pressure gradients and catheter peak instantaneous gradients in adults and adolescent children with dynamic obstruction from hypertrophic cardiomyopathy ($r = 0.89$ to 0.97) (349,350,357,368). The regression lines are close to unity in most of these studies. Those studies with simultaneous measurements showed improved results (357,368).

Studies in fixed discrete and tunnel subaortic stenoses comparing catheter and Doppler pressure gradients are limited (363,367). Linear regression analysis from these studies tended to include data from patients with valvar aortic stenosis.

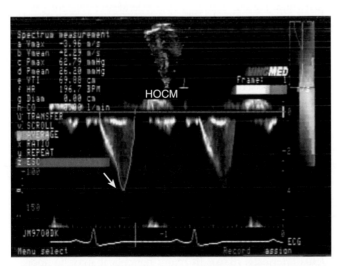

ECHO. 6-22. Doppler spectral velocity waveform in the left ventricular outflow tract of a patient with dynamic obstruction. As the obstruction increases with the emptying of the ventricle there is a late peaking *(arrow)* of the velocity waveform and the waveform takes on a characteristic "dagger" appearance. *HOCM,* hypertrophic obstructive cardiomyopathy.

Right Ventricular Outflow Tract Obstruction

Doppler studies of right ventricular outflow tract obstruction have mostly focused on the infundibular obstruction in patients with repaired and unrepaired tetralogy of Fallot and have included patients with the coexistence of valvar pulmonary stenosis (5,163,342,369).

Similar to subaortic obstruction where viscous effects can be neglected, surprisingly good correlations have been shown between Doppler peak instantaneous pressure gradients and catheter peak instantaneous gradients in children with infundibular and valvar obstruction with a regression line close to unity ($r = 0.90$) (369).

Supravalvar and Vascular Obstruction

Supravalvar Aortic Stenosis and Supravalvar Pulmonic Stenosis

There are a limited number of investigations that have evaluated the Doppler assessment of supravalvar aortic stenosis (163) and supravalvar pulmonic stenosis (163), especially those that single out comparisons of catheter and Doppler pressure gradients for the supravalvar lesion. There are generally three types of supravalvular stenosis: (a) discrete membranous type; (b) tubular hypoplastic type, where the great artery is small throughout; and (c) hourglass type (74).

Three generally accepted concepts regarding peak instantaneous Doppler and catheter gradients are important when considering these lesions. First, if there are multiple levels of obstruction the Doppler peak instantaneous gradient will overestimate the catheter peak instantaneous gradient due to pressure recovery similar to what we have described in subvalvular obstruction (77). Second, if a long supravalvar segment is present it is assumed viscous forces come into play (77) and the Doppler peak instantaneous gradient may underestimate the catheter peak instantaneous gradient. Third, the smooth transition of an hourglass lesion leads to a significant amount of pressure recovery leading to Doppler peak instantaneous pressure gradient overestimating the catheter peak instantaneous gradient. All of these general concepts need to be verified in further clinical studies.

One particular instance of supravalvar stenosis created surgically (used in patients with certain forms of congenital heart disease to limit pulmonary blood flow) is the supravalvar pulmonic stenosis created by a pulmonary artery band. Doppler pressure gradients across the band have correlated well with catheterization pressure gradients in this setting (343,370,371).

Peripheral Pulmonary Stenosis

Similar to supravalvar stenosis, peripheral pulmonary stenosis (or branch pulmonary stenosis) can occur in three types of lesions: (a) discrete membrane type; (b) tubular hypoplastic type; and (c) hourglass type. These lesions can be multiple in number. In newborns, it is quite common to note a velocity increase as the sample volume is moved from the main pulmonary artery to the branch pulmonary arteries (77,372). Transient peripheral pulmonary stenosis (PPS) occurs in premature infants and full-term neonates (373). Velocities above 2 m/s are considered unphysiologic at the branch pulmonary arteries by many pediatric echocardiographers.

Coarctation

Doppler echocardiography has become an important tool in the assessment of coarctation of the aorta (5,77,307,374–393). The general approach in the evaluation of the aorta for coarctation should begin with two-dimensional (see Echo. 28-1) and color flow imaging of the aortic arch. With color flow imaging, there may be significant flow disturbance in the region of the coarctation (see Echos. 28-3 and 28-4) (77). The PW Doppler sample can be "walked through the aortic arch," and significant changes in flow velocities can be recorded if present. The CW Doppler beam can then be directed through the descending aorta and through any suspicious areas. Depending on the severity of the obstruction, the CW Doppler velocity sampling through the coarctation (see Echos. 28-5 and 28-7) may show increased velocities and antegrade diastolic flow ("diastolic runoff") as well as a superimposition of the peak velocity in the precoarctation region (see Echo. 28-8). The antegrade diastolic flow (5,77,392) is due to the persistence of a pressure drop across the coarctation throughout diastole, with elevated systolic and diastolic pressures in the precoarctation region. In a patient with coarctation and a coexistent patent ductus arteriosus, normal Doppler velocity patterns may be obtained and can be misleading (77).

Pressure gradients are commonly used in the assessment of severity in coarctation. As with all the stenotic lesions we have discussed, it is important to remember that if cardiac output is low in a given patient, then pressure gradient alone will not be a good indicator of severity of coarctation (375). Additionally, in patients with a coexistent patent ductus arteriosus which may change the hemodynamics around the coarctation site, the lack of a pressure gradient across the coarctation site may be misleading. One study suggests considering a combination of factors (isthmus dimensions on two-dimensional imaging, presence or absence of continuous isthmus flow, direction of ductal flow) when diagnosing coarctation of the aorta in patents with a coexistent patent ductus arteriosus (376). In many patients it may be appropriate to wait for ductal closure prior to ruling out a coarctation lesion by Doppler and other means.

In addition to the issues of using the simplified echo Bernoulli equation (Eq. 14) in the Doppler estimation of pressure gradients, coarctation adds some considerations to the implementation of the Bernoulli equation. Coarctations can be discrete or long segment in nature. Viscous factors and factors related to multiple obstructions in series (162,347) may become important when using the simplified echo Bernoulli equation in long-segment coarctation lesions. The presence of collaterals may cause an accurate Doppler reading of pressure gradients but a poor estimation of coarctation severity (5). The ability to perform Doppler sampling through the affected region can be compromised in many patients (i.e., poor alignment), leading to an underestimation of peak velocities (5,77,377).

Another important factor to consider in the Doppler assessment of coarctation is the use of the precoarctation velocity in the simplified echo Bernoulli equation. The precoarctation velocity is often elevated, particularly if aortic stenosis is present, and, therefore, the full simplified echo Bernoulli equation (Eq. 13) should be used in most clinical settings:

$$\Delta P_{\text{peak instantaneous}}$$
$$= 4 \ (V^2_{\text{max - coarctation}} - V^2_{\text{max - precoarctation}}). \quad [50]$$

When comparing catheterization and Doppler pressure gradients, published studies showing poor linear correlations are generally those that have compared catheter pressure gradients to Doppler peak instantaneous pressure gradients derived ignoring the precoarctation velocities in the simplified echo Bernoulli equation (377,378,388). Studies have shown improved correlations by including the precoarctation velocities (382,384,386).

Good linear correlations have been found in several studies where the Doppler peak instantaneous gradient incorporating the precoarctation velocity has been compared to the catheter peak-to-peak pressure gradient ($r = 0.76$ to 0.98) (391) or the catheter peak instantaneous pressure gradient ($r = 0.94$) (382). As in other stenotic lesions, the Doppler peak instantaneous pressure gradient tends to overestimate the catheter peak-to-peak pressure gradient (377). The difference between catheter peak-to-peak and catheter peak instantaneous pressure gradients becomes less pronounced with increasing severity of the lesion (388) probably since the postcoarctation site pressure waveform becomes less pulsatile with severe coarctation. Mean Doppler and catheter pressure gradients have shown to have even better correlation ($r = 0.97$) (382). Interestingly, in one study worsening correlation was shown between Doppler and catheter pressure gradients after balloon valvuloplasty with the possible explanation of worsening Doppler alignment or variable collateral effects given as part of the explanation for this (384).

Despite these favorable results, the Doppler assessment of coarctation of the aorta is still used with some caution by many practicing echocardiographers (394), especially in evaluating the repaired patient with possible recoarcta-

tion. Further studies with current improved Doppler measuring devices are required.

REGURGITANT LESIONS

Atrioventricular Valve Regurgitation: Pressure Gradients

Tricuspid Regurgitation

Right heart systolic pressure is often estimated by techniques that use the simplified echo Bernoulli equation (Eq. 14) on the peak velocity of the tricuspid regurgitation Doppler waveform in patients of all ages (5,395–401). Since this regurgitation represents systolic flow between the right atrium and the right ventricle, the pressures obtained in this manner represent the systolic right ventricular to right atrial pressure gradient. Absolute right ventricular systolic pressure (RVSP) can be roughly estimated using assumed, measured, or approximated right atrial pressure (RAP) and adding that to the pressure gradient obtained by using the simplified echo Bernoulli equation (Eq. 14):

$$RVSP = 4 \ (V^2_{\text{max - tricuspid regurgitation}}) + RAP. \quad [51]$$

If there is no evidence of right ventricular outflow tract obstruction or pulmonary stenosis, this RVSP can be used as an estimate of systolic pulmonary artery pressure (77).

Issues such as pressure recovery, viscous losses, and the differences between peak instantaneous and peak-to-peak gradients appear to be much less of an issue when the simplified echo Bernoulli equation is used in this setting. Specifically, peak-to-peak pressure gradients and peak instantaneous pressure gradients are much closer in value with tricuspid regurgitation since the pressures in the "distal" chamber (the right atrium) are relatively much less pulsatile than the "proximal" chamber pressures (those in the right ventricle).

There have been several techniques used to estimate right atrial pressure in order to obtain an estimate of right ventricular pressures. Many echocardiographers simply use a right atrial pressure of 5 to 10 mmHg in children (76,77) and 10 to 15 in adults (200) if there is no suspicion of elevated pressures (77). Using jugular venous pressures in adults (usually not a practical measurement in children) has been shown to be a poor approximation to right atrial catheter pressure (74,396,397). Estimation of right atrial pressure from inferior vena caval diameter changes with respiration has been described in adults (74,402,403).

Not all patients have tricuspid regurgitation, while others have a weak Doppler signal. These signals can be enhanced using small amounts of contrast (404–409). Color Doppler can help in the proper alignment of the spectral Doppler beam parallel with the regurgitant flow for accurate peak velocity measurements (410).

Results comparing catheter pressure gradients to those estimated by Doppler show good correlation ($r = 0.87$ to 0.97) (5,395–400), especially when comparing simultaneous catheter and Doppler measurements.

Mitral Regurgitation

Left ventricular systolic pressure is less often estimated by techniques that use the simplified echo Bernoulli equation (Eq. 14) on the peak velocity of the mitral regurgitation Doppler waveform. The systolic pressure gradient obtained in this manner represents that between the left ventricle and the left atrium. If there is no evidence of LVOT obstruction and no aortic stenosis, LAP can be roughly estimated (300,200,411,412) using measured aortic systolic pressures (ASP) and the pressure gradient obtained by using the simplified echo Bernoulli equation (Eq. 14):

$$LAP = ASP - 4\ (V^2_{max - mitral\ regurgitation}). \qquad [52]$$

This method has been rejected by some (30,76) because (a) the absolute LAP is so much smaller than the systolic pressure gradient and systolic aortic pressure and small errors in measurement lead to large errors in the estimation of LAP; and (b) differences in cuff blood pressure versus central aortic pressure exist.

In adults, if the peak velocity of the mitral regurgitation Doppler signal is less than 4 m/s this most likely indicates a high LAP and a low left ventricular pressure (30).

Semilunar Valve Regurgitation: Pressure Gradients

Aortic Regurgitation

The end diastolic velocity of the aortic regurgitation Doppler waveform can be used in the simplified echo Bernoulli equation (Eq. 14) to estimate the instantaneous pressure gradient between the aorta and left ventricle at end diastole. Using the end diastolic cuff pressure as the aortic diastolic pressure, a rough estimate of the left ventricular end diastolic pressure can be obtained (30,412).

Pulmonic Regurgitation

Similar to aortic regurgitation, the end diastolic velocity of the pulmonic regurgitation Doppler waveform (Echo. 6-13) can be used in the simplified echo Bernoulli equation to estimate the pressure gradient between the right ventricle and pulmonary artery at end diastole. The right ventricular end diastolic pressure (or right atrial pressure) must be estimated and added to the pressure gradient obtained in order to estimate the end diastolic pulmonary artery pressure (413). A rough estimate of mean pulmonary artery pressure can be obtained from the average of estimated pulmonary artery systolic and diastolic pressures (30).

Atrioventricular Valve Regurgitation: Assessment of Severity

Mitral Regurgitation

We have previously introduced many of the methods of assessing regurgitant lesions which include (a) color Doppler flow mapping jet length and area (217,414–418); (b) CW Doppler signal strength (419); (c) width of the proximal color Doppler flow jet (234–237,420); and (d) venous flow patterns. These have been applied to the mitral valve and are still in general use today.

The technique of color flow mapping jet length and jet areas (216,217,414–418,420–422) uses methods derived from PW velocity mapping (213). In adults, jet length (Jet_{Length}) was shown to correlate well with angiographic determined severity ($r = 0.87$) (217,414) of mild regurgitation (less than 1.5 cm), moderate regurgitation (1.5 to 2.9 cm), moderately severe regurgitation (2.9 to 4.4 cm), and severe regurgitation (greater than 4.4 cm). Jet area (Jet_{area}) and the ratio of jet area to left atrial area (Jet_{ratio}), however, have shown improved correlation to angiographic data (415–417), classified in adults as mild regurgitation (Jet_{area} less than 4 cm^2; Jet_{ratio} less than 0.2), moderate regurgitation (Jet_{area} = 4 to 8 cm^2; Jet_{ratio} = 0.2 to 0.4), and severe regurgitation (Jet_{area} greater than 8 cm^2; Jet_{ratio} greater than 0.4) (216,414–416). Similar relationships have been developed using transesophageal echocardiography (418). In children, the classification is similar, but jet area is referenced to body surface area with mild regurgitation (Jet_{area} less than 4 cm^2/m^2; Jet_{ratio} less than 0.3), moderate regurgitation (Jet_{area} = 4 to 10 cm^2/m^2; Jet_{ratio} = 0.3 to 0.5), and severe regurgitation (Jet_{area} greater than 10 cm^2/m^2; Jet_{ratio} greater than 0.5) (420).

We have previously discussed some of the factors affecting jet area that may or may not be associated with the severity of the mitral regurgitation. These include (a) pressure, volume, and compliance of the receiving chamber; (b) instrumentation factors (226); (c) the effects of solid boundaries onto which the jet may impinge (228,422); and (d) interobserver (229) and day-to-day variability (423). One must remember the Doppler velocity image displays blood velocities, not blood flow, and the maximum jet area relates to peak flow rate rather than total regurgitant flow volume. Differences in pulmonary venous flows have been shown to be a potential source of variation in mitral regurgitant jet area (424).

Measuring the width of the color Doppler velocity image of the proximal flow jet is another technique developed to qualitatively assess the severity of mitral regurgitation (234–237). Many current studies report the best measurement of this width with multiplane transesophageal Doppler color flow imaging (234,235). Studies in adults (234–236) show good correlation to angiographic grades of regurgitation. Several of these studies also show a jet width greater than 5.5 to 6.5 mm correlated well with severe mitral regurgitation judged angiographically (234–236).

The presence and degree of reversed systolic flow in the pulmonary veins has been shown to correlate with the degree of mitral regurgitation (421,425–429). Just the presence of reversed systolic flow in the pulmonary veins may, in fact, indicate severe mitral regurgitation (421, 425,427,429). It is important to sample as many pulmonary veins as possible (430), and most current studies of pulmonary venous flow use transesophageal color Doppler for optimal imaging (421,425,427,429,430). The peak systolic forward pulmonary vein flow velocity has been shown to be inversely related to the degree of mitral regurgitation (427). The ratio of the VTI of the systolic pulmonary venous flow to the diastolic flow has been proposed as another means of assessing mitral regurgitation severity (428).

Mitral regurgitant jet direction can play an important role in pulmonary venous patterns and, therefore, can cause variations in the estimation of mitral regurgitation severity (431).

Investigators continue to strive to develop Doppler methods that quantitate flow volumes, regurgitant fractions, and regurgitant orifice areas to further quantitate the severity of regurgitation. Regurgitant stroke volume is obtained by measuring stroke volume (Eq. 3) at the regurgitant mitral valve ($SV_{mitral\ valve}$) and at a reference location ($SV_{reference}$) through a valve where there is no regurgitation (AOV or pulmonic valve) (148,149,432–435).

Regurgitant stroke volume (Eq. 8), for the mitral valve ($RSV_{mitral\ valve}$), is given as:

$$RSV_{mitral\ valve} = SV_{mitral\ valve} - SV_{reference}. \quad [53]$$

Regurgitant fraction (Eq. 9), for the mitral valve ($RF_{mitral\ valve}$), is given as:

$$RF_{mitral\ valve} = \frac{RSV}{SV_{mitral\ valve}}. \quad [54]$$

Clinical studies comparing these methods to angiographic methods have shown good correlation (148,433). However, similar to the problems with shunt calculations, these methods to calculate Doppler-derived flow rates have inherent errors, and the derived calculations could potentially magnify these errors manyfold (74).

We have previously introduced the flow convergence method (Eq. 5) and its use in estimating flow rates and orifice areas (Eqs. 24 and 25). These concepts have been used in the assessment of mitral regurgitation severity (118,185–187,436–446). Many of these studies have shown good correlation to quantitative angiographic measures of mitral regurgitation severity. Most studies of mitral regurgitation use the instantaneous peak flow rate (IFR_{peak}), where the isovelocity surface is chosen at a time of maximum regurgitant flow (Eq. 24).

Total regurgitant stroke volume has been estimated us-

ing the flow convergence method. The first aliased boundary can be sampled throughout the ejection cycle, and instantaneous flow rates (Eq. 5) can be summed to obtain an estimate of regurgitant stroke volume (436) (n = number of samples):

$$RSV = \Sigma IFR_i, i = 1, \ldots, n \quad [55]$$

Mean regurgitant flow rate (MRFR) can be measured using color M-mode to obtain a mean radius of the first aliased boundary through the ejection cycle, which is then used in the flow rate equation above (439). Another similar method of calculating the MRFR is to obtain the mean squared of the radii (MSR) throughout the ejection cycle by measuring the radius of the first aliased boundary in the color flow image sampled throughout the ejection phase (n = number of samples) (445):

$$MSR = \frac{r_1^2 + r_2^2 \ldots + r_n^2}{n}. \quad [56]$$

The MSR is then used in the flow convergence equation (Eq. 5) to calculate the MRFR:

$$MRFR = 2\pi * MSR^2 * V_{isovelocity}. \quad [57]$$

RSV can be calculated using ejection time (ET) with either of these methods that measure MRFR:

$$RSV = MRFR * T_{ejection}. \quad [58]$$

As we have previously discussed, the flow convergence method can be used to estimate regurgitant orifice areas. The orifice area at peak flow can be determined by first calculating the IFR_{peak} and obtaining the peak CW mitral regurgitant velocity (V_{peak}) (Eq. 25).

The average ROA can be determined using the RSV and the VTI of the mitral regurgitant flow:

$$Area_{orifice\ average} = \frac{RSV}{VTI}. \quad [59]$$

There is evidence that the mitral regurgitant orifice areas changes during the ejection cycle (438,443); therefore, the average regurgitant orifice area may be a more reliable index of severity. However, obtaining the regurgitant stroke volume by the flow convergence method can be quite cumbersome and may be clinically impractical. Investigators have obtained good results (185) using the RSV derived from Eq. 8.

Mitral regurgitant valves are sometimes found to have surrounding boundaries that form less than a 180-degree angle with the orifice (see Fig. 6-7) (109,113–115,192). As discussed, instead of a hemisphere, the isovelocity surface is the surface of a cone and peak instantaneous flow rate is shown in Eq. 6. The flow convergence method orifice area equation otherwise remains the same.

Tricuspid Regurgitation

The methods of assessing tricuspid regurgitant lesions include measuring regurgitant jet length and area (447), and CW Doppler signal strength. Severe tricuspid regurgitation (i.e., in need of repair) has been shown to correlate with a jet ratio (Jet$_{ratio}$ = the ratio of jet area to right atrial area) of less than 0.34 (216).

If systolic backflow is present in the inferior vena cava or hepatic veins, tricuspid regurgitation is considered to be at least moderate (216).

For a more quantitative assessment of tricuspid regurgitation severity, the flow convergence method has been used with some success (448,449) for regurgitant flow rates and regurgitant orifice areas.

The proximal jet size has been shown to be a good measure of tricuspid regurgitation severity with good correlation to other Doppler methods of assessment (450).

Semilunar Valve Regurgitation: Assessment of Severity

Aortic Regurgitation

Most of the methods used in the assessment of mitral regurgitation have been also used in the assessment of aortic regurgitation (451). These include (a) color Doppler flow mapping jet length and area; (b) CW Doppler signal strength (452); (c) width and cross-sectional area of the proximal color Doppler flow jet. In addition other indices used in the assessment of aortic regurgitation include (a) degree of reversal of flow in the aorta (ascending, descending, abdominal) (151,453–457) where the peak velocities, VTIs, and amplitude-weighted mean velocities of antegrade and retrograde aortic flow have been compared; (b) the slope of the deceleration phase of aortic regurgitation CW velocity waveform (458).

The technique of color flow mapping jet length and jet areas (215,230,459) has been shown to correlate with angiographic grades of aortic regurgitation but can be unreliable since the jets are often eccentric and coexist with mitral valve inflow (200). The width (Jet$_{width}$) and the cross-sectional area of the proximal color Doppler flow jet (Jet$_{CSA}$) have shown better correlation (230,414,460–462) and have been indexed (Jet$_{width.ratio}$ and Jet$_{CSA.ratio}$, respectively) to their respective measurements of the LVOT giving the following ratios:

$$\text{Jet}_{width.ratio} = \frac{\text{Jet}_{width}}{\text{LVOT}_{width}} \quad [60]$$

and

$$\text{Jet}_{CSA.ratio} = \frac{\text{Jet}_{CSA}}{\text{LVOT}_{CSA}} \quad [61]$$

where LVOT$_{width}$ is the width of the left ventricular outflow tract and LVOT$_{CSA}$ is the cross-sectional area of the left ventricular outflow tract. In adults, the jet width ratio (216,230,463) has been used to evaluate mild aortic regurgitation (Jet$_{width.ratio}$ < 25%), moderate aortic regurgitation (Jet$_{width.ratio}$ = 25% to 46%), moderately severe aortic re-

gurgitation (Jet$_{width.ratio}$ = 46% to 65%), and severe aortic regurgitation (Jet$_{width.ratio}$ greater than 65%) (230).

The slope of the deceleration phase (decay slope or DS) of the aortic regurgitant Doppler velocity waveform has been shown to correlate with the angiographic degree of disease (464). In adult studies, severe aortic regurgitation correlated with a decay slope of greater than 3 m/s^2 (461,464). In another study, mild aortic regurgitation correlated with a decay slope of less than 2 m/s^2 (201). However, significant overlap existed between various values of decay slope and angiographic grades of aortic regurgitation in these studies.

A different technique of evaluating the decay slope is to measure its pressure half-time. Pressure half-time is the time period from peak velocity (V_{peak}) to a velocity ($V_{pressure-half-time}$) where the pressure gradient is half the value of the peak gradient (Eq. 30). In adults, a pressure half-time below 300 to 400 ms correlates with severe aortic regurgitation (30,465).

Assessing severity of aortic regurgitation by measuring parameters related to the decay slope has limitations because the slope has been shown to depend not only on regurgitation severity but also on systemic vascular resistance, loading conditions, and left ventricular compliance (200,466–468).

As with mitral regurgitation, ongoing investigations continue to develop newer Doppler methods that quantitate flow volumes, regurgitant fractions, and regurgitant orifice areas more accurately. One such method measures regurgitant stroke volume (RSV) (Eq. 8). Stroke volume is calculated at the regurgitant aortic valve (SV$_{aortic valve}$) and at a reference location (SV$_{reference}$) through a valve where there is no regurgitation (mitral valve or pulmonic valve) (151). RSV (Eq. 8) for the aortic valve (RSV$_{aortic valve}$) is given as:

$$\text{RSV}_{aortic\ valve} = \text{SV}_{aortic\ valve} - \text{SV}_{reference}. \quad [62]$$

RF (Eq. 9) for the aortic valve (RF$_{aortic valve}$) is given as:

$$\text{RF}_{aortic\ valve} = \frac{\text{RSV}_{aortic\ valve}}{\text{SV}_{aortic\ valve}}. \quad [63]$$

ROA uses the VTI of the regurgitant signal and is given by:

$$\text{ROA} = \frac{\text{RSV}_{aortic\ valve}}{\text{VTI}}. \quad [64]$$

Clinical studies comparing these methods to angiographic methods have shown good correlation (148, 149,185,469–471). However, similar to the problems with shunt calculations, these methods to calculate Doppler-derived flow rates have inherent errors and perform calculations that could potentially magnify these errors (74). One method that has been proposed in an attempt to measure aortic regurgitant volume directly is to multiply the VTI of the aortic regurgitant signal by the cross-sectional area of the proximal jet; this has had promising results when compared to angiographic grading (472).

The flow convergence method is used in estimating aortic regurgitant flow rates and regurgitant orifice area (186,473). Most studies of aortic regurgitation and flow convergence use the instantaneous peak flow rate (IFR_{peak}), which is determined as previously shown in Eq. 24. The aortic regurgitant orifice area at peak flow can be determined (Eq. 25) by using the peak IFR and obtaining the peak CW aortic regurgitant velocity (V_{peak}), with peak orifice area ($Area_{orifice - peak}$).

There is debate whether the aortic ROA changes during the ejection cycle (474,475). In addition, the actual shapes of the isovelocity contours in the aortic regurgitant flow convergence region may represent ellipses rather than hemispheres (476,477) and modifications to the flow convergence equation have been proposed.

Pulmonic Regurgitation

Much less has been reported regarding assessing the severity of pulmonic regurgitation using Doppler techniques. The qualitative methods of assessing these regurgitant lesions include (a) regurgitant jet length and area; (b) CW Doppler signal strength (5); (c) the slope of the deceleration phase of pulmonic regurgitation CW velocity waveform (478); and (d) width of the proximal color Doppler flow jet.

A jet length greater than 20 mm in an early Doppler study has been shown to correlate with an audible regurgitant murmur (479). Jet area (Jet_{area}) indexed to body surface area has been shown to correlate with angiographic degrees of mild (0.64 ± 0.60 cm^2/m^2), moderate (1.07 ± 0.63 cm^2/m^2) and severe (2.2 ± 1.67 cm^2/m^2) regurgitation (74). These indicators have been studied in only a limited number of investigations and are most likely subject to the same inaccuracies as we have discussed with their use in aortic and mitral regurgitation.

Researchers have sought to quantitate flow volumes, regurgitant fractions, and ROAs to further quantitate the severity of regurgitation. Regarding regurgitant fractions, forward and reverse stroke volumes ($SV_{reverse}$ and $SV_{forward}$, respectively) are measured in the pulmonary artery by the method using the VTI of the forward and reverse Doppler velocity signals (151) (Eq. 3). Regurgitant fraction for the pulmonary valve ($RF_{pulm valve}$) is given as:

$$RF_{pulm valve} = \frac{SV_{reverse}}{SV_{forward}}. \qquad [65]$$

RSV can be determined (Eq. 8) using the stroke volume at the regurgitant pulmonic valve ($SV_{pulm valve}$) and at a reference location ($SV_{reference}$) through a valve where there is no regurgitation (mitral valve or aortic valve) (151). RSV is then given as the following:

$$RSV_{pulm valve} = SV_{pulm valve} - SV_{reference}. \qquad [66]$$

RF (Eq. 9) for the pulmonic valve ($RF_{pulm valve}$) is given as:

$$RF_{pulm valve} = \frac{RSV}{SV_{pulm valve}}. \qquad [67]$$

Regurgitant fractions have been shown to correlate with clinical severity of disease with mild regurgitation ($RF_{pulm valve}$ less than 40%), moderate regurgitation ($RF_{pulm valve} = 40\%$ to 60%), and severe regurgitation ($RF_{pulm valve}$ greater than 60%) (151,480), but significant crossover exists between disease states and various regurgitant fractions (74).

SHUNT LESIONS

Intracardiac Shunts

Prior to the development of color Doppler flow imaging, PW Doppler imaging used in conjunction with two-dimensional imaging offered many advantages over two-dimensional imaging alone in the echocardiographic detection of intracardiac shunts such as ventricular septal defects (VSDs) and atrial septal defects (ASDs) (5,481–487). Using the PW Doppler method, the area adjacent to the septum of interest was sampled. Areas found to have significant flow disturbance on the Doppler velocity waveform were then labeled as suspicious for septal defects. Practically, this was quite a time-consuming process. With the advent of color Doppler flow imaging, the diagnosis of such defects became more accurate, faster and easier (488–490). Color Doppler flow imaging can help determine the precise size of septal defects (491,492). Presently there is a role for all modalities of echocardiography in the diagnosis of intracardiac shunts including two-dimensional, PW and CW Doppler, and color flow imaging. Transesophageal echocardiography offers some additional advantages in certain situations as well, especially in adults (493–495).

We have already discussed calculating shunt flows by comparing flow rates through two different locations of the heart and we will not be discussing that further here.

Ventricular Septal Defects

PW Doppler and color Doppler flow imaging have been useful in understanding the hemodynamic changes that occur throughout the cardiac cycle in patients with a ventricular septal defect (VSD). Generally in most patients with isolated ventricular septal defects, there is left to right shunting throughout the systolic phase of the cardiac cycle, including during isovolumetric contraction. During isovolumetric relaxation there is right to left shunting. In early diastole, flow is right to left across the ventricular septal defect. Later in diastole flow is left to right (496,497). In patients with and without additional disease states these generalities may not hold true. One must remember the technical limitations of some of the current technology (frame rate of standard video tape recorders) when making judgments about shunt direction during limited time spans such as those during isovolumetric relaxation and contraction (498).

In patients with right ventricular volume overload and a ventricular septal defect, flow is generally right to left throughout diastole (496,499). In patients with concomitant elevated right ventricular pressures (e.g., significant pulmonary stenosis or pulmonary hypertension) flow in systole may start as left to right but then soon change to right to left shunting (500). These same patients may have diastolic flow which remains right to left through mid diastole (500).

Often the peak CW Doppler velocity obtained through a ventricular septal defect is used in the simplified echo Bernoulli equation (Eq. 14) to predict the pressure gradient between the left and right ventricles. One must remember the limitations of this technique. The peak pressure in the left and right ventricles may not occur simultaneously, making the catheter measured peak-to-peak gradient less than the instantaneous gradient measured by CW Doppler. The simplified echo Bernoulli equation applies to discrete fixed orifices and ventricular septal defects are not necessarily fixed or discrete (147). Setting the alignment of the CW sample beam directly parallel to the direction of jet flow may be difficult as well. At least one investigator has reported high-velocity CW Doppler jets in patients with equal right and left ventricular pressures; however, this was an early study (147).

With those limitations in mind, several studies have shown good correlation between catheter peak-to-peak pressure gradients and Doppler instantaneous pressure gradients from the left ventricle to right ventricle in infants, children, and adults ($r = 0.92$ to 0.98) (501–504). However, several studies reported poor correlation between the two gradients in children and adults with small defects (505–507) which may be in part due to the difficult alignment problems in such lesions (506).

In addition to calculating shunt flows by comparing flow rates through two different locations of the heart already discussed (see above), shunt flow has been estimated using the proximal flow convergence method (508). The peak instantaneous flow rate through the VSD ($IFR_{VSD\ peak}$) using the flow convergence method (Eq. 5) through the VSD is given as:

$$IFR_{VSD\ peak} = 2\pi r_{max}^2 * V_{isovelocity} \qquad [68]$$

where r_{max} = radius of hemisphere of first aliased boundary at peak flow, $2\pi r_{max}^2$ = the surface area of that hemisphere, and $V_{isovelocity}$ = the set aliased velocity (Nyquist limit). Peak instantaneous VSD flow rates were compared to mean VSD flow rates at catheterization (508); therefore, the accuracy of the flow convergence method was not tested (509). An approach using the flow convergence method in atrial septal defects may be applicable to certain ventricular septal defects (510). In the first step of

this method, VSD orifice area ($Area_{VSD\ orifice}$) is determined as previously described (Eq. 25), using the FCM:

$$Area_{VSD\ orifice} = \frac{IFR_{VSD\ peak}}{V_{peak}} \qquad [69]$$

where V_{peak} is the CW Doppler peak velocity through the VSD. In the second step of this method, VSD shunt flow (Q_{VSD}) is calculated by the following formula:

$$Q_{VSD} = Area_{VSD\ orifice} * TAV \qquad [70]$$

where TAV is as in Eq. 1.

Atrial Septal Defects

Spectral Doppler and color Doppler flow imaging have been useful in understanding the hemodynamic changes that occur throughout the cardiac cycle in patients with atrial septal defects as well. Some investigators feel there is no normal anatomic or physiologic setting where there is significant right to left atrial shunting (147). There probably exists some minor changes in direction of flow through most atrial septal defects; however, the preponderance of flow is left to right in most patients without concomitant disease (511–513). In patients with isolated atrial septal defects, significant right to left shunting typically indicates elevated right heart pressures (511).

In newborns with physiologically elevated right heart pressures a small right to left component has been demonstrated in the first day of life which subsequently disappears by four days of age (514).

Typically, the PW Doppler signals in patients with isolated defects have a characteristic pattern and detection of such a pattern is strongly suggestive of an atrial septal defect. Large defects may not show such a pattern since blood flow may not be as well directed as in smaller defects (76). The typical pattern includes a left to right shunt beginning in late systole with a rapid peak in velocity, the velocity then decreases during middiastole. Coinciding with atrial contraction the left to right shunt velocity increases again and peaks. The shunt then reverses to a right to left shunt early in systole (37). This pattern varies somewhat with respiration. In inspiration the pressure difference between the two atrial chambers is decreased leading to a decrease in left to right flow velocities (5,77). This fact can be used to distinguish flow through an atrial septal defect and flow from the superior vena cava. Superior vena cava flow has a similar velocity flow pattern compared to atrial septal defects except for the fact that velocities in the superior vena cava flow increase during inspiration (5).

Usually the peak velocity of the left to right shunt in late systole is 1 to 1.5 m/s, which translates to a peak pressure gradient (using the simplified echo Bernoulli equation) of around 5 mmHg (77).

In patients with certain types of congenital heart disease

atrial septal shunts may be necessary for survival: (a) right to left flow (e.g., tricuspid atresia, total anomalous pulmonary venous connection) (147); (b) bidirectional flow (e.g., complete transposition of the great arteries); (c) left to right flow (e.g., hypoplastic left-heart syndrome). Assessing the relative degree of obstruction at the atrial septal defect in patients with these congenital heart lesions often becomes critical in their proper clinical management. In the assessment of the degree of obstruction, the pressure gradient between atrial chambers is determined using the peak Doppler velocity across the shunt in the simplified echo Bernoulli equation (Eq. 14).

Extracardiac Shunts

Patent Ductus Arteriosus

Doppler technology has helped tremendously in the understanding of the normal and abnormal physiology of the ductus arteriosus. The normal and abnormal timing of ductus arteriosus closure has been studied extensively with the use of color and spectral Doppler (515–518).

Depending on the presence of structural abnormalities and/or the relative pressures between the pulmonary artery and the aorta, the patent ductus arteriosus may shunt predominantly left to right, bidirectionally, or right to left. The direct and indirect appearance of the color Doppler signals and the velocity waveforms associated with a patent ductus arteriosus may be quite different depending on the direction of shunting.

Indirect evidence of the existence of a patent ductus arteriosus can be seen with Doppler spectral and color flow patterns in the main pulmonary artery (519) and descending aorta (520,521). In the main pulmonary artery, if there is a notable left to right shunt, disturbed retrograde flow can be seen by color flow Doppler and detected by spectral Doppler at the distal end of the pulmonary artery near the origin of the left pulmonary artery. In the descending aorta below the ductus arteriosus, if there is a significant left to right shunt, there may be retrograde flow in the aorta in diastole reflecting the run-off lesion. The spectral diastolic signal in the descending aorta is usually M shaped with a peak in early diastole and after atrial contraction (77). The ratio of the retrograde VTI to the forward VTI of the Doppler velocity waveforms has been used to estimate shunt size (520,521). We have previously discussed other methods of calculating shunt flows and will not be discussing this further here (see above).

Direct interrogation of the color flow Doppler signal and the spectral Doppler signal of the patent ductus arteriosus provides enhanced sensitivity and specificity in detecting these lesions (see Echos. 30-1, 30-2, 30-4, 30-6, 30-7, and 30-8) (522). Patent ductus arteriosus with predominately left to right flow can be more easily

detected. Direct interrogation also allows for differentiation from lesions that also may cause disturbed flow in the pulmonary artery, such as aortopulmonary window and anomalous origin of a coronary artery from the pulmonary artery (77).

Spectral signals of the patent ductus arteriosus vary depending on the relative pulmonary pressures. In patients with an isolated patent ductus arteriosus and low pulmonary pressures (giving a left to right shunt), there is a continuous left to right velocity waveform with a peak in late systole and a gradual fall throughout diastole (Echo. 30.4) (523). With higher pulmonary artery pressures there is continuous left to right velocity waveform with a very low early diastolic velocity maintained throughout diastole (523).

Bidirectional shunting occurs with significant pulmonary hypertension (see Echos. 30-6 and 30-7) (524). The right to left velocity waveform occurs in systole and is followed by the left to right velocity waveform which begins in late systole and lasts into late diastole. The more severe the right to left shunting the later the right to left velocity waveform peaks in systole (77). With significant pulmonary hypertension the right to left velocity waveform may start in diastole interrupting the left to right diastolic flow (525–526). Care must be taken to ensure one is not misinterpreting what appears to be a right to left patent ductus arteriosus velocity waveform signal with a normal left pulmonary artery signal (77). Lastly, patients with isolated right to left shunting (severe pulmonary hypertension or interrupted arch) have a continuous right to left velocity signal which peaks in early systole (see Echo. 30-8) (524,527).

The peak CW Doppler velocity (V_{max}) obtained through a patent ductus arteriosus is used in the simplified echo Bernoulli equation (Eq. 11) to predict the pressure gradient between the aorta and pulmonary artery. The systemic peak systolic pressure (SYS_{SP}) is then used to estimate pulmonary artery peak systolic pressures (PA_{SP}):

$$PA_{SP} = SYS_{SP} - 4V_{max}^2 \qquad [71]$$

for left to right ductal flow, and

$$PA_{SP} = SYS_{SP} + 4V_{max}^2 \qquad [72]$$

for right to left ductal flow.

One might expect that this method would underestimate pressure gradients since viscous frictional forces may need to be considered in the Bernoulli equation as these are not discrete lesions. Other predicted sources of error include the fact that peak-to-peak pressure gradients are different from instantaneous pressure gradients. Also, precisely where along the ductus the velocities are recorded may give different results (528). This may be related to problems in locating the point of maximum jet flow (i.e., the narrowest part of the patent ductus arteriosus) and aligning the CW sample beam directly parallel to its flow direction as well as differing flow dynamics with different locations of the narrowest region which we will discuss with aortopulmonary shunts (529). Despite these limitations, studies have shown good correlation comparing Doppler peak instantaneous pressure gradients to catheter peak-to-peak pressure gradients (530,531) ($r = 0.97$) and to catheter peak instantaneous pressure gradients ($r = 0.94$) (528) between the aorta and pulmonary artery (401).

Surgical Shunts

Aortopulmonary Shunts

Spectral and color Doppler imaging have been instrumental in aiding the management of patients with aortopulmonary shunts. The most common of these aortopulmonary shunts is the Blalock–Taussig (BT) shunts (including modified BT shunts). Investigators have noted the ability of PW Doppler and color Doppler flow imaging to detect the presence of such shunts (532–535). The typical CW Doppler velocity waveform through such shunts is shown in Echo. 6-23. The maximum velocity through the shunt is highest early in systole and has a gradual decrease until the next systolic event (5).

The peak CW Doppler velocity (V_{max}) obtained through a shunt can be used in the simplified echo Bernoulli equation (Eq. 11) to predict the pressure gradient between the aorta and pulmonary artery. The systemic peak systolic pressure (SYS_{SP}) is then used to estimate pulmonary artery peak systolic pressures (PA_{SP}):

$$PA_{SP} = SYS_{SP} - 4V_{max}^2. \qquad [73]$$

As in the case of the ductus arteriosus, since these are not discrete lesions, one would expect there would be

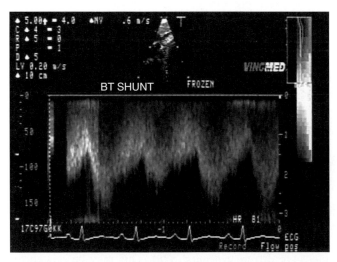

ECHO. 6-23. Typical CW Doppler spectral velocity waveform through a modified BT shunt showing maximum velocity through the shunt is highest early in systole and has a gradual decrease until the next systolic event.

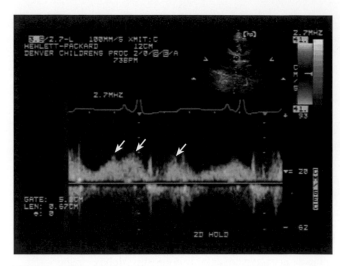

ECHO. 6-24. Typical Doppler spectral velocity waveform in normal functioning Fontan connection showing biphasic antegrade flow into the pulmonary artery beginning in early ventricular diastole *(first arrow)*, peaking during atrial systole *(second arrow)*, with a second peak in ventricular systole *(third arrow)*.

underestimation of pressure gradient when neglecting viscous effects. Studies have shown some overestimation (530) and underestimation (536) of pressure gradients with overall good correlation ($r = 0.94$) in animal models (537) and humans (530), with a tendency to underestimate pressure gradient (i.e., overestimate pulmonary artery peak systolic pressures) at lower velocities (530).

Preliminary work in our laboratory predicts differing flow dynamics through different anatomical types of obstructions (i.e., inlet, outlet, and diffuse) with identical obstructive cross-sectional areas (529). However, overall in these experiments, the Doppler pressure gradient showed good correlation with the actual pressure gradient with slight underestimation or overestimation depending on the site of obstruction.

Fontan Connections

Many variations exist to the originally described Fontan procedure and because of these variations it is critical to know the specific details of each surgical repair before a patient can be fully evaluated (74). Intraatrial baffles, atrial anastomoses, and extracardiac shunts are just some of the examples of markedly different surgical options.

Pulmonary artery spectral Doppler signals have a characteristic pattern in normally functioning Fontan connections (Echo. 6-24). There is biphasic antegrade flow into the pulmonary artery beginning in early ventricular diastole and peaking during atrial systole, with a second peak in ventricular systole (74,538–543). This peak during atrial systole occurs even in those patients where the right atrium is not part of the circuit to the pulmonary arteries (i.e., an extracardiac conduit) (543).

Overall, higher velocities are seen during inspiration (544,545). The atrial contribution to total pulmonary artery flow, assessed by velocity-time integrals, varied in one study between 22% and 73% (542).

Abnormal flow patterns can be seen with decreased ventricular function where the atrial waves are small and the respiratory variation in flow velocities is reduced (539). Poor outcome from the Fontan procedure has been predicted when there are diminished systolic velocities with late systolic reversal and delayed diastolic phase (541).

Similar flow patterns are seen in the pulmonary arteries of patients who have had a bidirectional Glenn procedure, where only the superior vena cava is anastomosed to the pulmonary arteries (546). Some patients, however, are left with some antegrade flow from the heart into the main pulmonary artery which obscures this biphasic pattern (546).

PROSTHETIC VALVES

Prosthetic valves are used less frequently in the pediatric population than in the adult population. Bioprosthetic and mechanical valves are the two categories of prosthetic valves. Bioprosthetic valves are made up partially or completely of biologic material.

Mechanical Valves

Probably the most frequently used mechanical valve in the pediatric-age patients is the St. Jude valve with bi-leaflet tilting hemidiscs. Others include the Starr–Edwards valve, which is a ball and cage valve, and the Bjork–Shiley valve, which is a tilting disc and cage valve. Many of the structures of the valves are strong reflectors of ultrasound signals and usually obscure the color Doppler flow image behind the valve itself.

Normal flow characteristics through these mechanical valves are much different from those of native valves. Flow characteristics have been studied extensively in mechanical valves in adults (547–553) but there have been only a limited number of studies in children (554). However, many children have adult-sized mechanical valves, and the data derived from adults can probably be applied to these cases (77).

The simplified echo Bernoulli equation (Eq. 11) has been used in the assessment of stenotic mechanical valves. Normal values for peak Doppler velocities, peak pressure gradients, and mean gradients have been established for most sizes and types of adult mechanical valves and these are different from velocities found in native valves (555) (Table 6-1). Mean gradients are felt by many to be more reliable than peak gradients since high velocities may be present transiently with normal mechanical valve opening (74).

We have previously discussed the phenomenon of pressure recovery with regards to native stenotic valve lesions and the discrepancies that occur between catheter- and Doppler-derived pressure gradients. Pressure recovery appears to be more pronounced and has been proposed as a significant cause of catheter and Doppler gradient

TABLE 6-1. *Normal Doppler values for mechanical prostheses according to size and position*

Prosthetis	Position	Size (mm)	No. patients	Peak velocity	Peak gradient	Mean velocity	Mean gradient
St. Jude Medical	Mitral	27	86	1.59 ± 0.27	10.11 ± 3.43		
			8			1.12 ± 0.22	5.00 ± 2.00
		29	25	1.54 ± 0.36	9.90 ± 4.49		
			79			0.82 ± 0.21	2.71 ± 1.36
		31	15			1.12 ± 0.34	5.00 ± 3.00
St. Jude Medical	Aortic	19	6	3.00 ± 0.77	31.2 ± 17.3		
			5			2.36 ± 0.58	22.2 ± 11.0
		21	14	2.70 ± 0.26	30.0 ± 5.7		
			11			1.89 ± 0.33	14.4 ± 5.0
		23	17	2.32 ± 0.60	23.2 ± 11.5		
			19			1.64 ± 0.48	10.8 ± 6.3
		25	12	2.20 ± 0.46	19.8 ± 8.2		
			9			1.24 ± 0.45	11.0 ± 6.0
Björk-Shiley	Aortic	21	4	2.76 ± 0.90	30.5 ± 19.9		
			1			2.0	16.0
		23	11	2.59 ± 0.42	27.29 ± 8.70		
			20			1.87 ± 0.33	14.0 ± 5.00
		25	13	2.14 ± 0.31	18.38 ± 5.31		
			13			1.82 ± 0.17	13.3 ± 2.53
		27	10	1.91 ± 0.20	14.55 ± 3.06		
			7			1.56 ± 0.20	9.7 ± 2.53
		29	2	1.87 ± 0.20	13.99 ± 2.54		
			2			1.32 ± 0.57	7.0 ± 6.00

Adapted from Reisner SA, Meltzer RS. Normal values of prosthetic valve Doppler echocardiographic parameters: a review. *J Am Soc Echocardiogr* 1988;1:201–210.

discrepancies (556,557) in St. Jude mechanical valves. The flow dynamics through each of the three orifices of this bileaflet valve have been shown to be dissimilar (556,558,559). Differing peak velocities are obtained when sampling through each orifice, and they may lead to disparate estimates of pressure gradient using the simplified echo Bernoulli equation (556).

As with native stenotic valves, the calculation of gradients with the simplified echo Bernoulli equation (Eq. 14) is flow-dependent and valve-type–dependent, with significant overlap observed in blood velocities and gradients across normally functioning valves (560). Doppler continuity equation–derived valve areas have been proposed as a potentially flow-independent assessment of mechanical valve stenosis (560,561). As in stenotic valve areas in native valves, investigators have noted discrepancies in area calculations for mechanical valves, including overestimation and significant dependence of Doppler-derived areas on flow rate and other hemodynamic factors (562,563).

There is still much that needs to be learned regarding the basic fluid dynamics around mechanical valves, and work is currently ongoing in many laboratories to improve the assessment of these valves using Doppler techniques (559,564,565).

Color Doppler images of flow through these valves may detect trivial valve regurgitation, which is common and in most cases normal (77). The St. Jude valve has a normal regurgitant backflow as back-pressure swings the leaflets through their closing arc (74). Once the St. Jude valve leaflets close, leakage occurs between the discs and the sewing ring, both peripherally and where the disks close centrally (74). This normal regurgitation must be differentiated from transvalvular regurgitation (i.e., valve malfunction) and paravalvular regurgitation (i.e., failure of valve apparatus fixation along the suture lines). Once the regurgitation is determined to be abnormal, clues suggesting paravalvular rather than transvalvular regurgitation include regurgitation seen outside the sewing ring, regurgitation originating from a point separate from the forward flow, and proximal flow convergence in the upstream chamber outside the sewing ring (74).

Bioprosthetic Valves

Probably the most frequently used bioprosthetic valves in pediatric patients are in aortic and pulmonary homografts placed in the aortic or pulmonary artery positions. There have been limited reports of Doppler assessment of homograft valves in adults and children. In an adult study, the investigators concluded that velocities across normally functioning homograft valves (1.8 ± 0.37 m/s) in the aortic position are slightly greater than velocities through native aortic valves (566). In one study of children immediately postoperatively with homografts in the

aortic position, peak velocities less than 2.6 m/s were considered normal, with a majority of patients (62%) having mild regurgitation (567).

SUMMARY

CW, PW, and color Doppler flow mapping have dramatically changed all aspects of pediatric cardiology. To many who have only recently entered the field, it is difficult to comprehend practicing pediatric cardiology without such tools.

Powerful diagnostic methods have been developed using these Doppler tools. Only after there is a firm understanding of the principles behind these methods should one feel comfortable using them. We hope we have provided some insight into many of those principles.

The use of these Doppler tools in two-dimensional echocardiography is currently close to, if not at, its full potential. Three-dimensional echocardiography offers the possibility of expanding Doppler methods in ways that are just begining to be realized.

REFERENCES

1. Hatle L. Maximal blood flow velocity: haemodynamic data obtained non-invasively with CW Doppler. *Ultrasound Med Biol* 1984;10:225–237.
2. Stevenson JG, Kawabori I. Noninvasive determination of pressure gradients in children: two methods employing pulsed Doppler echocardiography. *J Am Coll Cardiol* 1984;3:179–192.
3. Snider AR, Stevenson JG, French JW, et al. Comparison of high pulse repetition frequency and continuous-wave Doppler echocardiography for velocity measurement and gradient prediction in children with valvular and congenital heart disease. *J Am Coll Cardiol* 1986;7:873–879.
4. Sahn DJ. Real-time two-dimensional Doppler echocardiographic flow mapping. *Circulation* 1985;71:849–853.
5. Hatle L, Angelsen B. *Doppler ultrasound in cardiology.* 2nd ed. Philadelphia: Lea & Febiger, 1985.
6. Hatle L. Assessment of aortic blood flow velocities with continuous wave Doppler ultrasound in the neonate and young child. *J Am Coll Cardiol* 1985;5:113S–119S.
7. DeGroff CG, Baptista AM, Shiota T, Cable J, Foster L, Sahn DJ. A flow convergence method to quantitate regurgitant flow with a flail mitral valve leaflet: two-dimensional finite-element modeling and experimental studies. *J Am Coll Cardiol* 1995;25:398A(abst).
8. Walker PG, Cranney GB, Grimes RY, et al. Three-dimensional reconstruction of the flow in a human left heart by using magnetic resonance phase velocity encoding. *Ann Biomed Eng* 1996;24:139–147.
9. Segadal L, Matre K. Blood velocity distribution in the human ascending aorta. *Circulation* 1987;76:90–100.
10. Lighty GW, Gargiulo A, Kronzon I, Politzer F. Comparison of multiple views for the evaluation of pulmonary arterial blood flow by Doppler echocardiography. *Circulation* 1986;74:1002–1006.
11. Reynolds T, Appleton CP. Doppler flow velocity patterns of the superior vena cava, inferior vena cava, hepatic vein, coronary sinus, and atrial septal defect: a guide for the echocardiographer. *J Am Soc Echocardiogr* 1991;4:503–512.
12. Appleton CP, Hatle LK, Popp RL. Superior vena cava and hepatic vein Doppler echocardiography in healthy adults. *J Am Coll Cardiol* 1987;10:1032–1039.
13. Salim MA, DiSessa TG, Arheart KL, Alpert BS. Contribution of superior vena caval flow to total cardiac output in children: a

Doppler echocardiographic study. *Circulation* 1995;92:1860–1865.

14. Nishimura RA, Housmans PR, Hatle LK, Tajik AJ. Assessment of diastolic function of the heart: background and current applications of Doppler echocardiography. Part I. Physiologic and pathophysiologic features. *Mayo Clinic Proc* 1989;64:71–81.

15. Keren G, Sherez J, Megidish R, Levitt B, Laniado S. Pulmonary venous flow pattern—its relationship to cardiac dynamics: a pulsed Doppler echocardiographic study. *Circulation* 1985;71:1105–1112.

16. Rossvoll O, Hatle LK. Pulmonary venous flow velocities recorded by transthoracic Doppler ultrasound: relation to left ventricular diastolic pressures. *J Am Coll Cardiol* 1993;21:1687–1696.

17. Klein AL, Tajik AJ. Doppler assessment of pulmonary venous flow in healthy subjects and in patients with heart disease. *J Am Soc Echocardiogr* 1991;4:379–392.

18. Basnight MA, Gonzalez MS, Kershenovich SC, Appleton CP. Pulmonary venous flow velocity: relation to hemodynamics, mitral flow velocity and left atrial volume, and ejection fraction. *J Am Soc Echocardiogr* 1991;4:547–558.

19. Hoit BD, Shao Y, Gabel M, Walsh RA. Influence of loading conditions and contractile state on pulmonary venous flow, validation of Doppler velocimetry. *Circulation* 1992;86:651–659.

20. Agata Y, Hiraishi S, Oguchi K, et al. Changes in pulmonary venous flow pattern during early neonatal life. *Br Heart J* 1994;71:182–186.

21. Smallhorn JF, Freedom RM, Olley PM. Pulsed Doppler echocardiographic assessment of extraparenchymal pulmonary vein flow. *J Am Coll Cardiol* 1987;9:573–579.

22. Harada K, Suzuki T, Tamura M, Ito T, Shimada K, Takada G. Effect of aging from infancy to childhood on flow velocity patterns of pulmonary vein by Doppler echocardiography. *Am J Cardiol* 1996;77:221–224.

23. Masuyama T, Lee JM, Tamai M, Tanouchi J, Kitabatake A, Kamada T. Pulmonary venous flow velocity pattern as assessed with transthoracic pulsed Doppler echocardiography in subjects without cardiac disease. *Am J Cardiol* 1991;67:1396–1404.

24. Cohen GI, Pietrolungo JF, Thomas JD, Klein AL. A practical guide to assessment of ventricular diastolic function using Doppler echocardiography. *J Am Coll Cardiol* 1996;27.1753–1760.

25. Keren G, Sherez J, Megidish R, Levitt B, Laniado S. Pulmonary venous flow pattern—its relationship to cardiac dynamics. *Circulation* 1985;71:1105–1112.

26. Vick GW III, Murphy DJ, Ludomirsky A. Pulmonary venous and systemic ventricular inflow obstruction in patients with congenital heart disease. *J Am Coll Cardiol* 1987,9:580–587.

27. Sartori MP, Quinones MA, Kuo LC. Relation of Doppler derived left ventricular filling parameters to age and radius thickness ratio in normal and pathologic states. *Am J Cardiol* 1987;59:1179–1182.

28. Agata Y, Hiraishi S, Oguchi K, et al. Changes in pulmonary venous flow pattern during early neonatal life. *Br Heart J* 1994;71:182–186.

29. Appleton CP, Jensen JL, Hatle LK, Oh JK. Doppler evaluation of left and right ventricular diastolic function: a technical guide for obtaining optimal flow velocity recordings. *J Am Soc Echocardiogr* 1997;10:271–291.

30. Nishimura RA, Tajik AJ. Quantitative hemodynamics by Doppler echocardiography: a noninvasive alternative to cardiac catheterization. *Prog Cardiovasc Dis* 1994;36:309–342.

31. Courtois M, Kovacs SJ, Ludbrock PA. Transmitral pressure flow velocity relation: importance of regional pressure gradients in the left ventricle during diastole. *Circulation* 1988;78:661–671.

32. Utsunomiya T, Gardin JM. Observations on Doppler mid-diastolic mitral flow reversal. *J Am Soc Echocardiogr* 1991;4:361–366.

33. Thomas JD, Weyman AE. Echocardiographic Doppler evaluation of left ventricular diastolic function. Physics and physiology. *Circulation* 1991;84:977–990.

34. Riggs TW, Snider AR. Respiratory influence on right and left ventricular diastolic filling in normal children. *Am J Cardiol* 1989;63:858–861.

35. Bu Lock FA, Mott MG, Martin RP. Left ventricular diastolic function in children measured by Doppler echocardiography: normal values and relation with growth. *Br Heart J* 1995;73:334–339.

36. Grenadier E, Lima CO, Allen HD, et al. Normal intracardiac and great vessel Doppler flow velocities in infants and children. *J Am Coll Cardiol* 1984;4:343–350.

37. Emmanouilides GC, Riemenschneider TA, Allen HD, Gutgesell HP. *Heart disease in infants, children, and adolescents including the fetus and young adult.* 5th ed. Baltimore: Williams & Wilkins, 1995.

38. Harada K, Suzuki T, Tamura M, et al. Role of age on transmitral flow velocity patterns in assessing left ventricular diastolic function in normal infants and children. *Am J Cardiol* 1995;76:530–532.

39. Harada K, Shiota T, Takahashi Y, Tamura M, Toyono M, Takada G. Doppler echocardiographic evaluation of left ventricular output and left ventricular diastolic filling changes in the first day of life. *Pediatr Res* 1994;35:506–509.

40. Areias JC, Meyer R, Scott WA, Goldberg SJ. Serial echocardiographic and Doppler evaluation of left ventricular diastolic filling in full-term neonates. *Am J Cardiol* 1990;66:108–111.

41. Riggs TW, Rodriquez R, Snider AR, Batton D. Doppler echocardiographic evaluation of right and left ventricular diastolic function in normal neonates. *J Am Coll Cardiol* 1989;13:700–705.

42. Reed KL, Sahn DJ, Scagnelli, Anderson CF, Shenker L. Doppler echocardiographic studies of diastolic function in the human fetal heart: changes during gestation. *J Am Coll Cardiol* 1986;8:391–395.

43. Johnson GL, Moffett CB, Noonan JA. Doppler echocardiographic studies of diastolic ventricular filling patterns in premature infants. *Am Heart J* 1988;116:1568–1574.

44. Spirito P, Maron BJ. Influence of aging on Doppler echocardiographic indices of left ventricular diastolic function. *Br Heart J* 1988,59.672–679.

45. Kenny JF, Plappert T, Doubilet P, et al. Changes in intracardiac blood flow and right and left ventricular stroke volumes with gestational age in the normal human fetus: a prospective Doppler echocardiographic study. *Circulation* 1986;74:1208–1216.

46. Yock PG, Naaz C, Schnittger I, Popp RL. Doppler tricuspid and pulmonic regurgitation: is it real? *Circulation* 1984;70[Suppl 2]:40(abst).

47. Yoshida K, Yoshikawa J, Shakudo M, et al. Color Doppler evaluation of valvular regurgitation in normal subjects. *Circulation* 1988;78:840–847.

48. Sahn DJ, Maciel BC. Physiological valvular regurgitation. Doppler echocardiography and the potential for iatrogenic heart disease. *Circulation* 1988;78:1075–1077.

49. Maciel BC, Simpson IA, Valdes-Cruz LM, et al. Color flow mapping studies of physiologic pulmonary and tricuspid regurgitation: evidence for true regurgitation as opposed to a valve closing volume. *J Am Soc Echocardiogr* 1991;4:589–597.

50. Van Dijik APJ, Van Oort AM, Daniels O. Right-sided valvular regurgitation in normal children determined by combined colour-coded and continuous wave–Doppler echocardiography. *Acta Paediatr* 1994;83:200–203.

51. Brand A, Dollberg S, Keren A. The prevalence of valvular regurgitation in children with structurally normal hearts: a color Doppler echocardiographic study. *Am Heart J* 1992;123:177.

52. Feigenbaum H. *Echocardiography.* 4th ed. Philadelphia: Lea & Febiger, 1986.

53. Stevenson JG. Two-dimensional color Doppler estimation of the severity of atrioventricular valve regurgitation: important effects of instrument gain setting, pulse repetition frequency, and carrier frequency. *J Am Soc Echocardiogr* 1989;2:1.

54. Bucciarelli RL, Nelson RM, Egan EA III, Eitzman DV, Gessner IH. Transient tricuspid insufficiency of the newborn: a form of myocardial dysfunction in stressed newborns. *Pediatrics* 1977;59:330–337.

55. Freymann R, Kallfelz HC. Transient tricuspid incompetence in a newborn. *Eur J Cardiol* 1975;2/4:467–471.

56. Zhang Y, Nitter-Hauge S, Ihlen H, Myhre E. Doppler echocardiographic measurement of cardiac output using the mitral orifice method. *Br Heart J* 1985;53:130–136.

57. Goldberg SJ, Sahn DJ, Allen HD, Valdes-Cruz LM, Hoenecke H, Carnahan Y. Evaluation of pulmonary and systemic blood flow

by two-dimensional Doppler echocardiography using fast fourier transform spectral analysis. *Am J Cardiol* 1982;50:1394–1400.

58. Lighty GW, Gargiulo A, Kronzon I, Politzer F. Comparison of multiple views for the evaluation of pulmonary arterial blood flow by Doppler echocardiography. *Circulation* 1986;74:1002–1006.

59. Gardin JM, Tobis JM, Dabestani A, et al. Superiority of two-dimensional measurement of aortic vessel diameter in Doppler echocardiographic estimates of left ventricular stroke volume. *J Am Coll Cardiol* 1985;6:65–74.

60. Fisher DC, Sahn DJ, Friedman MJ, et al. The mitral valve orifice method for noninvasive two-dimensional echo-Doppler determinations of cardiac output. *Circulation* 1983;67:872–877.

61. Nicolosi GL, Pungercic E, Cervesato E, Modena L, Zanuttini D. Analysis of interobserver and intraobserver variation of interpretation of the echocardiographic and Doppler flow determination of cardiac output by the mitral orifice method. *Br Heart J* 1986;55:446–448.

62. De Zuttere D, Touche T, Saumon G, Nitenberg A, Prasquier R. Doppler echocardiographic measurement of mitral flow volume: validation of a new method in adult patients. *J Am Coll Cardiol* 1988;11:343–350.

63. Meijboom EJ, Horowitz S, Valdes-Cruz LM, Sahn DJ, Larson DF, Lima C. A Doppler echocardiographic method for calculating volume flow across the tricuspid valve: correlative laboratory and clinical studies. *Circulation* 1985;71:551–556.

64. Dubin J, Wallerson DC, Cody RJ, Devereux RB. Comparative accuracy of Doppler echocardiographic methods for clinical stroke volume determination. *Am Heart J* 1990;120:116–123.

65. Huntsman LL, Steward DK, Barnes SR, Franflin SB, Colocousis JS, Hessel EA. Noninvasive Doppler determination of cardiac output in man: clinical validation. *Circulation* 1983;67:593–602.

66. Ihlen H, Amlie JP, Dale J, et al. Determination of cardiac output by Doppler echocardiography. *Br Heart J* 1984;51:54–60.

67. Loeppky JA, Hoekenga DE, Greene ER, Luft UC. Comparison of noninvasive pulsed Doppler and Fick measurements of stroke volume in cardiac patients. *Am Heart J* 1984;107:339–346.

68. Chandraratna PA, Nanna M, McKay C, et al. Determination of cardiac output by transcutaneous continuous wave ultrasonic Doppler computer. *Am J Cardiol* 1984;53:234–237.

69. Bouchard A, Blumlein S, Schiller NB, et al. Measurement of left ventricular stroke volume using continuous-wave Doppler echocardiography of the ascending aorta and M-mode echocardiography of the aortic valve. *J Am Coll Cardiol* 1987;9:75–83.

70. Labovitz AJ, Buckingham TA, Habermehl K, Nelson J, Kennedy HL, Williams GA. The effects of sampling site on the two-dimensional echo-Doppler determination of cardiac output. *Am Heart J* 1985;109:327–332.

71. Valdes-Cruz LM, Sahn DJ. Two-dimensional echo Doppler for noninvasive quantification of cardiac flow: a status report. *Mod Concepts Cardiovasc Dis* 1982;51:123–128.

72. Lewis JF, Kuo LC, Nelson JG, Limacher MC, Quinones MA. Pulsed Doppler echocardiographic determination of stroke volume and cardiac output: clinical validation of two new methods using the apical window. *Circulation* 1984;70:425–431.

73. Goldberg SJ, Allen HD, Marx GR, Flinn CJ. *Doppler echocardiography.* Philadelphia: Lea & Febiger, 1985.

74. Weyman AE. *Principles and practice of echocardiography.* 2nd ed. Philadelphia: Lea & Febiger, 1994.

75. Nanda NC. *Doppler echocardiography.* 2nd ed. Philadelphia: Lea & Febiger, 1993.

76. Silverman NH. *Pediatric echocardiography.* Baltimore: Williams & Wilkins, 1993.

77. Snider AR, Serwer GA. *Echocardiography in pediatric heart disease.* Baltimore: Mosby-Year Book, 1990.

78. Dittman H, Voelker W, Karsch KR, Seipel L. Influence of sampling site and flow area on cardiac output measurements by Doppler echocardiography. *J Am Coll Cardiol* 1987;10:818–823.

79. Stewart WJ, Jiang L, Mich R, Pandian N, Guerrero JL, Weyman AE. Variable effects of changes in flow rate through the aortic, pulmonary and mitral valves on valve area and flow velocity: impact on quantitative Doppler flow calculations. *J Am Coll Cardiol* 1985;6:653–662.

80. Gill RW. Measurement of blood flow by ultrasound: accuracy and sources of error. *Ultrasound Med Biol* 1985;11:625–641.

81. Gardin JM. Estimation of volume flow by Doppler echocardiography. *Echocardiography* 1987;4:17–28.

82. Bojanowski LMR, Timmis AD, Najm YC, Gosling RG. Pulsed Doppler ultrasound compared with thermodilution for monitoring cardiac output responses to changing left ventricular function. *Cardiovasc Res* 1987;21:260–268.

83. Gardin JM, Dabestani A, Matin K, Allfie A, Rusell D, Henry WL. Area Doppler aortic blood flow velocity measurements reproducible? Studies on day to day and interobserver variability in normal subjects. *J Am Coll Cardiol* 1983;1:657(abst).

84. Morrow WR, Murphy DJ, Fisher DJ, Huhta JC, Jefferson LS, Smith EO. Continuous wave Doppler cardiac output: use in pediatric patients receiving inotropic support. *Pediatr Cardiol* 1988;9:131–136.

85. Mellander M, Sabel KG, Caidahl K, Solymar L, Eriksson B. Doppler determination of cardiac output in infants and children: comparison with simultaneous thermodilution. *Pediatr Cardiol* 1987;8:241–246.

86. Notterman DA, Castello FV, Steinberg C, Greenwald BM, O'Loughlin JE, Gold JP. A comparison of thermodilution and pulsed Doppler cardiac output measurement in critically ill children. *J Pediatr* 1989;115:554–560.

87. Sholler GF, Celermajer JM, Whight CM. Doppler echocardiographic assessment of cardiac output in normal children with and without innocent precordial murmurs. *Am J Cardiol* 1987;59:487–488.

88. Rein AJ, Hsieh KS, Elixson M, et al. Cardiac output estimates in the pediatric intensive care unit using a continuous-wave Doppler computer: validation and limitations of the technique. *Am Heart J* 1986;112:97–103.

89. Sholler GF, Whight CM, Celermajer JM. Pulsed Doppler echocardiographic assessment including use of aortic leaflet separation of cardiac output in children with structural heart disease. *Am J Cardiol* 1986;57:1195–1197.

90. Alverson DC, Eldridge M, Dillon T, Yabek SM, Berman W. Noninvasive pulsed Doppler determination of cardiac output in neonates and children. *J Pediatr* 1982;101:46–50.

91. Walther FJ, Siassi B, Ramadan NA, Wu PYK. Cardiac output in newborn infants with transient myocardial dysfunction. *J Pediatr* 1985;107:781–785.

92. Lucas CL, Keagy BA, Hsiao HS, Johnson TA, Henry GW, Wilcox BR. The velocity profile in the canine ascending aorta and its effects on the accuracy of pulsed Doppler determinations of mean blood velocity. *Cardiovasc Res* 1984;18:282–293.

93. Henry GW, Johnson TA, Ferreiro JI, et al. Velocity profile in the main pulmonary artery in a canine model. *Cardiovasc Res* 1984;18:620–625.

94. Kvitting P, Hessevik I, Matre K, Segadal L. Three-dimensional cross-sectional velocity distribution in the ascending aorta in cardiac patients. *Clin Physiol* 1996;16:239–258.

95. Kupari M, Koshinen P. Systolic flow velocity profile in the left ventricular outflow tract in persons free of heart disease. *Am J Cardiol* 1993;72:1172–1178.

96. Loeber CP, Goldberg SJ, Marx GR, Carrier M, Emery RW. How much does aortic and pulmonary artery area vary during the cardiac cycle? *Am Heart J* 1987;113:95–100.

97. Song JK, Handschumacher MD, Gilon D, et al. Improved proximal flow rate calculation using three-dimensional reconstruction of digital Doppler velocities and a control volume approach. *Circulation* 1996;94:I-335(abst).

98. Kim WY, Poulsen JK, Terp K, Staalsen NH. A new Doppler method for quantification of volumetric flow: in vivo validation using color Doppler. *J Am Coll Cardiol* 1996;27:182–192.

99. Fox RW, McDonald AT. *Introduction to fluid mechanics.* New York: John Wiley and Sons, 1992.

100. Sun JP, Stewart WJ, Fouad FM, Christian R, Klein AL, Thomas JD. Automated flow measurement using spatial and temporal integration of color Doppler data. *Circulation* 1995;92:I-15(abst).

101. Aida S, Shiota T, Tsujino H, Sahn DJ. Automated calculation of aortic regurgitant volume by a newly developed digital Doppler color flow mapping method: an in-vitro study. *J Am Coll Cardiol* 1996;27:269A(abst).

102. Krauzowicz B, Ludomirsky A, Nesser J, Denning K. Automatic on-line cardiac output measurement using color Doppler flow inte-

gration: in vivo validation in children. *Circulation* 1996;94:I-236(abst).

103. Van Camp G, Menassel M, Plein D, et al. Comparison of aortic and pulmonary flow in children, measured with the automatic cardiac output method. *Circulation* 1996;94:I-491(abst).

104. Tsujino H, Shiki E, Hirama M, Iiuma K. Quantitative measurement of volume flow rate (cardiac output) by the multibeam Doppler method. *J Am Soc Echocardiogr* 1995;8:621–630.

105. Sun JP, Fouad FM, Christian R, Stewart WJ, Thomas JD. Automated cardiac output measurement by spatiotemporal integration of color Doppler data. *Circulation* 1997;95:932–939.

106. Recusani F, Bargiggia GS, Yoganathan A, et al. A new method for quantification of regurgitant flow rate using color Doppler flow imaging of the flow convergence region proximal to a discrete orifice: an in vitro study. *Circulation* 1991;83:594–604.

107. Simpson IA, Shiota T, Gharib M, Sahn DJ. Current status of flow convergence for clinical applications: is it a leaning tower of Pisa? *J Am Coll Cardiol* 1996;27:504–509.

108. Shiota T, Teien D, Deng Y, et al. Estimation of regurgitant flow volume based on centerline velocity/distance profiles using digital color M-Q Doppler: application to orifices of different shapes. *J Am Coll Cardiol* 1994;24:440–445.

109. Vandervoort PM, Thoreau DH, Rivera M, Levine RA, Weyman AE, Thomas JD. Automated flow rate calculations based on digital analysis of flow convergence proximal to regurgitant orifices. *J Am Coll Cardiol* 1993;22:535–541.

110. Deng YB, Shiota T, Shandas R, Zhang J, Sahn DJ. Determination of the most appropriate velocity threshold for applying hemispheric flow convergence equations to calculate flow rate: selected according to the transorifice pressure gradient. *Circulation* 1993;88(part 1):1699–1708.

111. Rodriguez L, Anconina J, Flachskampf FA, Weyman AE, Levine RA, Thomas JD. Impact of finite orifice size on proximal flow convergence—implications for Doppler quantification of valvular regurgitation. *Circ Res* 1992;70:923–930.

112. Barclay SA, Eidenvall L, Karlsson M, et al. The shape of the proximal isovelocity surface area varies with regurgitant orifice size and distance from orifice: computer simulation and model experiments with color M-mode technique. *J Am Soc Echocardiogr* 1993;6:433–445.

113. Grimes RY, Burleson A, Levine RA, Yoganathan AP. Quantification of cardiac jets: theory and limitations. *Echocardiography* 1994;11:267–280.

114. DeGroff CG, Baptista AM, Sahn DJ. Evaluating the isovelocity surface area flow convergence method using finite element modeling. *J Am Soc Echocardiogr* (in press).

115. Ge S, Jones M, Shiota T, et al. Quantification of mitral flow by Doppler color flow mapping. *J Am Soc Echocardiogr* 1996;9:700–709.

116. Shandas R, Gharib M, Sahn DJ. Nature of flow acceleration into a finite-sized orifice: steady and pulsatile flow studies on the flow convergence region using simultaneous ultrasound Doppler flow mapping and laser Doppler velocimetry. *J Am Coll Cardiol* 1995;25:1199–1212.

117. Utsunomiya T, Ogawa T, Doshi R, et al. Doppler color flow "proximal isovelocity surface area" method for estimating flow rate: effects of orifice shape and machine factors. *J Am Coll Cardiol* 1991;17:1103–1111.

118. Schwammenthal E, Chen C, Giesler M, et al. New method for accurate calculation of regurgitant flow rate based on analysis of Doppler color flow maps of the proximal flow field. *J Am Coll Cardiol* 1996;27:161–172.

119. Shiota T, Sinclair B, Masahiro I, et al. Three-dimensional reconstruction of color Doppler flow convergence regions and regurgitant jets: an in vitro quantitative study. *J Am Coll Cardiol* 1996;27:1511–1518.

120. DeGroff CG, Baptista AM. Limitations of flow convergence methods when applied to finite size orifices: two-dimensional finite element modeling studies. *J Am Coll Cardiol* 1996;27:285A(abst).

121. Rodriguez L, Thomas JD, Monterroso V, et al. Validation of the proximal flow convergence method. Calculation of orifice area in patients with mitral stenosis. *Circulation* 1993;8:1157–1166.

122. Pu M, Vandervoort PM, Greenberg NL, Powell KA, Griffin BP, Thomas JD. Impact of wall constraint on velocity distribution in proximal flow convergence zone. *J Am Coll Cardiol* 1996;27:706–713.

123. Fleishman CE, Li J, Ota T, et al. Identification of congenital heart defects using real time three-dimensional echo in pediatric patients. *Circulation* 1996;94:I-416(abst).

124. Delabays A, Sugeng L, Pandian NG, et al. Dynamic three-dimensional echocardiographic assessment of intracardiac blood flow jets. *Am J Cardiol* 1995;76:1053–1058.

125. Belohlavek M, Foley DA, Gerber TC, Greenleaf JF, Seward JB. Three-dimensional reconstruction of color Doppler jets in the human heart. *J Am Soc Echocardiogr* 1994;7:553–560.

126. Minich LL, Snider AR, Meliones JN, Yanock C. In vitro evaluation of volumetric flow from Doppler power-weighted and amplitude-weighted mean velocities. *J Am Soc Echocardiogr* 1993;6:227–236.

127. Jenni R, Ritter M, Vieli A, et al. Determination of the ratio of pulmonary blood flow to systemic blood flow by derivation of amplitude weighted mean velocity from continuous-wave Doppler spectra. *Br Heart J* 1989;61:167–171.

128. Simpson IA, Valdes-Cruz LM, Sahn DJ, Murillo A, Tamura T, Chung KJ. Doppler color flow mapping of simulated in vitro regurgitant jets: evaluation of the effects of orifice size and hemodynamic variables. *J Am Coll Cardiol* 1989;13:1195–1207.

129. Bascom PAJ, Cobbold RSC. Origin of the Doppler ultrasound spectrum from blood. *IEEE Trans Biomed Eng* 1996;43:562–571.

130. MacIsaac AI, McDonald IG, Kirsner KL, Graham SA, Gill RW. Quantification of mitral regurgitation by integrated Doppler backscatter power. *J Am Coll Cardiol* 1994;24:690–695.

131. Enriquez-Sarano M, Kaneshige AM, Tajik AJ, Bailey KR, Seward JB. Amplitude-weighted mean velocity: clinical utilization for quantitation of mitral regurgitation. *J Am Coll Cardiol* 1993;22:1684–1690.

132. Magnin PA, Stewart JA, Myers S, von Ram MO, Kisslo JA. Combined Doppler and phased array echocardiographic estimation of cardiac output. *Circulation* 1981;63:388–392.

133. Caidahl K, Mellanger M, Sabel KG, Eriksson BO. Estimation of stroke volume using Doppler echocardiography and left ventricular echocardiographic dimensions in infants and children. *Acta Paediatr Scand* 1986;329[Suppl]:114–119.

134. Sahn DJ. Determination of cardiac output by echocardiographic Doppler methods: relative accuracy of various sites for measurement [Editorial]. *J Am Coll Cardiol* 1985;6:663–664.

135. Loeber CP, Goldberg SJ, Allen HD. Doppler echocardiographic comparison of flows distal to the four cardiac valves. *J Am Coll Cardiol* 1984;4:268–272.

136. Ascah KJ, Stewart WJ, Gillan CD, Trivizi MO, Newell JB, Weyman AE. Calculation of transmitral flow by Doppler echocardiography: a comparison of methods in a canine model. *Am Heart J* 1989;117:402–411.

137. Meijboom E, Horowitz S, Valdes-Cruz LM, et al. A simplified mitral valve method for two-dimensional echo Doppler blood flow calculation: validation in an open chest canine model and initial clinical studies. *Am Heart J* 1987;113:335–340.

138. Valdes-Cruz LM, Horowitz S, Mesel E, Sahn DJ, Fisher DC, Larson D. A pulsed doppler echocardiographic method for calculating pulmonary and systemic blood flow in atrial level shunts: validation studies in animals and initial human experience. *Circulation* 1984;69:80–86.

139. Sanders SP, Yeager S, Williams RG. Measurements of systemic and pulmonary blood flow and QP/QS ratio using Doppler and two-dimensional echocardiography. *Am J Cardiol* 1983;51:952–956.

140. Barron JV, Sahn DJ, Valdes-Cruz LM, et al. Clinical utility of two-dimensional Doppler echocardiographic techniques for estimating pulmonary to systemic blood flow ratios in children with left to right shunting atrial septal defect, ventricular septal defect, or patent ductus arteriosus. *J Am Coll Cardiol* 1984;3:169–178.

141. Kitabatake A, Inoue M, Asao M, et al. Noninvasive evaluation of the ratio of pulmonary to systemic flow in atrial septal defect by duplex Doppler echocardiography. *Circulation* 1984;69:73–79.

142. Sabry AF, Reller MD, Silberbach GM, Rice MJ, Sahn DJ. Comparison of four Doppler echocardiographic methods for calculating pulmonary to systemic shunt flow ratios in patients with ventricular septal defects. *Am J Cardiol* 1995;75:611–614.

143. Teien D, Karp K, Wendel H, Human DG, Nanton MA. Quantification of left to right shunts by echo Doppler cardiography in patients with ventricular septal defects. *Acta Paediatr Scand* 1991;80:355–360.

144. Goldberg SJ, Sahn DJ, Allen HD, Valdes-Cruz LM, Hoenecke H, Carnahan Y. Evaluation of pulmonary and systemic blood flow by two-dimensional Doppler echocardiography using fast Fourier transform spectral analysis. *Am J Cardiol* 1982;50:1394–1400.

145. Michelfelder EC, Vermilion RP, Ludomirsky A, Beekman RH, Lloyd TR. Comparison of simultaneous Doppler and catheter-derived right ventricular dP/dt in hypoplastic left heart syndrome. *Am J Cardiol* 1996;77:212–214.

146. Cloez JL, Schmidt KG, Silverman NH. Determination of pulmonary to systemic blood flow ratio in children by a simplified Doppler echocardiographic method. *J Am Coll Cardiol* 1988;11:825–830.

147. Stevenson JG. Doppler evaluation of atrial septal defect, ventricular septal defect, and complex malformations. *Acta Paediatr Scand* 1986;329[Suppl]:21–43.

148. Rokey R, Sterling LL, Zoghbi WA, et al. Determination of regurgitant fraction in isolated mitral or aortic regurgitation by pulsed Doppler two-dimensional echocardiography. *J Am Coll Cardiol* 1986;7:1273–1278.

149. Enriquez-Sarano M, Bailey KR, Seward JB, Tajik AJ, Krohn MJ, Mays JM. Quantitative Doppler assessment of valvular regurgitation. *Circulation* 1993;87:841–848.

150. Geisler M, Grossman G, Schmidt A, et al. Color Doppler echocardiographic determination of mitral regurgitant flow from the proximal velocity profile of the flow convergence region. *Am J Cardiol* 1993;71:217–224.

151. Goldberg SJ, Allen HD. Quantitative assessment of Doppler echocardiography of pulmonary or aortic regurgitation. *Am J Cardiol* 1985;56:131–135.

152. Holen J, Aaslid R, Landmark K, Simonsen S. Determination of pressure gradient in mitral stenosis with a non-invasive ultrasound Doppler technique. *Acta Med Scand* 1976;199:455–460.

153. Holen J, Aaslid R, Landmark K, Simonsen S, Ostrem T. Determination of the effective orifice area in mitral stenosis from noninvasive ultrasound Doppler data and mitral flow rate. *Acta Med Scand* 1977;201:83–88.

154. Hatle L, Angelsen BA, Tromsdal A. Non-invasive assessment of aortic stenosis by Doppler ultrasound. *Br Heart J* 1980;43:284–292.

155. Hatle L, Brubakk A, Tromsdal A, Angelsen BA. Noninvasive assessment of pressure drop in mitral stenosis by Doppler ultrasound. *Br Heart J* 1978;40:131–140.

156. Lima CO, Sahn DJ, Valdes-Cruz LM, et al. Noninvasive prediction of transvalvular pressure gradient in patients with pulmonary stenosis by quantitative two-dimensional echocardiographic Doppler studies. *Circulation* 1983;67:866–871.

157. Currie PJ, Steward JB, Reeder GS, et al. Continuous-wave Doppler echocardiographic assessment of severity of calcific aortic stenosis: a simultaneous Doppler-catheter correlative study in 100 adult patients. *Circulation* 1985;71:1162–1169.

158. Otto CM, Pearlman AS, Comess KA, Reamer RP, Janko CL, Huntsman LL. Determination of stenotic aortic valve area in adults using Doppler echocardiography. *J Am Coll Cardiol* 1986;7:509–517.

159. Valdes-Cruz LM, Yoganathan AP, Tamura T, Tomizuka F, Woo YR, Sahn DJ. Studies in vitro of the relationship between ultrasound and laser Doppler velocimetry and applicability of the simplified Bernoulli relationship. *Circulation* 1986;73:300–308.

160. Yoganathan AP, Cape EG, Sung HW, Williams FP, Jimoh A. Review of hydrodynamic principles for the cardiologist: applications to the study of blood flow and jets by imaging techniques. *J Am Coll Cardiol* 1988;12:1344–1353.

161. Levine RA, Jimoh A, Cape EG, McMillan S, Yoganathan AP, Weyman AE. Pressure recovery distal to a stenosis: potential cause of gradient overestimation by Doppler echocardiography. *J Am Coll Cardiol* 1989;13:706–715.

162. Yoganathan AP, Valdes-Cruz LM, Schmidt-Dohna J, et al. Continous wave-Doppler velocities and gradients across fixed tunnel obstructions: studies in vitro and in vivo. *Circulation* 1987;76:657–666.

163. Currie PJ, Hagler DJ, Seward JB, et al. Instantaneous pressure gradient: a simultaneous Doppler and dual catheter correlative study. *J Am Coll Cardiol* 1986;7:800–806.

164. Cape EG, Jones M, Yamada I, VanAuker MD, Valdes-Cruz LM. Turbulent/viscous interactions control Doppler/catheter pressure discrepancies in aortic stenosis: the role of the Reynolds number. *Circulation* 1996;94:2975–2981.

165. Lemler MS, Shaffer EM, Valdes-Cruz LM, Wiggins JW, Cape EG. Insights into catheter/Doppler discrepancies: a clinical study of congenital aortic stenosis. *Circulation* 1996;94:I-415(abst).

166. Baumgartner H, Schima H, Tulzer G, Kuhn P. Effect of stenosis geometry on the Doppler-catheter gradient relation in vitro: a manifestation of pressure recovery. *J Am Coll Cardiol* 1993;21:1018–1025.

167. Voelker W, Reul H, Stelzer T, Schmidt A, Karsch KR. Pressure recovery in aortic stenosis: an in vitro study in a pulsatile flow model. *J Am Coll Cardiol* 1992;20:1585–1593.

168. Levine RA, Cape EG, Yoganathan AP. Pressure recovery distal to stenoses: expanding clinical applications of engineering principles. *J Am Coll Cardiol* 1993;21:1026–1028.

169. Niederberger J, Schima H, Maurer G, Baumgartner. Importance of pressure recovery for the assessment of aortic stenosis by Doppler ultrasound. *Circulation* 1996;94:1934–1940.

170. Cape EG, Kelly DL, Ettedgui JA, Park SC. Influence of stenotic valve geometry on measured pressure gradients and ventricular work: the relationship between morphology and flow. *Pediatr Cardiol* 1996;17:155–162.

171. Agatston AS. Doppler diagnosis of valvular aortic stenosis. *Echocardiography* 1986;3:3–17.

172. Oshinski JN, Parks WJ, Markou CP, et al. Improved measurement of pressure gradients in aortic coarctation by magnetic resonance imaging. *J Am Coll Cardiol* 1996;28:1818–1826.

173. Weiss P. Doppler evaluation of aortic valve area in children with aortic stenosis [Letter]. *J Am Coll Cardiol* 1992;20:749.

174. Gorlin R, Gorlin SG. Hydraulic formula for calculation of the area of the stenotic mitral valve, other cardiac valves, and central circulatory shunts. *Am Heart J* 1951;41:1–29.

175. Segal J, Lerner DJ, Miller DC, Mitchell RS, Alderman EA, Popp RL. When should Doppler-determined valve area be better than the Gorlin formula? *J Am Coll Cardiol* 1987;9:1294–1305.

176. Dumesnil JG, Yoganathan AP. Theoretical and practical differences between the Gorlin formula and the continuity equation for calculating aortic and mitral valve areas. *Am J Cardiol* 1991;67:1268–1272.

177. Burwash IG, Thomas DD, Sadahiro M, et al. Dependence of Gorlin formula and continuity equation valve areas on transvalvular volume flow rate in valvular aortic stenosis. *Circulation* 1994;89:827–835.

178. Casale PN, Palacios IF, Abascal VM, Davidoff R, Weyman AE, Fifer MA. Effects of dobutamine on Gorlin and continuity equation valve areas and valve resistance in valvular aortic stenosis. *Am J Cardiol* 1992;70:1175–1179.

179. Kosturakis D, Allen HD, Goldberg SJ, Sahn DJ, Valdes-Cruz LM. Non-invasive quantification of stenotic semilunar valve areas by Doppler echocardiography. *J Am Coll Cardiol* 1984;3:1256–1262.

180. Skjaerpe T, Hegrenaes L, Hatle L. Noninvasive estimation of valve area in patients with aortic stenosis by Doppler ultrasound and two-dimensional echocardiography. *Circulation* 1985;72:810–818.

181. DeGroff CG, Shandas R, Valdes-Cruz L. Analysis of the effect of flow rate on the Doppler continuity equation for stenotic orifice area calculation: a numerical study. *Circulation* 1998;97:1597–1605.

182. Shandas R, Kwon J, Valdes-Cruz L. In vitro studies of velocity profiles within the proximal jet using digital particle image velocimetry: implications for clinical Doppler methods. *Circulation* 1996;94:I-492(abst).

183. Otto CM, Pearlman AS, Kraft CD, Miyake-Hull CY, Burwash IG, Gardner CJ. Physiologic changes with maximal exercise in asymptomatic valvular aortic stenosis assessed by Doppler echocardiography. *J Am Coll Cardiol* 1992;20:1160–1167.

184. Reimold SC, Ganz P, Bittl JA, et al. Effective aortic regurgitant orifice area: description of a method based on the conservation of mass. *J Am Coll Cardiol* 1991;18:761–768.

185. Enriquez-Sarano M, Seward JB, Bailey KR, Tajik AJ. Effective regurgitant orifice area: a noninvasive Doppler development of an old hemodyanamic concept. *J Am Coll Cardiol* 1994;23:443–451.

186. Vandervoort PM, Rivera JM, Mele D, et al. Application of color Doppler flow mapping to calculate effective orifice area: an in vitro study and initial clinical observations. *Circulation* 1993;88:1150–1156.

187. Enriquez-Sarano M, Miller FA, Hayes SN, Bailey KR, Tajik AJ, Seward JB. Effective mitral regurgitant orifice area: clinical use and pitfalls of the proximal isovelocity surface area method. *J Am Coll Cardiol* 1995;25:703–709.

188. Rodriquez L, Thomas JD, Monterroso V, et al. Validation of the proximal flow convergence method: calculation of orifice area in patients with mitral stenosis. *Circulation* 1993;88:1157–1166.

189. Rifkin RD, Harper K, Tighe D. Comparison of proximal isovelocity surface area method with pressure half-time and planimetry in evaluation of mitral stenosis. *J Am Coll Cardiol* 1995;26:458–465.

190. Shiota T, Jones M, Valdes-Cruz LM, Shandas R, Yamada I, Sahn DJ. Color flow Doppler determination of transmitral flow and orifice area in mitral stenosis: experimental evaluation of the proximal flow convergence method. *Am Heart J* 1995;129:114–123.

191. Deng YB, Matsumoto M, Wang XF, et al. Estimation of mitral valve area in patients with mitral stenosis by the flow convergence region method: selection of aliasing velocity. *J Am Coll Cardiol* 1994;24:683–689.

192. DeGroff CG, Baptista AM, Sahn DJ. Evaluating modifications to the flow convergence method for constrained regurgitant and stenotic orifices: finite element modeling. *Circulation* 1996;94:I-499(abst).

193. Thomas JD, Liu CM, Flachskampf FA, O'Shea JP, Davidoff R, Weyman AE. Quantification of jet flow by momentum analysis. *Circulation* 1990;81:247–259.

194. Ford LE, Feldman T, Carroll JD. Valve resistance. *Circulation* 1994;89:893–895.

195. Ford LE, Feldman T, Chiu YC, Carroll JD. Hemodynamic resistance as a measure of functional impairment in aortic valvular stenosis. *Circ Res* 1990;66:1–7.

196. Cannon JD, Zile MR, Crawford FA, Carabello BA. Aortic valve resistance as an adjunct to the Gorlin formula in assessing the severity of aortic stenosis in symptomatic patients. *J Am Coll Cardiol* 1992;20:1517–1523.

197. Burwash IG, Pearlman AS, Kraft CD, Miyake-Hull C, Healy NL, Otto CM. Flow dependence of measures of aortic stenosis severity during exercise. *J Am Coll Cardiol* 1994;24:1342–1350.

198. Ho PP, Pauls GL, Lamberton DF, Portnoff JS, Pai RG, Shah PM. Doppler derived aortic valve resistance in aortic stenosis: its hemodynamic validation. *J Heart Valve Dis* 1994;3:283–287.

199. Gardin JM, Burns CS, Childs WJ, Henry WL. Evaluation of blood flow velocity in the ascending aorta of normal subjects by Doppler echocardiography. *Am Heart J* 1984;107:310–318.

200. Feigenbaum H. *Echocardiography.* 5th ed. Philadelphia: Lea & Febiger, 1994.

201. Labovitz AJ, Ferrara RP, Kern MJ, Bryg RJ, Mrosek DG, Williams GA. Quantitative evaluation of aortic insufficiency by continuous wave Doppler echocardiography. *J Am Coll Cardiol* 1986;8:1341–1347.

202. Hatle L, Angelsen B, Tromsdal A. Noninvasive assessment of atrioventricular pressure half-time by Doppler ultrasound. *Circulation* 1979;60:1096–1104.

203. Myreng Y, Smiseth OA. Assessment of left ventricular relaxation by Doppler echocardiography. *Circulation* 1990;81:260–266.

204. Appleton CP, Hatle LK, Popp RK. Relation of transmitral flow velocity patterns to left ventricular diastolic function. *J Am Coll Cardiol* 1988;12:426–440.

205. Nishimura RA, Schwartz RS, Tajik AJ, Holmes DR. Noninvasive measurement of rate of left ventricular relaxation by Doppler echocardiography. *Circulation* 1993;88:146–155.

206. Chen C, Rodriguez L, Lethor JP, et al. Continuous wave Doppler echocardiography for noninvasive assessment of left ventricular dP/dt and relaxation time constant from mitral regurgitant spectra in patients. *J Am Coll Cardiol* 1994;23:970–976.

207. Scalia GM, Greenberg NL, McCarthy PM, Thomas JD, Vandervoort PM. Noninvasive assessment of the ventricular relaxation time constant in humans by Doppler echocardiography. *Circulation* 1997;95:151–155.

208. Bargiggia GS, Bertucci C, Recusani F, et al. A new method for estimating left ventricular dP/dt by continuous wave-Doppler echocardiography. *Circulation* 1989;80:1287–1292.

209. Chen C, Rodriquez L, Guerrero L, et al. Noninvasive estimation of the instantaneous first derivative of left ventricular pressure using continuous-wave Doppler echocardiography. *Circulation* 1991;83:2101–2110.

210. Imanishi T, Nakatani S, Yamada S, et al. Validation of continuous wave Doppler-determined right ventricular peak positive and negative dP/dt: effect of right atrial pressure on measurement. *J Am Coll Cardiol* 1994;23:1638–1643.

211. Sabbah HN, Khaja F, Brymer JF, et al. Noninvasive evaluation of left ventricular performance based on peak aortic blood acceleration measured with a continuous-wave Doppler velocity meter. *Circulation* 1986;74:323–329.

212. Bennett ED, Barclay SA, Davis AL, Mannering D, Mehta N. Ascending aortic blood velocity and acceleration using Doppler ultrasound in the assessment of left ventricular function. *Cardiovasc Res* 1984;18:632–638.

213. Abbasi AS, Allen MW, DeCristofaro D, Ungar I. Detection and estimation of the degree of mitral regurgitation by range-gated pulsed Doppler echocardiography. *Circulation* 1980;61:143–147.

214. Miyatake K, Kinoshita N, Nagata S, et al. Intracardiac flow pattern in mitral regurgitation studied with combined use of the ultrasonic pulsed Doppler technique and cross-sectional echocardiography. *Am J Cardiol* 1980;45:155–162.

215. Ciobanu M, Abbasi AS, Allen M, Hermer A, Spellberg R. Pulsed Doppler echocardiography in the diagnosis and estimation of severity of aortic regurgitation. *Am J Cardiol* 1982;49:339–343.

216. Cooper JW, Nanda NC, Philpot EF, Fan P. Evaluation of valvular regurgitation by color Doppler. *J Am Soc Echocardiogr* 1989;2:56–66.

217. Miyatake K, Izumi S, Okamoto M, et al. Semiquantitative grading of severity of mitral regurgitation by real-time two-dimensional Doppler flow imaging. *J Am Coll Cardiol* 1986;7:82–88.

218. Rivera JM, Vandervoort PM, Morris E, Weyman AE, Thomas JD. Visual assessment of valvular regurgitation: comparison with quantitative Doppler measurements. *J Am Soc Echocardiogr* 1994;7:480–487.

219. Smith MD, Kwan OL, Spain MG, DeMaria AN. Temporal variability of color Doppler jet areas in patients with mitral and aortic regurgitation. *Am Heart J* 1992;123:953–960.

220. Maciel BC, Moises VA, Shandas R, et al. Effects of pressure and volume of the receiving chamber on the spatial distribution of regurgitant jets as imaged by color Doppler flow mapping. *Circulation* 1991;83:605–613.

221. Krabill KA, Sung HW, Tamura T, Chung KJ, Yoganathan AP, Sahn DJ. Factors influencing the structure and shape of stenotic and regurgitant jets: an in vitro investigation using Doppler color flow mapping and optical flow visualization. *J Am Coll Cardiol* 1989;13:1672–1681.

222. Maciel BC, Moises VA, Shandas R, et al. Effects of pressure and volume of the receiving chamber on the spatial distribution of regurgitant jets as imaged by color Doppler flow mapping. *Circulation* 1991;83:605–613.

223. Sahn DJ. Instrumentation and physical factors related to visualization of stenotic and regurgitant jets by Doppler color flow mapping. *J Am Coll Cardiol* 1988;12:1354–1365.

224. Stewart WJ, Cohen GI, Salcedo EE. Doppler color flow image size: dependance on instrument settings. *Echocardiography* 1991;8:319–327.

225. Hoit BD, Jones M, Eidbo EE, Elias W, Sahn DJ. Sources of variability for Doppler color flow mapping of regurgitant jets in an animal model of mitral regurgitation. *J Am Coll Cardiol* 1989;13:1631–1636.

226. Stevenson JG. Two-dimensional color Doppler estimation of the severity of atrioventricular valve regurgitation: important effects of instrument gain setting, pulse repetition frequency, and carrier frequency. *J Am Soc Echocardiogr* 1989;2:1–10.

227. Cape EG, Yoganathan AP, Weyman AE, Levine RA. Adjacent solid boundaries alter the size of regurgitant jets on Doppler color flow maps. *J Am Coll Cardiol* 1991;17:1094–1102.

228. Chen C, Thomas JD, Anconina J, et al. Impact of impinging wall jet on color Doppler quantification of mitral regurgitation. *Circulation* 1991;84:712–720.

229. Smith MD, Grayburn PA, Spain MG, DeMaria AN. Observer variability in the quantitation of Doppler color flow jet areas for mitral and aortic regurgitation. *J Am Coll Cardiol* 1988;11:579–584.

230. Perry GJ, Helmcke F, Nanda NC, Byard C, Soto B. Evaluation of aortic insufficiency by Doppler color flow mapping. *J Am Coll Cardiol* 1987;9:952–959.

231. Switzer DF, Yoganathan AP, Nanda NC, Woo YR, Ridgway AJ. Calibration of color Doppler flow mapping during extremes of hemodynamic condition in vitro. *Circulation* 1987;75:837–846.

232. Reynolds T, Abate T, Tenney A, Warner MG. The JH/LVOH method in the quantification of aortic regurgitation: how the cardiac sonographer may avoid an important potential pitfall. *J Am Soc Echocardiogr* 1991;4:105–108.

233. Ishii M, Jones M, Shiota T, et al. Quantifying aortic regurgitation by using the color Doppler imaged vena contracta: a chronic animal model study. *Circulation* 1997;96:2009–2016.

234. Grayburn PA, Fehske W, Omran H, Bricker ME, Luderitz B. Multiplane transesophageal echocardiographic assessment of mitral regurgitation by Doppler color flow mapping of the vena contracta. *Am J Cardiol* 1994;74:912–917.

235. Tribouilloy C, Shen WF, Quere JP, et al. Assessment of severity of mitral regurgitation by measuring regurgitant jet width at its origin with transesophageal Doppler color flow imaging. *Circulation* 1992;85:1248–1253.

236. Fehske W, Omran H, Manz M, Kohler J, Hagendorff A, Luderitz B. Color-coded Doppler imaging of the vena contracta as a basis for quantification of pure mitral regurgitation. *Am J Cardiol* 1994;73:268–274.

237. Mele D, Vandervoort P, Palacios I, et al. Proximal jet size by Doppler color flow mapping predicts severity of mitral regurgitation. *Circulation* 1995;91:746–754.

238. Hall SA, Brikner E, Willett DL, Irani WN, Afridi I, Grayburn PA. Assessment of mitral regurgitation severity by Doppler color flow mapping of the vena contracta. *Circulation* 1997;95:636–642.

239. DeGroff CG, Shandas R, Valdes-Cruz LM. Utility of the proxmial color flow jet width in the assessment of regurgitant/stenotic orifices—effect of low velocity filter and comparison to actual vena contracta size: a numerical study. *J Am Coll Cardiol* 1998;31:475A(abst).

240. Shandas R, DeGroff CG, Kwon J, Valdes-Cruz LM. Relationship of color Doppler low velocity filter to vena contracta dimensions for regurgitant and stenotic jets: in vitro studies using laser flow visualization. *J Am Coll Echocardiogr* 1998;11:537(abst).

241. Shandas R, Kwon J, DeGroff C, Valdes-Cruz LM. Color Doppler imaging of the proximal jet is a good reflector of vena contracta area of regurgitant jets: in vitro studies using laser-induced fluorescence imaging. *J Am Coll Cardiol* 1997;29:341A(abst).

242. Brun P, Tribouilloy C, Duval AM, et al. Left ventricular flow propagation during early filling is related to wall relaxation. *J Am Coll Cardiol* 1992;20:420–432.

243. Takatsuji H, Mikami T, Urasawa K, et al. A new approach for evaluation of left ventricular diastolic function: spatial and temporal analysis of left ventricular filling flow propagation by color M-mode Doppler echocardiography. *J Am Coll Cardiol* 1996;27:365–371.

244. Stuggard M, Risoe C, Ihlen H, Smiseth OA. Intracavity filling pattern in the failing left ventricle assessed by color M-mode Doppler echocardiography. *J Am Coll Cardiol* 1994;24:663–670.

245. Duval-Moulin A-M, Dupouy P, Brun P, et al. Alteration of left ventricular diastolic function during coronary angioplasty-induced ischemia: a color M-mode Doppler study. *J Am Coll Cardiol* 1997;29:1246–1255.

246. Gardin JM, Iseri LT, Elkayam U, et al. Evaluation of dilated cardiomyopathy by pulsed Doppler echocardiography. *Am Heart J* 1983;106:1057–1065.

247. Harrison MR, Clifton GD, Berk MR, DeMaria AN. Effect of blood pressure and afterload on Doppler echocardiographic measurements of left ventricular systolic function in normal subjects. *Am J Cardiol* 1989;64:905–908.

248. Bedotto JB, Eichhorn EJ, Grayburn PA. Effects of left ventricular preload and afterload on ascending aortic blood velocity and acceleration in coronary artery disease. *Am J Cardiol* 1989;64:856–859.

249. Gardin JM. Doppler measurements of aortic blood flow velocity and acceleration: load-independent indexes of left ventricular performance? [Editorial]. *Am J Cardiol* 1989;64:935–936.

250. Harrison MR, Clifton GD, Sublett KL, DeMaria AN. Effect of heart rate on Doppler indexes of systolic function in humans. *J Am Coll Cardiol* 1989;14:929–935.

251. Kolettis M, Jenkins BS, Webb-Peploe MM. Assessment of left ventricular function by indices derived from aortic flow velocity. *Br Heart J* 1976;38:18–31.

252. Sabbah HN, Gheorghiade M, Smith ST, Frank DM, Stein PD. Serial evaluation of left ventricular function in congestive heart failure by measurement of peak aortic blood acceleration. *Am J Cardiol* 1988;61:367–370.

253. Hanseus K, Bjorkhem G, Lundstrom NR. Cardiac function in healthy infants and children: Doppler echocardiographic evaluation. *Pediatr Cardiol* 1994;15:211–218.

254. Harrison MR, Clifton GD, Sublett KL, DeMaria AN. Effect of heart rate on Doppler indexes of systolic function in humans. *J Am Coll Cardiol* 1989;14:929–935.

255. Isaaz K, Pasipoularides A. Noninvasive assessment of intrinsic ventricular load dynamics in dilated cardiomyopathy. *J Am Coll Cardiol* 1990;17:112–121.

256. Gutgesell HP, Paquet M, Duff DF, McNamara DG. Evaluation of left ventricular size and function by echocardiography. *Circulation* 1977;56:457–462.

257. Schmidt KG, Cloez JL, Silverman NH. Assessment of right ventricular performance by pulsed Doppler echocardiography in patients after intraatrial repair of aortopulmonary transposition in infancy and childhood. *J Am Coll Cardiol* 1989;13:1578–1585.

258. Elkayam U, Gardin J, Berkley R, Hughes CA, Henry WL. The use of Doppler flow velocity measurement to assess the hemodynamic response to vasodilators in patients with heart failure. *Circulation* 1983;67:377–383.

259. Pai RG, Bansal RC, Shah PM. Doppler-derived rate of left ventricular pressure rise: its correlation with the postoperative left ventricular function in mitral regurgitation. *Circulation* 1990;82:514–520.

260. Chung N, Nishimura RA, Holmes DR, Tajik AJ. Measurement of left ventricular dp/dt by simultaneous Doppler echocardiography and cardiac catheterization. *J Am Soc Echocardiogr* 1992;5:147–152.

261. Kawai H, Yokota Y, Yokoyama M. Noninvasive evaluation of contractile state by left ventricular dP/dt$_{max}$ divided by end-diastolic volume using continuous-wave Doppler and M-mode echocardiography. *Clin Cardiol* 1994;17:662–668.

262. Pai RG, Pai SM, Bodenheimer MM, Adamick RD. Estimation of rate of left ventricular pressure rise by Doppler echocardiography: its hemodynamic validation. *Am Heart J* 1993;126:240–242.

263. Kawai H, Yokota Y, Yokoyama M. Noninvasive evaluation of contractile state by left ventricular dP/dt$_{max}$ divided by end-diastolic volume using continuous-wave Doppler and M-mode echocardiography. *Clin Cardiol* 1994;17:662–668.

264. Anconina J, Danchin N, Selton-Suty C, et al. Noninvasive estimation of right ventricular dP/dt in patients with tricuspid valve regurgitation. *Am J Cardiol* 1993;71:1495–1497.

265. Pai RG, Bansal RC, Shah PM. Determinants of the rate of right ventricular pressure rise by Doppler echocardiography: potential value in the assessment of right ventricular function. *J Heart Valve Dis* 1994;3:179–184.

266. Appleton CP, Hatle LK, Popp RL. Relation of transmitral flow velocity patterns to left ventricular diastolic function: new insights from a combined hemodynamic and Doppler echocardiographic study. *J Am Coll Cardiol* 1988;12:426–440.

267. Nishimura RA, Abel MD, Hatle LK, Tajik AJ. Assessment of diastolic function of the heart: background and current applications of Doppler echocardiography. Part II. Clinical studies. *Mayo Clin Proc* 1989;64:71–81.

268. Thomas JD, Weyman AE. Echocardiographic Doppler evaluation of left ventricular diastolic function. *Circulation* 1991;84:977–990.

269. DeMaria AN, Wisenbaugh TW, Smith MD, Harrison MR, Berk

MR. Doppler echocardiographic evaluation of diastolic dysfunction. *Circulation* 1991;84[Suppl]:I288–I295(abst).

270. Giddings, Snider AR, Rocchini AP, Peters J, Fransworth R. Left ventricular diastolic filling in children with hypertrophic cardiomyopathy: assessment with pulsed Doppler echocardiography. *J Am Coll Cardiol* 1986;8:310–316.

271. Appleton CP, Galloway JM, Gonzalez MS, Gaballa M, Basnight MA. Estimation of left ventricular filling pressures using two-dimensional and Doppler echocardiography in adult patients with cardiac disease. *J Am Coll Cardiol* 1993;22:1972–1982.

272. Greenberg B, Chatterjee K, Parmley WM, Werner JA, Holly AN. The influence of left ventricular filling pressure on atrial contribution to cardiac output. *Am Heart J* 1979;98:742–751.

273. Channer KS, Culling W, Wilde P, Jones JV. Estimation of left ventricular end-diastolic pressure by pulsed Doppler ultrasound. *Lancet* 1986;1005–1007.

274. Bristow JD, Van Zee BE, Judkins MP. Systolic and diastolic abnormalities of the left ventricle in coronary artery disease. *Circulation* 1970;42:219–228.

275. Yu CM, Sanderson JE, Chan S, Yeung L, Hung YT, Woo KS. Right ventricular diastolic dysfunction in heart failure. *Circulation* 1996;93:1509–1514.

276. Vermilion RP, Snider R, Melioner JN, Peters J, Merida-Asmus L. Pulsed Doppler evaluation of right ventricular diastolic filling in children with pulmonary valve stenosis before and after balloon valvuloplasty. *Am J Cardiol* 1990;66:79–84.

277. Vermilion RP, Snider R, Bengur R, Meliones JN. Long-term assessment of right ventricular diastolic filling in patients with pulmonic valve stenosis successfully treated in childhood. *Am J Cardiol* 1991;68:648–652.

278. Lee CH, Vancheri F, Josen MS, Gibson DG. Discrepancies in the measurement of isovolumic relaxation time: a study comparing M-mode and Doppler echocardiography. *Br Heart J* 1990;64:214–218.

279. Frommelt MA, Snider AR, Crowley DC, Meliones JN, Heidelberger KP. Echocardiographic indexes of allograft rejection in pediatric cardiac transplant recipients. *J Am Soc Echocardiogr* 1992;5:41–47.

280. Goren A, Glaser J, Drukker A. Diastolic function in children and adolescents on dialysis and after kidney transplantation: an echocardiographic assessment. *Pediatr Nephrol* 1993;7:725–728.

281. Pai RG, Bucch GC. Newer Doppler measures of left ventricular diastolic function. *Clin Cardiol* 1996;19:277–288.

282. Chen C, Rodriquez L, Levine RA, Weyman AE, Thomas JD. Noninvasive measurement of the time constant of left ventricular relaxation using the continuous-wave Doppler velocity profile. *Circulation* 1992;86:272–278.

283. Yamamoto K, Masuyama T, Doi Y, et al. Noninvasive assessment of left ventricular relaxation using continuous-wave Doppler aortic regurgitant velocity curve. Its comparative value to the mitral regurgitation method. *Circulation* 1995;91:192–200.

284. Honda Y, Yokota Y, Yokoyama M. Evaluation of left ventricular relaxation using continuous wave Doppler velocity profile of aortic regurgitation: noninvasive measurement of left ventricular negative dP/dt and time constant. *Clin Cardiol* 1996;19:709–715.

285. Cetta F, O'Leary PW, Seward JB, Driscoll DJ. Idiopathic restrictive cardiomyopathy in childhood: diagnostic features and clinical course. *Mayo Clin Proc* 1995;70:634–640.

286. Garcia MJ, Ares MA, Asher C, Rodriguez L, Vandervoort P, Thomas JD. An index of early left ventricular filling that combined with pulsed Doppler peak E velocity may estimate capillary wedge pressure. *J Am Coll Cardiol* 1997;29:448–454.

287. Yang SS, Goldberg H. Simplified Doppler estimation of mitral valve area. *Am J Cardiol* 1985;56:488–489.

288. Thomas JD, Weyman AE. Doppler mitral pressure half-time: a clinical tool in search of a theoretical justification. *J Am Coll Cardiol* 1987;10:923–929.

289. Karp K, Teien D, Bjerle P, Eriksson P. Reassessment of valve area determinations in mitral stenosis by the pressure half-time method: impact of left ventricular stiffness and peak diastolic pressure difference. *J Am Coll Cardiol* 1989;13:594–599.

290. Chen C, Wang Y, Guo B, Lin Y. Reliability of the Doppler pressure half-time immediately after percutaneous mitral balloon valvuloplasty. *J Am Coll Cardiol* 1989;13:1309–1313.

291. Stamm RB, Martin RP. Quantification of pressure gradients across stenotic valves by Doppler ultrasound. *J Am Coll Cardiol* 1983;2:707–718.

292. Holen J, Aaslid R, Landmark K. Determination of pressure gradient in mitral stenosis with a non-invasive ultrasound Doppler technique. *Acta Med Scand* 1976;199:455–460.

293. Smith MD, Wisenbaugh T, Grayburn PA, Gurley JC, Spain MG, DeMaria AN. Value and limitations of Doppler pressure half-time in quantifying mitral stenosis: a comparison with micromanometer catheter recordings. *Am Heart J* 1991;121:480–488.

294. Banerjee A, Kohl T, Silverman NH. Echocardiographic evaluation of congenital mitral valve anomalies in children. *Am J Cardiol* 1995;76:1284–1291.

295. Nakatani S, Masuyama T, Kodama K, Kitabatake A, Fujii K, Kamadaz T. Value and limitations of Doppler echocardiography in the quantification of stenotic mitral valve area: comparison of the pressure half-time and the continuity equation methods. *Circulation* 1988;77:78–85.

296. Voelker W, Regele B, Dittmann H, et al. Effect of heart rate on transmitral flow velocity profile and Doppler measurements of mitral valve area in patients with mitral stenosis. *Eur Heart J* 1992;13:152–159.

297. Deng YB, Matsumoto M, Munehira J. Determination of mitral valve area in patients with mitral stenosis by the flow convergence region method during changing hemodynamic conditions. *Am Heart J* 1996;132:633–641.

298. Grenadier E, Sahn DJ, Valdes-Cruz LM, Allen HD, Oliveira Lima C, Goldberg SJ. Two-dimensional echo Doppler study of congenital disorders of the mitral valve. *Am Heart J* 1984;107:319–325.

299. Hatle L, Brubakk A, Tromsdal A. Noninvasive assessment of pressure drop in mitral stenosis by Doppler ultrasound. *Br Heart J* 1978;40:131–140.

300. Nishimura RA, Rihal CS, Tajik AJ, Holmes DR. Accurate measurement of the transmitral gradient in patients with mitral stenosis: a simultaneous catheterization and Doppler echocardiographic study. *J Am Coll Cardiol* 1994;24:152–158.

301. Pearlman AS. Role of echocardiography in the diagnosis and evaluation of severity of mitral and tricuspid stenosis. *Circulation* 1991;84[Suppl I]:I193–I197.

302. Veyrat C, Kalmanson D, Farjon M, Manin JP, Abitbol G. Noninvasive diagnosis and assessment of tricuspid regurgitation and stenosis using one- and two-dimensional echo pulsed Doppler. *Br Heart J* 1982;47:596–605.

303. Fawzy ME, Mercer EN, Dunn B, al-Amri M, Andaya W. Doppler echocardiography in the evaluation of tricuspid stenosis. *Eur Heart J* 1989;10:985–990.

304. Karp K, Teien D, Eriksson P. Doppler echocardiographic assessment of the valve area in patients with atrioventricular valve stenosis by application of the continuity equation. *J Intern Med* 1989;225:261–266.

305. Parris TM, Panidis JP, Ross J, Mintz GS. Doppler echocardiographic findings in rheumatic tricuspid stenosis. *Am J Cardiol* 1987;60:1414–1416.

306. Perez JE, Ludbrook PA, Ahumada GG. Usefulness of Doppler echocardiography in detecting tricuspid valve stenosis. *Am J Cardiol* 1985;55:601–602.

307. Hatle L. Assessment of aortic blood flow velocities with continuous wave Doppler ultrasound in the neonate and young child. *J Am Coll Cardiol* 1985;5:113S–119S.

308. Krafchek J, Robertson JH, Radford M, Adams D, Kisslo J. A reconsideration of Doppler assessed gradients in suspected aortic stenosis. *Am Heart J* 1985;110:765–773.

309. Hegrenaes L, Hatle L. Aortic stenosis in adults. Non-invasive estimation of pressure differences by continuous wave Doppler echocardiography. *Br Heart J* 1985;54:396–404.

310. Hatle L, Angelsen BA, Tromsdal A. Non-invasive assessment of aortic stenosis by Doppler ultrasound. *Br Heart J* 1980;43:284–292.

311. Taylor, R. Evolution of the continuity equation in the Doppler echocardiographic assessment of the severity of valvular aortic stenosis. *J Am Soc Echocardiogr* 1990;3:326–330.

312. Warth DC, Stewart WJ, Block PC, Weyman AE. A new method to calculate aortic valve area without left heart catheterization. *Circulation* 1984;70:978–983.

313. Panidis IP, Mintz GS, Ross J. Value and limitations of Doppler ultrasound in the evaluation of aortic stenosis: a statistical analysis of 70 consecutive patients. *Am Heart J* 1986;112:150–158.

314. Zoghbi WA, Farmer KL, Soto JG, Nelson JG, Quinones MA. Accurate noninvasive quantification of stenotic aortic valve area by Doppler echocardiography. *Circulation* 1986;73:452–459.

315. Otto CM, Pearlman AS, Comess KA, Reamer RP, Janko CL, Huntsman LL. Determination of the stenotic aortic valve area in adults using Doppler echocardiography. *J Am Coll Cardiol* 1986; 7:509–517.

316. Danielsen R, Nordrehaug JE, Stangeland L, Vik-Mo H. Limitations in assessing the severity of aortic stenosis by Doppler gradients. *Br Heart J* 1988;59:551–555.

317. Smith MD, Dawson PL, Elion JL, et al. Systematic correlation of continuous-wave Doppler and hemodynamic measurements in patients with aortic stenosis. *Am Heart J* 1986;111:245–252.

318. Wendel H, Teien D, Human DG, Nanton MA. Noninvasive estimation of aortic valve areas in children with aortic stenosis. *Acta Paediatr Scand* 1990;79:1112–1115.

319. Wright SB, Wienecke MM, Meyer KB, McKay CA, Wiles HB. Correlation of pediatric echocardiographic Doppler and catheter-derived valvar aortic stenosis gradients and the influence of regurgitation. *Am J Cardiol* 1996;77:663–665.

320. Simpson IA, Houston AB, Sheldon CD, Hutton I, Lawrie TD. Clinical value of Doppler echocardiography in the assessment of adults with aortic stenosis. *Br Heart J* 1985;53:636–639.

321. Garson A, Bricker JT, McNamara DG. *The science and practice of pediatric cardiology. Volume 1.* Malvern, PA: Lea & Febiger, 1990.

322. Berger M, Berdoff RL, Gallerstein PE, Goldberg E. Evaluation of aortic stenosis by continuous wave Doppler ultrasound. *J Am Coll Cardiol* 1984;3:150–156.

323. Danielsen R, Nordrehaug JE, Vik-Mo H. Factors affecting Doppler echocardiographic valve area assessment in aortic stenosis. *Am J Cardiol* 1989;63:1107–1111.

324. Yeager M, Yock PG, Popp RL. Comparison of Doppler-derived pressure gradient to that determined at cardiac catheterization in adults with aortic valve stenosis: implications for management. *Am J Cardiol* 1986;57:644–648.

325. Ohlsson J, Wranne B. Noninvasive assessment of valve area in patients with aortic stenosis. *J Am Coll Cardiol* 1986;7:501–508.

326. Teien D, Karp K, Eriksson P. Non-invasive estimation of the mean pressure difference in aortic stenosis by Doppler ultrasound. *Br Heart J* 1986;56:450–454.

327. Grayburn PA, Smith MD, Harrison MR, Gurley JC, DeMaria AN. Pivotal role of aortic valve area calculation by the continuity equation for Doppler assessment of aortic stenosis in patients with combined aortic stenosis and regurgitation. *Am J Cardiol* 1988; 61:376–381.

328. Oh JK, Taliercio CP, Holmes DR Jr, et al. Prediction of the severity of aortic stenosis by Doppler aortic valve area determination: prospective Doppler-catheterization correlation in 100 patients. *J Am Coll Cardiol* 1988;11:1227–1234.

329. Fan P-H, Kapur KK, Nanda NC. Color-guided Doppler echocardiographic assessment of aortic valve stenosis. *J Am Coll Cardiol* 1988;12:441–449.

330. Teirstein P, Yeager M, Yock PG, Popp RL. Doppler echocardiographic measurement of aortic valve area in aortic stenosis: a noninvasive application of the Gorlin formula. *J Am Coll Cardiol* 1986;8:1059–1065.

331. Bengur AR, Snider AR, Serwer GA, Peters J, Rosenthal A. Usefulness of the Doppler mean gradient in evaluation of children with aortic valve stenosis and comparison to gradient at catheterization. *Am J Cardiol* 1989;64:756–761.

332. Bengur AR, Snider AR, Meliones JN, Vermilion RP. Doppler evaluation of aortic valve area in children with aortic stenosis. *J Am Coll Cardiol* 1991;18:1499–1505.

333. Otto CM, Pearlman AS, Gardner CL, Kraft CD, Fujioka MC. Simplification of the Doppler continuity equation for calculating stenotic aortic valve area. *J Am Soc Echocardiogr* 1988;1:155–157.

334. Veyrat C, Gourtchiglouian C, Dumora P, Abitbol G, Sainte Beuve D. Kalmanson D. A new non-invasive estimation of the stenotic aortic valve area by pulsed Doppler mapping. *Br Heart J* 1987; 57:44–50.

335. Roger VL, Tajik AJ, Reeder GS, et al. Effect of Doppler echocardiography on utilization of hemodynamic cardiac catheterization in the preoperative evaluation of aortic stenosis. *Mayo Clin Proc* 1996;71:141–149.

336. Fischer JL, Haberer T, Dickson D, Henselmann L. Comparison of Doppler echocardiographic methods with heart catheterisation in assessing aortic valve area in 100 patients with aortic stenosis. *Br Heart J* 1995;73:293–298.

337. Berger M, Hecht SR. Doppler echocardiographic assessment of aortic stenosis using the peak velocity ratio. *Am J Cardiol* 1992; 70:536–537.

338. Blackshear JL, Kapples EJ, Lane GE, Safford RE. Beat-by-beat aortic valve area measurements indicate constant orifice area in aortic stenosis: analysis of Doppler data with varying RR intervals. *J Am Soc Echocardiogr* 1992;5:414–420.

339. Sjoberg BJ, Ask P, Loyd D, Wranne B. Subaortic flow profiles in aortic valve disease: a two-dimensional color Doppler study. *J Am Soc Echocardiogr* 1994;7:276–285.

340. Gutgesell HP, French M. Echocardiographic determination of aortic and pulmonary valve areas in subjects with normal hearts. *Am J Cardiol* 1991;68:773–776.

341. Frantz EG, Silverman NH. Doppler ultrasound evaluation of valvular pulmonary stenosis from multiple transducer positions in children requiring pulmonary valvuloplasty. *Am J Cardiol* 1988;61: 844–849.

342. Johnson GL, Kwan OL, Handshoe S, Noonan JA, DeMaria AN. Accuracy of combined two-dimensional echocardiography and continuous wave Doppler recordings in the estimation of pressure gradient in the right ventricular outlet obstruction. *J Am Coll Cardiol* 1984;3:1013–1018.

343. Houston AB, Sheldon CD, Simpson IA, Doig WB, Coleman EN. The severity of pulmonary valve or artery obstruction in children estimated by Doppler ultrasound. *Eur Heart J* 1985;6:786–790.

344. Goldberg SJ, Vasko SD, Allen HD, Marx GR. Can the technique for Doppler estimate of pulmonary stenosis gradient be simplified? *Am Heart J* 1986;111:709–713.

345. Aldousany AW, DiSessa TG, Dubois R, Alpert BS, Willey ES, Birnbaum SE. Doppler estimation of pressure gradient in pulmonary stenosis: maximal instantaneous vs peak to peak, vs. mean gradient. *Pediatr Cardiol* 1989;10:145–149.

346. Lim MK, Houston AB, Doig WB, Lilley S, Murtagh EP. Variability of the Doppler gradient in pulmonary valve stenosis before and after balloon dilatation. *Br Heart J* 1989;62:212–216.

347. Simpson IA, Valdes-Cruz LM, Yoganathan AP, Sung HW, Jimoh A, Sahn DJ. Spatial velocity distribution and acceleration in serial subvalve tunnel and valvular obstructions: an in vitro study using Doppler color flow mapping. *J Am Coll Cardiol* 1989;13:241–248.

348. Nishimura RA, Tajik AJ, Reeder GS, Seward JB. Evaluation of hypertrophic cardiomyopathy by Doppler flow imaging: initial observations. *Mayo Clin Proc* 1986;61:631–639.

349. Sasson Z, Yock PG, Hatle LK, Alderman EL, Popp RL. Doppler echocardiographic determination of the pressure gradient in hypertrophic cardiomyopathy. *J Am Coll Cardiol* 1988;11:752–756.

350. Stewart WJ, Schiavone WA, Salcedo EE, Lever HM, Cosgrove DM, Gill CC. Intraoperative Doppler echocardiography in hypertrophic cardiomyopathy: correlations with the obstructive gradient. *J Am Coll Cardiol* 1987;10:327–335.

351. Yock PG, Hatle L, Popp RL. Patterns and timing of Doppler detected intracavitary and aortic flow in hypertrophic cardiomyopathy. *J Am Coll Cardiol* 1986;8:1047–1058.

352. Boughner DR, Schuld RL, Persaud JA. Hypertrophic obstructive cardiomyopathy assessment by echocardiographic and Doppler ultrasound techniques. *Br Heart J* 1975;37:917–23.

353. Maron HJ, Gottdiener JS, Arce J, Rosing DR, Wesley YE, Epstein SE. Dynamic subaortic obstruction in hypertrophic cardiomyopathy: analysis by pulsed Doppler echocardiography. *J Am Coll Cardiol* 1985;6:1–15.

354. Gardin JM, Dabestani A, Glasgow GA, Butman S, Burn CS, Henry WL. Echocardiographic and Doppler flow observations in obstructed and nonobstructed hypertrophic cardiomyopathy. *Am J Cardiol* 1985;56:614–621.

355. Pasipoularides A. Clinical assessment of ventricular ejection dynamics with and without outflow obstruction. *J Am Coll Cardiol* 1990;15:859–882.

356. Rakowski H, Sasson Z, Wigle ED. Echocardiographic and Doppler assessment of hypertrophic cardiomyopathy. *J Am Soc Echocardiogr* 1988;1:31–47.

357. Panza JA, Petrone RK, Fananapazir L, Maron BJ. Utility of continuous wave Doppler echocardiography in the noninvasive assessment of left ventricular outflow tract pressure gradient in patients with hypertrophic cardiomyopathy. *J Am Coll Cardiol* 1992;19:91–99.

358. Sherrid MV, Chu CK, Delia E, Mogtader A, Dwyer EM. An echocardiographic study of the fluid mechanics of obstruction in hypertrophic cardiomyopathy. *J Am Coll Cardiol* 1993;22:816–825.

359. Bryg RJ, Pearson AC, Williams GA, Labovitz AJ. Left ventricular systolic and diastolic flow abnormalities determined by Doppler echocardiography in obstructive hypertrophic cardiomyopathy. *Am J Cardiol* 1987;59:925–931.

360. Barbier P, Bartorelli AL. Doppler evidence of abnormal intracavitary systolic and diastolic flow in hypertrophic cardiomyopathy with midventricular obstruction. *Am Heart J* 1993;126:483–487.

361. Joyner CR, Harrison FS, Gruber IW. Diagnosis of hypertrophic subaortic stenosis with a Doppler velocity flow detector. *Ann Intern Med* 1971;74:692–696.

362. Hoit BD, Penonen E, Dalton N, Sahn DJ. Doppler color flow mapping studies of jet formation and spatial orientation in obstructive hypertrophic cardiomyopathy. *Am Heart J* 1989;117:1119–1126.

363. Hatle L. Noninvasive assessment and differentiation of left ventricular outflow obstruction with Doppler ultrasound. *Circulation* 1981;64:381–387.

364. Valdes-Cruz LM, Jones M, Scagnelli S, Sahn DJ, Tomizuka FM, Pierce JE. Prediction of gradients in fibrous subaortic stenosis by continuous wave two-dimensional Doppler echocardiography: animal studies. *J Am Coll Cardiol* 1985;5:1363–1367.

365. Frommelt MA, Snider AR, Bove EL, Lupinetti FM. Echocardiographic assessment of subvalvular aortic stenosis before and after operation. *J Am Coll Cardiol* 1992;19:1018–1023.

366. Reeder GS, Danielson GK, Seward JB, Driscoll DJ, Tajik AJ. Fixed subaortic stenosis in atrioventricular canal defect: a Doppler echocardiographic study. *J Am Coll Cardiol* 1992;20:386–394.

367. Oliveira Lima C, Sahn DJ, Valdes-Cruz LM, et al. Prediction of the severity of left ventricular outflow tract obstruction by quantitative two-dimensional echocardiographic Doppler studies. *Circulation* 1983;68:348–354.

368. Schwammenthal E, Block M, Schwartzkopff B, et al. Prediction of the site and severity of obstruction in hypertrophic cardiomyopathy by color flow mapping and continuous wave Doppler echocardiography. *J Am Coll Cardiol* 1992;20:964–972.

369. Houston A, Simpson IA, Sheldon CD, Doig WB, Coleman EN. Doppler ultrasound in the estimation of the severity of pulmonary infundibular stenosis in infants and children. *Br Heart J* 1986;55:381–384.

370. Fyfe DA, Currie PJ, Seward JB, et al. Continuous wave Doppler determination of the pressure gradient across pulmonary artery bands: hemodynamic correlation in 20 patients. *Mayo Clin Proc* 1984;59:744–750.

371. Valdes-Cruz LM, Horowitz S, Sahn DJ, Larson D, Oliveira Lima C, Messel E. Validation of a Doppler echocardiographic method for calculating severity of discrete stenotic obstruction in a canine preparation with a pulmonary artery band. *Circulation* 1984;69:1177–1181.

372. Chatelain P, Oberhansli I, Friedli B. Physiologic pulmonary branch stenosis in newborns: two-dimensional echocardiographic and Doppler characteristics and follow up. *Eur J Pediatr* 1993;152:559–563.

373. Rodriguez RJ, Riggs TW. Physiologic peripheral pulmonic stenosis. *Am J Cardiol* 1990;66:1478–1481.

374. Guenthard J, Wyler F. Doppler echocardiography during exercise to predict residual narrowing of the aorta after coarctation resection. *Pediatr Cardiol* 1996;17:370–374.

375. Teien DE, Wendel H, Bjornebrink J, Ekelund L. Evaluation of anatomical obstruction by Doppler echocardiography and mag-netic resonance imaging in patients with coarctation of the aorta. *Br Heart J* 1993;69:352–355.

376. Ramaciotti C, Chin AJ. Noninvasive diagnosis of coarctation of the aorta in the presence of a patent ductus arteriosus. *Am Heart J* 1993;125:179–185.

377. Chan KC, Dickinson DF, Wharton GA, Gibbs JL. Continuous wave Doppler echocardiography after surgical repair of coarctation of the aorta. *Br Heart J* 1992;68:192–194.

378. Robinson PJ, Wyse RK, Deanfield JE, Franklin R, Macartney FJ. Continuous wave Doppler velocimetry as an adjunct to cross sectional echocardiography in the diagnosis of critical left heart obstruction in neonates. *Br Heart J* 1984;52:552–556.

379. Wyse RKH, Robinson PJ, Deanfield JE, Tunstall Pedoe DS, Macartney FJ. Use of continuous wave Doppler ultrasound velocimetry to assess the severity of coarctation of the aorta by measurement of aortic flow velocities. *Br Heart J* 1984;52:278–283.

380. Scott PJ, Wharton GA, Gibbs JL. Failure of Doppler ultrasound to detect coarctation of the aorta. *Int J Cardiol* 1990;28:379–381.

381. Carvalho JS, Redington AN, Shinebourne EA, Rigby ML, Gibson D. Continuous wave Doppler echocardiography and coarctation of the aorta: gradients and flow patterns in the assessment of severity. *Br Heart J* 1990;64:133–137.

382. Aldousany AW, DiSessa TG, Alpert BS, Birnbaum SE, Willey ES. Significance of the Doppler-derived gradient across a residual aortic coarctation. *Pediatr Cardiol* 1990;11:8–14.

383. Wilson N, Sutherland GR, Gibbs JL, Dickinson DF, Keeton BR. Limitations of Doppler ultrasound in the diagnosis of neonatal coarctation of the aorta. *Int J Cardiol* 1989;23:87–89.

384. Rao PS, Carey P. Doppler ultrasound in the prediction of pressure gradients across aortic coarctation. *Am Heart J* 1989;118:299–307.

385. Simpson IA, Sahn DJ, Valdes Cruz LM, Chung KJ, Sherman FS, Swensson RE. Color Doppler flow mapping in patients with coarctation of the aorta: new observations and improved evaluation with color flow diameter and proximal acceleration as predictors of severity. *Circulation* 1988;77:736–744.

386. Glaser J, Balkin JA. Doppler examination of aortic coarctation [Letter]. *Am Heart J* 1988;116:1659–1660.

387. George B, DiSessa TG, Williams R, Friedman WF, Laks H. Coarctation repair without cardiac catheterization in infants. *Am Heart J* 1987;114:1421–1425.

388. Houston AB, Simpson IA, Pollock JC, Jamieson MP, Doig WB, Coleman EN. Doppler ultrasound in the assessment of severity of coarctation of the aorta and interruption of the aortic arch. *Br Heart J* 1987;57:38–43.

389. Olsson B, Bjorkhem GE, Lundstrom NR. Diagnostic accuracy of two-dimensional echocardiography combined with Doppler echocardiography in neonates and infants with cardiac symptoms. *Acta Paediatr Scand* 1986;329[Suppl].111–113.

390. Hoadley SD, Duster MC, Miller JF, Murgo JP. Pulsed Doppler study of a case of coarctation of the aorta: demonstration of a continuous Doppler frequency shift. *Pediatr Cardiol* 1986;6:275–277.

391. Marx GR, Allen HD. Accuracy and pitfalls of Doppler evaluation of the pressure gradient in aortic coarctation. *J Am Coll Cardiol* 1986;7:1379–1385.

392. Sanders SP, MacPherson D, Yeager SB. Temporal flow velocity profile in the descending aorta in coarctation. *J Am Coll Cardiol* 1986;7:603–609.

393. Shaddy RE, Snider AR, Silverman NH, Lutin W. Pulsed Doppler findings in patients with coarctation of the aorta. *Circulation* 1986;73:82–88.

394. Gibbs JL. Ultrasound and coarctation of the aorta [Editorial]. *Br Heart J* 1990;64:109–110.

395. Berger M, Haimowitz A, Van Tosh A, Berdoff RL, Goldberg E. Quantitative assessment of pulmonary hypertension in patient with tricuspid regurgitation using continuous wave Doppler ultrasound. *J Am Coll Cardiol* 1985;6:359–365.

396. Yock PG, Popp RL. Noninvasive estimation of right ventricular systolic pressure by Doppler ultrasound in patients with tricuspid regurgitation. *Circulation* 1984;70:657–662.

397. Currie PJ, Seward JB, Chan K-L, et al. Continuous wave Doppler determination of right ventricular pressure: a simultaneous Doppler

catheterization study in 127 patients. *J Am Coll Cardiol* 1985;6: 750–756.

398. Chan KL, Currie PJ, Seward JB, Hagler DJ, Mair DD, Tajik AJ. Comparison of three Doppler ultrasound methods in the prediction of pulmonary artery pressure. *J Am Coll Cardiol* 1987;9:549–554.

399. Reller MD, Rice MJ, McDonald RW. Tricuspid regurgitation in newborn infants with respiratory distress: echo Doppler study. *J Pediatr* 1987;110:760–764.

400. Skjaerpe T, Hatle L. Noninvasive estimation of systolic pressure in the right ventricle in patients with tricuspid regurgitation. *Eur Heart J* 1986;7:704–710.

401. Skinner JR, Boys RJ, Heads A, Hey EN, Hunter S. Estimation of pulmonary artery pressure in the newborn: study of the repeatability of four Doppler echocardiographic techniques. *Pediatr Cardiol* 1996;17:360–369.

402. Simonson J, Schiller NZB. Sonospirometry: a new method for noninvasive estimation of mean right atrial pressure based on the two-dimensional echographic measurement of the inferior vena cava during measured inspiration. *J Am Coll Cardiol* 1988;11: 557–564.

403. Kircher BJ, Himelman RB, Schiller NB. Noninvasive estimation of right atrial pressure from the inspiratory collapse of the inferior vena cava. *Am J Cardiol* 1990;66:493–496.

404. Goldberg SJ. Range gated ultrasound detection of contrast echographic microbubbles for cardiac and great vessel flow patterns. *Am Heart J* 1981;101:793–796.

405. Waggoner AD, Barzilai B, Perez JE. Saline contrast enhancement of tricuspid regurgitant jets detected by Doppler color flow mapping. *Am J Cardiol* 1990;65:1368–1371.

406. Beppu S, Kazuaki T, Shimizu T, et al. Contrast enhancement of Doppler signals by sonicated albumin for estimating right ventricular pressure. *Am J Cardiol* 1991;67:1148–1150.

407. Torres F, Tye T, Gibbons R, Puryear J, Popp RL. Echocardiographic contrast increases the yield for right ventricular pressure measurement by Doppler echocardiography. *J Am Soc Echocardiogr* 1989;2:419–424.

408. Himmelman RB, Stulbarg MS, Lee E, Kuecherer HF, Schiller NB. Noninvasive evaluation of pulmonary artery systolic pressures during dynamic exercise by saline-enhanced Doppler echocardiography. *Am Heart J* 1990;119:685–688.

409. Beard JT, Byrd BF III. Saline contrast enhancement of trivial Doppler tricuspid regurgitation signals for estimating pulmonary artery pressure. *Am J Cardiol* 1988;62:486–488.

410. Hamer HPM, Takens BL, Posma JL, Lie KI. Noninvasive measurement of right ventricular systolic pressure by combined color-coded and continuous wave Doppler ultrasound. *Am J Cardiol* 1988;61:668–671.

411. Gorscan J, Snow FR, Paulsen W, Nixon JV. Noninvasive estimation of left atrial pressure in patients with congestive heart failure and mitral regurgitation by Doppler echocardiography. *Am Heart J* 1991;121:858–863.

412. Nishimura RA, Tajik AJ. Determination of left sided pressure gradients by utilizing Doppler aortic and mitral regurgitant signals. *J Am Coll Cardiol* 1988;11:317–321.

413. Masuyama T, Kodama K, Kitabatake A, Sato H, Nanto S, Inoue M. Continuous-wave Doppler echocardiographic detection of pulmonary regurgitation and its application to noninvasive estimation of pulmonary artery pressure. *Circulation* 1986;74:484–492.

414. Cujec B, David T, Wilansky S, Pollick C. Colour flow imaging in severe mitral and aortic regurgitation. *Can J Cardiol* 1988;4: 341–346.

415. Helmcke R, Nanda NC, Hsiung MC, et al. Color Doppler assessment of mitral regurgitation with orthogonal planes. *Circulation* 1987;75:175–183.

416. Spain MG, Smith MD, Grayburn PA, Harlamert EA, DeMaria AN. Quantitative assessment of mitral regurgitation by Doppler color flow imaging: angiographic and hemodynamic correlations. *J Am Coll Cardiol* 1989;13:585–590.

417. Galassi AR, Nihoyannopoulos P, Pupita G, Odawara H, Crea F, McKenna WJ. Assessment of colour flow imaging in the grading of valvular regurgitation. *Eur Heart J* 1990;11:1101–1108.

418. Castello R, Lenzen P, Aguirre F, Labovitz AJ. Quantitation of mitral regurgitation by transesophageal echocardiography with Doppler color flow mapping: correlation with cardiac catheterization. *J Am Coll Cardiol* 1992;19:1516–1521.

419. Utsunomiya T, Patel D, Doshi R, Quan M, Gardin JM. Can signal intensity of the continuous wave Doppler regurgitant jet estimate severity of mitral regurgitation? *Am Heart J* 1992;123:166–171.

420. Wu YT, Chang AC, Chin AJ. Semiquantitative assessment of mitral regurgitation by Doppler color flow imaging in patients aged <20 years. *Am J Cardiol* 1993;71:727–732.

421. Pieper EP, Hellemans IM, Hamer HP, et al. Value of systolic pulmonary venous flow reversal and color Doppler jet measurements assessed with transesophageal echocardiography in recognizing severe pure mitral regurgitation. *Am J Cardiol* 1996;78: 444–450.

422. Enriquez-Sarano M, Tajik AJ, Bailey KR, Seward JB. Color flow imaging compared with quantitative Doppler assessment of severity of mitral regurgitation: influence of eccentricity of jet and mechanism of regurgitation. *J Am Coll Cardiol* 1993;21:1211–1219.

423. Grayburn PA, Pryor SL, Levine BD, Klein MN, Taylor AL. Day to day variability of Doppler color flow jets in mitral regurgitation. *J Am Coll Cardiol* 1989;14:936–940.

424. Mizushige K, Shiota T, Paik J, et al. Effects of pulmonary venous flow direction on mitral regurgitation jet area as imaged by color Doppler flow mapping. *Circulation* 1995;91:1834–1839.

425. Kamp O, Huitink H, van Eenige MJ, Visser CA, Roos JP. Value of pulmonary venous flow characteristics in the assessment of severity of native mitral valve regurgitation: an angiographic correlated study. *J Am Soc Echocardiogr* 1992;5:239–246.

426. Castello R, Pearson AC, Lensen P, Labovitz AJ. Effect of mitral regurgitation on pulmonary venous velocities derived from transesophageal echocardiography color-guided pulsed Doppler imaging. *J Am Coll Cardiol* 1991;17:1499–1506.

427. Klein AL, Obarski TP, Stewart WJ, et al. Transesophageal Doppler echocardiography of pulmonary venous flow: a new marker of mitral regurgitation severity. *J Am Coll Cardiol* 1991;18:518–526.

428. Teien DE, Jones M, Shiota T, Yamada I, Sahn DJ. Doppler evaluation of severity of mitral regurgitation: relation to pulmonary venous blood flow patterns in an animal study. *J Am Coll Cardiol* 1995;25:264–268.

429. Klein AL, Stewart WJ, Bartlett J, et al. Effects of mitral regurgitation on pulmonary venous flow and left atrial pressure: an intraoperative transesophageal echocardiographic study. *J Am Coll Cardiol* 1992;20:1345–1352.

430. Klein AL, Bailey AS, Cohen GI, et al. Importance of sampling both pulmonary veins in grading mitral regurgitation by transesophageal echocardiography. *J Am Soc Echocardiogr* 1993;6:115–123.

431. Passafini A, Shiota T, Depp M, et al. Factors influencing pulmonary venous flow velocity patterns in mitral regurgitation: an in vitro study. *J Am Coll Cardiol* 1995;26:1333–1339.

432. Ascah KJ, Stewart WJ, Jian L, et al. A Doppler two-dimensional echocardiographic method for quantitation of mitral regurgitation. *Circulation* 1985;72:377–383.

433. Blumlein S, Bouchard A, Schiller NB, et al. Quantitation of mitral regurgitation by Doppler echocardiography. *Circulation* 1986;74: 306–314.

434. Enriquez-Sarano M, Bailey KR, Seward JB, Tajik AJ, Krohn MJ, Mays JM. Quantitative Doppler assessment of valvular regurgitation. *Circulation* 1993;87:841–848.

435. Zhang Y, Ihlen H, Myhre E, Levorstad K, Nitter-Hauge S. Measurement of mitral regurgitation by Doppler echocardiography. *Br Heart J* 1985;54:384–391.

436. Schwammenthal E, Chen C, Benning F, Block M, Breithardt G, Levine R. Dynamics of mitral regurgitant flow and orifice area. *Circulation* 1994;90:307–322.

437. Zhang J, Jones M, Shandas R, et al. Accuracy of flow convergence estimates of mitral regurgitant flow rates obtained by use of multiple color flow Doppler M-mode aliasing boundaries: an experimental animal study. *Am Heart J* 1993;125:449–458.

438. Shiota T, Jones M, Teien DE, et al. Dynamic change in mitral regurgitant orifice area: comparison of color Doppler echocardiographic and electromagnetic flowmeter-based methods in a chronic animal model. *J Am Coll Cardiol* 1995;26:528–536.

439. Chen C, Koschyk D, Brockhoff C, et al. Noninvasive estimation

of regurgitant flow rate and volume in patients with mitral regurgitation by Doppler color mapping of accelerating flow field. *J Am Coll Cardiol* 1993;21:374–383.

440. Xie G-Y, Berk MR, Hixson CS, Smith AC, DeMaria AN, Smith MD. Quantification of mitral regurgitant volume by the color Doppler proximal isovelocity surface area method: a clinical study. *J Am Soc Echocardiogr* 1995;8:48–54.

441. Rivera JM, Vandervoort PM, Thoreau DH, Levine RA, Weyman AE, Thomas JD. Quantification of mitral regurgitation with the proximal flow convergence method: a clinical study. *Am Heart J* 1992;124:1289–1296.

442. Grossman G, Giesler M, Schmidt A, et al. Quantification of mitral regurgitation—comparison of the proximal convergence method and the jet area method. *Clin Cardiol* 1995;18:512–518.

443. Enriquez-Sarano M, Sinak LJ, Tajik J, Bailey KR, Seward JB. Changes in effective regurgitant orifice throughout systole in patients with mitral valve prolapse. *Circulation* 1995;92:2951–2958.

444. Bargiggia GS, Tronconi L, Sahn DJ, et al. A new method for quantitation of mitral regurgitation based on color flow Doppler imaging of flow convergence proximal to regurgitant orifice. *Circulation* 1991;84:1481–1489.

445. Aotsuka H, Tobita K, Hamada H, et al. Validation of the proximal isovelocity surface area method for assessing mitral regurgitation in children. *Pediatr Cardiol* 1996;17:351–359.

446. Shiota T, Jones M, Teien DE, et al. Evaluation of mitral regurgitation using a digitally determined color Doppler flow convergence centerline acceleration method. Studies in an animal model with quantified mitral regurgitation. *Circulation* 1994;89:2879–2887.

447. Rivera JM, Vandervoort PM, Vazquez de Prada JA, et al. Which physical factors determine tricuspid regurgitation jet area in the clinical setting? *Am J Cardiol* 1993;72:1305–1309.

448. Rivera JM, Vandervoort PM, Mele D, et al. Quantification of tricuspid regurgitation by means of the proximal flow convergence method: a clinical study. *Am Heart J* 1994;127:1354–1362.

449. Rivera JM, Vandervoort PM, Morris E, Weyman AE, Thomas JD. Effective regurgitant orifice area in tricuspid regurgitation: clinical implementation and follow-up study. *Am Heart J* 1994;128:927–933.

450. Rivera JM, Vandervoort PM, Mele D, Weyman AE, Thomas JD. Value of proximal regurgitant jet size in tricuspid regurgitation. *Am Heart J* 1996;131:742–747.

451. Klein AL, Davison MB, Vonk G, Tajik AJ. Doppler echocardiographic assessment of aortic regurgitation: uses and limitations. *Cleve Clin J Med* 1992;59:359–368.

452. Wilkenshoff UM, Kruck I, Gast D, Schroder R. Validity of continuous-wave Doppler and colour Doppler in the assessment of aortic regurgitation. *Eur Heart J* 1994;15:1227–1234.

453. Boughner DR. Assessment of aortic insufficiency by transcutaneous Doppler ultrasound. *Circulation* 1975;52:874–879.

454. Touche T, Prasquier R, Nitenberg A, DeZuttere D, Gourgon R. Assessment and follow-up of patients with aortic regurgitation by an updated Doppler echocardiographic measurement of the regurgitant fraction in the aortic arch. *Circulation* 1985;72:819–824.

455. Diebold B, Peronneau P, Blanchard D, et al. Non-invasive quantification of aortic regurgitation by Doppler echocardiography. *Br Heart J* 1983;49:167–173.

456. Takenaka K, Dabestani A, Gardin JM, et al. A simple Doppler echocardiographic method for estimating severity of aortic regurgitation. *Am J Cardiol* 1986;57:1340–1343.

457. Hoppeler H, Jenni R, Ritter M, Krayenbuhl HP. Quantification of aortic regurgitation with amplitude-weighted mean flow velocity from continuous wave Doppler spectra. *J Am Coll Cardiol* 1990;15:1305–1309.

458. Masuyama T, Kodama K, Kitabatake A, et al. Noninvasive evaluation of aortic regurgitation by continuous-wave Doppler echocardiography. *Circulation* 1986;73:460–466.

459. Holm S, Eriksson P, Karp K, Osterman G, Teien D. Quantitative assessment of aortic regurgitation by combined two-dimensional, continuous-wave and colour flow Doppler measurements. *J Intern Med* 1992;231:115–121.

460. Tribouilloy C, Shen WF, Slama M, et al. Assessment of severity of aortic regurgitation by M-mode colour Doppler flow imaging. *Eur Heart J* 1991;12:352–356.

461. Dolan MS, Castello R, St. Vrain JA, Aguirre F, Labovitz AJ. Quantitation of aortic regurgitation by Doppler echocardiography: a practical approach. *Am Heart J* 1995;129:1014–1020.

462. Reimold SC, Thomas JD, Lee RT. Relation between Doppler color flow variables and invasively determined jet variables in patients with aortic regurgitation. *J Am Coll Cardiol* 1992;20:1143–1148.

463. Baumgartner H, Kratzer H, Helmreich G, Kuhn P. Quantitation of aortic regurgitation by colour-coded cross-sectional Doppler echocardiography. *Eur Heart J* 1988;9:380–387.

464. Grayburn PA, Handshoe R, Smith MD, Harrison MR, DeMaria AN. Quantitative assessment of the hemodynamic consequences of aortic regurgitation by means of continuous wave Doppler recordings. *J Am Coll Cardiol* 1987;10:135–141.

465. Teague SM, Heinsimer JA, Anderson JL, et al. Quantification of aortic regurgitation utilizing continuous wave Doppler ultrasound. *J Am Coll Cardiol* 1986;8:592–599.

466. Griffin BP, Flachskampf FA, Siu S, Weyman AE, Thomas JD. The effects of regurgitant orifice size, chamber compliance, and systemic vascular resistance on aortic regurgitant velocity slope and pressure half-time. *Am Heart J* 1991;122:1049–1056.

467. Samstad SO, Hegrenaes L, Skjaerpe T, Hatle L. Half-time of the diastolic aortoventricular pressure difference by continuous-wave Doppler ultrasound: a measure of the severity of aortic regurgitation? *Br Heart J* 1989;61:336–343.

468. Vanoverschelde JJ, Taymans-Robert AR, Raphael DA, Cosyns JR. Influence of transmitral filling dynamics on continuous-wave Doppler assessment of aortic regurgitation by half-time methods. *Am J Cardiol* 1989;64:614–619.

469. Kitabatake A, Ito H, Inoue M, et al. A new approach to noninvasive evaluation of aortic regurgitant fraction by two-dimensional Doppler echocardiography. *Circulation* 1985;72:523–529.

470. Xie GY, Berk MR, Smith MD, DeMaria AN. A simplified method for determining regurgitant fraction by Doppler echocardiography in patients with aortic regurgitation. *J Am Coll Cardiol* 1994;24:1041–1045.

471. Zhang Y, Nitter-Hauge S, Ihlen H, Rootwelt K, Mylhe E. Measurement of aortic regurgitation by Doppler echocardiography. *Br Heart J* 1986;55:32–38.

472. Dalal P, Nagv B, Berger M, Hecht S, Hunart P, Sherman W. Assessment of aortic regurgitation by color flow and continuous-wave Doppler echocardiography. *Am J Cardiol* 1996;77:661–663.

473. Shiota T, Jones M, Yamada I, et al. Evaluation of aortic regurgitation with digitally determined color Doppler-imaged flow convergence acceleration: a quantitative study in sheep. *J Am Coll Cardiol* 1996;27:203–210.

474. Shiota T, Jones M, Yamada I, et al. Effective regurgitant orifice area by the color Doppler flow convergence method for evaluating the severity of chronic aortic regurgitation. *Circulation* 1996;93:594–602.

475. Reimold SC, Maier SE, Fleischmann KE, et al. Dynamic nature of the aortic regurgitant orifice area during diastole in patients with chronic aortic regurgitation. *Circulation* 1994;89:2085–2092.

476. Shandas R, Yamata I, Solowiejcyk D, Manduley R, Jones M, Valdes-Cruz LM. A modified flow convergence equation for calculation of aortic regurgitant volume: studies in a quantified animal model. *J Am Coll Cardiol* 1996;27:396A(abst).

477. DeGroff CG, Shandas R, Valdes-Cruz LM. Analysis of a modified flow convergence equation for calculation of aortic regurgitant flow rate: a numerical study. *J Am Coll Cardiol* 1997;29:518A(abst).

478. Lei MH, Chen JJ, Ko YL, Cheng JJ, Kuan P, Lien WP. Reappraisal of quantitative evaluation of pulmonary regurgitation and estimation of pulmonary artery pressure by continuous wave Doppler echocardiography. *Cardiology* 1995;86:249–256.

479. Takao S. Clinical implications of pulmonary regurgitation in healthy individuals: detection by cross-sectional pulsed Doppler echocardiography. *Br Heart J* 1988;59:542–550.

480. Marx GR, Hicks RW, Allen HD, Goldberg SJ. Noninvasive assessment of hemodynamic response to exercise in pulmonary regurgitation after operations to correct pulmonary outflow obstruction. *Am J Cardiol* 1988;61:595–601.

481. Stevenson JG, Kawabori I, Dooley T, Guntheroth WG. Diagnosis

of ventricular septal defect by pulsed Doppler echocardiography. *Circulation* 1978;58:322–326.

482. Stevenson JG, Kawabori I, Stamm SJ, et al. Pulsed Doppler echocardiographic evaluation of ventricular septal defect patches. *Circulation* 1984;70[Suppl]:I38-I46.

483. Magherini A, Azzolina G, Wiechmann V, Fantini F. Pulsed Doppler echocardiography for diagnosis of ventricular septal defects. *Br Heart J* 1980;43:143–147.

484. Ludomirsky A, Huhta JC, Vick GW III, Murphy DJ Jr, Danford DA, Morrow WR. Color Doppler detection of multiple ventricular septal defects. *Circulation* 1986;74:1317–1322.

485. Hornberger LK, Sahn DJ, Krabill KA, et al. Elucidation of the natural history of ventricular septal defects by serial Doppler color flow mapping studies. *J Am Coll Cardiol* 1989;13:1111–1118.

486. Williams RG. Doppler color flow mapping and prediction of ventricular septal defect outcome [Editorial]. *J Am Coll Cardiol* 1989;13:1119–1121.

487. Minagoe S, Tei C, Kisanuki A, et al. Noninvasive pulsed Doppler echocardiographic detection of the direction of shunt flow in patients with atrial septal defect: usefulness of the right parasternal approach. *Circulation* 1985;71:745–753.

488. Ortiz E, Robinson PJ, Deanfield JE, Franklin R, Macartney FJ, Wyse RK. Localisation of ventricular septal defects by simultaneous display of superimposed colour Doppler and cross-sectional echocardiographic images. *Br Heart J* 1985;54:53–60.

489. Gnanapragasam JP, Houston AB, Doig WB, et al. Influence of colour Doppler echocardiography on the ultrasonic assessment of congenital heart disease: a prospective study. *Br Heart J* 1991;66:238–423.

490. Linker DT, Rossvoll O, Chapman JV, Angelsen BA. Sensitivity and speed of colour Doppler flow mapping compared with continuous wave Doppler for the detection of ventricular septal defects. *Br Heart J* 1991;65:201–203.

491. Faletra F, Scarpini S, Moreo A, et al. Color Doppler echocardiographic assessment of atrial septal defect size: correlation with surgical measurements. *J Am Soc Echocardiogr* 1991;4:429–434.

492. Godart F, Rey C, Francart C, Jarrar M, Vaksmann G. Two-dimensional echocardiographic and color Doppler measurements of atrial septal defect, and comparison with the balloon-stretched diameter. *Am J Cardiol* 1993;72:1095–1097.

493. Belkin RN, Pollack BD, Ruggiero ML, Alas LL, Tatini U. Comparison of transesophageal and transthoracic echocardiography with contrast and color flow Doppler in the detection of patent foramen ovale. *Am Heart J* 1994;128:520–525.

494. Hausmann D, Daniel WG, Mugge A, Ziemer G, Pearlman AS. Value of transesophageal color Doppler echocardiography for detection of different types of atrial septal defect in adults. *J Am Soc Echocardiogr* 1992;5:481–488.

495. Mehta RH, Helmcke F, Nanda NC, Hsiung M, Pacifico AD, Hsu TL. Transesophageal Doppler color flow mapping assessment of atrial septal defect. *J Am Coll Cardiol* 1990;16:1010–1016.

496. Sommer RJ, Golinko RJ, Ritter SB. Intracardiac shunting in children with ventricular septal defect: evaluation with Doppler color flow mapping. *J Am Coll Cardiol* 1990;16:1437–1444.

497. Webber SA, Sandor GGS, Patterson MWH. Doppler echocardiographic observations of diastolic trans-septal flow through small ventricular septal defects. *Eur Heart J* 1992;13:642–645.

498. Goldberg SJ. Relation between color Doppler-detected directional flow in a ventricular septal defect and frame rate [Editorial]. *J Am Coll Cardiol* 1990;16:1445.

499. Zeevi B, Keren G, Sherez J, Berant M, Blieden LC, Laniado S. Bidirectional flow in congenital ventricular septal defect: a Doppler echocardiographic study. *Clin Cardiol* 1987;10:143–146.

500. Stojnic B, Pavlovic P, Ponomarev D, Aleksandrov R, Prcovic M. Bidirectional shunt flow across a ventricular septal defect: pulsed Doppler echocardiographic analysis. *Pediatr Cardiol* 1995;16:6–11.

501. Marx GR, Allen HD, Goldberg SJ. Doppler echocardiographic estimation of systolic pulmonary artery pressure in pediatric patients with interventricular communications. *J Am Coll Cardiol* 1985;6:1132–1137.

502. Ge Z, Zhang Y, Kang W, Fan D, An F. Noninvasive evaluation of interventricular pressure gradient across ventricular septal defect:

503. Silbert DR, Brunson SC, Schiff R, Diamant S. Determination of right ventricular pressure in the presence of a ventricular septal defect using continuous wave Doppler ultrasound. *J Am Coll Cardiol* 1986;8:379–384.

504. Murphy DJ Jr, Ludomirsky A, Huhta JC. Continuous-wave Doppler in children with ventricular septal defect: noninvasive estimation of interventricular pressure gradient. *Am J Cardiol* 1986;57:428–432.

505. Otterstad JE, Simonsen S, Vatne K, Myhre E. Doppler echocardiography in adults with isolated ventricular septal defect. *Eur Heart J* 1984;5:332–337.

506. Garg A, Shrivastava S, Radhakrishnan S, Dev V, Saxena A. Doppler assessment of interventricular pressure gradient across isolated ventricular septal defect [Letter]. *Clin Cardiol* 1991;14:787.

507. Houston AB, Lim MK, Doig WB, Reid JM, Coleman EN. Doppler assessment of the interventricular pressure drop in patients with ventricular septal defects. *Br Heart J* 1988;60:50–56.

508. Moises VA, Maciel BC, Hornberger LK, et al. A new method for noninvasive estimation of ventricular septal defect shunt flow by Doppler color flow mapping: imaging of the laminar flow convergence region on the left septal surface. *J Am Coll Cardiol* 1991;18:824–832.

509. Levine RA. Doppler color mapping of the proximal flow convergence region: a new quantitative physiologic tool [Editorial]. *J Am Coll Cardiol* 1991;18:833–836.

510. Rittoo D, Sutherland GR, Shaw TR. Quantification of left-to-right atrial shunting and defect size after balloon mitral commissurotomy using biplane transesophageal echocardiography, color flow Doppler mapping, and the principle of proximal flow convergence. *Circulation* 1993;87:1591–1603.

511. Oki T, Iuchi A, Fukuda N, et al. Assessment of right-to-left shunt flow in atrial septal defect by transesophageal color and pulsed Doppler echocardiography. *J Am Soc Echocardiogr* 1994;7:506–515.

512. Hajduczok ZD, Winniford MD, Kerber RE. Sensitivity of contrast ultrasound in the detection of atrial septal defect with predominant left-to-right shunting. *J Am Soc Echocardiogr* 1992;5:475–480.

513. Lin FC, Fu M, Yeh SJ, Wu D. Doppler atrial shunt flow patterns in patients with secundum atrial septal defect: determinants, limitations, and pitfalls. *J Am Soc Echocardiogr* 1988;1:141–149.

514. Hiraishi S, Agata Y, Saito K, et al. Interatrial shunt flow profiles in newborn infants: a colour flow and pulsed Doppler echocardiographic study. *Br Heart J* 1991;65:41–45.

515. Reller MD, Rice MJ, McDonald RW. Review of studies evaluating ductal patency in the premature infant. *J Pediatr* 1993;122:59–62.

516. Roberson DA, Silverman NH. Color Doppler flow mapping of the patent ductus arteriosus in very low birthweight neonates: echocardiographic and clinical findings. *Pediatr Cardiol* 1994;15:219–224.

517. Shiraishi H, Yanagisawa M. Bidirectional flow through the ductus arteriosus in normal newborns: evaluation by Doppler color flow imaging. *Pediatr Cardiol* 1991;12:201–205.

518. Hiraishi S, Misawa H, Oguchi K, et al. Two-dimensional Doppler echocardiographic assessment of closure of the ductus arteriosus in normal newborn infants. *J Pediatr* 1987;111:755–760.

519. Liao PK, Su WJ, Hung JS. Doppler echocardiographic flow characteristics of isolated patent ductus arteriosus: better delineation by Doppler color flow mapping. *J Am Coll Cardiol* 1988;12:1285–1291.

520. Serwer GA, Armstrong BE, Anderson PW. Noninvasive detection of retrograde descending aortic flow in infants using continuous-wave Doppler ultrasonography. *J Pediatr* 1980;97:394–400.

521. Serwer GA, Armstrong BE, Anderson PA. Continuous wave Doppler ultrasonographic quantitation of patent ductus arteriosus flow. *J Pediatr* 1982;100:297–299.

522. Swensson RE, Valdes-Cruz LM, Sahn DJ, et al. Real-time Doppler color flow mapping for detection of patent ductus arteriosus. *J Am Coll Cardiol* 1986;8:1105–1112.

523. Houston AB, Lim MK, Doig WB, et al. Doppler flow characteristics in the assessment of pulmonary artery pressure in ductus arteriosus. *Br Heart J* 1989;62:284–290.

524. Cloez JL, Isaaz K, Pernot C. Pulsed Doppler flow characteristics of ductus arteriosus in infants with associated congenital anomalies of the heart or great arteries. *Am J Cardiol* 1986;57:845–851.

525. Stevenson JG, Kawabori I, Guntheroth WG. Noninvasive detection of pulmonary hypertension in patent ductus arteriosus by pulsed Doppler echocardiography. *Circulation* 1979;60:355–359.

526. Aziz K, Tasneem H. Evaluation of pulmonary artery pressure by Doppler colour flow mapping in patients with a ductus arteriosus. *Br Heart J* 1990;63:295–299.

527. Hiraishi S, Horiguchi Y, Misawa H, et al. Noninvasive Doppler echocardiographic evaluation of shunt flow dynamics of the ductus arteriosus. *Circulation* 1987;75:1146–1153.

528. Musewe NN, Smallhorn JF, Benson LN, Burrows PE, Freedom RM. Validation of Doppler-derived pulmonary arterial pressure in patients with ductus arteriosus under different hemodynamic states. *Circulation* 1987;76:1081–1091.

529. DeGroff CG, Shandas R, Moises VA, Valdes-Cruz LM. Accuracy of the Bernoulli equation for pressure gradient across Blalock-Taussig shunts: a numerical study. *J Am Soc Echocardiogr* 1998; 11:511(abst).

530. Marx GR, Allen HD, Goldberg SJ. Doppler echocardiographic estimation of systolic pulmonary artery pressure in patients with aortic-pulmonary shunts. *J Am Coll Cardiol* 1986;7:880–885.

531. Ge ZM, Zhang Y, Fan DS, et al. Reliability and accuracy of measurement of transductal gradient by Doppler ultrasound. *Int J Cardiol* 1993;40:35–43.

532. Stevenson JG, Kawabori I, Bailey WW. Noninvasive evaluation of Blalock-Taussig shunts: determination of patency and differentiation from patent ductus arteriosus by Doppler echocardiography. *Am Heart J* 1983;106:1121–1132.

533. Hofbeck M, Singer H, Wild F, Emde J. Color Doppler imaging of modified Blalock-Taussig shunts during infancy. *Pediatr Cardiol* 1994;15:163–166.

534. Horiguchi Y, Hiraishi S, Misawa H, Agata Y, Nakae S. Cross-sectional and Doppler echocardiographic evaluation of aortopulmonary shunts. *Br Heart J* 1992;67:312–315.

535. Allen HD, Sahn DJ, Lange L, Goldberg SJ. Noninvasive assessment of surgical systemic to pulmonary artery shunts by range-gated pulsed Doppler echocardiography. *J Pediatr* 1979;94:395–402.

536. Tacy TA, Whitehead KK, Cape EG. Reconciliation of Doppler predicted and actual pressure gradients in modified Blalock Taussig shunts. *J Am Coll Cardiol* 1996;27:212A(abst).

537. Meijboom EJ, Valdes-Cruz LM, Horowitz S, et al. A two dimensional Doppler echocardiographic method for calculation of pulmonary and systemic blood flow in a canine model with a variable-sized left-to-right extracardiac shunt. *Circulation* 1983; 68:437–445.

538. DiSessa TG, Child JS, Perloff JK, et al. Systemic venous and pulmonary arterial flow patterns after Fontan's procedure for tricuspid atresia or single ventricle. *Circulation* 1984;70:898–902.

539. Hagler DJ, Seward JB, Tajik AJ, Ritter DG. Functional assessment of the Fontan operation: combined M-mode, two-dimensional and Doppler echocardiographic studies. *J Am Coll Cardiol* 1984;4: 756–764.

540. Nakazawa M, Nakanishi T, Okuda H, et al. Dynamics of right heart flow in patients after Fontan procedure. *Circulation* 1984; 69:306–312.

541. Frommelt PC, Snider AR, Meliones JN, Vermilion RP. Doppler assessment of pulmonary artery flow patterns and ventricular function after the Fontan operation. *Am J Cardiol* 1991;68:1211–1215.

542. Qureshi SA, Richheimer R, McKay R, Arnold R. Doppler echocardiographic evaluation of pulmonary artery flow after modified Fontan operation: importance of atrial contraction. *Br Heart J* 1990; 64:272–276.

543. Giannico S, Corno A, Marino B, et al. Total extracardiac right heart bypass. *Circulation* 1992;86[Suppl]:II-110–II-117.

544. Penny DJ, Redington AN. Doppler echocardiographic evaluation of pulmonary blood flow after the Fontan operation: the role of the lungs. *Br Heart J* 1991;66:372–374.

545. Redington AN, Penny D, Shinebourne EA. Pulmonary blood flow after total cavopulmonary shunt. *Br Heart J* 1991;65:213–217.

546. Salzer-Muhar U, Marx M, Ties M, Proll E, Wimmer M. Doppler flow profiles in the right and left pulmonary artery in children with congenital heart disease and a bidirectional cavopulmonary shunt. *Pediatr Cardiol* 1994;15:302–307.

547. Holen J, Simonson S, Froysaker T. An ultrasound Doppler technique for the non-invasive determination of the pressure gradient in the Bjork-Shiley mitral valve. *Circulation* 1979;59:436–442.

548. Ramirez ML, Wong M, Sadler N, Shah PM. Doppler evaluation of 106 bioprosthetic and mechanical aortic valves. *J Am Coll Cardiol* 1985;5:527(abst).

549. Kotler MN, Mintz GS, Panidis IP, Morganroth J, Segal BL, Ross J. Noninvasive evaluation of normal and abnormal prosthetic valve function. *J Am Coll Cardiol* 1983;2:151–173.

550. Sagar KB, Wann LS, Paulsen WHJ, Romhilt DW. Doppler echocardiographic evaluation of Hancock and Bjork-Shiley prosthetic valves. *J Am Coll Cardiol* 1986;7:681–687.

551. Williams GA, Labovitz AJ. Doppler hemodynamic evaluation of prosthetic and bioprosthetic cardiac valves. *Am J Cardiol* 1985; 56:325–332.

552. Panidis IP, Ross J, Mintz GS. Normal and abnormal prosthetic valve function as assessed by Doppler echocardiography. *J Am Coll Cardiol* 1986;8:317–326.

553. Weinstein IR, Marbarger JP, Perez JE. Ultrasonic assessment of the St. Jude prosthetic valve: M-mode, two-dimensional, and Doppler echocardiography. *Circulation* 1983;68:897–905.

554. Martin GR, Galioto FM, Midgley FM. Doppler echocardiographic evaluation of tilting disc prosthetic heart valves in children. *Am J Cardiol* 1989;63:964–968.

555. Reisner SA, Meltzer RS. Normal values of prosthetic valve Doppler echocardiographic parameters: a review. *J Am Soc Echocardiogr* 1988;1:201–210.

556. Vandervoort PM, Greenberg NL, Powell KA, Cosgrove DM, Thomas JD. Pressure recovery in bileaflet heart valve prostheses. Localized high velocities and gradients in central and side orifices with implications for Doppler-catheter gradient relation in aortic and mitral position. *Circulation* 1995;92:3464–3472.

557. Baumgartner H, Khan S, DeRobertis M, Czer L, Maurer G. Discrepancies between Doppler and catheter gradients in aortic prosthetic valves in vitro. A manifestation of localized gradients and pressure recovery. *Circulation* 1990;82:1467–1475.

558. Shandas R, Kwon J. Digital particle image velocimetry (DPIC) measurements of the velocity profiles through bileaflet mechanical valves. *Biomed Sci Instrum* 1996;32:161–167.

559. Shandas R, Kwon J, Little E, et al. Three dimensional echocardiography and flow imaging of prosthetic heart valves. *J Am Coll Cardiol* 1996;27:233A(abst).

560. Chafizadeh ER, Zoghbi WA. Doppler echocardiographic assessment of the St. Jude medical prosthetic valve in the aortic position using the continuity equation. *Circulation* 1991;83:213–223.

561. Rothbart RM, Castriz JL, Harding LV, Russo CD, Teague SM. Determination of aortic valve area by two-dimensional and Doppler echocardiography in patients with normal and stenotic bioprosthetic valves. *J Am Coll Cardiol* 1990;15:817–824.

562. Baumgartner H, Khan SS, DeRobertis M, Czer LS, Maurer G. Doppler assessment of prosthetic valve orifice area. *Circulation* 1992;85:2275–2283.

563. Bitar JN, Lechin ME, Salazar G, Zoghbi WA. Doppler echocardiographic assessment with the continuity equation of St. Jude medical mechanical prostheses in the mitral valve position. *Am J Cardiol* 1995;76:287–293.

564. Solowiejczyk DE, Yamada I, Cape EG, Manduley RA, Gersony WM, Jones M, Valdes-Cruz LM. Simultaneous Doppler and catheter transvalvular pressure gradients across St. Jude bileaflet mitral valve prosthesis: in vivo study in a chronic animal model using pediatric valve sizes. *J Am Soc Echocardiogr* 1998 (in press).

565. Thomas JD, Vandervoort PM, Pu M, et al. Doppler/echocardiographic assessment of native and prosthetic heart valves: recent advances. *J Heart Valve Dis* 1995;4:S59–S63.

566. Jaffe WM, Coverdale HA, Roche AH, Brandt PW, Ormiston JA, Barratt-Boyes BG. Doppler echocardiography in the assessment of the homograft aortic valve. *Am J Cardiol* 1989;63:1466–1470.

567. Meliones JN, Snider AR, Bove EL, et al. Doppler evaluation of homograft valved conduits in children. *Am J Cardiol* 1989;64: 354–358.

CHAPTER 7

Three-dimensional Echocardiography: Technique and Clinical Applications

Kevin Y. Chung

As the field of echocardiography has evolved, the development of three-dimensional (3D) imaging has progressed rapidly as a clinical tool (1–4). The concept of 3D ultrasound imaging was first described by Baum and Greenwood in 1961 (5). Imaging was accomplished by acquiring serial parallel ultrasound images of the human orbit. The first 3D scans of the human heart were obtained in 1974 by Dekker and colleagues (6), who used a mechanical arm to locate spatial motion of the transducer as it moved across the chest. The data were then stored in a 3D computer matrix using the spatial information and physiologic gating. Recording of the 3D form and structure of the mitral valve was first reported by Levine and associates in 1989 (1). Since these early efforts, advances in acquisition, image processing, and display have greatly facilitated the use of 3D ultrasound imaging in the clinical setting.

Although two-dimensional (2D) echocardiography has greatly enhanced the ability to visualize the functioning heart, 3D interpretative mental skills are necessary to compile the 2D slices into a "mental picture" of the complex 3D anatomy, particularly in congenital heart disease. The fourth dimension (4D) is the temporal component, or the ability to show a structure in motion. Three-dimensional echocardiography offers the cardiologist a valuable tool to display and communicate anatomic relationships that may not be evident in 2D. For surgeons and others not specifically trained in echocardiography, it may be easier to understand images in 3D/4D.

TECHNIQUE

There are five major components in 3D echocardiography:

1. Image acquisition: 3D acquisition of a structure of interest

2. Geometric resampling: geometric conversion of the acquired images into a cubic data set
3. Image conditioning: reduction of noise and motion artifacts
4. Three-dimensional visualization: multiplanar and 3D surface reconstructions
5. Three-dimensional quantification: segmentation for volume or mass quantification

This chapter provides a detailed description of all the major components that relate to 3D echocardiography.

Acquisition Devices

The selection of the scanning devices is as important as the selection of the transducer. The scanning methods currently available include parallel scan, rotational scan, sweep/fan scan, and free-hand scan.

Parallel Scan

Parallel scanning shifts the attached probe parallel to the image plane. The attached probe can be tilted to a maximum of 30 degrees in each direction from the baseline. The benefit of parallel scanning is that the data set is acquired in an isotropic manner—that is, in slices that are equal in size and distance. Later re-formation of the data set is not necessary. The disadvantage is that a large acoustic window is needed. This acquisition method is recommended in areas of the abdomen, neck, and extremities where large acoustic windows are available (Fig. 7-1).

Rotational Scan

The rotational scanner rotates the attached probe around the center pivot point of the ultrasound scan plane.

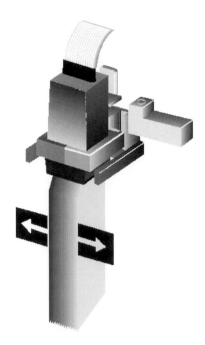

FIG. 7-1. Diagram of the TomTec parallel device (*TomTec Imaging Systems GMBH, Munich, Germany*) showing the direction of the ultrasound image plane.

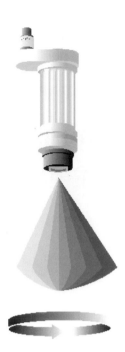

FIG. 7-2. Diagram of the transthoracic rotational device showing the rotation of the ultrasound plane.

The advantage of this method is that the acoustic window is only as big as the rotated diameter of the probe. Disadvantages are the nonisotropic acquisition and the necessity to complete 180 degrees of rotation to obtain a 3D data set. Therefore, any effort to improve the spatial or temporal resolution results in an increased acquisition time that cannot be compensated for through a smaller volume. In the future, integrated rotational probes, such as the multiplane transesophageal probes, will become more common for transthoracic imaging (Figs. 7-2, 7-3).

Sweep/Fan Scan

The sweep or fanlike scanner rotates the probe around an axis parallel to the ''x-axis'' of the image. The distance between this axis (pivot point) and the transducer tip determines the shape and size of the acoustic window. This method has the benefits of both the parallel and sweep devices. Although the acquisition is not parallel, less reformation is involved in this method because the images are close to parallel, unlike those obtained with the rotational scan. As in 2D ultrasound imaging, the resolution is decreased with increased depth. Thus, unnecessary oversampling in the far field is avoided. Nonetheless, it allows the user to reduce the scan range, which can increase the resolution without increasing the acquisition time. This feature is helpful in all cases in which high resolution is important. Also, the field of acquisition can be much broader in the far field, so the greater the depth, the greater the field of acquisition. This allows more data

or structure to be acquired in one acquisition; in contrast, the parallel device limits the width of the field and is not depth-dependent. Integrated sweep probes are available for general imaging and in the future should be available for cardiac use (Fig. 7-4).

Free-Hand Scanning Device

The free-hand scanning device uses a 3D position sensor device (e.g., an electromagnetic sensor that has three perpendicular coils for sending and receiving electromagnetic waves) that is attached to the ultrasound transducer, and for each acquired image the translational and rotational parameters are stored. The limitation with this acquisition technique is that electrocardiographic and respiration time intervals must be saved with the image to demonstrate temporal resolution. Gating with the free-hand technique has not been developed. Until electrocar-

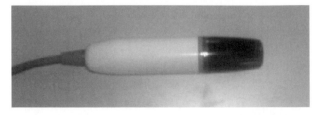

FIG. 7-3. Diagram of the TomTec integrated transthoracic probe (*TomTec Imaging Systems GMBH, Munich, Germany*).

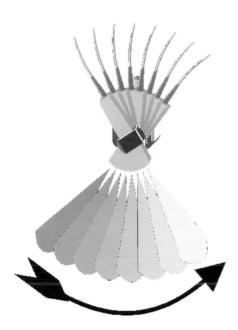

FIG. 7-4. Diagram showing the sweep/fanlike device with the sweeping of the ultrasound plane.

diographic and respiratory gating problems are solved, this technique cannot be used for acquiring images of the heart *in vivo*. The greatest potential for success of this device is in the general imaging arena, and it may one day make all other devices obsolete. In the future, this device will probably be integrated into transducers and ultrasound systems (Fig. 7-5).

Image Acquisition

Preparation of the Patient

The patient should be in a comfortable position and ideally should cooperate to slow or increase heart rate and to minimize movement, as patient movement during acquisition causes motion artifacts. If the patient is unable to cooperate, sedation may be necessary because the acquisition time can vary from 2 to 10 minutes.

Two-dimensional Image and Selection of Acoustic Window

The next step is to determine which cardiac structures will be displayed in 3D. Based on this information, the best possible acoustic window and most effective transducer must be selected.

Respiration and Electrocardiographic Gating

The setting of electrocardiographic and respiratory gating requires careful observation of the patient before ac-

quisition. A statistical trend of the patient's electrocardiographic and respiratory cycle must be estimated to set the gating limits for the acquisition. To determine these statistical values, the patient should be breathing normally, and adequate time should be allowed for the heart rate to stabilize.

Echocardiogram

Limits of the heart rate gating are set based on the RR interval. Although the difference between the upper and lower limits should not exceed 20%, in the presence of any rhythm disturbance the limits can be exceeded to allow for an acceptable acquisition time.

Respiration

Three methods are used to measure the respiratory cycle.

Chest Impedance Method. The impedance between two electrodes, mounted on the right and left sides of the chest, is measured. During inspiration, impedance increases, and in expiration, it decreases. Although this method of display shows no absolute respiratory position, it is effective under most circumstances. This is the respiratory monitoring method most commonly used.

Nasal Thermister Method. The nasal thermister measures the temperature change inside the nose or ventilator tubing. In inspiration, temperature decreases, and during expiration, it increases. The advantage of this method is its ease of use; also, there is no electric contact with the patient. A disadvantage is that it cannot be used in patients who cannot breathe through the nose.

Diaphragm Tension Method (Air Pressure). This relatively new method combines the advantages of both systems. A small "pair of bellows" is fixed with tape to the skin at the level of the diaphragm, where it measures the

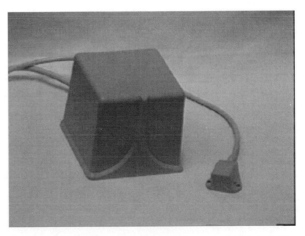

FIG. 7-5. Transmitter and position sensor displayed. Flock-of-birds technology.

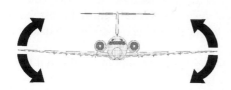

FIG. 7-6. Diagram illustrating alpha rotation of an airplane.

tension created through the changes in the chest circumference. Like the nasal thermister, this method does not require electric contact with the patient.

Image Processing

Calibration

Calibration of the acquired data is necessary if the video data have been acquired from an analog signal and digitized; however, if the data have been acquired digitally, no calibration is necessary. Calibration must be accomplished before any image processing can occur.

Geometric Resampling

The data are stored digitally. The algorithm used to review the data set requires a cartesian coordinate system in which all volume elements (voxels) are equal in size and distance; therefore, digital re-formation into cartesian coordinates is necessary. Gaps in the acquired volume must also be filled by means of interpolation algorithms. Once the raw data set has been reformatted, it can be stored for later review.

Image Conditioning

In the image-conditioning step, 3D/4D filters are applied to reduce noise and motion artifacts, as ultrasound images are not homogenous. Various filters can be applied, such as mean value, sigma, anisotropic diffusion, and median filters. Detailed discussion of these is beyond the scope of this chapter.

Three-dimensional Visualization of Volumetric Data

Three-dimensional data can be visualized in either of two ways: as a 2D multiplanar reconstructed cut plane (otherwise known as a reconstructed 2D image), or as a 3D surface reconstruction.

Multiplanar Reconstruction (Reconstructed Two-dimensional Image)

Multiplanar reconstruction allows the user to select any desired or imagined cut plane in space. The computer computes the desired cut plane from the originally acquired cut planes and displays them as a reconstructed 2D image. It is possible to move and rotate the cut plane in space by rotating around three axes. The three tools to accomplish this are called alpha, beta, and gamma.

Alpha, Beta, and Gamma

Before a 3D/4D image is created or a 3D volumetric measurement started, review of the data set is necessary to define a 2D cut plane. Defining this 2D plane can be difficult, as the only guide is a set of 3D/4D tools on a 2D format (cathode ray tube, CRT).

The anatomic structure of interest is suspended in space without any spatial orientation. This lack of spatial orientation makes review of the 3D/4D data difficult, like flying an airplane without knowing where the ground is. An airplane has tools to manipulate its plane through space; these rotations are called yaw, pitch, and roll. In 3D/4D echocardiography, the rotations are called alpha, beta, and gamma. However, unlike the pilot flying a plane, the user does not know where the ground is located, so a knowledge of cardiac anatomy is essential because the ground or landmark is the heart itself.

The alpha function rotates the plane in space as if the user were to tilt an airplane's wings up or down while facing the nose of the airplane on the ground (Fig. 7-6). The beta function rotates the plane in space as if the user were to tilt the nose or tail of the airplane up or down while facing the plane (Fig. 7-7). The gamma function does not change the orientation of the plane in the space

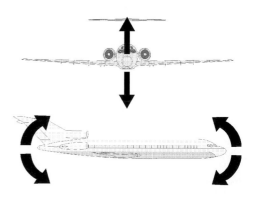

FIG. 7-7. Diagram illustrating beta rotation of an airplane.

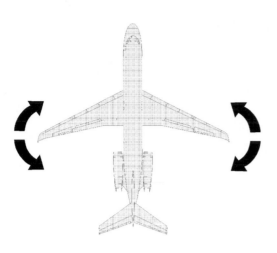

FIG. 7-8. Diagram illustrating gamma rotation of an airplane.

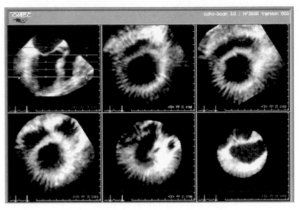

FIG. 7-10. Image representing paraplane mode. The image at the top left is the reference image.

that it occupies; rather, it rotates the plane clockwise or counterclockwise as seen from above (Fig. 7-8).

Modes of Review

The first step is to select the review mode. Several methods have been developed to manipulate a 2D plane in space.

In the *anyplane mode*, the selected cut plane can be rotated around three axes: alpha, beta, and gamma (Fig. 7-9).

In the *paraplane mode*, the same method is used as in the anyplane mode to rotate the plane in space. The difference is that this mode can calculate multiple parallel cut planes at the same time. This mode is extremely helpful when the image is difficult to understand or orientation

has been lost. The parallel images can be used to reestablish structures or orientation (Fig. 7-10).

In the *main plane mode*, the same method is used to rotate the plane in space. Additionally, there are two orthogonal cut planes that are perpendicular to the selected image. All cut planes are perpendicular to one another (Fig. 7-11).

In the *long-/short-axis mode*, an axis is defined along two points in space. All images with an orientation either along or perpendicular to this axis can be viewed. The images along the defined axis (long axis) are rotated around this axis. The images perpendicular to the defined axis (short axis) are parallel to each other (Figs. 7-12, 7-13).

The review mode most useful in congenital heart disease is the paraplane mode. It allows the user to see more of the heart at one time and provides a better view of the anatomy. This is accomplished by giving the user several parallel cut planes side by side, so that if the user cannot understand the image from one cut plane, reference can be made to another cut plane. Once the mode is chosen, the user must then create a start point. An analogy for

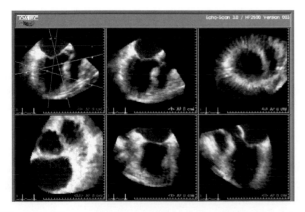

FIG. 7-9. Image representing anyplane mode. The image at the top left is the reference image.

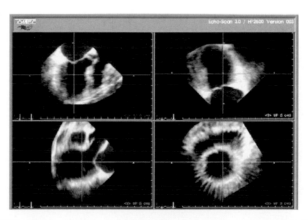

FIG. 7-11. Image representing main plane mode. The image at the top left is the reference image.

the start point is the ground when an airplane is flown; the airplane is the cut plane. The start point can be established by setting the alpha, beta, and gamma to zero. Once the settings are at zero, the user should study the anatomy, viewing the cut planes and their relationship to the reference image.

Selecting a reference image is like selecting a page from a book. Reference images are all parallel to one another in equal distances, just like the paraplane images, the only difference being that the reference image cannot be rotated in space. The purpose of the reference image is to provide the ability to travel to the object of interest by selecting a specific ''reference page.'' Once the user finds the reference page with the object of interest, a pivot point must be anchored near the object of interest. Alpha, beta, and gamma functions rotate off this pivot point. The reference image and the pivot point are probably the most important factors for the proper review of data. Selecting the wrong reference image or improper placement of the pivot point can impede the ability to achieve a desired cut plane in space.

When the alpha, beta, and gamma are to be used, it is recommended that the alpha function be used first. Manipulations with this function can be seen as a cut line on the reference image. In the first step, the user should achieve a view along the short or long axis of the structure. Then, by slight manipulation of the beta angle, the optimal short or long axis can be achieved. Using the beta function can be very confusing, as the cut line on the reference image does not move; therefore, spatial orientation can be easily lost if large manipulations are made with this function. It is useful to remember that the cut plane is perpendicular to the reference image if the beta function is set at zero degrees and is parallel to the reference image if beta is set at 90 degrees. The movements of alpha and beta are always perpendicular to each other. The gamma function should be used last, and only to rotate the plane to a proper spatial orientation for presen-

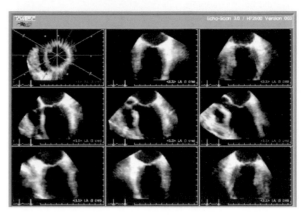

FIG. 7-13. Image representing the long-axis mode. The image at the top left is the reference image.

tation. Gamma does not change the cut plane angle in space; it only rotates it.

After a cut plane is chosen, the direction from which the structure will be viewed in 3D must be selected. For example, the parasternal short axis at the midventricular level can be viewed in the direction of the mitral valve or the left ventricular apex. Also, it is important to note that a plane that looks reversed on 2D is not always reversed in 3D. In the parasternal long axis, the apex is usually to the left; if it is to the right, this may mean that the plane is being viewed from a different direction. As an analogy, if one looks at a person's open right hand from the front, the thumb is to the right, but if one looks at it from the back, the thumb will be to the left.

A good display of the selected structure requires that there be no obstructions in the view or cavity between the chosen plane and the object. For example, a papillary muscle may obstruct the view of the mitral valve from a short-axis cut plane of the left ventricular apex. If speckles, artifacts, noise, or another structure obstructs the view to the object of interest from the chosen cut plane, then segmentation of the obstruction may be necessary to extract it from the data set. (See the section on quantification for details of segmentation.)

Three-dimensional Reconstruction

Visualization of medical image data in 3D has become possible in recent years with the development of advanced computers and image-processing methods. The two methods for 3D reconstruction are surface rendering and volumetric rendering.

The surface of an object can be determined by the *polygon (contour)* method or the *volume element (voxel)* method. In the polygon method, a contour-detection algorithm or manual tracing is used to create a contour-based (wire-frame) 3D model. This method was originally designed for computer-assisted design and manufacturing

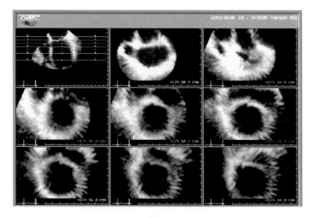

FIG. 7-12. Image representing the short-axis mode. The image at the top left is the reference image.

(CAD/CAM). In the volume element (voxel) method, an algorithm is used to find volumetric elements of one kind (texture). This technology was designed exclusively for medical tomographic data sets. The commonly used technique is called ray tracing, in which the user defines a viewpoint or plane from which the computer sends rays into the data set; the rays terminate when they arrive at the surface. The determination of surface is accomplished by selecting a certain echo density as surface (see below). In volumetric rendering the voxel information is taken into consideration, so that all the information inside the heart is included—the endocardium, myocardium, and epicardium.

The volume element (voxel) method is currently used for 3D reconstruction of 2D echocardiographic images. The following section focuses on this method, although the displaying techniques are similar in the polygon method. Information can be displayed in various forms. To visualize surface boundaries, a method to project information onto a 2D display must be selected. Two methods are available: the central projection method and the parallel projection method. In the central projection method, rays are sent out from one point to determine the surface of an object. Although the display of such reconstruction appears more realistic, the reconstruction can be distorted depending on the distance to the object, as when a fish-eye lens is used in photography. This technique is used to display objects from the inside (angioscopic view). In the parallel projection method, parallel rays are sent out from a plane to determine the surface of an object. This method creates no distortion; therefore, the images are more reliable. Because fewer rays are needed, this method of reconstruction is faster than the central projection method.

To give these projections a realistic 3D appearance, the algorithm applies surface shading. Four types of surface shading are used:

1. Distance shading. Brightness is applied depending on the distance from the object to the viewer. The closer the object is to the surface, the brighter it will appear. Distance shading results in smooth images with very few structural details, as small differences in distance result in only small differences in brightness, making it difficult to display details.

2. Gradient shading. In addition to distance shading, the algorithm applies a synthetic light source that shines from an imaginary point above the viewer. The shadows at the edges (gradient) enhance the visibility of small structures. However, enhancement of small structures also causes enhancement of artifacts.

3. Texture (voxel method only). Texture takes the most echo-dense volume element from the found surface and displays it at its position. With this method, the characteristics of the ultrasound data can be restored.

4. Maximum/minimum (voxel method only). Contrary to the surface-shading methods outlined above, the maximum/minimum method does not detect any surface; rather, the brightest and darkest gray values along each ray sent through the data volume are displayed. The result is a quasitransparent image in which a bright versus a dark structure is represented. The depth perception is rather poor, because no 3D information is available in a single image. The problem is similar to that seen in radiographic angiography, in which biplanar images are used to obtain 3D information.

Three-dimensional Quantification

When an object of complex geometry, such as a fetus, has to be visualized or its volume calculated, basic segmentation, such as is obtained with a cut plane, is not sufficient. In these cases, a more sophisticated segmentation is necessary.

Manual Polygon Segmentation

Manual segmentation is a labor-intensive, "slice-by-slice" method to trace the object of interest. Although relatively simple, it can be extremely time-consuming. In this method, the user must select a cut plane that is a cross section of the structure and select the paraplane mode to establish parallel cut planes. The user must also define the distance between each cut plane, as this will determine the amount of time needed and the accuracy of the quantification.

Automatic Segmentation

The automatic method of contour detection can be applied if the geometry of an object is known. A radial search for the boundary of an object can be performed from a user-defined point. This method is very difficult to apply in ultrasound data sets because the data contain too much noise and artifact.

Gray-level Thresholding (Semiautomatic Segmentation)

This method could be used for automatic segmentation, but because ultrasound is plagued with artifacts and dropouts, it must be combined with some manual segmentation techniques.

Gray-level thresholding is used to separate the object from the background. Gray values above the defined threshold belong to the object, and gray values below the defined threshold belong to the background. This difficult decision can be made somewhat easier by using a fuzzy segmentation. With a fuzzy segmentation, a gray-level window (gray-level range) is used. All voxels with gray values below the lower end of the window belong to the background, and all voxels above the upper end of the range belong to the object. Voxels with gray values within the gray-level range are assigned a certain probability for belonging to background or object.

CLINICAL APPLICATIONS

The potential future clinical applications of 3D echocardiography remain vast. Initial clinical trials indicate that 3D visualization of valves, vessels, and congenital defects and estimates of volume are among the first emerging applications (4,7).

Atrial Septal Defects

The 3D imaging and delineation of the site, size, shape, and dynamic geometry of atrial septal defects (Echo. 7-1) permit defects to be viewed from the right or left atrium as if seen through surgical atriotomies (8,9). These unique *en face* views of the atrial septum allow examination of the septum as a wall and of the defect as a window in the wall. Various unique multiplanar views also allow visualization of the site of pulmonary venous drainage, thus permitting detection of anomalous pulmonary venous return. Coexistent abnormalities such as enlarged chambers, cleft mitral valve, and altered chamber geometry can also be assessed.

This application has evolved to include assessment of the tissue surrounding an atrial septal defect for placement of occluder devices (10). Placement of certain devices, such as the Das-Angel Wings occluder, requires that all four corners be in apposition with the septum on both sides. Although 2D transesophageal and transthoracic im-

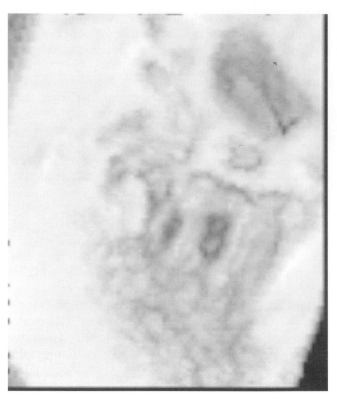

ECHO. 7-2. Three-dimensional reconstruction of two small muscular ventricular septal defects. (*Image courtesy of D. Fyfe, M.D., Ph.D., Egleston Children's Hospital at Emory University and the Children's Heart Center, Atlanta, Georgia.*)

ages are helpful, 3D *en face* views are needed to assess all four corners at once.

Ventricular Septal Defects

The visualization of ventricular septal defects is another emerging application (11,12). *En face* views and multiple projections and angles allow a ventricular septal defect to be visualized from both the left and right ventricular sides. The various locations of defects, such as within the perimembranous, muscular, or infundibular septum or in a doubly committed subarterial position, as well as their size, shape (circular, oval, or irregular), anatomic relationships, and dynamic geometry, can all be defined by 3D echocardiography (Echo. 7-2).

Evaluation of the Aorta

Another promising application of 3D imaging is the delineation of aortic coarctation, dissection, dilation, supravalvular stenosis, and atheromatosis (13) (Echos. 7-3,

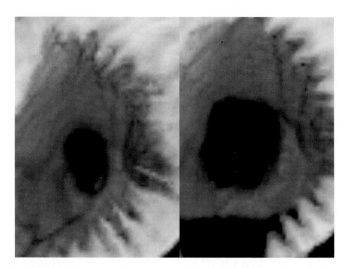

ECHO. 7-1. Three-dimensional reconstruction of an atrial septal defect shown from the right atrium in diastole. (*Image courtesy of H. Wollschlaeger, M.D., and A. Geibel, M.D., University Clinic, Freiburg, Germany.*)

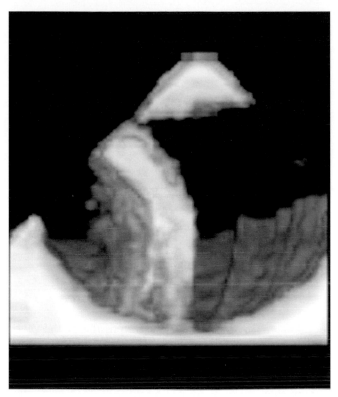

ECHO. 7-3. Three-dimensional reconstruction of an aortic dissection in the transverse arch. (*Image courtesy of I. Krontzon, M.D., New York University Medical Center, New York, New York.*)

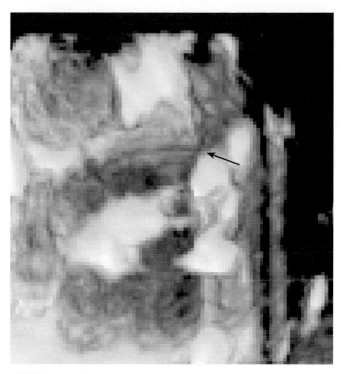

ECHO. 7-4. Three-dimensional reconstruction of an aortic coarctation (*arrow*). (*Image courtesy of F. Emge, M.D., Egleston Children's Hospital at Emory University and the Children's Heart Center, Atlanta, Georgia.*)

7-4). This application is uniquely suited for a rotational scan from the suprasternal notch; an annular array or mechanical transducer is used to facilitate fit in the suprasternal notch. Ideally, an internally rotating transducer or transesophageal probe would work best in pediatric applications.

Visualization of Coronary Arteries with Multiplanar Views

Two-dimensional imaging of the coronary arteries is accurate in children. Nonetheless, several problems are associated with 2D imaging of the coronary arteries because of their inherent 3D shape and motion during the cardiac cycle. Three-dimensional acquisition of the coronary arteries and review of the data set with multiplanar views have proved effective in allowing a greater length of the coronary arteries to be visualized. In a recent study, as much as 2.4 cm of the left anterior descending artery could be seen by means of 3D echocardiography (14). In this adult population, the left main coronary artery could be visualized in 84% of patients studied, the anterior descending branch in 80% of patients, and the circumflex branch in 26% of patients.

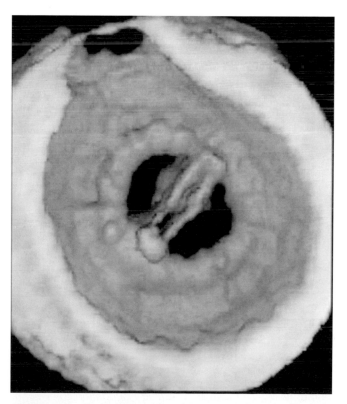

ECHO. 7-5. Three-dimensional reconstruction of a St. Jude prosthesis in the mitral valve position, displayed from the left atrial perspective during diastole, otherwise known as the surgeon's view. (*Image courtesy of the Coral Springs Medical Center, Coral Springs, Florida.*)

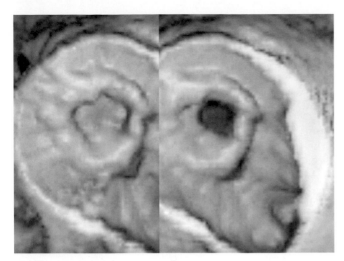

ECHO. 7-6. Three-dimensional reconstruction of a bioprosthetic mitral valve shown from the left atrial perspective in systole **(left)** and diastole **(right)**. (*Image courtesy of Professor Anguissola, M.D., University of Milan, 1st. Chir. Gen. Cardiov, Milan, Italy.*)

Evaluation of Cardiac Valves

The use of 3D echocardiography for the assessment of valvular, subvalvular, and annular morphology of the mitral valve is probably the leading emerging application (15–17). Multiplanar transesophageal technology provides an unobstructed view of the mitral valve from the esophagus through the left atrium, with the mitral valve in the focal zone. With image reconstruction, the left atrium can be "unroofed" so that the mitral valve can be visualized as by a surgeon (18). This "surgeon's view" can also be classified as an *en face* view of the

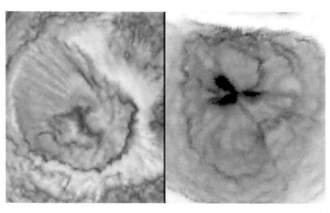

ECHO. 7-7. Left: Three-dimensional reconstruction of a mitral valve prolapse as seen from the left atrium (surgeon's view). (*Image courtesy of J. D. Thomas, M.D., and C. Breburda, M.D., The Cleveland Clinic Foundation, Cleveland, Ohio.*) **Right:** Three-dimensional reconstruction of mitral stenosis, enlarged left atrium, and mitral regurgitation shown from the left atrial perspective. Notice the regurgitant orifice. (*Image courtesy of J. Mathew, M.D., Yale University Medical Center, New Haven, Connecticut.*)

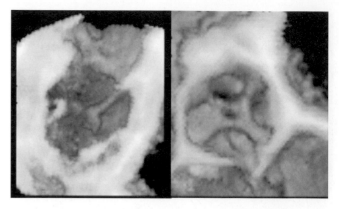

ECHO. 7-8. Left: Three-dimensional reconstruction of a tricuspid valve in systole. (*Image courtesy of I. Krontzon, M.D., New York University Medical Center, New York, New York.*) **Right:** Three-dimensional reconstruction of a quadricuspid tricuspid valve in systole. (*Image courtesy of Dr. Hsu, VGH, Taipei, Taiwan.*)

mitral valve. In cases of mitral valve prosthesis, the valve and perivalvular areas can be assessed without artifact because the shadowing is on the ventricular side or in the far field (Echos. 7-5, 7-6).

Transthoracic imaging can be utilized in children, but *en face* views are usually unobtainable. Nonetheless, reconstructions of the valve from different projections are still valuable in such conditions as mitral valve prolapse, stenosis (Echo 7-7), cleft, and parachute mitral valve.

Three-dimensional reconstruction has also been utilized for the assessment of other cardiac valves, such as the tricuspid and aortic valves; the presence of a normal or abnormal number of cusps can be determined (Echos. 7-8, 7-9), sometimes in association with more complex congenital cardiac malformations (Echo 7-10).

Three-dimensional Volumes

Three-dimensional imaging of ventricular volumes is useful to calculate the ejection fraction (2,19,20). Calcula-

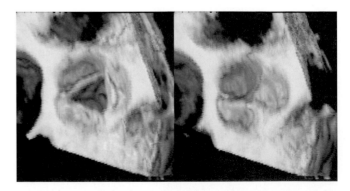

ECHO. 7-9. Three-dimensional reconstruction of an aortic valve in systole **(left)** and diastole **(right)**. (*Image courtesy of TomTec Imaging Systems, GMBH, Munich, Germany*)

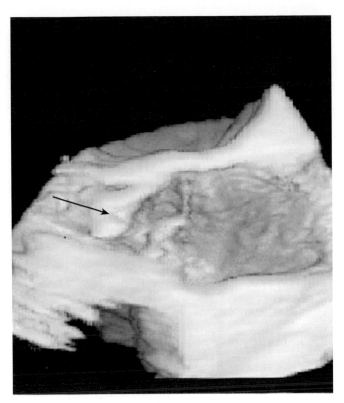

ECHO. 7-10. Three-dimensional reconstruction of a subaortic stenosis (*arrow*). (*Image courtesy of M. Vogel, M.D., Heart Center, Munich, Germany.*)

tion of left ventricular volumes by single or biplanar imaging techniques assumes a specific geometry and involves extrapolation for walls not visualized. Limitations of acoustic access and distortion of the ventricular shape may invalidate these assumptions and lead to errors. Three-dimensional echocardiography virtually eliminates such limitations. Two-dimensional measurement of right ventricular volumes is virtually impossible because of the asymmetric shape of the right ventricle (21,22). In malformations such as univentricular atrioventricular connections, the ventricular shape also precludes geometric assumptions (23). Three-dimensional measurement of ventricular volumes eliminates the need for geometric assumptions and takes into consideration all aspects of shape and geometry.

Various techniques and methods are available to obtain 3D volumes. A manual trace and segmentation is the most accurate and reliable method but is also the most tedious and time-consuming. It is also very difficult to trace the intricate details of the tissue manually, especially of the right ventricular trabeculae. Another method, which overcomes some of the limitations of the manual trace, is the threshold gray-scale tissue-depiction method; this identifies volume by selecting gray-value intensities. The limitation of this technique is that the ultrasound data are not homogenous and contain artifacts.

More simplified methods to measure the 3D volume of

the left ventricle have been developed. One method takes advantage of a number of apical views spanning the left ventricle and fits a surface to the traced endocardial borders by a cubic spline algorithm (24).

Three-dimensional Imaging of Flow Volumes

Three-dimensional imaging of flow volumes has been shown to provide valuable data in the assessment of color Doppler jet geometry and 3D propagation (25–31) (Echo. 7-11). Split or dual jets, flow convergence areas, and jet-wall interactions can be visualized with unique perspectives. Three-dimensional flows and flow orifices of atrial and ventricular septal defects provide a unique descriptor of shunt flow propagation.

Three-dimensional Intravascular Ultrasound

Two-dimensional intravascular ultrasound has proved to be an excellent technology to study the extent, distribution, and therapy of atherosclerotic plaques. It also has proved to be a valuable tool in intracardiac imaging. With

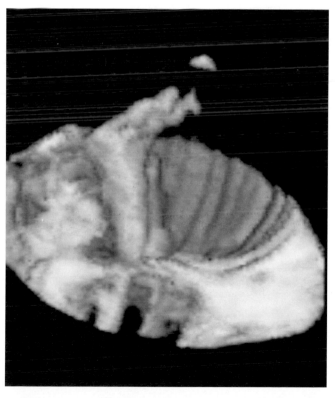

ECHO. 7-11. Three-dimensional reconstruction of a mitral regurgitant jet. (*Image courtesy of Dr. Hsu, VGH, Taipei, Taiwan.*)

the addition of 3D ultrasound (Fig. 7-14), increased diagnostic confidence can be offered to guide therapeutic decisions by providing accurate and reproducible area and volume measurements of the lumen and plaque (32) (Echo. 7-12). Additionally, 3D ultrasound provides unique longitudinal views, such as the "clam shell" view, in which the artery is pried open like a clam shell and the inside displayed, so that a better perception of the true size and extent of the plaque is obtained. In visualization of the inner lining of the vessel, the distensibility and compliance of the vessel wall can be assessed in a gated data set. Although on-line reconstruction is very valuable to guide therapeutic decisions during catheter-based interventions, off-line reconstruction can provide valuable information for studying progression and regression of atherosclerosis or restenosis. This technology also shows great potential for intracardiac reconstruction of vessels, as in stenosis of branch pulmonary arteries and coarctation of the aorta.

The current technology still has many limitations. Nongated acquisition, which is very practical during intervention because it can be accomplished quickly, does not provide accurate 3D displays of structures, and so the accuracy of the data is questionable. The integrity of gated acquisition data is clearly superior, but the increased acquisition and processing time are limiting factors.

Three-dimensional Echocardiography to Assist Electrophysiologic Interventions

The use of 3D echocardiography to guide electrophysiologic interventions for visualizing intracardiac anatomy, ablation catheter location, and pacer and defibrillator wire sites is another promising application (33). The ability to depict various catheter locations and anatomic relationships in one view could potentially reduce procedure time significantly.

Future Advances

The development of dedicated software packages for the various applications described above, integration of

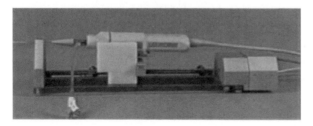

FIG. 7-14. Image of the TomTec intravascular pullback device with catheter handle mounted on the device (*TomTec Imaging Systems GMBH, Munich, Germany*).

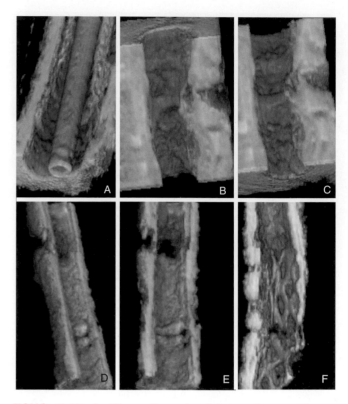

ECHO. 7-12. A: Three-dimensional long-axis reconstruction of a coronary artery tilted upward. Notice the catheter in the middle of the artery. **B:** Three-dimensional long-axis reconstruction of a coronary artery tilted down. Notice the narrowing in the center. **C:** Three-dimensional long-axis reconstruction of the same coronary artery tilted upward. Notice the narrowing in the center. **D:** Three-dimensional long-axis reconstruction of a coronary artery shown at an angle. Notice the two echogenic plaques. **E:** Three-dimensional long-axis reconstruction of the same coronary artery. This image is displayed with a different rotation. Notice the two echogenic plaques. **F:** Three-dimensional long-axis reconstruction of a stent placed inside a coronary artery. (*Images A–C courtesy of Professor J. Roelandt, M.D., Thorax Center, Rotterdam, The Netherlands. Images D–F courtesy of W. Fehske, M.D., University Clinic, Bonn, Germany.*)

acquisition technology into the standard 2D ultrasound system, and faster computation should contribute to ease of clinical use. Other advances, such as the integration of devices into the transducer housing (Fig. 7-3) and the development of spatial locating devices (Fig. 7-5) and transducers with a piezo-electric matrix alignment, will make real-time acquisition of cardiac images possible. Finally, virtual reality techniques should play a role in the visualization and manipulation of images.

If the historical progression of cardiac imaging technologies is any indication of the future, it is likely that once the quality of 3D imaging has been perfected, it will replace 2D imaging to a great extent.

REFERENCES

1. Levine RA, Handschumacher MD, Sanfilippo AJ, et al. Three-dimensional echocardiographic reconstruction of the mitral valve,

with implications for the diagnosis of mitral valve prolapse. *Circulation* 1989;80:589–598.

2. Emge FK, Chung KY, Parks WJ, Mukundan S Jr, Oshinski JN, Pettigrew RI. Three-dimensional echocardiographic measurement of left ventricular volume *in vivo*: validation with magnetic resonance imaging. *Circulation* 1994;90:I-337(abst).

3. Belohlavek M, Foley DA, Gerber TC, Kinter TM, Greenleaf JF, Seward JB. Three- and four-dimensional cardiovascular ultrasound imaging: a new era for echocardiography. *Mayo Clin Proc* 1993; 68:221–240.

4. Feigenbaum H. Evolution of echocardiography. *Circulation* 1996; 93:1321–1327.

5. Baum G, Greenwood I. Orbital lesion localization by three dimensional ultrasonography. *N Y State J Med* 1961;61:4149–4157.

6. Dekker DL, Piziali RL, Dong E Jr. A system for ultrasonically imaging the human heart in three dimensions. *Comput Biomed Res* 1974;7:544–553.

7. Roelandt JRTC, ten Cate FJ, Vletter WB, et al. Ultrasonic dynamic three-dimensional visualization of the heart with a multiplane transesophageal imaging transducer. *J Am Soc Echocardiogr* 1994;7: 217–229.

8. Marx G, Vogel M, Pandian N, et al. Delineation of the site, size, shape and dynamic geometry of atrial septal defects by real-time three-dimensional echocardiography using a tomographic ultrasound approach in in- and out-patients. *Circulation* 1993;88:I-409(abst).

9. Belohlavek M, Foley DA, Gerber TC, Greenleaf JF, Seward JB. Three-dimensional ultrasound imaging of the atrial septum: normal and pathologic anatomy. *J Am Coll Cardiol* 1993;22:1673–1678.

10. Magni G, Hijazi ZM, Marx G, et al. Utility of 3-D echocardiography in patient selection and guidance for atrial septal defect (ASD) closure by the new Das-Angel Wings occluder device. *J Am Coll Cardiol* 1995;27:190A.

11. Vogel M, Pandian N, Marx G, et al. Transthoracic real-time three-dimensional echocardiography in 100 pediatric and adult patients with heart disease: clinical utility of unique new views unavailable in 2-dimensional echocardiography. *Circulation* 1993;88[Suppl]:I-349(abst).

12. Rivera JM, Siu SC, Handschumacher MD, et al. Three-dimensional reconstruction of ventricular septal defects: validation studies and *in vivo* feasibility. *J Am Coll Cardiol* 1994;23:201–208.

13. Sugeng L, Cao Q-L, Delabays A, et al. Delineation of aortic coarctation, dissection and dilation, supravalvular stenosis, and atheromatosis in patients by volume-rendered three-dimensional echocardiography using multiplanar mode of data acquisition in the clinical scenario. *J Am Coll Cardiol* 1995;92:I-534(abst).

14. Hansen TH, Bates JR, Swanson ST, et al. Visualization of the left coronary artery using a transthoracic three-dimensional echocardiographic technique. *Circulation* 1995;92:I-534(abst).

15. Kanojia A, Mittal S, Kasliwal R, et al. Three-dimensional echocardiography is useful in the detailed assessment of valvular, subvalvular and annular morphology in rheumatic mitral valve disease: clinical experience in 130 cases. *J Am Coll Cardiol* 1995;27:296A(abst).

16. Pai RG, Azevedo J, Pandian N, et al. Delineation of the dynamic surgical anatomy of the diseased mitral valve by three-dimensional transesophageal echocardiography. *Circulation* 1993;88:I-349 (abst).

17. Pai RG, Tanimoto M, Jintapakorn W, Azevedo J, Pandian N, Shah PM. Volume rendered three dimensional anatomy of the mitral annulus using transesophageal echocardiography. *Circulation* 1993; 88:I-349(abst).

18. Foster E, Redberg RF, Schiller NB. Unroofing the heart and aorta

using 3-dimensional echocardiography. *Circulation* 1993;88:I-349(abst).

19. Legget ME, Martin RW, Sheehan FH, et al. Three dimensional reconstruction using a new dual axis multiplane transesophageal echo probe: calculation of left ventricular volume. *J Am Coll Cardiol* 1995;27:17A(abst).

20. Siu SC, Rivera JM, Guerrero JL, et al. Three-dimensional echocardiography. *In vivo* validation for left ventricular volume function. *Circulation* 1993;88:1715–1723.

21. Nesser HJ, Tkalec W, Niel J, Masani N, Pandian N. Accurate quantitation of right ventricular size and function by voxel-based 3-dimensional echocardiography in patients with normal and abnormal ventricles (3DE): comparison with magnetic resonance imaging. *J Am Coll Cardiol* 1995;27:149A(abst).

22. Jiang L, Handschumacher MD, Hibberd MG, et al. Three-dimensional echocardiographic reconstruction of right ventricular volume: *in vitro* comparison with two-dimensional methods. *J Am Soc Echocardiogr* 1994;7:150–158.

23. Cao Q-L, Marx G, Sugeng L, et al. Estimation of ventricular volumes, ejection fraction and cardiac output by automated acoustic quantification using transthoracic multiplane echocardiography in single ventricular morphology. *J Am Soc Echocardiogr* 1994;7: S25(abst).

24. Maehle J, Bjoernastad K, Aakhus S, Thorp HG, Angelsen BAJ. Three-dimensional echocardiography for quantitative left ventricular wall motion analysis: a method for reconstruction of endocardial surface and evaluation. *Echocardiography* 1994;11:397–408.

25. Sinclair BG, Teien D, Klas B, Derman R. Three-dimensional reconstruction of constrained flow convergence acceleration fields in an *in vitro* model of mitral valve prolapse. *Circulation* 1995;92:I-797(abst).

26. Shandas R, Kwon J, Little E, et al. Three-dimensional echocardiography and flow imaging of prosthetic valves: *in-vitro* studies. *J Am Coll Cardiol* 1995;27:233A(abst).

27. Shandas R, Kwon J, Knudson O, Valdes-Cruz L. Utility of three-dimensional ultrasound Doppler flow reconstruction of the proximal jet to quantify regurgitant orifice area: an *in-vitro* pulsatile flow study. *Circulation* 1995;92:I-797(abst).

28. Zhou X, Delabays A, Shiota T, et al. Effects of orifice shape, Nyquist limit and adjacent surfaces on three-dimensionally reconstructed color Doppler regurgitant jets: an *in vitro* study. *Circulation* 1995;92:I-722(abst).

29. Shiota T, Delabays A, Teien D, et al. Three dimensional reconstruction of color Doppler flow convergence regions for aortic and mitral regurgitation: an *in vitro* study. *Circulation* 1995;92:I-797(abst).

30. Delabays A, Shiota T, Teien D, Ge S, Sahn DJ, Pandian NG. Three-dimensional echocardiography allows accurate quantitation of the vena contracta and mitral regurgitation flow rates for asymmetric orifices: an *in vitro* validation study. *Circulation* 1995;92:I-798(abst).

31. Shiota T, Jones M, Delabays A, et al. 3D reconstruction of flow convergence and jets in aortic regurgitation: a chronic animal model study. *Circulation* 1995;92:I-797(abst).

32. Von Birgelen C, Erbel R, Di Mario C, et al. Three-dimensional reconstruction of coronary arteries with intravascular ultrasound. *Herz* 1995;230:277–289.

33. Delabays A, Pandian N, Cao Q-L, Sugeng L, Estes NAM III, Wang P. Three-dimensional echocardiographic visualization of intracardiac anatomy, ablation catheter location and pacer and defibrillator wire sites: *in vitro, in vivo* animal and clinical studies examining the potential of 3-D echo in guiding electrophysiologic interventions. *J Am Coll Cardiol* 1994;25:39A(abst).

PART II

Anomalies of Visceroatrial Situs

CHAPTER 8

Bilateral Right-sidedness and Left-sidedness Syndromes (Situs Ambiguus, Visceral Heterotaxies)

Lilliam M. Valdes-Cruz and Raul O. Cayre

In the majority of the population, the position of the thoracic and abdominal organs is normal in the system of bilateral symmetry, situs solitus. In a small group of fewer than one in 6,000 to 8,000 persons, the location of the thoracic and abdominal organs is the reverse or a mirror image of the normal, situs inversus (1). In 2.02% to 4.2% of patients with congenital cardiac anomalies, bilateral visceroatrial symmetry is present (2–4). This condition is situs ambiguus (indeterminate or uncertain) (5,6), which comprises the two syndromes of right isomerism, or bilateral right-sidedness, and left isomerism, or bilateral left-sidedness (7,8). These syndromes have also been referred to as visceral heterotaxies (9).

For years, the syndrome of bilateral right-sidedness has been associated with an absence of the spleen, or asplenia syndrome, and the syndrome of bilateral left-sidedness with the presence of many spleens, or polysplenia syndrome (5–17). However, rudimentary, multiple, or even normal spleens have been reported in cases of bilateral right-sidedness (4,5,7,9,18–20), absent spleen in bilateral left-sidedness (4), and multiple spleens in persons with structurally normal hearts (21). As such, the status of the spleen is of little value as a reference parameter in the diagnosis of congenital heart disease (4,20). Therefore, it is preferable to use the term bilateral right-sidedness rather than asplenia syndrome and bilateral left-sidedness instead of polysplenia syndrome.

EMBRYOLOGIC CONSIDERATIONS

In the early phases of embryologic development, the majority of structures from which the different organs and systems develop are located in the midline and have bilateral symmetry. Later in development, handed asymmetry is established; this determines specific differences between the right and left sides of certain organ systems, such as the nervous, digestive, circulatory, and respiratory systems. The direction of right- and left-handed asymmetry is genetically controlled, and three components have been suggested in its development: (a) a process of conversion through which molecular asymmetry is converted into cellular and multicellular asymmetry; (b) a maturation gradient determined by a reaction-diffusion mechanism that divides tissues in two regions, one with a higher molecular concentration than the other; and (c) a process of interpretation through which the embryonic cells recognize a difference in concentration of a substance on one side or the other (22). Freedom (23) considers that there is a persistence of the embryologic structures that are normally symmetric in the syndromes of visceral symmetry. Nonetheless, the mechanisms that establish handed asymmetry are still not definitively known (1,22,24,25). In the syndromes of visceral heterotaxy, characterized by a tendency toward right or left bilateral symmetry, there is a failure of the morphogenetic process that determines handed asymmetry. The cardiac anomalies seen in visceral heterotaxies are not primarily the result of abnormal gene activity, but rather are secondary to defective interactions during cardiac development (26).

ANATOMIC AND ECHOCARDIOGRAPHIC CONSIDERATIONS

Bilateral Right-sidedness Syndrome

In this syndrome, commonly called asplenia syndrome and also known as Ivemark syndrome (10), the visceroatrial situs is ambiguous; there is a tendency toward bilateral right-sidedness, with isomerism of the paired thoracoabdominal organs and midline location of the unpaired organs (see Fig. 2-4C). This syndrome usually includes splenic anomalies, cardiac malformations, absence of the coronary sinus, and abnormal drainage of the systemic, pulmonary, and coronary veins. Its incidence is approximately 1.9% of all cases of congenital cardiac anomalies (3).

Splenic Anomalies

Splenic anomalies seen in this syndrome consist of absence of the spleen in the majority of cases, although multiple spleens and even the presence of a normal spleen have been described (4,5,7,9,18–20). Usually, absence of the spleen is associated with cardiac malformations, so that establishing absence of the spleen is of great utility; however, its absence should not be considered pathognomonic for bilateral right-sidedness.

Liver

A symmetric liver positioned on the midline has been considered a roentgenographic sign of asplenia syndrome (12–14). However, this is not a rule in visceral heterotaxies, as a symmetric liver is not always present in this type of pathology (2,4,5,10,16,19,23,27). A symmetric, midline liver is found in 50% to 77% of cases of bilateral right-sidedness (4,5,7,19,28–31) (see Fig. 2-4C); in the remaining cases, the liver is found either on the right (situs solitus) or left (situs inversus) in equal numbers. The position of the liver is easily determined echocardiographically through a short-axis subcostal view of the abdomen (29) (see Figs. 4-12, 4-13) (Echo. 8-1).

Lungs and Tracheobronchial Tree

The lungs and tracheobronchial tree usually show bilateral symmetry in cases of visceral heterotaxy (5,11,12, 19,32–34). In bilateral right-sidedness, right isomerism of the lungs and tracheobronchial tree is almost a rule. Both lungs have the morphologic characteristics of a right lung, with three lobes, and the main bronchi are both right-sided (eparterial), shorter, and more vertical in orientation (see Fig. 2-4C). The morphologic characteristics of the bronchi have been considered pathognomonic parameters to determine visceroatrial situs (32–36), although there is discordance between the visceroatrial and tracheobronchial situs (4,17,28,30,31,37,38) in approximately 14.4% of cases of visceral heterotaxy (28). Nonetheless, the tracheobronchial morphology is still a fairly reliable indicator of bilateral isomerism syndromes. It cannot be determined echocardiographically but can be seen in a slightly overpenetrated plain film of the thorax (32,34).

Heart

Position of Heart in Thorax

In the bilateral right-sidedness syndromes, the position of the heart in the thorax has been variable in the series reported. In some, dextrocardia was found in 33% to 43% of cases (5,17,19,30,39); in others, there were equal numbers of cases of dextrocardia and levocardia (28,38), and in yet another series the incidence of dextrocardia was 69.2% (4). Mesocardia is very rare, occurring in about 3% of cases (17). The position of the heart in the thorax can be determined echocardiographically from the subcostal short-axis view of the abdomen with anterior or superior angulation of the transducer into the subcostal four-chamber view of the heart (Echo. 8-2).

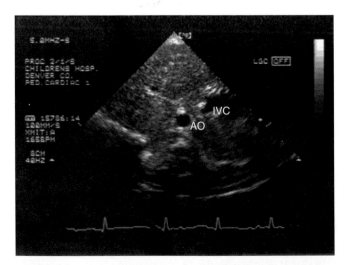

ECHO. 8-1. Subcostal short-axis view of the abdomen demonstrating midline liver. Note the aortocaval juxtaposition with vessels to the left of the spine. *AO*, aorta; *IVC*, inferior vena cava.

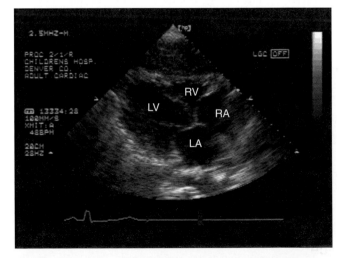

ECHO. 8-2. Subcostal four-chamber view of the position of the heart in the presence of dextrocardia. *RA*, right atrium; *LA*, left atrium; *RV*, right ventricle; *LV*, left ventricle.

Atrial Isomerism

For many years, a symmetric and midline liver, bronchial isomerism, and an absent or multiple spleens were all used to diagnose visceral heterotaxy. However, these features are not always present in bilateral right-sidedness syndromes. The morphology of the atrial appendages is the best guide to establish the atrial arrangement (1,3,4,28,30,38,39). The right atrial appendage is triangular, with a wide base and blunt border. The left atrial appendage has a narrow base, is fingerlike in appearance, and has a hooked apex. In bilateral right-sidedness syndromes, right atrial isomerism is present—that is, both atrial appendages are morphologically right (see Fig. 2-4C).

The right atrial appendage can be seen echocardiographically from the high parasternal long-axis view with angulation toward the right ventricular inflow (Echo. 8-3), from the subcostal sagittal short-axis view (Echo. 8-4), and from the right subclavicular sagittal view (Echo. 8-5). The left atrial appendage can be seen from the parasternal short-axis view at the level of the aortic valve with the transducer angulated slightly superiorly. It is observed at its attachment with the body of the left atrium just above the left upper pulmonary vein (see Fig. 4-7D, Echo. 8-9B). Transesophageal windows permit the best view of the atrial appendages (40,41), particularly in older patients. In the transverse view with the endoscope positioned behind the left atrium at the level of the left ventricular outflow tract and aortic valve, both the right and left atrial appendages can be imaged (see Fig. 4-29A,B, Echos. 4-17, 4-20).

Associated Cardiac Anomalies

In the majority of cases, the cardiac malformations associated with bilateral right-sidedness are complex and

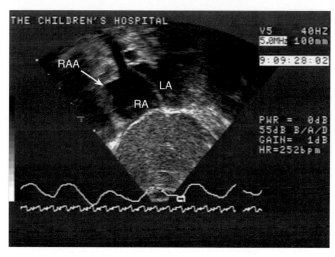

ECHO. 8-4. Subcostal sagittal view demonstrating the right atrial appendage. *RA*, right atrium; *LA*, left atrium, *RAA*, right atrial appendage.

wide-ranging. Anomalies of the interatrial septum are found, such as common atrium with virtual absence of the septum with or without a small remnant and atrial septal defect of the ostium secundum type. A patent foramen ovale or an intact interatrial septum has been seen in 9% of cases (28). Atrioventricular septal defects, partial or complete, are also associated, the latter being much more common. These are frequently accompanied by anomalies of the papillary muscles, such as displacement, hypoplasia, disproportion, or even absence (42). In more than half of cases, there is an atrioventricular univentricular connection of the double-inlet type through a common atrioventricular valve. Other associated cardiac malformations include perimembranous or muscular ventricular septal defects, isolated or multiple; complete transposition of the great arteries; double-outlet right ventricle; pulmo-

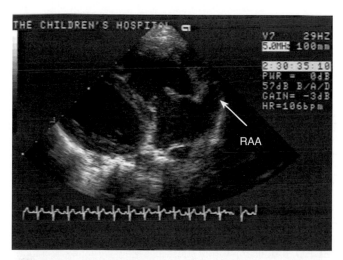

ECHO. 8-3. Parasternal long-axis view with angulation toward the right ventricular inflow demonstrating the right atrial appendage. It has a wide base and a blunt border. *RAA*, right atrial appendage.

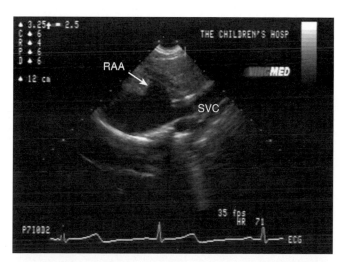

ECHO. 8-5. Right subclavicular sagittal view showing the right atrial appendage. *RAA*, right atrial appendage; *SVC*, superior vena cava.

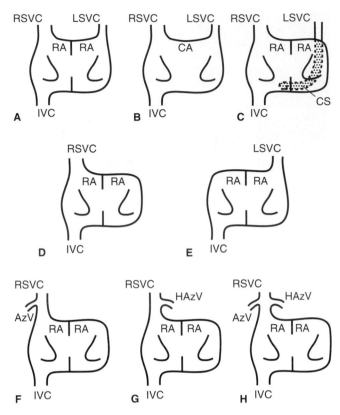

FIG. 8-1. A–H: Schematic drawings of the various types of systemic venous return seen in the bilateral right-sidedness syndromes. See text for details. *RA*, right atrium; *CA*, common atrium; *RSVC*, right superior vena cava; *LSVC*, left superior vena cava; *IVC*, inferior vena cava; *CS*, coronary sinus; *AzV*, azygous vein; *HAzV*, hemiazygous vein.

nary atresia; valvar or subvalvar pulmonic stenosis; valvar, subvalvar, or supravalvar aortic stenosis; aortic atresia; coarctation of the aorta with or without isthmic hypoplasia; and patent ductus arteriosus. The presence of a truncus arteriosus associated with bilateral right-sidedness, described by Ivemark (10), has been doubted (23). One case of interruption of the aortic arch has been reported by Berman et al. (43). The coronary sinus is typically absent (17,20,30,31,44–46), being present in only 3% of cases (46).

Systemic Venous Return

Abnormal systemic venous return is very frequent in visceral heterotaxy (4,5,19,20,28,30,31,38,44,46,47). In bilateral right-sidedness, bilateral superior venae cavae are seen in 52.8% to 86% of cases (4,5,19,20,30, 31,38,46,47). Each drains directly into the roof of one of the two morphologic right atria (Fig. 8-1A), or they drain into the right and left sides of a common atrium (Fig. 8-1B). If the coronary sinus is present, the right superior vena cava drains directly into the right atrium located to the right and the left superior vena cava drains into the

coronary sinus (31,46) (Fig. 8-1C). When a single superior vena cava is present, it is more commonly located on the right side (Fig. 8-1D) than on the left (Fig. 8-1E).

The echocardiographic views that permit visualization of the drainage of the right superior vena cava are the apical four-chamber view, subcostal long-axis view with superior transducer angulation, subcostal short-axis view, suprasternal view, and right subclavicular view (see Figs. 4-17D, 4-19A, 4-23, 4-25B). A left superior vena cava draining directly into the roof of the left-sided atrium or bilateral superior venae cavae can be seen from the parasternal short-axis view with the transducer tilted slightly superiorly and leftward, and from the suprasternal short-axis view with the transducer also directed leftward (Echo. 8-6).

In situs solitus, the descending aorta is in front or slightly to the left of the spine, and the inferior vena cava is on the right of the spine and anterior to the aorta. This can be seen readily from the subcostal abdominal short-axis view (29) (see Figs. 4-12, 4-13). In situs inversus, a mirror image of this arrangement is seen (Echo. 8-7). Because the aorta and inferior vena cava are located to the left and right of the spine, respectively, they cannot be seen simultaneously in the long-axis subcostal abdominal view. To follow the aorta cephalad, the transducer must be angled to the left, and to follow the inferior vena cava into the right atrium, the transducer must be angled to the right (see Figs. 4-14, 4-15). In bilateral right-sidedness, the inferior vena cava and abdominal aorta are found on the same side of the spine, either to the right or left; this has been called aortocaval juxtaposition (5,19,48). This relationship has been considered diagnostic of asplenia (5,19,48); however, similar findings have been observed in bilateral left-sidedness (23,29) and in the absence of the spleen and midline liver

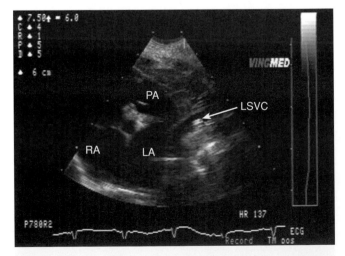

ECHO. 8-6. Parasternal short-axis view with the transducer tilted superiorly and leftward to demonstrate the presence of a left superior vena cava (*arrow*). Note the catheter inside the vessel. *PA*, pulmonary artery; *RA*, right atrium; *LA*, left atrium; *LSVC*, left superior vena cava.

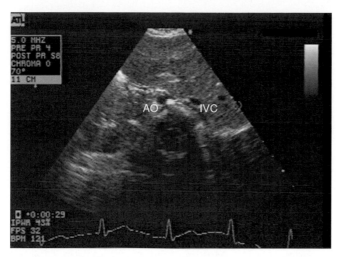

ECHO. 8-7. Abdominal short-axis view in the presence of situs inversus demonstrating the aorta on the right and the inferior vena cava on the left of the spine. *AO*, aorta; *IVC*, inferior vena cava.

but the usual atrial arrangement (49). Aortocaval juxtaposition can be seen from the subcostal short-axis and long axis views of the abdomen (see Figs. 4-12, 4-15) (Echo. 8-8). In the majority of cases of bilateral right-sidedness, there is no interruption of the hepatic portion of the inferior vena cava, which can be present with or without azygous and/or hemiazygous continuation (4,5,19,20,28,31,46) (Fig. 8-1F–H); however, isolated cases have been reported (27,30,38). An uninterrupted inferior vena cava with the presence of an azygous vein, hemiazygous vein, or both is seen in 8.3% of cases (46). Joined drainage of the inferior vena cava and hepatic vein into the atrium located to the right (Fig. 8-2A) or into the right side of a common atrium (Fig. 8-2B) is more commonly observed than drainage into

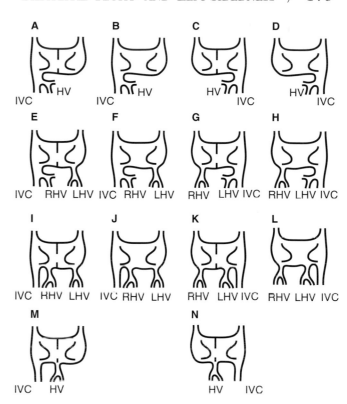

FIG. 8-2. A–N: Schematic drawings of the various types of hepatic venous return seen in the bilateral right-sidedness syndromes. All drawings are shown with bilateral superior venae cavae. See text for details. *IVC*, inferior vena cava; *HV*, hepatic veins; *RHV*, right hepatic vein; *LHV*, left hepatic vein.

the left-sided atrium (Fig. 8-2C) or into the left side of a common atrium (Fig. 8-2D). These four types are seen in 32% to 73% of cases reported (4,17,28,31,44,46). Less frequently, there can be joined drainage of the inferior vena cava and a hepatic vein on one side of the atrium and drainage of another hepatic vein on the contralateral side (Fig. 8-2E–H), or separate drainage of the inferior vena cava and a hepatic vein into the same atrium and drainage of another hepatic vein into the contralateral atrium (Fig. 8-2I,K) or into the same side of a common atrium (Fig. 8-2J,L). Rarely, there can be separate drainage of the inferior vena cava and the hepatic vein, with the latter overriding the interatrial septum (28) (Fig. 8-2M,N).

Pulmonary Venous Drainage

Anomalies of pulmonary venous drainage are the rule in bilateral right-sidedness because of the presence of two morphologic right atria or a common atrium with characteristics of a right atrium. Total anomalous pulmonary venous return to a systemic vein is seen in 61.5% to 88% of cases (4,5,19,30,31). Drainage can occur via a common collector into the right superior vena cava (Fig. 8-3A), left superior vena cava (Fig. 8-3B), innominate vein (Fig. 8-3C), inferior vena cava (Fig. 8-3D), azygous

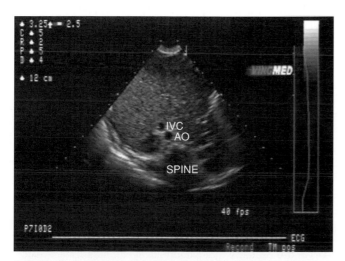

ECHO. 8-8. Abdominal short-axis view demonstrating aortocaval juxtaposition, with the inferior vena cava anterior to the aorta and both vessels located on the right side of the spine. *AO*, aorta; *IVC*, inferior vena cava.

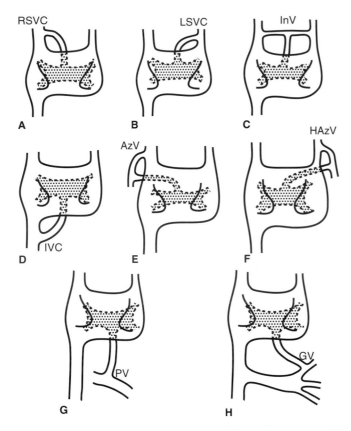

FIG. 8-3. A–H: Schematic drawings of the various types of total anomalous pulmonary venous connection to a systemic vein via a common collector seen in the bilateral right-sidedness syndromes. All drawings are shown with bilateral right superior venae cavae and normal drainage of the inferior venae cavae. The *shaded areas* indicate the sites of drainage of the pulmonary veins. See text for details. *RSVC*, right superior vena cava; *LSVC*, left superior vena cava; *InV*, innominate vein; *IVC*, inferior vena cava; *AzV*, azygous vein; *HAzV*, hemiazygous vein; *PV*, portal vein; *GV*, gastric vein.

vein (Fig. 8-3E), hemiazygous vein (Fig. 8-3F), portal vein (Fig. 8-3G), or gastric vein (Fig. 8-3H).

Drainage can be intracardiac through a wide range of connections. The four veins can drain separately into the anatomic right atrium located to the left (Fig. 8-4A) or to the right (Fig. 8-4C), or into the left or right side of a common atrium (Fig. 8-4B,D). Drainage of the veins through a common collector, which can be stenotic in up to 25% of cases, can be into the left-sided (Fig. 8-4E) or right-sided (Fig. 8-4G) atrium or into the left or right side of a common atrium (Fig. 8-4F,H). Occasionally, the right pulmonary veins drain directly or through a common vein into the right-sided atrium or right side of a common atrium, and the left pulmonary veins into the left-sided atrium or the left side of a common atrium (Fig. 8-4I–L).

Bilateral Left-sidedness Syndrome

In this syndrome, commonly called polysplenia syndrome, the visceroatrial situs is ambiguous and there is a

tendency toward bilateral left symmetry. Like the bilateral right-sidedness syndromes, it is characterized by isomerism of the paired thoracoabdominal organs, midline localization of the unpaired organs (see Fig. 2-4D), abnormalities of the spleen, cardiac malformations, and anomalous drainage of the systemic and pulmonary veins. Its incidence varies between 0.77% and 1.3% of all cases of congenital heart disease (3,4,31,50).

Splenic Anomalies

Splenic anomalies are usual; multiple spleens, between two and 16 in number, are located in the left or right upper quadrant of the abdomen or along the major curvature of the stomach (51). Multiple spleens are seen in 55% to 95.7% of published cases (3,4,20,28,30,42,50,51). The term polysplenia syndrome cannot always be applied to bilateral left-sidedness, as cases have been reported with only one spleen or with a bilobed (3,4,20,28,30,42,50,51)

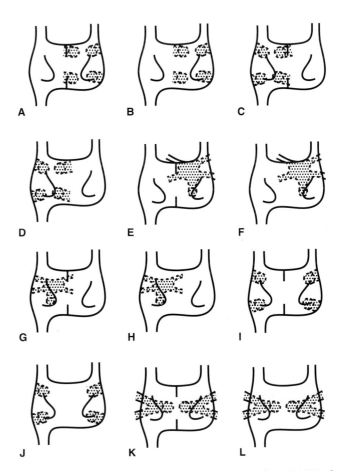

FIG. 8-4. A–L: Schematic drawings of the various types of intracardiac total anomalous pulmonary venous connection seen in the bilateral right-sidedness syndromes. See text for details. All drawings are shown with bilateral superior venae cavae and normal drainage of the inferior vena cava. The *shaded areas* indicate the sites of drainage of the pulmonary veins, separately or through a common collector.

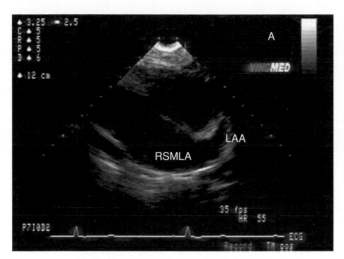
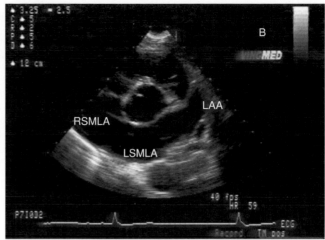

ECHO. 8-9. Echocardiographic demonstration of both left atrial appendages in bilateral left-sidedness syndrome. **A:** The right-sided morphologic left atrium is seen from the long-axis view with the transducer tilted toward the ventricular inflow. **B:** The left-sided morphologic left atrial appendage is seen from the parasternal short-axis view. *LAA*, left atrial appendage; *RSMLA*, right-sided morphologic left atrium; *LSMLA*, left-sided morphologic left atrium.

or absent spleen (4,42). Therefore, the term bilateral left-sidedness is more appropriate than polysplenia syndrome.

Liver

A symmetric liver positioned in the midline (see Fig. 2-4D) is not always present (4,28–31,38,51). In those cases in which the liver is not in the midline, it is found on the right (situs solitus) or left (situs inversus) of the abdomen with the same frequency.

Lungs and Tracheobronchial Tree

The lungs and tracheobronchial tree are in left isomerism in 62.3% to 100% of reported series (17,30,31, 38,50,51). Both lungs have the anatomic characteristics of a morphologic left lung—that is, they are bilobed, and both main bronchi are morphologically left-sided (hyparterial), longer, and more horizontally oriented (see Fig. 2-4D). In some cases of bilateral left-sidedness, no pulmonary or bronchial left isomerism is present (17,31,38,51). Tracheobronchial and pulmonary situs solitus has been found in 5.2% to 16% (31,38,51), situs inversus in 5.2% to 33.3% (17,31,38,51), and right isomerism in 6.9% to 15.7% (31,37,38) of cases in various series.

Heart

Position of Heart in Thorax

Among 227 cases of bilateral left-sidedness syndrome reported in the literature and reviewed by us,

levocardia was present in 139 (61.2%), dextrocardia in 87 (38.3%) (4,17,29,30,38,39,50,51), and mesocardia in only one case (0.5%) (51). The position of the heart in the thorax can be determined by echocardiography from the subcostal abdominal short-axis view with superior angulation into the long-axis subcostal view of the heart.

Atrial Isomerism

The morphology of the atrial appendages is the best guide to determine the atrial arrangement (1,3,4,28,30, 38,39). In the bilateral left-sidedness syndrome, both atrial appendages are morphologically of the left type — that is, narrow-based with a fingerlike appearance and a hooked apex (see Fig. 2-4D). The echocardiogram can demonstrate the atrial appendages from the same views described above under right-sidedness syndrome (Echo. 8-9).

Associated Cardiac Anomalies

The majority of cases of bilateral left-sidedness are associated with cardiac anomalies of a wide variety. Atrioventricular septal defects, partial or complete, have been reported in 40% to 65% of cases (5,28,30,38,39, 44,50,51). Obstruction of the right ventricular outflow tract has been seen in 35% to 66% of cases, mostly in the form of valvar and/or subvalvar stenosis (4,11,17, 38,44,51). Pulmonary atresia was found in 9% of 128 cases in a reported series (51). The ventriculoarterial connection is concordant in 50% to 84% of cases (4,17,20,29, 30,39,44,50,51), and the remaining cases are equally dis-

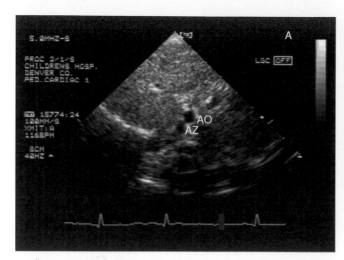
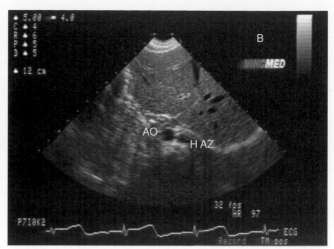

ECHO. 8-10. Subcostal abdominal short-axis view demonstrating the azygous **(A)** and hemiazygous **(B)** veins and their relationships to the aorta. *AO*, aorta; *AZ*, azygous; *HAZ*, hemiazygous.

tributed between discordant connection and double-outlet right ventricle. Other associated anomalies are ostium secundum atrial septal defect, sinus venosus type of atrial defect, patent foramen ovale, patent ductus arteriosus, perimembranous or muscular ventricular septal defects, univentricular atrioventricular connection, aortic valvar or subvalvar stenosis, coarctation of the aorta and/or isthmic hypoplasia, interrupted aortic arch, and tetralogy of Fallot (4,17,28–30,38,39,50,51).

Systemic Venous Drainage

The most common anomaly of systemic venous drainage seen in bilateral left-sidedness is absence of the hepatic segment of the inferior vena cava with azygous or hemiazygous continuation, which is seen in 55% to 91% of reported cases (4,5,17,19,20,28–31,38,44,47,50,51)

(Fig. 8-5A–C). Even though absence of the hepatic portion of the inferior vena cava is not always seen in bilateral left-sidedness, there should be a high index of suspicion any time this venous anomaly is observed. Continuity with the azygous vein located to the right and posterior to the aorta or with the hemiazygous vein located to the left and posterior to the aorta has a similar incidence. These can drain into the right, left, or bilateral superior venae cavae (Fig. 8-5A–C). If the inferior vena cava is not interrupted, it can drain directly into the morphologic left atrium located to the right (Fig. 8-5D) or into the right side of a common atrium (Fig. 8-5E). In one third of cases, the inferior vena cava drains into the atrium located on the left (Fig. 8-5F) or into the left side of a common atrium (Fig. 8-5G). Aortocaval juxtaposition is also seen in bilateral left-sidedness (5,23,29). The systemic venous drainage from the lower body (azygous vein, hemiazygous vein, and/or uninterrupted inferior

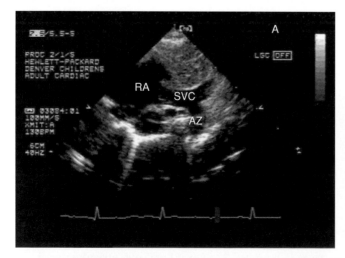
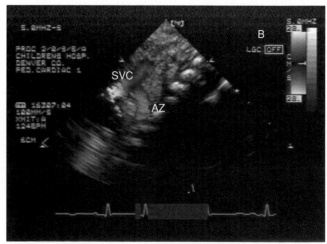

ECHO. 8-11. Drainage of the azygous vein into the posterior aspect of the right-sided superior vena cava. **A:** Anatomic image. **B:** Color Doppler flow image. *RA*, right atrium; *SVC*, superior vena cava; *AZ*, azygous vein.

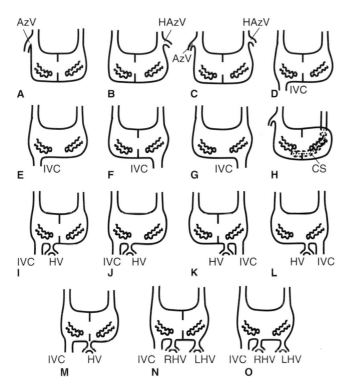

FIG. 8-5. A–O: Schematic drawings of the various types of systemic venous drainage seen in the bilateral left-sidedness syndrome. See text for details. All drawings are shown with bilateral superior venae cavae. *IVC*, inferior vena cava; *AzV*, azygous vein; *HAzV*, hemiazygous vein; *CS*, coronary sinus; *HV*, hepatic veins; *RHV*, right hepatic vein; *LHV*, left hepatic vein.

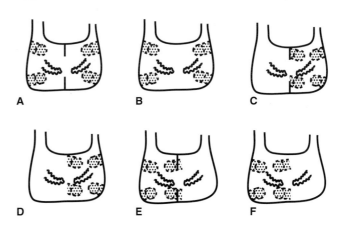

FIG. 8-6. A–F: Schematic drawings of the various types of pulmonary venous connections in the bilateral left-sidedness syndrome. See text for details. All drawings are shown with bilateral superior venae cavae and absence of the hepatic segment of the inferior vena cava. The *shaded areas* indicate the sites of drainage of the pulmonary veins.

overriding the atrial septum (Fig. 8-5M), or bilaterally into both atria (Fig. 8-5N) or both sides of a common atrium (Fig. 8-5O).

Pulmonary Venous Drainage

Most commonly, pulmonary venous drainage is bilateral—that is, the right pulmonary veins drain into the atrium located to the right or the right side of a common atrium, and the left pulmonary veins drain into the atrium located to the left or into the left side of a common atrium (Fig. 8-6A,B). Less frequently, the four pulmonary veins drain separately into the atrium located to the left or the left side of a common atrium (Fig. 8-6C,D), or into the atrium located to the right or the right side of a common atrium (Fig. 8-6E,F). Total anomalous drainage into a systemic vein has been reported in 21.7% of cases (31).

REFERENCES

1. Seo JW, Brown NA, Ho SY, Anderson RH. Abnormal laterality and congenital cardiac anomalies. Relations of visceral cardiac morphologies in the *iv/iv* mouse. *Circulation* 1992;86:642–650.
2. Fyler DC, Buckley LP, Hellenbrand WE, Cohn HE. Report of the New England Regional Infant Cardiac Program. *Pediatrics* 1980; 65[Suppl]:375–461.
3. Sharma S, Devine W, Anderson RH, Zuberbuhler JR. The determination of atrial arrangement by examination of appendage morphology in 1842 heart specimens. *Br Heart J* 1988;60:227–231.
4. Anderson C, Devine WA, Anderson RH, Debich DE, Zuberbuhler JR. Abnormalities of the spleen in relation to congenital malformations of the heart: a survey of necropsy findings in children. *Br Heart J* 1990;63:122–128.
5. Van Mierop LHS, Gessner IH, Schiebler GL. Asplenia and polysplenia syndromes. In: Bergsma D, ed. *Birth defects: original article series*, Vol 8. Baltimore: Williams & Wilkins, 1972:36–44.
6. Van Praagh R. Terminology of congenital heart disease. Glossary and commentary [Editorial]. *Circulation* 1977;56:139–143.
7. Van Mierop LHS, Wiglesworth FW. Isomerism of the cardiac atria in the asplenia syndrome. *Lab Invest* 1962;11:1303–1315.

vena cava) and its spatial relationship to the descending aorta are seen from the subcostal abdominal short- and long-axis views (see Figs. 4-12–4-15) (Echo. 8-10). Azygous and hemiazygous drainage to the superior vena cava can be seen from a right subclavicular position (Echo. 8-11; see color plate 8 following p. 364).

Bilateral superior venae cavae are seen in 44% to 70% of cases (5,17,20,28–30,44,51). The left superior vena cava can drain directly into the roof of the anatomic left atrium located to the left (Fig. 8-5D,F), into the left side of a common atrium (Fig. 8-5E,G), or into the coronary sinus (Fig. 8-5H). As stated above, the coronary sinus is usually absent in the bilateral right-sidedness syndromes; in contrast, the coronary sinus is present in 50% to 75% of cases of bilateral left-sidedness (17,20,30,31,44,50,51). The right and left superior venae cavae can be evaluated from the same echocardiographic views described for bilateral right-sidedness syndrome.

Anomalies of hepatic venous drainage are seen frequently (4,19,28–30,44,47,50). The hepatic vein usually drains separately from the inferior vena cava; it can drain directly into the atrium located on the right (Fig. 8-5I) or into the right side of a common atrium (Fig. 8-5J), into the atrium located on the left (Fig. 8-5K) or into the left side of a common atrium (Fig. 8-5L), at the midline

8. Moller JH, Nakib A, Anderson RC, Edwards JE. Congenital cardiac disease associated with polysplenia. A developmental complex of bilateral left-sidedness. *Circulation* 1967;36:789–799.

9. Freedom RM. The heterotaxy syndrome. *Circulation* 1971; 43[Suppl II]:II-115.

10. Ivemark BI. Implications of agenesis of the spleen on the pathogenesis of cono-truncus anomalies in childhood. An analysis of the heart malformations in the splenic agenesis syndrome, with fourteen new cases. *Acta Paediatr* 1955;44[Suppl 104]:1–110.

11. Brandt HM, Liebow AA. Right pulmonary isomerism associated with venous, splenic, and other anomalies. *Lab Invest* 1958;7:469–504.

12. Forde WJ, Finby N. Roentgenographic features of asplenia, a teratologic syndrome of visceral symmetry. *Am J Roentgenol* 1961;86:523–533.

13. Lucas RV, Neufeld HN, Lester RG, Edwards JE. The symmetrical liver as a roentgen sign of asplenia. *Circulation* 1962;25:973–975.

14. Ruttenberg HD, Neufeld HN, Lucas RV, et al. Syndrome of congenital cardiac disease with asplenia. Distinction from other forms of congenital cyanotic cardiac disease. *Am J Cardiol* 1964;13:387–406.

15. Van Mierop LHS, Patterson PR, Reynolds RW. Two cases of congenital asplenia with isomerism of the cardiac atria and the sinoatrial nodes. *Am J Cardiol* 1964;13:407–414.

16. Van Praagh R, Van Praagh S, Vlad P, Keith JD. Anatomic types of congenital dextrocardia. Diagnostic and embryologic implications. *Am J Cardiol* 1964;13:510–531.

17. Rose V, Izukawa T, Moes CAF. Syndromes of asplenia and polysplenia. A review of cardiac and non-cardiac malformations in 60 cases with special reference to diagnosis and prognosis. *Br Heart J* 1975;37:840–852.

18. Layman TE, Levine MA, Amplatz K, Edwards JE. Asplenic syndrome in association with rudimentary spleen. *Am J Cardiol* 1967;20:136–140.

19. Van Mierop LHS, Gessner IH, Schiebler GL. Asplenia and polysplenia syndromes. In: Bergsma D, ed. *Birth defects: original article series*, Vol 8. Baltimore: Williams & Wilkins, 1972:74–82.

20. Becker AE, Anderson RH. Isomerism of the atrial appendages—goodbye to asplenia and all that. In: Clark EB, Takao A, eds. *Developmental cardiology: morphogenesis and function*. Mount Kisco, NY: Futura Publishing, 1990:659–670.

21. Debich DE, Devine WA, Anderson RH. Polysplenia with normally structured hearts. *Am J Cardiol* 1990;65:1274–1275.

22. Brown NA, Wolpert L. The development of handedness in left/right asymmetry. *Development* 1990;109:1–9.

23. Freedom RM. Aortic valve and arch anomalies in the congenital asplenia syndrome. Case report, literature review and re-examination of the embryology of the congenital asplenia syndrome. *Johns Hopkins Med J* 1974;135:124–135.

24. Brown NA, McCarthy A, Wolpert L. The development of handed asymmetry in aggregation chimeras of situs inversus mutant and wild-type mouse embryo. *Development* 1990;110:949–954.

25. Morishima M, Miyagawa-Tomita S, Yasui H, Ando M, Nakasawa M, Takao A. Visceroatrial heterotaxy syndrome induced by maternal hyperthermia in the rat. *Cardiol Young* 1995;5:251–256.

26. Icardo JM, Sanchez de Vega MJ. Spectrum of heart malformations in mice with situs solitus, situs inversus, and associated visceral heterotaxy. *Circulation* 1991;84:2547–2558.

27. Freedom RM, Fellows KE Jr. Radiographic visceral patterns in the asplenia syndrome. *Radiology* 1973;107:387–391.

28. Macartney FJ, Zuberbuhler JR, Anderson RH. Morphological considerations pertaining to recognition of atrial isomerism. Consequences for sequential chamber localisation. *Br Heart J* 1980;44:657–667.

29. Huhta JC, Smallhorn JF, Macartney FJ. Two-dimensional echocardiographic diagnosis of situs. *Br Heart J* 1982;48:97–108.

30. Ho SY, Cook A, Anderson RH, Allan LD, Fagg N. Isomerism of the atrial appendages in the fetus. *Pediatr Pathol* 1991;11:589–608.

31. Van Praagh S, Kreutzer J, Alday L, Van Praagh R. Systemic and pulmonary venous connections in visceral heterotaxy, with emphasis on the diagnosis of the atrial situs: a study of 109 postmortem cases. In: Clark EB, Takao A, eds. *Developmental cardiology: morphogenesis and function*. Mount Kisco, NY: Futura Publishing, 1990:671–727.

32. Van Mierop LHS, Eisen S, Schiebler GL. The radiographic appearance of the tracheobronchial tree as an indicator of visceral situs. *Am J Cardiol* 1970;26:432–435.

33. Landing BH, Lawrence TK, Payne VC, Wells TR. Bronchial anatomy in syndromes with abnormal visceral situs, abnormal spleen and congenital heart disease. *Am J Cardiol* 1971;28:456–462.

34. Soto B, Pacifico AD, Souza AS, Bargeron LM Jr, Ermocilla R, Tonkin IL. Identification of thoracic isomerism from the plain chest radiograph. *Am J Roentgenol* 1978;131:995–1002.

35. Partridge JB, Scott O, Deverall PB, Macartney FJ. Visualization and measurement of the main bronchi by tomography as an objective indicator of thoracic situs in congenital heart disease. *Circulation* 1975;51:188–196.

36. Macartney FJ, Partridge JB, Shinebourne EA, Tynan MJ, Anderson RH. Identification of atrial situs. In: Anderson RH, Shinebourne EA, eds. *Paediatric cardiology 1977*. Edinburgh: Churchill Livingstone, 1978:16–26.

37. Caruso G, Becker AE. How to determine atrial situs? Considerations initiated by 3 cases of absent spleen with a discordant anatomy between bronchi and atria. *Br Heart J* 1979;41:559–567.

38. Sapire DW, Ho SY, Anderson RH, Rigby ML. Diagnosis and significance of atrial isomerism. *Am J Cardiol* 1986;58:342–346.

39. De Tommasi SM, Daliento L, Ho SY, Macartney FJ, Anderson RH. Analysis of atrioventricular junction, ventricular mass, and ventriculoarterial junction in 43 specimens with atrial isomerism. *Br Heart J* 1981;45:236–247.

40. Seward JB, Khandheria BK, Edwards WD, Oh JK, Freeman WK, Tajik AJ. Biplanar transesophageal echocardiography: anatomic correlations, image orientation, and clinical applications. *Mayo Clin Proc* 1990;65:1193–1213.

41. Stumper OFW, Sreeram N, Elzenga NJ, Sutherland GR. Diagnosis of atrial situs by transesophageal echocardiography. *J Am Coll Cardiol* 1990;16:442–446.

42. Uemura H, Anderson RH, Ho SY, et al. Left ventricular structures in atrioventricular septal defect associated with isomerism of atrial appendages compared with similar features with usual atrial arrangement. *J Thorac Cardiovasc Surg* 1995;110:445–452.

43. Berman W Jr, Yabek SM, Burstein J, Dillon T. Asplenia syndrome with atypical cardiac anomalies. *Pediatr Cardiol* 1982;3:35–38.

44. Kirklin JW, Barrat-Boyes BG. Atrial isomerism. In: Kirklin JW, Barrat-Boyes BG, eds. *Cardiac surgery*, Vol 2, 2nd ed. New York: Churchill Livingstone, 1993:1585–1596.

45. Uemura H, Ho SY, Anderson RH, et al. The surgical anatomy of coronary venous return in hearts with isomeric atrial appendages. *J Thorac Cardiovasc Surg* 1995;110:436–444.

46. Rubino M, Van Praagh S, Kadoba K, Pessotto R, Van Praagh R. Systemic and pulmonary venous connections in visceral heterotaxy with asplenia. Diagnostic and surgical considerations based on seventy-two autopsied cases. *J Thorac Cardiovasc Surg* 1995;110:641–650.

47. Huhta JC, Smallhorn JF, Macartney FJ, Anderson RH, De Leval M. Cross-sectional echocardiographic diagnosis of systemic venous return. *Br Heart J* 1982;48:388–403.

48. Elliot LP, Cramer GG, Amplatz K. The anomalous relationship of the inferior vena cava and abdominal aorta as a specific angiocardiographic sign in asplenia. *Radiology* 1966;87:859–863.

49. Radhakrishnan S, Singh M, Bajaj R. Discordance between abdominal and atrial arrangement in a case of complex congenital heart disease. *Int J Cardiol* 1992;36:361–363.

50. Sharma S, Devine W, Anderson RH, Zuberbuhler JR. Identification and analysis of the left atrial isomerism. *Am J Cardiol* 1987;60:1157–1160.

51. Peoples WM, Moller JH, Edwards JE. Polysplenia: a review of 146 cases. *Pediatr Cardiol* 1983;4:129–137.

PART III

Anomalies of Cardiac Septation

CHAPTER 9

Atrial Septal Defects

Lilliam M. Valdes-Cruz and Raul O. Cayre

The incidence of isolated atrial septal defects, excluding the partial atrioventricular septal defects of the ostium primum type, varies between 6% and 11% of all congenital cardiac anomalies in reported series (1–3).

EMBRYOLOGIC CONSIDERATIONS

The following structures contribute to the embryologic development of the interatrial septum complex: the septum primum, the inferior cushion of the atrioventricular canal, the septum secundum, and the left valve of the sinus venosus (4–6) (see Figs. 1-7, 1-8). The septum primum originates from the middorsal wall of the primitive atrium and grows toward the orifice of the atrioventricular canal, where the superior (or ventral) and inferior (or dorsal) endocardial cushions appear simultaneously (5) (see Fig. 1-7). The septum primum and superior and inferior cushions form the borders of an orifice called the ostium primum or foramen primum (see Fig. 1-7). The foramen primum is closed progressively by tissue from the septum primum and from the inferior cushion of the atrioventricular canal (5). While this is occurring, the ostium secundum, or foramen secundum, appears in the dorsocephalic area of the septum primum through a process of cellular death (see Fig. 1-8); the ostium secundum remains patent until after birth.

In the extreme cephalic end of the interseptovalvular space (4), limited by the right surface of the septum primum and the left surface of the left valve of the sinus venosus, a new septum appears, which is called the septum secundum (6) (see Fig. 1-8A). Its limbs grow toward the orifice of the inferior vena cava, outlining an incomplete oval ring called the limbus of the foramen ovale (see Fig. 1-8). The left valve of the sinus venosus progressively adheres to the right surface of the septum secundum and eventually disappears. Between the free border of the septum primum at the level of the foramen secundum on the left side and the free border of the septum secundum on the right side, a communication called the foramen ovale is established (see Fig. 1-8). After birth, the septum primum and septum secundum fuse, the foramen ovale disappears, and the limbus of the foramen ovale becomes the limbus of the fossa ovalis (see Fig. 1-8D).

Alterations in any of the basic developmental processes (7) that interfere with the normal development of the components of the atrial septal complex are expressed anatomically as one or more atrial septal defects, which can occur in isolation or in association with other malformations. These defects can also be transmitted as an autosomal dominant trait (8,9) or can be present in selected chromosomal aberrations (10,11), such as deletion of 4p (Wolf-Hirschhorn syndrome), deletion of 5p (cri du chat syndrome), trisomy 21, XO syndrome (Turner's syndrome), XXXXY syndrome (10), trisomy 13 (Patau's syndrome), and trisomy 22 (11).

Classically, atrial septal defects are divided into the following types: (a) patent foramen ovale, (b) ostium secundum or fossa ovalis defects, (c) ostium primum defects or persistent common atrioventricular canal, (d) sinus venosus defects of the superior vena caval type, (e) sinus venosus defects of the inferior vena caval type, and (f) defects involving the entire atrial septum or common atrium (2,12–15). Raghib et al. in 1965 (16) described a type of atrial septal defect associated with drainage of the left superior vena cava into the left atrium and absence of the coronary sinus. This defect has since been described by several authors (17–23) and has been variously called unroofed coronary sinus (17), left atrium-to-coronary sinus fenestration (20), atrial communication via the orifice of the coronary sinus (21), or coronary sinus defect (3,22,23). A rarer type of anomaly, called defect of the septum intermedium, true persistent ostium primum (22), or simple primum defect (24), can also occur (Fig. 9-1).

Persistent common atrioventricular canal of the partial type, or ostium primum defect, is a defect of the atrioventricular septum; therefore, it is not included in this chap-

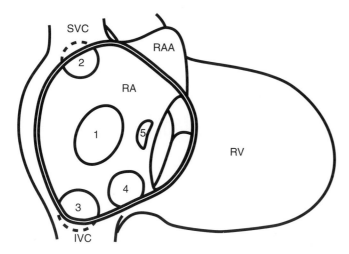

FIG. 9-1. Schematic drawing showing the different types of atrial septal defects. *1,* ostium secundum defect; *2,* sinus venosus defect of the superior vena caval type; *3,* sinus venosus defect of the inferior vena caval type; *4,* coronary sinus type; *5,* simple ostium primum type. *RA,* right atrium; *RAA,* right atrial appendage; *SVC,* superior vena cava; *IVC,* inferior vena cava; *RV,* right ventricle.

ter. The morphogenetic mechanisms, anatomic characteristics, and associated echocardiographic findings of this defect are covered in Chapter 11.

The foramen ovale is the communication that is established between the free border of the septum secundum on the right and the free border of the septum primum at the level of the ostium secundum. During fetal life, this communication permits the passage of blood from the right to the left atrium (see Fig. 1-8). After birth, the pressure in the left atrium rises above that of the right atrium and the septum primum abuts the septum secundum, causing the functional closure of the foramen ovale and thereby preventing the shunting of blood across the atrial septum. Later, the septum primum and septum secundum fuse, resulting in anatomic closure of the foramen ovale (25). In 20% to 30% of normal hearts, a patent foramen ovale may persist (14,26,27) because the septum primum and septum secundum fail to fuse.

The ostium secundum or fossa ovalis defect can result from abnormal development, abnormal resorption, or ectopic cellular death of the septum primum at the level of the fossa ovalis (2,3,22,24,28) (Fig. 9-1). If the septum secundum in the region adjacent to the fossa ovalis also develops abnormally, a larger defect results, which functionally behaves as a common atrium (22).

A variety of morphogenetic mechanisms have been proposed to explain sinus venosus defects of the superior vena caval type (3,22,27,29–32) (Fig. 9-1). These include excessive absorption of the sinus venosus (29), malposition of the orifice of the sinus venosus or sinoatrial orifice (30), excessive migration of the right upper pulmonary vein (31), and abnormal attachment of the right upper pulmonary vein to the wall of the superior vena cava with

reabsorption of the wall between them (3,27). Goor and Lillehei (22) propose that in those cases with normal drainage of the pulmonary veins, there could exist a failure of development of the septum secundum.

Sinus venosus atrial defects of the inferior vena caval type (Fig. 9-1), with anomalous return of the right lower pulmonary vein, would have the same morphogenetic mechanism as that causing defects of the superior vena caval type—namely, abnormal attachment of the right lower pulmonary vein to the wall of the inferior vena cava, with later reabsorption of the wall separating them (3,27). Cases with levoposition of the inferior vena cava and overriding of both atria have been described, and the same morphogenetic mechanism has been proposed (22,32).

Common or single atrium, frequently associated with heterotaxy syndrome (33) and with the autosomal recessive Ellis-van Creveld syndrome (2,10,11), is the result of failure of development of the embryologic components that contribute to the development of the atrial septal complex.

An abnormal development of the wall between the coronary sinus and the left atrium would be the morphogenetic mechanism causing atrial septal defects of the coronary sinus type (16,20,22,27,34) (Fig. 9-1).

Absence of that portion of the septum primum contributing to closure of the ostium or foramen primum (4,5) is expressed anatomically as a defect in the region of the foramen primum called true persistent ostium primum (22) or simple primum defect (24) (Fig. 9-1).

ANATOMIC AND ECHOCARDIOGRAPHIC CONSIDERATIONS

The echocardiographic evaluation of atrial septal defects should include the following: (a) determination of the location of the defect(s) and the relationship to the atrioventricular valves and drainage sites of the pulmonary and systemic veins, (b) estimation of the size of the defect(s) and assessment of the hemodynamic consequences, (c) assessment of associated anomalies, and (d) intraoperative and postoperative evaluation.

Location of Atrial Septal Defects

Determination of the location of the atrial septal defect(s) and the relationship to the atrioventricular valves and drainage sites of the pulmonary and systemic veins is discussed separately for each type of defect.

Patent Foramen Ovale

A patent foramen ovale, which is not considered a true atrial septal defect (21,27), is present in the first months of life in most infants and persists in 20% to 30% of normal hearts (14,26,27), permitting some shunting of blood between the two atria. For this reason, all echocardiographic studies should include a study of the interatrial septum. Anatomically, it is a tunnel whose floor is the septum primum, which makes up the valve of the foramen ovale. The entry orifice, on the right surface of the atrial septum, is located on the superior aspect of the limbus of the fossa ovalis and is limited by the free border of the septum secundum. The exit orifice, located on the left side, is bound by the free border of the septum primum at the level of the foramen secundum (see Fig. 1-8).

Echocardiographically, it is difficult to identify the presence of a foramen ovale because of its small anatomic size and the thinness of the septum primum at the level of the fossa ovalis, which can produce a false dropout of echoes at the midportion of the atrial septum corresponding to the region of the fossa ovalis. This echo dropout occurs most commonly in views in which the atrial septum is parallel to the echo beam, such as the parasternal short-axis and apical four-chamber views (35,36). The best visualization of the atrial septum is obtained from the subcostal views, and frequently, particularly in infants, the two components of the flap of the foramen (i.e., the septum primum on the left and the septum secundum on the right) can be seen from this view (Echo. 9-1). Shunting, if present, is best identified with the use of color Doppler flow mapping; it may vary with the respiratory cycle.

The presence of a patent foramen ovale with paradoxical right-to-left shunting has been implicated as a cause of strokes, especially in adults (2,14,27). Examination of the atrial septum from a transesophageal approach may be necessary in some of these patients, particularly adults, who may have poor parasternal and subcostal acoustic

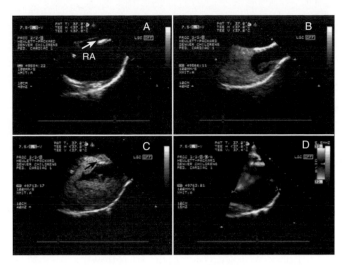

ECHO. 9-2. Transesophageal longitudinal view of the atria, emphasizing the atrial septum and right superior vena cava. **A:** Anatomic view. The *arrow* points to the flap of the foramen ovale. **B:** Peripheral venous contrast injection performed with the patient on room air. The right atrium is filled completely. Note the negative contrast of the superior vena caval inflow. No right-to-left shunting is seen. **C:** Peripheral venous contrast injection with the patient breathing 17% oxygen. The right atrium fills and there is right-to-left interatrial shunting. **D:** Color Doppler flow mapping of the right-to-left shunt. *RA*, right atrium.

windows (37). Commonly, peripheral venous contrast injections with and without Valsalva's maneuver or hypoxia are performed to establish definitively the presence of right-to-left shunting (38–40) (Echo. 9-2; see color plate 9 following p. 364). Van Hare and Silverman (40) found that 37% of 127 children tested had right-to-left shunting across a patent foramen ovale following a peripheral venous contrast injection.

Ostium Secundum Atrial Septal Defects

Ostium secundum atrial septal defects are the most common type of atrial communications, with an incidence of 62% to 78.7% among all atrial defects (2,22,41–43). These types of communications should be considered true atrial septal defects, as they are located within the anatomic limits of the true septum separating the right and left atria (3,23,44–46). They are found in the midportion of the interatrial septum, in the region of the fossa ovalis, and can include parts of the fossa ovalis itself (Fig. 9-1). As a result, the fossa ovalis can have one or multiple defects, or be totally absent. Very large defects can also extend to the adjacent atrial septum, resulting in a functional common atrium (22).

The proportion of connective tissue within the septum primum, which forms the floor or valve of the foramen ovale, increases progressively after birth (25), making it somewhat flaccid. This may allow a small amount of

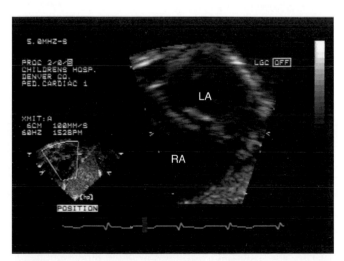

ECHO. 9-1. Subcostal view demonstrating the two components of the flap of the foramen ovale, the septum primum on the left and the septum secundum on the right. *LA*, left atrium; *RA*, right atrium.

shunting across a small defect of the fossa ovalis in infants with dilatation of the left atrium (23,47–49). Becker and Anderson (23) suggest that the flap of the valve of the fossa ovalis in these cases with left atrial dilatation can be stretched, and they therefore call this type of defect a fossa ovalis defect directly secondary to stretch.

The echocardiographic views that permit identification of an ostium secundum or fossa ovalis defect are primarily the subcostal four-chamber and short-axis views, which can be complemented by the parasternal short-axis and to a more limited extent by the apical four-chamber views. The subcostal views are the most useful, both for anatomic imaging and for demonstration of the flow by spectral and color Doppler, as the ultrasound beam is directly perpendicular to the atrial septum from this window (50–53) (Echo. 9-3; see color plate 10 following p. 364). It is important to sweep the transducer inferiorly and superiorly to visualize the entire atrial septum and rule out additional jets from a fenestrated defect or from associated defects located in other parts of the atrial septum (Echo. 9-4; see color plate 11 following p. 364). Rotation of the transducer to a short-axis or sagittal view of the atria also provides an excellent view of the septum and the systemic venous return (Echo. 9-5). In the apical four-chamber and parasternal short-axis views, the ultrasound beam is parallel to the atrial septum; consequently, there is commonly a false dropout of echoes from the atrial septum, especially in the area of the fossa ovalis, so care must be taken not to falsely diagnose atrial defects seen exclusively from these views (35,36,54). Nonetheless, these views permit definition of the relationship of the defect to the atrioventricular valves. Ostium secundum defects are far from the insertion of the mitral and tricuspid valves (Echo. 9-6; see color plate 12 following p. 364).

Even though only 3% of ostium secundum atrial septal defects are associated with anomalous drainage of one or

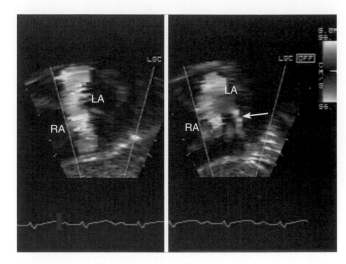

ECHO. 9-4. Color Doppler flow images of a fenestrated atrial septum with left-to-right shunting through several defects. The *arrow* points to one of the smaller defects. *RA*, right atrium; *LA*, left atrium.

more pulmonary veins (3), these should always be identified and the sites of drainage confirmed by the use of spectral and color Doppler. This is best accomplished from the apical and subcostal four-chamber views and from the suprasternal views (Echo. 9-7; see color plate 13 following p. 364).

Sinus Venosus Defects of the Superior Vena Caval Type

Sinus venosus defects of the superior vena caval type occur in 5.3% to 10% of all cases of atrial septal defects (13,22,55). They are located outside the limbus of the

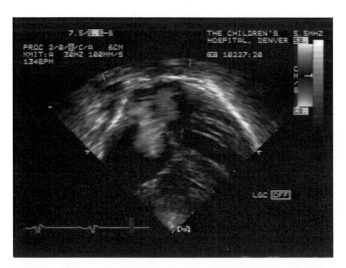

ECHO. 9-3. Color Doppler flow image from a subcostal long-axis view illustrating left-to-right shunting across an ostium secundum atrial septal defect.

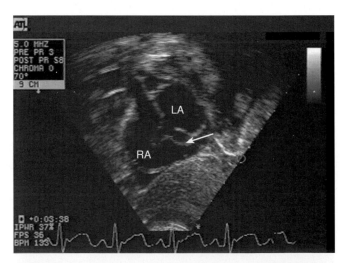

ECHO. 9-5. Subcostal sagittal view of the atria demonstrating a large aneurysmal atrial septum bulging from left to right (*arrow*). The effective defect is at the tip of the aneurysm. The superior and inferior venae cavae are seen connecting into the right atrium. *LA*, left atrium; *RA*, right atrium.

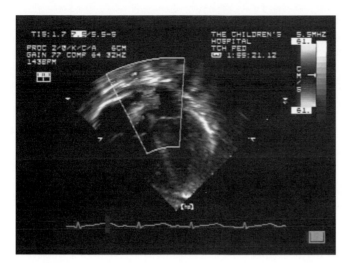

ECHO. 9-6. Apical four-chamber view demonstrating left-to-right shunting through an ostium secundum atrial septal defect. Note that the defect is far from the insertion of the tricuspid and mitral valves.

fossa ovalis, on the right septal surface adjacent to the drainage site of the superior vena cava (Fig. 9-1). This portion of the right atrial septal surface is not true atrial septum but rather an infolding of the roof of the atrium (21,44) that separates the superior vena cava from the right upper pulmonary vein. From an embryologic standpoint, these defects would not be considered true atrial septal defects (3,44,45). The superior vena cava usually overrides the defect (3,22,45), and commonly anomalies of pulmonary venous return are present (2,3,14,21,22,56).

The echocardiographic study of this type of defect is best accomplished from the subcostal approach (36,54,

56). Because the defect is located superiorly, it is necessary to sweep the transducer up from the standard four-chamber view to see the posterior wall of the right atrium and the drainage area of the superior vena cava. The transducer should also be rotated to a short axis and angled superiorly in a sagittal cut to image the superior vena cava overriding the defect and the site of connection of the right upper pulmonary vein (Echo. 9-8; see color plate 14 following p. 364). Sinus venosus defects of the superior vena caval type are also well demonstrated from the right infraclavicular sagittal view with the transducer aimed slightly to the left.

The sites of drainage of the four pulmonary veins must always be confirmed. This is best accomplished through four-chamber views from the apical and subcostal windows as well as through the suprasternal short-axis view. Flows from the four pulmonary veins should be sampled with pulsed-wave Doppler and color flow mapping to confirm their drainage; relying on two-dimensional anatomic imaging alone can sometimes be misleading (Echo. 9-9; see color plate 15 following p. 364).

Sinus Venosis Defects of the Inferior Vena Caval Type

Sinus venosus defects of the inferior vena caval type are very rare and make up only 2% of all atrial septal defects (42). These are located outside the limbus of the fossa ovalis, on the right atrial septal surface adjacent to the drainage site of the inferior vena cava (Fig. 9-1). From the embryologic standpoint, these also are not considered true defects of the atrial septum (3,44). Levoposition of the inferior vena cava with overriding of the defect (22) and anomalies of pulmonary venous drainage have been reported (14,22,32,44).

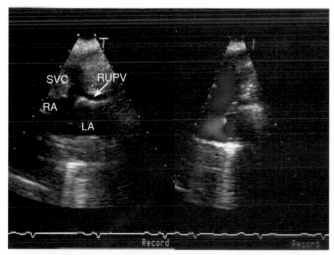

ECHO. 9-7. Suprasternal view tilted toward the superior vena cava demonstrating anomalous drainage of the right upper pulmonary vein at the junction of the right superior vena cava and right atrium. The color Doppler image also shows the superior vena caval inflow (*blue*) and the left-to-right atrial shunt (*red*). SVC, superior vena cava; RA, right atrium; LA, left atrium; RUPV, right upper pulmonary vein.

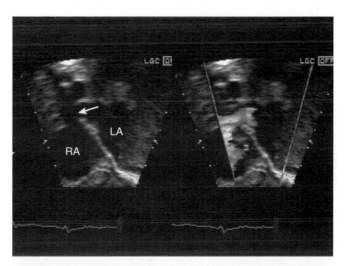

ECHO. 9-8. Anatomic and color flow image from the subcostal sagittal projection of the atrial septum demonstrating left-to-right shunting across a sinus venosus defect of the superior vena caval type (*arrow*). RA, right atrium; LA, left atrium.

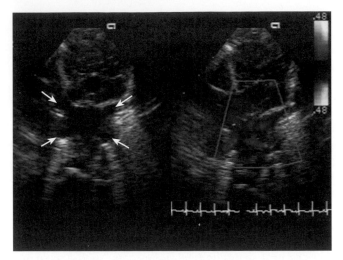

ECHO. 9-9. Suprasternal short-axis view of the four pulmonary veins connecting to the left atrium (*arrows*).

Echocardiographically, these defects are best seen from the subcostal views, starting with the four-chamber view and rotating the transducer approximately 90 degrees until the mouth of the inferior vena cava is seen, with the defect at its junction with the right atrium (57) (Echo. 9-10). The drainage sites of the four pulmonary veins should be confirmed with echocardiography as outlined above.

Common or Single Atrium

A common or single atrium implies complete absence of the interatrial septum. Usually, only a slight remnant is present on the posterior wall of the common chamber. This malformation is frequently associated with the heterotaxy syndromes (33) and with the Ellis-van Creveld syndrome (2,10,11). Echocardiographically, it is rela-

tively easy to demonstrate a virtually complete absence of the atrial septum. The parasternal short-axis view at the base, the apical and subcostal four-chamber views, and the subcostal short-axis view should all be diagnostic. The posterior septal remnant, if present, can also be seen from these projections (Echo. 9-11).

Atrial Septal Defects of the Coronary Sinus Type

An atrial septal defect of the coronary sinus type, also called unroofed coronary sinus, is a defect in the wall that separates the coronary sinus from the left atrium, which can be either fenestrated or totally absent (16–23). In the anatomic sense, it is not strictly speaking a defect in the atrial septum but rather a defect in the wall that separates the left atrium from the coronary sinus in the normal heart; an interatrial communication is the result. It is separated from the atrioventricular valve by a remnant of tissue (Fig. 9-1). It can occur as an isolated defect (18,20,34) or be associated with persistence of the left superior vena cava, which drains directly into the roof of the left atrium or into the coronary sinus (16,17,19,58). Echocardiographically, the views to demonstrate these defects would be those from which the coronary sinus is seen, most typically the four-chamber views (apical and subcostal), with the transducer angled posteriorly beyond the plane of the atrioventricular valves (54,59) (Echo. 9-12A). The coronary sinus may appear dilated if there is drainage of a persistent left superior vena cava. The parasternal long-axis view can also be used to visualize the coronary sinus and a defect in its wall (Echo. 9-12B). However, care must be taken in interpreting this view, as false echo dropouts in this region can lead to an erroneous diagnosis.

ECHO. 9-10. Subcostal sagittal view of the atria demonstrating a large sinus venosus defect of the inferior vena caval type. *RA*, right atrium; *LA*, left atrium.

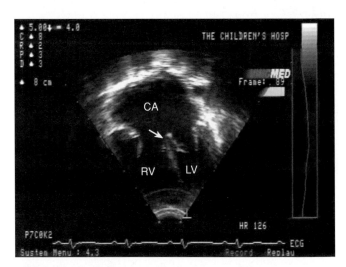

ECHO. 9-11. Apical four-chamber view of a single atrium. The *arrow* points to the atrioventricular septum, which causes the atrioventricular valves to insert at different levels.

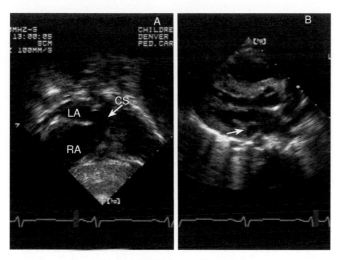

ECHO. 9-12. Echocardiogram of a patient with an atrial septal defect of the coronary sinus type (unroofed coronary sinus). The *arrows* point to the defect. **A:** Subcostal four-chamber view. **B:** Parasternal long-axis view. *LA*, left atrium; *RA*, right atrium; *CS*, coronary sinus.

Simple Ostium Primum Atrial Septal Defects

Simple ostium primum atrial septal defects are extremely rare; they were first described by Keith (60) and later by Goor and Lillehei (22) and Gosta Davidsen (24). These are located in the site corresponding to the embryologic ostium primum, adjacent to the septal leaflet of the mitral valve (Fig. 9-1). They are differentiated from a partial atrioventricular septal defect, ostium primum type, by the presence of the atrioventricular septum and normal atrioventricular valves, which insert at different levels.

Echocardiographically, the best views to locate these defects and determine their relationship to the atrioventricular septum and atrioventricular valves are the four-chamber views, both subcostal and apical, with the transducer swept from the crux cordis posteriorly and slowly anteriorly through the plane of the atrioventricular valves to the outflow tract of the left ventricle. The defect would be found on the lower portion of the atrial septum, adjacent to the septal leaflet of the mitral valve, which would have a normal insertion slightly superior to that of the septal leaflet of the tricuspid valve owing to the presence of a normal atrioventricular septum (Echo. 9-13).

Estimation of Defect Size

Defect size should be estimated and the hemodynamic consequences assessed. Anatomic sizing of the defect is important because of its implication for spontaneous closure (61–63). Recently, Radzik et al. (62) found that for atrial shunts, presumably of the ostium secundum type, diagnosed in the first 3 months of life, the incidence of spontaneous closure within 18 months was as follows:

100% for those measuring less than 3 mm, 87% for those 3 to 5 mm, 80% for those 5 to 8 mm, and no spontaneous closure for defects larger than 8 mm.

In newborn infants, shunting at the atrial level can be caused by a stretched valve of the foramen ovale, particularly in association with a patent ductus arteriosus and increased left atrial pressure and volume. In these instances, an aneurysm of the septum primum is often found bulging alternately into the right atrium and left atrium at different points in the cardiac cycle. These atrial shunts usually disappear after closure of the patent ductus and a lowering of left atrial pressure.

Small atrial septal defects have little if any hemodynamic consequences; therefore, the cardiac cavities are of normal size and the septal motion is also normal. In the presence of medium-sized and larger defects, the left-to-right shunting causes a volume overload of the right-sided cavities, which manifests as dilatation of the right atrium and ventricle (64) and of the pulmonary artery. The motion of the ventricular septum is also affected by the volume overload; it exhibits a flattened or frankly paradoxical motion (65–67). The abnormal systolic and diastolic septal motion can best be evaluated through M-mode traces derived from a short-axis, two-dimensional echocardiographic view at the level of the tips of the papillary muscles (67) (Echo. 9-14). This abnormal motion of the septum is not specifically caused by an atrial septal defect; rather, it is an indirect sign of right ventricular volume overload and can be seen with other lesions, such as tricuspid and/or pulmonary valve regurgitation and anomalous pulmonary venous return to the right atrium, and even postoperatively (68). Recently, Vincent et al. (69) and Vogel et al. (70) have suggested that the abnormal septal motion seen in patients with atrial septal

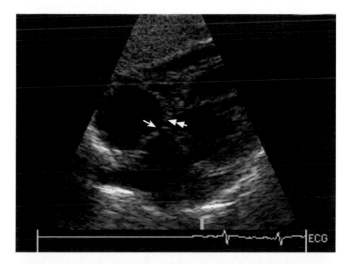

ECHO. 9-13. Subcostal four-chamber view of the atria in the presence of a simple ostium primum atrial septal defect. *Single arrow* points to the defect. *Double arrow* points to the atrioventricular septum, which is intact in this patient, so that the atrioventricular valves insert at different levels.

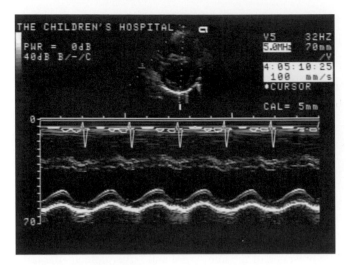

ECHO. 9-14. M-mode echocardiogram demonstrating paradoxical septal motion caused by right ventricular volume overload in the presence of an atrial septal defect.

defects is not related to a volume overload of the right side of the heart but is rather caused by an exaggerated anterior motion of the left ventricle (69) or of the entire heart relative to the fixed reference point of the M-mode recording line (70).

The dynamics of flow and resulting velocity patterns across atrial defects can be recorded with pulsed-wave Doppler, color flow mapping, and color M-mode traces. Usually, this is best accomplished for most atrial defects from the subcostal views, although in some older children and adults with poor subcostal windows, a parasternal short-axis view at the base can also allow fairly parallel positioning of the Doppler sample volume along the direction of flow. Left-to-right flow starts in early ventricular systole, peaks in late systole, and continues through diastole, with a second, smaller peak appearing in late diastole (atrial systole). Lin et al. have observed that even in predominantly left-to-right atrial shunts, there are short periods of right-to-left shunting during early ventricular systole or early ventricular diastole (71). Timing events can be best demonstrated with color M-mode and spectral Doppler tracings, which have a much better time resolution than two-dimensional color flow mapping (Echo. 9-15).

Several methods have been proposed for the estimation of shunt size, mostly related to the calculation of pulmonary and systemic flow ratios (72–76).

A simple and moderately accurate method of calculating shunt size in atrial defects involves estimation of the pulmonary-to-systemic flow ratio ($Qp{:}Qs$) through a combination of two-dimensional imaging and spectral Doppler techniques. Pulmonary blood flow is obtained by measuring the anatomic diameter of the main pulmonary artery and recording the velocity of flow at the same site, usually from a parasternal short-axis view. The vessel diameter is converted to area $[\pi(d/2)^2]$ and multiplied by

the velocity time integral (*VTI*) of the Doppler velocity curve to obtain the pulmonary artery stroke volume. Systemic blood flow is determined by measuring the ascending aorta and performing similar calculations. The aortic diameter is obtained from the parasternal long-axis view and the Doppler curves from the apical long-axis or outflow view. The ratio of the Doppler-calculated pulmonary blood flow to systemic blood flow provides an estimation of shunt size. The main drawback of this method involves errors in measurement of the anatomic diameter of the vessels, particularly of the pulmonary artery; these result from difficulties in imaging the outer vessel wall, especially in older children and adults. Errors may be compounded when the blood flow ratios are calculated. These methods are explained in detail in Chapter 6.

Pulmonary hypertension caused by shunting at the atrial level is rare in pediatric patients, but cases have been reported in infants and children (77–79) and in patients under 20 years of age living at altitudes over 4,000 ft (80). For these reasons, a complete evaluation of patients with atrial shunting should include attempts at estimating pulmonary arterial pressures (81–83). This can be accomplished most directly through measurement of the velocity of the tricuspid regurgitant jet, if present, and indirectly through calculation of the ratio of pulmonary acceleration time to ejection time (*AT:ET*), derived from the forward pulmonary artery velocity curves recorded with pulsed-wave Doppler. The size of the right ventricular wall and cavity, the thickness and motion of the interventricular septum, and the motion of the remaining atrial septum can serve as signs of increased right ventricular pressure and therefore of pulmonary arterial pressure in the absence of significant pulmonic valve stenosis. A

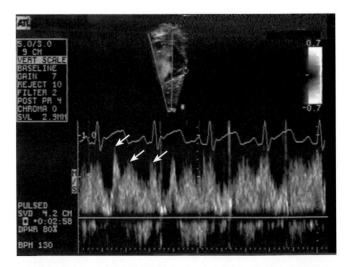

ECHO. 9-15. Spectral Doppler trace of the left-to-right flow across an atrial septal defect. *Arrows* point to the various timing events. The *first arrow* points to the shunt during early ventricular systole. The *second arrow* to the shunt during late systole. The *third arrow* indicates the shunt at atrial systole (a wave).

more detailed description of the methods to evaluate pulmonary artery pressure is given in Chapter 35.

Associated Anomalies

Atrial septal defects can exist as isolated lesions or in association with other cardiac pathologies, such as partial anomalous drainage of the pulmonary or systemic veins (see above), ventricular septal defects, patent ductus arteriosus, aortic coarctation, pulmonic stenosis, and atrioventricular septal defects. Prolapse of the mitral valve is found in 17% of cases of ostium secundum defects (84). In other, more complex cardiac anomalies, such as tricuspid atresia, complete transposition of the great arteries, and total anomalous pulmonary venous drainage, the atrial communication permits shunting, which is essential for survival. These are considered in the corresponding specific chapters.

INTRAOPERATIVE AND POSTOPERATIVE EVALUATION

We do not routinely perform intraoperative evaluation of simple, isolated atrial septal defects of the ostium secundum type in children at our institution. When the defects occur in adults or are found in more unusual locations, such as defects of the sinus venosus or coronary sinus type, intraoperative imaging may be performed, most commonly through a transesophageal approach (85–89). In these cases, the objectives of the study are to supplement the information obtained transthoracically, and special attention should be given to confirming the anatomic location and size of the defect, documenting

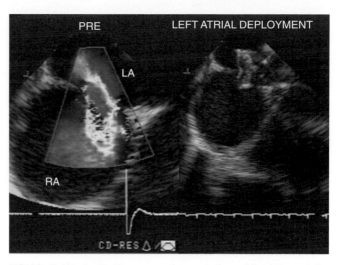

ECHO. 9-17. **Left:** Transesophageal view of the left-to-right shunt across an atrial septal defect immediately before deployment of a closure device under echocardiographic guidance. **Right:** View of the closure device as it is deployed through the left atrium. *RA*, right atrium; *LA*, left atrium.

the pulmonary and systemic venous return, and assessing ventricular function. Direction of shunting and drainage of the veins are confirmed with the adjunctive use of pulsed-wave and color flow Doppler.

The atrial septum is best seen transesophageally with the endoscope behind the left atrium and slightly withdrawn (see Fig. 4-30). Rotation from 0 to 120 degrees permits examination in the transverse and longitudinal planes (see Fig. 4-30A–D). Retroflexing and aiming the transducer toward the left atrium from the transverse four-chamber view is particularly useful to image coronary sinus defects (Echo. 9-16; see color plate 16 following p. 364). The transverse basal short-axis view, which is obtained by anteflexion and slight withdrawal of the trans-

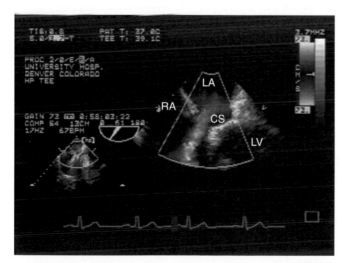

ECHO. 9-16. Transesophageal color Doppler image of the left-to-right flow across an atrial septal defect of the coronary sinus type. The endoscope must be retroflexed to image this portion of the atrial septum clearly. *LA*, left atrium; *RA*, right atrium; *CS*, coronary sinus; *LV*, left ventricle.

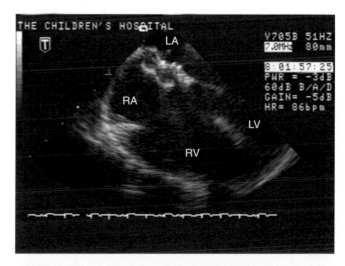

ECHO. 9-18. View of the device positioned on both sides of the atrial defect after deployment. *RA*, right atrium; *LA*, left atrium; *RV*, right ventricle; *LV*, left ventricle.

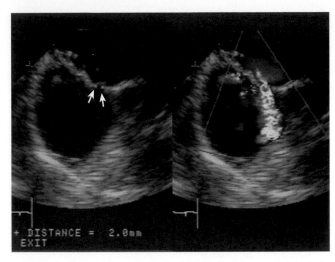

ECHO. 9-19. Transesophageal view of a tiny residual left-to-right shunt at the bottom edge of the closure device. *Arrows* point to the edges of the residual defect, which measured 2 mm.

ducer from a four-chamber orientation, is also useful to examine the atrial septum and the systemic and pulmonary veins (see Echos. 4-20, 4-21). Occasionally, all four pulmonary veins cannot be obtained transesophageally because of lack of resolution in the very near field; therefore, it is important that these be identified preoperatively from the transthoracic approach.

The evaluation immediately after bypass, if indicated, should address ventricular function, best assessed from transgastric views, and document the presence of any residual defects.

Closure of atrial septal defects through catheter deployment of devices has been possible for years. Usually, deployment in the cardiac catheterization laboratory is carried out under transesophageal echocardiographic guidance (Echos. 9-17, 9-18; see color plate 17 following p. 364). Echocardiographic criteria for successful deployment include the presence of tissue above and below the defect and a defect length of less than 15 mm as assessed from both the horizontal and longitudinal views. Residual defects, if present, are usually small and commonly seen at the bottom edge of the device (Echo. 9-19; see color plate 18 following p. 364).

The late follow-up of isolated atrial defects should be aimed mostly at documenting recovery of normal size and function of the right ventricle and return to normal ventricular septal motion.

REFERENCES

1. Fyler DC. Atrial septal defect secundum. In: Fyler DC, ed. *Nadas' pediatric cardiology.* Philadelphia: Hanley & Belfus, 1992:513–524.
2. Olsen EGJ. Atrial septal defects. In: Olsen EGJ, ed. *The pathology of the heart.* New York: Intercontinental Medical Book Corporation, 1973:113–119.
3. Beerman LB, Zuberbuhler FR. Atrial septal defect. In: Anderson RH, Macartney FJ, Shinebourne EA, Tynan M, eds. *Paediatric cardiology,* Vol 1. Edinburgh: Churchill Livingstone, 1987:541–562.
4. De la Cruz MV, Cayre R. Desarrollo embriologico del corazon y de las grandes arterias. In: Sanchez PA, ed. *Cardiologia pediatrica, clinica y cirugia,* Vol 1. Barcelona: Editorial Salvat, 1986:10–18.
5. De la Cruz MV, Gimenez-Ribotta M, Saravalli O, Cayre R. The contribution of the inferior endocardial cushion of the atrioventricular canal to cardiac septation and to the development of the atrioventricular valves: study in the chick embryo. *Am J Anat* 1983;166:63–72.
6. Odgers PNB. The formation of the venous valves, the foramen secundum and the septum secundum in the human heart. *J Anat* 1935;69:412–422.
7. Cayre R, Sanchez-Gomez C, Moreno-Rodriguez RA, De la Cruz MV. La teratologia y la epidemiologia en el estudio de los teratogenos ambientales. *Bol Med Hosp Infant Mex* 1992;49:397–403.
8. Holt M, Oram S. Familial heart disease with skeletal malformations. *Br Heart J* 1960;22:236–242.
9. Bizarro RO, Callahan JA, Feldt RH, Kurland LT, Gordon H, Brandenburg RO. Familial atrial septal defect with prolonged atrioventricular conduction. A syndrome showing the autosomal dominant pattern of inheritance. *Circulation* 1970;41:677–683.
10. Nora JJ. Etiologic aspects of heart diseases. In: Adams FH, Emmanouilides GC, Riemenschneider TA, eds. *Moss heart disease in infants, children, and adolescents,* 4th ed. Baltimore: Williams & Wilkins, 1989:15–23.
11. Rose V, Clark E. Etiology of congenital heart disease. In: Freedom RM, Benson LN, Smallhorn JF, eds. *Neonatal heart disease.* London: Springer-Verlag, 1992:3–17.
12. Bedford DE, Sellors TH, Somerville W, Belcher JR, Besterman EMM. Atrial septal defect and its surgical treatment. *Lancet* 1957;1:1255–1261.
13. Bedford DE. The anatomical types of atrial septal defect. Their incidence and clinical diagnosis. *Am J Cardiol* 1960;6:568–574.
14. Edwards JE. Congenital malformations of the heart and great vessels. A. Malformations of the atrial septal complex. In: Gould SE, ed. *Pathology of the heart and blood vessels.* Springfield, IL: Charles C Thomas Publisher, 1968:262–279.
15. Edwards JE, Carey LS, Neufeld HN, Lester RG. Atrial septal defect. In: Edwards JE, Carey LS, Neufeld HN, Lester RG, eds. *Congenital heart disease. Correlation of pathologic anatomy and angiocardiography.* Philadelphia: WB Saunders, 1965:191–207.
16. Raghib G, Ruttenberg HD, Anderson RC, Amplatz K, Adams P Jr, Edwards JE. Termination of left superior vena cava in left atrium, atrial septal defect, and absence of coronary sinus. A developmental complex. *Circulation* 1965;31:906–918.
17. Helseth HK, Peterson CR. Atrial septal defect with termination of left superior vena cava in the left atrium and absence of the coronary sinus. *Ann Thorac Surg* 1974;17:186–192.
18. Rose AG, Beckman CB, Edwards JE. Communication between coronary sinus and left atrium. *Br Heart J* 1974;36:182–185.
19. Bourdillon PD, Foale RA, Somerville J. Persistent left superior vena cava with coronary sinus and left atrial connections. *Eur J Cardiol* 1980;11:227–234.
20. Freedom RM, Culham JAG, Rowe RD. Left atrial to coronary sinus fenestration (partially unroofed coronary sinus). Morphological and angiocardiographic observations. *Br Heart J* 1981;46:63–68.
21. Becker AE, Anderson RH. Atrial septal defects. In: Becker AE, Anderson RH, eds. *Pathology of congenital heart disease. Postgraduate pathology series.* London: Butterworth-Heineman, 1981:67–75.
22. Goor DA, Lillehei CW. Septal defects. In: Goor DA, Lillehei CW, eds. *Congenital malformations of the heart. Embryology, anatomy, and operative considerations.* New York: Grune & Stratton, 1975:103–111.
23. Becker AE, Anderson RH. Atrial septal defects. In: Becker AE, Anderson RH, eds. *Cardiac pathology. An integrated text and colour atlas.* New York: Raven Press, 1982:10.13–10.16.
24. Gosta Davidsen H. Classification and embryological explanation of defects arising in the interatrial septum. In: Gosta Davidsen H, ed.

Atrial septal defect. An investigation into the natural history of a congenital heart disease. Copenhagen: J Jorgensen & Co, 1960: 25–30.

25. Patten BM. The closure of the foramen ovale. *Am J Anat* 1931;48: 19–44.

26. Hagen PT, Scholz DG, Edwards WD. Incidence and size of patent foramen ovale during the first 10 decades of life: an autopsy study of 965 normal hearts. *Mayo Clin Proc* 1984;59:17–20.

27. Vick GW III, Titus JL. Defects of the atrial septum including the atrioventricular canal. In: Garson A Jr, Bricker JT, McNamara DG, eds. *The science and practice of pediatric cardiology*, Vol II. Philadelphia: Lea & Febiger, 1990:1023–1054.

28. De la Cruz MV, Sanchez-Gomez C. Consideraciones embriologicas y anatomicas sobre la septacion cardiaca normal y patologica. I. Septum interauricular. *Bol Med Hosp Infant Mex* 1989;46:198–202.

29. Hudson R. The normal and abnormal inter-atrial septum. *Br Heart J* 1955;17:489–495.

30. Harley HRS. The sinus venosus type of interatrial septal defect. *Thorax* 1958;13:12–27.

31. Shaner RF. The high defect in the atrial septum. *Can Med Assoc J* 1958;78:688–690.

32. McCormack RJM, Pickering D, Smith II. A rare type of atrial septal defect. *Thorax* 1968;23:350–352.

33. Van Mierop LHS, Gessner IH, Schiebler GL. Asplenia and polysplenia syndrome. In Bergsma D, ed. *Birth defects: original article series*, Vol 8. Baltimore: Williams & Wilkins, 1972:74–82.

34. Kirklin JW, Barrat-Boyes BG. Unroofed coronary sinus syndrome. In: Kirklin JW, Barrat-Boyes BG, eds. *Cardiac surgery. Morphology, diagnostic criteria, natural history, techniques, results, and indications*, Vol 1, 2nd ed. New York: Churchill Livingstone, 1993: 683–692.

35. Bierman FZ, Williams RG. Subxiphoid two-dimensional imaging of the interatrial septum in infants and neonates with congenital heart disease. *Circulation* 1979;60:80–90.

36. Shub C, Dimopoulus IN, Seward JB, et al. Sensitivity of two-dimensional echocardiography in the direct visualization of atrial septal defect utilizing the subcostal approach: experience with 154 patients. *J Am Coll Cardiol* 1983;2:127–135.

37. Langholz D, Louie EK, Konstadt SN, Rao TLK, Scanlon PJ. Transesophageal echocardiographic demonstration of distinct mechanisms for right to left shunting across a patent foramen ovale in the absence of pulmonary hypertension. *J Am Coll Cardiol* 1991;18: 1112–1117.

38. Higgins JR, Sundstrom J, Gutman J, Schiller NB. Contrast echocardiography with quantitative Valsalva maneuver to detect patent foramen ovale. *Clin Res* 1982;30:12A (abst).

39. Dubourg O, Bourdarias JP, Farcot JC, et al. Contrast echocardiographic visualization of cough-induced right to left shunt through a patent foramen ovale. *J Am Coll Cardiol* 1984;4:587–594.

40. Van Hare GF, Silverman NH. Contrast two-dimensional echocardiography in congenital heart disease: techniques, indications and clinical utility. *J Am Coll Cardiol* 1989;13:673–686.

41. Keith JD. Atrial septal defect: ostium secundum, ostium primum, and atrioventricularis communis (common av canal). In: Keith JD, Rowe RD, Vlad P, eds. *Heart disease in infancy and childhood*, 3rd ed. New York: Macmillan, 1978:380–404.

42. Vazquez Perez J, Caffarena Raggio JM, Cordovilla Zurdo G. Comunicacion interauricular y drenaje venoso pulmonar anomalo parcial. In: Sanchez PA, ed. *Cardiologia pediatrica, clinica y cirugia*, Vol 1. Barcelona: Salvat Editores, 1986:245–257.

43. Silverman NH. Interatrial communications. In: Silverman NH, ed. *Pediatric echocardiography*. Baltimore: Williams & Wilkins, 1993: 109–121.

44. Soto B, Pacifico AD. Atrial septal defect. In: Soto B, Pacifico AD, eds. *Angiocardiography in congenital heart malformations*. Mount Kisco, NY: Futura Publishing, 1990:93–104.

45. Anderson RH, Ho SY. Tomographic anatomy of the normal and congenitally malformed heart. In: Higgins CB, Silverman NH, Kersting-Sommerhoff BA, Schmidt K, eds. *Congenital heart disease. Echocardiography and magnetic resonance imaging*. New York: Raven Press, 1990:1–35.

46. Sweeney LJ, Rosenquist GC. The normal anatomy of the atrial septum in the human heart. *Am Heart J* 1979;98:194–199.

47. Pagtakhan RD, Hartmann AF Jr, Goldring D, Kissane J. The valve-incompetent foramen ovale. A report on seven infants with left-to-right shunt. *J Pediatr* 1967;71:848–854.

48. Rudolph AM, Mayer FE, Nadas AS, Gross RE. Patent ductus arteriosus. A clinical and hemodynamic study of 23 patients in the first year of life. *Pediatrics* 1958;22:892–904.

49. Zhou TF, Guntheroth WG. Valve-incompetent foramen ovale in premature infants with ductus arteriosus: a Doppler echocardiographic study. *J Am Coll Cardiol* 1987;10:193–199.

50. Swensson RE, Sahn DJ, Valdes-Cruz LM. Color flow Doppler mapping in congenital heart disease. *Echocardiography* 1985;2:545–549.

51. Sherman FS, Sahn DJ, Valdes-Cruz LM, Chung KJ, Elias W, Swensson RE. Two-dimensional Doppler color flow mapping for detecting atrial and ventricular septal defects. *Echocardiography* 1986;3:527–531.

52. Reeder GS, Seward JB, Hagler DJ, Tajik AJ. Color flow imaging in congenital heart disease. *Echocardiography* 1986;3:533–540.

53. Sherman FS, Sahn DJ, Valdes-Cruz LM, Chung KJ, Elias W. Two-dimensional Doppler color flow mapping for detecting atrial and ventricular septal defects. Studies in an animal model and in the clinical setting. *Herz* 1987;12:212–216.

54. Sanders SP. Echocardiography and related techniques in the diagnosis of congenital heart defects. Part I: Veins, atria and interatrial septum. *Echocardiography* 1984;1:185–217.

55. Swan HJC, Kirklin JW, Becu LM, Wood EH. Anomalous connection of right pulmonary veins to superior vena cava with interatrial communications. Hemodynamic data in eight cases. *Circulation* 1957;16:54–66.

56. Nasser FN, Tajik AJ, Seward JB, Hagler DJ. Diagnosis of sinus venosus atrial septal defect by two-dimensional echocardiography. *Mayo Clin Proc* 1981;56:568–572.

57. Higgins CB, Silverman NH, Kersting-Sommerhoff B, Schmidt KG. Left-to-right shunt lesions. In: Higgins CB, Silverman NH, Kersting-Sommerhoff B, Schmidt KG, eds. *Congenital heart disease: Echocardiography and magnetic resonance imaging*. New York: Raven Press, 1990:99–133.

58. Cohen BE, Winer HE, Kronzon I. Echocardiographic findings in patients with left superior vena cava and dilated coronary sinus. *Am J Cardiol* 1979;44:158–161.

59. Yeager SB, Chin AJ, Sanders SP. Subxiphoid two-dimensional echocardiographic diagnosis of coronary sinus septal defects. *Am J Cardiol* 1984;54:686–687.

60. Keith A. The anatomy of valvular mechanism around the venous orifices of the right and left auricles with some observations on the morphology of the heart. *J Anat (Proceeding)* 1903;37:2. Cited by Goor DA, Lillehei CW. Septal defects. In: Goor DA, Lillehei CW, eds. *Congenital malformations of the heart. Embryology, anatomy, and operative considerations*. New York: Grune & Stratton, 1975: 103–111.

61. Brand A, Keren A, Branski D, Abrahamov A, Stern S. Natural course of atrial septal aneurysm in children and the potential for spontaneous closure of associated septal defect. *Am J Cardiol* 1989; 64:996–1001.

62. Radzik D, Davignon A, Van Doesburg N, Fournier A, Marchand T, Ducharme G. Predictive factors for spontaneous closure of atrial septal defects diagnosed in the first 3 months of life. *J Am Coll Cardiol* 1993;22:851–853.

63. Guntheroth W. Spontaneous closure of atrial septal defects [Letter to the Editor]. *J Am Coll Cardiol* 1994;23:828–829.

64. Hanseus K, Bjorkhem G, Lundstrom NR, Soeroso S. Cross-sectional echocardiographic measurement of right atrial and right ventricular size in children with atrial septal defect before and after surgery. *Pediatr Cardiol* 1988;9:231–236.

65. Diamond MA, Dillon JC, Haine CL, Chang S, Feigenbaum H. Echocardiographic features of atrial septal defects. *Circulation* 1971;43:129–135.

66. Tajik AJ, Gau GT, Ritter DG, Schattenberg TT. Echocardiographic pattern of right ventricular diastolic volume overload in children. *Circulation* 1972;46:36–43.

67. Weyman AE, Wann S, Feigembaum H, Dillon JC. Mechanism of abnormal septal motion in patients with right ventricular volume overload: a cross-sectional echocardiographic study. *Circulation* 1976;54:179–186.

68. Kerber R, Doty D. Abnormalities of interventricular septal motion following cardiac surgery. Cross-sectional echocardiographic studies. *Am J Cardiol* 1978;41:372(abst).

69. Vincent RN, Saurette RH, Pelech AN, Collins GF. Interventricular septal motion and left ventricular function in patients with atrial septal defect. *Pediatr Cardiol* 1988;9:143–148.

70. Vogel M, Schulze K, Buhlmeyer K. Assessment of interventricular septal motion by cross-sectional echocardiography in patients with isolated atrial septal defects within the oval fossa. *Cardiol Young* 1992;2:30–34.

71. Lin FC, Fú M, Yeh SJ, Wu D. Doppler atrial shunt flow patterns in patients with secundum atrial septal defect: determinants, limitations and pitfalls. *J Am Soc Echocardiogr* 1988;1:141–149.

72. Sanders SP, Yeager S, Williams RG. Measurement of systemic and pulmonary blood flow and Qp/Qs ratio using Doppler and two-dimensional echocardiography. *Am J Cardiol* 1983;51:952–956.

73. Valdes-Cruz LM, Horowitz S, Mesel E, Sahn DJ, Fisher DC, Larson D. A pulsed Doppler echocardiographic method for calculating pulmonary and systemic blood flow in atrial level shunts: validation studies in animals and initial human experience. *Circulation* 1984; 69:80–86.

74. Vargas Barron J, Sahn DJ, Valdes-Cruz LM, et al. Clinical utility of two-dimensional Doppler echocardiographic techniques for estimating pulmonary to systemic blood flow ratios in children with left to right shunting atrial septal defect, ventricular septal defect or patent ductus arteriosus. *J Am Coll Cardiol* 1984;3:169–178.

75. Kitabatake A, Inoue M, Asao M, et al. Noninvasive evaluation of the ratio of pulmonary to systemic flow in atrial septal defect by duplex Doppler echocardiography. *Circulation* 1984;69:73–79.

76. Cloez JL, Schmidt KG, Birk E, Silverman NH. Determination of pulmonary to systemic blood flow ratio in children by simplified Doppler echocardiographic method. *J Am Coll Cardiol* 1988;11:825–830.

77. Cabezuelo-Huerta G, Vazquez-Perez J, Frontera-Izquierdo P. Comunicacion interauricular con hipertension pulmonar en el lactante. *An Esp Pediatr* 1979;12:105–112.

78. Vazquez-Perez J, Quero M, Ardura J, Rey C, Frontera-Izquierdo P. Atrial septal defect with pulmonary hypertension in infancy. *Pediatr Cardiol* 1980;1:235(abst).

79. Haworth SG. Pulmonary vascular disease in secundum atrial septal defect in chilhood. *Am J Cardiol* 1983;51:265–272.

80. Dalen JE, Haynes FW, Dexter L. Life expectancy with atrial septal defect. Influence of complicating pulmonary vascular disease. *JAMA* 1967;200:442–446.

81. Kitabatake A, Inoue M, Asao M, et al. Noninvasive evaluation of pulmonary hypertension by a pulsed Doppler technique. *Circulation* 1983;68:302–309.

82. Dabestani A, Mahan G, Gardin JM, et al. Evaluation of pulmonary artery pressure and resistance by pulsed Doppler echocardiography. *Am J Cardiol* 1987;59:662–668.

83. Stevenson JG. Comparison of several noninvasive methods for estimation of pulmonary artery pressure. *J Am Soc Echocardiogr* 1989; 2:157–171.

84. Leachman RD, Cokkinos DV, Cooley DA. Association of ostium secundum atrial septal defects with mitral valve prolapse. *Am J Cardiol* 1976;38:167–169.

85. Cyran SE, Kimball TR, Meyer RA, et al. Efficacy of intraoperative transesophageal echocardiography in children with congenital heart disease. *Am J Cardiol* 1989;63:594–598.

86. Stumper OFW, Elzenga NJ, Hess J, Sutherland GR. Transesophageal echocardiography in children with congenital heart disease: an initial experience. *J Am Coll Cardiol* 1990;16:433–441.

87. Ritter SB. Transesophageal echocardiography in children: new peephole to the heart. *J Am Coll Cardiol* 1990;16:447–450.

88. Muhiudeen IA, Roberson DA, Silverman NH, Hass G, Turley K, Cahalan MK. Intraoperative echocardiography in infants and children with congenital cardiac shunt lesions: transesophageal versus epicardial echocardiography. *J Am Coll Cardiol* 1990;16:1687–1695.

89. Ritter SB. Transesophageal real-time echocardiography in infants and children with congenital heart disease. *J Am Coll Cardiol* 1991; 18:569–580.

CHAPTER 10

Ventricular Septal Defects

Lilliam M. Valdes-Cruz and Raul O. Cayre

Isolated ventricular septal defect is the most common type of congenital cardiac defect, excluding bicuspid aortic valve and prolapse of the mitral valve (1). Its incidence varies between 16% and 23% of all congenital heart disease (2–5).

EMBRYOLOGIC CONSIDERATIONS

As with the vast majority of congenital cardiac malformations, multiple etiologic factors contribute to the production of ventricular septal defects (6). These factors act on the embryo to alter one or several of the basic developmental processes, such as movement of cellular populations, cellular multiplication and differentiation, and cellular death (7). These alterations interfere in the normal development of the embryologic components of the heart and consequently in the development of the anatomic structures that originate from these components, resulting in a congenital malformation. Abnormal development of one or more of the embryologic components that contribute to the formation of the ventricular septum is expressed anatomically as ventricular septal defect(s), which can exist in isolation or in association with other congenital defects.

There are two recognizable portions of the interventricular septum: one composed of fibrous tissue, the membranous septum, and one of muscular tissue, the muscular septum (8). The muscular septum in turn has three parts: the inlet septum, which separates the ventricular inflows; the trabecular septum, located between the trabecular portion of both ventricles; and the outlet or infundibular septum, which separates the ventricular outflow tracts (8,9).

The inlet septum is derived from the inferior cushion of the atrioventricular canal and from tissue of the primitive interventricular septum (10–12). The trabecular septum originates from the primitive interventricular septum (13–15). The outlet or infundibular septum has a double embryologic origin; the right septal surface is derived from the dextrodorsal and sinistroventral conal crests (16), and the left septal surface is formed from the superior endocardial cushion (16,17) (see Fig. 1-13). The membranous septum is probably formed from tissue of the inferior endocardial cushion (10,16) (see Fig. 1-13). It corresponds to the point of closure of the secondary interventricular foramen by tissue originating from the inferior endocardial cushion, the primitive interventricular septum, and the dextrodorsal and sinistroventral conal crests (13,18).

The anatomic classification of ventricular septal defects proposed by Soto et al. (19) seems the most appropriate because it defines septal defects according to their location within the different portions of the ventricular septum (8,9) (Fig. 10-1), each of which has a different embryologic origin (10–18).

The term perimembranous ventricular septal defect is appropriate because in the majority of cases, septal defects located in the membranous septum extend to adjacent areas of the muscular septum (19–21). The inferior endocardial cushion and primitive interventricular septum are involved in the morphogenesis of perimembranous defects with inlet extensions and trabecular extensions (11). Abnormal development of the superior and inferior endocardial cushions and of the dextrodorsal and sinistroventral conal crests results in a perimembranous defect with outlet extensions (11).

Greater or lesser degrees of alteration of the embryologic components that form the muscular septum result in muscular ventricular septal defects (Fig. 10-1). As such, an alteration in the inferior endocardial cushion results in an inlet muscular defect. Abnormal development of the primitive interventricular septum results in a midtrabecular or apical defect. Alterations in the formation of the dextrodorsal and sinistroventral conal crests and in the superior cushion of the atrioventricular canal produce an outlet muscular defect (11).

An absence of the outlet septum resulting from an abnormality in the development of the conal crests and the

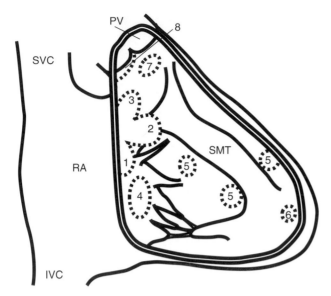

FIG. 10-1. Schematic drawing of the different types of ventricular septal defects. *1*, perimembranous with inlet extension; *2*, perimembranous with trabecular extension; *3*, perimembranous with outlet extension; *4*, inlet muscular; *5*, midtrabecular muscular; *6*, apical muscular; *7*, outlet muscular; *8*, doubly committed. *RA*, right atrium; *SMT*, septomarginal trabeculation; *PV*, pulmonic valve; *SVC*, superior vena cava; *IVC*, inferior vena cava.

septal portion of the superior endocardial cushion gives rise to a subarterial or doubly committed ventricular septal defect (Fig. 10-1). A purely subpulmonary or juxtapulmonary defect is uncommon (22) but probably arises from an abnormal development of the septal portion of the superior cushion of the atrioventricular canal, of the sinistroventral conal crest, and of the primitive interventricular septum.

ANATOMIC AND ECHOCARDIOGRAPHIC CONSIDERATIONS

The echocardiographic study of ventricular septal defects should include the following: (a) determination of the anatomic location of the defect(s), with definition of extension, borders, and relationship to the atrioventricular and semilunar valves; (b) estimation of defect size, recognition of signs of spontaneous closure, and assessment of hemodynamic consequences; (c) assessment of associated anomalies; and (d) intraoperative and postoperative evaluation.

Anatomic Location of Defects; Definition of Extension, Borders, and Relationship to Atrioventricular and Semilunar Valves

The interventricular septum occupies several spatial planes. In the frontal plane, it is convex to the right and

concave to the left; in the transverse plane, it is posterior to anterior, separating both inflow tracts, and then curves toward the front and right, making the outflow tract of the left ventricle. The membranous septum is found in this plane, immediately below the right anterior and the posterior noncoronary aortic cusps. Finally, the ventricular septum curves to the left, almost parallel to the frontal plane, separating the outflow tracts of the ventricles (Fig. 10-2). Because the spatial orientation of the septum varies, ventricular septal defects are located in various spatial planes, and various echocardiographic cuts are required for their visualization.

Perimembranous Ventricular Septal Defects

The membranous septum is one of the components of the ventricular septum (8) and is an integral part of the central fibrous body of the heart (22,23). It constitutes a small portion of the septum; when seen from the left, it is located below the middle posterior part of the right anterior coronary cusp and the posterior noncoronary cusp. The insertion of the septal leaflet of the tricuspid valve on the right side divides the membranous septum in two portions, an atrioventricular portion and an interventricular portion. The interventricular portion separates a part of the outflow tract of the left ventricle from a small part of the inflow of the right ventricle and is covered on the right side by the insertion of the septal leaflet of the tricuspid valve. The interventricular portion of the

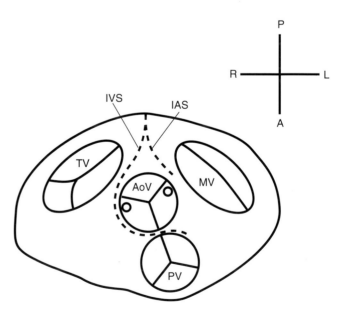

FIG. 10-2. Schematic drawing of the base of the heart illustrating the spatial orientation of the atrial and ventricular septa in the normal heart. *IAS*, interatrial septum; *IVS*, interventricular septum; *TV*, tricuspid valve; *MV*, mitral valve; *AoV*, aortic valve; *PV*, pulmonic valve. *R*, right; *L*, left; *A*, anterior; *P*, posterior.

membranous septum is of variable size, and it can be very small or even completely absent (24).

Perimembranous ventricular septal defects are located in the region of the membranous septum but almost always occupy an area larger than that of the membranous septum alone by extending into the adjacent inlet, trabecular, or outlet muscular septum (19–21,25) (Fig. 10-1); for this reason, they are called perimembranous defects (19). These are the most common type of ventricular septal defect, having an incidence of 60% to 75% of all isolated defects (2,3,26,27). They are adjacent to the central fibrous body of the heart, which comprises the fibrous continuity of the mitral, aortic, and tricuspid valves and includes the atrioventricular component of the membranous septum (28). Although Capelli et al. (29) reserve the term subaortic for defects resulting from malalignment of the infundibular septum with overriding of the aortic valve over the septum, it is important to note that because the aortic annulus is an integral part of the central fibrous body, a portion of the aortic valve forms the roof of all perimembranous septal defects. Therefore, perimembranous ventricular septal defects are necessarily subaortic.

Perimembranous Defects with Inlet Extensions

Perimembranous defects with inlet extensions are located in the membranous septum; the central fibrous body makes up one of the borders, and the major axis of these defects is directed toward the crux cordis (Fig. 10-1). Viewed from the right, the defect is covered by the septal leaflet of the tricuspid valve. The posterior or atrial border is formed by the mitral-tricuspid fibrous continuity; the inferior and anterior borders by the crests of the muscular inlet and trabecular septa; and the superior border by a portion of the infundibular septum anteriorly, which separates the right anterior aortic cusp from the defect, and by the noncoronary aortic cusp posteriorly, which is adjacent to the defect. The location of the medial papillary muscle is anterior and superior to the defect (8,11,19,28). Viewed from the left side, the defect is located under the posterior, noncoronary aortic cusp, which forms part of the roof of the defect (19). Its posterior border is made up of the aortic-mitral-tricuspid fibrous continuity. Its inferior and anterior borders are completely muscular.

These defects have been called isolated ventricular septal defects of the atrioventricular canal type because of their extensions toward the inlet septum (30). This terminology is erroneous from an anatomic standpoint because the atrioventricular septum is present and there is no atrioventricular communication (11). In addition, none of the other morphologic stigmata of atrioventricular septal defects are present, nor is the left-sided atrioventricular valve trileaflet (23,25,31).

Echocardiographically, perimembranous defects with inlet extensions can be visualized from the parasternal

long- and short-axis views and the apical and subcostal four-chamber and outflow views (29,32–35). In all these views, color Doppler flow mapping can be recorded to demonstrate the direction and extension of shunting.

The standard parasternal long-axis view of the left ventricle allows imaging of the trabecular and a portion of the outlet septum. Strictly speaking, neither the membranous nor the inlet muscular septum can be imaged from this position. The transducer has to be tilted slightly to the right and inferiorly toward the right ventricular inflow to demonstrate the membranous septum, where the defect would be seen under the right anterior coronary cusp (Echo. 10-1A, see color plate 19 following p. 364). The parasternal short-axis view, at the level of the aortic valve, allows imaging of the membranous septum and the insertion of the septal leaflet of the tricuspid valve. The defect, located under the right coronary cusp, is covered by the septal leaflet of the tricuspid valve (Echo. 10-1B). From the short-axis view, the transducer can be aimed slightly toward the apex to demonstrate the portion of the septum that separates the right ventricular inlet from the left ventricular outlet, and further to demonstrate the portion that separates both inlets. This scanning permits a limited illustration of the inlet extensions of the defect.

The membranous septum and trabecular septum can be imaged from the apical four-chamber view by tilting the transducer slightly anteriorly toward the left ventricular outflow tract and aortic root. A perimembranous defect can be seen from this projection (Echo. 10-2). Sweeping of the transducer posteriorly toward the crux cordis images the inlet septum in its entirety and allows determination of any inlet extension that may be present. It is important to note that in this projection it becomes clear that the atrioventricular septum is present and

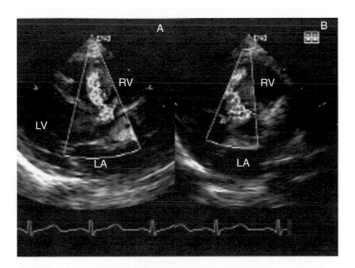

ECHO. 10-1. Echocardiograms demonstrating shunting through a perimembranous ventricular septal defect. **A:** Parasternal long-axis view with the transducer tilted toward the right ventricular inflow. **B:** Parasternal short-axis view. *RV,* right ventricle; *LV,* left ventricle; *LA,* left atrium.

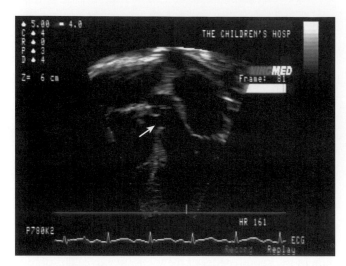

ECHO. 10-2. Apical view with the transducer tilted superiorly toward the left ventricular outflow tract, showing the presence of a perimembranous ventricular septal defect. Note that the aortic valve forms the roof of the defect.

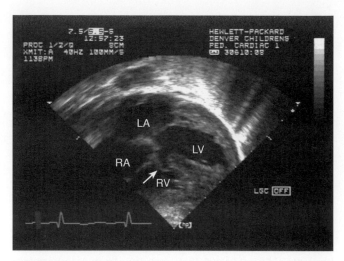

ECHO. 10-4. Subcostal four-chamber view demonstrating the inlet extensions of a perimembranous defect. The defect is covered by the septal leaflet of the tricuspid valve (*arrow*). *LA,* left atrium; *RA,* right atrium; *LV,* left ventricle; *RV,* right ventricle.

that the atrioventricular valves insert at different levels (Echo. 10-3).

The subcostal four-chamber view, similar to that obtained from the apical window, allows a posterior-to-anterior sweep from the crux cordis to the aortic root so that the membranous defect located under the aortic valve and covered by the septal leaflet of the tricuspid valve is seen as well as its inlet extensions (Echo. 10-4). By rotating the transducer 90 degrees and aiming it from the sagittal plane toward the left, the operator can sweep through the various short-axis cuts from the subcostal approach. This will again demonstrate the degree of inlet

extensions of the defect and its location under the septal leaflet of the tricuspid valve.

Perimembranous Defects with Trabecular Extensions

Perimembranous ventricular septal defects with trabecular extensions are located in the region of the membranous septum; the central fibrous body forms one of the borders, and the major axis of the defect is toward the cardiac apex (Fig. 10-1). Viewed from the right, its posterior border is formed by the central fibrous body with a remnant of the membranous atrioventricular septum and is covered by the septal leaflet of the tricuspid valve. Its inferior border is formed by the inlet septum, its anterior border by the trabecular septum at the level of the septo-marginal trabecula, and its superior border by the infundibular septum anteriorly and the noncoronary aortic cusp posteriorly. The medial papillary muscle, which is usually single but occasionally can be multiple (8,11), is located in front of the defect (8,11,19,28). Frequently, the septal leaflet of the tricuspid valve has a cleft at this point (8,11,28). Seen from the left side, its superior border is the noncoronary aortic cusp, which forms the roof of the defect. Its posterior border is the mitral-tricuspid fibrous continuity. The inferior and anterior borders are completely muscular, and the infundibular septum separates the right anterior aortic cusp from the defect.

The echocardiographic views that allow study of these defects are the same as those previously mentioned for defects with inlet extensions. However, the cuts that permit a better visualization of the trabecular septum are emphasized in this section.

The parasternal long-axis view tilted slightly toward the right ventricular inflow shows the defect immediately

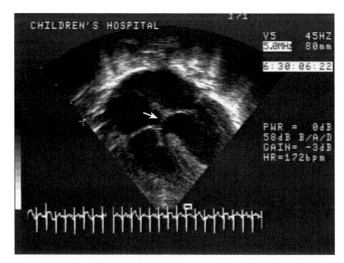

ECHO. 10-3. Four-chamber view with the transducer swept posteriorly toward the crux cordis. This image demonstrates the extensions of a perimembranous defect toward the inlet septum. The *arrow* points to the atrioventricular septum, which is intact, so that the atrioventricular valves insert at different levels.

below the right coronary aortic cusp in the region of the membranous septum. The extension of the defect toward the trabecular septum can be appreciated from the standard parasternal long-axis plane (Echo. 10-5; see color plate 20 following p. 364). The parasternal short-axis view at the level of the great vessels shows the defect under the right coronary cusp covered by the tricuspid leaflet. Its trabecular extensions are visualized by sweeping the transducer slowly toward the apex. Because the inlet and trabecular septa are located in the same plane of incidence of the ultrasound beam, the precise extensions of the defect, whether toward the inlet or toward the trabecular septum, cannot be determined from this particular view.

The apical and subcostal four-chamber views, with the transducer angled superiorly toward the left ventricular outlet and inferiorly toward the crux cordis, best define the defect underneath the aortic valve and its trabecular extensions.

Perimembranous Defects with Outlet Extensions

Perimembranous ventricular septal defects with outlet extensions are located at the level of the membranous septum. The central fibrous body forms one of the borders, and the major axis of these defects is toward the semilunar valves (Fig. 10-1). Viewed from the right side, the defect is located below the noncoronary cusp and below a portion of the right coronary cusp, both of which form its roof. The superior part of its anterior border is composed of the infundibular septum, which is often poorly developed. The inferior part of the anterior border and the inferior border are comprised of the trabecular septum and the septomarginal trabecula. The fibrous mitral-tricuspid continuity forms the posterior border of the defect. The medial papillary muscle is below the communication (8,11,19,36). Seen from the left side, the superior border is formed by the posterior noncoronary cusp and the posterior portion of the right anterior coronary cusp; the anterior border of the defect is the infundibular septum, which separates it from the anterior portion of the right coronary cusp. Both the anterior and inferior borders of the defect are completely muscular. The posterior border of the defect is formed by the central fibrous body.

Defects with outlet extensions are sometimes accompanied by prolapse of one of the aortic cusps, most commonly the right anterior coronary cusp, although the noncoronary cusp can also be involved (8,25,37,38). In these cases, the prolapsed cusp obstructs the defect, which can appear hemodynamically smaller. It is important to point out that prolapse of the aortic valve is progressive, eventually resulting in permanent damage to the aortic valve and aortic regurgitation, which is also progressive. Therefore, these defects should always be closed surgically, even though hemodynamically they may be small.

The echocardiographic cuts to visualize these defects are similar to those mentioned previously for the other types of perimembranous defects. The parasternal long-axis position with the transducer tilted toward the right-sided inflow shows the defect covered by the tricuspid leaflet. In these cases, however, the transducer should be swept from the inflow view through the standard long-axis view and leftward toward the outflow of the right ventricle to demonstrate the outlet extensions of the defect. This view also reveals prolapse of an aortic cusp if present (Echo. 10-6). The parasternal short-axis view at the level of the aortic valve is the best to demonstrate the

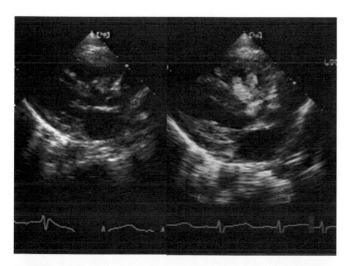

ECHO. 10-5. Parasternal long-axis view demonstrating a perimembranous defect with extension toward the trabecular septum.

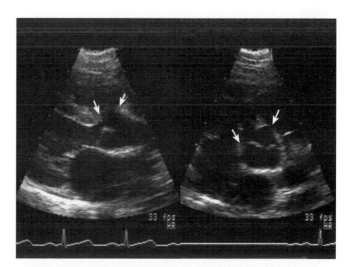

ECHO. 10-6. Parasternal long- and short-axis views demonstrating the presence of a perimembranous ventricular septal defect with extensions toward the outlet septum. There is prolapse of the right coronary cusp through the defect. *Arrows* point to the limits of the defect covered by the prolapsing aortic cusp.

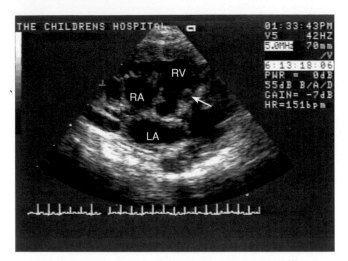

ECHO. 10-7. Short-axis parasternal view tilted leftward toward the right ventricular outflow tract to demonstrate the extensions of a perimembranous defect toward the outlet septum. The *arrow* points to the infundibular septum, which is intact. *RA*, right atrium; *RV*, right ventricle; *LA*, left atrium.

extensions toward the outlet septum (Echo. 10-7). The defect is seen under the septal leaflet of the tricuspid valve and extends toward the right ventricular outflow as the transducer is rotated leftward. It is important to attempt to visualize the entire length of the outlet septum by sweeping the transducer anteriorly, superiorly, and leftward from the plane of the aortic valve toward that of the pulmonary valve.

From the subcostal four-chamber view with the transducer aimed toward the aortic root, the defect can be observed immediately below the aortic valve and covered by the septal leaflet of the tricuspid valve. Because the outlet septum is almost parallel to the direction of the ultrasound beam in this view, the transducer should be rotated 90 degrees to a short axis to image the outflow tract of the right ventricle. From this projection, the defect can be seen extending in the direction of the pulmonic valve.

Muscular Ventricular Septal Defects

Muscular ventricular septal defects are characterized by the fact that all borders are muscular. They are classified according to their location in the various parts of the muscular ventricular septum as inlet muscular, trabecular muscular, and outlet muscular defects (19) (Fig. 10-1). They can occur singly or as multiple defects, which may be located within the same or different parts of the muscular septum. The incidence varies between 15% and 25% of all isolated ventricular septal defects (2,3,26,27).

Muscular Defects of the Inlet Septum

Muscular defects of the inlet septum are located within the portion of the ventricular septum that separates the inflow tracts of the ventricles (Fig. 10-1). Viewed from the right, the defect is underneath the septal leaflet of the tricuspid valve, and occasionally tendinous cords can be seen crossing in front of the defect and inserting directly on the right septal surface. It is separated from the fibrous annulus of the tricuspid valve by muscular tissue. The major axis of the defect is directed toward the crux cordis and therefore is perpendicular to the major axis of the heart (Fig. 10-1). These defects have also been named posterior (39–41) or juxtacrux (22) ventricular septal defects, and they can extend toward the areas adjacent to the posterior ventricular wall (41). Seen from the left side, they are located under the septal portion of the anterior mitral leaflet and separated from the mitral annulus by muscular tissue belonging to the inlet septum and the atrioventricular septum.

It is important to differentiate these defects from perimembranous defects with inlet extensions and from atrioventricular septal defects. They are different from perimembranous defects in that (a) the rim is totally muscular, (b) the central fibrous body does not form any of the borders, and (c) these defects never extend toward the membranous septum, which is always intact. They are differentiated from atrioventricular septal defects in that (a) the atrioventricular septum is always present, (b) the atrioventricular valves are at different levels, and (c) no other anatomic stigmata of an atrioventricular septal defect are present (42).

The parasternal long-axis view does not demonstrate these types of defects because the inlet septum is not seen from this perspective. In the rare cases in which an associated membranous defect might be present, such as in the case reported by Becu et al. (20), the membranous defect would be seen from this projection under the aortic valve by tilting the transducer slightly toward the inflow of the right ventricle, as described previously. In most instances, however, the membranous septum is intact. In the parasternal short-axis view, a scan from the base to the apex can demonstrate the inlet septal defect (Echo. 10-8; see color plate 21 following p. 364).

The apical four-chamber view in a scan beginning posteriorly at the crux cordis and sweeping toward the aortic outflow more anteriorly would show the inlet muscular defect. From this same view, the intact membranous septum can also be seen, and no relationship between the defect and the aortic valve can be established. The insertion of the atrioventricular valve leaflets at different levels and the muscular tissue separating this defect from the tricuspid valve would also serve to confirm the diagnosis of muscular septal defect of the inlet type (Echo. 10-9). The subcostal views also permit a similar posterior-to-anterior scan.

Muscular Defects of the Trabecular Septum

Muscular defects of the trabecular septum are also completely bordered by muscular tissue and can be located

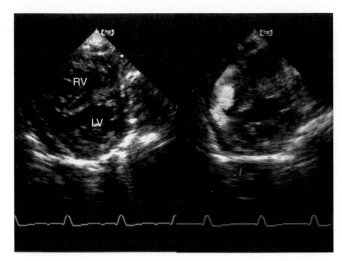

ECHO. 10-8. Short-axis view of the ventricles demonstrating the presence of a large ventricular septal defect in the muscular inlet septum. RV, right ventricle; LV, left ventricle.

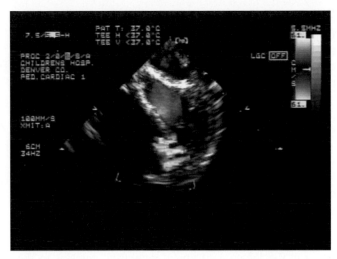

ECHO. 10-10. Color Doppler flow map obtained from a transesophageal horizontal view demonstrating left-to-right shunting across multiple small ventricular septal defects of the apical portion of the trabecular septum.

in any portion of the trabecular septum (Fig. 10-1). Those located in the midportion of the trabecular septum, classified as central or medial defects (22,29,41), are related to the septomarginal trabecula, can be in a location anterior or posterior to the moderator band, and can be single or multiple. If they are located more anteriorly, toward the cardiac apex, they are called apical (22,29) or marginal (41) (Fig. 10-1). If multiple small defects are seen, the term "Swiss cheese" defect has been used (Echo. 10-10; see color plate 22 following p. 364). Defects in the trabecular septum are frequently associated with additional defects in the perimembranous septum (8).

The echocardiographic study of trabecular defects should consider the anatomic characteristics of the sep-

tum, the spatial position of the trabecular septum, and the fact that these defects are often multiple. Therefore, a careful sweep of the ventricular septum should always be performed from all views (29,31–35).

The standard parasternal long-axis view, modified by tilting the transducer leftward toward the outflow of the right ventricle and rightward toward its inflow, scans the medial and apical portions of the interventricular septum and demonstrates the defect(s) in these areas, whether adjacent to the anterior or posterior ventricular wall (Echo. 10-11; see color plate 23 following p. 364). The parasternal and subcostal short-axis views, with scanning from apex to base, can also show trabecular muscular defects. In cases in which the defects are too small to

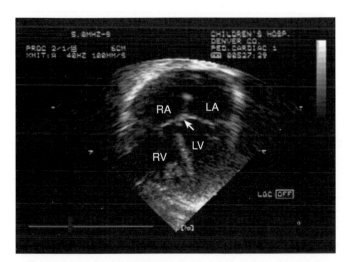

ECHO. 10-9. Four-chamber apical view at the level of the atrioventricular valves demonstrating the presence of a defect of the muscular inlet septum. The *arrow* points to the atrioventricular septum. RA, right atrium; LA, left atrium; RV, right ventricle; LV, left ventricle.

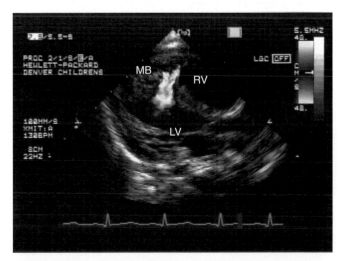

ECHO. 10-11. Parasternal long-axis view demonstrating the left-to-right shunt across a defect of the muscular trabecular ventricular septum adjacent to the moderator band. RV, right ventricle; LV, left ventricle; MB, moderator band.

be appreciated by two-dimensional imaging alone, color Doppler can aid in their recognition, particularly from these views. A careful sweep from apex to base with color Doppler can demonstrate defects(s) in the posterior portion of the septum adjacent to the posterior ventricular wall, in the middle portion of the septum, or in the anterior portion adjacent to the anterior ventricular wall (Echo. 10-12; see color plate 24 following p. 364).

The apical and subcostal four-chamber and outflow views with slow scanning from an inferior or posterior to an anterior or superior position also permit examination of the entire trabecular septum. The moderator band seen within the right ventricle from the four-chamber views can help differentiate central from apical defects. Central defects are located at or posterior to the moderator band, whereas the location of apical defects is anterior to the moderator band (Echo. 10-13; see color plate 25 following p. 364).

Muscular Defects of the Outlet Septum

Muscular defects of the outlet septum are also characterized by completely muscular borders. They are located within the outlet or infundibular septum and are separated from the semilunar valves by a portion of muscular tissue belonging to the outlet septum (11) (Fig. 10-1). They differ from perimembranous defects with outlet extensions in that (a) the central fibrous body does not form any of the borders, (b) the aortic valve does not form the roof, and (c) the membranous septum is intact. Muscular tissue formed by fusion of the posterior limb of the septomarginal trabecula and the ventriculoinfundibular fold separates these defects from the membranous septum (8).

The parasternal long-axis view of the right ventricular

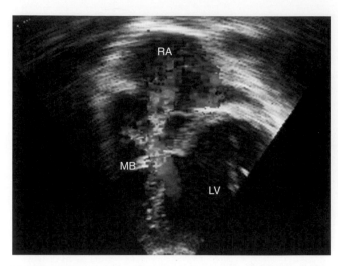

ECHO. 10-13. Apical four-chamber view modified to emphasize the shunt across a defect of the trabecular muscular ventricular septum, adjacent to the moderator band. *RA*, right atrium; *MB*, moderator band; *LV*, left ventricle.

outflow demonstrates defects of the outlet septum and the portion of muscular tissue separating the pulmonic valve from the interventricular communication. Tilting of the transducer to the right, toward the right ventricular inflow, confirms that the membranous septum is intact and that the defect is not related to the aortic valve. These observations permit clear differentiation from perimembranous defects with outlet extensions. Similarly, the parasternal short-axis view demonstrates the aortic valve, the intact membranous septum, and the location of the defect toward the pulmonic valve but separated from it by muscular tissue (Echo. 10-14; see color plate 26 following p. 364). The subcostal short-axis view is also very useful to

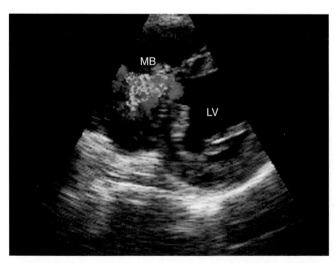

ECHO. 10-12. Parasternal short-axis view of the ventricles demonstrating left-to-right shunting across a defect of the muscular trabecular septum, adjacent to the moderator band. *LV*, left ventricle; *MB*, moderator band.

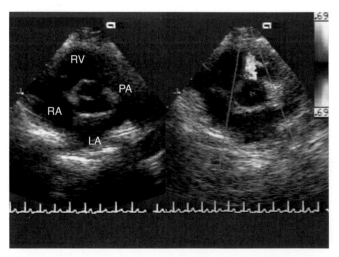

ECHO. 10-14. Parasternal short-axis view illustrating the presence of a defect of the outlet ventricular septum. There is muscular tissue separating the defect from both the tricuspid and pulmonic valves. *RV*, right ventricle; *RA*, right atrium; *LA*, left atrium; *PA*, pulmonary artery.

confirm these observations, showing that the defect is separated from both the tricuspid and pulmonic valves by muscular tissue.

Subarterial or Doubly Committed Ventricular Septal Defects

Subarterial or doubly committed ventricular septal defects are characterized by hypoplasia or absence of the infundibular or outlet septum, resulting in fibrous continuity between the aortic and pulmonic valves. Griffin et al. (43) point out that in addition to the outlet septum, the septal aspect of the subpulmonary infundibulum, which in the normal heart is not an integral part of the interventricular septum, is also absent. This determines that the semilunar valves are at the same level and in fibrous continuity. The border of the defect is fibromuscular. The fibrous portion is composed of the semilunar valves, which also form the roof of the defect (Fig. 10-1). A band of muscular tissue formed by fusion of the posterior limb of the septomarginal trabecula and the ventriculoinfundibular fold separates the membranous septum from the defect (8). These defects are differentiated from perimembranous defects with outlet extensions in that (a) the membranous septum is intact, and (b) the central fibrous body does not comprise any of its borders, despite the fact that the aortic valve is the roof of the defect. They are different from muscular outlet defects in that (a) they are adjacent to the semilunar valves and (b) the borders are fibromuscular rather than completely muscular.

Van Praagh and McNamara (37) mention that lack of support of the aortic valve apparatus resulting from hypoplasia or absence of the infundibular septum, along with a Venturi effect caused by flow through the defect, can result in prolapse of the aortic cusps with or without aortic regurgitation (8,25,37,38,43–46).

The incidence of this type of defect ranges from 3% to 6% of all ventricular septal defects (2,3,27), and they are more common in persons of Oriental descent (47). Generally, they occur as isolated defects, although they can be associated with tetralogy of Fallot (48–50).

Echocardiographically, the best projections to view this type of defect are the parasternal long-axis and short-axis views and the subcostal short-axis view. From the long-axis view, the defect can be seen immediately below the aortic valve, and the presence of aortic valve prolapse can also be evaluated. Tilting the transducer leftward toward the right ventricular outflow demonstrates that the semilunar valves are at the same level, that the infundibular septum is absent, and that the defect is related to both great arteries (Echo. 10-15; see color plate 27 following p. 364).

The echocardiographic image obtained by an intermediate rotation between a long and a short axis has been found to be very helpful to demonstrate the fibrous continuity between the two semilunar valves, which are seen at the

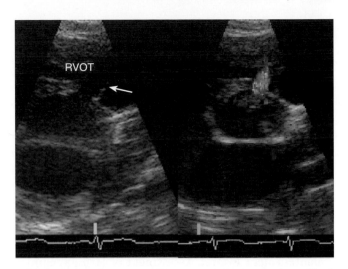

ECHO. 10-15. Parasternal long- and short-axis views tilted toward the right ventricular outflow showing a subarterial ventricular septal defect of moderate size immediately below the pulmonic valve, with absence of the infundibular septum. The *arrow* points to the pulmonic valve leaflets. *RVOT*, right ventricular outflow tract.

same level (51). Because of the spatial position of the right ventricular outflow tract, the parasternal and subcostal short-axis views permit visualization of the defect immediately below the pulmonic valve, without any tissue remnant separating them. These views also permit confirmation of an intact membranous septum (Echo. 10-15).

Color Doppler flow mapping is very useful to determine the location, size, and extensions of ventricular septal defects as well as shunt direction. This technique is particularly helpful in detecting small defects and in demonstrating multiple defects, particularly those in difficult-to-image areas of the muscular septum that may not be visualized by two-dimensional techniques alone. In these cases, the color jet of flow through any defects makes their presence evident.

The direction of flow of the color-encoded jet recorded from the parasternal short-axis view at the level of the aortic valve is also helpful in determining the extensions of perimembranous defects into adjacent areas of the septum. Jets from defects with inlet extensions are directed toward the right ventricle, more or less parallel to the plane of the tricuspid valve (Echo. 10-1). The direction of jets produced by defects with trabecular extensions is usually oblique to the plane of the tricuspid valve and toward the right ventricular body. In this type of defect, occasionally a jet is directed toward the right atrium through a cleft in the tricuspid valve, which is a common associated finding. Flow through perimembranous defects with outlet extensions is directed toward the outflow of the right ventricle. The pattern of jet flow on color Doppler allows differentiation of these defects from muscular defects of the outlet septum and from doubly committed, subarterial defects. In muscular outlet defects, the jet is directed toward the outflow of the right ventricle but is separated from the pulmonary valve by a remnant of outlet septum and is also far from the tricuspid valve because the membranous septum is intact (Echo. 10-14). In doubly committed defects, the jet is immediately below the pulmonic valve and is directed toward the right ventricular outflow tract and main pulmonary artery (26) (Echo. 10-15). In the four-chamber views, the colored jet from perimembranous defects with inlet extensions and from inlet and trabecular muscular defects is seen to be directed toward the right ventricular cavity, perpendicular to the plane of the ventricular septum.

Estimation of Defect Size; Recognition of Signs of Spontaneous Closure; Assessment of Hemodynamic Consequences

Anatomic sizing of ventricular septal defects requires careful imaging from the different views, as they are usually not circumferential and their size varies during the cardiac cycle. Defects are classified as small if the diameter is less than 5 mm, moderate if the diameter is 5 to 10 mm, and large if the diameter exceeds 10 mm. More commonly, the defect size is considered in relation to the aortic annular size; a defect is considered large if its size is greater than that of the aortic annulus, moderate if its diameter is between 50% and 100% of the annular diameter, and small if its diameter measures less than half the aortic annular diameter. The anatomic size and location of a defect are important factors related to reduction in size and/or complete spontaneous closure (52). All ventricular defects, whether perimembranous or muscular, that measure under 4 mm in diameter are thought to close spontaneously within 40 months (52). Large defects with extensions toward the inlet or outlet and subarterial, doubly committed defects do not close spontaneously (52,53). Hornberger et al. (52) compared defect size relative to the aortic root diameter with the presence of congestive heart failure and found that patients with heart failure had defects measuring 8.2 ± 1.9 mm on average and a ratio of defect size to aortic root diameter of 0.63 ± 0.18. Patients who did not have clinically evident heart failure had defects measuring 3.9 ± 1.7 mm in diameter and a ratio of defect size to aortic root diameter of 0.27 ± 0.10 (52).

The mechanisms of closure of perimembranous ventricular septal defects include reduplication of tricuspid valve tissue, adhesion of tricuspid valve leaflets around the defect (54,55), and prolapse of the aortic valve into the defect (54). Formation of a true aneurysm of the membranous septum is rare (54). Closure of small muscular defects is most likely a consequence of proliferation of endothelial tissue (27). Two-dimensional echocardiography is a sensitive technique to detect progressive spontaneous closure of ventricular defects, particularly perimembranous defects (55). For this purpose, the defect and its

adjacent structures should be studied carefully from several projections, including the parasternal long- and short-axis views and the apical and subcostal four-chamber and short-axis views (Echo. 10-16; see color plate 28 following p. 364).

Shunt size can be estimated directly by calculating the ratio of pulmonary to systemic flows through Doppler methods or indirectly from the hemodynamic consequences of the left-to-right shunt.

A variety of formulas has been proposed to estimate the ratio of pulmonary to systemic flow (Qp:Qs) by Doppler (56–61). As described for atrial septal defects, these methods combine two-dimensional imaging and Doppler measurement of velocity according to the general equation

$$\text{Flow} = \text{Area} \times \text{Velocity} \quad [1]$$

In its simplest format, the ratio of pulmonary to systemic flow is calculated with the same method described for atrial septal defects (56). Using the same principles, Vargas Barron et al. (58) combined measurements of all four intracardiac valves to arrive at a better estimation of pulmonary and systemic flows. In their method, pulmonary blood flow (Qp) is calculated as an average of the flows obtained at the pulmonary and mitral valves, and systemic blood flow (Qs) is derived from the average of flows obtained at the aortic and tricuspid valves in the absence of an atrial communication. Their formula is

$$\frac{Q\text{p}}{Q\text{s}} = \frac{[(\text{Area}_{PA} \times VTI_{PA}) + (\text{Area}_{MV} \times VTI_{MV})]/2}{[(\text{Area}_{AO} \times VTI_{AO}) + (\text{Area}_{TV} \times VTI_{TV})]/2} \quad [2]$$

where VTI is the velocity time integral in cm.

Cloez et al. (60) proposed a simplification of the conventional formula and used vessel diameter and peak velocity instead of areas and VTI:

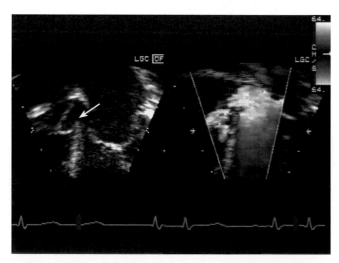

ECHO. 10-16. Magnified view of a perimembranous ventricular septal defect undergoing spontaneous closure. The *arrow* points to the defect partially covered by tricuspid valve tissue.

$$\frac{Qp}{Qs} = \frac{(\text{Luminal Diameter}_{PA})^2 \times \text{Peak Velocity}_{PA}}{(\text{Luminal Diameter}_{AO})^2 \times \text{Peak Velocity}_{AO}} \quad [3]$$

Tien et al. (61) calculated the systemic-to-pulmonary flow ratios using the cross-sectional area and velocity of the jet through the defect and of the left ventricular outflow tract as follows:

$$\frac{Qp}{Qs} = \frac{(\text{Area}_{jet} \times VTI_{jet}) + (\text{Area}_{LVOT} \times VTI_{LVOT})}{\text{Area}_{LVOT} \times VTI_{LVOT}} \quad [4]$$

Finally, Moises et al. (62) used the principles of flow convergence to calculate flow through the septal defect by visualizing the area of jet acceleration from the left ventricular side by means of color Doppler mapping. The radial distance from the point of aliasing to the orifice of the defect is measured and converted to surface area with a simple hemispheric geometric conversion formula (Area $= 2\pi r^2$). The aliasing velocity (Nyquist limit) is utilized as the velocity for the formula as follows:

$$Q \, (\text{L/min}) = \frac{2\pi r^2 \times \text{Aliasing Velocity} \times 60}{1000} \quad [5]$$

In addition to the quantitation of volume flows, estimation of pulmonary arterial pressures should also be attempted because increased pressure and resistance can be important hemodynamic consequences of the increased pulmonary blood flow.

By means of a simplification of the Bernoulli equation relating pressure drop to velocity, as proposed by Hatle,

$$P_2 - P_1 \, (\text{mmHg}) = 4 \times \text{Maximal Jet Velocity}^2 \quad [6]$$

an estimate of right ventricular pressure and therefore of the pulmonary artery pressure (in the absence of pulmonic stenosis) can be obtained. The maximal flow velocity across the ventricular septal defect is recorded with continuous-wave Doppler. The defect can be imaged from the parasternal long- and/or short-axis views with color Doppler flow mapping used to direct placement of the continuous-wave Doppler sampling line as nearly parallel as possible to the direction of the jet. Minor adjustments in transducer position are usually necessary until the cleanest audio and spectral Doppler signals are found (Echo. 10-17). From this maximal jet velocity, the gradient between the left and right ventricles can be calculated according to the Bernoulli equation. The systemic pressure is measured more or less simultaneously (63) with a blood pressure cuff, and the following relationship is then obtained:

$$\text{Pressure}_{RV} = \text{Systemic Systolic Pressure} \quad [7]$$

$$- \text{Peak Gradient}_{LV \, to \, RV}$$

The right ventricular peak systolic pressure can also be estimated from the velocity of the jet of tricuspid regurgitation, if present. This would represent the gradient between the right ventricle and right atrium (see Bernoulli

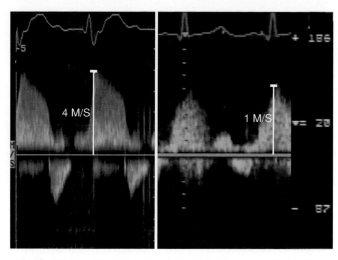

ECHO. 10-17. Continuous-wave Doppler recordings of the velocity across ventricular septal defects. The panel on the **left** demonstrates a velocity of 4 m/s across a restrictive defect. The panel on the **right** illustrates a velocity of 1 m/s through a nonrestrictive defect.

equation above) (63). In this instance, color flow mapping can also be used to guide the placement of the continuous-wave Doppler sampling line. To the calculated pressure drop between the right ventricle and right atrium must be added the estimate of right atrial pressure to arrive at an absolute right ventricular pressure. The right atrial pressure is assumed to be 5 mmHg in children and 10 mmHg in adults (63).

If there is no obstruction in the right ventricular outflow tract, the pulmonary arterial systolic pressure is the same as that of the right ventricle. The velocity across the right ventricular outflow tract should always be measured with pulsed-wave or continuous-wave Doppler, and if there is a gradient, it can be subtracted from the right ventricular pressure estimate to arrive at an approximation of peak systolic pulmonary artery pressure:

$$\text{Systolic Pressure}_{PA} \, (\text{mmHg})$$

$$= \text{Pressure}_{RV} - \text{Peak Gradient}_{RV \, to \, PA} \quad [8]$$

The diastolic pulmonary arterial pressure can be estimated from the end-diastolic velocity of a pulmonary regurgitant jet, if this is present (64). Color flow Doppler can again serve as a guide for positioning the pulsed-wave Doppler sample volume from a parasternal short-axis view. The velocity at the shoulder of the spectral waveform would correspond to the end-diastolic gradient between the pulmonary artery and right ventricle.

Indirect estimates of pulmonary artery pressure include measurement of the pulmonary arterial spectral Doppler tracing of the acceleration time and ejection time ($AT:ET$) and the isovolumetric relaxation time of the left ventricle (65), which is prolonged in the presence of pulmonary hypertension (63). A more detailed discussion of the

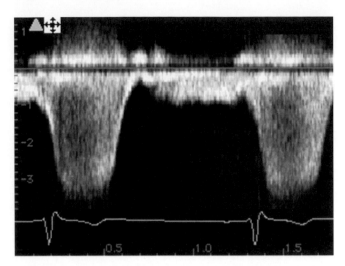

ECHO. 10-18. Continuous-wave Doppler recording of the velocity across a restrictive ventricular septal defect with left-to-right shunting during both systole and diastole.

methods to evaluate pulmonary arterial pressure is included in Chapter 35.

In small defects, in which the left ventricular pressure remains higher than the right ventricular pressure throughout the cardiac cycle, left-to-right shunt flow can be detected and recorded in both systole and diastole with color and spectral Doppler (63) (Echo. 10-18).

Associated Anomalies

Ventricular septal defects can be associated with a multitude of other cardiac anomalies. Typically, these can include valvar, subvalvar, and/or supravalvar pulmonic stenosis; branch pulmonary artery stenosis; aortic valvar, subvalvar, or supravalvar stenosis; aortic coarctation or interruption; patent ductus arteriosus; atrial septal defects; mitral stenosis and insufficiency; straddling of the mitral or tricuspid valves; anomalous systemic or pulmonary venous return; hypoplastic right ventricle; and unroofed coronary sinus. These defects can also exist as an integral part of a variety of congenital cardiac malformations, such as conotruncal malformations, tricuspid atresia, pulmonary valve atresia, and superoinferior ventricles. These malformations are discussed in detail in their respective chapters.

INTRAOPERATIVE AND POSTOPERATIVE EVALUATION

Intraoperative studies are conducted mostly through the transesophageal approach, which has been increasingly utilized, even in infants, since the advent of smaller single and biplane probes and most recently pediatric multiplane probes (66–74).

Intraoperative studies before bypass should be directed toward confirming the preoperative diagnosis, obtaining

baseline morphologic and hemodynamic information, and determining the surgical approach (66). In ventricular septal defects specifically, this would focus on confirming the location, size, and number of defects; determining the surgical approach to their closure (e.g., transatrial, transpulmonary); and evaluating ventricular function. The presence of multiple defects should be carefully ruled out before bypass because the surgical morbidity is increased (75).

Global ventricular systolic function is best assessed through the transverse, transgastric view (see Fig. 4-27A–B). Segmental wall motion can be studied through a combination of the transverse four-chamber view (see Fig. 4-28A–B) and the longitudinal two-chamber view and long-axis view (see Fig. 4-28C–D).

Ventricular septal defects in the perimembranous septum and in the inlet and midtrabecular muscular septum can be imaged from the transverse views, beginning with the transgastric position and carefully withdrawing the transducer into a four-chamber view and then further to the left ventricular outflow view (see Figs. 4-27A–B, 4-28A–B, 4-29A) (Echo. 10-19; see color plate 29 following p. 364). Slight retroflexion of the transducer may be necessary, in the four-chamber view particularly, to visualize the inlet and midtrabecular portions of the septum well (Echo. 10-20; see color plate 30 following p. 364). Anteflexion of the transducer will allow a short-axis sweep of the base of the heart from the transverse plane (slight withdrawal and advancement of the transducer) (76). Rotation of the array toward 100 to 120 degrees into a longitudinal plane will demonstrate the fibrous continuity between the pulmonary and aortic valves and the flows across doubly committed or subarterial communications (see Fig. 4-29D,E). Color Doppler can aid in localizing the primary defect and demonstrating

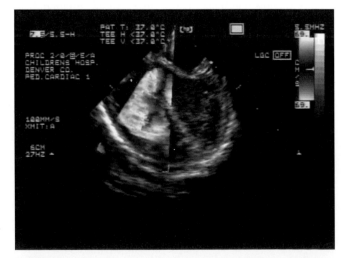

ECHO. 10-19. Transesophageal view of the ventricular septum from the horizontal plane. The endoscope is withdrawn slightly toward the left ventricular outflow, revealing the presence of a perimembranous defect immediately below the aortic valve.

additional defects that may have been missed transthoracically (Echo. 10-10). In perimembranous defects, the colored jet would be seen below the aortic valve directed toward the right ventricle below the septal leaflet of the tricuspid valve. Muscular inlet defects would be separated from the tricuspid valve by a remnant of muscular tissue (Echo. 10-20). In midtrabecular muscular defects, the flow would be detected in the midportion of the ventricular septum, behind the moderator band.

The apical trabecular septum is difficult to visualize from a transesophageal approach, so defects in this location can be missed intraoperatively; it is therefore important to examine this portion of the septum carefully during transthoracic preoperative studies.

The outlet septum is also difficult to visualize completely from the transesophageal window, although with the multiplane probes this is less of a problem. The longitudinal views behind the left atrium, obtained by withdrawing the transducer and rotating the endoscope progressively to the right until both outflow tracts and great vessels are seen, are the best to demonstrate defects in the outlet septum and subarterial or doubly committed defects (see Fig. 4-29D–F). Color Doppler can help define the extensions and locations of these difficult-to-image defects.

The gradient across the defect can be estimated by using continuous-wave Doppler in the same approach as that described above.

After bypass, the objectives should be to evaluate the effectiveness of the repair, estimate gradients (if pertinent), rule out significant residual shunts, assess ventricular function, and evaluate the fluid status of the patient (66). Ventricular systolic function and hypovolemia, if present, are evaluated initially from a transverse, transgastric approach (see Fig. 4-27A,B), followed by a study of regional wall motion from the four-chamber, outflow, and

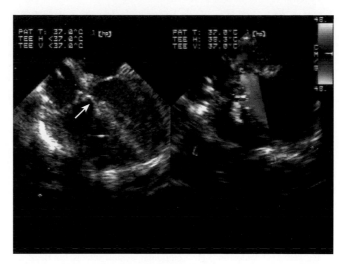

ECHO. 10-21. Transesophageal view of the ventricular septum from the horizontal plane demonstrating the surgical patch used to close a perimembranous ventricular septal defect (*arrow*). The color Doppler flow image reveals a tiny residual shunt detected immediately postoperatively, most likely through the patch itself.

two-chamber (longitudinal) views (see Fig. 4-28). Inflow velocities of the ventricles can be recorded from the four-chamber transverse view for evaluation of diastolic ventricular filling. Depending on the location of the defects, the various views described for the preoperative study can be used to assess the presence of significant residual shunts. Small residual shunts through the patches are always seen immediately postoperatively, particularly from the transesophageal position; these usually disappear with endothelialization of the patch and should not be confused with true residual defects (Echo. 10-21; see color plate 31 following p. 364).

In patients with subarterial, doubly committed defects or perimembranous defects with outlet extensions, special care should be taken to rule out aortic valve prolapse. This can be seen best from the longitudinal views of the outflow tracts (see Figs. 4-28D; 4-29E,F). If aortic prolapse is present, and particularly if it is associated with aortic regurgitation, it is important to note that these lesions are usually progressive, even after surgical repair of the defect with resuspension of the prolapsed cusps.

Recently, Van der Velde et al. (77) have used transesophageal echocardiography to guide transcatheter closure of ventricular septal defects in conjunction with fluoroscopy. This approach should be particularly useful because echocardiographic imaging affords a more detailed view of the intracardiac structures than can be obtained with fluoroscopy, so that erroneous placement of devices and/or interference with the valvular apparatus can be avoided.

REFERENCES

1. Roberts WC. The 2 most common congenital heart diseases [Editorial]. *Am J Cardiol* 1984;53:1198.

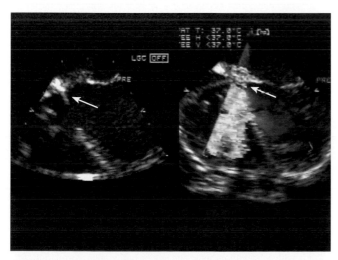

ECHO. 10-20. Transesophageal view of the ventricular septum from the horizontal plane demonstrating a ventricular septal defect of the inlet muscular septum. The *arrows* point to muscular tissue on the superior edge of the defect.

2. Roca Llop J, Casaldaliga Ferrer J, Cordovilla Zurdo G, Cabo Salvador J. Defectos interventriculares. In: Sanchez PA, ed. *Cardiologia pediatrica, clinica y cirugia*, Vol 1. Barcelona: Salvat Editores, 1986:284–315.

3. Fyler DC. Ventricular septal defect. In: Fyler DC, ed. *Nadas' pediatric cardiology*. Philadelphia: Hanley & Belfus, 1992:435–457.

4. Graham TP Jr, Bender HW, Spach MS. Ventricular septal defect. In: Adams FH, Emmanouilides GC, Riemenschneider TA, eds. *Moss heart disease in infants, children, and adolescents*, 4th ed. Baltimore: Williams & Wilkins, 1989:189–209.

5. Keith JD. Ventricular septal defect. In: Keith JD, Rowe RD, Vlad P, eds. *Heart disease in infancy and childhood*, 3rd ed. New York: Macmillan, 1978:320–379.

6. Nora JJ. Etiologic aspects of heart diseases. In: Adams FH, Emmanouilides GC, Riemenschneider TA, eds. *Moss heart disease in infants, children, and adolescents*, 4th ed. Baltimore: Williams & Wilkins, 1989:15–23.

7. Cayre R, Sanchez-Gomez C, Moreno-Rodriguez RA, De la Cruz MV. La teratologia y la epidemiologia en el estudio de los teratogenos ambientales. *Bol Med Hosp Infant Mex* 1992;49:397–403.

8. Becker AE, Anderson RH. Ventricular septal defect. In: Becker AE, Anderson RH, eds. *Pathology of congenital heart disease. Postgraduate pathology series*. London: Butterworth-Heineman, 1981:93–117.

9. Goor DA, Lillehei CW. The anatomy of the heart. In: Goor DA, Lillehei CW, eds. *Congenital malformations of the heart. Embryology, anatomy, and operative considerations*. New York: Grune & Stratton, 1975:1–37.

10. De la Cruz MV, Gimenez-Ribota M, Saravalli O, Cayre R. The contribution of the inferior endocardial cushion of the atrioventricular canal to cardiac septation and to the development of the atrioventricular valves: study in the chick embryo. *Am J Anat* 1983;166:63–72.

11. Sanchez-Gomez C, Cayre R, De la Cruz MV. Consideraciones embriologicas y anatomicas sobre la septacion cardiaca normal y patologica. II. Septum atrioventricular e interventricular. *Bol Med Hosp Infant Mex* 1990;47:51–58.

12. De la Cruz MV, Sanchez Gomez C, Cayre R. The developmental components of the ventricles: their significance in congenital cardiac malformations. *Cardiol Young* 1991;1:123–128.

13. Netter FH, Van Mierop LHS. Embryology. In: Netter FH, FF Yonkman FF, eds. *Heart*. Summit, NJ: Ciba Publications Department, 1969:112–130 (*The Ciba Collection of Medical Illustrations*, Vol 5).

14. Harth JY, Paul MH. Experimental cardiac morphogenesis. I. Development of the ventricular septum in the chick. *J Embryol Exp Morphol* 1975;33:13–28.

15. De la Cruz MV. Different concepts of univentricular heart. Experimental embryological approach. *Herz* 1979;4:67–72.

16. De la Cruz MV, Quero-Jimenez M, Arteaga Martinez M, Cayre R. Morphogenèse du septum interventriculaire. *Coeur* 1982;13:443–448.

17. Garcia Pelaez I, Diaz-Gongora G, Arteaga M. Contribution of the superior atrioventricular cushion to the left ventricular infundibulum. Experimental study on the chick embryo. *Acta Anat* 1984;118:224–230.

18. Domenech Mateu JM. Desarrollo del corazon. In: Soler Soler J, Bayes de Luna A, eds. *Cardiologia*. Barcelona: Editorial Doyma, 1986:3–13.

19. Soto B, Becker AE, Moulaert AJ, Lie JT, Anderson RH. Classification of ventricular septal defects. *Br Heart J* 1980;43:332–343.

20. Becu LM, Fontana RS, DuShane JW, Kirklin JW, Burchel HB, Edwards JE. Anatomic and pathologic studies in ventricular septal defect. *Circulation* 1956;14:349–364.

21. Hagler DJ, Edwards WD, Seward JB, Tajik AJ. Standardized nomenclature of the ventricular septum and ventricular septal defects, with applications for two-dimensional echocardiography. *Mayo Clin Proc* 1985;60:741–752.

22. Soto B, Pacifico AD. Ventricular septal defect. In: Soto B, Pacifico AD, eds. *Angiocardiography in congenital heart malformations*. Mount Kisco, NY: Futura Publishing, 1990:327–349.

23. Anderson RH. Ventricular septal defect: anatomical features as seen by the morphologist. In: Anderson RH, Park SC, Neches WH, Zuberbuhler JR, eds. *Perspectives in pediatric cardiology*, Vol 1. Mount Kisco, NY: Futura Publishing, 1988:9–24.

24. Allwork SP, Anderson RH. Developmental anatomy of the membranous part of the ventricular septum in the human heart. *Br Heart J* 1979;41:275–280.

25. Anderson RH, Macartney FJ, Shinebourne EA, Tynan M. Ventricular septal defect. In: Anderson RH, Macartney FJ, Shinebourne EA, Tynan M, eds. *Paediatric cardiology*, Vol 1. Edinburgh: Churchill Livingstone, 1987:615–642.

26. Helmcke F, De Souza A, Nanda NC, et al. Two-dimensional and color Doppler assessment of ventricular septal defect of congenital origin. *Am J Cardiol* 1989;63:1112–1116.

27. Silverman NH. Ventricular septal defects. In: Silverman NH, ed. *Pediatric echocardiography*. Baltimore: Williams & Wilkins, 1993:123–142.

28. Milo S, Ho SY, Wilkinson JL, Anderson RH. Surgical anatomy and atrioventricular conduction tissues of hearts with isolated ventricular septal defects. *J Thorac Cardiovasc Surg* 1980;79:244–255.

29. Capelli H, Andrade JL, Somerville J. Classification of the site of ventricular septal defect by 2-dimensional echocardiography. *Am J Cardiol* 1983;51:1474–1480.

30. Neufeld HN, Titus JL, DuShane JW, Burchel HB, Edwards JE. Isolated ventricular septal defect of the persistent common atrioventricular canal type. *Circulation* 1961;23:685–696.

31. Baker EJ, Leung MP, Anderson RH, Fischer DR, Zuberbuhler JR. The cross sectional anatomy of ventricular septal defects: a reappraisal. *Br Heart J* 1988;59:339–351.

32. Bierman FZ, Fellows K, Williams RG. Prospective identification of ventricular septal defects in infancy using subxiphoid two-dimensional echocardiography. *Circulation* 1980;62:807–817.

33. Canale JM, Sahn DJ, Allen HD, Goldberg SJ, Valdes-Cruz LM, Ovitt TW. Factors affecting real-time, cross-sectional echocardiographic imaging of perimembranous ventricular septal defects. *Circulation* 1981;63:689–697.

34. Cheatham JP, Latson LA, Gutgesell HP. Ventricular septal defect in infancy: detection with two-dimensional echocardiography. *Am J Cardiol* 1981;47:85–89.

35. Sutherland GR, Godman MJ, Smallhorn JF, Guiterras P, Anderson RH, Hunter S. Ventricular septal defects. Two-dimensional echocardiographic and morphological correlation. *Br Heart J* 1982;47:316–328.

36. Cabrera A, Velasco JV, Idigoras G, et al. Estudio de los defectos interventriculares por imagen y eco-Doppler color. *Rev Esp Cardiol* 1993;46:721–726.

37. Van Praagh RV, McNamara JJ. Anatomic types of ventricular septal defect with aortic insufficiency. Diagnostic and surgical considerations. *Am Heart J* 1968;75:604–619.

38. Rhodes LA, Keane JF, Keane JP, et al. Long follow-up (to 43 years) of ventricular septal defect with audible aortic regurgitation. *Am J Cardiol* 1990;66:340–345.

39. Warden HE, DeWall RA, Cohen M, Varco RL, Lillehei CW. A surgical-pathologic classification for isolated ventricular septal defects and for those in Fallot's tetralogy based on observation made on 120 patients during repair under direct vision. *J Thorac Cardiovasc Surg* 1957;33:21–44.

40. Edwards JE, Carey LS, Neufeld HN, Lester RG. In: Edwards JE, Carey LS, Neufeld HN, Lester RG, eds. *Congenital heart disease. Correlation of pathologic anatomy and angiocardiography*, Vol 1. Philadelphia: WB Saunders, 1965:95–97.

41. Wenink ACG, Oppenheimer-Dekker A, Moulaert AJ. Muscular ventricular septal defects: a reappraisal of the anatomy. *Am J Cardiol* 1979;43:259–264.

42. Anderson RH, Ebels TJ, Zuberbuhler JR, Silverman NH. Anatomical and echocardiographic features of the left valve in atrioventricular septal defect. In: Anderson RH, Neches WH, Park SC, Zuberbuhler JR, eds. *Perspectives in pediatric cardiology*, Vol 1. Mount Kisco, NY: Futura Publishing, 1988:299–310.

43. Griffin ML, Sullivan ID, Anderson RH, Macartney FJ. Doubly committed subarterial ventricular septal defect: new morphological criteria with echocardiographic and angiocardiographic correlation. *Br Heart J* 1988;59:474–479.

44. Keane JF, Plauth WH Jr, Nadas AS. Ventricular septal defect with aortic regurgitation. *Circulation* 1977;56[Suppl I]:I-72–I-77.

45. Craig BG, Smallhorn JF, Burrows P, Trusler GA, Rowe RD. Cross-

sectional echocardiography in the evaluation of aortic valve prolapse associated with ventricular septal defect. *Am Heart J* 1986; 112:800–807.

46. Schmidt KG, Cassidy SC, Silverman NH, Stanger P. Doubly committed subarterial ventricular septal defects: echocardiographic features and surgical implications. *J Am Coll Cardiol* 1988;12:1538–1546.

47. Ando M, Takao A. Pathological anatomy of ventricular septal defect associated with aortic valve prolapse and regurgitation. *Heart Vessels* 1986;2:117–126.

48. Ando M. Subpulmonary ventricular septal defect with pulmonary stenosis [Letters to the Editor]. *Circulation* 1974;50:412.

49. Neirotti R, Galindez E, Kreutzer G, Rodriguez Coronel A, Pedrini M, Becu L. Tetralogy of Fallot with subpulmonary ventricular septal defect. *Ann Thorac Surg* 1978;25:51–56.

50. Capelli H, Somerville J. Atypical Fallot's tetralogy with doubly committed subarterial ventricular septal defect. Diagnostic value of 2-dimensional echocardiography. *Am J Cardiol* 1983;51:282–285.

51. Fischer DR, Baker EJ, Anderson RH. Echocardiographic manifestations of ventricular septal defects. In: Anderson RH, Neches WH, Park SC, Zuberbuhler JR, eds. *Perspectives in pediatric cardiology*, Vol 1. Mount Kisco, NY: Futura Publishing, 1988:25–33.

52. Hornberger LK, Sahn DJ, Krabill KA, et al. Elucidation of the natural history of ventricular septal defects by serial Doppler color flow mapping studies. *J Am Coll Cardiol* 1989;13:1111–1118.

53. Williams RG. Doppler color flow mapping and prediction of ventricular septal defect outcome [Editorial Comment]. *J Am Coll Cardiol* 1989;13:1119–1121.

54. Anderson RH, Lenox CC, Zuberbuhler JR. Mechanisms of closure of perimembranous ventricular septal defect. *Am J Cardiol* 1983; 52:341–345.

55. Ramaciotti C, Keren A, Silverman NH. Importance of (perimembranous) ventricular septal aneurysm in the natural history of isolated perimembranous ventricular septal defect. *Am J Cardiol* 1986;57: 268–272.

56. Valdes-Cruz LM, Horowitz S, Mesel E, et al. A pulsed Doppler echocardiographic method for calculation of pulmonary and systemic flow: accuracy in a canine model with ventricular septal defect. *Circulation* 1983;68:597–602.

57. Sanders SP, Yeager S, Williams RG. Measurement of systemic and pulmonary blood flow and QP/QS ratio using Doppler and two-dimensional echocardiography. *Am J Cardiol* 1983;51:952–956.

58. Vargas Barron J, Sahn DJ, Valdes-Cruz LM, et al. Clinical utility of two-dimensional Doppler echocardiographic techniques for estimating pulmonary to systemic blood flow ratios in children with left to right shunting atrial septal defect, ventricular septal defect or patent ductus arteriosus. *J Am Coll Cardiol* 1984;3:169–178.

59. Sahn DJ. Determination of cardiac output by echocardiographic Doppler methods: relative accuracy of various sites of measurement. *J Am Coll Cardiol* 1985;6:663–664.

60. Cloez JL, Schmidt KG, Birk E, Silverman NH. Determination of pulmonary to systemic blood flow ratio in children by a simplified Doppler echocardiographic method. *J Am Coll Cardiol* 1988;11: 825–830.

61. Teien D, Karp K, Wendel H, Human DG, Nanton MA. Quantification of left-to-right shunts by echo Doppler cardiography in patients with ventricular septal defects. *Acta Paediatr Scand* 1991;80:355–360.

62. Moises VA, Maciel BC, Hornberger LK, et al. A new method for noninvasive estimation of ventricular septal defect shunt flow by Doppler color flow mapping: imaging of the laminar flow convergence region on the left septal surface. *J Am Coll Cardiol* 1991; 18:824–832.

63. Hatle L, Angelsen B. Pulsed and continuous wave Doppler in diagnosis and assessment of various heart lesions. In: Hatle L, Angelsen B, eds. *Doppler ultrasound in cardiology. Physical principles and clinical applications*, 2nd ed. Philadelphia: Lea & Febiger, 1985: 97–292.

64. Masuyama T, Kodama K, Kitabatake A, Sato H, Nanto S, Inoue M. Continuous-wave Doppler echocardiographic detection of pulmonary regurgitation and its application to noninvasive estimation of pulmonary artery pressure. *Circulation* 1986;74:484–492.

65. Burstin L. Determination of pressure in the pulmonary artery by external graphic recordings. *Br Heart J* 1967;29:396–404.

66. Sutherland GR, Quaegebeur J, van Daele MERM, Stumper OFW, Hess J. Intraoperative echocardiography in congenital heart disease: an overview. In: Erbel R, Khandheria BK, Brennecke R, Meyer J, Seward JB, Tajik AJ, eds. *Transesophageal echocardiography. A new window to the heart.* Berlin: Springer-Verlag, 1989:306–316.

67. Kasper W, Geibel A, Hofmann T, et al. Echocardiographic follow-up after surgery for congenital heart diseases. In: Erbel R, Khandheria BK, Brennecke R, Meyer J, Seward JB, Tajik AJ, eds. *Transesophageal echocardiography. A new window to the heart.* Berlin: Springer-Verlag, 1989:324–329.

68. Musewe NN, Smallhorn JF, Dyck J, Freedom RM. Transesophageal echocardiography in a pediatric population. *Circulation* 1989; 80[Suppl II]:II 186(abst).

69. Kyo S, Omoto R, Matsumura M, Shah P, Ito H. Intraoperative transesophageal Doppler-echo in pediatric congenital heart disease. *Circulation* 1989;80[Suppl II]:II-186(abst).

70. Cyran SE, Kimball TR, Meyer RA, et al. Efficacy of intraoperative transesophageal echocardiography in children with congenital heart disease. *Am J Cardiol* 1989;63:594–598.

71. Stumper OFW, Elzenga NJ, Hess J, Sutherland GR. Transesophageal echocardiography in children with congenital heart disease: an initial experience. *J Am Coll Cardiol* 1990;16:433–441.

72. Ritter SB. Transesophageal echocardiography in children: new peephole to the heart [Editorial Comment]. *J Am Coll Cardiol* 1990; 16:447–450.

73. Muhiudeen IA, Roberson DA, Silverman NH, Hass G, Turley K, Cahalan MK. Intraoperative echocardiography in infants and children with congenital cardiac shunt lesions: transesophageal versus epicardial echocardiography. *J Am Coll Cardiol* 1990;16:1687–1695.

74. Ritter SB. Transesophageal real-time echocardiography in infants and children with congenital heart disease. *J Am Coll Cardiol* 1991; 18:569–580.

75. Sutherland GR, Smyllie JH, Ogilvie BC, Keeton BR. Colour flow imaging in the diagnosis of multiple ventricular septal defects. *Br Heart J* 1989;62:43–49.

76. Seward JB, Khandheria BK, Oh JK, et al. Transesophageal echocardiography: technique, anatomic correlations, implementation, and clinical applications. *Mayo Clin Proc* 1988;63:649–680.

77. Van der Velde MA, Sanders SP, Keane JF, Perry SB, Lock JE. Transesophageal echocardiographic guidance of transcatheter ventricular septal defect closure. *J Am Coll Cardiol* 1994;23:1660–1665.

CHAPTER 11

Atrioventricular Septal Defects

Lilliam M. Valdes-Cruz and Raul O. Cayre

Atrioventricular septal defects, also called "atrioventricular canal defects" or "endocardial cushion defects," are one of the congenital cardiac malformations that have provoked the most controversy in terms of classification and anatomical types.

A case of an imperfection at the base of the heart in which the atria and ventricular septa are joined and the four cardiac cavities communicate was first reported in 1819, by M. Thibert (1). T. B. Peacock in 1846 (2) and 1858 (3) described a case of an imperfection of the atrial and ventricular septa. Anderson et al. (4) mention that Alexander Ecker of Freiberg described in his thesis an unequivocal case of atrioventricular septal defect, before the first publication by Peacock (2); however, they fail to mention the date of the thesis. Von Rokitanski in 1875 (5) reported the first description of atrioventricular septal defects with a common atrioventricular orifice and with two separate right and left atrioventricular valves and uses the term "ostium primum defect."

Failure of fusion of the endocardial cushions as the probable morphogenesis of atrioventricular defects was suggested by Keith in 1909 (6). Monckebert in 1924 (7) and Abbott in 1936 (8) mention that atrioventricular septal defects occur due to persistence of the embryonic atrioventricular canal; they called it "persistent ostium atrioventriculare commune." Gunn and Dieckmann in 1927 (9) called this malformation "common atrioventricular canal." The relationship between the persistent ostium atrioventriculare commune with Down's syndrome (then called "mongolism") was mentioned by Robson in 1931 (10). Rodgers and Edwards in 1948 (11) divided the persistent common atrioventricular ostium into partial and complete forms. The term "defect of the endocardial cushions" was first used by Watkins and Gross in 1955 (12) and later by Van Mierop et al. (13). Wakai and Edwards added a third type, the transitional or intermediate form, to the classification (14,15). Rastelli et al. (16) established a subclassification of the complete form based

on the presence or absence of a division in the anterior leaflet.

Ugarte et al. (17) determined that the division in the anterior leaflet proposed by Rastelli et al. (16) was in reality a commissure between the anterior leaflet of the left-sided valve (mitral valve) and the anterosuperior leaflet of the right-sided valve (tricuspid valve). The presence of a common orifice in the complete form and two orifices in the partial form was mentioned by Piccoli et al. (18,19). Recently, the presence of a single atrioventricular annulus in both the complete and partial forms was established, as well as the concept of small, moderate, or extreme bridging of the common anterior leaflet in the complete form (20–22).

The incidence of atrioventricular septal defects varies between 4% and 6.8% of all cases of congenital heart disease (23–25).

EMBRYOLOGIC CONSIDERATIONS

Factors to consider in the embryogenesis of atrioventricular septal defects are failure of development of the cushions of the atrioventricular canal, abnormal development of the interatrial septum in the region of the foramen primum, and the role of the ventricular myocardium, which participates in the morphogenesis of the atrioventricular valvular apparatus.

The atrioventricular canal initially has one orifice, which is subsequently divided by the atrioventricular septum into two separate orifices, each with a fibrous annulus (26,27) (see Figs. 1-7B and 1-12A,B). Failure of development of the inferior cushion of the atrioventricular canal results in absence of the atrioventricular septum, which originates from this cushion (28); therefore, in hearts with atrioventricular septal defects, whether in its complete or partial form, there is only a single fibrous annulus (29) (Figs. 11-1, 11-2). The septal portion of the anterior mitral leaflet and the septal leaflet of the tricuspid valve also arise from the inferior cushion of the atrioventricular canal (13,28,30) (see Fig. 1-13), and consequently these are also absent in atrioventricular septal defects. Instead, there is a common inferior leaflet with insertions in both ventricles (inferior bridging leaflet) (31) (Fig. 11-1) that originates from the ventricular myocardium through a process of delamination (31,32). The inferior cushion also participates in the development of the interventricular septum, which separates the inflow tracts of both ventricles, so its absence also results in a deficiency of the inlet septum (28,33). Additionally, the inferior cushion, along with the septum primum, is responsible for closure of the foramen primum (13,28,30,34).

Therefore, when the inferior cushion is missing, an interatrial communication of the ostium primum type occurs,

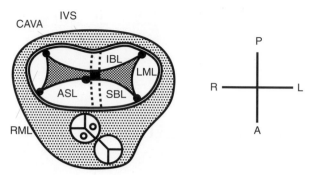

FIG. 11-2. Schematic drawing demonstrating the partial form of atrioventricular septal defect. See text for details. *CAVA,* common atrioventricular annulus; *SBL,* superior bridging leaflet; *IBL,* inferior bridging leaflet; *ASL,* anterosuperior leaflet; *LML,* left mural leaflet; *RML,* right mural leaflet; *IVS,* interventricular septum; *A,* anterior; *P,* posterior; *R,* right; *L,* left.

which is also contributed to by a deficiency of the atrial septum at the site of the embryonic ostium primum (35).

The right and left lateral cushions that give rise to the posterior tricuspid and posterior mitral leaflets (see Figs. 1-12B and 1-13) can be variously affected in atrioventricular septal defects. This is anatomically expressed in mural leaflets, which are smaller than the normal posterior tricuspid and mitral leaflets. The involvement of the right lateral cushion also results in the presence of a right anterosuperior leaflet, whose size is inversely proportional to that of the superior bridging leaflet (Fig. 11-1).

The superior cushion participates in the normal formation of the left ventricular infundibulum by contributing to the free portion of the anterior mitral leaflet, which is also the external wall of the left ventricular outflow tract (36–39) and to the left surface of the outlet septum (37) (see Fig. 1-13). The presence of a common atrioventricular annulus and the abnormal development of the superior cushion result in a superior and anterior displacement of the aortic valve as well as in an elongation of the left ventricular outflow tract compared to normal hearts, giving the classical goose-neck appearance. Further, absence of the superior cushion also results in the formation of a superior bridging leaflet (Fig. 11-1).

The two atrioventricular valvular orifices seen in the partial forms of atrioventricular septal defect are due to the presence of a tongue of leaflet tissue that joins the superior and inferior bridging leaflets at the midline (40) (Fig. 11-2) and that originates from the interventricular septal myocardium.

Absence of those embryologic structures that normally divide the atrioventricular canal and give rise to the atrioventricular valves, their chordae tendineae, and papillary muscles results in blood flow changes, whose morphogenetic effects express themselves in alterations in ventricular architecture with chordae and papillary muscles, which vary in form, size, and location.

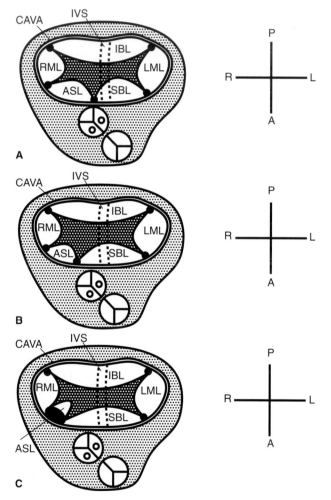

FIG. 11-1. Schematic drawings demonstrating the types of complete atrioventricular septal defects. See text for details. **A:** Mild bridging of the superior leaflet. **B:** Moderate bridging of the superior leaflet. **C:** Extreme bridging of the superior leaflet. *CAVA,* common atrioventricular annulus; *SBL,* superior bridging leaflet; *IBL,* inferior bridging leaflet; *LML,* left mural leaflet; *RML,* right mural leaflet; *ASL,* anterosuperior leaflet; *IVS,* interventricular septum; *A,* anterior; *P,* posterior; *R,* right; *L,* left.

ANATOMIC AND ECHOCARDIOGRAPHIC CONSIDERATIONS

The echocardiographic study of an atrioventricular septal defect, whether it is present in its complete or partial form, should include demonstration of (a) the anatomic consequences of absence of the atrioventricular septum; (b) a common atrioventricular annulus; (c) the anatomic and the functional characteristics of the atrioventricular valve; (d) the presence, location and shunting across intracardiac defects; (e) the anterior and slightly superior displacement of the aorta and disproportion between the inlet and outlet portions of the left ventricle; (f) any chamber dominance; (g) differential diagnosis; (h) associated anomalies; and (i) intra- and postoperative evaluation. Atrioventricular septal defects, if not associated with conotruncal malformations, usually have normal coronary anatomy.

Anatomic Consequences of Absence of the Atrioventricular Septum

The anatomic consequences of absence of the atrioventricular septum are an atrial septal defect ostium primum type, a deficiency of the inlet portion of the ventricular septum causing a variable "scooped out" appearance, and insertion of the right and left components of the atrioventricular valve at the same level. Shunting across the atrial and ventricular septal defects depends on the attachments of the atrioventricular valve leaflets. The four-chamber apical and subcostal views, sweeping the transducer anterior to posterior, usually clearly demonstrate these anatomical features, although other views provide additional important information.

An ostium primum defect is located in the lower portion of the atrial septum limited by the free border of the atrial septum superiorly and the atrioventricular valve inferiorly (Echo. 11-1). The actual size of the interatrial communication depends on additional coexisting deficiencies of the adjacent atrial septum as well as on the insertions of the atrioventricular valve to the underside of the septum. Uncommonly, these insertions may result in shunting only at the ventricular level. Since there can be septal dropout from an apical window, the presence and size of the atrial septal defect should be verified from the subcostal approach. Beginning from the four-chamber position, the two-dimensional ultrasound beam is aimed perpendicular to the atrial septal structures (see Fig. 4-17C) (Echo. 11-2); with 90 degrees of rotation to a short axis of the atria, the systemic venous drainage and the atrial septum can be seen (see Fig. 4-19A).

A deficiency of the inlet portion of the ventricular septum is seen between the crest of the interventricular septum and the atrioventricular valve. The presence and size of the interventricular communication depends on the in-

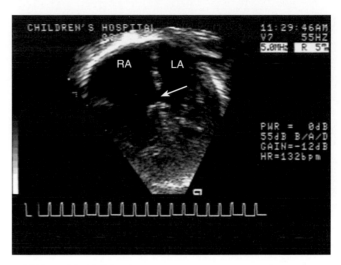

ECHO. 11-1. Apical four-chamber view of an ostium primum atrial septal defect *(arrow)*. Note that the atrioventricular valves insert at the same level due to the absence of the atrioventricular septum. *RA,* right atrium; *LA,* left atrium.

sertions of the atrioventricular valve to the ventricular septum as well as on concomitant deficiencies in the adjacent septum (41). A ventricular septal defect is almost always present in the complete form of atrioventricular septal defect but is generally absent in the partial form (42). To establish the presence, exact location, and extensions of a ventricular septal defect, it is necessary to thoroughly scan the area normally occupied by the atrioventricular septum from apical and subcostal four-chamber views by sweeping the probe anteroposteriorly from the outflow tract to the crux cordis (Echo. 11-3). The connections between the atrioventricular valve leaflets and their attachments to the interventricular septum are

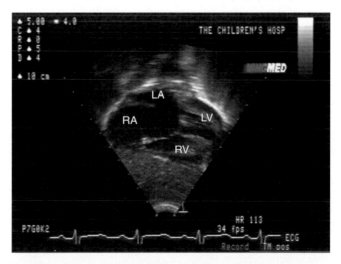

ECHO. 11-2. Subcostal four-chamber view of a large ostium primum atrial septal defect. Note the small left-sided structures due to the disposition of the atrioventricular annulus mainly over the right ventricle. *RA,* right atrium; *LA,* left atrium; *RV,* right ventricle; *LV,* left ventricle.

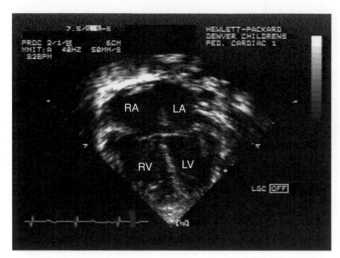

ECHO. 11-3. Apical four-chamber view of a complete atrioventricular septal defect with atrial and ventricular components. Note that the atrioventricular valves insert at the same level. *RA*, right atrium; *LA*, left atrium; *RV*, right ventricle; *LV*, left ventricle.

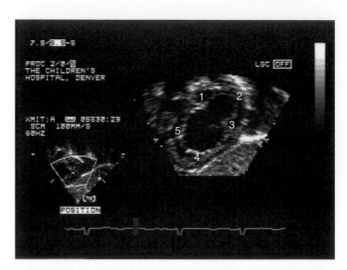

ECHO. 11-4. Magnified subcostal short-axis view demonstrating the common atrioventricular annulus and five-leaflet atrioventricular valve, hallmarks of an atrioventricular septal defect. The numbers *(1–5)* point to the five leaflets of the common valve.

also evident in this scan. Generally, the apical view is preferred for analysis of anterior septal structures, whereas the subcostal view is better for posterior structures, although this is very dependent on the patient's age and individual physical characteristics.

Insertion of the right and left components of the atrioventricular valve at the same level is considered one of the hallmarks of an atrioventricular septal defect. Echocardiographic definition of their relative levels of insertion is accomplished by sweeping the transducer anteroposteriorly from the aortic outflow to the crux in an apical view (Echo. 11-3). It is important to note that in the normal heart the apical displacement of the septal leaflet of the tricuspid valve is more evident posteriorly near the crux, whereas anteriorly, this displacement is less distinct.

A Common Atrioventricular Annulus

A common atrioventricular annulus is a consequence of the lack of contiguity of atrial and ventricular septal structures, which also results from the absent atrioventricular septum (41) (Figs. 11-1, 11-2). The common atrioventricular annulus is an ovoid-shaped single atrioventricular junction, which, according to the observations of Carpentier (43), has the greater axis of the left valvular orifice pointing towards the aorta irrespective of whether there is one common orifice or two distinct orifices. Echocardiographically, the short-axis view of the ventricles obtained either from a parasternal or a subcostal window will best reveal the common valve ring guarded by a five-leaflet valve (Echo. 11-4).

Anatomic and Functional Characteristics of the Atrioventricular Valve

Currently, most investigators agree that the atrioventricular valve in atrioventricular septal defects is basically constituted by five leaflets and bears little resemblance to either the tricuspid or mitral valves found in the normal heart (2,43,44). This justifies the use of the terms "left and right valvular components" when describing the atrioventricular valve in atrioventricular septal defect.

The left side of the valve is almost always trileaflet (44), with superior (or anterior) and inferior (or posterior) leaflets that have insertions in both ventricles; they are consequently called "bridging leaflets" (Fig. 11-1). Following the suggestions of Kirklin et al. (45–47), we prefer the use of superior and inferior terminology for the bridging leaflets because of its greater correlation with the surgeon's view, even though, in strict echocardiographic orientation, the relationship is more anteroposterior. A third left mural (or lateral) leaflet is usually smaller than normal. While the mural leaflet of a normal mitral valve occupies two-thirds of the annular circumference, in atrioventricular septal defects it usually makes up less than one-third of the orifice (21) (Echo. 11-5). The right valve shares the superior and inferior bridging leaflets and additionally has an anterosuperior and a mural leaflet (8,21,48,49) (Fig. 11-1) (Echo. 11-6). The right mural leaflet usually differs little from that found in the normal heart, although it can be somewhat smaller. In complete atrioventricular septal defect, the superior bridging and the right anterosuperior leaflet form an anatomical unit in terms of their size and insertions. This forms the basis for the classic differentiation originally proposed by Ras-

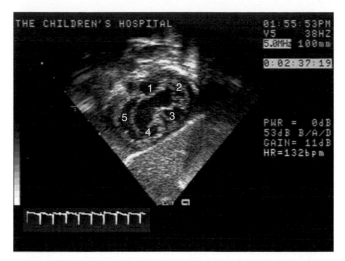

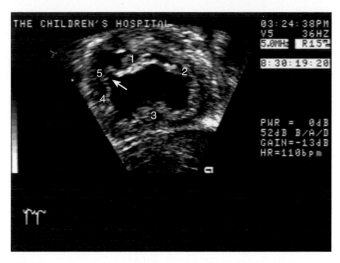

ECHO. 11-5. Subcostal short-axis view demonstrating the five leaflets of a common atrioventricular valve in a patient with mild bridging of the superior bridging leaflet (Rastelli type A). The superior leaflet attaches to the superior papillary muscle of the left ventricle and to a normally placed medial papillary muscle of the right ventricle. Leaflet *1,* superior bridging leaflet; *2,* left mural leaflet; *3,* inferior bridging leaflet, *4,* right mural leaflet; *5,* right anterosuperior leaflet.

ECHO. 11-7. Subcostal short-axis view demonstrating the five-leaflet arrangement in a patient with extreme bridging of the superior bridging leaflet (Rastelli type C). The superior bridging leaflet attaches to the right anterior papillary muscle directly *(arrow).* The anterosuperior leaflet is very small and the anterior papillary muscle supports the attachment of the superior bridging leaflet as well as the commissure between the anterosuperior and right mural leaflets. For leaflet numbers, see Echo. 11-5.

telli et al. (16), which in actuality is related to the degree of commitment of the superior bridging leaflet to the right ventricle (Fig. 11-1) (Echos. 11-5–11-7). As such, the Rastelli type A refers to a situation with minimal bridging of the superior leaflet, which attaches to the superior papillary muscle of the left ventricle and to the normally placed medial papillary muscle in the right ventricle. The

right anterosuperior leaflet is normal in size and inserts into the medial and anterior papillary muscles of the right ventricle (Fig. 11-1A) (Echo. 11-5). The Rastelli B comprises moderate bridging of the superior leaflet into the right ventricle, where it inserts into an anomalously located medial papillary muscle, which is either displaced partly down the septomarginal trabecula or adjacent to the anterior papillary muscle. The right anterosuperior leaflet is smaller, whereas the superior bridging leaflet is proportionately larger in size (Fig. 11-1B) (Echo. 11-6). Rastelli C includes extreme bridging of the superior leaflet. The medial papillary muscle is not apparent; rather, the superior bridging leaflet is attached to the anterior papillary muscle directly, which supports not only its commissure with the small anterosuperior leaflet but also the commissure between the anterosuperior and the right mural leaflet (21) (Fig. 11-1C) (Echo. 11-7). The inferior bridging leaflet has insertions in both ventricles, into the inferior papillary muscle of the left ventricle, and into the posterior papillary muscle of the right ventricle (Fig. 11-1). It exhibits variability in its overall size, and its insertions to the ventricular septum can be firmly anchored to the septum or attached through multiple chordae, or the leaflet can be totally free floating.

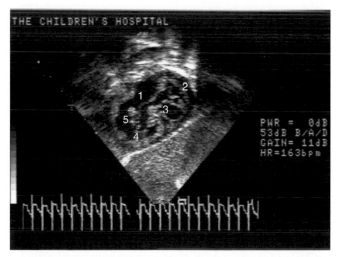

ECHO. 11-6. Subcostal short-axis view demonstrating the five leaflets of a common atrioventricular valve in a patient with moderate bridging of the superior bridging leaflet (Rastelli type B). The superior bridging leaflet attaches to a displaced medial papillary muscle. The right anterosuperior leaflet is proportionately smaller while the superior bridging leaflet is proportionately larger in size. For leaflet numbers, see Echo. 11-5.

In both complete and partial forms of atrioventricular septal defect, when the inferior and left mural leaflets are smaller than expected, there can be a lack of coaptation of the superior and inferior bridging leaflets (44). The insertions of the superior and inferior bridging leaflets to the interventricular septum typically mimic each other whether they are attached directly, through chordae, or free floating; shunting through a ventricular septal defect is related to these insertions, being almost always greater under the superior than the inferior leaflet (21).

The left ventricular papillary muscles in the normal heart are of equal size and are located obliquely within the ventricle in an anterolateral and posteromedial position. In both common and partial forms of atrioventricular septal defect, the papillary muscles are shifted in position so they hold a more superior and inferior relationship on the left ventricular free wall (4,21) (Figs. 11-1, 11-2) (Echo. 11-8). This is the result mostly of a shift in the position of the posteromedial papillary muscle rather than of the anterolateral papillary muscle. The superior papillary muscle supports the commissure between the superior bridging and the left mural leaflet, whereas the inferior one supports the commissure between the left mural and the inferior bridging leaflet (Fig. 11-1). In the right ventricle, there are normally three papillary muscles: an anterior or anterolateral muscle inserted at the anterior free wall of the right ventricle and joined with the apical end of the septomarginal trabecula by the moderator band, a posterior muscle located juxtaseptally, and a medial (conal) papillary muscle inserted in the ventricular septum and related with the posterior limb of the septomarginal trabecula. In partial atrioventricular septal defects, these are normal in shape and position. In the complete form, the anterior papillary muscle is positioned normally, but its shape is unusual, being bifid and having a wider base. It supports either the commissure between the anterosuperior and the right mural leaflet (Rastelli A and B), or it incorporates the attachments of the superior bridging leaflet (Rastelli C) (Fig. 11-1). The posterior papillary muscle is positioned normally and supports the commissure between the right mural and inferior bridging leaflets.

The medial papillary muscle is more variable. It is normally located in Rastelli type A, anomalously placed in Rastelli type B, and absent in Rastelli type C (4,21,22,44) (Fig. 11-1).

In arriving at a logical and clinically useful nomenclature for the leaflets composing this valve, a point of controversy has been the actual nature of the so-called "cleft of the anterior mitral leaflet." It is presently agreed that the area of separation between the left-sided superior and inferior bridging leaflets traditionally named "cleft of the anterior mitral leaflet" is more a true commissure than a cleft even if it lacks commissural chords (40,50). This more functional denotation adopted for atrioventricular septal defect is justified in the living heart since the space between the superior and inferior leaflets is part of the orifice (20,22) and not merely a gap in an otherwise structurally single leaflet (a true cleft) (Echo. 11-9). The other area of separation between the superior bridging leaflet and the anterosuperior leaflet of the right component, which has been termed "cleft or division of the common anterior leaflet," is less of a conceptual problem. Even in their original description, Rastelli et al. (16) recognized the similarity between this "cleft" and the anteroseptal commissure of the normal tricuspid valve. Later, several authors emphasized this similarity (17,45,51), particularly since this "cleft" has commissural chordae attached to papillary muscles (40,50). As such, then, this gap should also be considered a commissure both in anatomic and functional terms (20) (Echo. 11-7). This apparently academic controversy acquires clinical, echocardiographic, and surgical importance in its differentiation from cases

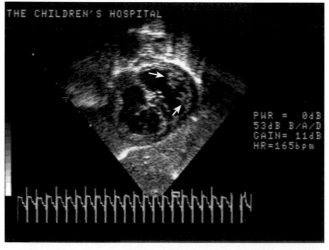

ECHO. 11-8. Subcostal short-axis view in a repaired complete atrioventricular septal defect. The arrows point to the two left-sided papillary muscles that are displaced into a more superior and inferior relationship on the left ventricular free wall.

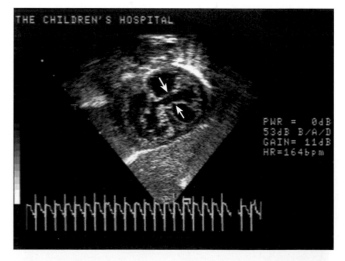

ECHO. 11-9. Subcostal short-axis view demonstrating the commissure between the superior and inferior bridging leaflets (arrows), commonly called the "cleft of the anterior mitral leaflet." Note that the space between the bridging leaflets is part of the valve orifice itself and not merely a gap in an otherwise single leaflet. Further, the space points towards the interventricular septum and not towards the left ventricular outflow as would be seen in a true isolated cleft of the mitral valve. (Compare to Echo. 13-11.)

of isolated clefts of the anterior mitral leaflet (discussed below), as well as in the surgical approach required to maintain left valve integrity (16,43,52,53). The abnormal disposition of the left-sided papillary muscles determines the vertical orientation of the left valvular orifice, different from the oblique direction seen in the normal mitral valve. Therefore, the commissure between the two bridging leaflets points to the interventricular septum rather than towards the aortic outflow tract, as seen in isolated clefts of the anterior mitral leaflet (21,54,55) (see Echo. 13-11).

The basic difference between the common and partial forms of atrioventricular septal defects is in the anatomy of the two bridging leaflets. While in the complete defect the two bridging leaflets are separate entities giving origin to one orifice, in the partial form (ostium primum atrial septal defect) the bridging leaflets are joined by a connecting tongue of leaflet tissue running along the plane of the ventricular septum and usually adherent to its crest, thereby resulting in two distinct orifices, albeit with one common ring (48,56) (Figs. 11-1, 11-2) (Echo. 11-10). Often a ''gap in the septal leaflet of the tricuspid valve'' is described with this form of atrioventricular septal defect. This is, in reality, the result of a curved attachment of the superior bridging leaflet to the right side of the ventricular septum, producing an apparent lack of valvar tissue (17,21). This line of attachment can also appear as a bulge or ''pouch,'' which has resulted in its being called ''tricuspid pouch'' by some authors (57). When present, this pouch usually prevents shunting from the left ventricle into the right atrium (Echo. 11-11).

The echocardiographic analysis of the atrioventricular valvular apparatus in these lesions centers around the

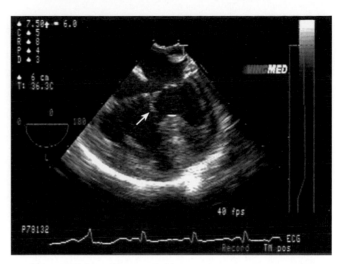

ECHO. 11-11. Transesophageal horizontal four-chamber view demonstrating a tricuspid pouch that is the result of a curved attachment of the superior bridging leaflet onto the right side of the ventricular septum (arrow). This pouch often prevents shunting across the ventricular defect.

parasternal and subcostal short-axis views. With posterior orientation of the transducer, the papillary muscle arrangement comes into view, and the abnormal superior-inferior position of the left-sided papillary muscles is evident (Echo. 11-8). Sweeping anteriorly towards the valve reveals its five-leaflet configuration, the position and size of the commissure between the two bridging leaflets, and the definition as to whether the defect is complete or partial (Echos. 11-5–11-7, 11-12). The orientation of the commissure facing the interventricular septum is also seen in this sweep.

The four-chamber apical and subcostal views reveal the degree of bridging of the superior and inferior leaflets,

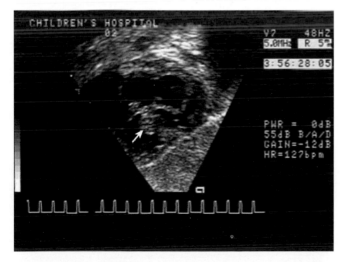

ECHO. 11-10. Subcostal short-axis view in a partial atrioventricular septal defect illustrating the tongue of leaflet tissue running along the interventricular septum (arrow). This connecting tissue tongue joins the superior and inferior bridging leaflets, giving origin to two distinct orifices while still with one common annulus.

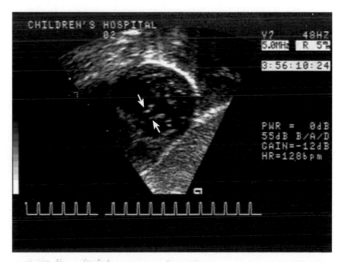

ECHO. 11-12. Subcostal short-axis view emphasizing the commissure between the superior and inferior bridging leaflets (arrow) in a partial form of atrioventricular septal defect.

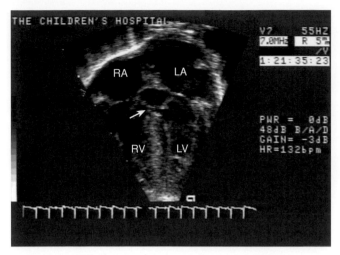

ECHO. 11-13. Apical four-chamber view revealing the superior bridging leaflet firmly attached to the underside of the atrial septum. There is a ventricular septal defect *(arrow)* underneath the inferior bridging leaflet. *RA*, right atrium; *LA*, left atrium; *RV*, right ventricle; *LV*, left ventricle.

the presence of a ventricular septal defect under both leaflets, and the right ventricular anatomy—usually not available from a short axis view (Echos. 11-1, 11-3, 11-13). The site of attachment of the superior bridging leaflet in the right ventricle—to the normally placed medial papillary muscle (Rastelli A) (Echo. 11-11), to an anomalously displaced medial papillary muscle (Rastelli B) (Echo. 11-14), or to the anterior papillary muscle (Rastelli C) (Echo. 11-15)—is determined by angling the transducer anteroposteriorly and left to right. The size of the different leaflets can also be measured from a combination of the short-axis and four-chamber views, and particular emphasis should be placed on the size of the inferior and left

mural leaflets and on the separation between the bridging leaflets because of their obvious surgical implications.

In the partial form, a short-axis sweep from parasternal or subcostal positions demonstrates the two separate orifices (Echos. 11-10, 11-12). The four-chamber apical or subcostal views also show the apparent gap in the "septal" component of the right valve due to the attachment of the superior bridging leaflet along the right border of the interventricular septum. The nature of the septal attachments of both bridging leaflets can be defined in detail in these views so that a defect underneath either leaflet can be identified preoperatively (Echos. 11-1, 11-3, 11-13). Color Doppler flow mapping can aid in the identification of small ventricular septal defects, which may be hidden under chordal attachments (see below).

Even without additional anomalies, the usual arrangement of the left atrioventricular valve in atrioventricular septal defects tends towards dysfunction because of the abnormal papillary muscle position, the deficit in leaflet tissue, the abnormal chordae tendineae, and the trifoliate valve format (58). The echocardiographic study will be approached sequentially for the separate components of the valvular system: leaflets, chordae tendineae, and papillary muscles.

Leaflets

The deficit in leaflet tissue is most evident in two areas of the left valve, at the site of the commissure between the bridging leaflets (so-called "cleft" of the anterior mitral leaflet) and at the commissure between the inferior bridging and the left mural leaflets. Predictably, regurgitation is seen most commonly at these two points. The regurgitant jet occurring through the commissure of the

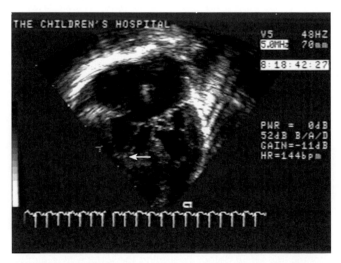

ECHO. 11-14. Apical four-chamber view demonstrating moderate bridging of the superior bridging leaflet attaching onto a displaced medial papillary muscle (Rastelli type B) *(arrow)*.

ECHO. 11-15. Apical four-chamber view demonstrating extreme bridging of the superior bridging leaflet (Rastelli type C). The attachment of the leaflet to the anterior papillary muscle is shown *(arrow)*.

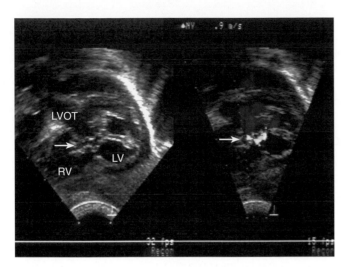

ECHO. 11-16. Left: Subcostal view illustrating the commissure between the bridging leaflets *(arrow)*. **Right:** The color Doppler flow map of the regurgitation through the commissural space is shown *(arrow)*. *LV,* left ventricle; *RV,* right ventricle; *LVOT,* left ventricular outflow tract.

bridging leaflets should be evaluated from the parasternal and apical long-axis and the apical and subcostal four- and two-chamber views; it is usually medial and is almost universally present in different grades of severity, which explains the tendency of most surgeons to attempt closure of this commissure, with mixed results (59,60) (Echo. 11-16; see color plate 32 following p. 364). Regurgitation around the inferior bridging and left mural leaflets is localized centrally within the valve orifice or at either one of its commissures (Echo. 11-17; see color plate 33 following p. 364). It has been suggested that, in partial atrioventricular septal defect, when the inferior bridging leaflet is small relative to the size of the left mural leaflet, regurgitation is more likely

to occur postoperatively (58). Valvular dysplasia can be a factor in regurgitation. However, echocardiographically, this is seen merely as tissue thickening; a specific correlation with regurgitation has not been established to date.

Most commonly, as has been stated, the left valve in both forms of atrioventricular septal defect is trifoliate, but occasionally anomalies are found, including a dual or accessory orifice, two leaflets, one leaflet, and an imperforate orifice. Based on findings in an autopsy series of 151 hearts with atrioventricular septal defect, Ebels et al. (44) have suggested an explanation of these anomalies in terms of a spectrum of diminishing commissural formation, particularly frequent in the partial form of atrioventricular septal defect. A dual left-sided orifice was most commonly the result of partial fusion of the commissure between the inferior bridging and the left mural leaflets, rarely involving the superior bridging leaflet and having a smaller but fully formed papillary muscle supporting the "extra" orifice. These observations were confirmed in the study by Draulans-Noe et al. (61). A bileaflet left valve resulted from lack of formation of the commissure between the inferior and mural leaflets and was supported by a single papillary muscle. A single leaflet left valve had no recognizable commissures, was supported by a single papillary muscle, and was associated with hypoplastic left ventricle. Imperforate valves were found also in association with hypoplastic left ventricles and, predictably, supporting structures were not definable. The ventricular architecture in these hearts with left atrioventricular valve anomalies had greater inlet to outlet disproportion and a greater degree of ventricular septal scooping than other hearts with atrioventricular septal defect (44). By far the most common anomaly of leaflet formation is the dual orifice left valve, usually of the inferior bridging leaflet (44,62,63) (Echo. 11-18).

Although its preoperative identification is reassuring to

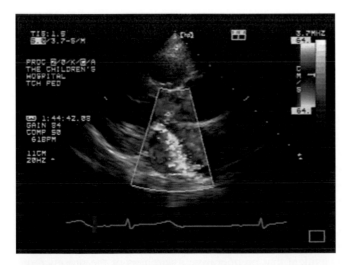

ECHO. 11-17. Color Doppler flow map from a parasternal long-axis view demonstrating a central regurgitant jet most likely originating around the inferior bridging and left mural leaflets.

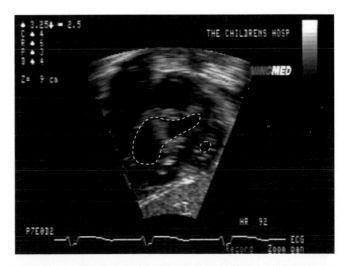

ECHO. 11-18. Subcostal view demonstrating the presence of dual orifices of the left atrioventricular valve, with major and minor orifices outlined *(dotted lines)*.

both the echocardiographer and the surgeon, in effect any attempt to open the partially fused commissure at surgery results in severe regurgitation so that currently published surgical series suggest leaving the dual orifice intact because results are comparable to those in patients without this valve anomaly, even if the combined size of the two orifices appears smaller than usual (60,63,64). Echocardiographically, anomalies of the left valve leaflets should be detected from the short-axis views (parasternal and subcostal combined) by slowly scanning from the ventricular apex to the valve annulus (Echo. 11-18). Since abnormalities of the papillary muscles are commonly found in association with unusual leaflet anatomy, their detection during the scan should alert the examiner to a more careful review of leaflet structure. Nonetheless, it should be noted that since a dual orifice left valve in atrioventricular septal defect may be the result of fusion of leaflet tissue partially obliterating a commissure, its supporting valvular structures are usually close to those expected in atrioventricular septal defect, which compounds the diagnostic problem for the examiner, particularly in the young infant or if the "extra" orifice is small (44,61,65–68). With the advent of color Doppler flow mapping, the diagnosis of dual orifice valves has been facilitated. Forward flow across the atrioventricular valves is particularly amenable to interrogation from the apical four-chamber view, and with the current spatial resolution of color encoding, flow through the two orifices may be seen as a double jet entering the left ventricle in diastole, although angling of the transducer slightly anteroposteriorly and right to left is necessary since the two orifices are usually in different planes. Guided by the color image, it may be possible to differentiate the major and minor orifices, and obtain a semiquantitative estimate of their effective areas. This approach is also suitable for detecting other leaflet anomalies and should be considered an integral part of the complete echocardiographic assessment of the left valve pre- and postoperatively.

Stenosis of the left atrioventricular valve, if hemodynamically significant, is usually found in association with left ventricular underdevelopment, although isolated annular hypoplasia can also be seen (54). Evaluation of annular and ventricular size is best accomplished starting from a parasternal long-axis view followed by clockwise rotation of the transducer to a short axis, where serial cuts from annulus to apex permit sequential measurements of chamber size for comparison with normal values (69). The four-chamber apical and subcostal views will also serve to confirm the site(s) and degree of hypoplasia. Depending on the patient's age and physique, a subcostal short-axis view can provide additional important information on the size of the left heart structures. The Doppler study is best conducted from the apical window in a four-chamber view, which permits direct alignment of the interrogating beam with flow across the valve. A higher than expected velocity will most likely be recorded due

to the presence of significant valve regurgitation and a shunt. This makes the estimation of the transvalvular peak and mean gradient and the effective valvular area difficult to relate specifically to the presence of left-sided valve stenosis. Therefore, a critical examination of the anatomy of the valve becomes essential.

Chordae Tendineae

Chordal malattachment and presence of short, fused, or elongated chordal support, even in the presence of otherwise usual leaflet arrangement, can lead to regurgitation or, less commonly, stenosis of the left valve in atrioventricular septal defect. Usually, anomalies of the tensor apparatus are compounded by alterations in the papillary muscle structure, although situations occur when all chords of the left valve insert into one papillary muscle, even though two papillary muscle groups are present, thereby creating a potentially parachute-like functional situation (62). The echocardiographic assessment of the tensor apparatus is conducted simultaneously with the overall study of the leaflets and papillary muscles. The parasternal, apical, and subcostal long-axis views are particularly useful for evaluation of the chordae and their relationship to the left ventricular outflow tract. As has been previously emphasized, chords of the left valve can be anomalously attached to the outflow tract and can cause obstruction. Chordal anatomy is also well seen from four-chamber views, the apical position being particularly helpful for evaluating those of the superior leaflet and the subcostal position for the inferior and mural leaflets. The Doppler evaluation of secondary regurgitation or stenosis of the valve is similar to that described above.

Papillary Muscles

Anomalies of the left papillary muscle in atrioventricular septal defect can, if unrecognized, cause important problems, particularly in the postoperative period. The presence of a single papillary muscle is relatively frequent in hearts with atrioventricular septal defect, particularly with common atrioventricular orifice (17,61). In this setting it has been called "potentially parachute" since the orifice becomes overtly stenotic if the commissure between the bridging leaflets ("cleft") is sutured at surgery, especially if the left mural leaflet is very small or totally absent (60,61). The orifice, however, may be restrictive even prior to surgery depending on the morphology of the chords and the location of the single papillary muscle. Carpentier has advocated splitting the single papillary muscle, thereby creating two muscles from one (43). It is evident that preoperative awareness of the presence of a single papillary muscle is essential for adequate planning, and echocardiography is ideally suited for this assessment. The short-axis views (parasternal and subcostal) permit detailed study by sequentially "cutting" the ventricle from apex to base. A single papillary muscle has been likened to a solitary tooth in the mouth, with its position being usually central within the ventricle (65). Other abnormalities that require echocardiographic identification, since they can functionally mimic a single papillary muscle, are single-focus left ventricular chordal attachment; a so-called "dominant papillary muscle group," where one is much larger than the other; abnormal proximity of the two papillary muscles; and presence of three papillary muscles, which can join in a common base on the ventricular wall (58,62,65,68). Doppler study of transvalvular flow is best accomplished from the apical four-chamber view where, following the same techniques explained previously, both forward velocities and presence and location of regurgitation can be assessed.

Presence, Location, and Shunting Across Intracardiac Defects

In all types of atrioventricular septal defects, intracardiac shunts vary, depending on the nature of the attachments of the bridging leaflets to the ventricular septal crest and/or the underside of the atrial septum. We will consider these possibilities firstly when two separate valve orifices are present (partial form) and secondly when only one common atrioventricular valve orifice exists (complete form).

In the vast majority of cases of atrioventricular septal defect with two separate valve orifices, there is shunting at the atrial level (ostium primum atrial septal defect). The spectral and color Doppler demonstration of the direction and velocity of shunting through the atrial defect is accomplished through the complementary use of the apical and subcostal four-chamber views, positioning the transducer as much as possible along the presumed direction of flow (Echo. 11-19; see color plate 34 following p. 364). Shunting is usually holodiastolic, laminar, and of low velocity, seen on the color Doppler map as a band of deep red or orange left-to-right flow. Actual velocity measurement across the defect itself can be obtained by placing the pulsed Doppler sample volume within the defect guided by the two-dimensional image and the color flow map. These can be somewhat elevated, resulting in aliasing depending on the size of the defect and the amount of blood shunting across it. The combination of the color flow pattern and the spectral velocities along with other indirect anatomical and functional indicators can give a fairly accurate qualitative measure of the amount of shunting. Depending on hemodynamics and other associated malformations, there can also be reversal of flow direction (i.e., right-to-left atrial shunting) during short periods of the cardiac cycle, which can be confirmed by careful frame-by-frame analysis of the two-dimensional color Doppler flow images and by recording

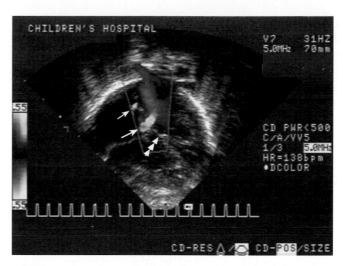

ECHO. 11-19. Color Doppler flow map of the left-to-right shunt across an ostium primum atrial septal defect *(large arrow)*. Note the presence of a smaller shunt across a patent foramen ovale *(small arrow)*. The ventricular septum, through which there is no shunt, is shown *(triple arrows)*.

of pulsed-wave and color M-mode traces of the flow across the defect since these have a better time resolution. A parasternal short-axis view at the level of the aortic root angling the transducer towards the crux cordis can also demonstrate shunting through an atrial septal defect on the color Doppler flow map. This view is useful as an indirect indicator of an atrial defect when there is a difficult apical or subcostal window.

In most instances of separate atrioventricular valve orifices, the bridging leaflets and their connecting tissue tongue are firmly attached to the crest of the ventricular septum so that no shunting occurs at the ventricular level. If shunting across a ventricular septal defect is present, it is usually small and located under the inferior bridging leaflet through its chordal insertions to the ventricular septum. There are rare cases of atrioventricular septal defect with two orifices in which the bridging leaflets and their connecting tissue tongue are firmly attached to the underside of the atrial septum so that shunting is only present at the ventricular level (Echo. 11-13). In these instances, the diagnosis of atrioventricular septal defect requires confirmation of other anatomical stigmata of the lesion since these could represent a perimembranous ventricular septal defect with inlet extensions (see "Differential Diagnosis"). As with the common form, in atrioventricular septal defect with two orifices, a ventricular septal defect under the inferior bridging leaflet is best visualized from a subcostal four-chamber view, while an apical four-chamber view is preferred for identifying defects under the superior bridging leaflet. Color Doppler flow mapping in these views demonstrates the extent, direction, and point of origin of the shunting. In most instances a jet is seen to originate within the left ventricle and cross the septum in a left-to-right direction towards the right ventricular and/or right atrial cavities during systole. This is confirmed by identifying the region of laminar rapid flow acceleration (flow convergence zone) within the left ventricle while the turbulent decelerating jet, seen as color variance on the flow map, is noted within the right heart cavities. The overall width of the jet at the point of crossing of the actual defect can serve as an indirect indicator of the anatomic size of the defect.

In atrioventricular septal defect with one common orifice, almost invariably there is shunting at both atrial and ventricular levels (Echo. 11-20; see color plate 35 following p. 364). The atrial shunting is of the ostium primum type and of variable size. The ventricular defect is located beneath the superior leaflet in all cases, and generally the shunt size is larger, with greater degrees of bridging. Depending on the size of the inferior bridging leaflet, its degree of septal attachments, and the thickness of its supporting chords, there can also be a shunt posteriorly, although the anatomic demonstration of this defect itself by two-dimensional echocardiography alone can be difficult in some cases, thereby requiring the use of color Doppler flow imaging.

The echocardiographic and Doppler approaches to the study of shunting patterns across the atrial and ventricular septa in atrioventricular septal defect with common orifice is similar to that in the partial form. In the presence of a common orifice, however, the size of the interventricular shunt is usually larger and consequently of greater hemodynamic importance. A left ventricular to right atrial shunt, when present, is also larger, and, depending on right-sided hemodynamics, there can be right ventricular to left atrial shunting and flow reversal across the ventricular defect during certain points in systole. Due to the typically short duration of these flow reversals, coupled with the frame rate limitations imposed by the two-

dimensional color flow mapping technique, they can be missed during routine examination. The color M-mode format is a more accurate and sensitive means of visualizing the direction of flow throughout the cardiac cycle without acquisition time limitations; it should be used for the conclusive demonstration of the direction and duration of shunting. Recording of a clean velocity trace with pulsed-wave or continuous wave Doppler should also be attempted across a ventricular septal defect of any significant size in order to derive the interventricular pressure gradient. The four-chamber views usually do not permit orientation of the spectral Doppler interrogating beam along the actual direction of flow across the ventricular defect; this is best accomplished from the parasternal long-axis view. Care should be exercised so that the velocity trace reflects true interventricular flow without contamination from either a left ventricular to right atrial shunt or a jet of valvular regurgitation, which would result in an erroneous gradient estimation. A clean spectral velocity trace can also serve as an adjunct to the color M-mode study to determine the direction of shunting throughout the cardiac cycle.

As a result of the greater volume load imposed on the left ventricle in the presence of left-to-right shunting, diminished function can occur in these patients, manifesting clinically as congestive heart failure. Measurements of left ventricular function, estimation of left-to-right shunting at different sites qualitatively with the use of color flow mapping as explained above, and assessment of valvular regurgitation using a combination of two-dimensional imaging, and color and spectral Doppler are all pertinent parameters of utility in the clinical management and surgical planning for these patients. In addition, due to the risk of pulmonary hypertension, particularly in patients with associated Down's syndrome, measurement of velocities across the ventricular septal defect, of the tricuspid regurgitant jet, and of the pulmonary valve using pulsed-wave and/or continuous wave Doppler is useful in estimating pulmonary artery pressure using the Bernoulli equation and should be attempted routinely (see Chapter 35).

Anterior and Slightly Superior Displacement of the Aorta and Disproportion Between the Inlet and Outlet Portions of the Left Ventricle

This anatomical finding results from the single atrioventricular junction universally present in atrioventricular septal defect and contributes to the characteristic so-called "goose neck" deformity. As a consequence, the fibrous ventriculoinfundibular fold, which would constitute the aortic-left atrioventricular valve continuity, is lengthened and separates the junction point of the leaflets, giving rise to an elongated and narrowed appearance of the left ventricular outflow tract (4,70). Despite this anatomical appearance, actual obstruction is rare, particularly preop-

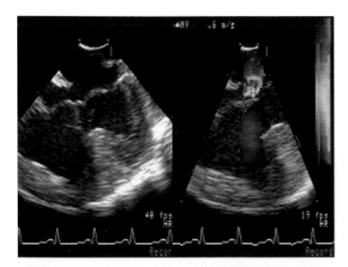

ECHO. 11-20. Transesophageal horizontal four-chamber view of a complete atrioventricular septal defect with atrial and ventricular defects. There is mild bridging of the superior leaflet and left-to-right shunting across both defects.

eratively (65,71). Predicting preoperatively the risk of postoperative left ventricular outflow tract obstruction is not obvious from the echocardiogram. However, most authors agree that short and thickened chordal attachments of the superior bridging leaflet to the crest of the ventricular septum is a major factor in creating postoperative obstruction (71), especially in the partial forms of atrioventricular septal defect since in the common form the superior leaflet is usually free floating (72,73). In the partial form of atrioventricular septal defect, Ebels et al. (72) found other causes of left ventricular outflow tract obstruction such as abnormal insertions of the superior bridging leaflet rarely, different degrees of malalignment of the aorta in up to 62% of cases (as a function of the rightward aortic root displacement), and passive muscular obstruction of the outflow tract in 71% of cases, which manifested on the echocardiogram as premature closure of the aortic valve in 28% of patients in their series. Other mechanisms responsible for obstruction of the outflow tract seen in both common and partial forms of atrioventricular septal defect are malposition of the left-sided papillary muscles, accessory chords or tissue tags within the outflow tract, fibromuscular obstruction, aneurysms or remnants of the membranous septum protruding into the outflow tract, and hypoplasia of left-sided structures seen in dominant right forms of atrioventricular septal defect (65,72,73).

Echocardiographically, the left ventricular outflow tract is best studied from the long-axis views obtained from the parasternal, apical, and/or subcostal approaches. In these views, its elongated and narrowed appearance is readily seen, contributing to the typical "goose neck" deformity (74) (Echo. 11-21). The movement of the superior bridging leaflet relative to the outflow tract is well seen also in these views; usually this leaflet is seen to encroach into the outflow tract in diastole and can even touch the interventricular septum, giving the impression of obstruction. However, careful examination demonstrates a free outflow tract in systole (Echo. 11-22). The anterior displacement of the aorta (appearance of malalignment) can also be evaluated in these views.

Assessment of flows through the left ventricular outflow tract using spectral and color Doppler flow mapping requires alignment with the direction of flow. This is best accomplished from an apical window, with the transducer directed anteriorly and superiorly, bringing into view the entire subaortic area. Mapping of velocities using a combination of pulsed-wave and high PRF Doppler would reveal any specific area of obstruction. Velocities can be verified from a suprasternal and a right parasternal or infraclavicular window with an independent Pedof probe to avoid possible underestimation of actual velocities.

The disproportion between the inlet and outlet portions of the left ventricle seen in atrioventricular septal defects is accentuated by the elongation of the left ventricular outflow tract and unwedging of the aorta. It occurs to the same extent in both the complete and partial forms (4,21,22). In addition, the deficiency of the inlet portion of the ventricular septum gives the septum a "scooped" appearance, which tends to be more marked in the complete than the partial form of the defect, as demonstrated by the "scoop"/outlet ratio described by Penkoske et al. (21) and Anderson et al. (4,75).

Echocardiographically, the inlet/outlet disproportion is evident from a parasternal, an apical, or a subcostal long-axis view, although actual measurements are not commonly performed (Echo. 11-21). The deficiency in the mid portion of the ventricular septum is also seen from the apical four-chamber view. Gutgesell and Huhta (76)

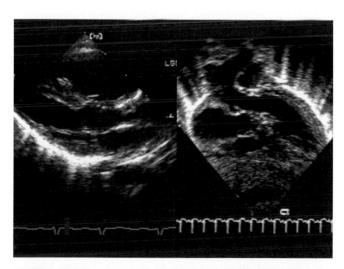

ECHO. 11-21. Long-axis parasternal **(left)** and subcostal **(right)** views demonstrating the elongated and narrowed left ventricular outflow tract, giving the typical goose neck deformity.

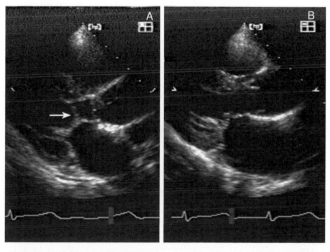

ECHO. 11-22. Parasternal long-axis view in diastole **(left)** and systole **(right)** illustrating the movement of the superior leaflet encroaching into the left ventricular outflow tract in diastole *(arrow)*. In systole, the outflow tract is free.

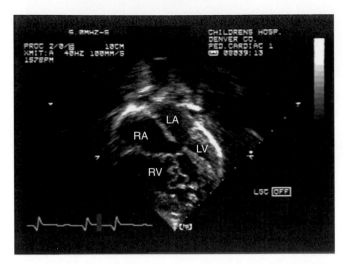

ECHO. 11-23. Apical four-chamber view of a right dominant form of complete atrioventricular septal defect. *RA,* right atrium; *LA,* left atrium; *RV,* right ventricle; *LV,* left ventricle.

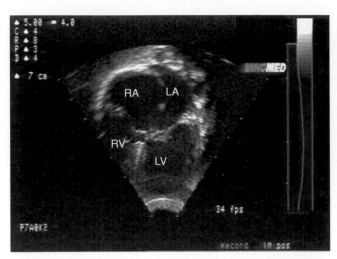

ECHO. 11-24. Apical four-chamber view of a left dominant type of complete atrioventricular septal defect. *RA,* right atrium; *LA,* left atrium; *RV,* right ventricle; *LV,* left ventricle.

measured the atrial and ventricular septum from this view in patients with atrioventricular septal defect (common and partial forms) and compared their results with normals and with patients having other lesions. They demonstrated a deficiency in atrioventricular and ventricular septal tissue, which was greater in the common form (76). These findings correspond to those of Penkoske et al. (21,75).

Chamber Dominance

In both forms of atrioventricular septal defect, ventricular chamber dominance is determined by the disposition of the single atrioventricular annulus relative to the ventricles. In the balanced form (the most usual), the atrioventricular annulus is equally committed over both ventricles, which are then of equal size (Echo. 11-3). A right dominant form exists when the atrioventricular annulus is primarily committed to the right ventricle, resulting in small left-sided structures (Echos. 11-2, 11-23). A left dominant type is present when the atrioventricular annulus is related mainly with the left ventricle, leading to an underdevelopment of the right-sided components (77) (Echo. 11-24). Malalignment of atrial and ventricular septa is frequently present when there is chamber dominance in the face of a common orifice type of atrioventricular septal defect. In these cases, the inlet ventricular septum does not extend to the crux cordis and, therefore, resembles those associated with straddling tricuspid valve (Echo. 11-24) (see "Differential Diagnosis"). The concept of chamber dominance can be applied to the atria when the atrioventricular annulus is equally connected to both ventricles, which are of comparable size, but the atrial septum is malaligned

with respect to the ventricular septum; this is named "double outlet atrium."

Echocardiographically, the best approach to assess chamber dominance is the four-chamber view from the apical and the subcostal windows. Scanning the transducer right to left and anteroposteriorly, the examiner can determine the position of the atrial and ventricular septa, detect any malalignment between them, and assess the size of the four cardiac chambers, possible hypoplasia of their components, and the disposition of the atrioventricular annulus with respect to the ventricles (Echos. 11-2, 11-23, 11-24). Actual measurements of ventricular cavities should be made from the parasternal short-axis view and compared to the established normals for body surface area (69).

In cases of right ventricular dominance, the left-sided structures, usually small, must be evaluated from multiple echocardiographic cuts. The long-axis views (parasternal, apical, and subcostal) can be used for assessing left atrioventricular valve stenosis or hypoplasia and for estimating the size of the left ventricular outflow tract and the aortic annulus and valve, and the dimensions of the ascending aorta. The suprasternal and right parasternal views supplemented by the subcostal long-axis view in infants, are useful for examination of the ascending, transverse arch and descending aorta, and detection of the presence of coarctation of the aorta or arch interruption. Doppler study of flow velocities from these views, using color and spectral formats, facilitates the diagnosis and allows determination of the severity of obstruction. The echocardiographic and color Doppler appearance in aortic arch interruption is quite specific, with the head and neck vessels directed almost superiorly without the usual curvature, which normally forms the shape of the connection between the ascending and the descending aorta.

In left ventricular dominance, the right-sided structures

are small. Besides the four-chamber views, the parasternal short-axis sweep from apex to base permits not only assessment of the size of the right ventricular cavity for comparison to normals but also evaluation of the size of the right ventricular outflow, pulmonary annulus, and valve and pulmonary arterial bifurcation. Doppler velocities across the right ventricular outflow tract and pulmonic valve can be used to estimate any gradient. The color Doppler study demonstrates the amount of forward transvalvular flow and aids in the differentiation from valve atresia. The suprasternal short-axis and left high parasternal windows can be used to visualize and measure the size of the confluence and the distal pulmonary arteries. The color flow map also facilitates the diagnosis of extracardiac shunts, which can be present, such as patent ductus arteriosus.

In atrial dominance, it is important to determine the outlet of the nondominant atrium. This is best accomplished from four-chamber views using two-dimensional imaging as well as Doppler. If the left atrial outlet is inadequate there can be resultant pulmonary hypertension similar to that found in other forms of obstruction to left ventricular inflow, with devastating consequences.

Differential Diagnosis

An atrioventricular septal defect must be differentiated from a perimembranous ventricular septal defect with inlet extensions; from a left ventricular to right atrial communication through the membranous portion of the atrioventricular septum; from a straddling tricuspid valve; and from an isolated cleft in an otherwise normal mitral valve. It is important to emphasize that, in all these circumstances, the atrioventricular septum is present; consequently, these all lack the anatomical stigmata of true atrioventricular septal defects.

A perimembranous ventricular septal defect with inlet extensions is located in the region of the membranous septum roofed by the central fibrous body of the heart, partially covered by the septal leaflet of the tricuspid valve and more or less extended into the right ventricular inlet. In this type of defect, erroneously called "ventricular septal defect, canal type" (78), there are two separate atrioventricular valvular annuli, normally configured mitral and tricuspid valves with the aorta wedged between them. These features are clearly seen echocardiographically through the long-axis, short-axis, and four-chamber views obtained parasternally, apically, and subcostally.

A left ventricular to right atrial defect ("Gerbode defect") is very uncommon; it is small and located in the membranous portion of the atrioventricular septum (79). Echocardiographically, it can be seen from an apical approach angling the transducer anteriorly and superiorly towards the left ventricular outflow tract. Color Doppler flow mapping can demonstrate the presence of these de-

fects, even if very small, where two-dimensional imaging alone may miss them.

A straddling tricuspid valve complex comprises a ventricular defect in the inlet portion of the septum, malalignment between the atrial and ventricular septa, and attachment of the tricuspid valve chords to the left ventricle. At the level of the atrioventricular junction, the ventricular septum is far from the crux to an extent proportional to the degree of straddle (80). Despite the straddling, there are still two separate atrioventricular valves that insert at different levels; consequently, this would not fulfill the criteria for an atrioventricular septal defect. These anatomical details can be observed best from the four-chamber views.

As has been stated in previous sections of this chapter, the left atrioventricular valve in atrioventricular septal defect is trileaflet and the so-called "cleft of the anterior mitral valve" is truly the commissure between the superior and inferior bridging leaflets. This commissure points to the interventricular septum and is part of the orifice of the valve itself. Isolated clefts of the mitral valve point to the left ventricular outflow tract and resemble an artificial cut made with a surgical scalpel dividing the free portion of the anterior mitral leaflet and resulting in a flail, grossly regurgitant valve (20,48,51). The best echocardiographic views to evaluate a mitral valve cleft are the short-axis views. In a base-to-apex sweep, the bileaflet mitral valve is seen (and differentiated from the trileaflet one seen in atrioventricular septal defects) and the orientation of the cleft towards the outflow is confirmed (see Echo. 13-11). Spectral and color Doppler flow mapping obtained from the parasternal long-axis and the apical four-chamber, long-axis, and two-chamber views demonstrate the presence and location of the regurgitation and permit estimation of its severity.

Associated Anomalies

Atrioventricular septal defects can be found in association with other types of atrial and ventricular septal defects, most notably defects in the fossa ovalis and muscular septum, respectively, as well as patent ductus arteriosus, anomalous pulmonary venous drainage, and unroofed coronary sinus. Echocardiographically, the diagnosis of additional muscular ventricular defects has been facilitated by the use of color Doppler flow mapping, which helps bring into evidence the additional shunts typically seen from the short-axis and four-chamber views, even when these are small. The echocardiographic diagnosis of anomalous pulmonary venous drainage is established from a combination of the apical and subcostal four-chamber views, and the suprasternal and high parasternal long- and short-axis cuts. Details of this examination will be covered in the corresponding chapter. An unroofed coronary sinus is best seen from four-chamber apical and subcostal views tilting the transducer posteriorly; pulsed and color Doppler flow mapping would demonstrate the coronary sinus drainage into the left atrium.

Ebstein's malformation of the right-sided atrioventricular valve is a rare association of atrioventricular septal defect described generally in relation to the partial form. In these cases, the anterosuperior leaflet is downwardly displaced (81,82). The echocardiographic views best suited to uncover this anomaly are the four-chamber apical and subcostal views, which would demonstrate the downward displacement of the anterosuperior leaflet of the right-sided valve, the "atrialized" portion of the right ventricle, and the enlarged "right atrium."

A common atrioventricular valve can be found in association with double inlet ventricles, with concordant, discordant, or ambiguous atrioventricular connections. Because the anatomy in double inlet and discordant connections is otherwise quite different from that in atrioventricular septal defect, Anderson et al. (41) suggest not including these within "atrioventricular septal defects," but rather reserving this term exclusively for instances with concordant and ambiguous connections. The echocardiographic diagnosis of visceral and atrial situs has been covered in detail in Chapter 8. However, it should be noted at this point that the appendages characterize the atria as right or left and that the presence and position of the vena cava and other systemic veins are also of diagnostic importance. These require several tomographic scanning planes, primarily from a subcostal approach.

Ventriculoarterial connections in atrioventricular septal defect are usually concordant, but complete transposition of the great arteries (ventriculoarterial discordance), double outlet right ventricle, and truncus arteriosus can also be found. Tetralogy of Fallot, pulmonary infundibular, and/or valvar stenosis or atresia are other associated lesions of the right ventricular outflow tract. Left outflow obstructions are particularly common and have been covered in detail above.

INTRAOPERATIVE AND POSTOPERATIVE EVALUATION

The pre-bypass intraoperative evaluation of complete atrioventricular septal defects should begin with global assessment of systolic ventricular function from the transgastric transverse short-axis view of the ventricles (see Fig. 4-27A). Withdrawing the transducer to a four-chamber view behind the left atrium, still in a transverse plane (see Fig. 4-28A), would reveal the absence of the atrioventricular septum and permit detailed confirmation of the anatomy of the superior and inferior bridging leaflets and their attachments as well as the degree of bridging of the anterior leaflet (Echos. 11-11, 11-20). The size of the left mural leaflet, which is essential in the surgical procedure, would be best studied from the short-

axis transgastric view (see Fig. 4-27B). A small left mural leaflet increases the difficulty of the surgery and the incidence of significant regurgitation in the postoperative period. The size and extent of the ostium primum atrial defect can also be assessed from the transverse four-chamber view rotated to image the atrial septum; additional atrial defects can also be detected from this position. Presence of atrioventricular valve regurgitation should be studied carefully from the four-chamber view as well. The longitudinal plane would allow examination of the outflow tract of the ventricles and detection of any chordal attachments into the left ventricular outflow tract that could result in obstruction postoperatively (see Fig. 4-29). The velocity across the outflow tracts is best measured from the transgastric longitudinal plane (see Fig. 4-27D,E), and this should be assessed pre-bypass, particularly of the left side.

The post-bypass assessment of atrioventricular septal defect, whether with one or two atrioventricular orifices, requires evaluation of possible residual shunts, integrity of the atrioventricular valve, patency of the left ventricular outflow tract, function of the left ventricle, and estimation of the pulmonary resistance.

Residual shunting of any significance can be relatively easily ruled out from the transverse four-chamber view, which also permits visualization of the surgical patches and their relationships to the bridging leaflets (see Fig. 4-28A,B) (Echo. 11-25; see color plate 36 following p. 364). Residual shunting across additional defects can also be evaluated from this view, although the apical muscular ventricular septum is foreshortened from this plane.

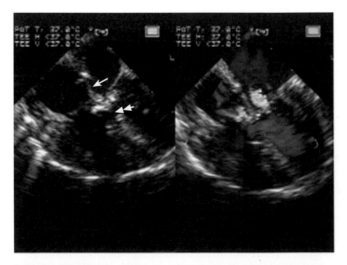

ECHO. 11-25. Transesophageal four-chamber views obtained immediately post repair of complete atrioventricular septal defect. **Left:** The atrial patch *(single arrow)* and the presence of a small residual ventricular septal defect *(double arrow)* are demonstrated. **Right:** The color Doppler flow map shows mild atrioventricular valve regurgitation.

Evaluation of the integrity of the repair of the atrioventricular valve, particularly the left side, can also be accomplished from the transverse four-chamber plane (Echo. 11-25). The inferior and left mural leaflets are best seen as the probe is retroflexed and withdrawn into the esophagus from the stomach. With further withdrawal and some forward flexion, the superior bridging leaflet and the right-sided valve come into view. The longitudinal views display the left ventricular two-chamber and long-axis views, the left-sided valve, and the left atrium (see Fig. 4-28C,D), and with rightward rotation of the transducer, the right ventricular inflow. From these views, the examiner can visually inspect the movement of both valves and, with the aid of Doppler techniques, can determine the presence and location of (as well as evaluate semiquantitatively the severity of) any residual regurgitation. Care must be taken not to overestimate the severity of residual regurgitation, a particularly frequent tendency when color Doppler images are obtained from a transesophageal window. Forward velocities can be measured with pulsed Doppler to rule out inflow obstruction after valve reconstruction, although mild stenosis may be masked in the operating room by a relatively reduced cardiac output immediately post-bypass. The velocity of the regurgitation of the right-sided atrioventricular valve measured with continuous wave Doppler offers a fairly accurate measure of pulmonary systolic pressure if there is no right ventricular outflow tract obstruction.

When anomalies of the left valve make it necessary to replace it with a prosthesis, problems peculiar to atrioventricular septal defect are encountered that raise the operative mortality substantially. The most important one is the potential for left ventricular outflow tract obstruction, especially compounded by the elongated plane of the left atrioventricular valve-aortic continuity (14). Ebels (60) has proposed inserting the prosthesis at the level of the aortic valve and reconstructing the posteroinferior wall of the outflow tract, thereby removing the potential obstruction.

Evaluation of the left ventricular outflow tract can be started from the transverse plane by slight forward flexion and withdrawal of the transducer from a four-chamber view (see Fig. 4-29A). Because of the elongation of the outflow in atrioventricular septal defect, it appears somewhat foreshortened in this plane. The longitudinal view offers a much better image of both outflow tracts in their entire length (see Fig. 4-29E). Gradual rightward rotation of the transducer from a low esophageal, left ventricular two-chamber view (see Fig. 4-28C) permits visualization of the right and then left ventricular outflow tracts (see Fig. 4-29D,F), although imaging of the entire aortic arch is not possible. Demonstration of the possible sites of obstruction, be it from accessory or anomalous insertions of the superior bridging leaflet, from discrete subaortic shelves, from dynamic contraction of the inferoposterior wall of the outflow tract, or from placement of a prosthe-

sis, should be evident from these views. Color flow mapping and direct velocity interrogation of the entire length of the outflow tract and across the aortic valve using pulsed-wave and continuous wave Doppler are best performed from the longitudinal transgastric views (see Fig. 4-27D,E) since these afford better positioning of the Doppler sample line along the direction of flow across the outflow tracts.

Ventricular function can be evaluated globally in the operating room from the transgastric short-axis view (see Fig. 4-27A,B). The main drawback to this approach is the lack of standardized values for left ventricular size and function to date. Recently, parameters of left ventricular function have been evaluated within 1 month preoperatively in infants with common atrioventricular septal defect through a combination of echocardiographic and angiographic measurements in an attempt to predict surgical outcome and tailor postoperative management. Volume characteristics of the left ventricle such as end diastolic volume, ejection fraction, thickness of the left ventricular free wall, left ventricular mass, and predicted wall stress appear to have prognostic value for successful surgical outcome (83). Increased predicted wall stress is largely due to a mismatch between ventricular volume and free wall thickness, which can occur in the presence of large left-to-right ventricular shunts and/or severe left valve regurgitation. This becomes critical postoperatively with the sudden rise in systemic resistance, so the use of vasodilator therapy immediately postoperatively can prove life saving in these patients.

Long-term follow-up of patients after surgery for atrioventricular septal defects centers around issues that are

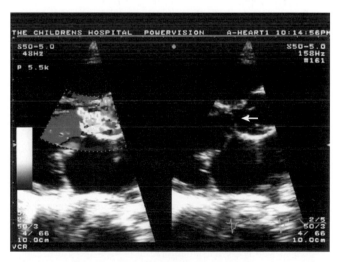

ECHO. 11-26. Parasternal long-axis view of residual left ventricular outflow tract obstruction following repair of a complete atrioventricular septal defect. **Right:** The site of encroachment of the left-sided valve into the outflow tract is shown *(arrow).* **Left:** Color aliasing due to flow velocity acceleration at that same site is shown.

also of importance in the immediate postoperative period (Echo. 11-26; see color plate 26 following p. 364). Late functional capacity and survival are mostly related to the function of the left atrioventricular valve and its hemodynamic consequences. Echocardiography offers the optimal technique for serial long-term assessment through the combined use of transthoracic and transesophageal techniques, the choice guided by the size of the patient and the quality of the transthoracic windows as adolescence and adulthood are reached. It is important to note that, even though left valve and ventricular function may be adequate early on, dysfunction can occur in the long term in some patients, especially in atrioventricular septal defect with two orifices (partial form). Meijboom et al. (58) have attempted to relate abnormal papillary muscle architecture to the presence of regurgitation late postoperatively, without success. As with most instances of complex congenital cardiac malformations, surgery does not offer a final cure, and these patients require periodic evaluations throughout adulthood as a new "natural history" unfolds postoperatively.

REFERENCES

1. Thibert M. *J Gen Med* 2me Serie 1819;8:254. Cited by Peacock TB. Heart consisting of four cavitites—one or both of the septa imperfect. In: Peacock TB, ed. *On malformations, and cavities, of the human heart. With original cases.* [Rpt. of 1858 ed.] Boston, MA. Mildford House, 1973: 21–25.
2. Peacock TB. Malformation of the heart consisting in an imperfection of the auricular and ventricular septa. *Trans Pathol Soc Lond* 1846;1:61–62.
3. Peacock TB. Heart consisting of four cavities—one or both of the septa imperfecta. In: Peacock TB, ed. *On malformations, and cavities, of the human heart. With original cases* [Rpt. of 1858 ed.]. Boston: Mildford House, 1973:21–25.
4. Anderson RH, Baker EJ, Ho SY, Rigby ML, Ebels T. The morphology and diagnosis of atrioventricular septal defects. *Cardiol Young* 1991;1:290–305.
5. Rokitanski CF von. *Die defect der scheidewande des herzens.* Pathologisch-anatomische Vienna: Wilhelm Braumuller, 1875;27–36.
6. Keith A. The Hunterian Lectures on malformations of the heart. Lecture II. *Lancet* 1909;2:433–435.
7. Monckebert JG. Das Verhalten des Atrioventrikularsystems bei persistierendem Ostium atrioventriculare commune. *Zentralbl All Pathol* 1923–1924;34:139.
8. Abbott ME. A. Persistent ostium atrio-ventriculare commune. In: Abbot ME, ed. *Atlas of congenital cardiac disease.* New York: American Heart Association, 1936:50–51.
9. Gunn FD, Dieckmann JM. Malformations of the heart including two cases with common atrioventricular canal and septum defects and one with defect of the atrial septum (cor triloculare biventriculosum). *Am J Pathol* 1927;3:595–615.
10. Robson GM. Congenital heart disease. A persistent ostium atrioventriculare commune with septal defects in a Mongolian idiot. *Am J Pathol* 1931;7:229–236.
11. Rogers HM, Edwards JE. Incomplete division of the atrioventricular canal with patent interatrial foramen primum (persistent common atrioventricular ostium). Report of five cases and review of the literature. *Am Heart J* 1948;36:28–54.
12. Watkins E Jr, Gross RE. Experiences with surgical repair of atrial septal defects. *J Thorac Cardiovasc Surg* 1955;30:469–491.
13. Van Mierop LHS, Alley RD, Kausel HW, Stranahan A. The anatomy and embryology of endocardial cushion defects. *J Thorac Cardiovasc Surg* 1962;43:71–83.
14. Wakai CS, Edwards JE. Developmental and pathologic considerations in persistent common atrioventricular canal. *Proc Staff Meet Mayo Clin* 1956;31:487–500.
15. Wakai CS, Edwards JE. Pathologic study of persistent common atrioventricular canal. *Am Heart J* 1958;56:779–794.
16. Rastelli G, Kirklin JW, Titus JL. Anatomic observations on complete form of persistent common atrioventricular canal with special reference to atrioventricular valves. *Mayo Clin Proc* 1966;41:296–308.
17. Ugarte M, Enriquez de Salamanca F, Quero M. Endocardial cushion defects. An anatomical study of 54 specimens. *Br Heart J* 1976;38:674–682.
18. Piccoli GP, Gerlis LM, Wilkinson JL, Lozsadi K, Macartney FJ, Anderson RH. Morphology and classification of atrioventricular defects. *Br Heart J* 1979;42:621–632.
19. Piccoli GP, Wilkinson Jl, Macartney FJ, Gerlis LM, Anderson RH. Morphology and classification of complete atrioventricular defects. *Br Heart J* 1979;42:633–639.
20. Anderson RH, Zuberbuhler JR, Penkoske PA, Neches WH. Of cleft, commisures, and things. *J Thorac Cardiovasc Surg* 1985;90:605–610.
21. Penkoske PA, Neches WH, Anderson RH, Zuberbuhler JR. Further observations on the morphology of atrioventricular septal defects. *J Thorac Cardiovasc Surg* 1985;90:611–622.
22. Anderson RH, Ebels TJ, Zuberbuhler JR, Silverman NH. Anatomical and echocardiographic features of the left valve in atrioventricular septal defect. In: Anderson RH, Neches WH, Park SC, Zuberbuhler JR, eds. *Perspectives in pediatric cardiology.* Volume 1. Mount Kisco, NY: Futura Publishing, 1988:299–310.
23. Hoffman JIE, Christianson R. Congenital heart disease in a cohort of 19,502 births with long-term follow-up. *Am J Cardiol* 1978;42:641–647.
24. Fyler DC, Buckley LP, Hellenbrand WE, Cohn HE. Report of the New England Regional Infant Cardiac Program. *Pediatrics* 1980;65[Suppl]:375–461.
25. Samanek M, Slavik Z, Zborilova B, Hrobonova V, Voriskova M, Skovranek J. Prevalence, treatment, and outcome of heart disease in live-born children: a prospective analysis of 91,823 live-born children. *Pediatr Cardiol* 1989;10:205–211.
26. Davis CL. Development of the human heart from its first appearance to the stage found in embryos of twenty paired somites. *Contrib Embryol* 1927;19:245–284.
27. De la Cruz MV, Cayre R. Desarrollo embriologico del corazon y de las grandes arterias. In: Sanchez PA, ed. *Cardiologia pediatrica. Clinica y cirugia.* Volume 1. Barcelona: Editorial Salvat, 1986:10–18.
28. De la Cruz MV, Gimenez-Ribotta M, Saravalli O, Cayre R. The contribution of the inferior endocardial cushion of the atrioventricular canal to cardiac septation and to the development of the atrioventricular valves: study in the chick embryo. *Am J Anat* 1983;166:63–72.
29. Quero-Jimenez M. Atrioventricular canal defects. Round table discussion on the correlations between experimental cardiac embryology and teratology and congenital cardiac defects. In: Aranega A, Pexieder T, eds. *Correlations between experimental cardiac embryology and teratology and congenital cardiac defects.* Granada: Universidad de Granada, 1989:299–317.
30. Netter FH, Van Mierop LHS. Formation of the cardiac septa. In: Netter FH, Yonkman FF, eds. *The Ciba collection of medical illustrations. Heart.* Volume 5. Summit, NJ: CIBA Publications Department, 1969:119–126.
31. Anderson RH, Shinebourne EA, Macartney FJ, Tynan M. Atrioventricular septal defects. In: Anderson RH, Shinebourne EA, Macartney FJ, Tynan M, eds. *Paediatric cardiology.* Volume 1. London: Churchill Livingstone, 1987:571–613.
32. Anderson RH, Wenink ACG. Thoughts on concepts of development of the heart in relation to the morphology of congenital malformations. *Experientia* 1988;44:951–960.
33. De la Cruz MV, Sanchez Gomez C, Cayre R. The developmental components of the ventricles: their significance in congenital cardiac malformations. *Cardiol Young* 1991;1:123–128.
34. Sadler TW. Abnormalities of atrioventricular canal. In: Tracy TM, ed. *Langman's medical embryology.* 5th ed. Baltimore: Williams & Wilkins, 1985:182–184.

35. Feldt RH, Porter CJ, Edwards WD, Puga FJ, Seward JB. Defects of the atrial septum and the atrioventricular canal. In: Adams FH, Emmanouilides GC, Riemenschneider TA, eds. *Moss heart disease in infants, children, and adolescents.* 4th ed. Baltimore: Williams & Wilkins, 1989:170–189.

36. Diaz G, Garcia-Pelaez I, Arteaga M, De la Cruz MV. Importance of the ventral cushion of the atrioventricular canal in the normal morphogenesis of the left ventricular infundibulum. *Proc World Congress Paediatr Cardiol* 1980:406.

37. De la Cruz MV, Quero-Jimenez M, Arteaga M, Cayre R. Morphogenese du septum interventriculaire. *Coeur* 1982;13:443–448.

38. Garcia-Pelaez I, Diaz-Gongora G, Arteaga M. Contribution of the superior atrioventricular cushion to the left ventricular infundibulum. *Acta Anat* 1984;118:224–230.

39. Walmsley R. Anatomy of the left ventricular outflow tract. *Br Heart J* 1979;41:263–267.

40. Anderson RH. The present day place of correlations between embryology and anatomy in the understanding of congenitally malformed hearts. In: Aranega A, Pexieder T, eds. *Correlations between experimental cardiac embryology and teratology and congenital cardiac defects.* Granada: Universidad de Granada, 1989:265–295.

41. Anderson RH, Ho SY, Macartney FJ, Becker AE. The anatomy of atrioventricular septal defects. In: Quero-Jimenez M, Arteaga M, eds. *Pediatric cardiology. Atrioventricular septal defects.* Madrid: Doyma, 1988:132–150.

42. Becker AE, Anderson RH. *Pathology of congenital heart disease.* London: Butterworth, 1981:77–92.

43. Carpentier A. Surgical anatomy and management of the mitral component of atrioventricular canal defects. In: Anderson RH, Shinebourne EA, eds. *Paediatric cardiology 1977.* Edinburgh: Churchill Livingston, 1978:477–490.

44. Ebels T, Anderson RH, Devine WA, Debich DE, Penkoske PA, Zuberbuhler JR. Anomalies of the left atrioventricular valve and related ventricular septal morphology in atrioventricular septal defects. *J Thorac Cardiovasc Surg* 1990;99:299–307.

45. Kirklin JW, Barratt-Boyes BG. Atrioventricular canal defect. In: Kirklin JW, Barratt-Boyes BG, eds. *Cardiac surgery. Morphology, diagnostic criteria, natural history, techniques, results and indications.* Volume 1. 2nd ed. New York: Churchill Livingstone, 1993:693–747.

46. Berger TJ, Kirklin JW, Blackstone EH, Pacifico AD, Kouchoukos NT. Primary repair of complete atrioventricular canal in patients less than 2 years old. *Am J Cardiol* 1978;41:906–913.

47. Studer M, Blackstone EH, Kirklin JW, et al. Determinants of early and late results of repair of atrioventricular septal (canal) defects. *J Thorac Cardiovasc Surg* 1982;84:523–542.

48. Becker AE, Anderson RH. Atrioventricular septal defects: what's in a name? *J Thorac Cardiovasc Surg* 1982;83:461–469.

49. Silverman NH, Ho SY, Anderson RH, Smith A, Wilkinson JL. Atrioventricular septal defect with intact atrial and ventricular septal structures. *Int J Cardiol* 1984;5:567–572.

50. Ranganathan N, Lam JHC, Wigle ED, Silver MD. Morphology of the human mitral valve. II. The valve leaflets. *Circulation* 1970;41:459–467.

51. McGoon DC, Puga FJ, Danielson GK. Atrioventricular canal. In: Sabiston DC Jr, Spencer FC, eds. *Gibbon's surgery of the chest.* 4th ed. Philadelphia: WB Saunders, 1983:1051–1066.

52. Frater RWM. Persistent common atrioventricular canal. Anatomy and function in relation to surgical repair. *Circulation* 1961;32:120–129.

53. Van Mierop LHS, Alley RD. The management of the cleft mitral valve in endocardial cushion defects. *Ann Thorac Surg* 1966;2:416–423.

54. Smallhorn JF, Tommasini G, Anderson RH, Macartney FJ. Assessment of atrioventricular septal defects by two dimensional echocardiography. *Br Heart J* 1982;47:109–121.

55. Smallhorn JF, de Leval M, Stark J, et al. Isolated anterior mitral cleft. Two dimensional echocardiographic assessment and differentiation from clefts associated with atrioventricular septal defect. *Br Heart J* 1982;48:109–116.

56. Anderson RH, Becker AE, Lucchese FA, Meier MA, Rigby ML, Soto B. Atrioventricular septal defects. In: Anderson RH, Becker AE, Lucchese FA, Meier MA, Rigby ML, Soto B, eds. *Morphology of congenital heart disease. Angiocardiographic, echocardiographic and surgical correlates.* Baltimore: University Park Press, 1983:65–83.

57. Kudo T, Yokoyama M, Imai Y, Konno S, Sakakibara S. The tricuspid pouch in endocardial cushion defect. *Am Heart J* 1974;87:544–549.

58. Meijboom EJ, Ebels T, Anderson RH, et al. Left atrioventricular valve after surgical repair in atrioventricular septal defect with separate valve orifices ("ostium primum atrial septal defect"): an echo-Doppler study. *Am J Cardiol* 1986;57:433–436.

59. McGoon DC, Rastelli GC. Operation for persistent atrioventricular canal. In: Feldt RH, ed. *Atrioventricular canal defects.* Philadelphia: WB Saunders, 1976:119–138.

60. Ebels T. Surgery of the left atrioventricular valve and of the left ventricular outflow tract in atrioventricular septal defect. *Cardiol Young* 1991;1:344–355.

61. Draulans-Noe HAY, Wenink ACG, Quaegebeur J. Single papillary muscle ("parachute valve") and double-orifice left ventricle in atrioventricular septal defect convergence of chordal attachment: surgical anatomy and results of surgery. *Pediatr Cardiol* 1990;11:29–35.

62. David I, Castaneda AR, Van Praagh R. Potentially parachute mitral valve in common atrioventricular canal. *J Thorac Cardiovasc Surg* 1982;84:178–186.

63. Lee CN, Danielson GK, Schaff HV, Puga FJ, Mair DD. Surgical treatment of double-orifice mitral valve in atrioventricular canal defects. Experience in 25 patients. *J Thorac Cardiovasc Surg* 1985;90:700–705.

64. Warnes C, Sommerville J. Double mitral valve orifice in atrioventricular defects. *Br Heart J* 1983;49:59–64.

65. Freedom RM, Smallhorn JF. A review of those morphological variables influencing competence of the valve and modalities of clinical investigation. In: Anderson RH, Neches WH, Park SC, Zuberbuhler JR, eds. *Perspectives in pediatric cardiology.* Volume 1. Mount Kisco, NY: Futura Publishing, 1988:311–327.

66. Rowe DW, Desai B, Bezmalinovic Z, Desai JM, Wessel RJ, Grayson LH. Two-dimensional echocardiography in double orifice mitral valve. *J Am Coll Cardiol* 1984;4:429–433.

67. Trowitzsch E, Bano-Rodrigo A, Burger BM, Colan SD, Sanders SP. Two-dimensional echocardiographic findings in double orifice mitral valve. *J Am Coll Cardiol* 1985;6:383–387.

68. Chin AJ, Bierman FZ, Sanders SP, Williams RG, Norwood WI, Castaneda AR. Subxyphoid two-dimensional echocardiographic identification of left ventricular papillary muscle anomalies in complete common atrioventricular canal. *Am J Cardiol* 1983;51:1695–1699.

69. Mehta S, Hirschfeld S, Riggs T, Liebman J. Echocardiographic estimation of ventricular hypoplasia in complete atrioventricular canal. *Circulation* 1979;59:888–893.

70. Ebels TJ, Ho SY, Anderson RH, Meijboom EJ, Eijgelaar A. The surgical anatomy of the left ventricular outflow tract in atrioventricular septal defect. *Ann Thorac Surg* 1986;41:483–488.

71. Lecompte Y, Crupi G. Atrioventricular septal defect—the need for a flexible surgical approach in a lesion with markedly individual features. *Cardiol Young* 1991;1:261–263.

72. Ebels T, Meijboom EJ, Anderson RH, et al. Anatomic and functional "obstruction" of the outflow tract in atrioventricular septal defects with separate valve orifices ("ostium primum atrial septal defect"): an echocardiographic study. *Am J Cardiol* 1984;54:843–847.

73. Piccoli GP, Ho SY, Wilkinson JL, Macartney FJ, Gerlis LM, Anderson RH. Left-sided obstructive lesions in atrioventricular septal defects. An anatomic study. *J Thorac Cardiovasc Surg* 1982;83:453–460.

74. Yoshida H, Funabashi T, Nakaya S, Maeda T, Taniguchi N. Subxiphoid cross-sectional echocardiographic imaging of the "gooseneck" deformity in endocardial cushion defect. *Circulation* 1980;62:1319–1323.

75. Anderson RH, Neches WH, Zuberbuhler JR, Penkoske PA. Scooping of the ventricular septum in atrioventricular septal defect [Letter]. *J Thorac Cardiovasc Surg* 1988;95:146.

76. Gutgesell HP, Huhta JC. Cardiac septation in atrioventricular canal defect. *J Am Coll Cardiol* 1986;8:1421–1424.
77. Bharati S, Lev M. The spectrum of common atrioventricular orifice (canal). *Am Heart J* 1973;86:553–561.
78. Neufeld HN, Titus JL, DuShane JW, Burchell HV, Edwards JE. Isolated ventricular septal defect of the persistent common atrioventricular canal type. *Circulation* 1961;23:685–696.
79. Gerbode F, Hultgren H, Melrose D, Osborne J. Syndrome of left ventricular-right atrial shunt. Successful surgical repair of defect in five cases with observation of bradycardia on closure. *Ann Surg* 1958;148:433–446.
80. Anderson RH. Ventricular septal defect: anatomical features as seen by the morphologist. In: Anderson RH, Neches WH, Park SC, Zuberbuhler JR, eds. *Perspectives in pediatric cardiology.* Mount Kisco, NY: Futura Publishing, 1988:9–24.
81. Zuberbuhler JR, Becker AE, Anderson RH, Lenox CC. Ebstein's malformation and the embryological development of the tricuspid valve. *Pediatr Cardiol* 1984;5:289–296.
82. Caruso G, Losekoot TG, Becker AE. Ebstein's anomaly in persistent common atrioventricular canal. *Br Heart J* 1978;40:1275–1279.
83. Seguchi M, Nakazawa M, Oyama K, Kawada M, Kurosawa H, Imai Y. Significance of left ventricular wall stress in infants with atrioventricular septal defect, common atrioventricular orifice and regurgitation across the left atrioventricular valve. *Cardiol Young* 1991;1:390–395.

PART IV

Anomalies of the Atrioventricular Valves

CHAPTER 12

Anomalies of the Tricuspid Valve and Right Atrium

Lilliam M. Valdes-Cruz and Raul O. Cayre

Anomalies involving the tricuspid valve and right atrium include cor triatriatum dexter, anomalies of the tricuspid valve apparatus (which involve the valve annulus, valve leaflets, chordae tendineae, and papillary muscles) and left juxtaposition of the atrial appendages.

COR TRIATRIATUM DEXTER

Cor triatriatum dexter is a rare anomaly characterized by a membrane that divides the right atrium into two chambers. The first mention of a membrane dividing the right atrium into an anterior and a posterior chamber was by Lauenstein in 1876 (1), and the term "cor triatriatum dextrum," or "dexter," was first coined by Doucette in 1963 (2). This has been the most commonly used term since (3–9). Other names that have been applied to this malformation have been "anomalies of the venous valves of the right atrium" (10), "persistent right valve of the sinus venosus" (2,11), "anomalous septum in the right atrium" (12), "persistent venous valves" (13), "supravalvular tricuspid stenosis" (14,15), "persistence of the right sinus venosus valve" (16), "persistent right sinus venosus valve" (17), and "divided right atrium" (18). The real incidence of this malformation is not known, but an incidence one-fourth that of cor triatriatum sinister has been quoted (19).

EMBRYOLOGIC CONSIDERATIONS

The sinus venosus initially connects with the primitive atrium and later with the right atrium through the sinoatrial orifice, which is guarded by two valves, a right and a left sinus venosus valve, which are fused at their cephalic end and constitute the septum spurium (10,20,21) (see Figs. 1-8A and 1-9B). The valves of the sinus veno-

sus progressively diminish in size. The left valve and the septum spurium become attached to the right surface of the interatrial septum. The superior portion of the right valve disappears, and the inferior portion divides into two parts; one forms the Eustachian valve of the inferior vena cava, and the other the Thebesian valve of the coronary sinus.

There is a general agreement that persistence of the right valve of the sinus venosus due to failure in its normal regression process results in cor triatriatum dexter (2–8,10–18).

ANATOMIC AND ECHOCARDIOGRAPHIC CONSIDERATIONS

The echocardiographic study of cor triatriatum dexter should consider the following: (a) the anatomic characteristics of the malformation; (b) the presence of obstruction to right ventricular inflow; and (c) associated anomalies. The intraoperative and postoperative evaluation is presented below.

Anatomic Characteristics of the Malformation

Persistence of the right valve of the sinus venosus determines the presence of a membrane that is directed from the crista terminalis to the lower portion of the interatrial septum, immediately above the tricuspid valve annulus. It has a posterior-to-anterior and a right-to-left orientation, thus dividing the right atrial cavity into an anterolateral and a posteromedial chamber (Fig. 12-1). The anterolateral chamber corresponds to the trabeculated portion of the right atrium and is related with the right atrial appendage and the tricuspid valve. The posteromedial chamber corresponds to the smooth or sinusal portion of the right

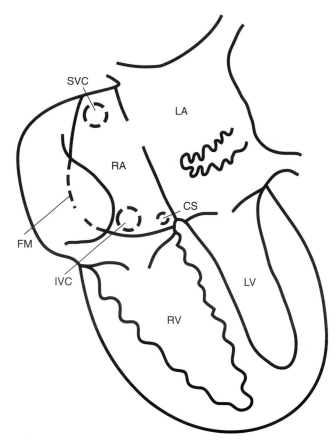

FIG. 12-1. Schematic drawing of cor triatriatum dexter. *RA,* right atrium; *LA,* left atrium; *RV,* right ventricle; *LV,* left ventricle; *SVC,* superior vena cava; *IVC,* inferior vena cava; *CS,* coronary sinus; *FM,* fibrous membrane.

atrium and receives the drainage of the superior and inferior vena cavae. The coronary sinus can be related to either the anterolateral (4,5,11,16) or the posteromedial (2,7,8) chamber. Usually, there are one (5,7,11,13,15,18) or more perforations of the membrane, which permit communication between the two atrial chambers (2,8,12,14). At the level of the interatrial septum, there is commonly an atrial septal defect of the ostium secundum type (5,6,11,14,15,18) or a patent foramen ovale (2,7–9,12,13) connecting the left atrium to the posteromedial chamber. In the case reported by Hansing et al. (4), there was a patent foramen ovale and a small atrial septal defect. Cases with intact atrial septum have been reported as well (3,12,19).

The echocardiographic views that permit the study of cor triatriatum dexter are the parasternal long-axis view tilted towards the right ventricular inflow, the parasternal and subcostal short-axis views, and the apical and subcostal four-chamber views. In the parasternal and subcostal short-axis views, the membrane is seen crossing the right atrium diagonally. In the four-chamber views, the membrane is seen in a more or less oblique direction with respect to the interatrial septum (Echo. 12-1). These views also allow demonstration of the vena caval connection to

the posteromedial chamber. Color Doppler flow mapping confirms the flow of the vena cavae into the posteromedial chamber and also the right-to-left atrial level shunting if present. The flow across the orifice(s) of the membrane can be seen on color Doppler and the velocity recorded with spectral Doppler to determine the presence of obstruction.

Presence of Obstruction to Right Ventricular Inflow

Usually, there is obstruction to tricuspid flow and underdevelopment of the right side of the heart. The tricuspid annulus is frequently small, but the valve itself can be small though anatomically normal or have thickened leaflets with fused commissures and shortened papillary muscles (4,12,14,15). Cases with a normal tricuspid annulus and a morphologically normal tricuspid valve have been reported (6,7). The membrane that divides the right atrium can be convex towards the orifice of the tricuspid valve or partially cover the tricuspid orifice with variable degrees of obstruction. Occasionally, the membrane can be aneurysmal, prolapsing through the tricuspid orifice into the right ventricular cavity and outflow tract, and sometimes even crossing the pulmonic valve, causing obstruction (14–17).

The parasternal and subcostal short-axis and the apical and subcostal four-chamber views are the best to demonstrate the presence of obstruction to right ventricular inflow. Analysis of the tricuspid valve apparatus should be undertaken from these projections so as to define the presence of anomalies of the leaflets, chordae, and papil-

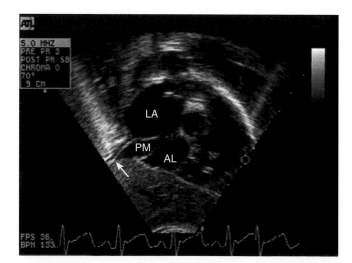

ECHO. 12-1. Subcostal four-chamber view in the presence of cor triatriatum dexter. The membrane is directed from posterior to anterior and with a right-to-left angulation dividing the right atrium into a posteromedial and an anterolateral chamber. The superior vena cava is committed to the posteromedial atrial chamber *(arrow). PM,* posteromedial right atrial chamber; *AL,* anterolateral right atrial chamber; *LA,* left atrium.

lary muscles. Spectral and color Doppler flow mapping should be used from these projections to assess the presence and severity of flow obstruction.

Associated Anomalies

There have been various malformations associated with cor triatriatum dexter. These include patent ductus arteriosus (2,5,7,11,13–15), tricuspid atresia (11), Ebstein's anomaly of the tricuspid valve (8), imperforate Ebstein's anomaly (5), valve pulmonic stenosis (7,14), pulmonary atresia with intact ventricular septum (5,13,14), ventricular septal defect (7,10,15), supravalve mitral ring (7), coronary artery-right ventricular communications (13), unroofed coronary sinus (14), and atresia of the superior vena caval–right atrial junction (18).

ANOMALIES OF THE TRICUSPID VALVE APPARATUS

The anomalies of the tricuspid valve apparatus comprise a series of malformations, including Ebstein's anomaly, tricuspid valve dysplasia, tricuspid valve prolapse, double orifice tricuspid valve, parachute deformity, unguarded tricuspid orifice, tricuspid atresia due to imperforate valve, and overriding and straddling of the tricuspid valve.

EMBRYOLOGIC CONSIDERATIONS

In the early postloop stage, the superior, inferior, right, and left lateral cushions of the atrioventricular canal appear within its orifice (22–26) (see Fig. 1-13). Simultaneously, the dextrodorsal and sinistroventral conal crests also appear (26,27) (see Fig. 1-12). The superior and inferior cushions divide the orifice of the atrioventricular canal into a left and a right orifice (see Fig. 1-12B). The cushions of the atrioventricular canal, the dextrodorsal conal crest and the ventricular walls all participate in the embryologic development of the atrioventricular valves (22–25,28,29) (see Fig. 1-13). The posterior leaflet of the tricuspid valve originates from the right lateral cushion (23,25,30) and the septal leaflet from the inferior cushion (25). The anterolateral leaflet has a dual embryologic origin: the medial portion adjacent to the septal leaflet originates from the dextrodorsal conal crest and the lateral portion from the right lateral cushion (23,25). The leaflet tissue is initially muscular and transforms into connective tissue through a process of cellular differentiation while the chordae tendineae and the papillary muscles develop through a process of diverticulation and undermining of the ventricular walls (22). Any anomaly in the origin or development of the inferior and right lateral cushion of the atrioventricular canal and in the dextrodorsal conal

crest, as well as any failure in the process of diverticulation and undermining of the ventricular walls, will result in an abnormal development of the tricuspid valve apparatus.

ANATOMIC AND ECHOCARDIOGRAPHIC CONSIDERATIONS

The echocardiographic study of the tricuspid valve apparatus should include the following considerations: (a) the anatomic characteristics of the various malformations; (b) presence of stenosis and/or regurgitation; and (c) associated anomalies.

Anatomic Characteristics of the Various Malformations

Ebstein's anomaly of the tricuspid valve was first described by Ebstein in 1866. It was reported as the presence of an abnormally low situation of fused anterior and posterior tricuspid leaflets that ballooned into the right ventricle, a rudimentary septal leaflet, absence of the Thebesian valve, and patent foramen ovale (31). The term "Ebstein's disease," applied to the congenital displacement of the tricuspid valve, was proposed by Arnstein in 1927 (32). The incidence of this malformation varies between 0.03% and 0.6% of all congenital heart disease (33–37).

Ebstein's anomaly comprises a wide spectrum of variations in the morphology of the tricuspid valve that is characterized by adherence of the posterior and septal leaflets to the subjacent myocardium, redundancy and fenestration of the anterosuperior leaflet, and downward displacement of the valve orifice with atrialization of a portion of the right ventricle and dilatation of the right atrioventricular junction or tricuspid annulus (35,37–48) (Fig. 12-2).

Almost all cases of Ebstein's malformation of the tricuspid valve present with situs solitus, atrioventricular concordance, and ventriculoarterial concordance, with normally related great vessels. Those presenting with atrioventricular discordance and ventriculoarterial discordance are discussed in Chapter 15.

The entire valvular apparatus is dysplastic, and some authors consider this an integral part of the anomaly (39,43). The tricuspid annulus is almost always dilated. The degree of displacement of the valve can range from minimal to severe. In the presence of minimal displacement, only the posterior leaflet is usually involved, although there can also be mild displacement of the posterior portion of the septal leaflet. The anterosuperior leaflet is normal. In severe Ebstein's anomaly, which is more common, there is displacement of the posterior leaflet (which is plastered to the ventricular wall), there is a rudimentary septal leaflet, and the anterosuperior leaflet

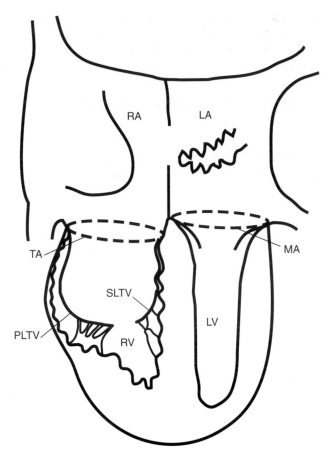

FIG. 12-2. Schematic drawing of Ebstein's anomaly of the tricuspid valve. *RA,* right atrium; *LA,* left atrium; *RV,* right ventricle; *LV,* left ventricle; *TA,* tricuspid annulus; *SLTV,* septal leaflet tricuspid valve; *PLTV,* posterior leaflet tricuspid valve; *MA,* mitral annulus.

is sail-like, attached to the tricuspid annulus. The displacement reaches the union of the inlet and trabecular portions of the right ventricle. Intermediate levels of severity can exist, with involvement of the posterior leaflet, the septal leaflet, or both. The commissure between the septal and mural leaflet or inferior commissure marks the point of maximal displacement, which never extends beyond the union between the inlet and trabecular portions of the right ventricle (41–43).

Even though there is dysplasia of the entire tricuspid valve apparatus, the anterosuperior leaflet is usually the least involved, although it rarely is completely normal. Even when maintaining its normal attachment to the tricuspid annulus, it is adherent to the ventricular wall through abnormal chordae tendineae and papillary muscles. It can have a sail-like appearance, be redundant, cause a variable degree of right ventricular obstruction, and be joined to the posterior or septal leaflet as a hammock-like structure (43,46). It can be fenestrated, causing obstruction to right ventricular inflow and/or outflow. The posterior and septal leaflets present various degrees of dysplasia with thickened and rolled edges and

excrescences similar to a cauliflower. Cases with focal agenesis of one leaflet (39), and complete absence of the posterior (44), the septal (44,47), or both leaflets (44) have also been reported.

The downward displacement of the valve determines the presence of an atrialized portion of the right ventricle, which is limited between the true tricuspid annulus and the tricuspid orifice, at the union between the inlet and trabecular portions of the right ventricle (Fig. 12-2). This atrialized or proximal portion of the right ventricle, which corresponds to the inlet of the ventricle, is usually dilated or aneurysmal, with thin walls and reduced or even absent muscular fibers in the myocardium; in this latter situation, the walls are formed by fibrous tissue only (40,42). The endocardium is thickened, fibrous, and smooth (40). The distal or functional right ventricle is dilated and also has thin walls in approximately two-thirds of cases of Ebstein's anomaly (40,42), so that this has been considered an integral component of this malformation (49). As in the atrialized portion, there is a reduction in the amount of myocardial fibers found within the distal portion of the right ventricle (50).

Ten percent of cases of Ebstein's are imperforate, with a muscular partition between the inlet and trabecular portions of the right ventricle, and an unguarded tricuspid orifice in which there is either a small remnant or total absence of valvular tissue (5,41,42,51).

Presence of an atrial septal defect is seen in 65% to 93% of cases (36,40–43). The majority are a patent foramen ovale or small ostium secundum type of defect. Cases with multiple fenestrations in the floor of the fossa ovalis have been reported (38,44,49). The origin and distribution of the coronary arteries are normal except in the region of the posterior ventricular wall, which can be supplied by the posterior descending branch of the right coronary artery, by the circumflex, or by vessels originating from both coronary arteries (40,42).

The echocardiographic study of Ebstein's malformation is best accomplished from the parasternal long-axis view tilted towards the inflow of the right ventricle, the parasternal short-axis view, the apical four-chamber view, and the subcostal four-chamber and short-axis views. The characteristics of the anterosuperior leaflet, the downward displacement of the posterior and septal leaflets, the atrialized portion of the right ventricle, and the functional right ventricular chamber can best be analyzed from the parasternal long axis of the right ventricle, using the parasternal short-axis and apical four-chamber views (Echo. 12-2). The apical four-chamber is the view of choice for assessing the degree of septal leaflet displacement into the right ventricular cavity (Echo. 12-3). A displacement of more than 8 mm/m^2 has been found to be a sensitive indicator of Ebstein's anomaly (52). The parasternal and subcostal short-axis views are helpful in cases where the anterosuperior leaflet causes obstruction to the right ventricular outflow. Displacement of the posterior leaflet can

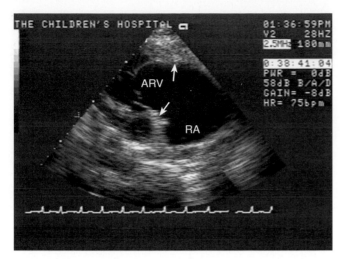

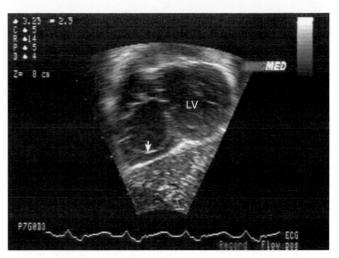

ECHO. 12-2. Parasternal long-axis view of the right ventricular inflow demonstrating the downward displacement of the septal leaflet of the tricuspid valve and the atrialized portion of the right ventricle in the presence of Ebstein's anomaly of the tricuspid valve. The position of the annulus is shown (arrows). ARV, atrialized right ventricle; RA, right atrium.

ECHO. 12-4. Subcostal short-axis view in the presence of Ebstein's anomaly of the tricuspid valve demonstrating the degree of displacement of the posterior leaflet (arrow). LV, left ventricle.

be seen from the subcostal four-chamber and short-axis views (53) (Echo. 12-4).

Evaluation of the tricuspid valve for surgical repair or replacement in Ebstein's malformation is accomplished well with echocardiography. The main criterion for plastic repair of the valve is the presence of a good-sized, mobile anterior leaflet that can be modified into a unicuspid valve (Echos. 12-2, 12-3). Plication of the tricuspid annulus and of the atrialized chamber is also performed if necessary. Tethering of the anterior leaflet to the ventricular walls and a dilated, noncontractile atrialized portion of the right ventricle are unfavorable characteristics for repair of the valve and suggest the need for replacement.

Doppler study with color and spectral modes demonstrates the presence of regurgitation of the tricuspid valve (Echo. 12-5; see color plate 38 following p. 364). In the presence of fenestrations of the anterior leaflet, more than one regurgitant jet may be seen. Stenosis of the tricuspid valve can be diagnosed and its severity estimated with spectral Doppler. The various Doppler techniques used to estimate the severity of tricuspid valve stenosis and regurgitation are discussed in detail in Chapter 6. Color Doppler can show the presence of right-to-left atrial shunting, which is almost always found in Ebstein's anomaly.

Ebstein's anomaly has been associated with ventricular septal defect (37,39–45,46,51), patent ductus arteriosus (37,41,51), the partial form of atrioventricular septal de-

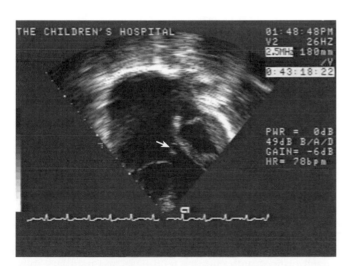

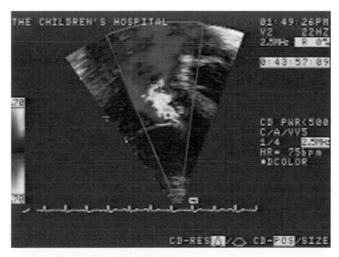

ECHO. 12-3. Apical four-chamber view in Ebstein's malformation of the tricuspid valve showing the degree of displacement of the septal leaflet (arrow).

ECHO. 12-5. Color Doppler flow map demonstrating the jet of tricuspid valve regurgitation in Ebstein's anomaly. Note the point of origin of the regurgitant jet.

fect (51), valve pulmonic stenosis (39,40,42–44,46), aortic valve stenosis (43), pulmonary atresia (39,40–42,44–46), bicuspid pulmonic valve (39), bicuspid aortic valve (39), mitral valve prolapse (54), persistent left superior vena cava (40,41), coarctation of the aorta (41,43), cor triatriatum dexter (44), and partial anomalous pulmonary venous connection (44).

Dysplasia of the tricuspid valve affects the entire valvular apparatus. The valve annulus can be of normal size, be dilated, or be small. The leaflets can have focal nodular or diffuse thickening, with rolled edges and commissural fusion. They can also be elongated, irregular in shape with infiltration by mucoid tissue. They can be fenestrated with small portions of valvular tissue adherent to the ventricular endocardium or have focal agenesis of valvular tissue (39). The chordae tendineae and papillary muscles have fibrous thickening, shortened chordae, and obliterated interchordal spaces. In the rare cases of isolated congenital tricuspid stenosis, the anomalies of the tricuspid valve are accompanied by underdevelopment of the inlet and trabecular portions of the right ventricle (55,56). Gerlis et al. (57) published a rare case of dysplasia of the anterosuperior leaflet of the tricuspid valve that caused right ventricular outflow tract obstruction. The right atrium is almost always dilated. Occasionally, tricuspid valve dysplasia can be accompanied by dysplasia of other cardiac valves (58). There can be various grades of valvular regurgitation. It is important to note that it is common to find a redundant, dysplastic-looking, regurgitant tricuspid valve in some neonates that resolves with development. This transitory valvular regurgitation has been attributed to late development of the septal leaflet of the tricuspid valve (59,60). This type of tricuspid regurgitation should be differentiated from that secondary to right ventricular dysfunction due to neonatal asphyxia.

The echocardiographic views allowing examination of a dysplastic tricuspid valve are the parasternal long-axis view of the right ventricular inflow, the parasternal and subcostal short-axis views, and the apical and subcostal four-chamber views. From these views, the morphology of the entire tricuspid valve apparatus can be evaluated, along with the presence of regurgitation and/or stenosis (Echo. 12-6). In neonates with severe tricuspid regurgitation, there can be functional pulmonary atresia with little or no forward flow across the right ventricular outflow tract. Imaging of normal-appearing pulmonary leaflets and identification of even small amounts of forward and/or regurgitant pulmonary flows can establish the differential diagnosis with anatomical pulmonary atresia.

Associated anomalies that have been reported include pulmonic stenosis (39,44,58), ventricular septal defect (39,44,57,58), pulmonary atresia (39,44), atrial septal defect (39,44,58,61,62), patent ductus arteriosus (58), bicuspid aortic valve (58), and single coronary artery (58).

Tricuspid valve prolapse is rare as an isolated lesion, being more commonly seen in association with mitral valve

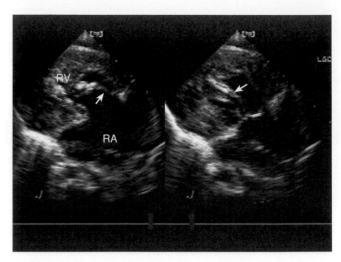

ECHO. 12-6. Parasternal views of the right ventricular inflow showing the presence of a dysplastic and thickened tricuspid valve apparatus. Thickened chords and papillary muscles are shown *(arrows). RA,* right atrium.

prolapse (63–65). Similar to mitral prolapse, there is a primary myxomatous transformation of the tricuspid valve with myxomatous proliferation of the spongiosa and collagen, and mucopolysaccharide deposits in the pars fibrosa of the valve. The leaflets appear lucid and redundant, and the chords are thinned and elongated (66–68). This myxomatous transformation causes one or more leaflets to move upwards during systole into the right atrium, beyond the line that connects the basal attachment of the leaflets (65). Brown and Anderson (65), in an echocardiographic study of 13 patients with tricuspid valve prolapse, found that there was prolapse of both the anterior and septal leaflets in 46%, of the anterior and posterior leaflets in 23%, of the septal leaflet alone in 15%, of the anterior leaflet only in 8% and of the three leaflets in 8%.

The echocardiographic study of tricuspid valve prolapse is initiated from the long-axis parasternal view of the right ventricular inflow, which permits visualization of the septal and posterior leaflets (Echo. 12-7). The anterior and septal leaflets are best evaluated from the parasternal short-axis and from the apical and subcostal four-chamber views. Color and spectral Doppler reveal the presence and severity of regurgitation.

In 40% to 48% of cases, there was associated mitral valve prolapse (63–65). Double orifice tricuspid valve has also been found associated with tricuspid prolapse (69).

Double orifice tricuspid valve is a very rare lesion that can be seen in isolation or associated with double orifice of the mitral valve. There are two types of double orifice. One is called "bridge type," in which there is a fusion or band between the anterosuperior and the septal leaflets dividing the tricuspid orifice into two more or less equal-sized orifices with chordae tendineae and papillary muscles present in each orifice. The other is called "hole type," in which a discrete orifice in the septal leaflet is

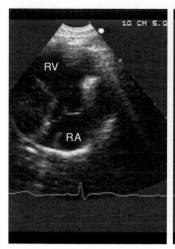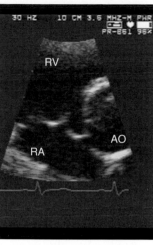

ECHO. 12-7. Parasternal long-axis view of the right ventricular inflow **(left)** and short-axis view **(right)** demonstrating prolapse of the tricuspid valve. *RA,* right atrium; *RV,* right ventricle; *AO,* aorta.

seen supported by chordae tendineae (69–72). The valvular components of both valve orifices can be competent or regurgitant.

The two orifices of a double orifice tricuspid valve can be visualized echocardiographically from a modified apical four-chamber view rotating the transducer 30 degrees clockwise (72), aiming towards the tricuspid valve. Other views such as a parasternal inflow and short-axis view and the subcostal four-chamber and short-axis view are also helpful in visualizing the orifices and evaluating for the presence of regurgitation with the use of color Doppler flow mapping. The transducer may need to be positioned slightly off the plane of the valve leaflets themselves in order to demonstrate the orifices on the leaflet surface.

Lesions found in association with double tricuspid orifice include valve pulmonic stenosis (71), prolapse of the tricuspid valve (69), double orifice mitral valve (72,73), ostium primum atrial septal defect, persistent left superior vena cava, and absence of the coronary sinus (72).

Parachute tricuspid valve is extremely rare. We have found only two reported cases in the literature (74,75). As described, the leaflets and chords showed variable degrees of dysplasia and all inserted into one single papillary muscle.

The best echocardiographic views to demonstrate the presence of one single papillary muscle would be the parasternal inflow view of the right ventricle, the apical and subcostal four-chamber views. We have not seen any case of this malformation.

Associated lesions that have been reported are tetralogy of Fallot (74), double outlet right ventricle, ventricular septal defect, and straddling mitral valve (75).

Unguarded tricuspid orifice is used to describe a type of malformation in which there is a normal orifice between the right atrium and right ventricle but absence of

the tricuspid valve apparatus. The first case of this anomaly was reported by Klein in 1938 (76). The tricuspid orifice is present, but there is either complete absence or only remnants of valvular tissue present (77–79). The right atrium is dilated and the right ventricle is hypoplastic.

The echocardiographic views to evaluate unguarded tricuspid orifice are the parasternal long-axis view of the right ventricular inflow, the parasternal short-axis view, and the apical and subcostal four-chamber views. Color Doppler flow mapping demonstrates free flow between the right atrium and ventricle during atrial contraction and between the right ventricle and right atrium in systole (80) (Echo. 12-8; see color plate 39 following p. 364).

Associated anomalies reported have been Ebstein's anomaly (5,41,42,51), pulmonary atresia with intact ventricular septum (5,77,80), atrial septal defect (5,41, 51,77,80), patent ductus arteriosus (5,51,77,80), double chambered right ventricle (78), cor triatriatum dexter (5), ventricular septal defect (41,51,78), Uhl's malformation (80), and left superior vena cava draining into the right atrium (41).

Tricuspid atresia due to imperforate valve is characterized by a fibrous membrane separating the right atrium and right ventricle (see Fig. 2-7A). In this malformation, a potential connection exists between the right atrium and ventricle as opposed to the situation in absent right atrioventricular connection in which there is no potential connection present (81,82) (see Fig. 2-6B). The right atrium is dilated and separated by the imperforate membrane from a right ventricle, which is hypoplastic, but in which can be recognized an inlet, a trabecular and an outlet portion, and the presence of a rudimentary valvular apparatus. The septal insertion of the membrane divides the ventricular septum into an atrioventricular and an in-

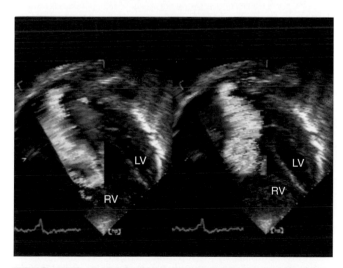

ECHO. 12-8. Color Doppler flow map of the free flow between the right atrium and right ventricle in diastole **(left)** and systole **(right)** in the presence of an unguarded tricuspid orifice. *RV,* right ventricle; *LV,* left ventricle.

terventricular portion (see Fig. 2-7A). Occasionally, the right ventricle can be normal in size (84). Ottenkamp et al. (85) have reported a case of tricuspid atresia due to imperforate membrane of the Ebstein type and four cases with overriding imperforate membrane.

The presence of an imperforate membrane at the level of the valve orifice can be demonstrated from the long-axis inflow view of the right ventricle, the parasternal short-axis view, and the four-chamber apical and subcostal views (Echo. 12-9; see color plate 40 following p. 364). From these views, the potential connection between the right atrium and ventricle can be recognized as well as the presence of two ventricular chambers. The ventriculoarterial connection can be evaluated from the parasternal short-axis view and from the apical and subcostal four-chamber views with anterior sweeping of the transducer. The spatial relationship of the great vessels can be established from the parasternal short-axis view. Color Doppler flow mapping aids in the demonstration of the flow pattern in this lesion, namely absence of antegrade flow from right atrium to right ventricle and the presence of right-to-left shunting at the atrial level (Echo. 12-9).

Associated malformations that have been reported include ventricular septal defect (82–84), complete transposition of the great arteries (82), atrial septal defect (83,84), patent foramen ovale (83), subpulmonic stenosis (83), pulmonary atresia (83,85), juxtaposition of the atrial appendages (85), and right aortic arch (85).

Overriding and Straddling of the Tricuspid Valve. Overriding tricuspid valve is characterized by a tricuspid orifice that is related to both ventricles (see Fig. 2-7D), whereas a straddling tricuspid valve is one in which there are chordae tendineae inserted on both sides of the ventricular septum (see Fig. 2-7E). Overriding and straddling of the tricuspid valve can be present individually or combined in the same heart. As a result, there can be overriding without straddling, straddling without overriding, overriding and straddling together, and overriding and straddling of both atrioventricular valves.

Overriding of the tricuspid valve is mild if the valve overrides the ventricular septum less than 50%. In this case, overriding exists within the context of two ventricles with concordant atrioventricular connection. As the spectrum of overriding becomes more extreme, the tricuspid valve is progressively committed to the left ventricle and the right ventricle becomes progressively more hypoplastic, which can result in double inlet left ventricle. The tricuspid valve always overrides the posterior septum, which rarely reaches the crux cordis (86).

Straddling can be classified according to the site(s) of insertion of the tensor apparatus. Type A straddling defines chordal insertions into the contralateral ventricle close to the crest of the ventricular septum, near its midline. Type B refers to insertions in the contralateral ventricle, along the septum, distant from its midline. Type C is present when the chords insert in the free wall or papillary muscles of the contralateral ventricle (87).

Echocardiographically, overriding and straddling of the tricuspid valve is best evaluated from the apical four-chamber view. The degree of override should be always evaluated at the level of the crux cordis where the atrial and ventricular septa are best aligned. In overriding, there is a degree of malalignment between the atrial and ventricular septa, proportional to the severity of the overriding; however, this should always be determined from a true apical four-chamber view to avoid misdiagnosis (Echo. 12-10). The tricuspid valve straddles the posterior portion of the ventricle, so the ventricular septal defect is located posteriorly. As a result, the atrioventricular septum is defective, so the normal offsetting between the atrioventricular valves may be lost. This is best identified from the four-chamber views, tilting the transducer inferiorly (Echo. 12-11).

Tricuspid valve overriding and straddling does not occur as an isolated lesion but in association with atrioventricular septal defects, conotruncal abnormalities, and univentricular atrioventricular connection.

INTRAOPERATIVE AND POSTOPERATIVE EVALUATION

The intraoperative pre-bypass evaluation of tricuspid valve anomalies is directed towards confirmation of the morphology of the valve and establishing a baseline assessment of the degree of stenosis and/or regurgitation under intraoperative hemodynamic conditions for comparison to the immediate post-bypass study. Ventricular

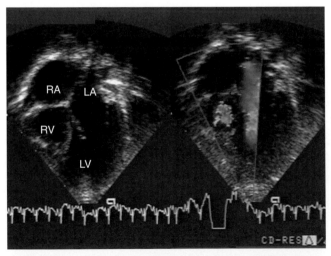

ECHO. 12-9. Left: Apical four-chamber view demonstrating the presence of tricuspid atresia due to an imperforate valve; the right ventricle is hypoplastic. **Right:** Normal inflow through the mitral valve; the blue color Doppler signal in the right ventricle represents low velocity swirling flow within the right ventricle from a small ventricular septal defect. *RA,* right atrium; *RV,* right ventricle; *LA,* left atrium; *LV,* left ventricle.

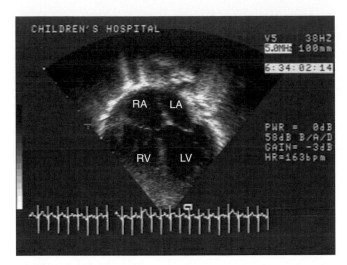

ECHO. 12-10. Apical four-chamber view of an overriding tricuspid valve. Note the malalignment between the atrial and ventricular septa. *RA*, right atrium; *RV*, right ventricle; *LA*, left atrium; *LV*, left ventricle.

size and function are best evaluated from the transgastric horizontal view (see Fig. 4-27A). Withdrawal of the endoscope into a horizontal four-chamber position behind the left atrium (see Fig. 4-28A,B) reveals the anterior and septal leaflets of the tricuspid valve and portions of its subvalve apparatus; the posterior leaflet can be seen with slight retroflexion of the transducer tip. The presence and degree of stenosis and regurgitation can be ascertained from this view, which allows fairly good orientation of the Doppler beam. From this view also, presence of the intraatrial membrane in cor triatriatum dexter can be seen. The longitudinal view behind the left atrium with rightward rotation from the two-chamber view of the left ventricle affords another look at the tricuspid valve and

subvalve apparatus as well as additional evaluation of the functional status of the valve. A double orifice valve can be demonstrated from this orientation since the leaflets are seen slightly *en face*. In Ebstein's malformation, the pre-bypass study acquires major importance since the decision for an attempt at repair versus replacement is made based on the echocardiographic appearance of the valve. Although most details pertaining to the anatomic characteristics of the valve can be unequivocally established in the transthoracic study, the transesophageal, intraoperative examination would allow a final confirmation of critical anatomic details such as the size and mobility of the anterior leaflet of the tricuspid valve, the size and contractility of the atrialized portion of the right ventricle, the functional capacity of the right ventricle, and the severity of regurgitation (Echo. 12-12).

Post-bypass, the intraoperative evaluation should begin with assessment of ventricular size and function from the transgastric horizontal position (see Fig. 4-27A). From the retrocardiac horizontal and longitudinal views with the endoscope positioned behind the left atrium, the tricuspid valve should be examined carefully, as in the pre-bypass study, for residual stenosis and/or regurgitation. If valve replacement has been performed with a mechanical prosthesis, usually with a bileaflet valve, the velocities across each orifice should be recorded with pulsed wave Doppler and the presence of any regurgitant leaks should be confirmed for later comparison during early and late follow-up.

The late postoperative follow-up after repair of the tricuspid valve should involve detailed anatomic examination of the valve and subvalve apparatus from the parasternal, apical, and subcostal windows. From these positions, assessment of the presence and degree of resid-

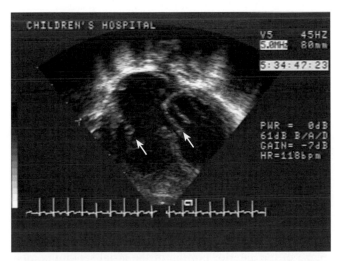

ECHO. 12-11. Apical four-chamber view in the presence of straddling of the tricuspid valve. The anterosuperior and septal leaflets are shown *(arrows)*. The septal leaflet inserts on the left side of the interventricular septum.

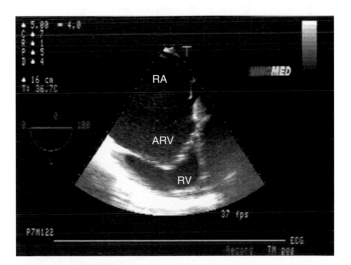

ECHO. 12-12. Transesophageal horizontal view in the presence of Ebstein's anomaly of the tricuspid valve. Note the displaced valve and enlarged right atrium due to the atrialized portion of the right ventricle. *RA*, right atrium; *ARV*, atrialized right ventricle; *RV*, right ventricle.

ual or recurrent stenosis and/or regurgitation with spectral and color Doppler should be undertaken. If a prosthetic valve has been implanted, the peak velocity across the valve is be measured most reliably from the apical position. Regurgitation of the prosthetic valve can be demonstrated from the parasternal inflow view of the right ventricle, from where shadowing from the prosthetic valve ring is least. The evaluation of prosthetic valves with Doppler is discussed in detail in Chapter 6.

LEFT JUXTAPOSITION OF THE ATRIAL APPENDAGES

Left juxtaposition of the atrial appendages is much more common than right juxtaposition, comprising 93% of all cases of atrial appendage juxtaposition (88). Both atrial appendages are found side by side to the left of the great vessels (Fig. 12-3). The first case of left juxtaposition of the atrial appendages was reported by Birmingham in 1893 (89). The term "left juxtaposition of the atrial appendages" was suggested by Dixon in 1954 (90).

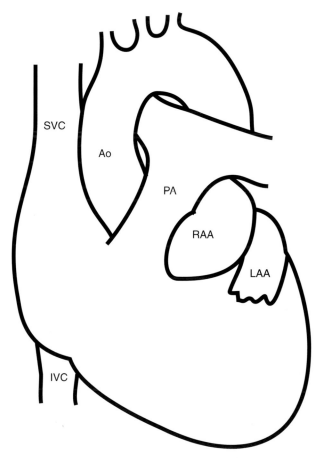

FIG. 12-3. Schematic drawing of a heart with left juxtaposition of the atrial appendages. *RAA,* right atrial appendage; *LAA,* left atrial appendage; *SVC,* superior vena cava; *IVC,* inferior vena cava; *Ao,* aorta; *PA,* pulmonary artery.

EMBRYOLOGIC CONSIDERATIONS

Wenner postulated in 1909 that juxtaposition of the atrial appendages was a consequence of underdevelopment of the process of torsion of the primitive cardiac tube and called it "undertorsion of the primitive cardiac tube" (90,91). Mathew (92) considers that undertorsion is present in cases with D bulboventricular loop, whereas there is an overtorsion in those with L bulboventricular loop.

ANATOMIC AND ECHOCARDIOGRAPHIC CONSIDERATIONS

The echocardiographic study in left juxtaposition of the atrial appendages should include the following: (a) position of the heart in the thorax; (b) visceroatrial situs; (c) position of the atrial appendages; (d) atrioventricular connection; (e) ventriculoarterial connection and spatial position of the great vessels; and (f) associated anomalies.

Position of the Heart in the Thorax

Of the 75 cases of left juxtaposition of the atrial appendages reported in the literature and reviewed by us, the heart was in levocardia in 63 cases (84%) and in dextrocardia in 12 cases (16%) (88,90,93–99).

Visceroatrial Situs

The visceroatrial situs was situs solitus in 73 cases (99%) (88,90,93–99), situs inversus in one case (0.5%) (88), and situs ambiguus in one case (0.5%) (88).

Position of the Atrial Appendages

The atrial appendages are found side by side to the left of the great vessels. The right atrial appendage crosses behind the aorta and is situated in front of the left atrial appendage (Fig. 12-3). In some cases, the right atrial appendage is bifid, with its right portion normally positioned and its left portion juxtaposed. These cases have been called "partial left-sided juxtaposition of the atrial appendages" and have been found in 60% of left juxtaposition (93). The juxtaposed right appendage does not lose its connection with the right atrium; rather, there is a distortion of the internal morphology of the atrial septum, which acquires an abnormal position. The orifice that communicates the right atrium with the right atrial appendage is found in front of the oval fossa. The major plane of the anterior portion of the atrial septum is more parallel to the frontal plane and directed from right to left. This abnormal position of the atrial septum reduces the volume of the right atrium.

Atrioventricular Connection

In 69 of the 75 cases in the literature reviewed by us, the atrioventricular connection was concordant (92%) (88,90,93–99); it was discordant in five cases (7%) (88,93) and double inlet in one case (1%) (99). Anomalies of the atrioventricular valves are common in left juxtaposition; tricuspid valve atresia was seen in 21 cases (28%) (88,93,96,99), tricuspid stenosis in five cases (7%) (88,95), mitral atresia in one case (1.3%) (88), mitral stenosis in one case (1.3%) (88), straddling tricuspid valve in one case (1.3%) (99), and common atrioventricular valve in one case (1.3%) (88).

Ventriculoarterial Connection and Spatial Position of the Great Vessels

The ventriculoarterial connection was discordant in 52 of the 75 cases reviewed. There was complete transposition of the great arteries in 63% (88,94,95,98,99) and corrected transposition in four cases (5%) (88). Concordant ventriculoarterial connection was found in nine cases, five had normal spatial relation of the great arteries (7%) (88,93) and four had anatomically corrected malposition of the great arteries (5%) (88,96). Double outlet right ventricle was seen in 12 cases (15.5%) (88,90, 93,99), truncus arteriosus in two cases (3%) (97,98), and double-outlet outlet chamber in one case (1.5%) (99).

The echocardiographic demonstration of left juxtaposition of the atrial appendages is accomplished from the parasternal short-axis, the apical four-chamber and the subcostal four-chamber views (99). The parasternal short-axis view permits the visualization of the abnormal position of the atrial septum, which is found behind the posterior great vessel and parallel to its posterior wall. This view also shows the right atrial appendage positioned to the left and in front of the left atrial appendage. The four-chamber apical view also permits examination of the plane of the atrial septum and of the position of the right atrial appendage behind and to the left of the great vessels.

The echocardiographic study of the visceroatrial situs, the atrioventricular and ventriculoarterial connections, and the spatial position of the great vessels are discussed in detail in Chapter 4.

Associated Anomalies

In addition to those mentioned above, left juxtaposition of the atrial appendages can be seen in association with ventricular septal defect, ostium secundum atrial septal defect, patent foramen ovale, atrioventricular septal defects, patent ductus arteriosus, common atrium, valve pulmonic stenosis, infundibular pulmonic stenosis isolated or combined with valve pulmonic stenosis, pulmonic atresia, subvalve aortic stenosis, aortic atresia, coarctation of the aorta, univentricular atrioventricular connection, left superior vena cava draining into the coronary sinus, absent coronary sinus, common pulmonary vein draining into the left atrium, and single coronary artery (88,90,93–99).

INTRAOPERATIVE AND POSTOPERATIVE EVALUATION

Intraoperative evaluation in the presence of left juxtaposition of the atrial appendages is directed towards the study of the associated malformation requiring surgical repair. Left juxtaposition can be seen from the transesophageal transverse four-chamber view (see Fig. 4-28A) and the transverse view at the level of the great vessels (see Fig. 4-29B). It can also be demonstrated from the longitudinal view similar to the parasternal short-axis view. From these views, the right atrial appendage can be seen crossing behind the great arteries and situated to their left side. The abnormal spatial position of the atrial septum can also be demonstrated.

The immediate and late postoperative evaluation is directed towards the surgical repair of the associated lesions.

REFERENCES

1. Lauenstein C. Varietat der klappen des rechten atrium. *Virchows Arch* 1876;68:632–633.
2. Doucette J, Knoblich R. Persistent right valve of the sinus venosus: so-called cor triatriatum dextrum. Review of the literature and report of a case. *Arch Pathol* 1963;75:105–112.
3. Verel D, Pilcher J, Hynes DM. Cor triatriatum dexter. *Br Heart J* 1970;32:714–716.
4. Hansing CE, Young WP, Rowe GG. Cor triatriatum dexter. Persistent right sinus venosus valve. *Am J Cardiol* 1972;30:559–564.
5. Gerlis LM, Anderson RH. Cor triatriatum dexter with imperforate Ebstein's anomaly. *Br Heart J* 1976;38:108–111.
6. Burton DA, Chin A, Weinberg PM, Pigott JD. Identification of cor triatriatum dexter by two-dimensional echocardiography. *Am J Cardiol* 1987;60:409–410.
7. Alboliras ET, Edwards WD, Driscoll DJ, Seward JB. Cor triatriatum dexter: two-dimensional echocardiographic diagnosis. *J Am Coll Cardiol* 1987;9:334–337.
8. Trakhtenbroit A, Majid P, Rokey R. Cor triatriatum dexter: antemortem diagnosis in an adult by cross-sectional echocardiography. *Br Heart J* 1990;63:314–316.
9. Savas V, Samyn J, Schreiber TL, Hauser A, O'Neill WW. Cor triatriatum dexter: recognition and percutaneous transluminal correction. *Cathet Cardiovasc Diagn* 1991;23:183–186.
10. Yater WM. Variations and anomalies of the venous valves of the right atrium of the human heart. *Arch Pathol* 1929;7:418–441.
11. Jones RN, Niles NR. Spinnaker formation of sinus venosus valve. Case report of a fatal anomaly in a ten-year-old boy. *Circulation* 1968;38:468–473.
12. Dubin IN, Hollinshead WH. Congenitally insufficient tricuspid valve accompanied by an anomalous septum in the right atrium. *Arch Pathol* 1944;38:225–228.
13. Kauffman SL, Andersen DH. Persistent venous valves, maldevelopment of the right heart, and coronary artery-ventricular communications. *Am Heart J* 1963;66:664–669.
14. Folger GM. Supravalvular tricuspid stenosis. Association with developmental abnormalities of the right heart and derivatives of the sixth aortic arch. *Am J Cardiol* 1968;21:81–87.
15. Nakano S, Kawashima Y, Miyamoto T, Kitamura S, Manabe H.

Supravalvular tricuspid stenosis resulting from persistent right sinus venosus valve. A report of successful correction. *Ann Thorac Surg* 1974;17:591–595.

16. Battle-Diaz J, Stanley P, Kratz C, Fouron JC, Guerin R, Davignon A. Echocardiographic manifestations of persistence of the right sinus venosus valve. *Am J Cardiol* 1979;43:850–853.

17. Gussenhoven WJ, Essed CE, Bos E. Persistent right sinus venosus valve. *Br Heart J* 1982;47:183–185.

18. Muhler EG. Franke A, Messmer BJ. Divided right atrium ("cor triatriatum dexter") with azygous drainage of the superior caval vein. *Cardiol Young* 1996;6:80–83.

19. Gharagozloo F, Bulkley BH. Hutchins GM. A proposed pathogenesis of cor triatriatum: impingement of the left superior vena cava on developing left atrium. *Am Heart J* 1977;94:618–626.

20. Odgers PNB. The formation of the venous valves, the foramen secundum and the septum secundum in the human heart. *J Anat* 1935;69:412–422.

21. Arey LB. The heart and circulation changes. In: Arey LB, ed. *Developmental anatomy. A textbook and laboratory manual of embryology.* 7th ed. Philadelphia: WB Saunders, 1966:375–395.

22. Van Mierop LHS, Alley RD, Kausel HW, Stranahan A. The anatomy and embryology of endocardial cushion defects. *J Thorac Cardiovasc Surg* 1962;43:71–83.

23. Netter FH, Van Mierop LHS. Embryology. In: Netter FH, Yonkman FF, eds. *The Ciba collection of medical illustrations. Heart.* Volume 5. Summit, NJ: CIBA Publications Department, 1969:112–130.

24. De la Cruz MV, Quero-Jimenez M, Arteaga Martinez M, Cayre R. Morphogenese du septum interventriculaire. *Coeur* 1982;13:443–448.

25. De la Cruz MV, Gimenez-Ribotta M, Saravalli O, Cayre R. The contribution of the inferior endocardial cushion of the atrioventricular canal to cardiac septation and to the development of the atrioventricular valves: study in the chick embryo. *Am J Anat* 1983;166:63–72.

26. De la Cruz MV, Cayre R. Desarrollo embriologico del corazon y las grandes arterias. In: Sanchez PA, ed. *Cardiologia pediatrica. Clinica y cirugia.* Volume 1. Barcelona: Editorial Salvat, 1986:10–18.

27. De la Cruz MV, Munoz Armas S, Castellanos L. *Development of the chick heart.* Baltimore: The Johns Hopkins Press, 1971.

28. Garcia-Pelaez I, Diaz-Gongora G, Arteaga Martinez M. Contribution of the superior atrioventricular cushion to the left ventricular infundibulum. Experimental study on the chick embryo. *Acta Anat* 1984;118:224–230.

29. Domenech Mateu JM. Desarrollo del corazon. In: Soler J, Bayes de Luna A, eds. *Cardiologia.* Barcelona: Editorial Doyma, 1986:3–13.

30. Thompson RP, Losada Cabrera MA, Fitzharris TP. Embryology of cardiac cushion tissue. In: Aranega A, Pexieder T, eds. *Correlations between experimental cardiac embryology and teratology and congenital cardiac defects.* Granada: Universidad de Granada, 1989:147–169.

31. Ebstein W. Uber einen schr seltenen fall von insufficienz der valvula tricuspidalis, bedingt durch eine angeborene hochgradige missbildung derselben. *Arch Anat Physiol Wissensch Med* 1866;33:238–254. Cited by Schiebler GL, Gravenstein JS, Van Mierop LHS. Ebstein's anomaly of the tricuspid valve. [Translation of original description with comments.] *Am J Cardiol* 1968;22:867–873.

32. Arnstein A. Eine seltene Missbildung der Trikuspidalklappe ("Ebsteinsche Krankheit"). *Virchows Arch* 1927;266:247–254.

33. Simcha A, Bonham-Carter RE. Ebstein's anomaly: clinical study of 32 patients in childhood. *Br Heart J* 1971;33:46–49.

34. Fyler DC, Buckley LP, Hellenbrand WE, Cohn HE. Report of the New England Regional Infant Cardiac Program. *Pediatrics* 1980;65[Suppl]:377–461.

35. Freedom RM, Benson LN. Ebstein's malformation of the tricuspid valve. In: Freedom RM, Benson LN, Smallhorn JF, eds. *Neonatal heart disease.* London: Springer-Verlag, 1992:471–483.

36. Vacca JB, Bussmann DW, Mudd JG. Ebstein's anomaly. Complete review of 108 cases. *Am J Cardiol* 1958;2:210–226.

37. Genton E, Blount SG. The spectrum of Ebstein's anomaly. *Am Heart J* 1967;73:395–425.

38. Schiebler GL, Gravenstein JS, Van Mierop LHS. Ebstein's anomaly of the tricuspid valve. Translation of original description with comments. *Am J Cardiol* 1968;22:867–873.

39. Becker AE, Becker MJ, Edwards JE. Pathologic spectrum of dysplasia of the tricuspid valve. Features in common with Ebstein's malformation. *Arch Pathol* 1971;91:167–178.

40. Anderson KR, Lie JT. Pathologic anatomy of Ebstein's anomaly of the heart revisited. *Am J Cardiol* 1978;41:739–745.

41. Zuberbuhler JR, Allwork SP, Anderson RH. The spectrum of Ebstein's anomaly of the tricuspid valve. *J Thorac Cardiovasc Surg* 1979;77:202–211.

42. Anderson KR, Zuberbuhler JR, Anderson RH, Becker AE, Lie JT. Morphologic spectrum of Ebstein's anomaly of the heart. *Mayo Clin Proc* 1979;54:174–180.

43. Zuberbuhler JR, Anderson RH. Ebstein's malformation of the tricuspid valve: Morphology and natural history. In: Anderson RH, Neches WH, Park SC, Zuberbuhler JR, eds. *Perspectives in pediatric cardiology.* Volume 1. Mount Kisco, NY: Futura Publishing, 1988:99–112.

44. Lang D, Oberhoffer R, Cook A, et al. Pathologic spectrum of malformations of the tricuspid valve in prenatal and neonatal life. *J Am Coll Cardiol* 1991;17:1161–1167.

45. Celermajer DS, Dood SM, Greenwald SE, Wyse RKH, Deanfield JE. Morbid anatomy in neonates with Ebstein's anomaly of the tricuspid valve: pathophysiologic and clinical implications. *J Am Coll Cardiol* 1992;19:1049–1053.

46. Edwards WD. Embryology and pathologic features of Ebstein's anomaly. *Prog Pediatr Cardiol* 1993;2:5–15.

47. Freedom RM, Benson LN. Neonatal expression of Ebstein's anomaly. *Prog Pediatr Cardiol* 1993;2:22–27.

48. Chavaud SM, Mihaileanu SA, Gaer JAR, Carpentier AC. Surgical treatment of Ebstein's malformation—the "Hopital Broussais" experience. *Cardiol Young* 1996;6:4–11.

49. Edwards JE. Pathologic features of Ebstein's malformation of the tricuspid valve. *Proc Staff Meet Mayo Clin* 1953;28:89–94.

50. Anderson KR, Lie JT. The right ventricular myocardium in Ebstein's anomaly. A morphometric histopathologic study. *Mayo Clin Proc* 1979;54:181–184.

51. Zuberbuhler JR, Becker AE, Anderson RH, Lenox CC. Ebstein's malformation and the embryological development of the tricuspid valve. With a note on the nature of "clefts" in the atrioventricular valves. *Pediatr Cardiol* 1984;5:289–296.

52. Hagler DJ. Echocardiographic assessment of Ebstein's anomaly. *Prog Pediatr Cardiol* 1993;2:28–37.

53. Silverman NH, Birk E. Ebstein's malformation of the tricuspid valve: cross-sectional echocardiography and Doppler. In: Anderson RH, Neches WH, Park SC, Zuberbuhler JR, eds. *Perspectives in pediatric cardiology.* Volume 1. Mount Kisco, NY: Futura Publishing, 1988:113–125.

54. Roberts WC, Glancy DL, Seningen RP, Maron BJ, Epstein SE. Prolapse of the mitral valve (floppy valve) associated with Ebstein's anomaly of the tricuspid valve. *Am J Cardiol* 1976;38:377–382.

55. Becker AE, Becker MJ, Moller JH, Edwards JE. Hypoplasia of right ventricle and tricuspid valve in three siblings. *Chest* 1971;60:273–277.

56. Freedom RM, Culham JAG, Moes CAF. The straddling tricuspid valve; congenital tricuspid stenosis; congenital tricuspid regurgitation. In: Freedom RM, Culham JAG, Moes CAF, eds. *Angiocardiography of congenital heart disease.* New York: Macmillan, 1984:99–110.

57. Gerlis LM, Ho SY, Rigby ML. Right ventricular outflow obstruction by anomalies of the tricuspid valve: report of a windsock diverticulum. *Pediatr Cardiol* 1992;13:59–62.

58. Hyams VJ, Manion WC. Incomplete differentiation of the cardiac valves. A report of 197 cases. *Am Heart J* 1968;76:173–182.

59. Freymann R, Kallfelz HC. Transient tricuspid incompetence in a newborn. *Eur J Cardiol* 1975;2:467–471.

60. Carpentier A. Malformations of the tricuspid valve and Ebstein's anomaly. In: Stark J, De Leval M, eds. *Surgery for congenital heart defects.* 2nd ed. Philadelphia: WB Saunders, 1994:615–622.

61. Dimich I, Goldfinger P, Steinfeld L, Lukban SB. Congenital tricuspid stenosis. Case treated by heterograft replacement of the tricuspid valve. *Am J Cardiol* 1973;31:89–92.

62. Cohen ML, Spray T, Gutierrez F, Barzilai B, Bauwens D. Congeni-

tal tricuspid valve stenosis with atrial septal defect and left anterior fascicular block. *Clin Cardiol* 1990;13:497–499.

63. Mardelli TJ, Morganroth J, Chen CC, Naito M, Vergel J. Tricuspid valve prolapse diagnosed by cross-sectional echocardiography. *Chest* 1981;79:201–205.

64. Ogawa S, Hayashi J, Sasaki H, et al. Evaluation of combined valvular prolapse syndrome by two-dimensional echocardiography. *Circulation* 1982;65:174–180.

65. Brown AK, Anderson V. Two-dimensional echocardiography and the tricuspid valve. Leaflet definition and prolapse. *Br Heart J* 1983; 49:495–500.

66. Read RC, Thal AP, Wendt VE. Symptomatic valvular myxomatous transformation (the floppy valve syndrome). A possible forme fruste of the Marfan syndrome. *Circulation* 1965;32:897–910.

67. Pomerance A. Ballooning deformity (mucoid degeneration) of atrioventricular valves. *Br Heart J* 1969;31:343–351.

68. Roberts WC. Morphologic aspects of cardiac valve dysfunction. *Am Heart J* 1992;123:1610–1632.

69. Pignoni P, Carraro R, Nicolosi GL. Prolapse of atrioventricular valve leaflets in the setting of double orifice. *Int J Cardiol* 1988; 19:115–119.

70. Sanchez Cascos A, Rabago P, Sokolowski M. Duplication of the tricuspid valve. *Br Heart J* 1967;29:943–946.

71. Lynch TG, Doty DB. Duplication of the tricuspid valve. *Cardiovasc Dis* 1980;7:159–164.

72. Honnekeri ST, Tendolkar AG, Lokhandwala YY. Double-orifice mitral and tricuspid valves in association with the Raghib complex. *Ann Thorac Surg* 1993;55:1001–1002.

73. Bano-Rodrigo A, Van Praagh S, Trowitzsch E, Van Praagh R. Double-orifice mitral valve: a study of 27 postmortem cases with developmental, diagnostic and surgical considerations. *Am J Cardiol* 1988;61:152–160.

74. Ariza S, Cintado C, Castillo JA, et al. Valvule tricuspide en parachute associee a une tetrulogie de Fallot. *Arch Mal Coeur* 1979,72. 317–320.

75. Milo S, Stark J, Macartney FJ, Anderson RH. Parachute deformity of the tricuspid valve. *Thorax* 1979;34:543–546.

76. Klein H. Uber einen seltenen fall von herzmissbildung mit rudimentarer entwicklung des rechten ventrikels und defekt der tricuspidalklappen. *Virchows Arch* 1938;301:1–16.

77. Kanjuh VI, Stevenson JE, Amplatz K, Edwards JE. Congenitally unguarded tricuspid orifice with coexistent pulmonary atresia. *Circulation* 1964;30:911–917.

78. Gussenhoven EJ, Essed CE, Bos E. Unguarded tricuspid orifice with two-chambered right ventricle. *Pediatr Cardiol* 1986;7:175–177.

79. Anderson RH, Silverman NH, Zuberbuhler JR. Congenitally unguarded tricuspid orifice: its differentiation from Ebstein's malformation in association with pulmonary atresia and intact ventricular septum. *Pediatr Cardiol* 1990;11:86–90.

80. Agarwala B, Waldman JD, Carbone M. Unguarded tricuspid orifice with Uhl's malformation. *Cardiol Young* 1996;6:177–180.

81. Anderson RH, Wilkinson JL, Gerlis ML, Smith A, Becker AE. Atresia of the right atrioventricular orifice. *Br Heart J* 1977;39: 414–428.

82. Dickinson DF, Wilkinson JL, Smith A, Anderson RH. Atresia of the right atrioventricular orifice with atrioventricular concordance. *Br Heart J* 1979;42:9–14.

83. Rigby ML, Gibson DG, Joseph MC, et al. Recognition of imperforate atrioventricular valves by two-dimensional echocardiography. *Br Heart J* 1982;47:329–336.

84. Crupi G, Villani M, Di Benedetto G, et al. Tricuspid atresia with imperforate valve: Angiographic findings and surgical implications in two cases with AV concordance and normally related great arteries. *Pediatr Cardiol* 1984;5:49–54.

85. Ottenkamp J, Wenink ACG, Rohmer J, Gittenberger–de Groot A. Tricuspid atresia with overriding imperforate tricuspid membrane: an anatomic variant. *Int J Cardiol* 1984;6:599–609.

86. Anderson RH, Ho SY. Straddling and overriding valves-segmental morphology. In: Wenink ACG, Oppenheimer-Dekker A, Moulaert AJ, eds. *The ventricular septum of the heart.* The Hague, The Netherlands: Leiden University Press, 1981:157–173.

87. Rice MJ, Seward JB, Edwards WD, et al. Straddling atrioventricular valve: Two-dimensional echocardiographic diagnosis, classification and surgical implications. *Am J Cardiol* 1985;55:505–513.

88. Melhuish BPP, Van Praagh R. Juxtaposition of the atrial appendages. A sign of severe cyanotic congenital heart disease. *Br Heart J* 1968;30:269–284.

89. Birmingham A. Extreme anomaly of the heart and great vessels. *J Anat Physiol* 1893;27:139. Cited by Melhuish BPP, Van Praagh R. Juxtaposition of the atrial appendages. A sign of severe cyanotic congenital heart disease. *Br Heart J* 1968;30:269–284.

90. Dixon ASJ. Juxtaposition of the atrial appendages: two cases of an unusual congenital cardiac deformity. *Br Heart J* 1954;16:153–164.

91. Wenner O. Beitrage zur Lehre der Herzmissbildungen. *Virchows Arch* 1909;196:127–168. Cited by Mathew R, Replogle R, Thilenius OG, Arcilla RA. Right juxtaposition of the atrial appendages. *Chest* 1975;67:483–486.

92. Mathew R, Replogle R, Thilenius OG, Arcilla RA. Right juxtaposition of the atrial appendages. *Chest* 1975;67:483–486.

93. Charuzi Y, Spanos PK, Amplatz K, Edwards JE. Juxtaposition of the atrial appendages. *Circulation* 1973;47:620–627.

94. Moene RJ, Brom AG. Anastomosis between the atrial appendages in a patient with juxtaposition. *Chest* 1971;59:583–586.

95. Ellis K, Jameson G. Congenital levoposition of the right atrial appendage. *Am J Roentgenol* 1963;89:984–988.

96. Freedom RM, Harrington DP. Anatomically corrected malposition of the great arteries. Report of two cases, one with congenital asplenia; frequent association with juxtaposition of atrial appendages. *Br Heart J* 1974;36:207–215.

97. Park MK, Chang CHJ, Vaseenon T. Congenital levojuxtaposition of the right atrial appendage. Association with persistent truncus arteriosus type 4. *Chest* 1976;69:550–552.

98. Allwork SP, Urban AE, Anderson RH. Left juxtaposition of the auricles with l-position of the aorta. Report of six cases. *Br Heart J* 1977;39:299–308.

99. Rice MJ, Seward JB, Hagler DJ, Edwards WD, Julsrud PR, Tajik AJ. Left juxtaposed atrial appendages: diagnostic two-dimensional echocardiographic features. *J Am Coll Cardiol* 1985;1:1330–1336.

CHAPTER 13

Anomalies of the Mitral Valve and Left Atrium

Lilliam M. Valdes-Cruz and Raul O. Cayre

The congenital anomalies of the mitral valve and left atrium comprise a spectrum of deformities that includes cor triatriatum sinister, supravalve mitral ring, and malformations of the mitral valvular apparatus. These latter can be divided into anomalies of the annulus, of the leaflets, of the chordae tendineae, and of the papillary muscles. Right juxtaposition of the atrial appendages is also included in this chapter.

COR TRIATRIATUM SINISTER

Cor triatriatum sinister is a rare cardiac malformation characterized by the presence of a fibromuscular membrane that divides the left atrium into a distal chamber (which is the true left atrium and is related to the left atrial appendage and the mitral valve) and a proximal chamber or accessory left atrium (which is related to the pulmonary veins) (1) (Fig. 13-1). The first description of this malformation was by Church in 1868 (2); however, Andral in 1829 mentions having seen a triatrial heart with a right atrium that received the systemic venous return, a left atrium that received the pulmonary veins, and a middle atrium (3). The term "cor triatriatum" was used first by Borst-Gottinger in 1905 (4). The adjective "sinister" is used to differentiate this particular left atrial partition from partitions of the right atrium or cor triatriatum dexter and from other triatrial hearts such as the case reported by Patten and Taggart (5).

The incidence of cor triatriatum sinister varies between 0.1% and 0.3% of all congenital cardiac malformations (6–8).

EMBRYOLOGIC CONSIDERATIONS

Several theories have been proposed to explain the morphogenesis of cor triatriatum. These include malseptation due to overgrowth of the valve of the foramen ovale (9); "failure in the complete amalgamation of that part of the auricle which is said to be derived from the confluent portions of the pulmonary veins and that derived from the left-hand division of the common auricle of the embryonic heart" (10); displacement of the pulmonary venous trunk towards the right with drainage between the septum primum and the septum secundum (4); entrapment of the common pulmonary vein by tissue of the sinus venosus from which the septum primum develops (11); and impingement of the left superior vena cava on the developing left atrium (12). Nonetheless, there is a general consensus that this malformation is due to failure in the process of absorption of the common pulmonary vein into the left atrium (13–19).

ANATOMIC AND ECHOCARDIOGRAPHIC CONSIDERATIONS

The echocardiographic study of cor triatriatum sinister should include the following: (a) anatomic characteristics; (b) presence of obstruction to pulmonary venous flow; and (c) associated anomalies. The intraoperative and postoperative evaluation will be discussed at the end of the chapter.

Anatomic Characteristics of the Anomaly

In the classic form of cor triatriatum sinister, also called diaphragmatic type (17), there is a fibromuscular membrane that divides the left atrium into a proximal chamber or accessory left atrium and a distal chamber or true left atrium (1,8,16–20) (Fig. 13-1). The membrane has a slight oblique orientation from posterior-left to anterior-right and is composed of myocardial tissue covered by a layer of thickened endocardial tissue (17,21). The accessory or proximal atrial chamber corresponds to a dilated common pulmonary vein and is located posteriorly, supe-

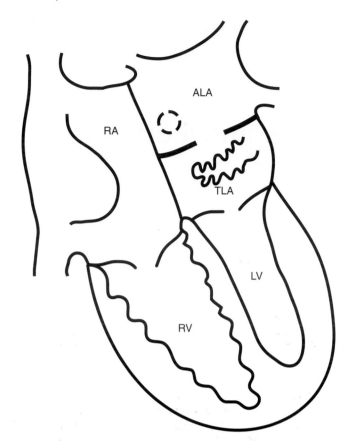

FIG. 13-1. Schematic representation of a cor triatriatum sinister. *RA*, right atrium; *ALA*, accessory left atrium; *TLA*, true left atrium; *RV*, right ventricle; *LV*, left ventricle.

riorly, and to the right of the distal or true left atrial chamber. The accessory chamber usually receives the four pulmonary veins (Fig. 13-1). Its walls are composed of myocardial tissue covered by a very thickened endocardial layer (18). The distal atrial chamber or true left atrium occupies an anterior, inferior, and leftward position with respect to the accessory atrial chamber. Its walls are thinner, and it is related to the left atrial appendage, the mitral valve, and the foramen ovale. The rest of the fossa ovalis can be above or below the fibromuscular membrane (17,18). Usually, there is communication between both atrial chambers through an orifice in the fibromuscular membrane, which can vary from 3 to 15 mm in diameter (17). Less commonly, there can be two or more orifices of variable sizes (17,19–22). Rarely, there is atresia of the orifice (1,14,21,23–25).

The atrial septum is intact in 17% to 50% of cases (1,17,21,26). In those with atrial septal defects, it is usually of the ostium secundum type or is a patent foramen ovale that communicates the right atrium with the distal or true left atrial cavity. Rarely, the communication is to the proximal or accessory atrial chamber (1,6,8,17, 19,21,27,28). Atrioventricular septal defects, partial type, between the right atrium and the distal atrial chamber have been reported either in isolation (17,29) or associated

with an additional atrial septal defect between the right atrium and the proximal atrium (1,22).

The pulmonary veins usually connect into the accessory proximal chamber, but there can also be anomalous connections. Some of those described in the literature include connection of the right pulmonary veins and the left upper pulmonary vein to the accessory chamber and the left lower pulmonary vein to the distal or true left atrium (30); connection of the right upper pulmonary vein to the vena cava, the right lower pulmonary vein to the right atrium, the left upper pulmonary vein to the proximal atrial chamber, and the left lower pulmonary vein to the distal atrial chamber (25); connection of a vein draining the upper and middle right lobes and of another vein draining the lower half of the right lower lobe into the accessory atrial chamber and connection of the veins draining the left lung and one vein draining the upper half of the right lower lobe into the innominate vein (31); connection of the right pulmonary veins to the proximal atrial chamber and the left pulmonary veins to the innominate vein (1,17,21); connection of the left upper pulmonary vein to the right atrium via a left superior vena cava-innominate vein-right superior vena cava (11); connection of the upper pulmonary veins to the distal atrial chamber and of the lower pulmonary veins to the accessory atrial cavity (17); and connection of one right and one left pulmonary vein to the right atrium and to the accessory left atrial chamber, respectively (23).

In addition to the classic or diaphragmatic type, there are two variants of cor triatriatum that have been described: an hourglass type in which there is a narrowing seen externally at the point of union of the accessory and true left atrial chambers without a membrane; and a tubular type in which the accessory chamber has a tubular form without a membrane at its point of union with the left atrium (17).

The echocardiographic views that allow examination of cor triatriatum are the parasternal long-axis and short-axis views, the apical and subcostal four-chamber views, and the apical two-chamber view. In the parasternal long-axis view, the membrane dividing the left atrium crosses the cavity more or less diagonally. In the apical and subcostal views, the intraatrial membrane is perpendicular to the atrial septum and more or less parallel to the plane of the mitral valve (Echo. 13-1; see color plate 41 following p. 364; Echo. 13-2). It can also be funnel-shaped, with its vertex directed towards the mitral valve, from which it is separated by a variable distance. In the parasternal short-axis view, the membrane is seen behind the aortic root and perpendicular to the interatrial septum. In this view, the left atrial appendage can also be seen related to the distal or true left atrial cavity and the pulmonary veins related to the accessory or distal chamber. Color Doppler flow mapping is helpful in demonstrating the flow between the two atrial chambers and through the mitral valve, which, along with the left atrial appendage,

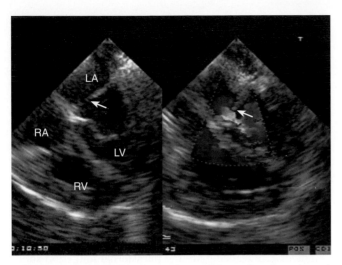

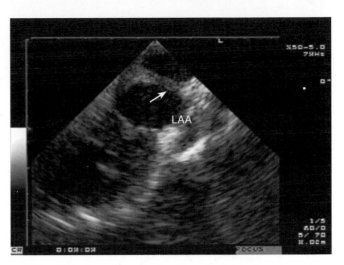

ECHO. 13-1. Left: Transesophageal four-chamber view of cor triatriatum sinister. The membrane is perpendicular to the atrial septum and more or less parallel to the plane of the mitral valve, dividing the left atrium into a proximal or accessory chamber, which receives the pulmonary veins, and a distal or true chamber. **Right:** The color Doppler map of the flow between the two chambers through an orifice in the membrane *(arrow)*. *RA,* right atrium; *RV,* right ventricle; *LA,* left atrium; *LV,* left ventricle.

ECHO. 13-2. Transesophageal longitudinal view in cor triatriatum sinister demonstrating the membrane *(arrow)*. Note that the mitral valve and left atrial appendage are related to the distal or true left atrium. *LAA,* left atrial appendage.

is always related to the distal or true left atrium (Echo. 13-1). Color Doppler can also be useful in demonstrating the presence of several orifices in the membrane. In addition, if there is atresia of the orifice, color Doppler would establish the presence of shunting between the proximal chamber and the right atrium without flow into the distal or true left atrium. The pulmonary veins can be seen from the apical and subcostal four-chamber views and from the suprasternal short-axis view. The adjunctive use of spectral and color Doppler can confirm the site(s) of connection of the veins in a manner similar to that employed to visualize the pulmonary venous connections in the absence of cor triatriatum sinister.

Presence of Obstruction to Pulmonary Venous Flow

Almost always the orifice(s) within the intra-atrial membrane are restrictive, resulting in a degree of pulmonary venous obstruction. Color Doppler flow mapping shows the site of obstructive flow, and the actual velocities can be recorded with spectral Doppler. The views permitting demonstration of the obstructive flows are the fourchamber apical and subcostal views and the two-chamber apical view because these allow the best alignment of the Doppler with the direction of flow.

Associated Anomalies

In addition to atrial septal defects and anomalous pulmonary venous connections, other malformations re-

ported in association with cor triatriatum sinister have been tetralogy of Fallot (1,11,17); double outlet right ventricle (1); coarctation of the aorta (1,11,12,17); bicuspid aortic valve (1,11,12,17); aortic stenosis (1); subaortic stenosis (17); patent ductus arteriosus (1,8,11,12,21,25); ventricular septal defect (1,11,12,17); bicuspid pulmonic valve (1,11,12,17); pulmonic stenosis (1,31); supravalve mitral ring (17); parachute mitral valve (17); mitral stenosis (14); tricuspid stenosis (1); tricuspid atresia (11,19); Ebstein's anomaly (17,32); complete transposition of the great arteries (11); corrected transposition of the great arteries (17); univentricular atrioventricular connection (12); endocardial fibroelastosis (21); persistent left superior vena cava draining into the coronary sinus (1,11,12,17), hypoplastic left ventricle (25), hypoplastic aortic arch (17); and right aortic arch (1,17).

SUPRAVALVE MITRAL RING

Supravalve mitral ring is another rare anomaly characterized by the presence of a membrane within the left atrium. It is different from cor triatriatum sinister in that the membrane is found immediately above the mitral valve and does not divide the left atrium into two chambers (Fig. 13-2). The first description was by Fischer in 1902 (33). In the majority of reported cases, supravalve mitral ring is included in the group of congenital mitral stenoses; therefore, its true incidence is not known exactly. It varies between 9% and 20% of reported cases of congenital mitral stenosis (34–37).

EMBRYOLOGIC CONSIDERATIONS

The morphogenetic process that results in a supravalve mitral ring is not known. It has been mentioned that it

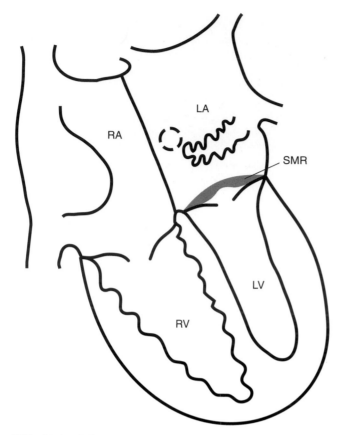

FIG. 13-2. Schematic drawing of a supravalve mitral ring. *RA*, right atrium; *LA*, left atrium; *SMR*, supravalve mitral ring; *RV*, right ventricle; *LV*, left ventricle.

could be a result of a congenital lesion of the atrial endocardium, an abnormal atrial septation, or a defect in the division of the endocardial cushions during early cardiac development (38–40).

ANATOMIC AND ECHOCARDIOGRAPHIC CONSIDERATIONS

The echocardiographic study of supravalve mitral ring should define the following: (a) anatomic characteristics; (b) presence of obstruction to left ventricular inflow; and (c) associated anomalies.

Anatomic Characteristics

A supravalve mitral ring is characterized by the presence of a shelf-like partial or complete ring composed of connective tissue located immediately above the mitral valve (Fig. 13-2). This ring originates from the area adjacent to the fibrous mitral annulus and inserts into the base of the atrial surface of the mitral leaflets. It has a central orifice of variable size. The left atrial appendage is above the ring, and this anatomical characteristic allows differentiation with cor triatriatum sinister, in which the left

atrial appendage is below the intraatrial membrane (Figs. 13-1, 13-2). Histologically, the ring shows a high grade of organization and is formed by collagenous fibers that appear to originate from the substance of the atrium (41). According to Anderson et al. (26) and Becker and Anderson (42), the supravalve ring is a concentric thickening of the left atrial endocardium immediately above the valve annulus.

The supravalve mitral ring is usually associated with parachute mitral valve in isolation or as part of the complex described by Shone et al. (43), which includes supravalve mitral ring, parachute mitral valve, subaortic stenosis, and coarctation of the aorta (Fig. 13-3). Only in 4% of cases is this an isolated malformation (44).

The echocardiographic views that allow the study of a supravalve mitral ring are the parasternal long- and short-axis, the apical and subcostal four-chamber, and the apical two-chamber views. The ring is seen immediately above the mitral annulus (Echo. 13-3). There are two echocardiographic variants: one in which there is a small separation between the mitral valve and the ring seen during diastole; and another in which the membrane is firmly adhered to the mitral leaflets and is difficult to visualize in real time but is detected in slow frame-by-frame playback (45). The first type can be confused with cor triatriatum;

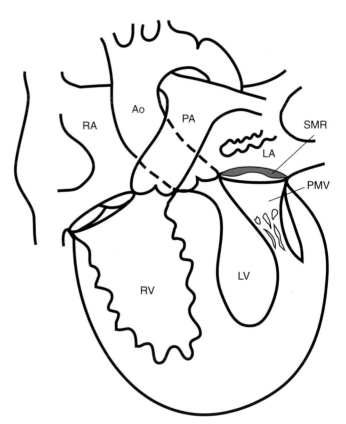

FIG. 13-3. Schematic drawing of a Shone's heart. *RA*, right atrium; *LA*, left atrium; *SMR*, supravalve mitral ring; *PMV*, parachute mitral valve; *RV*, right ventricle; *LV*, left ventricle; *Ao*, aorta; *PA*, pulmonary artery.

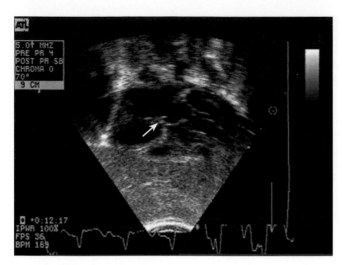

ECHO. 13-3. Subcostal four-chamber view showing the presence of a supravalve mitral ring *(arrow)*. Note that there is a small separation between the ring and the mitral leaflets. The left atrial appendage is above the membrane, differentiating this from cor triatriatum sinister.

however, demonstration of the left atrial appendage above the membrane in this case would establish the differential diagnosis between the lesions.

Presence of Obstruction to Left Ventricular Inflow

In the majority of cases, the supravalve mitral ring does not produce obstruction to left ventricular inflow (34). However, there can be obstruction in cases where the orifice of the ring is small or the ring is associated with anomalies of the mitral valve such as small mitral annulus, fusion of the valve commissures, accessory mitral tissue, parachute mitral valve, and thickened or myxomatous leaflets (34–36,45–48).

Using the echocardiographic views mentioned above, the mitral valve area can be examined carefully, and the spectral and color Doppler can demonstrate the presence and degree of obstruction. Color Doppler is particularly useful in demonstrating the site of the obstruction that would be identified as flow acceleration. Guided by that image, spectral Doppler interrogation can measure the actual flow velocities from which the gradient can be estimated.

Associated Anomalies

A supravalve mitral ring has been seen with the following associated lesions: coarctation of the aorta (34–37,39,45,49); ventricular septal defect (16,34,35,37, 41,45,48–50); double outlet right ventricle (34,45,48); tetralogy of Fallot (35,51); subaortic stenosis (34,35,37, 45,48,50); bicuspid aortic valve (45); valve aortic stenosis (37); rolled mitral valve leaflets with shortened chords

(52); complete atrioventricular septal defect (53); patent ductus arteriosus (35,37,45,52); bicuspid pulmonic valve (46); atrial septal defect (45); patent foramen ovale (46); abnormal tricuspid valve (48); persistent left superior vena cava draining into the coronary sinus (39,45,48); partial anomalous pulmonary venous connection (45); endocardial fibroelastosis (46); double aortic arch (37); hypoplastic left ventricle (37); and coronary anomalies (54).

MALFORMATIONS OF THE MITRAL VALVE APPARATUS

The spectrum of congenital anomalies of the mitral valve apparatus comprises those with predominant stenosis, those with predominant regurgitation, and those with both. Anatomically, these include hypoplastic mitral valve annulus, anomalies of the valve leaflets, double orifice mitral valve, accessory mitral orifice, mitral atresia due to imperforate valve, Ebstein's anomaly of the mitral valve, mitral arcade, parachute mitral valve, and overriding and straddling of the mitral valve.

EMBRYOLOGIC CONSIDERATIONS

In the early post loop stage, the superior or ventral, the inferior or dorsal, and the right and left lateral cushions of the atrioventricular canal appear inside the orifice of the atrioventricular canal (see Fig. 1-12B). The superior and inferior cushions divide the canal into a right and a left orifice (see Fig. 1-12B). The cushions of the atrioventricular canal, the dextrodorsal conal crest, and the ventricular walls all participate in the development of the atrioventricular valves (55–60). The posterior mitral leaflet originates from the left lateral cushion (56,58); the anterior mitral leaflet has a dual embryologic origin: the septal portion arises from the inferior cushion (56,58) and the free portion from the superior cushion of the atrioventricular canal (see Fig. 1-13) (55–58). The leaflet tissue is initially muscular and transforms into connective tissue through a process of cellular differentiation (55). The chordae tendineae and the papillary muscles originate from a process of diverticulation and undermining of the ventricular walls (55). Any anomaly in the origin or in the development of the cushions of the canal as well as any failure in the diverticulation and undermining process of the ventricular walls will result in malformations of the mitral apparatus.

ANATOMIC AND ECHOCARDIOGRAPHIC CONSIDERATIONS

The echocardiographic study of anomalies of the mitral apparatus should determine the following features: (a) the anatomic characteristics of the various malformations; (b) presence and degree of stenosis and/or regurgitation; and (c) associated anomalies.

Anatomic Characteristics of the Various Malformations

These will be outlined for each individual malformation.

Normal but small mitral apparatus describes a situation where all of the components of the mitral apparatus are normal morphologically but small in relation to the size of the tricuspid valve and to the length of the left ventricle (61). It is rarely associated with coarctation of the aorta (61).

Hypoplastic mitral valve annulus is always present in the syndrome of hypoplastic left heart and so is discussed in Chapter 21.

Dysplasia of the mitral valve includes the entire mitral apparatus and is characterized by thickening of the leaflets with rolled edges, fused commissures, anomalous development of the chordae tendineae with short chordae and obliterated interchordal spaces, and poorly developed papillary muscles (42,62,63). This type of anomaly, termed typical congenital mitral stenosis by Ruckman and Van Praagh (36), has been seen in 49% of cases of congenital mitral stenosis.

Mucoid dysplasia involves a mucoid thickening of the mitral valve leaflets with excrescences of mucoid tissue (63). These can be nodular and of variable size and can also be found in the tricuspid and aortic leaflets, thereby forming part of a polyvalvular mucoid congenital disease (63) or congenital polyvalvular disease (64). This mucoid tissue may cause obstruction to left ventricular inflow or outflow.

Echocardiographically, a dysplastic mitral valve has echodense thickened leaflets with limited excursion, shortened chordae, and poorly developed papillary muscles (Echo. 13-4; see color plate 42 following p. 364; Echo. 13-5). In the presence of associated stenosis, the valve would be domed in the open position. In the presence of mucoid dysplasia, the nodules would be seen adhered to the leaflets on the atrial or ventricular aspect of the valve. The latter may cause left ventricular outflow tract obstruction.

Accessory mitral orifice is a result of a circular deficiency of leaflet tissue. Its size can vary, and the borders of the accessory orifice can be free of chordae tendineae or can insert into an independent papillary muscle (34,63).

Double orifice mitral valve describes an anomaly in which there are two orifices with leaflets, chordae tendineae, and papillary muscles. The first report was in 1876 by Greenfield (65), who described two competent orifices of unequal size and postulated an adhesion between the two leaflets at one point. In 85% of cases, the orifices are unequal in size, with the smaller orifice positioned close to the anterolateral commissure in 41% and close to the posteromedial commissure in 44% (66). In the majority of cases, there are two mitral orifices, each with its own tensor apparatus, and normal chords and papillary mus-

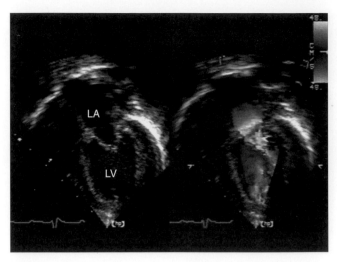

ECHO. 13-4. Apical views showing a dysplastic, stenotic mitral valve that is domed in the open position **(left)** and showing flow acceleration through it in diastole **(right)**. *LA,* left atrium; *LV,* left ventricle.

cles. Less commonly, there is a fibrous bridge between two normal leaflets. The number of papillary muscles is variable, and there can be two, three, or four. A double orifice mitral valve can be found as an isolated abnormality or in association with other malformations (42,63,65–73). The most common associated anomaly is atrioventricular septal defect of the complete or partial type, which can be seen in 38% to 56% of cases of double mitral orifice (66,69).

Echocardiographically, a double orifice mitral valve is best demonstrated on the parasternal and subcostal short-axis views and the apical four-chamber and/or two-chamber views (74) tilting the transducer anteroposteriorly, slightly off the plane of the leaflets themselves to show the orifices (Echo. 13-6). Color Doppler flow mapping is useful to demonstrate the flow through the orifices and the presence of any regurgitation. Directed by the color images, the pulsed-wave sample volume can be placed through the orifices to measure the inflow velocities.

Ebstein's anomaly of a morphologic mitral valve was first described by Edwards in 1954 (74). Since then, 11 cases of this rare anomaly have been reported (76–84). This anomaly should not be confused with Ebstein's malformation of a morphologic tricuspid valve located to the left in the setting of atrioventricular discordance and ventriculoarterial discordance, that is, congenitally corrected transposition of the great arteries. The left atrium is dilated, and there is normal pulmonary venous connection. There is downward displacement of the markedly dysplastic posterior leaflet of the mitral valve, which is adherent to the ventricular wall and has thickened free borders and short and thick chordae tendineae. The anterior mitral leaflet is not displaced, thereby marking the normal level of insertion of the mitral valve into the ven-

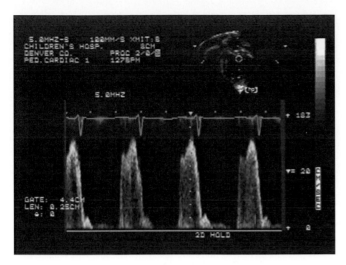

ECHO. 13-5. Spectral Doppler velocity traces in the presence of mitral stenosis showing an increased velocity.

tricular septum in a more superior position with respect to that of the septal leaflet of the tricuspid valve. The downward displacement of the posterior leaflet divides the left ventricle into a proximal "atrialized" chamber and a distal chamber. The "atrialized" portion was thinned in only one reported case (77). The distal portion of the left ventricle is reduced in size, and its wall is thinner than normal. In two reported cases, there was also Ebstein's anomaly of the tricuspid valve (81,83).

The best echocardiographic views to demonstrate Ebstein's anomaly of the mitral valve are the apical and subcostal four-chamber views and the apical two-chamber view. These show the downward displacement of the posterior mitral leaflet, the normal position of the anterior mitral leaflet with respect to the tricuspid valve, the presence of the "atrialized" proximal ventricular chamber, and the smaller than normal distal ventricular cavity. Regurgitation is a common finding, and this is best detected with color Doppler flow mapping and confirmed with spectral Doppler.

The differentiation between Ebstein's malformation of a left-sided morphologic mitral valve and Ebstein's malformation of a left-sided morphologic tricuspid valve with corrected transposition of the great arteries can be accomplished echocardiographically. If the tricuspid valve is located on the left side (atrioventricular discordance), the offsetting between the two atrioventricular valves is reversed. If the tricuspid valve is located on the right (atrioventricular concordance), even if there is Ebstein's malformation of the morphologic mitral valve, the normal offsetting between the septal insertion of both valves is preserved since the anterior mitral leaflet is not displaced downward.

Mitral atresia due to an imperforate valve is characterized by the presence of a membrane that separates the left atrium and the left ventricle (see Fig. 2-7B). These

cases must be differentiated from those associated with aortic atresia, discussed in Chapter 21, and from those with absent left atrioventricular connection, discussed in Chapter 17. In absent left atrioventricular connection (classic mitral atresia), there is only one ventricle and one accessory chamber within the ventricular mass. Further, there is no potential connection between the left atrium and the accessory left ventricular chamber (see Fig. 2-6C). In mitral atresia due to imperforate valve (see Fig. 2-7B), there are two separate, identifiable ventricles with inlet, trabecular, and outlet portions. Also, there is a potential connection between the left atrium and the left ventricle. The left atrium ends blindly, and there is an interatrial communication that allows passage of blood from the pulmonary veins into the right atrium. The left ventricle is usually hypoplastic except in cases where there is overriding and straddling of the tricuspid valve (85). The aortic valve is patent and can be normal or hypoplastic (85–87). The ventriculoarterial connection can be concordant, but most frequently there is double outlet right ventricle.

In mitral atresia due to an imperforate valve, the thin membrane separating the left atrium and ventricle and the small left ventricular cavity are best appreciated from the apical two- and four-chamber and the subcostal four-chamber views, complemented by the parasternal long- and short-axis view (Echo. 13-7). From these views, presence of any subvalvular mitral apparatus may also be detected (87).

Mitral arcade or hammock valve was first described in 1967 by Layman and Edwards (87), who used the term "anomalous mitral arcade." Seen from the atrial side, the mitral valve has the shape of a funnel, with absent commissures and a central orifice of variable size in which are seen crossed chordae tendineae, giving the appearance of a hammock (89). It can also be partially obstructed

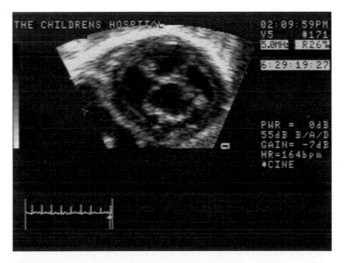

ECHO. 13-6. Subcostal short-axis view of a double orifice mitral valve. One orifice is superior and the other inferior.

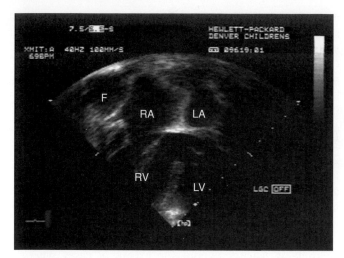

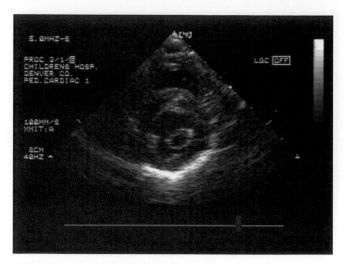

ECHO. 13-7. Apical four-chamber view of mitral atresia due to an imperforate valve. This patient has undergone a Fontan type of operation. The presence of a large ventricular septal defect allowed for an adequately sized left ventricular cavity. *RA,* right atrium; *RV,* right ventricle; *F,* Fontan connection; *LA,* left atrium; *LV,* left ventricle.

ECHO. 13-8. Parasternal short-axis view demonstrating the presence of a parachute mitral valve. Note that the valve is related to the anterolateral papillary muscle without attachments to the small posteromedial papillary muscle.

by thickened papillary muscles (90). Seen from the left ventricle, there is a bridge of fibrous tissue in the shape of an arcade below the anterior mitral leaflet that extends from the anterolateral to the posteromedial papillary muscle. The leaflets insert directly into the papillary muscles or through short, thick chords (34,42,63,88–92).

Echocardiographically, the direct insertion of the leaflets into the papillary muscles or through short, thick chords as well as the presence of a fibrous tissue bridge adhered to the inferior aspect of the anterior mitral leaflet can be best demonstrated from the apical and subcostal four- and two-chamber views. The parasternal short-axis view angling the transducer anteroposteriorly through the mitral apparatus can also demonstrate these anomalies as well as the extension of the fibrous tissue between both papillary muscles (93).

Parachute mitral valve was first described in 1961 by Schiebler et al. (94), who applied this term to characterize an anomaly of the mitral apparatus in which all the chordae tendineae were inserted into one papillary muscle. Later, Shone et al. (43) used the same term to describe a complex that included supravalve mitral ring, parachute mitral valve, subaortic stenosis, and coarctation of the aorta (Fig. 13-3). In Schiebler's publication (92) and in seven of the eight cases reported by Shone et al. (43), there was only one papillary muscle present into which all chordae tendineae converged. In the remaining case, there were two papillary muscles immediately adjacent to each other so that functionally the chordal insertions produced the effect of a single papillary muscle. Adjacent papillary muscles were also observed by Davachi et al. (34) and by Rosenquist (61), who considers that these cases in which there is failure of development of the space

between the anterolateral and posteromedial papillary muscles should be considered a variant of parachute mitral valve. For Ruckman and Van Praagh (36), parachute mitral valve implies the presence of one posteromedial papillary muscle into which all chords insert with absence of the anterolateral papillary muscle. In both cases, either with adjacent papillary muscles or with one single papillary muscle, there is obstruction to mitral inflow, and the only passage of blood from the left atrium is across interchordal spaces and short, thickened chords.

The number and disposition of the papillary muscles and the chordal insertions to a single or to two adjacent papillary muscles can be evaluated echocardiographically from a slow sweep along the parasternal short axis (Echo. 13-8). The obstruction to mitral inflow can be estimated through spectral Doppler techniques, aided with the use of color Doppler flow mapping to guide positioning of the sample volume from the apical four- and two-chamber views.

Overriding and Straddling of the Mitral Valve. Overriding of an atrioventricular valve is present when the valvular orifice is related with both ventricles (Figs. 13-4, 13-5). Straddling is present when the tensor apparatus of an atrioventricular valve has insertions into both sides of the interventricular septum (95) (Figs. 13-5, 13-6). Both anomalies can coexist in the same heart or be present independently. As such, there can be overriding without straddling (Fig. 13-4), overriding with straddling (Fig. 13-5), and straddling without overriding (Fig. 13-6). In addition, there can also be overriding and straddling of both atrioventricular valves. As described for the tricuspid valve, overriding is mild if it is less than 50% and severe if it is greater than 50% over the ventricular septum. Straddling is classified as Type A, B, or C depending on the site of insertion of the tensor apparatus within the

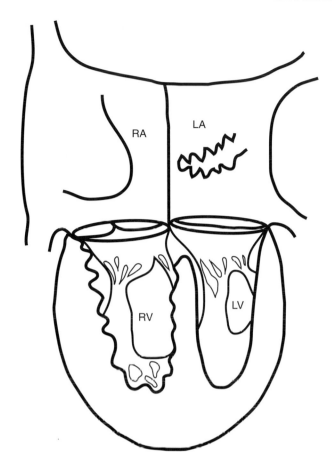

FIG. 13-4. Schematic drawing of an overriding mitral valve without straddling. *RA,* right atrium; *LA,* left atrium; *RV,* right ventricle; *LV,* left ventricle.

contralateral ventricle (see Chapter 12). The mitral valve straddles the anterior portion of the ventricular septum; therefore, the ventricular septal defect is located in the anterior septum. The ventricular septum reaches the crux cordis, and the atrioventricular valves maintain the normal offsetting of the septal insertions.

The best echocardiographic approach to evaluate the presence and degree of overriding and/or straddling of the mitral valve is the apical four-chamber view (Echo. 13-9). This permits examination of the site(s) of the chordal insertions into the contralateral ventricle. It is important to consider overriding of the valve relative to its position at the crux cordis since the atrial and ventricular septa are aligned at this point. As the transducer is swept superiorly towards the left ventricular outflow tract, the atrial and ventricular septa become somewhat malaligned even in normal hearts, so errors in diagnosis can occur. Other echocardiographic views are complementary to the complete evaluation of overriding and straddling of the mitral valve; these include the subcostal four-chamber view and the parasternal long- and short-axis views.

Overriding and straddling of the mitral apparatus do not occur as isolated lesions; rather, they are associated with atrioventricular septal defects or with conotruncal

abnormalities such as double outlet right ventricle with subpulmonary ventricular septal defect, complete transposition of the great arteries, or corrected transposition of the great arteries, or with criss-cross hearts and hearts with univentricular atrioventricular connection. These are discussed in their corresponding chapters.

Floppy mitral valve syndrome describes a primary myxomatous transformation of the mitral valve (96–99). Histologically, there is myxomatous proliferation of the spongiosa layer of the valve with increased mucopolysaccharides and degeneration of the collagen of the fibrous portion of the valve (96–101). This myxomatous transformation of the mitral valve, which occurs most frequently on the posterior rather than the anterior leaflet, causes a translucent thickening of the valve leaflets, which acquire a redundant appearance and balloon into the left atrium during systole (97). The leaflets do not appose correctly so that one or both leaflets cross into the left atrium during systole, causing prolapse of the valve (100). The myxomatous transformation affects the tendinous chords, which become thin and elongated. The annulus is dilated, contributing to the valve prolapse. The etiology of the floppy mitral valve syndrome is not known, although it

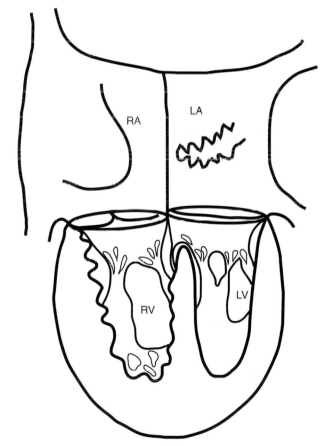

FIG. 13-5. Schematic drawing of overriding and straddling of the mitral valve. *RA,* right atrium; *LA,* left atrium; *RV,* right ventricle; *LV,* left ventricle.

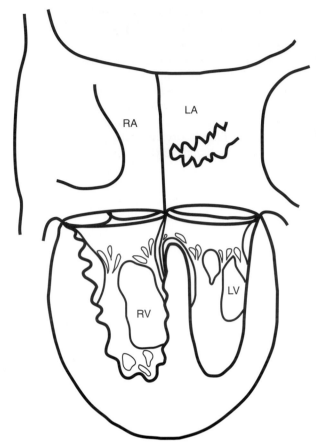

FIG. 13-6. Schematic drawing of straddling of the mitral valve without overriding. *RA,* right atrium; *LA,* left atrium; *RV,* right ventricle; *LV,* left ventricle.

has been considered a forme fruste of the Marfan syndrome (96).

Prolapse of the mitral valve can be seen echocardiographically from various views, including the parasternal long-axis and short-axis, the apical four-chamber, two-

chamber and long-axis, and from the subcostal long- and short-axis views. The two-dimensional echocardiographic diagnosis of mitral valve prolapse is based on the demonstration of motion of one or both mitral leaflets posterior to the plane of the mitral annulus into the left atrium during systole (Echo. 13-10). The M-mode recording of the leaflet motion obtained from the parasternal long- and/ or short-axis views is also diagnostic of mitral prolapse (Echo. 13-10). Occasionally, prolapse of the valve becomes more evident during Valsalva maneuver.

Isolated cleft of the mitral valve is rare, with a reported incidence of 15% of all congenital anomalies of the mitral valve (102). Generally, the cleft is seen in the anterior leaflet, but cases of isolated cleft of the posterior leaflet have been reported (103). The cleft extends from the free border of the leaflet towards the fibrous annulus of the mitral valve and divides the anterior leaflet into two parts, which, in the majority of cases, are of equal size (34,63,104,105). The leaflets can be normal or demonstrate a degree of dysplasia with thickened and rolled edges. The borders of the cleft can be free or have chords inserting into the interventricular septum or anterior ventricular wall. The long axis of the cleft is directed towards the outflow tract of the left ventricle.

The major differential diagnosis of isolated clefts of the mitral valve are the so-called "clefts" of the anterior mitral leaflet seen in atrioventricular septal defects. These, however, are not clefts within the anterior mitral leaflet but rather a true commissure between the anterior and the posterior bridging leaflets. As such, their major axis is not directed towards the left ventricular outflow tract but rather towards the interventricular septum. Further, in the presence of isolated clefts of the mitral valve, there are none of the other stigmata of atrioventricular septal defects. These are discussed in detail in Chapter 11.

The echocardiogram demonstrates isolated clefts of the

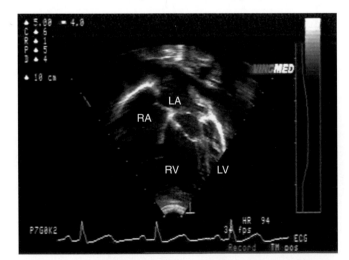

ECHO. 13-9. Apical four-chamber view of a straddling and overriding mitral valve. Note the very small left ventricle. *RA,* right atrium; *RV,* right ventricle; *LA,* left atrium; *LV,* left ventricle.

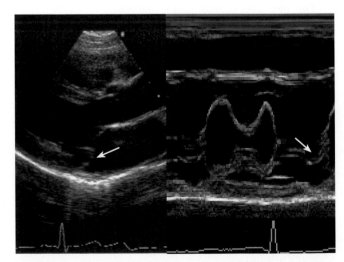

ECHO. 13-10. Parasternal long-axis view and M-mode trace of a prolapsed posterior mitral valve leaflet *(arrows).*

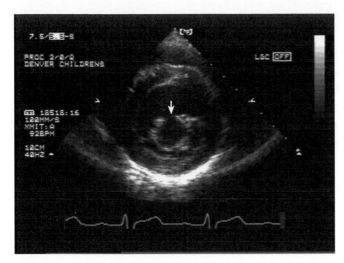

ECHO. 13-11. Parasternal short-axis view of an isolated cleft of the anterior mitral leaflet *(arrow)*. Note that the cleft points towards the left ventricular outflow tract.

mitral valve from the parasternal short-axis view and the subcostal short-axis view. The direction of the cleft within the anterior leaflet is clearly seen pointing towards the left ventricular outflow tract (Echo. 13-11). Presence and severity of regurgitation can be evaluated from the spectral and color Doppler. The parasternal long-axis view, the apical four- and two-chamber views, and the subcostal views should all be recorded for assessment of regurgitation.

Presence and Degree of Stenosis and/or Regurgitation

Mitral valve stenosis can be diagnosed and its severity estimated by recording the transvalvular velocities with spectral Doppler and estimating the pressure gradient using the simplified Bernoulli equation. Valve area can be estimated from the pressure half-time method with moderately good results (106).

There have been numerous methods proposed for estimating the severity of mitral valve regurgitation. Detection of the regurgitant jet is fairly easy with the use of color Doppler flow mapping recorded from orthogonal planes. These include the parasternal long-axis, the apical four-chamber, two-chamber, and long-axis views, and the subcostal long-axis view. Accurate quantitation of severity involves a combination of spectral and color Doppler methods, two-dimensional imaging, and evaluation of systolic and diastolic left ventricular function.

Methods used to evaluate and grade mitral valve stenosis and regurgitation are discussed in detail in Chapter 6.

Associated Anomalies

There is a wide spectrum of anomalies associated with malformations of the mitral valve apparatus.

A normal but small mitral apparatus has been associated with bicuspid aortic valve, valve aortic stenosis, patent foramen ovale, patent ductus arteriosus, atrial septal defect, ventricular septal defect, partial atrioventricular septal defect, tubular aortic hypoplasia, coarctation of the aorta, and endocardial fibroelastosis (36,61).

Dysplasia of the mitral valve has been associated with valve aortic stenosis, subvalve aortic stenosis, valve pulmonic stenosis, patent ductus arteriosus, ventricular septal defect, coarctation of the aorta, tetralogy of Fallot, double outlet right ventricle, tricuspid stenosis, persistent left superior vena cava, Ebstein's anomaly of the tricuspid valve, and hypoplastic left ventricle (16,18,34–37,89,92).

Mucoid dysplasia has been seen in association with atrial septal defect, ventricular septal defect, patent ductus arteriosus, and bicuspid aortic valve (63,64).

Accessory mitral tissue has been seen with coarctation of the aorta, parachute mitral valve, endocardial fibroelastosis, supravalve mitral ring, and hypoplastic left ventricle (34). Accessory mitral tissue can cause left ventricular outflow tract obstruction (Echo. 13-12; see color plate 43 following p. 364).

Accessory mitral orifice can be seen in transposition of the great arteries with ventricular septal defect, partial atrioventricular septal defect, and interruption of the inferior vena cava (63,92).

Mitral arcade can be found in association with atrial septal defect, patent ductus arteriosus, aortic stenosis due to nodular mucoid dysplasia, subvalve aortic stenosis, and coarctation of the aorta (34,63,89,92).

Double orifice mitral valve can be seen in combination with coarctation of the aorta, bicuspid aortic valve, subaortic stenosis, bicuspid pulmonic valve, patent ductus arteriosus, Ebstein's malformation of the tricuspid valve, tricuspid stenosis, double orifice of the tricuspid valve, ostium secundum atrial septal defect, common atrium,

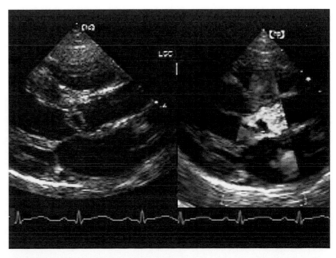

ECHO. 13-12. Parasternal long-axis view of accessory mitral valve tissue, causing left ventricular outflow tract obstruction.

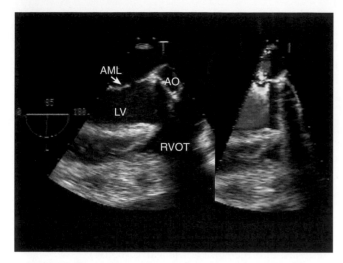

ECHO. 13-13. Transesophageal longitudinal view of the left ventricle demonstrating the presence of a perforation of the anterior mitral leaflet (**left**, *arrow*) and regurgitation through the defect in the leaflet tissue (**right**). AML, anterior mitral leaflet; *LV*, left ventricle; *AO*, aorta; *RVOT*, right ventricular outflow tract.

ventricular septal defect, mitral stenosis, parachute mitral valve, mitral valve regurgitation, complete transposition of the great arteries, tetralogy of Fallot, double outlet right ventricle, type I truncus arteriosus, left superior vena cava draining into the roof of the left atrium and absence of the coronary sinus, mitral valve prolapse, and hypoplastic left heart syndrome (37,53,66,70–74).

Ebstein's anomaly of the mitral valve can be found with dilatation of the ascending aorta (Marfan syndrome), double outlet right ventricle with subaortic ventricular septal defect, partial mitral arcade, fossa ovalis type of atrial septal defect, patent foramen ovale, patent ductus arteriosus, coarctation of the aorta, hypoplasia of the ascending aorta, and valvular aortic stenosis (77,79,80,84).

An imperforate mitral valve can be associated with atrial septal defect, ventricular septal defect, and patent foramen ovale (87).

Parachute mitral valve has been seen in association with ventricular septal defect, valvular pulmonic stenosis, right ventricular outflow tract obstruction, double outlet right ventricle, patent ductus arteriosus, complete transposition of the great arteries, corrected transposition of the great arteries, aortic regurgitation, ostium secundum atrial septal defect, persistent left superior vena cava, bicuspid aortic valve, valve aortic stenosis, tetralogy of Fallot, and endocardial fibroelastosis (34,36,37,47,48,63,89,92,107).

Floppy mitral valve syndrome is seen with mitral regurgitation, aortic regurgitation, ostium secundum atrial septal defect, tricuspid regurgitation, and rupture of a tendinous chord (96,100,101).

Isolated clefts of the mitral valve can be associated with ventricular septal defects, complete transposition of the great arteries, tetralogy of Fallot, double outlet right

ventricle with subpulmonary ventricular septal defect, left ventricular outflow tract obstruction secondary to anomalous insertions of the mitral valve into the interventricular septum, and ostium secundum atrial septal defects (34,63,102).

INTRAOPERATIVE AND POSTOPERATIVE EVALUATION

The intraoperative study of mitral valve anomalies prebypass should be directed towards confirming the type of lesion previously diagnosed and obtaining a baseline estimate of the severity of the stenosis and/or regurgitation immediately prior to intervention when the hemodynamics may be different from those present during the transthoracic study. There are several transesophageal views to evaluate the anatomy and function of the mitral valve. The horizontal four-chamber view obtained behind the left atrium is a good starting point for assessment of the valve (see Fig. 4-28A,B). This view allows examination of both leaflets and the chordae, and the size of the left atrium and ventricle. Color Doppler is usually well aligned for detection of regurgitation, and the spectral Doppler can offer clean velocity signals of forward and reverse flows. The left ventricular outflow tract can be evaluated for any obstruction due to intrinsic associated malformations or due to accessory mitral tissue by slight withdrawal of the transducer from this same orientation (see Fig. 4-29A). The longitudinal views (see Figs. 4-28C, 4-29E,F) allow visualization of the mitral apparatus and examination for the presence of regurgitation from an orthogonal plane. From these views, the mitral valve can be carefully examined for most anomalies described

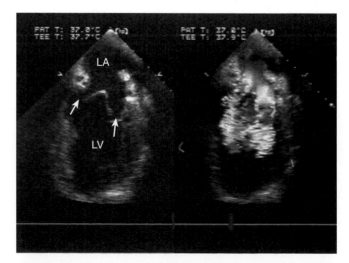

ECHO. 13-14. Transesophageal longitudinal view of a double orifice mitral valve. **Left:** Anatomic image of the two orifices. The major and minor orifices are indicated *(arrows)*. **Right:** Color Doppler flow map demonstrating the flow through the two orifices. *LA*, left atrium; *LV*, left ventricle.

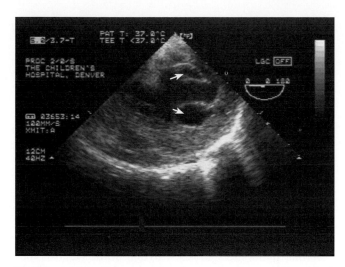

ECHO. 13-15. Transgastric short-axis view of the mitral valve in the presence of a double orifice (same patient as in Echo 13-14). The two orifices are indicated *(arrows)*.

previously. Presence and site of origin of valve regurgitation can be easily detected (Echo. 13-13; see color plate 44 following p. 364). Also, deformities such as double orifice, dysplastic, or parachute valves can be visualized from the longitudinal planes (Echo. 13-14; see color plate 45 following p. 364). The left ventricle and mitral apparatus can be evaluated in a short axis from the transgastric approach (see Fig. 4-27A,B). Withdrawal and advancement of the transducer permits recording of views equivalent to a short-axis sweep through the mitral apparatus from which the anatomy of the valve can be further elucidated (Echo. 13-15). This sweep is usually the preferred view for estimating left ventricular size and function.

Immediately post-bypass, the left ventricular size and function should be evaluated from the transgastric views as outlined above (see Fig. 4-27A,B). The repair of the mitral lesion would be assessed from views similar to those described for the pre-bypass study. A thorough assessment of the repair should be performed from all available views to determine if further intervention is required prior to termination of the surgical procedure.

The late postoperative evaluation of repair or replacement of the mitral valve entails a similar approach to that described for the transthoracic studies. Depending on the age of the child, repairs may require revisions and even valve replacement later in life. Serial assessment of these patients is imperative since a complete resolution of the valve problem is rarely accomplished, especially in the small child. A detailed discussion of the Doppler methods to estimate mitral stenosis and regurgitation is included in Chapter 6.

RIGHT JUXTAPOSITION OF THE ATRIAL APPENDAGES

Right juxtaposition of the atrial appendages is a very rare malformation in which both atrial appendages are

situated side by side, to the right of the great vessels (Fig. 13-7). The first case was reported by Saphir and Lev in 1941 (108). The term "right juxtaposition" was proposed by Dixon in 1954 (109). Its incidence is not known. To our knowledge, there have been 13 cases reported in the literature (108–117).

EMBRYOLOGIC CONSIDERATIONS

Wenner proposed that left juxtaposition of the atrial appendages is due to an underdevelopment of the process of torsion of the primitive cardiac tube (118). Based on this theory, Dixon (109) considers that right juxtaposition may be the result of an overdevelopment or overtorsion of the primitive cardiac tube in cases with D bulboventricular loop and undertorsion in cases with L loop. Melhuish and Van Praagh (111) consider that, from the morphogenetic standpoint, juxtaposition of the atrial appendages would be secondary to an associated anomaly rather than a primary cardiac malformation per se.

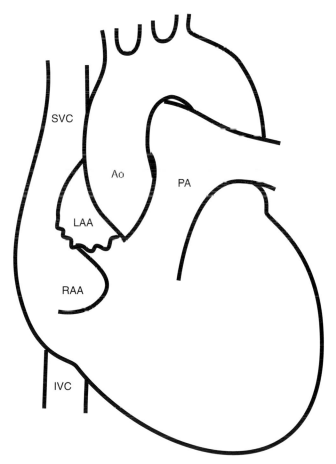

FIG. 13-7. Schematic drawing of a heart with right juxtaposition of the atrial appendages. *RAA*, right atrial appendage; *LAA*, left atrial appendage; *SVC*, superior vena cava; *IVC*, inferior vena cava; *Ao*, aorta; *PA*, pulmonary artery.

ANATOMIC AND ECHOCARDIOGRAPHIC CONSIDERATIONS

The echocardiographic study of right juxtaposition of the atrial appendages should consider the following: (a) position of the heart in the thorax; (b) visceroatrial situs; (c) position of the atrial appendages; (d) atrioventricular connection; (e) ventriculoarterial connection; and (f) associated anomalies.

Position of the Heart in the Thorax

Of the 13 cases reported in the literature, the heart was in levocardia in 11 cases (87%) (108–110,112–117); in mesocardia in one case (6.5%) (111); and in dextrocardia in one case (6.5%) (111).

Visceroatrial Situs

Situs solitus was found in 11 cases (87%) (108–117), and, in the two remaining cases, the situs was ambiguous (13%) (117).

Position of the Atrial Appendages

In the normal heart, the atrial appendages are situated on both sides of the great vessels. In right juxtaposition, both appendages are side by side, to the right of the great vessels (Fig. 13-7).

Atrioventricular Connection

The atrioventricular connection was concordant in seven cases (54%) (108,110,112–117); discordant in three cases (23%) (109,111); and ambiguous in two cases (15%) (117); and was a univentricular atrioventricular connection in one case (8%) (114).

Ventriculoarterial Connection

The ventriculoarterial connection was concordant in six cases (45%) (110–112,115–117); double outlet right ventricle in three cases (23%) (108,109,117); discordant in one case (corrected transposition) (8%) (111); concordant with levo malposition of the aorta in one case (8%) (113); concordant with dextro malposition of the aorta in one case (8%) (117); and indeterminate in one case with the aorta anterior and to the right (8%) (114).

The echocardiographic determination of the position of the heart in the thorax, the visceroatrial situs, the atrioventricular and ventriculoarterial connections, and the spatial position of the great vessels are covered in detail in Chapter 4. The echocardiographic demonstration of right juxta-position of the atrial appendages is extremely difficult and is generally an incidental finding at surgery or autopsy.

Associated Anomalies

Right juxtaposition of the atrial appendages can be found in association with simpler forms of congenital cardiac malformations. Those reported in the literature have been ventricular septal defect, atrial septal defect, atrioventricular septal defect, common atrium, pulmonic stenosis, patent ductus arteriosus, total anomalous pulmonary venous return, tricuspid atresia, univentricular atrioventricular connection, hypoplasia of the tricuspid valve, hypoplasia of the mitral valve, bicuspid pulmonic valve, valvular pulmonic stenosis, valvular aortic stenosis, persistent left superior vena cava, inferior vena cava draining into the left atrium, and coarctation of the aorta (108–117).

REFERENCES

1. Thilenius OG, Bharati S, Lev M. Subdivided left atrium: an expanded concept of cor triatriatum sinistrum. *Am J Cardiol* 1976; 37:743–752.
2. Church WS. Congenital malformation of the heart; abnormal septum in the left auricle. *Trans Pathol Soc Lond* 1868;19:188–190.
3. Andral G. *Exces de developpement du coeur. Precis d'anatomie pathologique.* Vol. 2. Paris: Gabon, 1829:313–314.
4. Borst-Gottingen M. Ein cor triatriatum. *Verh Dtsch Ges Pathol* 1905;9:178–192.
5. Patten BM, Taggart WB. An unusual type of triatrial heart. *Arch Pathol* 1929;8:894–905.
6. Ostman-Smith I, Silverman NH, Oldershaw P, Lincoln C, Shinebourne EA. Cor triatriatum sinistrum. Diagnostic features on cross sectional echocardiography. *Br Heart J* 1984;51:211–219.
7. Fyler DC, Buckley LP, Hellenbrand WE, Cohn HE. The New England Regional Infant Cardiac Program. *Pediatrics* 1980; 65[Suppl]:375–461.
8. Rodefeld MD, Brown JW, Heimansohn DA, et al. Cor triatriatum: clinical presentation and surgical results in 12 patients. *Ann Thorac Surg* 1990;50:562–568.
9. Fowler JK. Membranous band in the left auricle. *Trans Pathol Soc Lond* 1882;33:77–78.
10. Griffith TW. Note on a second example of division of the cavity of the left auricle into two compartments by a fibrous band. *J Anat Physiol* 1902;37:255–257.
11. Van Praagh R, Corsini I. Cor triatriatum: pathologic anatomy and a consideration of morphogenesis based on 13 postmortem cases and a study of the normal development of the pulmonary vein and atrial septum in 83 human embryos. *Am Heart J* 1969;78:379–405.
12. Gharagozloo F, Bulkley BH, Hutchins GM. A proposed pathogenesis of cor triatriatum: impingement of the left superior vena cava on the developing left atrium. *Am Heart J* 1977;94:618–626.
13. Loeffler E. Unusual malformation of the left atrium: pulmonary sinus. *Arch Pathol* 1949;48:371–376.
14. Parsons CG. Cor triatriatum. Concerning the nature of an anomalous septum in the left auricle. *Br Heart J* 1950;12:327–337.
15. Edwards JE. Congenital stenosis of pulmonary veins. Pathologic and developmental considerations. *Lab Invest* 1960;9:46–66.
16. Lucas RV Jr, Anderson RC, Amplatz K, Adams P Jr, Edwards JE. Congenital causes of pulmonary venous obstruction. *Pediatr Clin North Am* 1963;10:781–836.
17. Marin-Garcia J, Tandon R, Lucas RV, Edwards JE. Cor triatriatum: study of the 20 cases. *Am J Cardiol* 1975;35:59–66.
18. Glancy DL, Roberts WC. Congenital obstructive lesions involving

the major pulmonary veins, left atrium, or mitral valve: a clinical, laboratory, and morphologic survey. *Cathet Cardiovasc Diagn* 1976;2:215–252.

19. Jacobstein MD, Hirschfeld SS. Concealed left atrial membrane: pitfalls in the diagnosis of cor triatriatum and supravalve mitral ring. *Am J Cardiol* 1982;49:780–786.

20. Potter P, Ranson SW. A heart presenting a septum across the left auricle. *J Anat Physiol* 1904;39:69–73.

21. Niwayama G. Cor triatriatum. *Am Heart J* 1960;59:291–317.

22. Edwards BS, Edwards WD, Bambara JF, van der Bel-Kahn J, Bove KE, Edwards JE. Anomalies of the left atrium and mitral valve. Cords, flaps, and duplication of valve. *Arch Pathol Lab Med* 1983;107:29–33.

23. Stoeber H. Ein weiterer fall von cor triatriatum mit eigenarting gekreuzter mundung der lungenvenen. *Virchows Arch* 1908;193:252–257.

24. Pedersen A, Therkelsen F. Cor triatriatum: a rare malformation of the heart, probably amenable to surgery. Report of a case, with review of literature. *Am Heart J* 1954;47:676–691.

25. Wilson JW, Graham TP, Gehweiler JA, Canent RV. Cor triatriatum with intact subdividing diaphragm and partial anomalous pulmonary venous connection to the proximal left atrial chamber (an unreported type). *Pediatrics* 1971;47:745–750.

26. Anderson RH, Macartney FJ, Shinebourne EA, Tynan M. Partitioning of atrial chamber ("cor triatriatum"). In: Anderson RH, Macartney FJ, Shinebourne EA, Tynan M, eds. *Paediatric cardiology.* Volume 1. Edinburgh: Churchill Livingstone, 1987:563–570.

27. Somerville J. Masked cor triatriatum. *Br Heart J* 1966;28:55–61.

28. Marin-Garcia J, Amplatz K, Moller JH, Tandon R, Edwards JE. Clinical pathologic conference. *Am Heart J* 1974;87:238–245.

29. Gahagan T, Ziegler RF. Triatrial heart with persistent ostium primum and cleft mitral valve. *J Thorac Cardiovasc Surg* 1967;3:231–234.

30. Donatelli R, Meriggi A, Santoli C, Mombelloni G. Il "cor triatriatum." *Minerva Cardioangiol* 1969;17:651–664.

31. Shone JD, Anderson RC, Amplatz K, Varco RL, Leonard AS, Edwards JE. Pulmonary venous obstruction from two separate coexistent anomalies. Subtotal pulmonary venous connection to cor triatriatum and subtotal pulmonary venous connection to left innominate vein. *Am J Cardiol* 1963;2:525–531.

32. From AHL, Mazzitello WF, Judd AS, Edwards JE. Ebstein's malformation of the tricuspid valve associated with valvular stenosis and cor triatriatum. *Chest* 1973;64:248–251.

33. Fisher T. Two cases of congenital disease of the left side of the heart. *BMJ* 1902;1:639–641.

34. Davachi F, Moller JH, Edwards JE. Diseases of the mitral valve in infancy. An anatomic analysis of 55 cases. *Circulation* 1971;43:565–579.

35. Collins-Nakai RL, Rosenthal A, Castaneda AR, Bernhard WF, Nadas AS. Congenital mitral stenosis. A review of 20 years' experience. *Circulation* 1977;56:1039–1047.

36. Ruckman RN, Van Praagh RN. Anatomic types of congenital mitral stenosis: report of 49 autopsy cases with consideration of diagnosis and surgical implications. *Am J Cardiol* 1978;42:592–601.

37. Moore P, Adatia I, Spevak PJ, et al. Severe congenital mitral stenosis in infants. *Circulation* 1994;89:2099–2106.

38. Stretton TB, Fentem PH. Stenosis of the left atrio-ventricular canal. *Br Heart J* 1962;24:237–240.

39. Cassano GB. Congenital annular stenosis of the left atrioventricular canal. So-called supravalvular mitral stenosis. *Am J Cardiol* 1964;13:708–713.

40. Srinivassan V, Lewin NA, Pieroni D, Levinsky L, Gomez Alicea JR, Subramanian S. Supravalvular stenosing ring of the left atrium: case report and review of the literature. *Cardiovasc Dis Bull* 1980;7:149–158.

41. Manubens R, Krovetz LJ, Adams P Jr. Supravalvular stenosing ring of the left atrium. *Am Heart J* 1960;60:286–295.

42. Becker AE, Anderson RH. Atrioventricular valve malformations. In: Becker AE, Anderson RH, eds. *Pathology of congenital heart disease.* London: Butterworth, 1981:137–163.

43. Shone JD, Sellers RD, Anderson RC, Adams P Jr, Lillehei CW, Edwards JE. The developmental complex of "parachute mitral

valve," supravalvular ring of left atrium, subaortic stenosis, coarctation of aorta. *Am J Cardiol* 1963;11:714–725.

44. Chung KJ, Manning JA, Lipchick EO, Gramiak R, Mahoney EB. Isolated supravalvular stenosing ring of the left atrium: diagnosis before operation and successful surgical treatment. *Chest* 1974;65:25–28.

45. Sullivan ID, Robinson PJ, De Leval M, Graham TP Jr. Membranous supravalvular mitral stenosis: a treatable form of congenital heart disease. *J Am Coll Cardiol* 1986;8:159–164.

46. Mehrizi A, Hutchins GM, Wilson EF, Breckinridge JC, Rowe RD. Supravalvular mitral stenosis. *J Pediatr* 1965;67:1141–1149.

47. Glancy DL, Chang MY, Dorney ER, Roberts WC. Parachute mitral valve. Further observations and associated lesions. *Am J Cardiol* 1971;27:309–313.

48. Macartney FJ, Scott O, Ionescu MI, Deverall PB. Diagnosis and management of parachute mitral valve and supravalvular mitral ring. *Br Heart J* 1974;36:641–652.

49. Neirotti R, Kreutzer G, Galindez E, Becu L, Ross D. Supravalvular mitral stenosis associated with ventricular septal defect. *Am J Dis Child* 1977;131:862–865.

50. Snider AR, Roge CL, Schiller NB, Silverman NH. Congenital left ventricular inflow obstruction evaluated by two-dimensional echocardiography. *Circulation* 1980;61:848–855.

51. Benrey J, Leachman RD, Cooley DA, Klima T, Lufschanowski R. Supravalvular mitral stenosis associated with tetralogy of Fallot. *Am J Cardiol* 1976;37:111–114.

52. Johnson NJ, Dodd K. Obstruction to left atrial outflow by a supravalvular stenosing ring. *J Pediatr* 1957;51:190–193.

53. Strasburger JF. Cor triatriatum, pulmonary vein obstruction, supravalvar mitral stenosis, and congenital mitral valve disease. In: Garson A Jr, Bricker JT, McNamara DG, eds. *The science and practice of pediatric cardiology.* Volume 2. Philadelphia: Lea & Febiger, 1990:1308–1315.

54. Huhta JC, Edwards WD, Danielson GK. Supravalvular mitral ridge containing the dominant left circumflex coronary artery. *J Thorac Cardiovasc Surg* 1981;81:577–579.

55. Van Mierop LHS, Alley RD, Kausel HW, Stranahan A. The anatomy and embryology of endocardial cushion defects. *J Thorac Cardiovasc Surg* 1962;43:71–83.

56. Netter FH, Van Mierop LHS. Embryology. In: Netter FH, Yonkman FF, eds. *The Ciba collection of medical illustrations. Heart.* Volume 5. Summit, NJ: CIBA Publications Department, 1969:112–130.

57. De la Cruz MV, Quero-Jimenez M, Arteaga Martinez M, Cayre R. Morphogenese du septum interventriculaire. *Coeur* 1982;13:443–448.

58. De la Cruz MV, Gimenez-Ribotta M, Saravalli O, Cayre R. The contribution of the inferior endocardial cushion of the atrioventricular canal to cardiac septation and to the development of the atrioventricular valves: study in the chick embryo. *Am J Anat* 1983;166:63–72.

59. Garcia-Pelaez I, Diaz-Gongora G, Arteaga Martinez M. Contribution of the superior atrioventricular cushion to the left ventricular infundibulum. Experimental study on the chick embryo. *Acta Anat* 1984;118:224–230.

60. Domenech Mateu JM. Desarrollo del corazon. In: Soler J, Bayes de Luna A, eds. *Cardiologia.* Barcelona: Editorial Doyma, 1986:3–13.

61. Rosenquist GC. Congenital mitral valve disease associated with coarctation of the aorta. A spectrum that includes parachute deformity of the mitral valve. *Circulation* 1974;49:985–993.

62. Becker AE, Becker MJ, Edwards JE. Pathologic spectrum of dysplasia of the tricuspid valve. *Arch Pathol* 1971;91:167–178.

63. Thiene G, Frescura C, Daliento L. The pathology of the congenitally malformed mitral valve. In: Marcelletti C, Anderson RH, Becker AE, Corno A, Di Carlo D, Mazzera E, eds. *Paediatric cardiology 6.* Edinburgh: Churchill Livingstone, 1986:225–239.

64. Bharati SD, Lev M. Congenital polyvalvular disease. *Circulation* 1973;47:575–586.

65. Greenfield WS. Double mitral valve. *Trans Pathol Soc Lond* 1876;27:128–129.

66. Bano-Rodrigo A, Van Praagh S, Trowitzsch E, Van Praagh R. Double-orifice mitral valve: a study of 27 postmortem cases with

developmental, diagnostic and surgical considerations. *Am J Cardiol* 1988;61:152–160.

67. Schraft WC Jr, Lisa JR. Duplication of the mitral valve. Case report and review of the literature. *Am Heart J* 1950;39:136–140.

68. Edwards JE, Burchell HB. Pathologic anatomy of mitral insufficiency. *Proc Staff Meet Mayo Clin Proc* 1958;33:497–509.

69. Rosenberg J, Roberts WC. Double orifice mitral valve. Study of the anomaly in two calves and a summary of the literature in humans. *Arch Pathol* 1968;86:77–80.

70. Di Segni E, Lew S, Shapira H, Kaplinsky E. Double mitral valve orifice. *Pediatr Cardiol* 1986;6:215–217.

71. Pignoni P, Carraro R, Nicolosi GL. Prolapse of atrioventricular valve leaflets in the setting of double orifice. *Int J Cardiol* 1988; 19:115–119.

72. Honnekeri ST, Tendolkar AG, Lokhandwala YY. Double-orifice mitral and tricuspid valves in association with Raghib complex. *Ann Thorac Surg* 1993;55:1001–1002.

73. Goldenberg N, Schifter D, Aron M, Shapiro RS, Krasnow N, Stein RA. Double orifice mitral and tricuspid valve. *Echocardiography* 1996;13:85–90.

74. Edwards JE. Differential diagnosis of mitral stenosis. A clinico-pathologic review of simulating conditions. *Lab Invest* 1954;3:89–115.

75. Actis-Dato A, Milocco I. Anomalous attachment of the mitral valve to the ventricular wall. *Am J Cardiol* 1966;17:278–281.

76. Ruschhaupt DG, Bharati S, Lev M. Mitral valve malformation of Ebstein type in absence of corrected transposition. *Am J Cardiol* 1976;38:109–112.

77. Anderson KR, Zuberbuhler JR, Anderson RH, Becker AE, Lie JT. Morphologic spectrum of Ebstein's anomaly of the heart. A review. *Mayo Clin Proc* 1979;54:174–180.

78. Leung M, Rigby ML, Anderson RH, Wyse RKH, Macartney FJ. Reversed offsetting of the septal attachments of the atrioventricular valves and Ebstein's malformation of the morphologically mitral valve. *Br Heart J* 1987;57:184–187.

79. Caruso G, Cifarelli A, Balducci G, Facilone F. Ebstein's malformation of the mitral valve in atrioventricular and ventriculoarterial concordance. *Pediatr Cardiol* 1987;8:209–210.

80. Dusmet M, Oberhaensli I, Cox JN. Ebstein's anomaly of the tricuspid and mitral valves in otherwise normal heart. *Br Heart J* 1987; 58:400–404.

81. Jacob JLB, Sobrinho SH, Lorga AM, et al. Anomalia de Ebstein da valva mitral: uma rarissima malformacao congenita do coracao: relato de caso. *Arq Bras Cardiol* 1989;53:283–285. Cited by Erickson LC, Cocalis MW. Ebstein's malformation of the mitral valve: association with aortic obstruction. *Pediatr Cardiol* 1995; 16:45–47.

82. Ferreira SMF, Ebaid M, Aiello VD. Ebstein's malformation of the tricuspid and mitral valves associated with hypoplasia of the ascending aorta. *Int J Cardiol* 1991;33:170–172.

83. Erickson LC, Cocalis MW. Ebstein's malformation of the mitral valve: association with aortic obstruction. *Pediatr Cardiol* 1995; 16:45–47.

84. Rosenquist GC. Overriding right atrioventricular valve in association with mitral atresia. *Am Heart J* 1974;87:26–32.

85. Moreno F, Quero M, Diaz LP. Mitral atresia with normal aortic valve. A study of eighteen cases and a review of the literature. *Circulation* 1976;53:1004–1010.

86. Rigby ML, Gibson DG, Joseph MC, et al. Recognition of imperforate atrioventricular valves by two dimensional echocardiography. *Br Heart J* 1982;47:329–336.

87. Layman TE, Edwards JE. Anomalous mitral arcade. A type of congenital mitral insufficiency. *Circulation* 1967;35:389–395.

88. Carpentier A, Branchini B, Cour JC, et al. Congenital malformations of the mitral valve in children. Pathology and surgical treatment. *J Thorac Cardiovasc Surg* 1976;72:854–866.

89. Castaneda AR, Anderson RC, Edwards JE. Congenital mitral stenosis resulting from anomalous arcade and obstructing papillary muscles. Report of correction by use of ball valve prothesis. *Am J Cardiol* 1969;24:237–240.

90. Frech RS, White RI Jr, Bessinger FB, Alplatz K. Anomalous mitral arcade with enlarged papillary muscles. Angiocardiographic study of two cases. *Radiology* 1972;103:633–636.

91. Macartney FJ, Brain HH, Ionescu MI, Deverrall PB, Scott O.

92. Schiebler GL, Edwards JE, Burchell HB, DuShane JW, Ongley PA, Wood EH. Congenital corrected transposition of the great vessels. A study of 33 cases. *Pediatrics* 1961;27[Suppl]:851–888.

93. Milo S, Ho SY, Macartney FJ, et al. Straddling and overridng atrioventricular valves: morphology and classification. *Am J Cardiol* 1979;44:1122–1134.

94. Read RC, Thal AP, Wendt VE. Symptomatic valvular myxomatous transformation (the floppy valve syndrome). A possible forme fruste of the Marfan syndrome. *Circulation* 1965;32:897–910.

95. Pomerance A. Ballooning deformity (mucoid degeneration) of atrioventricular valves. *Br Heart J* 1969;31:343–351.

96. Guthrie RB, Edwards JE. Pathology of the myxomatous mitral valve. *Minn Med* 1976;59:637–647.

97. Lucas RV Jr, Edwards JE. The floppy mitral valve. *Curr Probl Cardiol* 1982;7:1–48.

98. Roberts WC. Morphologic aspects of cardiac valve dysfunction. *Am Heart J* 1992;123:1610–1632.

99. Agozzino L, Falco A, De Vivo F, et al. Surgical pathology of the mitral valve: gross and histological study of 1288 surgically excised valves. *Int J Cardiol* 1992;37:79–89.

100. Trowitzsch E, Bano-Rodrigo A, Burger BM, Colan SD, Sanders SP. Two-dimensional echocardiograhic findings in double orifice mitral valve. *J Am Coll Cardiol* 1985;6:383–387.

101. Grenadier E, Sahn DJ, Valdes-Cruz LM, Allen HD, Oliveira Lima C, Goldberg SJ. Two-dimensional echo Doppler study of congenital disorders of the mitral valve. *Am Heart J* 1984;107:319–325.

102. Banerjee A, Kohl T, Silverman NH. Echocardiographic evaluation of congenital mitral valve anomalies in children. *Am J Cardiol* 1995;76:1284–1291.

103. Creech O, Ledbetter MK, Reemtsma K. Congenital insufficiency with a cleft in the posterior leaflet. *Circulation* 1962;25:390–394.

104. Di Segni E, Edwards JE. Cleft anterior leaflet of the mitral valve with intact septa. A study of twenty cases. *Am J Cardiol* 1983; 51:919–922.

105. Di Segni E, Bass JL, Lucas RV Jr, Einzig S. Isolated cleft mitral valve: a variety of congenital mitral regurgitation identified by two-dimensional echocardiography. *Am J Cardiol* 1983;51:927–931.

106. Hatle L, Angelsen B, Tromsdal A. Noninvasive assessment of atrioventricular pressure half-time by Doppler ultrasound. *Circulation* 1979;60:1096–1104.

107. Schachne A, Varsano I, Levy MJ. The parachute mitral valve complex. Case report and review of the literature. *J Thorac Cardiovasc Surg* 1975;70:451–457.

108. Saphir O, Lev M. The tetralogy of Eisenmenger. *Am Heart J* 1941; 21:31–46.

109. Dixon ASJ. Juxtaposition of the atrial appendages. Two cases of an unusual congenital cardiac deformity. *Br Heart J* 1954;16:153–164.

110. Edwards JE. Congenital malformations of the heart and great vessels. D. Malformation of cardiac chambers and myocardium. In: Gould SE, ed. *Pathology of the heart and blood vessels*. 3rd ed. Springfield, IL: Charles C. Thomas Publisher, 1968:352.

111. Melhuish BPP, Van Praagh R. Juxtaposition of the atrial appendages. A sign of severe cyanotic congenital heart disease. *Br Heart J* 1968;30:269–284.

112. Becker AE, Becker MJ. Juxtaposition of atrial appendages associated with normally oriented ventricles and great arteries. *Circulation* 1970;41:685–688.

113. Wagner HR, Alday LE, Vlad P. Juxtaposition of the atrial appendages: a report of six necropsied cases. *Circulation* 1970;42:157–163.

114. Charuzi Y, Spanos PK, Amplatz K, Edwards JE. Juxtaposition of the atrial appendages. *Circulation* 1973;47:620–627.

115. Deutsch V, Shem-Tov A, Yahini JH, Neufeld HN. Juxtaposition of atrial appendages: angiocardiographic observations. *Am J Cardiol* 1974;34:240–244.

116. Mathew R, Replogle R, Thilenius OG, Arcilla RA. Right juxtaposition of the atrial appendages. *Chest* 1975;67:483–486.

117. Anderson RH, Smith A, Wilkinson JL. Right juxtaposition of the auricular appendages. *Eur J Cardiol* 1976;4:495–503.

118. Wenner O. Beitrage zur lehre der herzmissbildungen. *Virchows Arch* 1909;196:127–168. Cited by Mathew R, Replogle R, Thilenius O, Arcilla RA. Right juxtaposition of the atrial appendages. *Chest* 1975;67:483–486.

PART V

Anomalies of Ventricular Looping

CHAPTER 14

Isolated Ventricular Inversion

Lilliam M. Valdes-Cruz and Raul O. Cayre

Isolated ventricular inversion is an extremely rare cardiac malformation characterized by atrioventricular discordance with ventriculoarterial concordance (1). It was originally described by Ratner et al. in 1921 (2). Since then, several cases have been reported with situs solitus and situs inversus, and in the presence of levocardia or dextrocardia (3–17).

EMBRYOLOGIC CONSIDERATIONS

Atrioventricular discordance with ventriculoarterial concordance implies the presence of two atria, one morphologically right and one morphologically left; two ventricles, one morphologically right and one morphologically left; and two great arteries, each connected to their usual corresponding ventricle. Therefore, instances with situs ambiguus, univentricular atrioventricular connection, criss-cross atrioventricular discordance, superoinferior ventricles, double outlet right or left ventricles, or single outlet ventricle are not considered in this chapter.

In this malformation, the anatomic right atrium is connected with an anatomic left ventricle from which emerges the aorta. The anatomic left atrium is connected with the anatomic right ventricle, which gives rise to the pulmonary artery (Fig. 14-1). It is similar to corrected transposition of the great arteries in that there is atrioventricular discordance, but in this case there is ventriculoarterial concordance, so the great arteries are normally related (cf. Fig. 14-1A and Fig. 15-1A).

The morphogenesis of this lesion should include consideration of the situs, the bulboventricular looping, and the conal, truncal, and aortopulmonary septation.

Visceroatrial Situs and Bulboventricular Looping

The situs can be solitus or inversus, and the bulboventricular looping can be D or L (18). Since there is atrio-ventricular discordance, in situs solitus the anatomic right atrium is located to the right and is connected to a morphologic left ventricle located to the right (L bulboventricular looping) (Fig. 14-1A). The anatomic left atrium is located to the left and is connected with the morphologic right ventricle located to the left. In cases of situs inversus, there is a D bulboventricular loop with the heart in mirror image of that seen in situs solitus (Fig. 14-1B).

Conal Septation

In the majority of cases, the conal septation is similar to that found in corrected transposition. The conal crests develop abnormally, so there is a dextroventral and a sinistrodorsal conal crest (Fig. 14-2A), which upon fusion give origin to a conal septum that is abnormally directed from left to right and posterior to anterior. The single conus, which is originally connected to the primordium of the trabecular portion of the right ventricle, located to the left, is divided into an anterolateral and a posteromedial conus by the conal septum (Fig. 14-2A). The anterolateral conus remains connected to the morphologic right ventricle located to the left (left-sided ventricle), and the posteromedial conus is incorporated into the anatomic left ventricle located to the right (right-sided ventricle) (Fig. 14-2A). Cases with situs inversus are in mirror image to those in situs solitus (Fig. 14-2B).

Truncal Septation

Truncal swellings appear in the caudal end of the truncus in a position similar to that found in the normal heart—i.e., one dextrosuperior and one sinistroinferior (Fig. 14-2A). The intercalated truncal swellings also appear in the right and the left sides of the truncus, respectively. The dextrosuperior and sinistroinferior truncal swellings fuse to form the truncal septum, which is di-

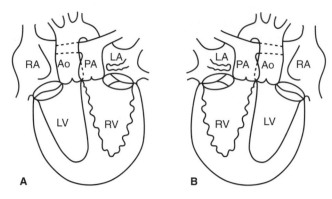

FIG. 14-1. Schematic drawings of hearts with isolated ventricular inversion. **A:** Situs solitus and L bulboventricular loop. **B:** Situs inversus and D bulboventricular loop. *RA,* right atrium; *LA,* left atrium; *RV,* right ventricle; *LV,* left ventricle; *Ao,* aorta; *PA,* pulmonary artery.

rected from left to right and posterior to anterior (Fig. 14-2A). They also give rise to the posterior right and left pulmonary valve leaflets, and to the anterior right and left aortic leaflets (Fig. 14-2A). The right intercalated swelling gives rise to the posterior noncoronary aortic cusp and

the left intercalated swelling to the anterior pulmonary leaflet. In situs inversus, the relationships are in mirror image (Fig. 14-2B).

Aortopulmonary Septation

The aortopulmonary septum develops normally, being directed at its cephalic end from right to left and from posterior to anterior (Fig. 14-2A) and at its caudal end from left to right and from posterior to anterior. This determines that the aorta will be connected with the posteromedial conus and therefore to the morphologic left ventricle located to the right, whereas the pulmonary artery will be connected with the anterolateral infundibulum and consequently to the morphologic right ventricle located to the left (Fig. 14-2A). Situs inversus is in mirror image (Fig. 14-2B).

There have been cases reported with different spatial relationships of the great arteries (6,7,19). In the cases with situs inversus reported by Clarkson et al. (7) and by Espino-Vela et al. (6), the aortopulmonary septum, the truncal septum, and the conal septum all had an abnormal

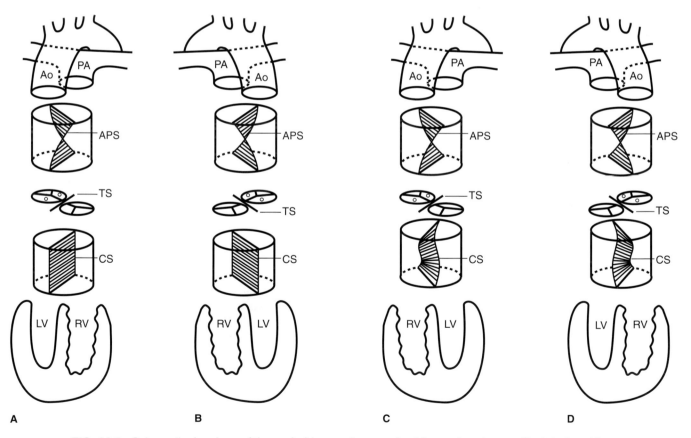

FIG. 14-2. Schematic drawings of the probable morphogenesis of the various types of isolated ventricular inversion. **A:** Situs solitus and L loop. **B:** Situs inversus and D loop. **C:** Cases reported by Clarkson et al. (7) and by Espino-Vela et al. (6) with situs inversus and D loop. **D:** Case reported by Pasquini et al. (19) with situs solitus and L loop. See text for details. *Ao,* aorta; *PA,* pulmonary artery; *RV,* right ventricle; *LV,* left ventricle; *CS,* conal septum; *TS,* truncal septum; *APS,* aortopulmonary septum.

position for situs inversus (cf. Figs. 14-2B,C). In these cases at the cephalic end, the aortopulmonary septum was directed from right to left and posterior to anterior, the truncal septum was directed from left to right and posterior to anterior, and the aortic valve was posterior and to the right of the pulmonary valve, which was anterior and to the left (Fig. 14-2C). The dextrosuperior truncal swelling was in continuity with the sinistroventral conal crest and the sinistroinferior truncal swelling with the dextrodorsal conal crest (Fig. 14-2C). This resulted in the great arteries having a spatial position similar to that seen in the normal heart but not corresponding to what should be found in situs inversus. In the case reported by Pasquini et al. (19) as situs solitus with "inverted normally related great arteries," the pulmonary artery was anterior and rightward with respect to the aorta. The morphogenesis of this case could be that the aortopulmonary septum in its cephalic end does not have the spatial position corresponding to situs solitus in that it is directed from left to right and from posterior to anterior (cf. Figs. 14-2A,D). This septum would not have the normal complete spiral; rather, it would be semispiral and in continuity with the truncal septum, which also would not have the normal orientation for situs solitus in that it would be directed from right to left and posterior to anterior (Fig. 14-2D). In the caudal end of the truncus, there would be a dextroinferior truncal swelling, which would be continuous with an abnormally positioned sinistrodorsal conal crest, whereas the sinistrosuperior truncal swelling would be in continuity with a dextroventral conal crest (Fig. 14-2D). This case would be mirror image to the other two described previously (6,7).

ANATOMIC AND ECHOCARDIOGRAPHIC CONSIDERATIONS

This malformation has been called by names that have created confusion, such as mixed levocardia with ventricular inversion (3), isolated ventricular inversion (4,10,11), ventricular inversion without transposition of the great arteries (6,13), isolated atrial inversion (7), atrioventricular discordance with ventriculoarterial concordance (1,14,17,18), isolated atrioventricular discordance (15,16), ventricular inversion with normally related great vessels (12), isolated atrial noninversion (20), or ventricular inversion with inverted normally related great arteries in situs solitus (20). We have used isolated ventricular inversion (4,10,11) because this is the fundamental alteration, and also atrioventricular discordance with ventriculoarterial concordance (1,14,17,18) because it allows definition and segmental analysis of this malformation.

Physiologically, venous blood returns to the morphologic right atrium and flows through a mitral valve to a morphologic left ventricle, which is connected to the aorta (Fig. 14-1). The pulmonary venous blood returns to a left atrium and flows through a tricuspid valve to a morphologic right ventricle, which is connected to the pulmonary artery. Consequently, the circulations are in parallel, and the physiology is similar to that in complete transposition of the great arteries.

The echocardiographic study of isolated ventricular inversion should include definition of (a) visceroatrial situs; (b) atrioventricular discordance; (c) ventriculoarterial concordance; (d) the spatial relationship of the great vessels; (e) origin and distribution of the coronary arteries; (f) associated anomalies; and (g) intra- and postoperative follow-up. The first case of an echocardiographic diagnosis of isolated ventricular inversion was described by Snider et al. in 1984 (21).

Visceroatrial Situs and Atrioventricular Discordance

The anatomic characteristics and echocardiographic determination of visceroatrial situs and atrioventricular connection are discussed in depth in Chapters 2 and 4. The echocardiographic diagnosis of atrioventricular discordance is addressed specifically in Chapter 15. The reader is referred to those chapters for details.

Briefly, the four-chamber views are most suitable for the demonstration of atrioventricular discordance. In the presence of situs solitus, the anatomic left ventricle is located to the right and receives right atrial blood through its mitral valve, which is inserted superiorly. The anatomic right ventricle is seen to the left, connected to the left atrium (Echo. 14-1).

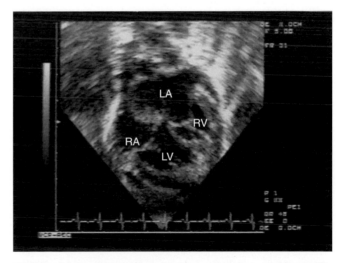

ECHO. 14-1. Apical four-chamber view in a patient with isolated ventricular inversion. Note that the morphologic left ventricle is located to the right and the morphologic right ventricle to the left (atrioventricular discordance). *RA*, right atrium; *LV*, left ventricle; *LA*, left atrium; *RV*, right ventricle. *(Echocardiogram courtesy of Dr. Mario Cazzaniga, Pediatric Cardiology Service, Hospital Ramon y Cajal, Madrid, Spain.)*

Ventriculoarterial Concordance

In contrast to corrected transposition, in isolated ventricular inversion there is concordance between the ventricular and the arterial connection. The aorta emerges from the morphologic left ventricle and the pulmonary artery from the morphologic right ventricle (Fig. 14-1). The ventricles are located spatially strictly side by side (11,19), whereas in corrected transposition they have a slightly more anteroposterior relationship.

The aorta emerges from a posterior rightward infundibulum and is in fibrous continuity with the septal leaflet of the mitral valve (mitral-aortic continuity). The pulmonary artery emerges from a totally muscular anterior leftward infundibulum and is separated from the tricuspid valve by the muscular ventriculoinfundibular fold (pulmonary-tricuspid discontinuity). However, Pasquini et al. (19) have described a case of isolated ventricular inversion in which there was aortic-mitral discontinuity and pulmonary-tricuspid continuity.

Echocardiographically, the ventriculoarterial concordance can be demonstrated from the apical and subcostal views. The transducer should be tilted superiorly towards the outflow tracts of both ventricles. This permits demonstration of the aorta emerging from the infundibulum of the morphologic left ventricle (located to the right) and the fibrous continuity between the aorta and the septal portion of the anterior leaflet of the mitral valve (Echo. 14-2). With further superior and anterior angulation, the pulmonary artery can be seen emerging from the anterior infundibulum of the morphologic right ventricle (located to the left) and to be discontinuous with the tricuspid

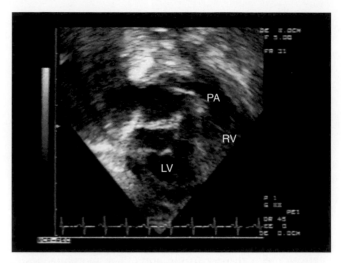

ECHO. 14-3. Apical view tilted superiorly to demonstrate the pulmonary artery emerging from the right ventricular outflow tract. Note the bifurcation of the pulmonary artery into right and left branches. *LV,* left ventricle; *RV,* right ventricle; *PA,* pulmonary artery. *(Echocardiogram courtesy of Dr. Mario Cazzaniga, Pediatric Cardiology Service, Hospital Ramon y Cajal, Madrid, Spain.)*

valve (Echo. 14-3). From the subcostal window, the same findings can be confirmed. A standard parasternal long-axis view is difficult to obtain since the ventricles are side by side, but it can be modified somewhat to visualize the ventricles and their respective great vessels and to serve as an adjunctive view to those described above. The parasternal and subcostal short-axis views can help identify the anatomy and spatial location of the ventricles and further establish the ventriculoarterial connection by sweeping the transducer from apex to base (Echos. 14-4, 14-5).

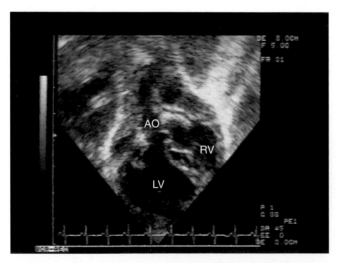

ECHO. 14-2. Apical view tilted superiorly to visualize the aorta emerging from the left ventricular outflow tract (ventriculoarterial concordance). Note the right coronary artery, which serves to identify the aorta. *LV,* left ventricle; *AO,* aorta; *RV,* right ventricle. *(Echocardiogram courtesy of Dr. Mario Cazzaniga, Pediatric Cardiology Service, Hospital Ramon y Cajal, Madrid, Spain.)*

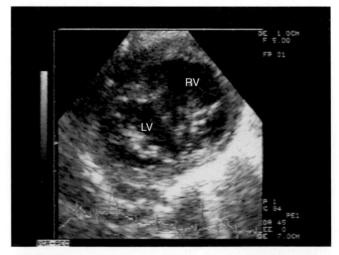

ECHO. 14-4. Parasternal short-axis view showing the anatomy and spatial location of the right and left ventricles. *LV,* left ventricle; *RV,* right ventricle. *(Echocardiogram courtesy of Dr. Mario Cazzaniga, Pediatric Cardiology Service, Hospital Ramon y Cajal, Madrid, Spain.)*

Color Doppler mapping can help identify the direction of blood flow and confirm the relationships defined with two-dimensional imaging.

Spatial Relationship of the Great Vessels

In the majority of cases with situs solitus, the aorta is posterior and to the right and the pulmonary artery anterior and to the left (Fig. 14-3) (Echo. 14-5). This can be best defined from the parasternal short-axis plane at the level of the semilunar valves, which demonstrates the normal great vessel relationship. In situs inversus, the relationship is in mirror image.

Origin and Distribution of the Coronary Arteries

The coronary arteries originate from the cusps of the aorta facing the pulmonary artery; their distribution corresponds to that seen in atrioventricular discordance and is that which is appropriate to the corresponding ventricle (4,22–24). The right-sided coronary artery (3) originates from the right anterior aortic cusp and divides into the anterior descending and circumflex (anatomically a left coronary artery), whereas the left-sided coronary artery (3) originates from the left anterior aortic cusp and follows the atrioventricular sulcus, frequently giving rise to the posterior descending (anatomically a right coronary artery) (Fig. 14-3A). In situs inversus, the origin and distribution is similar to that found in the normal heart; i.e., the right-sided coronary artery is an anatomic right coronary, whereas the left-sided coronary artery is an anatomic left coronary artery (Fig. 14-3B). The origin

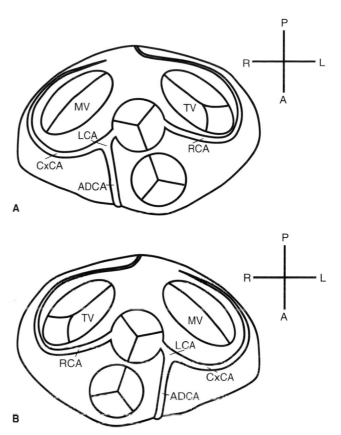

FIG. 14-3. Schematic drawing showing the origin and distribution of the coronary arteries in isolated ventricular inversion. See text for details. **A:** Situs solitus and L loop. **B:** Situs inversus and D loop. *TV*, tricuspid valve; *MV*, mitral valve; *RCA*, right coronary artery; *LCA*, left coronary artery; *ADCA*, anterior descending coronary artery; *CxCA*, circumflex coronary artery; *R*, right; *l*, left; *A*, anterior; *P*, posterior.

and distribution of the coronary arteries are best evaluated from a parasternal short axis view with the transducer positioned either slightly higher or lower than usual in order to see their branching.

Associated Anomalies

The most frequently found associated anomaly is a ventricular septal defect, which can be subaortic (4,11,19,21,23) and can be associated with one or several additional muscular defect(s) (4,11,25). The echocardiographic demonstration of the ventricular septal defect(s) is performed from the parasternal short-axis view and the apical and subcostal four-chamber and short-axis views. The subaortic defects can be seen immediately below the aortic valve and covered by the septal leaflet of the mitral valve. Color Doppler would demonstrate flow from the left ventricle (right-sided) to the right ventricle (left-sided). Use of color Doppler flow mapping can also aid in the identification of multiple defects, particularly of the muscular septum. The velocity recorded across the

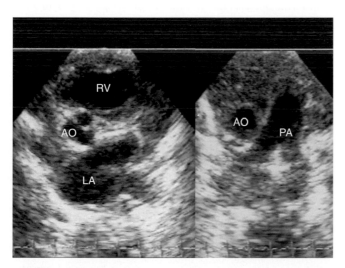

ECHO. 14-5. Parasternal short-axis views at the level of the great vessels demonstrating the normal spatial position of the aorta and pulmonary artery. *RV*, right ventricle; *AO*, aorta; *LA*, left atrium; *PA*, pulmonary artery. *(Echocardiogram courtesy of Dr. Mario Cazzaniga, Pediatric Cardiology Service, Hospital Ramon y Cajal, Madrid, Spain.)*

septal defect with continuous wave Doppler can serve to calculate the gradient between both ventricles and therefore estimate the pulmonary artery pressure in the absence of pulmonic stenosis.

Other associated anomalies that have been reported are ostium secundum atrial septal defects (6,19), patent ductus arteriosus (5,8,11), pulmonic stenosis (3,6), coarctation of the aorta (3,4), hypoplasia of the tricuspid valve (11), and right ventricular hypoplasia (11).

INTRAOPERATIVE AND POSTOPERATIVE EVALUATION

The objective of the surgical repair of this defect is to correct the transposition physiology and any associated anomalies. Since the morphologic left ventricle is the systemic ventricle in this case, the operation usually consists of an atrial switch of the Mustard or Senning type (7,14,23–27).

Pre-bypass, the transesophageal study should establish the ventricular size and function, typically from the transgastric short-axis view (see Fig. 4-27A). From the transverse four-chamber view (see Fig. 4-28A), the atrioventricular discordance would be seen clearly as well as any ventricular septal defect. Also from this view the anatomy and function of the atrioventricular valves can be assessed. The longitudinal views would provide an alternate site to examine the atrioventricular valves (see Figs. 4-28C,D) and provide a view of the outflow of the ventricles and any outlet ventricular defects and possible obstruction (see Figs. 4-29A,D–F). It is important to remember that certain parts of the ventricular septum are difficult to examine from the transesophageal approach, most importantly the apical and outlet muscular portions.

Post-bypass, the objectives would be to reassess the ventricular size and function as in the pre-bypass study. In addition, specific attention should be directed toward detecting any residual ventricular or atrial shunts that can be accomplished from the transverse four-chamber and the atrial views (see Fig. 4-30). If an atrial switch operation has been performed, the systemic and pulmonary venous baffles should be examined for leaks and for obstruction. This is best accomplished from the transverse four-chamber views and from the longitudinal views of the inflows and the atria.

The late postoperative follow-up in these patients would be directed towards the function of the baffles, assuming no significant residual ventricular shunts or outflow tract stenoses. This would specifically include any baffle obstruction that may develop with time. The baffles are best evaluated from the apical and subcostal four-chamber views with the aid of color Doppler flow mapping. The velocities of the venous connections, both systemic and pulmonary, should be recorded with spectral Doppler throughout their length to permit accurate diagnosis of any obstruction.

Further details on the immediate and late postoperative assessment of the atrial switch procedure are discussed in Chapter 24.

REFERENCES

1. Kirklin JW, Pacifico AD, Bargeron LM Jr, Soto B. Cardiac repair in anatomically corrected malposition of the great arteries. *Circulation* 1973;48:153–159.
2. Ratner B, Abbott ME, Beattie WW. Rare cardiac anomaly. Cor triloculare biventriculare in mirror-picture dextrocardia with persistent omphalo-mesenteric bay, right aortic arch and pulmonary artery forming descending aorta. *Am J Dis Child* 1921;22:508–515.
3. Lev M, Rowlatt UF. The pathologic anatomy of mixed levocardia. A review of thirteen cases of atrial or ventricular inversion with or without corrected transposition. *Am J Cardiol* 1961;8:216–263.
4. Van Praagh R, Van Praagh S. Isolated ventricular inversion. A consideration of the morphogenesis, definition and diagnosis of nontransposed and transposed great arteries. *Am J Cardiol* 1966;17:395–406.
5. Martinez Pico A, Munoz A. Inversion ventricular. Transposicion fisiologica de la circulacion y relacion aorto-pulmonar normal. *Bol Asoc Med P R* 1967;59:26–33.
6. Espino-Vela J, De la Cruz MV, Munoz-Castellanos L, Plaza L, Attie F. Ventricular inversion without transposition of the great vessels in situs inversus. *Br Heart J* 1970;32:292–303.
7. Clarkson PM, Brandt PWT, Barrat-Boyes BG, Neutze JM. "Isolated atrial inversion." Visceral situs solitus, visceroatrial discordance, discordant ventricular d loop without transposition, dextrocardia: diagnosis and surgical correction. *Am J Cardiol* 1972;29:877–881.
8. Perez Trevino C, Hurtado del Rio D, Holden AM. Inversion ventricular aislada. *Arch Inst Cardiol Mex* 1972;42:966–973.
9. Anderson RH, Arnold R, Jones RS. D-bulboventricular loop with l-transposition in situs inversus. *Circulation* 1972;46:173–179.
10. Anderson RH, Wilkinson JL. Isolated ventricular inversion with situs solitus. *Br Heart J* 1975;37:1202–1204.
11. Quero-Jimenez M, Raposo-Sonnenfeld I. Isolated ventricular inversion with situs solitus. *Br Heart J* 1975;37:293–304.
12. Tandon R, Moller JH, Edwards JE. Ventricular inversion associated with normally related great vessels. *Chest* 1975;67:98–100.
13. Dunkman WB, Perloff JK, Roberts WC. Ventricular inversion without transposition of the great arteries. *Am J Cardiol* 1977;39:226–231.
14. Leijala MA, Lincoln CR, Shinebourne EA, Nellen M. A rare congenital cardiac malformation with situs inversus and discordant atrioventricular and concordant ventriculoarterial connections: diagnosis and surgical treatment. *Am Heart J* 1981;101:355–356.
15. Calabro R, Marino B, Marsico F. A case of isolated atrioventricular discordance. *Br Heart J* 1982;47:400–403.
16. Ostermeyer J, Bircks W, Krian A, Sievers G, Hilgenberg F. Isolated atrioventricular discordance. Report of two surgical cases with isolated ventricular inversion. *J Thorac Cardiovasc Surg* 1983;86:926–929.
17. Tandon R, Heineman RP, Edwards JE. Ventricular inversion with normally connected great vessels in situs solitus (atrioventricular discordance with ventriculoarterial concordance). *Pediatr Cardiol* 1986;7:107–109.
18. Van Praagh R. The segmental approach to diagnosis in congenital heart disease. In: Bergsma D, ed. *Birth defects. Original article series.* Volume 8. Baltimore: Williams & Wilkins, 1972:4–23.
19. Pasquini L, Sanders SP, Parness I, et al. Echocardiographic and anatomic findings in atrioventricular discordance with ventriculoarterial concordance. *Am J Cardiol* 1988;62:1256–1262.
20. Van Praagh R. Segmental approach to diagnosis. In: Fyler DC, ed. *Nadas pediatric cardiology.* Philadelphia: Hanley & Belfus, 1992:27–35.
21. Snider AR, Enderlein MA, Teitel DF, Hirji M, Heymann MA. Isolated ventricular inversion: two-dimensional echocardiographic findings and a review of the literature. *Pediatr Cardiol* 1984;5:27–33.

22. Neufeld HN, Schneeweiss A. Isolated ventricular inversion. In: Neufeld HN, Schneeweiss A, eds. *Coronary artery disease in infants and children.* Philadelphia: Lea & Febiger, 1983:92–94.

23. Arciprete P, Macartney FJ, De Leval M, Stark J. Mustard's operation for patients with ventriculoarterial concordance. Report of two cases and a cautionary tale. *Br Heart J* 1985;53:443–450.

24. Kirklin JW, Barratt-Boyes BG. Atrioventricular discordant connection. In: Kirklin JW, Barratt-Boyes BG, eds. *Cardiac surgery. Morphology, diagnostic criteria, natural history, techniques, results and indications.* Volume 2. 2nd ed. New York: Churchill Livingstone, 1993:1535–1547.

25. Baudet EM, Hafez A, Choussat A, Roques X. Isolated ventricular inversion with situs solitus: successful surgical repair. *Ann Thorac Surg* 1986;41:91–94.

26. Mullins CE. Ventricular inversion. In: Garson A Jr, Bricker JT, McNamara DG, eds. *The science and practice of pediatric cardiology.* Volume II. Philadelphia: Lea & Febiger, 1990:1233–1245.

27. Freedom RM. Double-outlet left ventricle; isolated atrioventricular discordance; anatomically corrected malposition of the great arteries; and syndrome of juxtaposition of the atrial appendages. In: Freedom RM, Benson LN, Smallhorn JF, eds. *Neonatal heart disease.* London: Springer-Verlag, 1992:561–569.

CHAPTER 15

Congenitally Corrected Transposition of the Great Arteries

Lilliam M. Valdes-Cruz and Raul O. Cayre

Congenitally corrected transposition of the great arteries was first described in 1875 by von Rokitansky (1) in two infants who had the right ventricle and tricuspid valve located to the left and the left ventricle and mitral valve located to the right. The aorta emerged from the anatomic right ventricle (left-sided ventricle), and its location was anterior and to the left of the pulmonary artery. The pulmonary artery emerged from the anatomic left ventricle (right-sided ventricle), and its location was posterior and to the right of the aorta. The incidence of this condition is between 0.5% and 1.3% of cases of congenital heart disease (2–10).

EMBRYOLOGIC CONSIDERATIONS

Congenitally corrected transposition consists of atrioventricular discordance and ventriculoarterial discordance. Atrioventricular discordance implies the presence of a morphologic right atrium and a morphologic left atrium; therefore, it can exist in situs solitus or situs inversus but not in situs ambiguus. Atrioventricular discordance also implies the presence of a morphologic right ventricle and a morphologic left ventricle; therefore, it cannot occur with a univentricular atrioventricular connection. Ventriculoarterial discordance indicates that an anatomic left ventricle is connected to a pulmonary artery and that an anatomic right ventricle is connected to the aorta. The heart can be in levocardia, mesocardia, or dextrocardia. Cases of crisscross atrioventricular discordance are discussed in Chapter 16.

To understand the probable morphogenesis of this cardiac malformation, we should consider the following: visceroatrial situs, bulboventricular looping, conal septation, truncal septation, and aorticopulmonary septation.

Visceroatrial Situs

Situs solitus is present in 90% to 95% of cases of corrected transposition of the great arteries (11–13). The morphologic right atrium is located to the right and the morphologic left atrium to the left (Fig. 15-1A). In cases of situs inversus, the structures are positioned in a mirror image—that is, the anatomic right atrium is located to the left and the anatomic left atrium to the right (Fig. 15-1B).

Bulboventricular Looping

The primitive cardiac tube, which initially is straight in the preloop stage, acquires a shape that is convex to the right and concave to the left during the looping stage. This determines a D (dextro) loop (14), in which the primordium of the trabecular portion of the right ventricle is to the right and the primordium of the trabecular portion of the left ventricle is to the left (Fig. 15-2A). If L (levo) looping (14) occurs instead, the anatomic right ventricle will be to the left and the anatomic left ventricle will be to the right (Fig. 15-2B).

In corrected transposition with situs solitus, the looping is to the left (L loop) (5,15–20). This determines that the atrioventricular connection will be discordant—that is, the anatomic right atrium, located to the right, will be connected to the morphologic left ventricle, also located to the right, and the anatomic left atrium, located to the left, will be connected to the morphologic right ventricle, located to the left (Fig. 15-1A). In corrected transposition with visceroatrial situs inversus, the looping is to the right (D loop) (5), also resulting in atrioventricular discordance. The anatomic right atrium, located to the left, is connected to the morphologic left ventricle, located to the left, and the anatomic left atrium, located to the right, is connected to the morphologic right ventricle, located to the right (Fig. 15-1B) (Echo. 15-1).

Conal Septation

The conus or primordium of the infundibula of both ventricles appears in the loop stage (21); it forms the

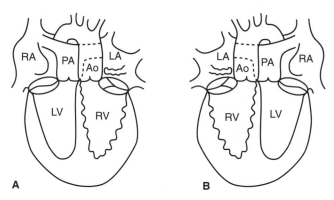

FIG. 15-1. Schematic drawings of hearts with congenitally corrected transposition of the great arteries. **A:** Situs solitus and L loop. **B:** Situs inversus and D loop. *RA*, right atrium; *LA*, left atrium; *RV*, right ventricle; *LV*, left ventricle; *Ao*, aorta; *PA*, pulmonary artery.

extreme cephalic portion of the heart (22) and is in continuity with the primordium of the trabeculated portion of the right ventricle caudally (Fig. 15-2). In the early postloop stage, the truncus appears and is in continuity with the conus caudally and with the aortic sac cephalically (21) (see Fig. 1-5C). At this stage, cardiac septation begins (22). The dextrodorsal and sinistroventral conal

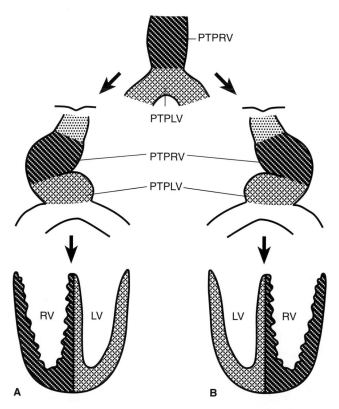

FIG. 15-2. Schematic representation of the spatial position of the ventricles according to the bulboventricular loop. **A:** D loop. **B:** L loop. *PTPRV*, primordium of the trabeculated portion of the right ventricle; *PTPLV*, primordium of the trabeculated portion of the left ventricle; *RV*, right ventricle; *LV*, left ventricle.

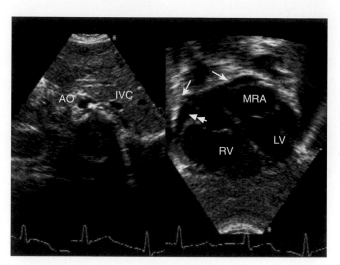

ECHO. 15-1. **Left:** Subcostal abdominal view demonstrating the position of the aorta (*to the right*) and inferior vena cava (*to the left*) in situs inversus. **Right:** Subcostal four-chamber view showing atrioventricular discordance in situs inversus with levocardia, implying a D loop. Note the left atrial appendage with its fingerlike appearance (*double arrows*), identifying the right-sided morphologic left atrium, and the pulmonary venous return (*single arrows*) to that atrium. *RV*, right ventricle; *MRA*, morphologic right atrium; *LV*, left ventricle.

crests appear within the conus and divide it into an anterolateral and a posteromedial conus (23) (see Figs. 1-12, 1-14A). Eventually, the anterolateral conus connects exclusively with the right ventricle and the posteromedial conus with the left ventricle (see Fig. 1-5D,E).

In corrected transposition with situs solitus, the conus is related with the primordium of the trabeculated portion of the right ventricle, which in this case is located to the left. The conal crests appear within the conus in an abnormal position—that is, in a dextroventral and sinistrodorsal orientation (16,24) (Fig. 15-3A). Upon fusion, the conal crests form the conal septum, which is positioned from posterior to anterior and from left to right (25) (Figs. 15-3B, 15-4A), thereby dividing the conus into an anterolateral and a posteromedial conus. The anterolateral conus is connected with the anatomic right ventricle, located to the left, and the posteromedial conus with the anatomic left ventricle, located to the right (Fig. 15-4A). In corrected transposition with situs inversus, the position of the conal crests and conal septum is a mirror image of that found in situs solitus (Figs. 15-3C, 15-4B).

Truncal Septation

The truncus appears in the early postloop stage, at the cephalic end of the heart in continuity with the aortic sac (21) (see Fig. 1-5C). Within its caudal end, the dextrosuperior and sinistroinferior truncal swellings as well as the right and left intercalated truncal swellings appear. These give rise to the aortic and pulmonary leaflets and to the truncal septum (see Fig. 1-14B).

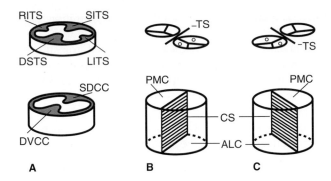

FIG. 15-3. Schematic drawings of conal and truncal septation in congenitally corrected transposition of the great arteries. **A:** Location of the conal crests and truncal swellings in hearts with situs solitus. **B:** Spatial position of the conal and truncal septa in hearts with situs solitus. **C:** Spatial position of the conal and truncal septa in hearts with situs inversus. *DVCC*, dextroventral conal crest; *SDCC*, sinistrodorsal conal crest; *DSTS*, dextrosuperior truncal swelling; *SITS*, sinistroinferior truncal swelling; *RITS*, right intercalated truncal swelling; *LITS*, left intercalated truncal swelling; *CS*, conal septum; *TS*, truncal septum; *ALC*, anterolateral conus; *PMC*, posteromedial conus.

In corrected transposition with situs solitus, the truncal swellings maintain a location similar to that in the normal heart and give rise to the posterior aortic leaflets and anterior pulmonary leaflets (Fig. 15-3A,B). The left intercalated swelling develops into the anterior aortic leaflet and the right intercalated swelling into the posterior pulmonary leaflet (Fig. 15-3A,B). Fusion of the dextrosuperior truncal swelling and the sinistroinferior truncal swelling give rise to the truncal septum, which has an orientation similar to that of the conal septum—that is,

from posterior to anterior and from left to right (Figs. 15-3B, 15-4A). In situs inversus, the position of these structures is a mirror image of that in situs solitus (Figs. 15-3C, 15-4B).

Aorticopulmonary Septation

The aorticopulmonary septum originates from cells that migrate from the neural crest (26) and divides the truncus into the ascending aorta and pulmonary trunk. At its cephalic end, it has a posterior-to-anterior and a right-to-left orientation (see Fig. 1-14C), whereas at its caudal end, its position is posterior to anterior and left to right (see Fig. 1-14B2). This spiral shape of the aorticopulmonary septum determines the normal spatial relation of the great arteries.

In hearts with corrected transposition in situs solitus, the direction of the aorticopulmonary septum at its cephalic end is posterior to anterior and left to right; this direction is maintained at its caudal extreme, where it becomes continuous with the truncal septum (Fig. 15-4A). This straight position of the aorticopulmonary septum, truncal septum, and conal septum (16) results in an aorta situated to the left and anteriorly with respect to the pulmonary artery and connected with the anatomic right ventricle located to the left. Similarly, the pulmonary artery, which is posterior and to the right of the aorta, connects with the anatomic left ventricle, located to the right (Fig. 15-4A). In cases with situs inversus, the orientation is a mirror image of that in situs solitus (Fig. 15-4B).

Allwork et al. (12) described two cases of corrected transposition with situs solitus in which the location of

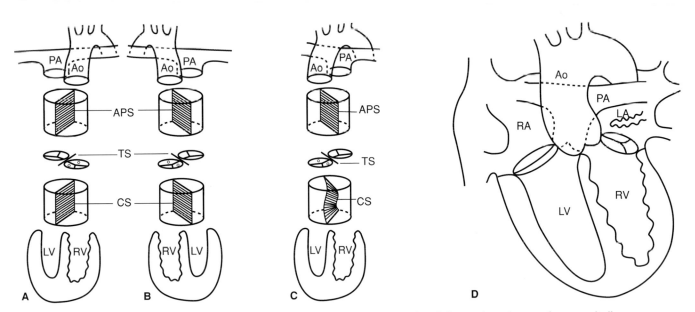

FIG. 15-4. Schematic drawings of the probable morphogenesis of the various types of congenitally corrected transposition of the great arteries. **A:** Situs solitus. **B:** Situs inversus. **C,D:** Case of Allwork et al. (12) with situs solitus, aorta to the right and anterior, and pulmonary artery to the left and posterior. *RV*, right ventricle; *LV*, left ventricle; *CS*, conal septum; *TS*, truncal septum; *APS*, aorticopulmonary septum; *Ao*, aorta; *PA*, pulmonary artery; *RA*, right atrium; *LA*, left atrium.

the aorta was anterior and to the right of the pulmonary artery (Fig. 15-4C,D). In these cases, the probable morphogenesis could be an anomalous development of the aorticopulmonary septum, truncal septum, and conal septum as well as an alteration in the spatial position of the ventricles. The aorticopulmonary and truncal septa would develop in a manner similar to that in complete transposition with an anterior and rightward aorta. The aorticopulmonary septum would be straight—that is, directed posteriorly to anteriorly and from right to left at its cephalic end, resulting in the ascending aorta and aortic valve occupying a rightward and anterior location with respect to the pulmonary trunk and pulmonary valve (Fig. 15-4C). The conal septum would develop abnormally and have a semispiral spatial disposition. Additionally, the ventricles would also have an abnormal spatial situation, with the morphologic right ventricle occupying an anterior and leftward location and the morphologic left ventricle a posterior and rightward one (Fig. 15-4D).

ANATOMIC AND ECHOCARDIOGRAPHIC CONSIDERATIONS

Corrected transposition of the great arteries has received various names in the literature: congenitally corrected transposition (5,10–13), mixed levocardia with corrected transposition (27), inverted transposition (28), L transposition (29,30), and atrioventricular discordance with ventriculoarterial discordance (6). The terms mixed levocardia with corrected transposition and inverted transposition should not be used because they are confusing. The term L transposition was used in reference to the anterior and leftward position of the aorta (29,30) that is usually seen in corrected transposition (Fig. 15-4A). This terminology, however, would not be valid in the presence of corrected transposition with situs solitus and an anterior and rightward aorta (12,31) (Fig. 15-4C,D), or in those cases with situs inversus in which the aorta is also anterior and to the right (Fig. 15-4B). Consequently, this term should be used with caution. We use the term atrioventricular discordance with ventriculoarterial discordance, which is applicable to all cases irrespective of the spatial position of the great arteries.

In this malformation, systemic venous return is into an anatomic right atrium, which is connected to the anatomic left ventricle and the pulmonary artery. The pulmonary venous return is into an anatomic left atrium, which is connected to the anatomic right ventricle and the aorta; therefore, the circulation is in series, not in parallel, as is found in complete transposition (Fig. 15-1). This justifies the terminology of congenitally corrected transposition of the great arteries (1). In the same manner, the segmental analysis approach denominates this malformation as atrioventricular and ventriculoarterial discordances (14,29) and adds descriptions of the spatial relation of the cardiac structures and of the type and mode in which they are connected

(32,33), thereby also providing a clear definition of the defect.

Echocardiographic studies in corrected transposition should define (a) visceroatrial situs, (b) atrioventricular discordance, (c) ventriculoarterial discordance, (d) spatial relation of the great arteries, (e) origin and distribution of the coronary arteries, (f) ventricular function, and (g) associated anomalies, and intraoperative and postoperative evaluations should be included.

Visceroatrial Situs

In corrected transposition, the anatomic characteristics of the atria are similar to those in the normal heart. The anatomic right atrium, which receives the blood flow from the systemic veins and coronary sinus, whether located to the right in situs solitus or to the left in situs inversus, has a broad base and a blunt edge. Its internal characteristics include the fossa ovalis, limbus of the fossa ovalis, crista terminalis, and pectinate muscles extending from the crista terminalis to the base of the atrial appendage. The anatomic left atrium receives the pulmonary venous return, whether it is located to the left in situs solitus or to the right in situs inversus. It also maintains its normal anatomic characteristics, having an appendage with a thin base and a fingerlike appearance and lacking pectinate muscles.

Situs can be determined echocardiographically from a short-axis subcostal abdominal view (34) (see Figs. 4-12, 4-13). In situs solitus, the aorta is to the left and the inferior vena cava is to the right of the spine. Rotating the transducer 90 degrees counterclockwise permits imaging from a long axis (see Figs. 4-14, 4-15). The long axis of the aorta is obtained by slight orientation of the transducer leftward until the characteristic systolic pulsations are detected and the origins of the hepatic and superior mesenteric arteries are identified (see Fig. 4-15A). Rightward orientation permits imaging of the long axis of the inferior vena cava with its characteristic venous pulsations. Tilting the transducer cephalically demonstrates the drainage of the right hepatic vein into the inferior vena cava and the caval drainage into the right atrium (see Fig. 4-15B). Also from this view, the drainage of the superior vena cava into the right atrium can be seen. Color and spectral Doppler interrogation facilitates identification of the flows into the heart and permits analysis of their direction and characteristics. In infants and occasionally in older children with easy subcostal windows, the abdominal and thoracic portions of the descending aorta as well as the aortic arch and the ascending aorta can be visualized with further cephalic and leftward angulation of the transducer from the long axis. Situs inversus is a mirror image of situs solitus.

The left atrial appendage is identified from a parasternal short-axis view, with the transducer angled superiorly and slightly to the left (see Fig. 4-7D). Pulmonary venous drainage can be confirmed with imaging and spectral and color Doppler interrogation from the parasternal long-axis, apical four-chamber, subcostal four-chamber, and suprasternal short-axis views. The right atrial appendage can be visualized from a parasternal long-axis view of the right ventricular inflow (see Fig. 4-5B) and from a high right parasternal sagittal view (see Figs. 4-24B, 4-25B).

Atrioventricular Discordance

Corrected transposition implies the presence of atrioventricular discordance. In patients with situs solitus, the anatomic right atrium is located to the right; it connects, via a bileaflet atrioventricular valve with characteristics similar to those of a mitral valve, to a ventricle that has the morphologic markers of a left ventricle but is located to the right. The anatomic left atrium is located to the left and connects, through a trileaflet atrioventricular valve similar to a tricuspid valve, to a morphologic right ventricle located to the left (Fig. 15-1A).

The anatomic left ventricle has the same characteristics as in the normal heart—namely fine trabeculations in its body and two papillary muscles, one anterolateral and one posteromedial. In corrected transposition, although at the level of the crux cordis posteriorly the interventricular septum is aligned with the atrial septum, anteriorly it deviates toward the left; the atrial septum, on the other hand, deviates toward the right, resulting in a malalignment between the atrial and ventricular septa (12,35,36) (Fig. 15-5). The resulting gap between the atrial and ventricular septa is closed by tissue from the membranous septum, which as a consequence is larger than in the normal heart (6,36), and by the left ventricular or subpulmonary outflow tract, which is wedged within this space or gap (6,36,37). The mitral valve, located on the right, is composed of a mural

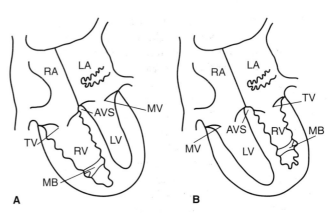

FIG. 15-6. Schematic drawings of the spatial position of the cardiac chambers and atrioventricular septum in hearts with situs solitus. **A:** Atrioventricular concordance (normal heart). Note that the atrioventricular septum separates the right atrium from the left ventricle. **B:** Atrioventricular discordance. Note that the atrioventricular septum separates the left atrium from the left ventricle. *RA*, right atrium; *LA*, left atrium; *RV*, right ventricle; *LV*, left ventricle; *TV*, tricuspid valve; *MV*, mitral valve; *AVS*, atrioventricular septum; *MB*, moderator band.

leaflet and a septal leaflet that is in fibrous continuity with the pulmonary valve and makes up one of the walls of the left (subpulmonary) ventricular outflow tract, which consequently is fibromuscular. The muscular portion of the left ventricular outflow tract is made up of the interventricular septum inferiorly, the free wall of the left ventricle, and the infundibular septum superiorly. The septal leaflet of the mitral valve and the membranous septum constitute its fibrous portion. Between the left ventricular free wall and the pulmonary outflow tract is a recess called the anterior recess or anterior diverticulum (12,38,39); this forms as a result of the wedged position of the pulmonary valve between the mitral and tricuspid valves, and it becomes more prominent with an increasingly wedged position of the pulmonary valve (6).

The morphologic right ventricle, located on the left, does not differ substantially from the right ventricle in the normal heart. The septomarginal trabecula, the moderator band, and the crista supraventricularis, which separates the tricuspid valve from the aorta, are present. This ventricle also has a conal or medial papillary muscle, an anterolateral papillary muscle, and one or more posterior papillary muscles. Its outflow tract is completely muscular, having as its walls the infundibular septum, the free wall of the ventricle, and the ventriculoinfundibular fold. The outflow tract is anterior and to the left and emerges in a straight direction parallel to the pulmonary outflow. The tricuspid valve has three leaflets: septal, anterior, and posterior. The septal leaflet insertion is inferior to that of the mitral valve because of the presence of an atrioventricular septum that is part of the larger membranous septum seen in corrected transposition (Fig. 15-6B). However, because of atrioventricular discordance in this malformation, the atrioventricular septum separates the anatomic left ventricle from the anatomic left atrium (Fig. 15-6B), whereas

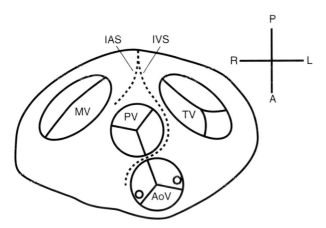

FIG. 15-5. Schematic drawing of the base of the heart showing the spatial orientation of the interatrial and interventricular septa in hearts with congenitally corrected transposition of the great arteries and situs solitus. *TV*, tricuspid valve; *MV*, mitral valve; *AoV*, aortic valve; *PV*, pulmonary valve; *IAS*, interatrial septum; *IVS*, interventricular septum. *R*, right; *L*, left; *A*, anterior; *P*, posterior.

in the normal heart the atrioventricular septum separates the left ventricle from the right atrium (Fig. 15-6A). As previously mentioned, the malalignment between the atrial and ventricular septa creates a gap occupied by a larger-than-normal membranous septum. It has two portions: a smaller atrioventricular portion separating the left ventricle from the left atrium and a larger interventricular portion separating the left ventricular outflow tract from the morphologic right ventricle (36). The relationship of the ventricles is more side by side than anteroposterior (the normal relationship); therefore, the ventricular septum is more perpendicular to the frontal plane.

The echocardiographic views that allow identification of atrioventricular discordance are the apical and subcostal four-chamber and the parasternal and subcostal short-axis views. From the four-chamber views, the anatomic characteristics of the ventricles and the systemic and pulmonary venous drainage are seen. The smoother-walled ventricle with a higher insertion of its atrioventricular valve (markers of an anatomic left ventricle) is located to the right and is connected to the atrium that receives the systemic venous return, also located to the right (in situs solitus) (Fig. 15-6B). A moderator band and the lower insertion of the septal leaflet of the atrioventricular valve, hallmarks of an anatomic right ventricle, are identified in the ventricle located to the left (Fig. 15-6B) (Echo. 15-2). From these same views, the pulmonary veins can be identified entering the left-sided atrium, thereby further confirming the atrioventricular discordance. The atrioventricular septum is seen to separate the anatomic left ventricle (located to the right) from the anatomic left atrium (located to the left) (Echo. 15-2). From the short-axis views, further morphologic characterization of the ventri-

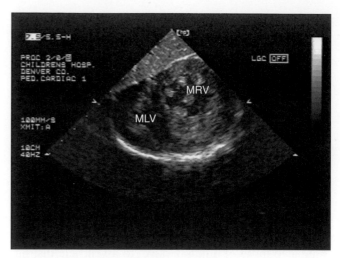

ECHO. 15-3. Short-axis views of the ventricles. The morphologic left ventricle is located to the right and the morphologic right ventricle to the left. *MLV*, morphologic left ventricle; *MRV*, morphologic right ventricle.

cles is possible (Echo. 15-3). The ventricle on the right is seen to have two papillary muscles, one anterolateral and one posteromedial, and its atrioventricular valve is bileaflet, with a "fish-mouth" appearance; the ventricle located on the left has a trileaflet atrioventricular valve. Because the ventricular septum is more perpendicular to the frontal plane, it is difficult to obtain a standard parasternal long-axis view.

Spectral and color Doppler interrogation of the systemic and pulmonary veins will confirm the connections and drainage to the right and left atria, respectively. The atrioventricular valves should also be interrogated from the four-chamber views to detect presence of high forward velocities, which are suggestive of restrictive inflows and/or regurgitation of either valve.

Ventriculoarterial Discordance

In corrected transposition, ventriculoarterial discordance is present in addition to atrioventricular discordance. In situs solitus and L loop, the pulmonary artery, identified echocardiographically by its immediate bifurcation into a right and left branch, emerges from an infundibulum located posteriorly and rightward and connected to an anatomic left ventricle on the right. The aorta, identified echocardiographically by its lack of bifurcation and the presence of coronary ostia, emerges from an infundibulum located anteriorly and leftward and connected to a morphologic right ventricle on the left (Echo. 15-4). In situs inversus with D loop, the relationships are in mirror image (Echo. 15-5).

The mitral valve is in fibrous continuity with the pulmonary artery. The mitral-pulmonary continuity can be seen from an apical or subcostal view by sweeping the transducer from a four-chamber position inferiorly near the crux cordis toward a superior or anterior position at the level

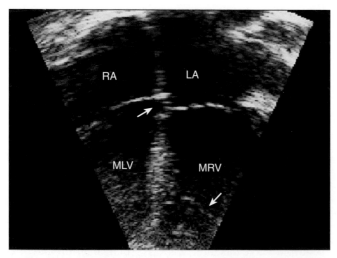

ECHO. 15-2. Apical four-chamber view demonstrating the presence of a moderator band (*lower arrow*) and the apical displacement of the insertion of the left-sided atrioventricular valve, distinguishing the left-sided ventricle as a morphologic right ventricle (atrioventricular discordance). The atrioventricular septum is indicated by the *upper arrow*. *RA*, right atrium; *MLV*, morphologic left ventricle; *LA*, left atrium; *MRV*, morphologic right ventricle.

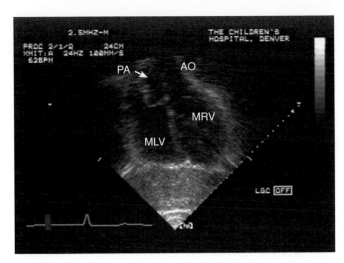

ECHO. 15-4. Subcostal view with the transducer aimed superiorly to demonstrate the ventriculoarterial connection. The pulmonary artery emerges from the morphologic left ventricle located to the right, and the aorta from the morphologic right ventricle located to the left (ventriculoarterial discordance). *PA*, pulmonary artery; *MLV*, morphologic left ventricle; *AO*, aorta; *MRV*, morphologic right ventricle.

of the great vessels (Echos. 15-4, 15-5). Inferiorly at the crux cordis, the atrial and ventricular septa are aligned, but they become malaligned anteriorly, and this gap is occupied by the subpulmonary infundibulum. The apical long-axis view of the morphologic left ventricle, obtained by angling the transducer superiorly and to the right, is also useful to demonstrate these anatomic findings (40).

The subcostal long axis view, obtained by sweeping the transducer from an inferior to a superior position with slight rotation rightward, manifests the discordant connec-

tion between the anatomic left ventricle (on the right) and the pulmonary artery and between the morphologic right ventricle (on the left) and the aorta. This view can also demonstrate the discontinuity between the tricuspid valve and aortic valve, separated by the ventriculoinfundibular fold. These outflow views also permit Doppler interrogation of the velocities of the pulmonary and systemic outflow tracts with spectral and color flow mapping to rule out obstruction (see Associated Anomalies).

Spatial Relation of the Great Arteries

In the vast majority of cases of corrected transposition of the great arteries with situs solitus, the aorta occupies an anterior and leftward position relative to the pulmonary artery, which is posterior and rightward (Fig. 15-1A). In a few cases with situs solitus, the aorta has been described as being anterior and to the right (12,31). In the presence of situs inversus, the aorta is usually anterior and to the right of the pulmonary artery (Fig. 15-1B). The spatial relationship of the great arteries is established from a parasternal short-axis view, which allows localization in both the anterior and posterior as well as right and left planes (Echos. 15-6, 15-7).

Origin and Distribution of the Coronary Arteries

In situs solitus, the aortic valve usually occupies an anterior and leftward position; its nonfacing sinus is anterior, and the facing cusps are posterior right and left, respectively (Fig. 15-7A). The pulmonic valve is located posteriorly and to the right; its facing cusps are anterior right and left, respectively, and its nonfacing sinus is posterior.

The coronary arteries originate from the facing sinuses of Valsalva, as in the normal heart (41), and their distribu-

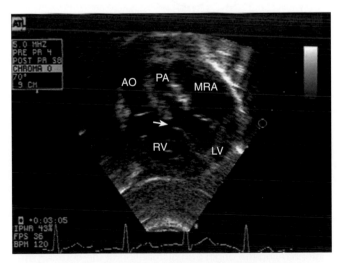

ECHO. 15-5. Subcostal view with the transducer aimed superiorly in the presence of situs inversus and D loop. The anterior mitral leaflet is in fibrous continuity with the pulmonary artery. Note the presence of a ventricular septal defect (*arrow*) and narrowing of the pulmonary outflow tract. *AO*, aorta; *RV*, morphologic right ventricle; *PA*, pulmonary artery; *MRA*, morphologic right atrium; *LV*, morphologic left ventricle.

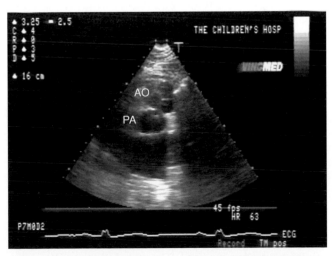

ECHO. 15-6. Parasternal short-axis view of the great vessels. The aorta is anterior and slightly to the left of the pulmonary artery. *AO*, aorta; *PA*, pulmonary artery.

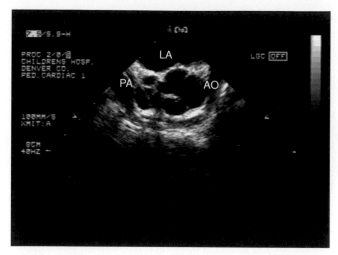

ECHO. 15-7. Transesophageal horizontal short-axis view of the great vessels. The great arteries are in a strictly side-by-side relationship, with the aorta to the left of the pulmonary artery. *PA*, pulmonary artery; *AO*, aorta; *LA*, left atrium.

tion follows the anatomy of their respective morphologic ventricles (11,12,39,41–45). Therefore, because of the presence of atrioventricular discordance, the distribution of the coronary arteries can be said to be a mirror image of that seen in the normal heart (Fig. 15-7A).

To define the origin and distribution of the coronary arteries in corrected transposition, we use the terms right-sided and left-sided coronary arteries, as proposed by Lev and Rowlatt (27). The right-sided coronary artery originates from the right posterior aortic cusp and has a distribution corresponding to that of an anatomic left coronary artery—namely, a short common trunk dividing into anterior descending and circumflex branches (Fig. 15-7A). The anterior descending branch is directed toward the front of the heart and courses along the interventricular sulcus, whereas the circumflex branch runs along the right-sided atrioventricular sulcus. The left-sided coronary artery has a morphology similar to that of the right coronary artery in the normal heart. It emerges from the posterior left aortic cusp and courses along the left-sided atrioventricular sulcus toward the crux cordis, where it usually gives rise to the posterior descending branch (Fig. 15-7A). In situs inversus with corrected transposition, the distribution of the coronary arteries is similar to that in the normal heart—that is, the right-sided coronary artery is anatomically a right coronary artery and the left-sided coronary artery is anatomically a left coronary artery (11,12) (Fig. 15-7B). The echocardiographic view that permits definition of the origin and proximal distribution of the coronary arteries is the parasternal short-axis view, obtained from a somewhat lower transducer position but aimed superiorly at the level of the valve leaflets.

Anomalies in origin and distribution of the coronary arteries have been reported. These include the following: origin of the anterior descending and circumflex branches from separate ostia of the right posterior cusp (12), ab-

sence of the circumflex branch (12), origin of the left-sided (anatomic right) coronary artery and anterior descending branch from two separate ostia of the posterior left aortic cusp (12), and single coronary artery emerging from the posterior right aortic cusp with division into three branches: circumflex, anterior descending, and anatomic right coronary (44,45).

Ventricular Function

The fact that the systemic ventricle in corrected transposition is a morphologic right ventricle poses the problem of whether it can adequately tolerate systemic resistance for a long time. Several reports in the literature imply that the morphologic right ventricle in corrected transposition is adapted to the systemic resistance and can function normally (46–48). Nonetheless, with longer survival following repair of associated anomalies, a deterioration of ventricular function can be seen (46), especially in the presence of tricuspid regurgitation, which usually progresses with time (49).

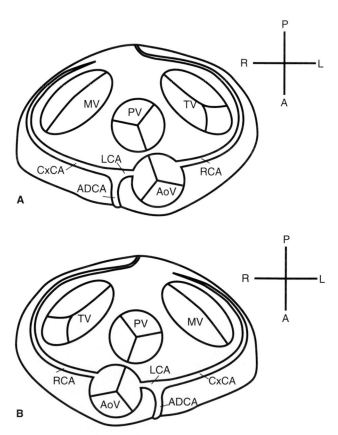

FIG. 15-7. Schematic drawings of the base of the heart demonstrating the origin and distribution of the coronary arteries in congenitally corrected transposition of the great arteries. See text for details. **A:** Situs solitus. **B:** Situs inversus. *TV*, tricuspid valve; *MV*, mitral valve. *AoV*, aortic valve; *PV*, pulmonic valve; *RCA*, right coronary artery; *LCA*, left coronary artery; *ADCA*, anterior descending coronary artery; *CxCA*, circumflex coronary artery. *A*, anterior; *P*, posterior; *R*, right; *L*, left.

Systolic ventricular function can be evaluated from the short-axis views and from a derived M mode. The diastolic function can be assessed from the pulsed-wave Doppler velocities of the atrioventricular inflows and from the systemic and pulmonary venous velocities, which are best recorded from a four-chamber apical view; the isovolumic relaxation time of the systemic ventricle can also be obtained from this position. Ideally, recording of these traces should be performed with a respirometer and completed within a few minutes to ensure measurements in inspiration and under a more or less stable hemodynamic condition.

Segmental wall motion should also be included in a complete evaluation of ventricular function. This should be assessed from the parasternal short-axis view, the apical four- and two-chamber views, and the apical long-axis view.

Associated Anomalies

Only 1% of identified cases of corrected transposition fail to have an associated anomaly (5,13,45). The most common ones, which according to Van Praagh (50) should be considered integral components of this malformation, are interventricular communications, obstruction of the pulmonary outflow tract, and anomalies of the tricuspid valve.

Interventricular Communications

These are the most common associated anomalies and are found in 60% to 87% of identified cases of corrected transposition of the great arteries (6,10,13,36,51). These can occur alone or in combination with other anomalies.

The most common type of ventricular septal defect is in the perimembranous septum, with posterior extension toward the inlet septum (6,39). The pulmonary valve in these cases overrides the ventricular septum and forms the roof of the defect, which is covered by the septal leaflet of the morphologic mitral valve. The anterosuperior border of the septal defect is composed of the infundibular or outlet septum, and the anteroinferior and inferior borders are formed by the trabecular septum and the free border of the inlet septum, respectively. The posterior border is fibrous and corresponds to the mitral-pulmonary-tricuspid continuity. The level of the aortic valve is higher than that of the pulmonary valve (52), and it is separated from the septal defect by the infundibular or outlet septum. Losekoot et al. (6) report that on rare occasions there can be a muscular subpulmonary infundibulum with mitral-pulmonary discontinuity caused by the presence of a muscular ventriculoinfundibular fold. In these cases, the ventricular septal defect is also subpulmonary, but its borders are totally muscular. Occasionally, the perimembranous defect can extend toward the trabecular portion or toward the outlet portion of the ventricular septum (39).

The juxtaarterial or doubly committed type of ventricular septal defect can occur rarely in corrected transposition (6,12,39,52). In these cases, the infundibular septum is hypoplastic or absent, and both semilunar valves are at the same level, overriding the septal defect. Even more rarely, a ventricular septal defect can be located in the middle or apical portion of the muscular septum.

Straddling of the atrioventricular valves is rare in corrected transposition (53), but some cases have been reported involving either the morphologic mitral or tricuspid valve (6,10,54–56). In straddling or overriding of the tricuspid valve, the ventricular septal defect has inlet extensions, whereas in mitral straddling or overriding, the defect extends anteriorly toward the outlet septum (6,10,56).

The echocardiographic apical and subcostal four-chamber views allow definition of the perimembranous ventricular septal defect immediately below the pulmonary valve and covered by the septal leaflet of the morphologic mitral valve. Sweeping the transducer from the crux cordis posteriorly slowly toward a more anterior plane demonstrates any extensions the defect may have toward the inlet or outlet septa (Echo. 15-5) as well as any morphologic tricuspid valve straddling or overriding that may exist. Color flow Doppler facilitates identification of the ventricular defect and demonstration of the direction of flow. From a modified long-axis parasternal view and from a subcostal four-chamber view, the velocity across the defect can be measured with spectral Doppler so that the interventricular gradient can be estimated. The parasternal short-axis view also may be useful to align the spectral Doppler sampling line for measurement of velocities; in addition, this view can demonstrate any trabecular extensions of the defect (57). The apical and subcostal four-chamber views with superior and anterior transducer angulation can illustrate a doubly committed defect with the aortic and pulmonary leaflets at the same level and overriding the septal defect.

Obstruction of the Pulmonary Outflow Tract

This associated anomaly has been observed in 30% to 57% of reported cases of corrected transposition of the great arteries (5,12,13,36,51,58,59), and in 80% of these, an associated ventricular septal defect is present (60).

Obstruction of the pulmonary outflow tract can be valvular, subvalvular, or mixed. Subvalvular obstruction can be caused by hypertrophy of the anterior ventricular wall (36), which can be dynamic when hypertrophy of the anterior portion of the trabecular septum is also present (6,61); by an aneurysm of the membranous septum (36,59); by accessory tissue of the mitral valve (58,61), tricuspid valve (36), or pulmonary valve (36); and by a subvalvar fibrous membrane or ring (6,61). Isolated stenosis of the pulmonic valve is rare but can occur in the presence of a trileaflet, bileaflet, or unicuspid pulmonic valve (6,39,45).

The apical and subcostal views of the morphologic left ventricle, obtained by angling the transducer toward the pulmonary outflow tract superiorly, permit imaging of the subpulmonary area and identification of any obstruction, whether subvalvar or valvar (40) (Echo. 15-5). Color Doppler imaging allows visualization of any velocity aliasing and aids in the positioning of the Doppler sampling line in continuous-wave and/or high pulsed repetition frequency (PRF) mode for actual gradient estimation.

Anomalies of the Morphologic Tricuspid Valve

Anomalies of the tricuspid valve (located to the left in the systemic ventricle) can be found in up to 90% of reported cases of corrected transposition (10,12), and they are the cause of the systemic atrioventricular valve regurgitation seen in 48% of cases (62). Valvar regurgitation can be absent in infancy and present in adulthood.

The tricuspid valve can be dysplastic (10,38,39,57,63) with thickened and shortened leaflets and chords (11,16,38,64) or exhibit downward displacement of the leaflet attachments, particularly of the septal and posterior leaflets, as in Ebstein's malformation (63–66); however, a true atrialized portion of the morphologic right ventricle is rarely present (6,57). The tricuspid valvar and subvalvar anatomy can be seen in detail from the four-chamber apical and subcostal views (Echo. 15-8; see color plate 46 following p. 364). Doppler recording of the forward velocities should be performed to determine the presence of possible restricted inflows. More commonly, regurgitation of the tricuspid valve can be diagnosed, its severity estimated, and the direction of the regurgitant jet determined from spectral and color Doppler velocity recordings.

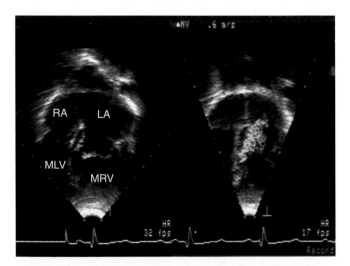

ECHO. 15-8. Apical four-chamber view of Ebstein's malformation of the left-sided tricuspid valve. The **right** panel shows tricuspid regurgitation originating from the inferiorly displaced septal and posterior leaflets. *RA*, right atrium; *MLV*, morphologic left ventricle; *LA*, left atrium; *MRV*, morphologic right ventricle.

Other Associated Anomalies

Other anomalies have been associated much less frequently with corrected transposition. Some that have been reported include atrial septal defect (45,62), patent ductus arteriosus (45,62), interrupted aortic arch (66), subaortic membrane (67), subaortic obstruction resulting from hypertrophy of the infundibular septum (68), supravalvar tricuspid ring (68), and coarctation of the aorta (68).

The specific echocardiographic approach to the detection of these defects is covered under their corresponding chapters. Nonetheless, it is important to note that the subcostal short-axis view and the subcostal left oblique view are particularly useful in the study of subaortic obstructions. Because of the anterior and leftward position of the aorta, it is sometimes difficult to image the transverse arch from a suprasternal long-axis view. In these instances, a high left parasternal projection from the left subclavicular position can be useful.

INTRAOPERATIVE AND POSTOPERATIVE EVALUATION

Surgical treatment in corrected transposition of the great arteries is directed toward correction of the associated anomalies.

The intraoperative transesophageal study performed before bypass should confirm the presence and location of any ventricular septal defect(s) and the relationship to the atrioventricular and semilunar valves. This is best accomplished from the transverse four-chamber view by withdrawing the transducer until the aortic valve is seen emerging from the left-sided morphologic right ventricle (see Figs. 4-28A,B; 4-29A). The relationship of the defect to the pulmonary valve can be best studied from the longitudinal views (see Fig. 4-29D–F).

The transverse four-chamber views should also permit visualization of the atrioventricular valves and demonstration by spectral and color flow Doppler of the presence and degree of regurgitation, particularly of the left-sided tricuspid valve. The presence of chordal abnormalities, valvular dysplasia, and/or Ebstein-like inferior displacement of the septal and posterior leaflets of the tricuspid valve would be evident. In these cases, and particularly if tricuspid regurgitation is severe, it is important to note the degree of displacement of the septal and posterior leaflets as well as the size and mobility of the anterosuperior leaflet to determine whether the valve can be repaired rather than replaced.

The outflow tracts can be examined from longitudinal views by withdrawing and rotating the transducer until the semilunar valves are evident (see Fig. 4-29D–F). The subpulmonary area should be studied carefully anatomically as well as with Doppler for the presence of obstruction, especially if a ventricular septal defect is present. This should be possible from the modified retrocardiac longitudinal views, especially with the use of a multiplane probe, and from the transgastric longitudinal view for better positioning of the Doppler sampling line (see Fig. 4-27D,E).

The intraoperative post-bypass study should begin with a thorough evaluation of ventricular function, both systolic and diastolic, and of the various wall segments from the transgastric short- and long-axis views and from the various transverse and longitudinal views.

The ventricular septum should be imaged for possible residual defects—from the transverse four-chamber view for the perimembranous, inlet, and trabecular septa and from the longitudinal views for the outlet septum.

Residual outflow tract obstruction is best ruled out from the longitudinal views, particularly in the subpulmonary area. Actual recordings of Doppler velocities are difficult to obtain from this approach and usually require interrogation from the longitudinal transgastric position.

Patients with ventricular septal defects and pulmonary outflow obstruction may require implantation of an external conduit between the morphologic left ventricle and the pulmonary artery (62,69,70). In these instances, an attempt should be made to visualize the conduit, record forward velocities throughout the conduit, and assess the presence and degree of conduit valve regurgitation.

The accurate post-bypass evaluation of the left-sided tricuspid valve is critical to the immediate and long-term outcome of these patients. If the tricuspid valve has undergone repair, it is important to record the inflow velocities with pulsed-wave Doppler to determine if any stenosis is present; this is best accomplished from a transverse four-chamber view. Further, the presence of residual regurgitation must be established and its degree estimated before it is decided whether the repair has been satisfactory or a replacement is necessary at this point. This analysis is best started from a transverse four-chamber view with color Doppler and continuous-wave Doppler. Once the direction of the jet is observed, it is necessary to turn to the longitudinal views, progressively if a multiplane probe is being used, to ensure that other regurgitant jets directed along different planes are not missed.

The late follow-up of these patients centers mostly around the functional status of the systemic morphologic right ventricle and the tricuspid valve. Serial studies should be performed on these patients as they grow into adulthood, even if initially the function is normal, as late dysfunction is possible (46,49).

REFERENCES

1. Von Rokitansky KF. *Die defecte der scheidewande des herzens.* Vienna: W Braumuller, 1875:83–86.
2. Abbott ME. *Atlas of congenital cardiac disease.* New York: American Heart Association, 1936.
3. Fontana RS, Edwards JE. Corrected transposition of the great vessels associated with various other cardiovascular malformations: age at death and distribution according to sex of patients in the pathologic material of the Mayo Clinic. In: Fontana RS, Edwards JE, eds. *Congenital cardiac disease: a review of 357 cases studied pathologically.* Philadelphia: WB Saunders, 1962:180–186.
4. Stanger P, Rudolph AM, Edwards JE. Cardiac malposition. An overview based on study of sixty-five necropsy specimens. *Circulation* 1977;56:159–172.
5. Kidd BSL. Congenitally corrected transposition of the great arteries. In: Keith JD, Rowe RD, Vlad P, eds. *Heart disease in infancy and childhood*, 3rd ed. New York: Macmillan, 1978:612–627.
6. Losekoot TG, Anderson RH, Becker AE, Danielson GK, Soto B. *Congenitally corrected transposition.* Edinburgh: Churchill Livingstone, 1983.
7. Freedom RM, Benson LN, Smallhorn JF. Congenitally corrected transposition of the great arteries. In: Moller JH, Neal WA, eds. *Fetal, neonatal, and infant cardiac disease.* Norwalk, CT: Appleton & Lange, 1990:555–570.
8. Mullins CE. Ventricular inversion. In: Garson A Jr, Bricker JT, McNamara DG, eds. *The science and practice of pediatric cardiology*, Vol II. Philadelphia: Lea & Febiger, 1990:1233–1245.
9. Fyler DC. Corrected transposition of the great arteries. In: Fyler DC, ed. *Nadas' pediatric cardiology.* Philadelphia: Hanley & Belfus, 1992:701–706.
10. Freedom RM, Benson LN. Congenitally corrected transposition of the great arteries. In Freedom RM, Benson LN, Smallhorn JF, eds. *Neonatal heart disease.* London: Springer-Verlag, 1992:523–542.
11. Schiebler GL, Edwards JE, Burchell HB, DuShane JW, Ongley PA, Wood EH. Congenital corrected transposition of the great vessels: a study of 33 cases. *Pediatrics* 1961;27:851–888.
12. Allwork SP, Bentall HH, Becker AE, et al. Congenitally corrected transposition of the great arteries: morphologic study of 32 cases. *Am J Cardiol* 1976;38:910–923.
13. Bjarke BB, Kidd BSL. Congenitally corrected transposition of the great arteries. *Acta Paediatr Scand* 1976;65:153–160.
14. Van Praagh R. The segmental approach to diagnosis in congenital heart disease. In: Bergsma D, ed. *Birth defects: original article series*, Vol 8. Baltimore: Williams & Wilkins, 1972:4–23.
15. Anderson RC, Lillehei CW, Lester RG. Corrected transposition of the great vessels of the heart. A review of 17 cases. *Pediatrics* 1957;20:626–646.
16. De la Cruz MV, Anselmi G, Cisneros F, Reinhold M, Portillo B, Espino-Vela J. An embryologic explanation for the corrected transposition of the great vessels: additional description of the main anatomic features of this malformation and its varieties. *Am Heart J* 1959;57:104–117.
17. De la Cruz MV, Polansky BJ, Navarro-Lopez F. The diagnosis of corrected transposition of the great vessels. *Br Heart J* 1962;24:483–497.
18. Anselmi G, Munoz S, Machado I, Blanco P, Espino-Vela J. Complex cardiovascular malformations associated with the corrected type of transposition of the great vessels. *Am Heart J* 1963;66:614–626.
19. Van Mierop LHS, Wiglesworth FW. Pathogenesis of transposition complexes. III. True transposition of the great vessels. *Am J Cardiol* 1963;12:233–239.
20. Grant RP. The morphogenesis of corrected transposition and other anomalies of cardiac polarity. *Circulation* 1964;29:71–83.
21. De la Cruz MV, Sanchez Gomez C, Arteaga M, Arguello C. Experimental study of the development of the truncus and the conus in the chick embryo. *J Anat* 1977;123:661–686.
22. De la Cruz MV, Cayre R. Desarrollo embriologico del corazon y de las grandes arterias. In: Sanchez PA, ed. *Cardiologia pediatrica, clinica y cirugia*, Vol 1. Barcelona: Editorial Salvat, 1986:10–18.
23. De la Cruz MV, Munoz Armas S, Munoz-Castellanos L. *Development of the chick heart.* Baltimore: The Johns Hopkins Press, 1971.
24. Barthel H. Teratologische entwicklungsreihe der missbildungen des arteriellen herzendes. In: Barthel H, ed. *Missbildungen Des Menschlichen Herzens.* Stuttgart: Georg Thieme Verlag, 1960:153–181.
25. Anderson RH, Wilkinson JL, Arnold R, Becker AE, Lubkiewicz K. Morphogenesis of bulboventricular malformations. II. Observations on malformed hearts. *Br Heart J* 1974;36:948–970.
26. Kirby ML, Gale TF, Stewart DE. Neural crest cells contribute to normal aorticopulmonary septation. *Science* 1983;220:1059–1061.
27. Lev M, Rowlatt UF. The pathologic anatomy of mixed levocardia. A review of thirteen cases of atrial or ventricular inversion with or without corrected transposition. *Am J Cardiol* 1961;8:216–263.
28. Lev M, Vass A. *Spitzer's architecture of normal and malformed hearts.* Springfield, IL: Charles C Thomas Publisher, 1951:72.
29. Van Praagh R, Van Praagh S, Vlad P, Keith JD. Anatomic types

of congenital dextrocardia. Diagnostic and embryologic implications. *Am J Cardiol* 1964;13:510–531

30. Paul MH, Van Praagh S, Van Praagh R. Transposition of the great arteries. In: Watson H, ed. *Paediatric cardiology*. London: Lloyd-Luke (Medical Books) Ltd, 1968:576–610.

31. Van Praagh R, Layton WM, Van Praagh S. The morphogenesis of normal and abnormal relationships between the great arteries and the ventricles: pathologic and experimental data. In: Van Praagh R, Takao A, eds. *Etiology and morphogenesis of congenital heart disease*. Mount Kisco, NY: Futura Publishing, 1980:271–316.

32. Shinebourne EA, Macartney FJ, Anderson RH. Sequential chamber localization—logical approach to diagnosis in congenital heart disease. *Br Heart J* 1976;38:327–340.

33. Tynan MJ, Becker AE, Macartney FJ, Quero-Jimenez M, Shinebourne EA, Anderson RH. Nomenclature and classification of congenital heart disease. *Br Heart J* 1979;41:544–553.

34. Huhta JC, Smallhorn JF, Macartney FJ. Two dimensional echocardiographic diagnosis of situs. *Br Heart J* 1982;48:97–108.

35. Anderson RH, Becker AE, Arnold R, Wilkinson JL. The conducting tissues in congenitally corrected transposition. *Circulation* 1974; 50:911–923.

36. Becker AE, Anderson RH. Conditions with discordant atrioventricular connexions—anatomy and conducting tissues. In: Anderson RH, Shinebourne EA, eds. *Paediatric cardiology 1977*. Edinburgh: Churchill Livingstone, 1978:184–197.

37. Anderson RH, Becker AE, Gerlis LM. The pulmonary outflow tract in classically corrected transposition. *J Thorac Cardiovasc Surg* 1975;69:747–757.

38. Casanova Gomez M, Cazzaniga Bullon M, Arciniegas E. Transposicion corregida de las grandes arterias. In: Sanchez PA, ed. *Cardiologia pediatrica, clinica y cirugia*, Vol 1. Barcelona: Editorial Salvat, 1986:547–560.

39. Soto B, Pacifico AD. Atrioventricular discordant connection. In: Soto B, Pacifico AD, eds. *Angiocardiography in congenital heart malformations*. Mount Kisco, NY: Futura Publishing, 1990:239–271.

40. Hagler DJ, Tajik AJ, Seward JB, Edwards WD, Mair DD, Ritter DG. Atrioventricular and ventriculoarterial discordance (corrected transposition of the great arteries). Wide-angle two-dimensional echocardiographic assessment of ventricular morphology. *Mayo Clin Proc* 1981;56:591–600.

41. Anderson RH, Becker AE. Coronary arterial patterns: a guide to the identification of congenital heart disease. In: Becker AE, Losekoot TG, Marcelleti C, eds. *Paediatric cardiology*, Vol 3. Edinburgh: Churchill Livingstone, 1979:251–262.

42. Shea PM, Lutz JF, Vieweg WVR, Corcoran FH, Van Praagh R, Hougen TJ. Selective coronary arteriography in congenitally corrected transposition of the great arteries. *Am J Cardiol* 1979;44:1201–1206.

43. Neufeld HN, Schneeweiss A. Corrected transposition of the great arteries. In: Neufeld HN, Schneeweiss A, eds. *Coronary artery disease in infants and children*. Philadelphia: Lea & Febiger, 1983:91–92.

44. Dabizzi RP, Barletta GA, Capriolo G, Baldrighi G, Baldrighi V. Coronary artery anatomy in corrected transposition of the great arteries. *J Am Coll Cardiol* 1988;12:486–491.

45. Kirklin JW, Barrat-Boyes BG. Congenitally corrected transposition of the great arteries. In: Kirklin JW, Barrat-Boyes BG, eds. *Cardiac surgery. Morphology, diagnostic criteria, natural history, techniques, results, and indications*, Vol 2, 2nd ed. New York: Churchill Livingstone, 1993:1511–1533.

46. Graham TP, Parrish MD, Boucek RJ, et al. Assessment of ventricular size and function in congenitally corrected transposition of the great arteries. *Am J Cardiol* 1983;51:244–251.

47. Benson LN, Burns R, Schwaiger M, et al. Radionuclide angiographic evaluation of ventricular function in isolated congenitally corrected transposition of the great arteries. *Am J Cardiol* 1986;58:319–324.

48. Dimas AP, Moodie DS, Sterba R, Gill CC. Long-term function of the morphologic right ventricle in adult patients with corrected transposition of the great arteries. *Am Heart J* 1989;118:526–530.

49. Lam D, Cheitlin MD, Popper RW, Szarnicki RJ. Rapid development of biventricular heart failure in corrected transposition of the great arteries during pregnancy. *Am Heart J* 1988;116:1111–1115.

50. Van Praagh R. What is congenitally corrected transposition? *New Engl J Med* 1970;282:1097–1098.

51. Egloff M, Rothlin J, Schneider G, et al. Congenitally corrected transposition of the great arteries: a clinical and surgical study. *J Thorac Cardiovasc Surg* 1980;28:228–232.

52. Okamura K, Konno S. Two types of ventricular septal defect in corrected transposition of the great arteries: reference to surgical approaches. *Am Heart J* 1973;85:483–489.

53. Quero Jimenez M, Perez Martinez VM, Maitre Azcarate MJ, Merino Batres G, Moreno Granados F. Exaggerated displacement of the atrioventricular canal towards the bulbus cordis (rightward displacement of the mitral valve). *Br Heart J* 1973;35:65–74.

54. Becker AE, Ho SY, Caruso G, Milo S, Anderson RH. Straddling right atrioventricular valves in atrioventricular discordance. *Circulation* 1980;61:1133–1141.

55. Kurosawa H, Imai Y, Becker AE. Congenitally corrected transposition with normally positioned atria, straddling mitral valve, and isolated posterior atrioventricular node and bundle. *J Thorac Cardiovasc Surg* 1990;99:312–313.

56. Milo S, Ho SY, Macartney FJ, et al. Straddling and overriding atrioventricular valves: morphology and classification. *Am J Cardiol* 1979;44:1122–1134.

57. Anderson RH, Becker AE, Lucchese FA, Meier MA, Rigby ML, Soto B. Congenitally corrected transposition. In: Anderson RH, Becker AE, Lucchese FA, Meier MA, Rigby ML, Soto B, eds. *Morphology of congenital heart disease. Angiocardiographic, echocardiographic and surgical correlates*. Kent, England: Castle House Publications Ltd, 1983:101–120.

58. Levy MJ, Lillehei CW, Elliot LP, Carey LS, Adams P Jr, Edwards JE. Accessory valvular tissue causing subpulmonary stenosis in corrected transposition of great vessels. *Circulation* 1963;27:494–502.

59. Krongrad E, Ellis K, Steeg CN, Bowman FO Jr, Malm JR, Gersony WM. Subpulmonary obstruction in congenitally corrected transposition of the great arteries due to ventricular membranous septal aneurysms. *Circulation* 1976;54:679–683.

60. Losekoot TG, Becker AE. Discordant atrioventricular connexion and congenitally corrected transposition. In: Anderson RH, Macartney FJ, Shinebourne EA, Tynan M, eds. *Paediatric Cardiology*, Vol 1. Edinburgh: Churchill Livingstone, 1987:867–887.

61. Edwards JE, Carey LS, Neufeld HN, Lester RG. Corrected transposition, ventricular septal defect and obstruction to pulmonary flow. In: Edwards JE, Carey LS, Neufeld HN, Lester RG, eds. *Congenital heart disease. Correlation of pathologic anatomy and angiocardiography*, Vol II. Philadelphia: WB Saunders, 1965:491–512.

62. Danielson GK, McGoon DC, Wallace RB, Fiddler GI, Maloney JD. Surgery of corrected transposition. In: Anderson RH, Shinebourne EA, eds. *Paediatric Cardiology 1977*. Edinburgh: Churchill Livingstone, 1978:224–230.

63. Becu LM, Swan HJC, DuShane JW, Edwards JE. Ebstein malformation of the left atrioventricular valve in corrected transposition of the great vessels with ventricular septal defect. *Proc Staff Meet Mayo Clin* 1955;30:483–490.

64. Jaffe RB. Systemic atrioventricular valve regurgitation in corrected transposition of the great vessels. Angiographic differentiation of operable and nonoperable valve deformities. *Am J Cardiol* 1976;37:395–402.

65. Van Mierop LHS, Alley RD, Kausel HW, Stranahan A. Ebstein's malformation of the left atrioventricular valve in corrected transposition, with subpulmonary stenosis and ventricular septal defect. *Am J Cardiol* 1961;8:270–274.

66. Celermajer DS, Cullen S, Deanfield JE, Sullivan ID. Congenitally corrected transposition and Ebstein's anomaly of the systemic atrioventricular valve: association with aortic arch obstruction. *J Am Coll Cardiol* 1991;18:1056–1058.

67. Ross-Ascuitto NT, Ascuitto RJ, Kopf GS, et al. Discrete subaortic obstruction in a patient with corrected transposition of the great arteries. *Pediatr Cardiol* 1987;8:147–149.

68. Marino B, Sanders SP, Parness IA, Colan SD. Obstruction of right ventricular inflow and outflow in corrected transposition of the great arteries (S,L,L): two-dimensional echocardiographic diagnosis. *J Am Coll Cardiol* 1986;8:407–411.

69. Hwang B, Bowman F, Malm J, Krongrad E. Surgical repair of congenitally corrected transposition of the great arteries: results and follow-up. *Am J Cardiol* 1982;50:781–785.

70. Westerman GR, Lang P, Castaneda AR, Norwood WI. Corrected transposition and repair of associated intracardiac defects. *Circulation* 1982;66[suppl I]:I-197–I-202.

CHAPTER 16

Superoinferior Ventricles and Crisscross Heart

Lilliam M. Valdes-Cruz and Raul O. Cayre

Superoinferior ventricles and crisscross heart constitute a group of malformations resulting from an abnormal rotation of the ventricular mass on its longitudinal axis and a deviation in the spatial position of the ventricles from what would be expected for the particular atrioventricular connection present. There has been controversy regarding both the nomenclature and the morphology of these anomalies.

The first description of a heart with an abnormal spatial position of the ventricles and crossed atrioventricular connection was published in 1961 by Lev and Rowlatt (1) under the name of mixed levocardia. Since then, various names have been utilized, such as corrected transposition of the great arteries with extreme counterclockwise torsion of the heart and crossing of the inflow tracts (2), crisscross atrioventricular relationships or crisscross heart (3), corrected transposition of the great arteries associated with ventricular rotation (4), crossing atrioventricular valves (5), upstairs-downstairs ventricles (6), superoinferior ventricular heart (7), uncorrected levotransposition with horizontal ventricular septum (8), crossed atrioventricular connections (9), and superoinferior ventricles (10).

The terms superoinferior ventricles and crisscross heart are frequently used synonymously. The two situations coexist in cases with crossed atrioventricular connection because superoinferior ventricles are always present in these instances. However, not all cases of superoinferior ventricles present with crossed atrioventricular connections; therefore, the terms should not be used interchangeably.

Superoinferior ventricles are characterized by an abnormal spatial relationship of the ventricles, in which they are situated one on top of the other instead of side by side and are separated by an interventricular septum that is more or less horizontal (10). In crisscross heart, the systemic and pulmonary venous flows cross at the atrioventricular level but do not mix (3).

The actual incidence of these types of malformations is not known.

EMBRYOLOGIC CONSIDERATIONS

The anatomic characteristics of the ventricles depend on the primordia of the trabecular portions, whereas the spatial position is related to bulboventricular looping. In hearts with situs solitus and a D (dextro) bulboventricular loop (Fig. 16-1B), the morphologic right ventricle is located to the right and the morphologic left ventricle to the left, resulting in a concordant atrioventricular connection (Fig. 16-1D). On the other hand, in cases of an L (levo) bulboventricular loop (Fig. 16-1C), the morphologic right ventricle is on the left and the morphologic left ventricle is on the right, resulting in atrioventricular discordance (Fig. 16-1E).

In hearts with situs solitus and concordant crisscross, a D bulboventricular loop develops, and, after cardiac septation, a clockwise rotation of the ventricular mass occurs on its long axis (3,4,7,9,11–14). This determines that the anatomic right atrium, located on the right, connects with an anatomic right ventricle that is located above and leftward; the anatomic left atrium, located on the left, connects with an anatomic left ventricle that is located below the right ventricle (Fig. 16-1D,F).

Discordant crisscross with situs solitus occurs as a result of development of an L bulboventricular loop and counterclockwise rotation of the ventricular mass along its long axis after cardiac septation (2–4,9,12–14). As a consequence, the anatomic right atrium, located to the right, connects with an anatomic left ventricle located inferiorly and leftward, and the anatomic left atrium, located on the left, connects with an anatomic right ventricle located to the right and superior to the left ventricle (Fig. 16-1E,G).

Cases with situs inversus would be a mirror image of those with situs solitus.

Hearts with superoinferior ventricles without crisscross atrioventricular connection develop as the result of displacement of the ventricular mass along the horizontal plane of its long axis rather than rotation on its long axis (13,14).

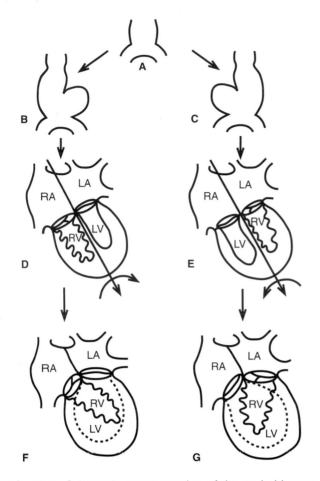

FIG. 16-1. Schematic representation of the probable morphogenesis of superoinferior ventricles in situs solitus with concordant and discordant crisscross. **A:** Straight-tube heart. **B:** D bulboventricular loop. **C:** L bulboventricular loop. **D:** Atrioventricular concordance. The *curved arrow* indicates the clockwise rotation of the ventricular mass over the long axis of the heart. **E:** Atrioventricular discordance. The *curved arrow* indicates the counterclockwise rotation of the ventricular mass over the long axis of the heart. **F:** Spatial position of the ventricles in cases of concordant crisscross. **G:** Spatial position of the ventricles in cases of discordant crisscross. *RA*, right atrium; *LA*, left atrium; *RV*, right ventricle; *LV*, left ventricle.

ANATOMIC AND ECHOCARDIOGRAPHIC CONSIDERATIONS

The echocardiographic study of crisscross heart should determine (a) the spatial position of the heart in the thorax, and the visceroatrial situs; (b) the atrioventricular connection, spatial position of the ventricles and interventricular septum, and spatial position and any anomalies of the atrioventricular valves; (c) the presence of any ventricular septal defect; (d) the presence of outflow tract obstruction; (e) the ventriculoarterial connection and spatial relationship of the great arteries; and (f) the presence of associated anomalies. Intraoperative and postoperative evaluation should also be included.

Spatial Position of the Heart in the Thorax and Visceroatrial Situs

In a total of 83 cases of crisscross heart reported in the literature and reviewed by us, the position of the heart in the thorax was mentioned in only 75. Levocardia was present in 80%, mesocardia in 7%, and dextrocardia in 13% (1–4,7–9,11,12,15–29).

Among the 83 cases of crisscross heart reviewed, situs solitus was seen in 96.3% (1–4,7–9,11,12,15–21,23–29). Situs inversus was found in only two cases (2.4%) (9,22), and situs ambiguus in only one case (1.3%) (7).

The position of the heart in the thorax and the visceroatrial situs can be determined echocardiographically most rapidly from the subcostal and the abdominal long- and short-axis views. These techniques were covered in detail in Chapters 2 and 4.

Atrioventricular Connection, Spatial Position of the Ventricles and Interventricular Septum, Spatial Position and Anomalies of the Atrioventricular Valves

In 81% of the cases reviewed in the literature (67 of 83), the atrioventricular connection was concordant (3–5,7–9,11,12,15,19–22,25–29). In hearts with situs solitus, the morphologic right atrium, located to the right, was connected with the morphologic right ventricle, which was positioned superiorly and leftward. The morphologic left atrium, located to the left, was connected to the morphologic left ventricle, positioned inferiorly and to the right (Fig. 16-1F). The two cases reported with situs inversus also had concordant atrioventricular connection (9,22). In this arrangement, the morphologic right atrium was located to the left and connected to the morphologic right ventricle, situated to the right and superiorly, whereas the morphologic left atrium, located on the right, connected to the morphologic left ventricle, which was situated to the left and inferiorly (9,22).

Rarely, the concordant atrioventricular connection is incompletely or partially crossed (25). In these cases, the anatomic right atrium is connected to the anatomic right ventricle, located superiorly and to the left, and the anatomic left atrium is connected to the anatomic left ventricle, which is situated in a normal inferior relationship to the right ventricle. In these instances, only the connection of the right atrium to the right ventricle is crossed.

In 16 (19%) of the cases reviewed, the atrioventricular connection was discordant; all presented in situs solitus (1–5,9,12,16–19,23,24,26,27). The anatomic right atrium, located on the right, connected to an anatomic left ventricle, located inferiorly and to the left. The anatomic right ventricle was situated superiorly and to the right and was connected to the anatomic left atrium, located on the left (Fig. 16-1G).

Hypoplasia of the morphologic right ventricle is common in crisscross hearts and involves the inlet and trabecular portions of the right ventricle, whereas the infundibular portion is normal. Marino et al. (27), in an echocardiographic study of 14 cases of crisscross heart, found that the infundibular portion of the right ventricle is significantly larger than normal in these patients. The left ventricle is usually of normal size.

In the majority of cases with situs solitus and atrioventricular concordance, the interventricular septum has a more or less horizontal position in space with a superior-right to inferior-left inclination (Fig. 16-2). In situs solitus and atrioventricular discordance, however, the septum has a superior-left to inferior-right inclination.

The spatial rotation of the ventricular mass over its long axis determines an abnormal spatial position not only of the ventricles but also of the atrioventricular valves. The tricuspid valve has a more anterior and superior position with respect to the mitral valve, which is more posteriorly and inferiorly located. In situs solitus and atrioventricular concordance, the tricuspid valve has an anterior-right orientation and connects the anatomic right atrium on the right with the anatomic right ventricle situated to the left and superiorly. The mitral valve has a posterior-left orientation and connects the morphologic left atrium on the left with the morphologic left ventricle situated inferiorly and to the right (Fig. 16-1F). In situs solitus with discordant atrioventricular connection, the tricuspid valve has an anterior-left position and connects the anatomic left atrium on the left with the anatomic right ventricle located superiorly and rightward. The mitral valve has a posterior-right orientation and connects

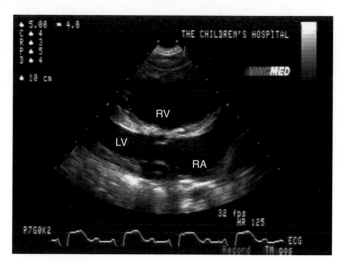

ECHO. 16-1. Parasternal long-axis view in discordant atrioventricular connection. *RV*, right ventricle; *RA*, right atrium; *LV*, left ventricle.

the morphologic right atrium on the right with the morphologic left ventricle located inferiorly and to the left (Fig. 16-1G).

In a large percentage of cases, anomalies of the tricuspid valve are present, with variable degrees of stenosis, hypoplasia, and dysplasia, such as Ebstein's anomaly, overriding, straddling, and atresia (7,8,15,16,21,22,27–29). Anomalies of the mitral valve are less frequent, but regurgitation, overriding, and straddling have all been reported (22,28,29).

The type of atrioventricular connection (discordant or concordant) and the spatial position of the ventricles and interventricular septum can be established from the parasternal long-axis and apical four-chamber views, complemented by the subcostal long- and short-axis views (Echos. 16-1–16-4). Because of the different spatial posi-

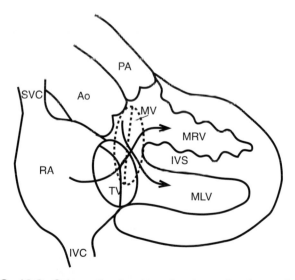

FIG. 16-2. Schematic drawing of a heart in situs solitus with superoinferior ventricles and concordant atrioventricular connection, demonstrating the horizontal position of the interventricular septum. The *arrows* indicate the concordant atrioventricular connection. *RA*, right atrium; *MRV*, morphologic right ventricle; *MLV*, morphologic left ventricle; *IVS*, interventricular septum; *TV*, tricuspid valve; *MV*, mitral valve; *PA*, pulmonary artery; *Ao*, aorta; *SVC*, superior vena cava; *IVC*, inferior vena cava.

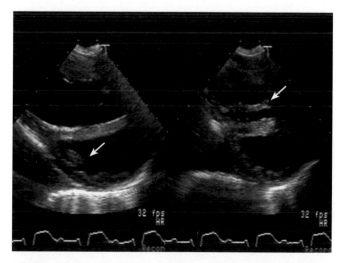

ECHO. 16-2. Parasternal short-axis views in discordant atrioventricular connection. **Left:** The location of the left ventricle posteriorly (*arrow* points to the papillary muscle). **Right:** The moderator band within the anatomic right ventricle (*arrow*).

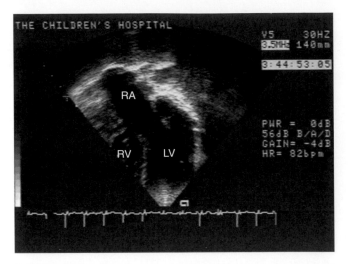

ECHO. 16-3. Apical view demonstrating the discordant crisscross atrioventricular connection between the right atrium on the right and the left ventricle on the left through a mitral valve that is oriented posteriorly and rightward. *RA,* right atrium; *RV,* right ventricle; *LV,* left ventricle.

tions of the cardiac structures, the transducer must be tilted anteroposteriorly and from right to left to define them clearly. Color Doppler flow mapping can be helpful by demonstrating the direction of flow from the atria to the ventricles, whether crisscross or superoinferior.

Anomalies of the atrioventricular valves can be studied from the subcostal long-axis and the apical four-chamber views, with anteroposterior and right-left angulation of the transducer because the valves are in different planes. Color Doppler can aid in demonstrating any regurgitation, and spectral Doppler velocities can verify any gradient across the valve(s).

Ventricular Septal Defect

A ventricular septal defect is almost always present in cases of crisscross heart and superoinferior ventricles (Fig. 16-2). Only one case has been reported of superoinferior ventricle with an intact ventricular septum (30). The defect is always large and can be located in any portion of the septum, although usually it is perimembranous with inlet, trabecular, or outlet extensions. Nonetheless, isolated muscular defects in the inlet, trabecular, or outlet portion of the septum have been reported. Atrioventricular septal defects are very rare. In the majority of cases of double-outlet right ventricle, the septal defect is caused by malalignment.

The echocardiographic study of interventricular septal defects can be accomplished through the subcostal long- and short-axis views with superior-inferior angulation of the transducer, and from the parasternal long- and short-axis views and apical views with anterior-posterior sweep of the transducer (Echo. 16-5). Color Doppler flow mapping demonstrates the site and direction of shunting and aids in the positioning of the spectral Doppler along the line of flow for recording of velocities.

Outflow Tract Obstruction

Obstruction of the pulmonary outflow tract is common, seen in 55% of cases (2–5,7–9,11,12,14,16,18,21,23,25, 27,28). In 66% of these cases, subvalvular stenosis was present as a result of hypertrophy of the infundibular septum, a muscular subpulmonary infundibulum, or accessory tissue of the atrioventricular valves. Among the remaining cases, valvular pulmonic stenosis was present in 17%, pulmonic valve atresia in 15%, and stenosis of the branch pulmonary arteries in 2%.

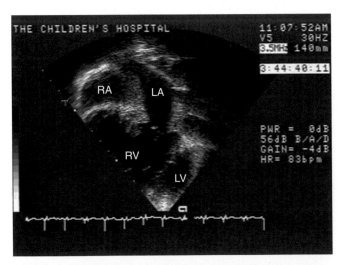

ECHO. 16-4. Apical view showing the discordant crisscross connection between the left atrium on the left and the right ventricle on the right. The tricuspid valve has an anterior-left orientation. *RA,* right atrium; *RV,* right ventricle; *LA,* left atrium; *LV,* left ventricle.

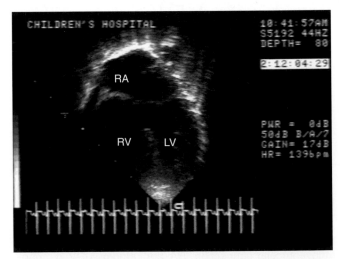

ECHO. 16-5. Apical view demonstrating the presence of a large ventricular septal defect. Note the right atrial-to-left ventricular connection through a mitral valve oriented leftward. *RA,* right atrium; *RV,* right ventricle; *LV,* left ventricle.

Aortic outflow obstruction was seen in 10% of the cases of crisscross heart reviewed in the literature: subaortic stenosis in two cases, hypoplastic aortic annulus in one, hypoplasia of the aortic arch in two, and coarctation of the aorta in three (7,12,15,21,22,28).

The outflow tracts can be seen from the subcostal long- and short-axis views, with modifications to adjust for the different orientations of the right and left outflow tracts. These views allow a full examination of the outflow tracts, so the subvalvar, valvar, and supravalvar regions are seen. The long- and short-axis parasternal views and apical outflow views are also important (Echo. 16-6). Spectral Doppler is used to measure the velocity across the outflow tracts and estimate the gradient.

Ventriculoarterial Connection and Spatial Relationship of the Great Arteries

A discordant ventriculoarterial connection with the aorta positioned to the right and anteriorly, strictly anteriorly, to the left and anteriorly, or side by side and to the left of the pulmonary artery was seen in 54% of cases reported in the literature. Double-outlet right ventricle was seen in 30% of cases, concordant ventriculoarterial connection with normally related great arteries in 11%, and single-outlet, pulmonary atresia type in 5% (1–5,7–9,11,12,15–29). We have not found any case reported with single-outlet, truncus arteriosus type or single-outlet, aortic atresia type.

The echocardiographic views that help establish the ventriculoarterial connections are the long- and short-axis parasternal views, apical outflow and long-axis views, and subcostal outflow and short-axis views (Echo. 16-7). The best view to determine the spatial relationship of the great vessels is the parasternal short axis view.

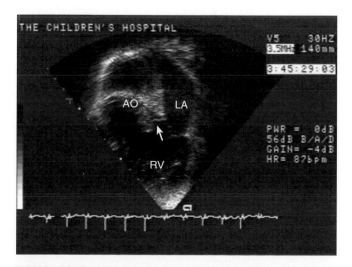

ECHO. 16-6. Apical view illustrating the presence of subvalvar pulmonary stenosis in discordant crisscross connection. *Arrow* points to the subpulmonic area. *AO*, aorta; *LA*, left atrium; *RV*, right ventricle.

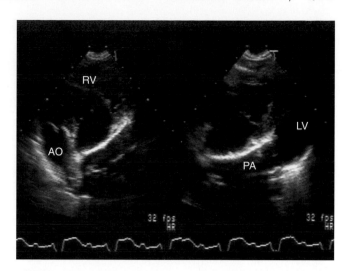

ECHO. 16-7. Apical views of discordant ventriculoarterial connections in the presence of crisscross heart. **Left:** The aorta emerging from the right ventricle. **Right:** The pulmonary artery connected to the left ventricle. *RV*, right ventricle; *AO*, aorta; *LV*, left ventricle; *PA*, pulmonary artery.

Associated Anomalies

Anomalies associated with crisscross heart have been patent ductus arteriosus (3,4,11,20,21,23,25); atrial septal defect, ostium secundum type (11,15,21,25,28); patent foramen ovale (3,4,23); left juxtaposition of the atrial appendages (2,7,9,21); right juxtaposition of the atrial appendages (15); left superior vena cava draining into the coronary sinus (2,7); bicuspid pulmonic valve (4,18); right aortic arch (3,11); azygous vein continuation (7); and cor triatriatum (14).

INTRAOPERATIVE AND POSTOPERATIVE EVALUATION

The intraoperative pre-bypass evaluation of crisscross and superoinferior ventricles is directed toward confirmation of the type of atrioventricular connection and any associated anomalies. The views permitting examination of the spatial ventricular relationship and position of the interventricular septum are the transverse four-chamber views (see Fig. 4-28A,B) with anteflexion and retroflexion of the endoscope as well as right and left manipulation. These views should also clarify the morphologic characteristics of the atrioventricular valves and ventricles and the presence and location of a ventricular septal defect (Echo. 16-8). A transverse short-axis view of the great vessels (see Fig. 4-29A–C) demonstrates the relationship of the great arteries. Obstruction of either outflow tract is best illustrated from the transgastric and retrocardiac longitudinal views of the outflow tracts (see Figs. 4-27D,E; 4-29D–F). The transgastric longitudinal approach is the most appropriate for recording spectral

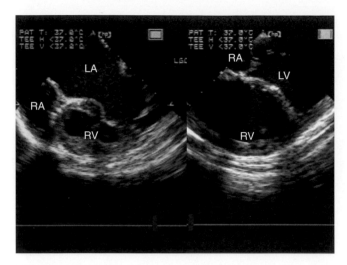

ECHO. 16-8. Left: Transesophageal four-chamber view demonstrating the relationship between the left atrium and right ventricle in a discordant crisscross connection. Note that the right atrium is not related to the right ventricle. **Right:** Transesophageal view illustrating the spatial relationship and connection between the right atrium and left ventricle. Note that the right atrium and right ventricle are not connected. *RA*, right atrium; *LA*, left atrium; *RV*, right ventricle; *LV*, left ventricle.

Doppler velocities along the direction of flow (see Fig. 4-27E).

After bypass and in the late postoperative period, the echocardiographic evaluation is directed toward evaluation of the repair of the ventricular defect and any outflow obstruction or anomalies of the atrioventricular valves.

REFERENCES

1. Lev M, Rowlatt UF. The pathologic anatomy of mixed levocardia. A review of thirteen cases of atrial or ventricular inversion with or without corrected transposition. *Am J Cardiol* 1961;8:216–263.
2. Franco-Vazquez JS, Perez-Trevino C, Gaxiola A. Corrected transposition of the great arteries with extreme counter-clockwise torsion of the heart. *Acta Cardiol* 1973;28:636–643.
3. Anderson RH, Shinebourne EA, Gerlis LM. Criss-cross atrioventricular relationships producing paradoxical atrioventricular concordance or discordance. Their significance to nomenclature of congenital heart disease. *Circulation* 1974;50:176–180.
4. Kinsley RH, McGoon DC, Danielson GK. Corrected transposition of the great arteries. Associated ventricular rotation. *Circulation* 1974;49:574–578.
5. Ando M, Takao A, Nihmura I, Mori K. Crossing atrioventricular valves. Clinical study of 8 cases. *Circulation* 1976;53/54 [Suppl II]:II-90(abst).
6. Van Praagh R, Weinberg PM, Van Praagh S. Malposition of the heart. In: Moss AJ, Adams FH, Emmanouilides GC, eds. *Heart disease in infants, children and adolescents.* Baltimore: Williams & Wilkins, 1977:395–399.
7. Freedom RM, Culhman G, Rowe RD. The criss-cross and superoinferior ventricular heart: an angiocardiographic study. *Am J Cardiol* 1978;42:620–628.
8. Guthaner D, Higgins CB, Silverman JF, Hayden WG, Wexler L. An unusual form of the transposition complex. Uncorrected levo-

transposition with horizontal ventricular septum: report of two cases. *Circulation* 1976;53:190–195.
9. Attie F, Munoz-Castellanos L, Ovseyevitz J, et al. Crossed atrioventricular connections. *Am Heart J* 1980;99:163–172.
10. Van Praagh S, LaCorte M, Fellows KE, et al. Supero-inferior ventricles: anatomic and angiocardiographic findings in ten postmortem cases. In: Van Praagh R, Takao A, eds. *Etiology and morphogenesis of congenital heart disease.* Mount Kisco, NY: Futura Publishing, 1980:317–378.
11. Zach M, Singer H, Loser H, Hagel KJ. The horizontal interventricular septum. Three cases with different ventriculoarterial connections. *Eur J Cardiol* 1980;11:269–282.
12. Tadavarthy SM, Formanek A, Castaneda-Zuniga W, Moller JH, Edwards JE, Amplatz K. The three types of criss-cross heart: a simple rotational anomaly. *Br J Radiol* 1981;54:736–743.
13. Anderson RH. A question of definition. Criss-cross hearts revisited. *Pediatr Cardiol* 1982;3:305–313.
14. Freedom RM. Supero-inferior ventricle and criss-cross atrioventricular connections: an analysis of the myth and mystery. *Mod Probl Paediatr* 1983;22:48–62.
15. Wagner HR, Alday LE, Vlad P. Juxtaposition of the atrial appendages. A report of six necropsied cases. *Circulation* 1970;42:157–163.
16. Symons JC, Shinebourne EA, Joseph MC, Lincoln C, Ho Y, Anderson RH. Criss-cross heart with congenitally corrected transposition: report of a case with d-transposed aorta and ventricular preexcitation. *Eur J Cardiol* 1977;5/6:493–505.
17. Waldhausen JA, Pierce WS, Whitman V. Horizontal interventricular septum in congenital heart disease: surgical considerations. *Ann Thorac Surg* 1977;23:271–275.
18. Anderson KR, Lie JT, Sieg K, Hagler DJ, Ritter DG, Davis GD. A criss-cross heart. Detailed anatomic description and discussion of morphogenesis. *Mayo Clin Proc* 1977;52:569–575.
19. Sieg K, Hagler DJ, Ritter DG, et al. Straddling right atrioventricular valve in criss-cross atrioventricular relationship. *Mayo Clin Proc* 1977;52:561–568.
20. Sato K, Ohara S, Tsukaguchi I, et al. A criss-cross heart with concordant atrioventriculo-arterial connections. Report of a case. *Circulation* 1978;57:396–400.
21. Otero-Coto E, Wilkinson JL, Dickinson DF, Rufilanchas JJ, Marquez J. Gross distortion of atrioventricular and ventriculo-arterial relations associated with left juxtaposition of atrial appendages. Bizarre form of atrioventricular criss-cross. *Br Heart J* 1979;41:486–492.
22. Danielson GK, Tabry IF, Ritter DG, Fulton RE. Surgical repair of criss-cross heart with straddling atrioventricular valve. *J Thorac Cardiovasc Surg* 1979;77:847–851.
23. Marino B, Chiariello L, Bosman C, et al. Criss-cross heart with discordant atrioventricular connections. *Pediatr Cardiol* 1982;3:315–318.
24. Van Mill G, Moulaert A, Harinck E, Wenink A, Oppenheimer-Dekker A. Subcostal two-dimensional echocardiographic recognition of a criss-cross heart with discordant ventriculo-arterial connection. *Pediatr Cardiol* 1982;3:319–323.
25. Scheeweiss A, Shem-Tov A, Blieden LC, Deutsch V, Neufeld HN. Criss-cross heart—a case with horizontal septum, complete transposition, pulmonary atresia and ventricular septal defect. *Pediatr Cardiol* 1982;3:325–328.
26. Robinson PJ, Kumpeng V, Macartney FJ. Cross sectional echocardiographic and angiocardiographic correlation in criss cross hearts. *Br Heart J* 1985;54:61–67.
27. Marino B, Sanders SP, Pasquini L, Giannico S, Parness IA, Colan SD. Two-dimensional echocardiographic anatomy in crisscross heart. *Am J Cardiol* 1986;58:325–333.
28. Hery E, Jimenez M, Didier D, et al. Echocardiographic and angiographic findings in supero-inferior cardiac ventricles. *Am J Cardiol* 1989;63:1385–1389.
29. Geva T, Van Praagh S, Sanders SP, Mayer JE, Van Praagh R. Straddling mitral valve with hypoplastic right ventricle, crisscross atrioventricular relations, double outlet right ventricle and dextrocardia: morphologic, diagnostic and surgical considerations. *J Am Coll Cardiol* 1991;17:1603–1612.
30. Santos MA, Simoes LC. Paroxysmal supraventricular tachycardia in supero-inferior ventricles with intact ventricular septum. *Int J Cardiol* 1987;14:232–235.

PART VI

Anomalies of the Ventricles

CHAPTER 17

Univentricular Atrioventricular Connection

Lilliam M. Valdes-Cruz and Raul O. Cayre

Controversy has existed regarding the most appropriate terminology to be used for hearts in which both atria connect with a single ventricular chamber (1–6). This rare cardiac malformation, in a case with normally related great arteries, was originally described by Holmes in 1824 (7); it is classically known as Holmes' heart. Peacock in 1855 (8) published a case with complete transposition of the great arteries. Since then, various denominations have been used in the literature: cor triloculare biatriatum (9–11), three-chambered heart (12), single ventricle with diminutive outlet chamber (13), single ventricle with rudimentary outlet chamber (14), single or common ventricle (3,10,11,13–24), primitive ventricle (1,20,25), double-inlet left ventricle (26–32), double-inlet right ventricle (33,34), univentricular heart (2,4,35–42), and univentricular atrioventricular connection (6,43–45).

The type of atrioventricular connection can be either biventricular (two atria connected with two separate ventricles through separate atrioventricular valves) or univentricular (two atria connected with only one ventricle). The terms univentricular atrioventricular connection and double-inlet ventricle have clarified to some extent the confusion created by the innumerable names previously used to describe the malformation in which both atria connect with one ventricle (6,26–34,43–46).

There are various modes of univentricular atrioventricular connections: (a) two separate, perforated atrioventricular valves; (b) two separate atrioventricular valves, one perforated and one absent (classic tricuspid or mitral atresia); (c) one common atrioventricular valve; (d) overriding atrioventricular valve; and (e) straddling atrioventricular valve (44–49).

If two ventricular chambers are present within the ventricular mass, as is usual, the ventricle that receives both atrial connections is called the main chamber or dominant ventricle, and the ventricle that is lacking an inlet portion is called the rudimentary ventricular chamber or rudimentary ventricle (6,43,44,46–48). If the rudimentary ventric-

ular chamber has a trabecular portion and one or both outlet portions, it is called an outlet chamber; if it has only a trabecular portion, it is called a trabecular pouch (47–49). The characteristics of the trabecular portion usually permit anatomic identification of the main chamber and rudimentary chamber as morphologically right and left ventricles. Rarely, only one ventricular chamber is present in the main ventricular mass, with no identifiable right or left ventricular morphologic characteristics; in these cases, the ventricular chamber is called a solitary or morphologically indeterminate ventricle (45,47), or true single ventricle (50).

The true incidence of this anomaly is difficult to know because opinions differ as to which types of malformations are to be included, particularly when univentricular atrioventricular connection with absent right or left connection is considered. The incidence varies between 1% and 4.3% of all congenital cardiac malformations (10,11,19,20,51–54).

DOUBLE-INLET VENTRICLE

Situations in which two atria connect with one ventricle through two separate, perforated atrioventricular valves or through a common atrioventricular valve with or without overriding and/or straddling are discussed in this section (Fig. 17-1). Atrioventricular connection through one perforated and one atretic valve is considered under the sections on atresia of the right-sided or left-sided atrioventricular valve (see below).

There are three anatomic types of double-inlet atrioventricular connection: (a) double-inlet left ventricle with rudimentary right ventricular chamber (Fig. 17-1A,B,G,H); (b) double-inlet right ventricle with rudimentary left ventricular chamber (Fig. 17-1C,D,I,J); and (c) double-inlet solitary or indeterminate ventricle (Fig. 17-1E,F). Each one can present with situs solitus, situs inversus, or situs ambiguus with levocardia, dextrocar-

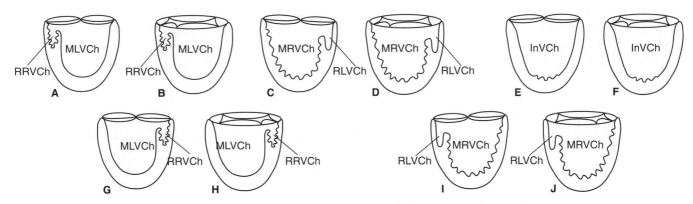

FIG. 17-1. Schematic drawings of the different types of double-inlet ventricles. **A:** Double-inlet left ventricle with D loop and two perforated atrioventricular valves. **B:** Double-inlet left ventricle with D loop and one common atrioventricular valve. **C:** Double-inlet right ventricle with D loop and two perforated atrioventricular valves. **D:** Double-inlet right ventricle with D loop and one common atrioventricular valve. **E:** Double-inlet indeterminate ventricle with two perforated atrioventricular valves. **F:** Double-inlet indeterminate ventricle and one common atrioventricular valve. **G:** Double-inlet left ventricle with L loop and two perforated atrioventricular valves. **H:** Double-inlet left ventricle with L loop and one common atrioventricular valve. **I:** Double-inlet right ventricle with L loop and two perforated atrioventricular valves. **J:** Double-inlet right ventricle with L loop and one common atrioventricular valve. *MLVCh*, main left ventricular chamber; *MRVCh*, main right ventricular chamber; *RLVCh*, rudimentary left ventricular chamber; *RRVCh*, rudimentary right ventricular chamber; *InVCh*, indeterminate ventricular chamber.

dia, or mesocardia. Cases in which two ventricular chambers can be identified within the ventricular mass can present without ventricular inversion (morphologic right ventricle to the right) (Fig. 17-1A–D) or with ventricular inversion (morphologic right ventricle to the left) (Fig. 17-1G–J).

EMBRYOLOGIC CONSIDERATIONS

A discussion of the morphogenesis of double-inlet ventricles should consider the visceroatrial situs, development of the bulboventricular loop, septation of the atrioventricular canal, development of the ventricular chambers and intercameral septum, septation and incorporation of the conus, and aorticopulmonary septation.

Visceroatrial Situs and Bulboventricular Looping (Spatial Position of the Ventricular Chambers)

Double-inlet ventricle, left or right ventricular type, can present with situs solitus, inversus, or ambiguus; in levocardia, dextrocardia, or mesocardia; and with D (dextro), L (levo), or anterior bulboventricular looping.

In double-inlet left ventricle with rudimentary right ventricular chamber, situs solitus, and levocardia, a D bulboventricular loop results in ventricular chambers that

are not inverted (Fig. 17-2A). The main chamber or left ventricle is located to the left and posteriorly, and the rudimentary right ventricle is located to the right and anteriorly. On the contrary, L bulboventricular looping gives rise to inverted ventricles, so that the left ventricle

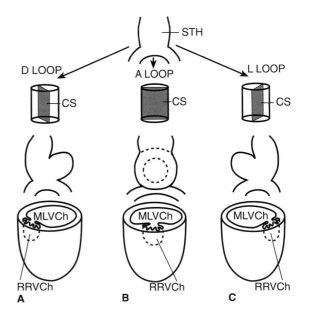

FIG. 17-2. Schematic representation of the probable morphogenesis of double-inlet left ventricle. **A:** D bulboventricular loop. **B:** Anterior bulboventricular loop. **C:** L bulboventricular loop. *STH*, straight-tube heart; *CS*, conal septum; *MLVCh*, main left ventricular chamber; *RRVCh*, rudimentary right ventricular chamber.

or main chamber is situated to the right and posteriorly and the rudimentary right ventricular chamber is situated to the left and anteriorly (Fig. 17-2C). Very rarely, the location of the main left ventricular chamber is strictly posterior and that of the rudimentary right ventricle strictly anterior as the result of an anterior bulboventricular loop (Fig. 17-2B).

In double-inlet right ventricle with rudimentary left ventricle, situs solitus, and levocardia, a D loop results in the right or main ventricle being located to the right and anteriorly and the rudimentary left ventricular chamber to the left and posteriorly (Fig. 17-3A). An L loop gives rise to ventricular inversion, with the location of the main right ventricle to the left of and anterior to the rudimentary left ventricular chamber, which is situated to the right and posteriorly (Fig. 17-3C). With an anterior loop, the right ventricle is directly anterior to the posteriorly located left ventricular rudimentary chamber (Fig. 17-3B).

In levocardia with situs inversus, the ventricular chambers have the same spatial position as in levocardia with situs solitus. However, there is ventricular inversion in D loop, and in L loop there is not. An anteroposterior ventricular relationship is also possible if the looping is anterior. Hearts with dextrocardia in situs inversus are a mirror image of those in situs solitus with levocardia. Those with dextrocardia in situs solitus are a mirror image of those with levocardia in situs inversus.

Septation of the Atrioventricular Canal

The superior and inferior endocardial cushions divide the orifice of the atrioventricular canal into a right and a

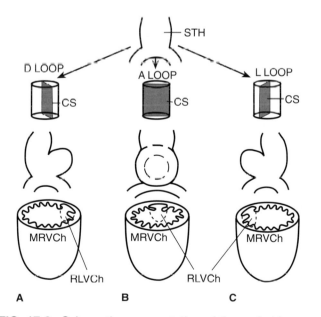

FIG. 17-3. Schematic representation of the probable morphogenesis of double-inlet right ventricle. **A:** D bulboventricular loop. **B:** Anterior bulboventricular loop. **C:** L bulboventricular loop. *STH*, straight-tube heart; *CS*, conal septum; *MRVCh*, main right ventricular chamber; *RLVCh*, rudimentary left ventricular chamber.

left atrioventricular orifice and, along with the ventricular walls, participate in the formation of the atrioventricular valves (55–57) (see Figs. 1-7, 1-12B, 1-13). In double-inlet ventricle, normal septation of the canal gives rise to two atrioventricular valves, whereas failure of development of the cushions results in a common atrioventricular valve, with an absent right and absent left atrioventricular valve (58).

Development of Ventricular Chambers and Intercameral Septum

The normal development of the primordia of the trabecular portion of both ventricles determines the normal growth or expansion of the trabecular portion of the ventricles and of the trabecular portion of the interventricular septum. Failure of a balanced expansion of the primordia of the trabecular portions of the ventricles leads to the abnormal development of one or the other ventricular chamber and a malalignment of the interventricular septum with the atrioventricular and atrial septa. This failure of balanced ventricular development and consequent malalignment between the interventricular septum, atrioventricular canal, and atrial septum results in a spectrum of malformations, which include double-inlet left ventricle, straddling of the tricuspid valve, straddling of the mitral valve, and double-inlet right ventricle. Rychter et al. (59) also feel that double-inlet left or double-inlet right ventricle is caused by hypoplasia of the right or left ventricular anlage or primordium, and that severe hypoplasia of both the right and left ventricular anlagen results in double-inlet indeterminate or solitary ventricle. Studies in experimental embryology on the contribution of the cushions of the atrioventricular canal (56,60) support this theory because from the moment the cushions of the atrioventricular canal appear, they are aligned with the interatrial and interventricular septa (see Figs. 1-7A; 1-12A,B). Consequently, there is no moment in development when the atrioventricular canal migrates to the right. An exaggerated rightward expansion of the atrioventricular canal has been mentioned as the morphogenetic mechanism for double-inlet right ventricle (33,61), whereas failure of rightward expansion has been thought to be the cause of double-inlet left ventricle (25–27,61,62). Both of these mechanisms lack embryologic evidence.

Septation and Incorporation of the Conus

The conus or primordium of the ventricular infundibula appears in the loop stage at the cephalic end of the heart and is continuous caudally with the primordium of the trabecular portion of the morphologic right ventricle (57,63) (see Fig. 1-5B). In the normal heart, fusion of the dextrodorsal and sinistroventral conal crests gives rise to the infundibular or conal septum; its posterior-to-anterior, right-to-left spatial orientation divides the conus into an anterolateral right and a posteromedial left conus (see Figs. 1-12, 1-14A). The latter becomes incorporated into the left ventricle during the late postloop stage and constitutes its outflow tract (see Fig. 1-5D,E).

In hearts with univentricular atrioventricular connection, situs solitus, and D loop, the conal septation can be similar to that of the normal heart, resulting in an anterolateral right and posteromedial left conus (Figs. 17-2A, 17-3A). If the conal crests are located to the right and left, the infundibular septum will be directed from left to right parallel to the frontal plane and will divide the conus into an anterior and a posterior conus. Conal crests can also develop in a dextroventral and sinistrodorsal position and at fusion give rise to a posterolateral right and an anteromedial left conus. In hearts with situs solitus and L loop, the conal crests are dextroventral and sinistrodorsal, and their fusion results in an infundibular septum directed posteriorly to anteriorly and from left to right, so that the conus is divided into an anterolateral left and a posteromedial right conus (Figs. 17-2C, 17-3C). The fusion of a right and a left conal crest will result in a septum parallel to the frontal plane and an anterior and a posterior conus. If conal crests are positioned in a dextrodorsal and sinistroventral position, the coni will be in an anteromedial right and posterolateral left orientation.

In hearts with double-inlet left ventricle and rudimentary right ventricular chamber, incorporation of a medial or posterior conus into the main chamber causes the great vessel emerging from this conus to be connected with the main chamber, whereas the other great vessel remains connected to the rudimentary right ventricular outlet chamber (Fig. 17-4A). Failure of incorporation of a me-

dial or a posterior conus into the main left ventricle results in the formation of a double-outlet rudimentary chamber from which both great vessels emerge; this is termed double-outlet outlet chamber (Fig. 17-4B). If both coni become incorporated into the main left ventricular chamber, a double outlet of the main ventricle and a right ventricular trabecular pouch are the result (Fig. 17-4C).

In the presence of double-inlet right ventricle with rudimentary left ventricular chamber (Fig. 17-5), failure of incorporation of a medial or a posterior conus into the rudimentary chamber causes the great vessel emerging from that conus to remain related to the main right ventricular chamber; consequently, there is a double outlet from the main ventricle and a rudimentary left ventricular trabecular pouch (Fig. 17-5C). If, on the contrary, the medial or posterior conus becomes incorporated into the left ventricular rudimentary chamber, the great vessel emerging from it is related to the left ventricular outlet chamber, whereas the other great vessel remains connected with the main right ventricle (Figs. 17-5A,B). Incorporation of both coni into the rudimentary left ventricular chamber results in double-outlet outlet chamber (Fig. 17-5D).

Aorticopulmonary Septation

The aorticopulmonary and truncal septa divide the truncus and aortic sac into the ascending aorta and pulmonary arterial trunk. The way these septa develop determines the spatial relationship of the great arteries and, along with the conal incorporation, the ventriculoarterial connection as well.

In hearts with double-inlet left ventricle with rudimentary right ventricular chamber, situs solitus, and D loop, if the aorticopulmonary and truncal septa develop normally, the great arteries will be normally related. The incorporation of the coni determines which chamber they will be connected to. If the medial or posterior conus is incorporated into the main left ventricle, there will be ventriculoarterial concordance—that is, the posterior and rightward aorta will emerge from the left ventricle, and the anterior and leftward pulmonary artery will emerge from the rudimentary right ventricular outlet chamber (Fig. 17-4A). If, on the other hand, the medial or posterior conus is not incorporated into the left ventricle, then both great arteries, although normally related, will emerge from the right ventricular outlet chamber (double-outlet outlet chamber) (Fig. 17-4B). If both coni are incorporated into the left ventricle, there will be a double-outlet main left ventricular chamber (Fig. 17-4C).

If the aorticopulmonary septum does not develop its normal spiral shape but rather is semispiral, and the truncal septum acquires an abnormal spatial orientation from right to left, the location of the great vessels will be anterior (aorta) and posterior (pulmonary artery). If the posterior conus becomes incorporated into the main left

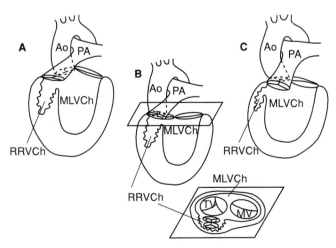

FIG. 17-4. Schematic drawings of double-inlet left ventricle with normally related great arteries. **A:** Ventriculoarterial concordance. **B:** Double-outlet outlet chamber. **C:** Double-outlet main left ventricular chamber. *MLVCh,* main left ventricular chamber; *RRVCh,* rudimentary right ventricular chamber; *Ao,* aorta; *PA,* pulmonary artery; *TV,* tricuspid valve; *MV,* mitral valve.

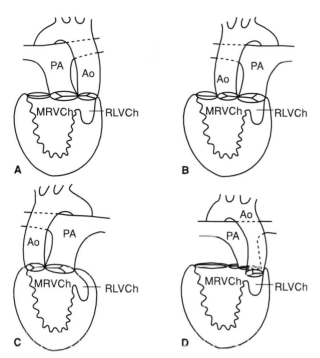

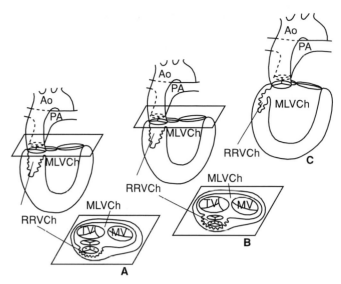

FIG. 17-5. Schematic drawings of the different types of ventriculoarterial connection and spatial relationship of the great arteries in double-inlet right ventricle. **A:** Ventriculoarterial concordance and side by side great arteries with aorta to the left. **B:** Atrioventricular discordance and side-by-side great arteries with aorta to the right. **C:** Double-outlet main right ventricular chamber and side-by-side great arteries with aorta to the right. **D:** Double-outlet outlet chamber, with aorta anterior and to the left and pulmonary artery posterior and to the right. *MRVCh,* main right ventricular chamber; *RLVCh,* rudimentary left ventricular chamber; *Ao,* aorta; *PA,* pulmonary artery.

FIG. 17-6. Schematic drawings of double-inlet left ventricle with strictly anterior and posterior relationship of great arteries. **A:** Ventriculoarterial discordance. **B:** Double-outlet outlet chamber. **C:** Double-outlet main left ventricular chamber. *MLVCh,* main left ventricular chamber; *RRVCh,* rudimentary right ventricular chamber; *Ao,* aorta; *PA,* pulmonary artery; *TV,* tricuspid valve; *MV,* mitral valve.

ventricle, then the pulmonary artery, which is related to that conus, will emerge from the left ventricle, and ventriculoarterial discordance will result. The aorta will maintain an anterior position and emerge from the rudimentary right ventricular chamber (Fig. 17-6A). Failure of the posterior conus to become incorporated into the left ventricle will result in both great vessels emerging from the rudimentary right ventricular outlet chamber (double-outlet outlet chamber) in an anterior-posterior relationship (Fig. 17-6B). Similarly, if both coni are incorporated into the main left ventricular chamber, there will be a double-outlet left ventricle with anteroposterior great vessels. The rudimentary right ventricle is then only a trabecular pouch (Fig. 17-6C).

Development of a straight rather than spiral aorticopulmonary septum, with the truncal septum in a posterior to anterior and right to left direction, will result in the aorta having an anterior and rightward position relative to the pulmonary artery, which will be in a leftward and posterior location. If the posteromedial conus is incorporated into the main left ventricular chamber, there will be ventriculoarterial discordance, with the pulmonary artery,

which is committed to the posteromedial conus, emerging from the left ventricle and the aorta from the right ventricular outlet chamber (Fig. 17-7A). Failure of incorporation of the posteromedial conus results in double outlet of the rudimentary right ventricular outlet chamber, with the aorta anterior and to the right (Fig. 17-7B). Incorporation of both coni into the main chamber gives rise to double-outlet left ventricle, with the aorta positioned anteriorly

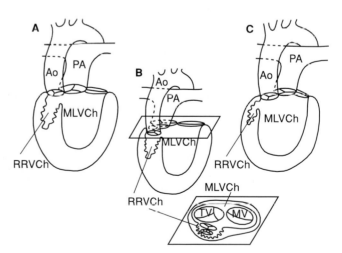

FIG. 17-7. Schematic drawings of double-inlet left ventricle with aorta anterior and to the right and pulmonary artery posterior and to the left. **A:** Ventriculoarterial discordance. **B:** Double-outlet outlet chamber. **C:** Double-outlet main left ventricular chamber. *MLVCh,* main left ventricular chamber; *RRVCh,* rudimentary right ventricular chamber; *Ao,* aorta; *PA,* pulmonary artery; *TV,* tricuspid valve; *MV,* mitral valve.

and to the right and the pulmonary artery posteriorly and to the left (Fig. 17-7C).

Double-inlet left ventricle with rudimentary right ventricle in situs solitus with L loop can have any of these same ventriculoarterial connections, but the positions will be a mirror image of those with D loop.

In hearts with double-inlet right ventricle, rudimentary left ventricular chamber, situs solitus, and D loop, the same ventriculoarterial connections and great arterial spatial relations can exist. As in double-inlet left ventricle, the shape and orientation of the aorticopulmonary and truncal septa determine the spatial relationship of the great arteries. The incorporation of the coni, on the other hand, determine the ventriculoarterial connection: concordant (Fig. 17-5A), discordant (Fig. 17-5B), double-outlet main right ventricular chamber (Fig. 17-5C), or double-outlet left ventricular outlet chamber (Fig. 17-5D).

The mirror-image relationships exist in double-inlet right ventricle with rudimentary ventricular chamber, left situs solitus, and L loop.

Double inlet into a solitary or indeterminate ventricle can be seen with any of the types of spatial relationships of the great vessels described. In these cases, however, the ventriculoarterial connection is not denominated as concordant or discordant because there is only one ventricular chamber within the ventricular mass (Fig. 17-8A–C).

ANATOMIC AND ECHOCARDIOGRAPHIC CONSIDERATIONS

The echocardiographic study of double-inlet ventricle, in addition to establishing the visceroatrial situs and systemic and pulmonary venous drainage, should determine the following: (a) morphology and location of the ventricular chambers and location and size of the ventricular septal or intercameral defect; (b) morphology of the atrioventricular valves or of the common valve; (c) the ventriculoarterial connection and spatial position of the great arteries; (d) obstruction of either outflow tract; (e) origin and distribution of the coronary arteries; and (f) any associated anomalies. Intraoperative and postoperative evaluation is discussed at the end of the chapter, along with with that for the other types of univentricular atrioventricular connections.

Morphology and Location of the Ventricular Chambers; Location and Size of Septal or Intercameral Defect

Double-inlet left ventricle is the most common type of double-inlet ventricle, with an incidence of approximately 61% to 80% of all cases (24,32,47,49). Two ventricular chambers can be recognized within the ventricular mass. The main chamber, which receives flow from both atria

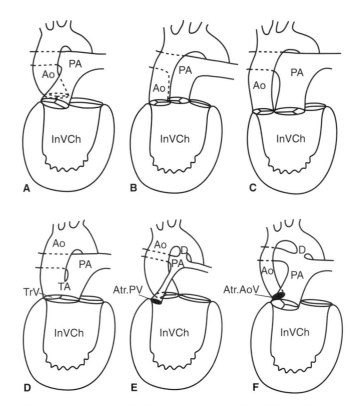

FIG. 17-8. Schematic drawings showing the different types of ventriculoarterial connection and spatial relationship of the great arteries in double-inlet indeterminate ventricle. **A:** Normally related great arteries. **B:** Aorta anterior and to the right and pulmonary artery posterior and to the left. **C:** Side-by-side great arteries and aorta to the right. **D:** Single outlet, truncus arteriosus type. **E:** Single outlet, pulmonary atresia type. **F:** Single outlet, aortic atresia type. *InVCh,* indeterminate ventricular chamber; *Ao,* aorta; *PA,* pulmonary artery; *TA,* truncus arteriosus; *TrV,* truncal valve; *Atr PV,* atretic pulmonic valve; *Atr AoV,* atretic aortic valve; *D,* ductus arteriosus.

through two separate, perforated atrioventricular valves or through one common valve, has trabeculations with morphologic characteristics typical of a left ventricle. It occupies a posterior and inferior position within the ventricular mass, and its location can be to the left of and posterior, strictly posterior, or to the right of and posterior to the rudimentary chamber (Fig. 17-2). The rudimentary chamber lacks an inlet, and its trabecular portion has the characteristics of a morphologic right ventricle. Its location is anterior and superior within the ventricular mass and can be to the right of and anterior, strictly anterior, or to the left of and anterior to the main ventricular chamber (Fig. 17-2). The trabecular portion of the rudimentary right chamber is separated from the trabecular portion of the main chamber by a trabecular septum that hardly ever extends into the crux cordis (64) (Fig. 17-2). The trabecular and interatrial septa are malaligned, as are also, in cases with two separate atrioventricular valves, the trabecular septum and a posterior portion of the inlet septum located between the two atrioventricular valves. The spatial position of the trabecular septum varies according to the spatial position of the ventricular chambers. When the rudimentary right chamber is anterior and to the right, the trabecular septum is directed from posterior to anterior and from right to left; when the orientation of the ventricles is strictly anteroposterior, the septum is parallel to the frontal plane, and when the rudimentary right chamber is anterior and to the left with respect to the main chamber, the septum is directed from posterior to anterior and from left to right (Fig. 17-2). The septal defect is located within the trabecular septum and allows communication between the two ventricular chambers. It is totally muscular, being formed by the free border of the trabecular septum and the interinfundibular septum. Frequently, its shape is elliptical, similar to that of a buttonhole, and it usually tends to diminish in size with time, particularly if it is small initially. Occasionally, there can be more than one defect, either because a muscular band divides it, as is common in the presence of a rudimentary chamber located to the right with ventriculoarterial discordance (32), or because an additional apical trabecular defect is present (49).

Double-inlet right ventricle with a rudimentary left ventricular outlet chamber is seen in 12% to 27% of all cases of double-inlet ventricle (24,32,47,49). Two ventricular chambers are present within the ventricular mass. A main one, which receives flow from both atria through either two separate atrioventricular valves or through one common valve, has the characteristics of a right ventricle, with coarse trabeculations and a septomarginal trabecula on its septal surface. The location of the rudimentary left ventricular chamber is always posterior and inferior to the main ventricle. Usually, it is to the left of the main ventricle, but more rarely its location can be strictly posterior or posterior and to the right of the main ventricle (34,39,40,47,64–66) (Fig. 17-3). The trabecular septum, which separates the main right ventricle from the rudimentary left chamber, is posterior, and its spatial orientation depends on the location of the left ventricle within the ventricular mass. If the small left ventricular chamber is located posteriorly and leftward, the orientation of the septum is posterior to anterior and from right to left; when the rudimentary left ventricle is strictly posterior, the septum is parallel to the frontal plane; and when the left ventricular chamber is posterior and to the right, the direction of the septum is posterior to anterior and from left to right (Fig. 17-3). No matter what the location of the rudimentary left ventricular chamber, the septum almost always extends to the crux cordis (39,64). As in double-inlet left ventricle, the defect is totally muscular and in the majority of cases is located between the limbs of the septomarginal trabecula (47,65,67).

Double-inlet solitary or indeterminate ventricle has an incidence between 3% and 19% of all cases of double-inlet ventricle (24,32,47,49). Only one ventricular chamber is present, with coarse trabeculations but without clear morphologic characteristics of either an anatomic left or anatomic right ventricle.

Hearts with huge ventricular septal defects are not considered to have a univentricular atrioventricular connection because the trabecular characteristics of a right and left ventricle are recognizable within the apical portions of the ventricular chambers, which are separated by a remnant of trabecular septum. Consequently, these hearts have a biventricular atrioventricular connection (67).

The echocardiographic views that permit identification of the characteristics of the ventricular chambers and their spatial positions are the parasternal long-axis and short-axis views, the apical four-chamber and outflow views, and the subcostal four-chamber, short-axis, and outflow views. Visualization of the ventricular trabeculations, whether fine or coarse, and the presence of papillary muscles or of a septomarginal trabecula and a moderator band can aid in the definition of an anatomic left or right ventricle, respectively (Echos. 17-1–17-3). However, echocardiographically it is not always possible to clearly establish the distinction between the ventricles based solely on trabecular patterns. The location of the rudimentary chamber, whether anterior or posterior to the main chamber, and the orientation of the trabecular septum and its relationship to the atrioventricular valves permit inference of the ventricular chamber morphology (68) (Echos. 17-2, 17-4–17-6).

The same echocardiographic views permit examination of the septal or intercameral defect(s) and establishment of its location and size. The size of the defect is important in the overall clinical prognosis if one or both great vessels emerge from an outlet chamber. Subaortic stenosis has been shown to develop in neonates with double-inlet

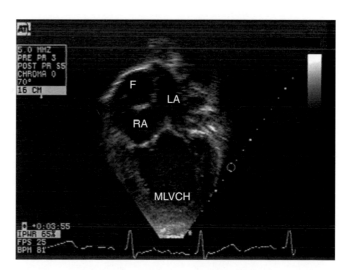

ECHO. 17-1. Apical view of a double-inlet left ventricle. Note the presence of two atrioventricular valves connecting to a single morphologic left ventricle. The Fontan connection is visible within the right atrium. *RA,* right atrium; *LA,* left atrium; *F,* Fontan connection; *MLVCH,* main left ventricular chamber.

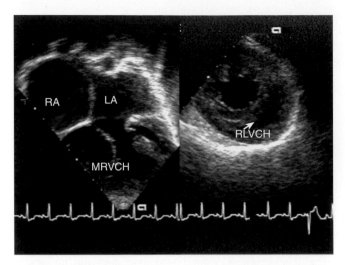

ECHO. 17-2. Left: Apical view of a double-inlet right ventricle. Note the small left ventricular chamber. **Right:** Parasternal short-axis view demonstrating the large anterior right ventricle and the very small posterior left ventricle. *RA*, right atrium; *LA*, left atrium; *MRVCH*, main right ventricular chamber; *RLVCH*, rudimentary left ventricular chamber.

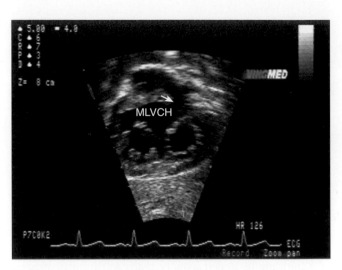

ECHO. 17-4. Subcostal short-axis view of the two atrioventricular valve orifices opening into a morphologic left ventricle. There is L looping with resulting atrioventricular and ventriculoarterial discordance. The left ventricle is located posteriorly and rightward and the right ventricle anteriorly and leftward. The *arrow* points to the bulboventricular foramen connecting the large left ventricle to the smaller anterior right ventricular chamber. *MLVCH*, main left ventricular chamber.

left ventricle, transposition of the great arteries, and defects measuring less than 2 cm²/m² (69); therefore, it is important to establish the size of the defect relative to body surface area and follow it closely by echocardiography. Spectral Doppler also allows estimation of the gradient across the defect, which can be used clinically to determine whether the defect is physiologically restrictive and to follow patients with one or both great arteries emerging from an outlet chamber. The best views to measure the velocity across the defect are the long- and short-

axis views, modified to allow interrogation in an orientation as parallel as possible to the direction of flow. This study can be greatly aided by the complementary use of color Doppler flow mapping (Echos. 17-4 – 17-7; see color plate 47 following p. 364).

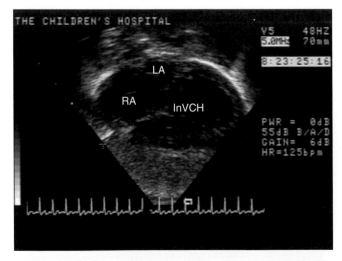

ECHO. 17-3. Subcostal four-chamber view in a patient with a double-inlet indeterminate ventricle. The left-sided atrioventricular valve is severely hypoplastic. Note the attachments of the right-sided atrioventricular valve to the same area at the ventricular apex. *LA*, left atrium; *RA*, right atrium; *InVCH*, indeterminate ventricular chamber.

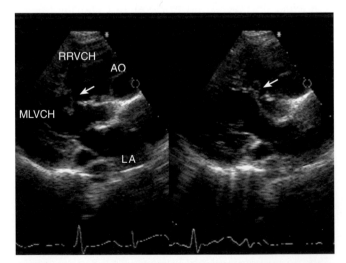

ECHO. 17-5. Left: Parasternal view demonstrating the bulboventricular foramen and straddling of the left-sided atrioventricular valve (*arrow*). A main left ventricular chamber gives rise to the pulmonary artery, and the aorta originates from an anterior rudimentary right ventricle. **Right:** Parasternal view with the transducer tilted to the right and inferiorly to better demonstrate the straddling of the left atrioventricular valve (*arrow*). *RRVCH*, rudimentary right ventricular chamber; *MLVCH*, main left ventricular chamber; *AO*, aorta; *LA*, left atrium.

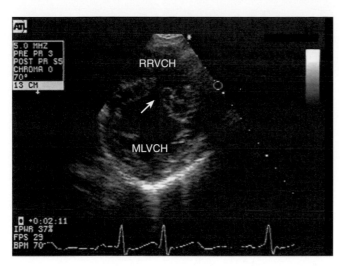

ECHO. 17-6. Parasternal short-axis view showing a main left ventricular chamber posteriorly and a rudimentary right ventricular chamber anteriorly connected through a bulbo-ventricular foramen (*arrow*). *RRVCH*, rudimentary right ventricular chamber; *MLVCH*, main left ventricular chamber.

Morphology of the Atrioventricular Valves or the Common Valve

In double-inlet ventricle, the connection of both atria to a single ventricle can be across two perforated atrioventricular valves or one common valve (Fig. 17-1). Double-inlet left ventricles are more commonly associated with two atrioventricular valves (Echo. 17-1), whereas a single, common atrioventricular valve is more frequently found in double-inlet right or double-inlet solitary or indeterminate ventricle.

It is often impossible to identify the morphologic characteristics of the atrioventricular valves; therefore, it is more convenient to use the terminology right and left atrioventricular valves in cases with two separate valves and right and left valvular components in cases with a common atrioventricular valve (49). However, it is important to point out that in double-inlet left ventricle with rudimentary right ventricular chamber, both atrioventricular valves usually have two leaflets, similar to a mitral valve (61).

Straddling or overriding of one of the atrioventricular valves or of the common valve can be seen with relative frequency. In the presence of straddling or overriding of either the right or left atrioventricular valve, if less than 50% of the annulus of the overriding valve is committed to the ventricle that receives the other valve, then the condition is not considered univentricular atrioventricular connection (47,70) (see Fig. 2-7D,E). In double-inlet left ventricle, straddling of the right atrioventricular valve is more common, although rarely there can be straddling of the left valve or of the common valve (Echo. 17-5). In a series of 137 cases of double-inlet ventricle, left ventricular type, Anderson et al. (47) found 17 cases of right

valve straddling (14%) and 13 cases of left valve straddling (8%) in the 126 cases with two perforated valves, and two cases of common atrioventricular valve straddling (18%) in the 11 instances of a common atrioventricular valve. Straddling of the right, left, or common atrioventricular valve in double-inlet ventricle, right ventricular type, is rare.

Other anomalies of the atrioventricular valves, such as stenosis, hypoplasia, or insufficiency, have been reported, but without relationship to the type of double-inlet ventricle or to the spatial orientation of the great arteries (37).

The echocardiographic views that are best for the study of the atrioventricular valve morphology are the parasternal long-axis and the apical and subcostal four-chamber views, as well as the short-axis projections from the parasternal and subcostal positions. From these, the presence of one common or of two separate valves can be determined (Echos. 17-1–17-4), as well as the presence of straddling or overriding (Echo. 17-5). The spatial relationship between the atrioventricular valves and the trabecular septum can also be studied from these views, particularly from the parasternal views, and can be used to infer the morphology of the ventricular chambers. In double-inlet left ventricle, the atrioventricular valves are located behind the trabecular septum (Echo. 17-4), whereas in double-inlet right ventricle, they are located in front of the septum (68) (Echo. 17-2). Doppler color flow mapping is useful in demonstrating the pattern of blood flow from the atria into the main and accessory ventricles, the relative streaming that may be present with straddling or overriding valves, and the existence of regurgitation. The forward flow and regurgitant jet velocities can be mea-

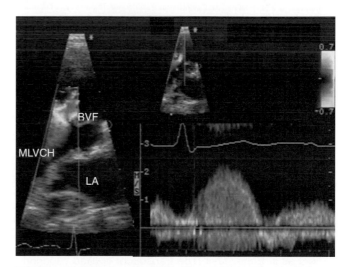

ECHO. 17-7. Color Doppler flow map and spectral recording of velocities across a mildly restrictive bulboventricular foramen connecting a main left ventricular chamber to an anterior rudimentary right ventricular chamber. *BVF*, bulboventricular foramen; *MLVCH*, main left ventricular chamber; *LA*, left atrium.

sured with spectral Doppler, and the appropriate gradients calculated.

Ventriculoarterial Connection and Spatial Position of the Great Arteries

When two ventricular chambers are present within the ventricular mass in cases of double-inlet ventricle, there can be any type of ventriculoarterial connection: concordant, discordant, double outlet of the main chamber (left or right type), double outlet of the rudimentary outlet chamber (right or left), and single outlet of one or the other chamber, which can be the of truncus arteriosus type or an absence of one of the semilunar valves. In double-inlet solitary or indeterminate ventricle, there can be only a double outlet or single outlet from that ventricle, the latter being either of the truncus arteriosus type or an absence of one of the semilunar valves (1,71).

In *double inlet, left ventricular type*, the most common ventriculoarterial connection is discordant, with the aorta emerging from the rudimentary right ventricle and the pulmonary artery from the main left ventricle (Figs. 17-6A, 17-7A) (Echos. 17-8, 17-9). This type of connection is found in 65% to 91% of cases of this malformation (18,24,38,47,72,73). Concordant connection—that is, origin of the pulmonary artery from the rudimentary chamber and of the aorta from the main one—is seen in 9% to 16% of cases (18,24,38,47,72,73) (Fig. 17-4A) (Echos. 17-10, 17-11). Double outlet from the main chamber is found in 5% to 17% of cases (Figs. 17-4C, 17-6C, 17-7C); double outlet from the rudimentary chamber in

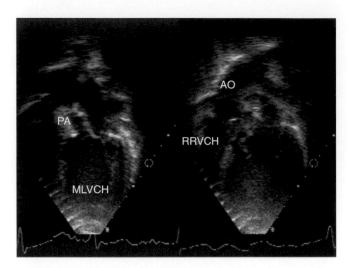

ECHO. 17-9. Apical views with the transducer tilted superiorly to demonstrate the ventriculoarterial connections. The main left ventricular chamber **(left)** is connected to the pulmonary artery, which in this case is stenotic. The rudimentary right ventricular chamber **(right)** is connected to the aorta. Discordant ventriculoarterial connection is the most common in double-inlet left ventricle. *PA*, pulmonary artery; *MLVCH*, main left ventricular chamber; *AO*, aorta; *RRVCH*, rudimentary right ventricular chamber.

4.3% to 4.5% (Figs. 17-4B, 17-6B, 17-7B); and single outlet from either the main or the rudimentary chamber in 8.5% (47,72) (Fig. 17-9).

In *double inlet, right ventricular type*, the most common ventriculoarterial connection is the double outlet from the main chamber, which has been seen in 40% to

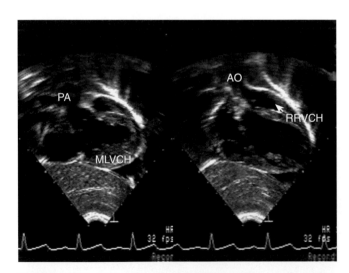

ECHO. 17-8. Subcostal four-chamber views in the same patient as in Echo. 17-4. The transducer is tilted superiorly to visualize the ventriculoarterial connections. The large morphologic left ventricular chamber **(left)** gives rise to the pulmonary artery. The small, rudimentary right ventricular chamber **(right)** gives rise to the aorta. *PA*, pulmonary artery; *MLVCH*, main left ventricular chamber; *AO*, aorta; *RRVCH*, rudimentary right ventricular chamber.

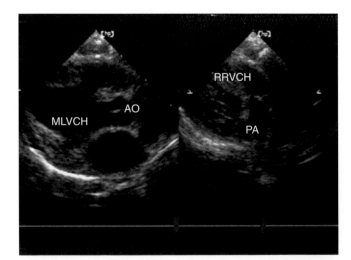

ECHO. 17-10. Left: Parasternal long-axis view in double-inlet left ventricle with concordant ventriculoarterial connection. **Right:** Parasternal view with the transducer tilted toward the right ventricular outflow tract demonstrating the connection between the rudimentary right ventricular chamber and the pulmonary artery. *MLVCH*, main left ventricular chamber; *AO*, aorta; *RRVCH*, rudimentary right ventricular chamber; *PA*, pulmonary artery.

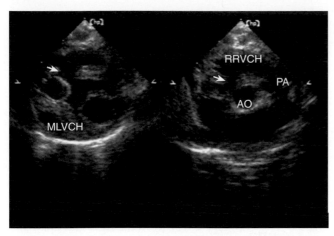

ECHO. 17-11. Parasternal short-axis views of concordant ventriculoarterial connection in double-inlet left ventricle. Short-axis view at the level of the ventricle (left) showing the two atrioventricular valve orifices opening into the main left ventricular chamber. The *arrow* points to the posterior extensions of the bulboventricular foramen. Short-axis view at the level of the great vessels (right) showing the pulmonary artery arising from the rudimentary right ventricular chamber. *Arrow* points to the superior-anterior extensions of the bulboventricular foramen. *MLVCH,* main left ventricular chamber; *RRVCH,* rudimentary right ventricular chamber; *PA,* pulmonary artery; *AO,* aorta.

100% of cases in various series (24,39,40,47,65,72) (Fig. 17-5C). It is followed in frequency by single outlet, with an incidence of 25% to 42% (24,40,45,47,65,72) (Fig. 17-10), and finally by concordant connection—that is, pulmonary artery from the main right ventricle and aorta from the rudimentary left ventricle, which has been seen in 9% to 32% of cases (40,47,65) (Fig. 17-5A).

Double inlet, indeterminate ventricular type, presents with double outlet in 85% of cases (Fig. 17-8A–C) and single outlet in 15% (47) (Fig. 17-8D–F). The great vessels can be side by side in double outlet, and there can be

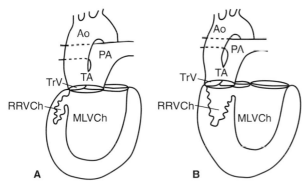

FIG. 17-9. Schematic drawings of double-inlet left ventricle and single outlet, truncus arteriosus type. A: Single-outlet main left ventricular chamber. B: Single-outlet outlet chamber. *MLVCh,* main left ventricular chamber; *RRVCh,* rudimentary right ventricular chamber; *TA,* truncus arteriosus; *TrV,* truncal valve; *Ao,* aorta; *PA,* pulmonary artery.

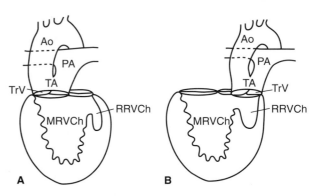

FIG. 17-10. Schematic drawings of double-inlet right ventricle with single outlet, truncus arteriosus type. A: Single-outlet main right ventricular chamber. B: Single-outlet outlet chamber. *MRVCh,* main right ventricular chamber; *RRVCh,* rudimentary left ventricular chamber; *TA,* truncus arteriosus; *TrV,* truncal valve; *Ao,* aorta; *PA,* pulmonary artery.

discontinuity between the semilunar and atrioventricular valves because of the presence of a bilateral muscular ventriculoinfundibular fold.

In all types of double-inlet ventricle (left, right, or indeterminate), the spatial relationship of the great arteries can have a wide variation. They can be normally related, with a posterior and rightward aorta and anterior and leftward pulmonary artery; side by side; with the aorta anterior and to the right; with the aorta strictly anterior; or with aorta anterior and to the left (Echos. 17-11, 17-12).

The ventriculoarterial connection can be seen from the parasternal long-axis view and the four-chamber apical and subcostal views with the transducer angled superiorly

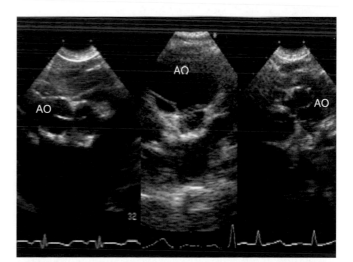

ECHO. 17-12. Parasternal short-axis views of various possible spatial relationships of the great vessels in double-inlet ventricle. Left: Strictly side-by-side relationship of the great vessels, with aorta to the right of the pulmonary artery. Middle: Aorta directly anterior to the smaller pulmonary artery. Right: Aorta to the left of and slightly anterior to the pulmonary artery. *AO,* aorta.

or anteriorly toward the outflow tracts (Echos. 17-5, 17-8–17-11). The spatial relationship of the great arteries is best appreciated from the parasternal short-axis view (Echos. 17-11, 17-12).

Outflow Tract Obstruction

In double-inlet ventricle, one can observe obstruction to the outflow tracts at the subvalvular or valvular level with a bicuspid valve. The size of the ventricular septal defect or intercameral communication and the type of ventriculoarterial connection should be considered in the study of these obstructions.

In double inlet, left ventricular type, obstruction at the intercameral communication, whether present at birth or appearing later, plays an important role in the development of infundibular obstruction of the vessel emerging from the outlet chamber. In cases of discordant connection in which the aorta is connected to the outlet chamber, the resulting subaortic obstruction is usually associated with aortic isthmic hypoplasia, coarctation, or aortic arch interruption. Obstruction of the infundibulum of the vessel emerging from the main chamber is rare and is usually subpulmonary; it can occur because of a posterior displacement of the outlet septum, the presence of a tissue tag, or abnormal implantation of an atrioventricular valve leaflet (67). On occasion, there may be atresia of either the subaortic or subpulmonary infundibulum; the latter is most commonly seen in hearts with ventriculoarterial discordance.

In double-inlet right ventricle with an accessory left ventricular chamber, there can be subvalvar aortic or pulmonary stenosis, especially when the great vessels are in an anteroposterior relationship (71).

Subvalvar aortic or pulmonary obstructions can also be found in double-inlet ventricle, indeterminate type. These can result from muscle bands producing subvalvar obstruction of either great vessel.

The echocardiographic views best suited to demonstrate outflow tract obstructions are the same as those used to study the ventriculoarterial connections—namely, the parasternal long- and short-axis views and the four-chamber views obtained from the apex and from the subcostal approach, with the transducer angled anteriorly or superiorly to reveal the outflow tracts and great vessels (Echos. 17-5, 17-9). The use of Doppler from these views permits estimation of the severity and determination of the site(s) of obstruction. Mapping the velocities across the outflow tracts with pulsed-wave and high pulsed repetition frequency (PRF) techniques demonstrates the gradient across the obstruction(s). Color flow mapping also aids in demonstrating the sites of obstruction (Echo. 17-7). Continuous-wave Doppler can be used to measure the highest velocity across the entire outflow tract, from which the total gradient can be calculated (Echo. 17-7).

Origin and Distribution of the Coronary Arteries

Anomalies in the origin and distribution of the coronary arteries vary according to the ventricular disposition (inverted or not) and the ventriculoarterial connection (concordant or not).

In double-inlet left ventricle without ventricular inversion (accessory right ventricular chamber located anterosuperiorly and to the right), the coronary pattern depends on the ventriculoarterial connection. If the great vessels are normally related, the coronary arteries have an origin and distribution that is similar to normal (21,23,74). The left coronary artery originates from the left anterior cusp and the right coronary artery from the right anterior cusp. The coronary branches that delimit the outlet chamber, called right and left delimiting coronary arteries (20), originate from the right and left coronary arteries, respectively. If the great vessels are transposed, with the aorta situated anteriorly and to the right, the coronary pattern is similar to that found in ventriculoarterial discordance, with the aorta anterior and to the right (74,75); the left coronary artery emerges from the right-sided cusp or sinus No. 1 and the right coronary artery from the left-sided cusp or sinus No. 2 (see Chapter 24).

Two coronary arterial patterns have been reported in double-inlet left ventricle with ventricular inversion and ventriculoarterial discordance (aorta emerging from right ventricular accessory chamber located anterosuperiorly and to the left) (75,76). There has been some confusion regarding the terminology used to describe the coronary patterns in this setting; we have found the one proposed by Lev and Rowlatt to be the most helpful—that is, left-sided and right-sided coronary artery (see Chapter 15). The most common pattern is that in which the left-sided coronary artery is an anatomic left coronary emerging from the left posterior cusp and the right-sided coronary artery is an anatomic right coronary emerging from the right posterior cusp. The other pattern described is similar to that found in congenitally corrected transposition of the great arteries.

In double-inlet right ventricle, the origin and distribution of the coronaries is similar to normal. The accessory left ventricular chamber, situated posteroinferiorly, is delimited by the anterior and posterior descending coronary arteries (67).

The echocardiographic short-axis views best demonstrate the origin and proximal distribution of the coronary arteries. From the parasternal window, the transducer may have to be positioned lower on the chest to obtain a better image of the proximal distribution of these arteries.

Associated Anomalies

Associated malformations include multiple ventricular septal defects; straddling and overriding of the atrioventricular valves; bicuspid aortic or pulmonary valves; single-outlet heart of the truncus arteriosus, pulmonary atresia, or aortic atresia type; coarctation of the aorta; and hypoplasia or interruption of the aortic arch. All these have been mentioned previously. In addition, there can be patent ductus arteriosus, atrial septal defect, parachute mitral valve, and anomalous systemic or pulmonary venous drainage, particularly in cases of situs ambiguus and right isomerism.

UNIVENTRICULAR ATRIOVENTRICULAR CONNECTION WITH ATRESIA OF ONE ATRIOVENTRICULAR VALVE

In a heart with univentricular atrioventricular connection, it is usually difficult to recognize the morphologic characteristics of a tricuspid or mitral valve; therefore, it is more appropriate to refer to such valves as right- or left-sided atrioventricular valves rather than tricuspid or mitral valves.

Atresia of one atrioventricular valve can be the result of either an imperforate valve or an absence of the atrioventricular connection. This can occur with either the right- or left-sided atrioventricular valve.

ATRESIA OF THE RIGHT-SIDED ATRIOVENTRICULAR VALVE

In this type of atrioventricular connection, there is no direct communication between the right atrium and the ventricular mass because of atresia of the tricuspid or right-sided atrioventricular valve. Such atresia is generally secondary to an absence of the right atrioventricular connection (classic tricuspid atresia), and rarely to the presence of an imperforate valvular membrane (tricuspid atresia with imperforate valve) (49,77,78). The first type represents a univentricular atrioventricular connection, with a main ventricular chamber and an accessory chamber present within the ventricular mass. There is a potential connection between the blind-ending right atrium and the main chamber but no potential connection with the rudimentary chamber (77) (see Fig. 2-6B). In the second type of atresia, with imperforate valve, there is a clear potential connection between the blind right atrium and the right ventricle because in these rare cases two ventricles are present with three recognizable ventricular components (inlet, trabecular, and outlet portions) (77,78) (see Fig. 2-7A). Therefore, this type of tricuspid atresia represents a biventricular atrioventricular connection and is discussed in Chapter 12.

The first description of a heart with absent right atrioventricular connection was made by Kreysig in 1817 (79); this case had associated complete transposition of the great arteries and coarctation of the aorta. The term

atresia was first proposed for this lesion by Schuberg in 1861 (80).

Atresia of the right-sided atrioventricular valve can present with different types of visceroatrial situs and bulboventricular looping.

Situs Solitus and D Looping. The morphologic right atrium is located to the right and ends blindly, communicating with the left atrium through a patent foramen ovale or atrial septal defect. The rudimentary right ventricular chamber is located anterosuperiorly and to the right, and the right-sided atrioventricular valve (''tricuspid valve'') is atretic. The anatomic left atrium is located on the left and communicates through a left-sided atrioventricular valve (''mitral valve'') with a dominant left ventricle, located posteroinferiorly and to the left. This type of atresia of the right-sided atrioventricular valve is called classic tricuspid atresia (see Fig. 2-6B).

Situs Solitus and L Looping. The morphologic right atrium, located to the right, is a blind-ending chamber that communicates with the left atrium through a patent foramen or atrial septal defect. A rudimentary left ventricular cavity is located to the right (ventricular inversion), and the right-sided atrioventricular valve (''mitral valve'') is atretic (mitral atresia). The anatomic left atrium, located to the left, communicates through a left-sided atrioventricular valve (''tricuspid valve'') with a dominant right ventricular chamber, located to the left (Fig. 17-11A).

Situs Inversus with L Looping. The morphologic right atrium is located to the left and communicates with a dominant right ventricle, located on the left, through a left-sided atrioventricular valve (''tricuspid valve''). The anatomic left atrium, located to the right, ends blindly and communicates with the right atrium through a patent foramen or atrial septal defect. The rudimentary left ventricular chamber is located to the right, and the right-sided atrioventricular valve (''mitral valve'') is atretic (mitral atresia) (Fig. 17-11B).

Situs Inversus and D Looping. The morphologic right atrium is located to the left and communicates with the main anatomic left ventricular chamber, located on the left (ventricular inversion), through a left-sided atrioventricular valve (''mitral valve''). The morphologic left atrium ends blindly and communicates with the right atrium through an atrial defect or patent foramen ovale. The rudimentary right ventricular chamber is located to the right, and the right-sided atrioventricular valve (''tricuspid valve'') is atretic (tricuspid atresia) (Fig. 17-11C).

Situs Ambiguus and D Looping. The ventricular chambers are normally related, with the right ventricle on the right and the left ventricle on the left. The right-sided atrioventricular valve is atretic (tricuspid atresia) (Fig. 17-11D).

Situs Ambiguus and L Looping. The right ventricular chamber is located to the left and the left ventricular cavity is on the right (ventricular inversion). The right-

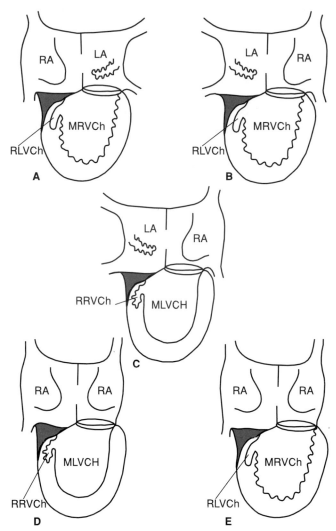

FIG. 17-11. Schematic drawings demonstrating the various types of absent right atrioventricular connection. The *shaded area* indicates the fibrofatty tissue in the right atrioventricular sulcus. **A:** Situs solitus and L loop. **B:** Situs inversus and L loop. **C:** Situs inversus and D loop. **D:** Situs ambiguus, bilateral right-sidedness, and D loop. **E:** Situs ambiguus, bilateral right-sidedness, and L loop. *RA*, right atrium; *LA*, left atrium; *MRVCh*, main right ventricular chamber; *RLVCh*, rudimentary left ventricular chamber; *MLVCh*, main left ventricular chamber; *RRVCh*, rudimentary right ventricular chamber.

sided atrioventricular valve is atretic (mitral atresia) (Fig. 17-11E).

Hearts with situs solitus and D looping, situs inversus and D looping, and situs ambiguus and D looping represent types of "tricuspid atresia." Those with situs solitus and L looping, situs inversus and L looping, and situs ambiguus and L looping correspond to types of "mitral atresia." All these are considered types of absent right atrioventricular connection, irrespective of the morphology of the valve.

The first classification of tricuspid atresia was by Kuhne in 1906 (81), who established two groups, one with normally related great arteries and one with transposition of the great vessels. Edwards and Burchell (82) utilized the same criteria of the ventriculoarterial connection for their classification into type I, with normally related great arteries, and type II, with transposed great arteries. In each of these two types, they recognized three subtypes based on obstruction to pulmonary flow: subtype A, with pulmonary atresia; subtype B, with pulmonary hypoplasia or stenosis; and subtype C, without pulmonary stenosis. A modification of these classifications was proposed by Vlad (83), who used type II of Edwards and Burchell as tricuspid atresia with complete transposition of the great arteries and aorta located anteriorly and to the right (D transposition) and created a type III as tricuspid atresia with ventricular inversion and aorta positioned anteriorly and to the left (L transposition of the great arteries). This latter type included two subtypes: subtype A, with pulmonary or subpulmonary stenosis, and subtype B, with aortic stenosis. This author includes in type III a case of situs solitus and L looping with absent right atrioventricular connection (right-sided mitral valve).

Inclusion of the various types of ventriculoarterial connections and great vessel malpositions was proposed by Rao (84). In his classification, there are four types of tricuspid atresia. Types I and II are the same as in the Edwards and Burchell (82) and Vlad (83) classifications. Type III, with malposed great arteries, includes five subtypes: subtype 1, with L transposition of the great arteries; subtype 2, with double-outlet right ventricle; subtype 3, with double-outlet left ventricle; subtype 4, with D malposition of the great arteries; and subtype 5, with L malposition of the great arteries. Type IV includes cases with persistent truncus arteriosus, and along with the subtypes in type III, these are further divided into three subgroups: subgroup A, with pulmonary atresia; subgroup B, with pulmonary hypoplasia or stenosis; and subgroup C, without pulmonary stenosis. In the reevaluation of the classification of tricuspid atresia of Tandon and Edwards (85), cases of tricuspid atresia with situs solitus and L looping are included. These cases, in which a right atrium is connected with a dominant left ventricular chamber, located to the right, and the left atrium ends blindly and has no connection with the rudimentary right ventricular chamber, located to the left, should be considered as absent left atrioventricular connection and not as "tricuspid atresia" (Fig. 17-12A).

EMBRYOLOGIC CONSIDERATIONS

Several theories attempt to explain the morphogenesis of univentricular atrioventricular connection with absent right atrioventricular connection. The morphogenetic mechanisms would be the same as those mentioned under double-inlet ventricle but would also include anomalous development of the right atrioventricular valve. The failure of a balanced expansion of the ventricles, resulting in

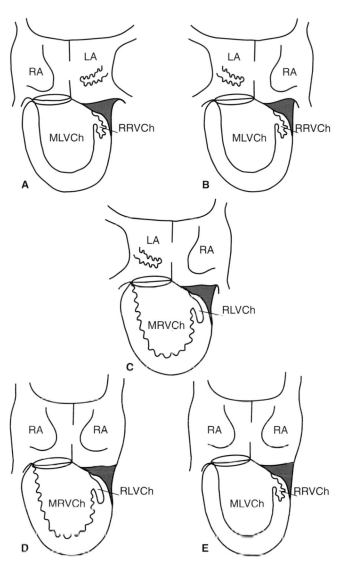

FIG. 17-12 Schematic drawing of the various types of absent left atrioventricular connection. The *shaded areas* indicate the fibrofatty tissue in the left atrioventricular sulcus. **A:** Situs solitus and L loop. **B:** Situs inversus and L loop. **C:** Situs inversus and D loop. **D:** Situs ambiguus, bilateral right-sidedness, and D loop. **E:** Situs ambiguus, bilateral right-sidedness, and L loop. *RA*, right atrium; *LA*, left atrium; *MLVCh*, main left ventricular chamber; *RRVCh*, rudimentary right ventricular chamber; *MRVCh*, main right ventricular chamber; *RLVCh*, rudimentary left ventricular chamber.

malalignment between the interventricular and interatrial septa and abnormality of the endocardial cushions, has been mentioned by Ando et al. (58) in the explanation of a spectrum of malformations that would include tricuspid atresia. Other authors consider that the absence of a right atrioventricular connection is caused by a fusion of tissue surrounding the right atrioventricular orifice, resulting in atresia of that orifice (62,86,87). The absence of a subvalvular apparatus or of remnants of that apparatus, seen in this anomaly, would occur as a result of early closure of the right atrioventricular orifice, preventing the later delamination and undermining of the ventricular walls, which normally form the subvalvular apparatus.

ANATOMIC AND ECHOCARDIOGRAPHIC CONSIDERATIONS

The echocardiographic examination in absent right atrioventricular connection should include, in addition to determination of visceroatrial situs and systemic and pulmonary drainage, the following: (a) morphology of the cardiac chambers; (b) ventricular septal or intercameral defect; (c) outflow tract obstruction; (d) ventriculoarterial connection and spatial relationship of the great vessels; (e) origin and distribution of the coronary arteries; and (e) associated anomalies.

Morphology of the Cardiac Chambers

In absent right atrioventricular connection, considered classic tricuspid atresia, the morphologic right atrium is almost always dilated, located to the right (visceroatrial situs solitus), and separated from the rudimentary right ventricular chamber by fibrofatty tissue occupying the right atrioventricular sulcus. This tissue separates the atrial from the ventricular myocardium so that there is no continuity between them along the atrioventricular sulcus, but only at the level of the central fibrous body of the heart (88) (see Fig. 2-6B). The floor of the right atrium is completely muscular, and in 25% of cases a dimple appears at the site where the right atrioventricular valve should be (89). At this point, a potential connection with the main left ventricular chamber can be established, but not with the rudimentary right ventricular chamber (77). The right atrium communicates with the morphologic left atrium, located on the left, through a patent foramen ovale or, more frequently, across an ostium secundum atrial septal defect. The left atrium is morphologically normal and connects through a mitral valve with the main left ventricular chamber, located to the left and posteriorly in respect to the rudimentary chamber, which is in an anterosuperior and rightward position (see Fig. 2-6B). Rarely, the mitral valve can straddle the intercameral septum. The septum separating the ventricular chambers does not extend to the crux cordis, similar to the situation in double-inlet left ventricle (64). The rudimentary right ventricular chamber lacks an inlet portion and is composed of only a trabecular and an outlet portion. No subvalvular apparatus or remnants of such an apparatus are present. Rarely, the rudimentary right ventricular chamber can be located in a strictly anterior or anterior and leftward position (77).

The echocardiographic four-chamber views, apical or subcostal, demonstrate clearly the absence of a right atrioventricular connection. The right atrium is separated from the rudimentary right ventricle by a thick band of tissue corresponding to the muscular floor of the right atrium and to the fibrofatty tissue of the right atrioventricular sulcus (Echo. 17-13). These views also reveal the presence of a patent foramen ovale or atrial septal defect as well as the bulging of atrial septum to the left when the defect is restrictive. Doppler color flow mapping demonstrates the right-to-left shunting across the atrial communication. Spectral Doppler is used to measure the velocity of flow as an estimate of the gradient between the two atria, which is of clinical importance.

The parasternal and subcostal short-axis views are the most helpful to demonstrate the spatial position of the main ventricle and rudimentary chamber. The presence of an anterior rudimentary chamber implies that it is morphologically of the right type and that the main ventricle is of the left ventricular type.

Ventricular Septal or Intercameral Defect

In the majority of cases of absent right atrioventricular connection, a ventricular septal defect connects the main left ventricular chamber with the rudimentary right ventricular chamber. It is a totally muscular defect, frequently located between the trabecular portion and outlet portion of the septum. Its size is variable and should be analyzed carefully because a restrictive defect can close functionally or anatomically, with clinical consequences to the patient (90,91). Hypoxic crises, typical of tetralogy of Fallot, have also been seen in absent right atrioventricular connection and have been related to functional closure of the septal defect (90). The definitive anatomic closure of these defects can be caused by progressive muscular

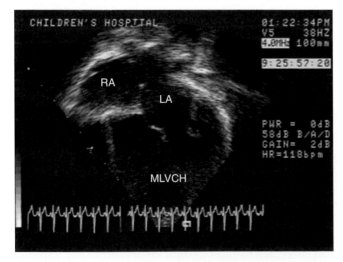

ECHO. 17-13. Apical view of univentricular atrioventricular connection resulting from atresia of the right-sided atrioventricular valve. Note that there is no potential connection between the right atrium and rudimentary right ventricle. *RA*, right atrium; *LA*, left atrium; *MLVCH*, main left ventricular chamber.

encroachment along its borders, with fibrosis and endocardial proliferation (91). Multiple ventricular septal defects can also occur with tricuspid atresia (92).

The echocardiographic views that best allow demonstration and sizing of the defect are the parasternal long-axis, apical and subcostal four-chamber, and short-axis views. Color Doppler defines the site(s) of shunting, which can be from left to right or bidirectional. Spectral Doppler recording of the shunt flow velocity is essential for assessing the possible progressive closure of the defect.

Outflow Tract Obstruction

In approximately half of cases of absent right atrioventricular connection with normally related great vessels, the pulmonary flow is obstructed at the level of the intercameral defect or at the subvalvular level. The pulmonary valve is usually normal, but even in the presence of a bicuspid valve, there is usually no stenosis at the valvular level. Pulmonary valve atresia is seen in approximately 10% of cases of absent right atrioventricular connection with normally related great arteries; in these instances, the rudimentary chamber is very hypoplastic and can even be limited to a small, endothelialized cavity within the ventricular mass (93).

In the presence of ventriculoarterial discordance, there can be obstruction to the systemic flow at the level of the ventricular septal or intercameral defect. This defect tends toward progressive spontaneous closure and is usually associated with a variable degree of aortic isthmic hypoplasia or aortic coarctation. Subpulmonary stenosis, caused by displacement of the outlet septum into the main left ventricular chamber, can also be present (88).

The echocardiographic evaluation of these obstructions is similar to the technique described for obstructions in double-inlet ventricles (see above).

Ventriculoarterial Connection and Spatial Relationship of the Great Vessels

In absent right atrioventricular connection, termed classic tricuspid atresia, a concordant ventriculoarterial connection is most common, seen in 60% to 70% of cases (83,86,93). The pulmonary artery emerges from the rudimentary right ventricular chamber and is located anteriorly and to the left with respect to the aorta, which emerges from the main left ventricular chamber. There is usually fibrous continuity between the aortic and mitral valves. The rudimentary right ventricular chamber is almost always of an acceptable size when ventriculoarterial concordance is present, irrespective of the size of the ventricular septal defect (88). As mentioned above, in the presence of pulmonary atresia and normally related great arteries, the rudimentary right ventricular chamber is usually very small.

In rare instances, a concordant ventriculoarterial connection can be seen with the aorta emerging from the main left ventricular chamber but occupying an anterior and leftward position (anatomically corrected malposition of the great arteries).

The second most common type of ventriculoarterial connection is a discordant ventriculoarterial connection in which the aorta is located anteriorly and rightward. In these cases, the rudimentary right ventricular chamber is less developed and its outlet portion is shorter (89). The ventricular defect is usually small and tends toward progressive spontaneous closure. The aorta can also be located anteriorly or anteriorly and to the left, but this is rare.

Other types of ventriculoarterial connection, such as double outlet of the right or left ventricular type and single outlet of the truncus arteriosus type, can also be seen.

The ventriculoarterial connection can be defined echocardiographically through the parasternal and apical long-axis views and the four chamber apical and subcostal views, with angulation of the transducer superiorly toward the outflows. Color Doppler demonstrates the origin and preferential direction of flow into the great vessels and the relation of the intercameral defect to the semilunar valves. The spatial relationship of the great vessels can be defined best through the parasternal and subcostal short-axis views.

Origin and Distribution of the Coronary Arteries

The origin and distribution of the coronary arteries in absent right atrioventricular connection are not substantially different from those of double-inlet left ventricle (94). The patterns are related to the types of ventriculoarterial connection, which have been covered in the preceding section on double-inlet ventricle. The short-axis views from parasternal and subcostal windows are the best to define the coronary arteries.

Associated Anomalies

In addition to the associations mentioned above, tricuspid atresia can be seen in association with juxtaposition of the atrial appendages; abnormal systemic or pulmonary venous drainage, especially a persistent left superior vena cava; Ebstein's anomaly; unroofed coronary sinus; and patent ductus arteriosus.

ATRESIA OF THE LEFT-SIDED ATRIOVENTRICULAR VALVE

In this type of univentricular atrioventricular connection, there is no direct connection of the morphologic left atrium with the ventricular mass because of atresia of the left-sided atrioventricular valve. As in tricuspid atresia, in the majority of cases this is secondary to an absence of the left atrioventricular connection (classic mitral atresia). Much more rarely, it is secondary to an imperforate valvular membrane (mitral atresia due to imperforate valve) (49,64,92,95–98). In the first case, a main ventricular chamber and an accessory chamber are present within the ventricular mass, and there is no potential connection between the blind-ending morphologic left atrium and the rudimentary ventricular chamber (see Fig. 2-6C). In the second type, a potential connection between the blind left atrium and the left ventricle can be established, and consequently the atrioventricular connection is biventricular (see Fig. 2-7B). This situation is considered in Chapter 13.

Like atresia of the right-sided atrioventricular valve, atresia of the left-sided valve can be found with different types of visceroatrial situs and bulboventricular loop.

Situs Solitus and D Looping. The morphologic right atrium is located on the right and connects with a main right ventricular chamber, located on the right, through a patent right-sided valve ("tricuspid valve"). The morphologic left atrium, located on the left, is blind and communicates with the right atrium through a patent foramen ovale or atrial septal defect. The rudimentary left ventricular chamber is located on the left, and the left-sided atrioventricular valve ("mitral valve") is atretic (classic mitral atresia) (see Fig. 2-6C).

Situs Solitus and L Looping. The morphologic right atrium is located to the right and communicates through a right-sided atrioventricular valve ("mitral valve") with a main left ventricular chamber that is located to the right (ventricular inversion). The morphologic left atrium is a blind-ending chamber that communicates through a patent foramen ovale or atrial septal defect with the right atrium. The rudimentary right ventricle is located on the left, and the left-sided atrioventricular valve ("tricuspid valve") is atretic (tricuspid atresia) (Fig. 17-12A).

Situs Inversus and L Looping. The morphologic left atrium is located to the right and communicates through a right-sided atrioventricular valve ("mitral valve") with a dominant left ventricular chamber. The anatomic right atrium is located on the left and communicates with the anatomic left atrium through a patent foramen ovale or atrial septal defect. The rudimentary right ventricular chamber is located on the left, and the left-sided atrioventricular valve ("tricuspid valve") is atretic (tricuspid atresia) (Fig. 17-12B).

Situs Inversus with D Looping. The morphologic left atrium is located to the right and connects through the right-sided atrioventricular valve ("tricuspid valve") with a dominant right ventricular chamber, located on the right. The anatomic right atrium, located on the left, is blind-ending and communicates with the anatomic left atrium through a patent foramen ovale or atrial septal defect. The rudimentary left ventricular chamber is located on the left, and the left-sided atrioventricular valve ("mitral valve") is atretic (mitral atresia) (Fig. 17-12C).

Situs Ambiguus with D Looping. The ventricular chambers are normally related, with the main right ventricular chamber located on the right and the rudimentary left ventricular cavity on the left. The left-sided atrioventricular valve ("mitral valve") is atretic (mitral atresia) (Fig. 17-12D).

Situs Ambiguus and L Looping. The dominant left ventricle is on the right and the rudimentary right ventricular chamber is on the left (ventricular inversion). The left-sided atrioventricular valve ("tricuspid valve") is atretic (tricuspid atresia) (Fig. 17-12E).

Hearts with situs solitus and D looping, situs inversus and D looping, and situs ambiguus and D looping can be considered to have "mitral atresia." Those with situs solitus and L looping, situs inversus and L looping, and situs ambiguus and L looping can be considered to have "tricuspid atresia." All these types are considered to have an absent left atrioventricular connection, irrespective of the morphology of the valves.

Most cases of univentricular atrioventricular connection with absent left atrioventricular connection are associated with aortic atresia and fall within the spectrum of hypoplastic left ventricle or hypoplastic left-heart syndrome when hypoplasia of the aortic arch is present. This type of mitral atresia is discussed in Chapter 21.

Cases of univentricular atrioventricular connection with an absent left atrioventricular connection but a patent aortic valve are the topic of this section. In this type of univentricular atrioventricular connection, the right atrium connects with a main morphologic right ventricular chamber, and the left atrium has no potential connection with the rudimentary left ventricular chamber. These cases are described in the literature as mitral atresia with a patent or normal aortic valve (97,99,100).

EMBRYOLOGIC CONSIDERATIONS

The morphogenetic mechanisms causing this anomaly are the same as those described for double-inlet ventricle (see above), along with an abnormality in the development of the left atrioventricular valve. Mechanisms similar to those for tricuspid atresia—failure of a balanced expansion of the ventricles, consequent malalignment of the interventricular and interatrial septa, and an associated anomaly of the tissues of the endocardial cushions—have been implicated as causes of mitral atresia (58). An exaggerated growth, or alternately a fusion of tissues of the endocardial cushions at the level of the left atrioventricular orifice, has also been mentioned (99,101).

ANATOMIC AND ECHOCARDIOGRAPHIC CONSIDERATIONS

The echocardiographic study of mitral atresia with patent aortic valve should define the visceroatrial situs and systemic and pulmonary venous drainage and should also determine the following: (a) morphology of the cardiac chambers; (b) ventricular septal or intercameral defect; (c) outflow tract obstructions; (d) ventriculoarterial connection and spatial relationship of the great vessels; (e) origin and distribution of the coronary arteries; and (f) associated anomalies.

Morphology of the Cardiac Chambers

The morphologic right atrium is usually dilated and located to the right (in situs solitus); it connects through a right-sided atrioventricular valve (tricuspid valve) with a main right ventricular chamber, located anteriorly and to the right. Rarely, the right-sided atrioventricular valve can straddle the intercameral septum. The morphologic left atrium, usually small in size, is located on the left and communicates with the right atrium through a patent foramen ovale or atrial septal defect. Its floor is totally muscular, with a dimple at the site where the left atrioventricular valve would be located. It is separated from the rudimentary left ventricular chamber by fibrofatty tissue occupying the left atrioventricular sulcus. The rudimentary left ventricular chamber is usually hypoplastic and occupies a posterior and leftward position; it has a trabecular and an outlet portion but no inlet portion and no subvalvular apparatus (95). In cases of double outlet from the main chamber, the rudimentary left ventricle is only a trabecular pouch. The ventricular or intercameral septum almost always extends to the crux cordis, as in double-inlet right ventricle (49,95,97). However, Anderson et al. (64) described a case of univentricular atrioventricular connection of the right ventricular type with absent left atrioventricular connection and straddling and overriding of the right atrioventricular valve in which the trabecular septum did not extend to the crux cordis.

The same echocardiographic views utilized in absent right-sided atrioventricular connection are also useful in the visualization of an absent left connection. These include the long-axis parasternal view and the four-chamber apical and subcostal views (Echo. 17-14). The left atrium is seen to be separated from the rudimentary left ventricle by a thick band of tissue corresponding to the floor of the left atrium and to the fibrofatty tissue of the left atrioventricular sulcus. The four-chamber subcostal views also permit evaluation of the atrial septum for the presence of a patent foramen ovale or atrial septal defect and sizing of any communication. Bulging of the septum to the right suggests a restrictive defect. Color Doppler flow mapping shows the obligatory left-to-right shunting, and pulsed-

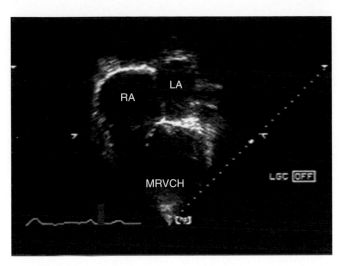

ECHO. 17-14. Apical view of univentricular atrioventricular connection resulting from atresia of the left-sided atrioventricular valve. Note the thick band of tissue corresponding to the muscular floor of the left atrium and the lack of a potential connection between the left atrium and a rudimentary left ventricular chamber. *RA*, right atrium; *LA*, left atrium; *MRVCH*, main right ventricular chamber.

wave Doppler sampling of velocities allows evaluation of any gradient between the atria.

The short-axis views from parasternal and subcostal positions allow inference of the morphology of the ventricular chambers according to their spatial positions. A rudimentary right ventricular chamber is located anteriorly, and a rudimentary left ventricular cavity posteriorly.

Ventricular Septal or Intercameral Defect

Almost always, a ventricular septal defect, which can be perimembranous or muscular, isolated or multiple, is present. In perimembranous defects, the roof of the defect is one of the semilunar valves, either the aortic or the pulmonary valve. When the defect is totally muscular, all its borders are muscular, and it is separated from the semilunar valves. In the rare instances of intact ventricular septum, usually a double outlet from the main ventricular chamber is seen (95).

The echocardiographic views that best analyze the ventricular or intercameral septum are the parasternal long- and short-axis and the apical and subcostal four-chamber views. These views demonstrate the presence and location of the defect and the relationship to the semilunar valves. Doppler color flow mapping aids in the demonstration of the site(s) of shunting, particularly if the defect(s) is anatomically small. Color Doppler also helps in the alignment of the spectral (pulsed- or continuous-wave) Doppler sampling line for recording of velocities and calculation of the gradient across the defect.

Outflow Tract Obstructions

Various degrees of aortic arch obstruction are seen in cases of absent left atrioventricular connection, particularly in the presence of concordant ventriculoarterial connection and normally related great arteries. Less commonly, aortic obstruction is present with anatomically corrected malposition of the great arteries or with ventriculoarterial discordance. In cases of double outlet from the main right ventricular chamber, aortic coarctation or aortic arch hypoplasia is also common (95,97).

Subpulmonary obstruction is also frequently seen in cases with double outlet from the dominant right ventricle and in cases with transposition of the great arteries. Pulmonary atresia is more common in double outlet from the dominant right chamber than in the presence of ventriculoarterial concordant or discordant connections.

Occasionally, the ventricular septal or intercameral defect can be restrictive, causing subaortic obstruction in cases of ventriculoarterial concordance or subpulmonary obstruction in cases of double outlet from the dominant right ventricular chamber or of ventriculoarterial discordance (95).

The outflow tracts are studied echocardiographically from the long-axis and four-chamber views, with the transducer angled toward the ventricular outflows. Mapping of velocities with pulsed-wave and high PRF Doppler reveals the level(s) and site(s) of obstruction; this can be facilitated with the use of color Doppler flow mapping, which demonstrates aliasing of velocities at the obstruction. The total gradient can be estimated from the velocities recorded with continuous-wave Doppler.

Ventriculoarterial Connection and Spatial Relationship of the Great Arteries

The ventriculoarterial connection in hearts with absent left atrioventricular connection and patent aortic valve can be concordant, discordant, double-outlet of the main chamber, or single-outlet of the pulmonary atresia type. The most commonly seen type is double-outlet from the main right ventricular chamber, which is found in 46.5% to 55% of cases (95,97). The next most commonly found type is the concordant ventriculoarterial connection, with an incidence of 40% to 45% (95,97). Most rarely, discordant connection occurs in 6% of cases (95).

Echocardiographically, the parasternal long-axis view and the four-chamber views obtained from the apex or subcostal approach with the transducer angled superiorly to the outflow tracts can demonstrate the ventriculoarterial connection. Color Doppler can aid in determining the direction and preferential flow of blood into the great arteries. The parasternal and subcostal short-axis views serve to demonstrate the spatial relationship of the great vessels.

Origin and Distribution of the Coronary Arteries

The origin and distribution of the coronaries in this type of univentricular atrioventricular connection are not substantially different from those seen in double-inlet ventricle. These have already been discussed in that section (see above).

Associated Anomalies

Associated anomalies found in absent left atrioventricular connection, in addition to those already mentioned, are bicuspid aortic and pulmonary valve, patent ductus arteriosus, persistent left superior vena cava draining into the coronary sinus, partial anomalous pulmonary venous drainage, and cor triatriatum.

INTRAOPERATIVE AND POSTOPERATIVE EVALUATION

Palliative operations in these complex lesions vary according to the underlying physiology. In the presence of increased pulmonary blood flow, banding of the pulmonary artery should be performed within the first 3 months of life to prevent an increase in pulmonary resistances (Echo. 17-15; see color plate 48 following p. 364). This should be followed by a superior vena cava-to-pulmonary artery anastomosis by 6 to 8 months of age to control the pulmonary flows further and protect the main ventricular chamber from volume overload and dilatation. In the presence of severe cyanosis resulting from obstruction of the pulmonary outflow, a systemic-to-pulmonary anastomosis of the modified Blalock-

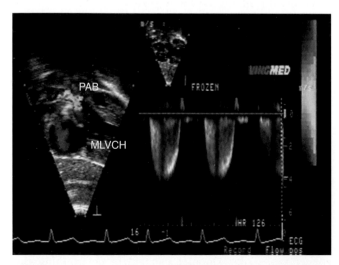

ECHO. 17-15. Subcostal view tilted superiorly to image the banded pulmonary artery emerging from a main left ventricular chamber. Note the aliasing of the color Doppler flow and the high velocity spectral signal across the band. *PAB*, pulmonary artery band; *MLVCH*, main left ventricular chamber.

Taussig type would be performed in the early newborn period (71,102,103), when cavopulmonary anastomoses are still not feasible physiologically. The interatrial communication should be evaluated carefully and if judged restrictive should be increased by balloon or blade septostomy in the cardiac catheterization laboratory (71) or by septectomy at surgery (71,104). In cases of obstruction of the systemic outflow tract, several options are available: (a) increasing the ventricular septal or intercameral defect with banding of the pulmonary artery (105); (b) palliative arterial switch operation, resulting in physiologic pulmonary banding (106); (c) creation of an anastomosis between the pulmonary artery and aorta, with transection of the pulmonary trunk and creation of a systemic-pulmonary, cavopulmonary, or atriopulmonary shunt (107–109); and (d) placement of a conduit between the ventricular apex and descending aorta (110). Correction of any associated aortic arch anomalies, such as coarctation or arch interruption, usually needs to be performed soon after birth. In these palliative operations, the use of intraoperative echocardiographic monitoring is limited. In atrial septostomies conducted in the catheterization laboratory, transesophageal or transthoracic echocardiographic monitoring can be very useful to ensure correct localization of the atrial septum, which can be in unusual orientations because of malalignment with the ventricular septum and hypoplasia of one of the atrial cavities. The serial evaluations after palliative surgery should address those issues of importance in preparation for additional procedures. These include determination of the size of the interatrial and intercameral communications and estimation of the gradients across the defects, determination of the adequacy of the pulmonary arterial banding, estimation of pulmonary arterial pressures through Doppler techniques, evaluation of the presence and severity of atrioventricular valvar regurgitation and systolic and diastolic dominant ventricular function, and assessment of the adequacy of the aortic arch repairs if these have been required.

The objective of the more definitive surgical procedures for these defects is the separation of the pulmonary and systemic circulations. In double-inlet ventricle, septation has been suggested (111), consisting of dividing the main ventricular chamber into two chambers of adequate size and function.

The other alternatives are the so-called right-heart bypass operations. The first right-heart bypass was reported by Fontan and Baudet in 1971 for the treatment of tricuspid atresia (112). Originally, the technique consisted of performing a Glenn type of anatomosis between the superior vena cava and right pulmonary artery, placing a valve at the inferior vena caval-right atrial junction, closing the atrial communication, transecting the pulmonary trunk with oversewing of the proximal end, and placing a valved conduit between the right atrium and distal pulmonary artery. In 1973, Kreutzer et al. (113) proposed two variations of the technique for tricuspid atresia. One included partial closure of the foramen ovale, transection of the pulmonary trunk with closure of the proximal end, and placement of a pulmonary homograft between the right atrial appendage and distal pulmonary artery. The second variation consisted of anatomosing the pulmonary artery proper, including its valve, to the right atrial appendage. Since then, several modifications have been made to the technique, known as atriopulmonary connection or Fontan-Kreutzer operation. This surgical approach, originally proposed for tricuspid atresia, is now used commonly in absent left atrioventricular connection and in double-inlet right and double-inlet left ventricle.

The various modifications now generally used include the bidirectional Glenn anastomosis, the atrioventricular anastomosis, the total cavopulmonary anastomosis, and the fenestrated Fontan operation. The Glenn anastomosis or cavopulmonary shunt (114), originally used in the Fontan operation, consists of an anastomosis between the superior vena cava and the distal right pulmonary artery, with closure of the proximal end of the right pulmonary artery. All the superior vena caval flow is directed into the right lung; therefore, flow is unidirectional. The bidirectional cavopulmonary shunt, or bidirectional Glenn operation, consists of an end-to-side anastomosis of the superior vena cava, transected just above its junction to the right atrium, into the superior surface of the right pulmonary artery; the anatomic integrity of the pulmonary branches is maintained (115) (Echo. 17-16; see color plate 49 following p. 364). From the physiologic standpoint, the

cavopulmonary shunt presents several advantages over a systemic-to-pulmonary shunt. First, it allows more desaturated blood to reach the lungs, thereby increasing the systemic oxygen saturation; second, by directing a part of the systemic venous return directly into the lungs, the volume overload of the heart is reduced; in contrast, a systemic-to-pulmonary shunt increases it (109).

In some cases of tricuspid atresia with ventriculoarterial concordance and an acceptable subpulmonary chamber judged to be of sufficient size to contribute to pulmonary blood flow, an atrioventricular anastomosis has been proposed. This technique consists of closure of the atrial and ventricular communications and placement of a valved conduit between the right atrial appendage and rudimentary right ventricular chamber. The advantage of a direct atriopulmonary anastomosis is that a valved conduit between the right atrium and pulmonary artery is not used (Echo. 17-17; see color plate 50 following p. 364). This technique includes closure of the septal defects and creation of an anastomosis between the roof of the right atrium and inferior surface of the right pulmonary branch or distal end of the main pulmonary trunk, which is completed with a Dacron patch. On occasion, a bidirectional Glenn has been performed in conjunction with a direct atriopulmonary anastomosis (109). The total cavopulmonary anastomosis includes a bidirectional Glenn and placement of an intraatrial conduit or baffle to connect the inferior and superior venae cavae.

In cases of absent left atrioventricular connection, the atrial defect is not closed; rather, it is sometimes augmented to prevent obstruction of the pulmonary venous return into the right atrioventricular valve.

A total cavopulmonary anastomosis and fenestration of the intraatrial baffle, known as the fenestrated Fontan operation (116), or the creation of an adjustable atrial septal defect, the partial Fontan operation (117,118), has as its objective the creation of a right-to-left shunt to diminish the systemic venous pressure in cases of transitory increase in pulmonary resistances or ventricular dysfunction following the Fontan operation. The adjustable atrial defect is later closed surgically (117), and the fenestration can be closed with a device in the cardiac catheterization laboratory (116).

The intraoperative evaluation of these patients with transesophageal echocardiography (119–122) has as its main objective the assessment of ventricular function and the detection of regurgitation of the atrioventricular valve(s) and residual outflow tract obstructions. Ventricular function is best evaluated from the transverse transgastric views (see Fig. 4-27A) and from the transverse retrocardiac views, with anteflexion of the transducer into a short-axis-equivalent view. The presence of atrioventricular valve regurgitation is best assessed from the transverse four-chamber view and from the longitudinal inflow views, with the transducer aimed leftward (see Fig. 4-28). Systemic outflow tract obstruction is evaluated from vari-

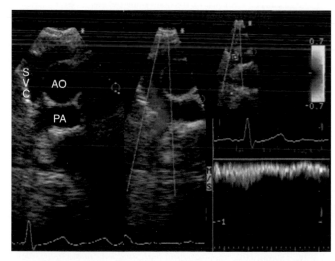

ECHO. 17-16. Right subclavicular view of a bidirectional Glenn connection between the superior vena cava and the right pulmonary artery. **Left:** Anatomic view of the superior vena cava-pulmonary artery connection. **Middle:** Color Doppler map of the unrestricted superior vena cava-to-pulmonary artery flow. **Right:** Spectral Doppler velocity recording of the low-velocity flow with accentuation in inspiration. *SVC,* superior vena cava; *AO,* aorta; *PA,* pulmonary artery.

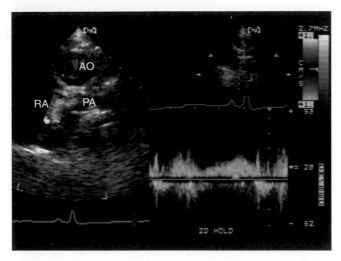

ECHO. 17-17. Right subclavicular view demonstrating the Fontan connection between the right atrium and pulmonary artery. **Left:** Color Doppler flow map. **Right:** Spectral Doppler recording of velocities through the Fontan connection. Note the biphasic velocity curves with peaks in middle-late systole and diastole. *AO*, aorta; *RA*, right atrium; *PA*, pulmonary artery.

ous views. The transverse four-chamber view with withdrawal of the transducer permits visualization of the systemic outflow (see Fig. 4-29A). The longitudinal views obtained from the same transducer location allow evaluation of both pulmonary and systemic outflow (see Figs. 4-29D–F). None of these approaches, however, permits correct alignment of the Doppler sampling line, so the longitudinal transgastric view should be attempted, which may result in positioning of the Doppler beam in a direction somewhat parallel to the flow (see Fig. 4-27D,E).

The objectives of the long-term echocardiographic evaluation of these patients are similar to those of the immediate intraoperative study. The chief long-term complications are main ventricular dysfunction, atrioventricular valve regurgitation, and to a lesser extent recurrent systemic outflow obstruction. At altitude, or if the pulmonary resistances were borderline at the time of surgery, systemic venous congestion and various degrees of superior and inferior vena caval syndromes can develop. The dynamics of the cavopulmonary flows should be assessed serially with pulsed-wave Doppler. Normal waveforms are of low velocity; respiratory variations indicate increased forward flows into the pulmonary artery in inspiration (Echos. 17-16, 17-17). Frommelt et al. (123) studied a group of patients after they had undergone the Fontan operation for various types of univentricular atrioventricular connection. Diastolic function of the main ventricular chamber assessed by Doppler velocities was impaired, demonstrating a compromised ventricular relaxation and a diminished early diastolic flow velocity. These factors were evidenced by reduced early filling and a more dominant late atrial (A wave-dominant) pattern.

The spectral velocity curves of the pulmonary artery reflected the systolic function of the ventricle. In the presence of a normal ventricular ejection fraction, the forward pulmonary velocity curves were biphasic, peaking in middle-late systole and middiastole. With lower ejection fractions, the forward pulmonary flow in systole and early diastole was diminished to absent, and flow reversal was noted in late systole and early diastole. The long-term follow-up of patients after the Fontan operation should include serial echocardiographic evaluation of systolic and diastolic ventricular function and Doppler recording of the pulmonary arterial velocities, which appear to have predictive clinical value.

REFERENCES

1. Anderson RH, Wilkinson JL, Macartney FJ, et al. Classification and terminology of primitive ventricle. In: Anderson RH, Shinebourne EA, eds. *Paediatric Cardiology 1977*. Edinburgh: Churchill Livingstone, 1978:311–322.
2. Anderson RH, Becker AE, Macartney FJ, Shinebourne EA, Wilkinson JL, Tynan MJ. Is tricuspid atresia a univentricular heart? *Pediatr Cardiol* 1979;1:51–56.
3. Bharati S, Lev M. The concept of tricuspid atresia complex as distinct from that of the single ventricle complex. *Pediatr Cardiol* 1979;1:57–62.
4. Anderson RH, Shinebourne EA, Becker AE, Macartney FJ, Wilkinson JL, Tynan MJ. Tricuspid atresia and univentricular heart [Letters to the Editor]. *Pediatr Cardiol* 1979/80;1:165–166.
5. Van Praagh R, David I, Van Praagh S. What is a ventricle? The single-ventricle trap. *Pediatr Cardiol* 1982;2:79–84.
6. Anderson RH, Macartney FJ, Tynan M, et al. Univentricular atrioventricular connection: the single ventricle trap unsprung. *Pediatr Cardiol* 1983;4:273–280.
7. Holmes WF. Case of malformation of the heart. *Trans Med Chir Soc Edinburgh* 1824;1:252–259.
8. Peacock TB. Case of malformation of the heart. Both auricles opening into the left ventricle, and transposition of the aorta and pulmonary artery. *Trans Pathol Soc London* 1855;6:117–119.
9. Mann JD. Cor triloculare biatriatum. *Br Med J* 1907;1:614–616.
10. Abbott ME. Cor triloculare biatriatum and biventriculare. In: *Atlas of congenital cardiac disease*. New York: American Heart Association, 1936:50–51.
11. Dry TJ, Edwards JE, Parker RL, Burchell HB, Rogers HM, Bulbulian AH. Cor triloculare biatriatum. In: Dry TJ, Edwards JE, Parker RL, Burchell HB, Rogers HM, Bulbulian AH, eds. *Congenital anomalies of the heart and great vessels. Clinicopathologic study of 132 cases*. Springfield, IL: Charles C Thomas Publisher, 1948:5–7.
12. Young AH. Rare anomaly of the human heart—a three-chambered heart in an adult aged thirty-five years. *J Anat Physiol London* 1907;41:190–197.
13. Taussig HB. Cardiovascular anomalies. A single ventricle with a diminutive outlet chamber. *J Tech Methods* 1939;19:120–128.
14. Lambert EC. Single ventricle with a rudimentary outlet chamber. Case report. *Bull Johns Hopkins Hosp* 1951;88:231–238.
15. Taussig HB. A single ventricle and a rudimentary outlet chamber. In: Taussig HB, ed. *Congenital malformations of the heart*. New York: The Commonwealth Fund, 1947:278–296.
16. Rogers HM, Edwards JE. Cor triloculare biatriatum: an analysis of the clinical and pathologic features of nine cases. *Am Heart J* 1951;41:299–310.
17. Megevand RP, Paul RN, Parker J. Single ventricle with diminutive outlet chamber. Associated with coarctation of the aorta and other cardiac anomalies. *J Pediatr* 1953;43:687–694.
18. Van Praagh R, Ongley PA, Swan HJC. Anatomic types of single or common ventricle in man. Morphologic and geometric aspects of 60 necropsied cases. *Am J Cardiol* 1964;13:367–386.

19. Gasul BM, Arcilla RA, Lev M. Single (common) ventricle. In: Gasul BM, Arcilla RA, Lev M, eds. *Heart disease in children. Diagnosis and treatment.* Philadelphia: JB Lippincott Co, 1966: 289–309.

20. Lev M, Liberthson RR, Kirkpatrick JR, Eckner FA, Arcilla RA. Single (primitive) ventricle. *Circulation* 1969;39:577–591.

21. Marin-Garcia J, Tandon R, Moller JH, Edwards JE. Common (single) ventricle with normally related great vessels. *Circulation* 1974;49:565–573.

22. Marin-Garcia J, Tandon R, Moller JH, Edwards JE. Single ventricle with transposition. *Circulation* 1974;49:994–1004.

23. Macartney FJ, Partridge JB, Scott O, Deverall PB. Common or single ventricle. An angiocardiographic and hemodynamic study of 42 patients. *Circulation* 1976;53:543–554.

24. Van Praagh R, Plett JA, Van Praagh S. Single ventricle. Pathology, embryology, terminology and classification. *Herz* 1979;4:113–150.

25. Liberthson RR, Paul MH, Muster AJ, Arcilla RA, Eckner FA, Lev M. Straddling and displaced atrioventricular orifices and valves with primitive ventricles. *Circulation* 1971;43:213–226.

26. Mehrizi A, McMurphy DM, Ottesen OE, Rowe RD. Syndrome of double inlet left ventricle. Angiocardiographic differentiation from single ventricle with rudimentary outlet chamber. *Bull Johns Hopkins Hosp* 1966;119:255–267.

27. De la Cruz MV, Miller BL. Double-inlet left ventricle. Two pathological specimens with comments on the embryology and on its relation to single ventricle. *Circulation* 1968;37:249–260.

28. Tandon R, Becker AE, Moller JH, Edwards JE. Double inlet left ventricle. Straddling tricuspid valve. *Br Heart J* 1974;36:747–759.

29. Anderson RH, Arnold R, Thapar MK, Jones RS, Hamilton DI. Cardiac specialized tissue in hearts with an apparently single ventricular chamber (double inlet left ventricle). *Am J Cardiol* 1974;33:95–106.

30. Freedom RM, Nanton M, Dische MR. Isolated ventricular inversion with double inlet left ventricle. *Eur J Cardiol* 1977;5:63–86.

31. Anderson RH, Lenox CC, Zuberbuhler JR, Ho SY, Smith A, Wilkinson JL. Double-inlet left ventricle with rudimentary right ventricle and ventriculoarterial concordance. *Am J Cardiol* 1983;52:573–577.

32. Anderson RH, Penkoske PA, Zuberbuhler JR. Variable morphology of ventricular septal defect in double inlet left ventricle. *Am J Cardiol* 1985;55:1560–1565.

33. Munoz-Castellanos L, De la Cruz MV, Cieslinski A. Double inlet right ventricle. Two pathological specimens with comments on embryology. *Br Heart J* 1973;35:292–297.

34. Keeton BR, Macartney FJ, Rees PG, et al. Double inlet right ventricle. *Br Heart J* 1977;39:930–931.

35. Anderson RH, Becker AE, Wilkinson JL, Gerlis LM. Morphogenesis of univentricular hearts. *Br Heart J* 1976;38:553–572.

36. Anderson RH, Becker AE, Freedom RM, et al. Problems in the nomenclature of the univentricular heart. *Herz* 1979;4:97–106.

37. Quero-Jimenez M, Cameron AH, Acerete F, Quero-Jimenez C. Univentricular hearts: pathology of the atrioventricular valves. *Herz* 1979;4:161–165.

38. Ritter DG, Seward JB, Moodie D, Danielson GK. Univentricular heart (common ventricle): preoperative diagnosis. Hemodynamic, angiocardiographic and echocardiographic features. *Herz* 1979;4:198–205.

39. Soto B, Bertranou EG, Bream PR, Souza A Jr, Bargeron LM Jr. Angiographic study of univentricular heart of right ventricular type. *Circulation* 1979;60:1325–1334.

40. Shinebourne EA, Lau K, Calcaterra G, Anderson RH. Univentricular heart of right ventricular type: clinical, angiographic and electrocardiographic features. *Am J Cardiol* 1980;46:439–445.

41. Freedom RM, Picchio F, Duncan WJ, Harder JR, Moes CAF, Rowe RD. The atrioventricular junction in the univentricular heart: a two-dimensional echocardiographic analysis. *Pediatr Cardiol* 1982;3:105–117.

42. Moodie DS, Ritter DG, Tajik AJ, O'Fallon WM. Long-term follow-up in the unoperated univentricular heart. *Am J Cardiol* 1984;53:1124–1128.

43. Anderson RH, Becker AE, Lucchese FA, Meier MA, Rigby ML, Soto B. Hearts with univentricular atrioventricular connexion. In: Anderson RH, Becker AE, Lucchese FA, Meier MA, Rigby ML, Soto B, eds. *Morphology of congenital heart disease. Angiocardiographic, echocardiographic and surgical correlates.* London: Castle House Publications, 1983:121–143.

44. Anderson RH, Becker AE, Tynan M, Macartney FJ, Rigby ML, Wilkinson JL. The univentricular atrioventricular connection: getting to the root of a thorny problem. *Am J Cardiol* 1984;54:822–828.

45. Freedom RM, Smallhorn JF. Hearts with a univentricular atrioventricular connection. In: Freedom RM, Benson LN, Smallhorn JF, eds. *Neonatal heart disease.* London: Springer-Verlag, 1992:497–521.

46. Wilkinson JL, Becker AE, Tynan M, et al. Nomenclature of the univentricular heart. *Herz* 1979;4:107–112.

47. Anderson RH, Tynan M, Freedom RM, et al. Ventricular morphology in the univentricular heart. *Herz* 1979;4:184–197.

48. Tynan MJ, Becker AE, Macartney FJ, Quero Jimenez M, Shinebourne EA, Anderson RH. Nomenclature and classification of congenital heart disease. *Br Heart J* 1979;41:544–553.

49. Ho SY, Zuberbuhler JR, Anderson RH. Pathology of hearts with a univentricular atrioventricular connection. In: Rosenberg HS, Bernstein J, eds. *Cardiovascular diseases. Perspectives in pediatric pathology,* Vol 12. Basel: Karger, 1988:69–99.

50. Thies WR, Soto B, Diethelm E, Bargeron LM Jr, Pacifico AD. Angiographic anatomy of hearts with one ventricular chamber: the true single ventricle. *Am J Cardiol* 1985;55:1363–1366.

51. Anderson RH, Macartney FJ, Shinebourne EA, Tynan M. Double inlet ventricle. In: Anderson RH, Macartney FJ, Shinebourne EA, Tynan M, eds. *Paediatric Cardiology,* Vol 1. Edinburgh: Churchill Livingstone, 1987;643–673.

52. Bound JP, Logan WFWE. Incidence of congenital heart disease in Blackpool 1957–1971. *Br Heart J* 1977;39:445–450.

53. Hoffman JIE, Christianson R. Congenital heart disease in a cohort of 19,502 births with long-term follow-up. *Am J Cardiol* 1978;42:641–647.

54. Hoffman JIE. Incidence of congenital heart disease: I. Postnatal incidence. *Pediatr Cardiol* 1995;16:103–113.

55. Netter FH, Van Mierop LHS. Embryology. In: Netter FH, Yonkman FF, eds. *Heart.* Summit, NJ: Ciba Publications Department, 1969:112–130 (*The Ciba collection of medical illustrations,* Vol 5).

56. De la Cruz MV, Gimenez-Ribotta M, Saravalli O, Cayre R. The contribution of the inferior endocardial cushion of the atrioventricular canal to cardiac septation and to the development of the atrioventricular valves: study in the chick embryo. *Am J Anat* 1983;166:63–72.

57. De la Cruz MV, Cayre R. Desarrollo embriologico del corazon y las grandes arterias. In: Sanchez PA, ed. *Cardiologia pediatrica, clinica y cirugia.* Barcelona: Salvat Editores SA, 1986:10–18.

58. Ando M, Satomi G, Takao A. Atresia of tricuspid or mitral orifice: anatomic spectrum and morphogenetic hypothesis. In: Van Praagh R, Takao A, eds. *Etiology and morphogenesis of congenital heart disease.* Mount Kisco, NY: Futura Publishing, 1980:421–487.

59. Rychter Z, Rychterova V, Lemez L. Formation of the heart loop and proliferation structure of its wall as a base for ventricular septation. *Herz* 1979;4:86–90.

60. Arteaga M, Garcia Pelaez I. Nomenclature in the embryonic heart. In: Aranega A, Pexieder T, eds. *Correlations between experimental cardiac embryology and teratology and congenital cardiac defects.* Granada, Spain: Universidad de Granada, 1989:17–35.

61. Van Mierop LHS. Embryology of the univentricular heart. *Herz* 1979;4:78–85.

62. Van Mierop LHS. Pathology and pathogenesis of the common cardiac malformations. *Cardiovasc Clin* 1970;2:27–59 (Brest AN, ed. *Congenital heart disease*).

63. De la Cruz MV, Sanchez Gomez C, Arteaga MM, Arguello C. Experimental study of the development of the truncus and the conus in the chick embryo. *J Anat* 1977;123:661–686.

64. Anderson RH, Ho SY, Becker AE. The morphology of septal structures in univentricular hearts. In: Wenink ACG, Oppenheimer-Dekker A, Moulaert AJ, eds. *The ventricular septum of the heart. Boerhaave series for postgraduate medical education,* Vol 21. The Hague: Leiden University Press, 1981:203–224.

65. Wilkinson JL, Keeton B, Dickinson DF, Tynan M, Macartney FJ,

Anderson RH. Morphology and conducting tissue in univentricular hearts of right ventricular type. *Herz* 1979;4:151–160.

66. Rigby ML, Anderson RH, Gibson D, Jones ODH, Joseph MC, Shinebourne EA. Two dimensional echocardiographic categorization of the univentricular heart. Ventricular morphology, type, and mode of atrioventricular connection. *Br Heart J* 1981;46:603–612.

67. Becker AE, Anderson RH, Penkoske PA, Zuberbuhler JR. Morphology of double inlet ventricle. In: Anderson RH, Crupi G, Parenzan L, eds. *Double inlet ventricle. Anatomy, diagnosis and surgical management.* New York: Elsevier Science, 1987:36–71.

68. Carminati M, Valsechi O, Borghi A, et al. Cross-sectional echocardiography. In: Anderson RH, Crupi G, Parenzan L, eds. *Double inlet ventricle. Anatomy, diagnosis and surgical management.* New York: Elsevier Science, 1987:122–132.

69. Matitiau A, Geva T, Colan SD, et al. Bulboventricular foramen size in infants with double-inlet left ventricle or tricuspid atresia with transposed great arteries: influence of initial palliative operation and rate of growth. *J Am Coll Cardiol* 1992;19:142–148.

70. Soto B, Pacifico AD, eds. *Angiocardiography in congenital heart malformations.* Mount Kisco, NY: Futura Publishing, 1990:291–307.

71. Quero Jimenez M, Perez Martinez VM, Arteaga Martinez M, Puga FJ. Corazon univentricular. In: Sanchez PA, ed. *Cardiologia pediatrica, clinica y cirugia,* Vol 1. Barcelona: Salvat Editores SA, 1986:600–619.

72. Kirklin JW, Barrat-Boyes BG, eds. *Cardiac surgery. Morphology, diagnosis criteria, natural history, techniques, results and indications,* Vol 2. New York: Churchill Livingstone, 1993:1549–1580.

73. Huhta JC, Seward JB, Tajik AJ, Hagler DJ, Edwards WD. Two-dimensional echocardiographic spectrum of univentricular atrioventricular connection. *J Am Coll Cardiol* 1985;5:149–157.

74. Keeton BR, Lie JT, McGoon DC, Danielson GK, Ritter DG, Wallace RB. Anatomy of coronary arteries in univentricular hearts and its surgical implications. *Am J Cardiol* 1979;43:569–580.

75. Neufeld HN, Schneeweiss A, eds. *Coronary artery disease in infants and children.* Philadelphia: Lea & Febiger, 1983:96–102.

76. Elliot LP, Amplatz K, Edwards JE. Coronary arterial patterns in transposition complexes. Anatomic and angiocardiographic studies. *Am J Cardiol* 1966;17:362–378.

77. Anderson RH, Wilkinson JL, Gerlis LM, Smith A, Becker AE. Atresia of the right atrioventricular orifice. *Br Heart J* 1977;39:414–428.

78. Crupi G, Villani M, Di Benedetto G, et al. Tricuspid atresia with imperforate valve: angiographic findings and surgical implications in two cases with AV concordance and normally related great arteries. *Pediatr Cardiol* 1984;5:49–54.

79. Kreysig FL. Die krankheiten des herzens. Dritte Thiel. Berlin: AW Hayn, 1817:104. Cited by Rashkind WJ. Tricuspid atresia: a historical review. *Pediatr Cardiol* 1982;2:85–88(ref 17).

80. Schuberg W. Beobachtung von Verkummerung des rechten herzventrikels in folge von atresie des ost. venos. dextr.; Perforation des herzscheidewand und dadurch bildung eines canales, der durch den rudimentaren rechtaen ventrikel in die art. pulmon. fuhrt. *Virchows Arch Pathol Anat* 1861;20:294–296. Cited by Rashkind WJ. Tricuspid atresia: a historical review. *Pediatr Cardiol* 1982;2:85–88(ref. 24).

81. Kuhne M. Uber zwei falle von kongenitaler atresie des ostium venosum dextrum. *Jahresb Kinderheile* 1906;63:235–249. Cited by Lev M, Liberthon RR, Kirkpatrick JR, Eckner FA, Arcilla RA. Single (primitive) ventricle. *Circulation* 1969;39:577–591.

82. Edwards JE, Burchell HB. Congenital tricuspid atresia: a classification. *Med Clin North Am* 1949;33:1177–1196.

83. Vlad P. Tricuspid atresia. In: Keith JD, Rowe RD, Vlad P, eds. *Heart disease in infancy and childhood,* 3rd ed. New York: Macmillan, 1978:518–541.

84. Rao PS. A unified classification for tricuspid atresia. *Am Heart J* 1980;99:799–804.

85. Tandon R, Edwards JE. Tricuspid atresia. A re-evaluation and classification. *J Thorac Cardiovasc Surg* 1974;67:530–542.

86. Perez Martinez VM, Rodriguez Coronel A, Sanchez PA, Kreutzer GO, Vargas FJ, Laura JP. Atresia tricuspidea. In: Sanchez PA, ed. *Cardiologia pediatrica, clinica y cirugia,* Vol 1. Barcelona: Salvat Editores SA, 1986:458–474.

87. Gessner IH. Embryology of atrioventricular valve formation and embryogenesis of tricuspid atresia. In: Syamasundar Rao P, ed. *Tricuspid atresia,* 2nd ed. Mount Kisco, NY: Futura Publishing, 1992:39–57.

88. Anderson RH, Macartney FJ, Shinebourne EA, Tynan M, eds. *Paediatric Cardiology,* Vol 1. Edinburgh: Churchill Livingstone, 1987:675–696.

89. Scalia D, Russo P, Anderson RH, et al. The surgical anatomy of hearts with no direct communication between the right atrium and the ventricular mass—so-called tricuspid atresia. *J Thorac Cardiovasc Surg* 1984;87:743–755.

90. Rao PS, Linde LM, Liebman J, Perrin E. Functional closure of physiologically advantageous ventricular septal defects: observations in three cases with tricuspid atresia. *Am J Dis Child* 1974;127:36–40.

91. Rao PS. Natural history of the ventricular septal defect in tricuspid atresia and its surgical implications. *Br Heart J* 1977;39:276–288.

92. Soto B, Pacifico AD, eds. *Angiocardiography in congenital heart malformations.* Mount Kisco, NY: Futura Publishing, 1990:213–238.

93. Kirklin JW, Barrat-Boyes BG, eds. *Cardiac surgery. Morphology, diagnosis criteria, natural history, techniques, results and indications,* Vol 2. New York: Churchill Livingstone, 1993:1055–1104.

94. Deanfield JE, Tommasini G, Anderson RH, Macartney FJ. Tricuspid atresia: analysis of coronary artery distribution and ventricular morphology. *Br Heart J* 1982;48:485–492.

95. Thiene G, Daliento L, Frescura C, De Tommasi M, Macartney FJ, Anderson RH. Atresia of left atrioventricular orifice. Anatomical investigation in 62 cases. *Br Heart J* 1981;45:393–401.

96. Shore D, Jones O, Rigby ML, Anderson RH, Lincoln C. Atresia of left atrioventricular connection. Surgical considerations. *Br Heart J* 1982;47:35–40.

97. Mickell JJ, Mathews RA, Anderson RH, et al. The anatomical heterogeneity of hearts lacking a patent communication between the left atrium and the ventricular mass (''mitral atresia'') in presence of a patent aortic valve. *Eur Heart J* 1983;4:477–486.

98. Gittenberger-de Groot AC, Wenink ACG. Mitral atresia. Morphological details. *Br Heart J* 1984;51:252–258.

99. Watson DG, Rowe RD, Conen PE, Duckworth JWA. Mitral atresia with normal aortic valve. Report of 11 cases and review of the literature. *Pediatrics* 1960;25:450–467.

100. Moreno F, Quero M, Perez Diaz L. Mitral atresia with normal aortic valve. A study of eighteen cases and a review of the literature. *Circulation* 1976;53:1004–1010.

101. Manhoff LJ, Howe JS. Congenital heart disease: tricuspid atresia and mitral atresia associated with transposition of the great vessels. *Am Heart J* 1945;29:90–98.

102. Crupi G, Pignatelli R, Carminati M, et al. Palliative surgery. In: Anderson RH, Crupi G, Parenzan L, eds. *Double inlet ventricle.* New York: Elsevier Science, 1987:165–173.

103. Franklin RCG, Spiegelhalter DJ, Anderson RH, et al. Double-inlet ventricle presenting in infancy. II. Results of palliative operations. *J Thorac Cardiovasc Surg* 1991;101:917–923.

104. Stefanelli G, Kirklin JW, Naftel DC, et al. Early and intermediate-term (10-year) results of surgery for univentricular atrioventricular connection (''single ventricle''). *Am J Cardiol* 1984;54:811–821.

105. Cheung HC, Lincoln C, Anderson RH, et al. Options for surgical repair in hearts with univentricular atrioventricular connection and subaortic stenosis. *J Thorac Cardiovasc Surg* 1990;100:672–681.

106. Karl TR, Watterson KG, Sano S, Mee RBB. Operation for subaortic stenosis in univentricular hearts. *Ann Thorac Surg* 1991;52:420–428.

107. Mayer JE Jr. Surgical aortico-pulmonary anastomosis for a complex aortic obstruction with single ventricle. *Prog Pediatr Cardiol* 1994;3:106–111.

108. Castaneda AR, Jonas RA, Mayer JE, Hanley FL, eds. *Cardiac surgery of the neonate and infant.* Philadelphia: WB Saunders, 1994:249–272.

109. De Leval M. Right heart bypass operations. In: Stark J, de Leval M, eds. *Surgery for congenital heart defects,* 2nd ed. Philadelphia: WB Saunders, 1994:565–585.

110. Penkoske PA, Freedom RM, Williams WG, Trusler GA, Rowe RD. Surgical palliation of subaortic stenosis in the univentricular heart. *J Thorac Cardiovasc Surg* 1984;87:767–781.

111. McGoon DC, Danielson GK, Ritter DG, Wallace RB, Maloney JD, Marcelletti C. Correction of the univentricular heart having two atrioventricular valves. *J Thorac Cardiovasc Surg* 1977;74: 218–226.

112. Fontan F, Baudet E. Surgical repair of tricuspid atresia. *Thorax* 1971;26:240–248.

113. Kreutzer G, Galindez E, Bono H, De Palma C, Laura JP. An operation for the correction of tricuspid atresia. *J Thorac Cardiovasc Surg* 1973;66:613–621.

114. Glenn WWL. Circulatory bypass of the right side of the heart. IV. Shunt between superior vena cava and distal right pulmonary artery—report of clinical application. *N Engl J Med* 1958;259: 117–120.

115. Azzolina G, Eufrate S, Pensa P. Tricuspid atresia: experience in surgical management with a modified cavopulmonary anastomosis. *Thorax* 1972;27:111–115.

116. Danielson GK. Surgical management of double inlet ventricle. In: Anderson RH, Crupi G, Parenzan L, eds. *Double inlet ventricle. Anatomy, diagnosis and surgical management.* New York: Elsevier Science, 1987:174–182.

117. Bridges ND, Lock JE, Castaneda AR. Baffle fenestration with subsequent transcatheter closure. Modification of the Fontan operation for patients at increased risk. *Circulation* 1990;82:1681–1689.

118. Laks H, Pearl JM, Haas GS, et al. Partial Fontan: advantages of an adjustable interatrial communication. *Ann Thorac Surg* 1991; 52:1084–1095.

119. Seward JB, Khandheria BK, Edwards WD, Oh JK, Freeman WK, Tajik AJ. Biplanar transesophageal echocardiography: anatomic correlations, image orientation, and clinical applications. *Mayo Clin Proc* 1990;65:1193–1213.

120. Fyfe DA, Kline CH, Sade RM, Greene CA, Gillette PC. The utility of transesophageal echocardiography during and after Fontan operations in small children. *Am Heart J* 1991;122:1403–1415.

121. Stumper O, Sutherland GR, Geuskens R, Roelandt JRTC, Bos E, Hess J. Transesophageal echocardiography in evaluation and management after a Fontan procedure. *J Am Coll Cardiol* 1991; 17:1152–1160.

122. Fyfe DA, Kline CH, Sade RM, Gillette PC. Transesophageal echocardiography detects thrombus formation not identified by transthoracic echocardiography after the Fontan operation. *J Am Coll Cardiol* 1991;18:1733–1737.

123. Frommelt PC, Snider AR, Meliones JN, Vermilion RP. Doppler assessment of pulmonary artery flow patterns and ventricular function after the Fontan operation. *Am J Cardiol* 1991;68:1211–1216.

Part VII

Anomalies of the Ventricular Outflows

CHAPTER 18

Anomalies of the Right Ventricular Outflow Tract and Pulmonary Arteries

Lilliam M. Valdes-Cruz and Raul O. Cayre

The anomalies of the right ventricular outflow tract make up a series of malformations that include those generally called "pulmonary stenoses," i.e., valvular pulmonic stenosis and subvalvular pulmonary stenosis (infundibular pulmonary stenosis and double-chamber right ventricle); pulmonary atresia with intact ventricular septum; and pulmonary valvular insufficiency. The supravalve obstructions at the level of the trunk and branches of the pulmonary artery are discussed below in "Anomalies of the Pulmonary Artery and its Branches." Obstructions caused by displacement of the infundibular or outlet septum to the right and anterior such as seen in tetralogy of Fallot, double outlet right ventricle, and transposition of the great arteries are discussed in Chapters 22, 23, and 24, respectively. Pulmonary atresia with ventricular septal defect is considered a severe form of tetralogy of Fallot and is discussed in that chapter (Chapter 22).

ANOMALIES OF THE RIGHT VENTRICULAR OUTFLOW TRACT

The incidence of anomalies included within the term "pulmonary stenosis" (valvular and subvalvular) varies between 10.7% and 30% of all congenital cardiac anomalies (1–5).

VALVULAR PULMONIC STENOSIS

Approximately 80% to 90% of cases of pulmonary stenosis are due to isolated stenosis at the valvular level (4–6). Its incidence varies between 3.1% and 10% of all congenital heart disease (2,6,7–13). The first description of this malformation was by Morgagni in 1761 (14). Similar cases were reported later by Ogle in 1854 (15), Peacock in 1858 (16) and 1859 (17), Andrew in 1865 (18), and Peacock in 1879 (19). In that same year, Barlow (20)

and Finlay (21) described the dilatation of the pulmonary artery above the valvular obstruction. Fallot in 1888 (22) separated the cases of pulmonary stenosis with ventricular septal defect and dextroposition of the aorta (tetralogy of Fallot) from those with pulmonary stenosis, intact ventricular septum, and patent foramen ovale, calling these "trilogy." Since then, a series of terms has been used to describe this malformation: "pulmonary stenosis with closed septa" (23), "pulmonary stenosis with patent foramen ovale and closed ventricular septum" (23–25), "pulmonary stenosis with intact ventricular septum" (26), "syndrome of pulmonary stenosis with patent foramen ovale" (27), "pure congenital pulmonary stenosis" (28), "congenital pulmonary stenosis with closed ventricular septum" (29), "simple pulmonary valvular stenosis with closed septa" (30), "pulmonary stenosis with normal aortic root" (6), "congenital valvular pulmonary stenosis with or without intratrial communication" (7), "isolated pulmonary stenosis" (7), "simple pulmonary stenosis" (8), and "pulmonary valvar stenosis with normal aortic root" (31).

EMBRYOLOGIC CONSIDERATIONS

The semilunar valves of the great arteries originate from the truncal swellings and from the intercalated swellings (see Fig. 1-14B). The anterior leaflet of the pulmonic valve is derived from the dorsal or left intercalated swelling and the posterior, noncoronary aortic leaflet from the ventral or right intercalated swelling (32,33). The posterior right and left leaflets of the pulmonic valve and the anterior right and left aortic leaflets originate from the dextrosuperior and sinistroinferior truncal swellings, respectively (32,33) (Fig. 18-1A). The valve commissures are the result of the separation of these embryologic structures. The separation of the dextrosuperior and sinistroinferior truncal swellings give rise to the commissure be-

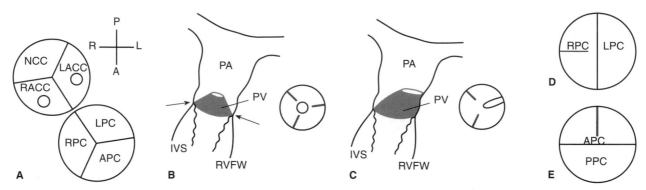

FIG. 18-1. Schematic drawings of the different types of pulmonary valve. **A:** Normal pulmonary valve and its anatomic relationship to the aortic valve. **B:** Acommissural pulmonary valve. The raphes are located at the point of fusion of the commissures. The arrows indicate the right ventricular-pulmonary artery junction. **C:** Unicommissural pulmonary valve. The raphes are located at the point of fusion of the commissures. **D:** Bicuspid pulmonic valve with one right and one left cusp. **E:** Bicuspid pulmonic valve with one anterior and one posterior cusp. *APC,* anterior pulmonic valve cusp; *RPC,* right posterior pulmonic valve cusp; *LPC,* left posterior pulmonic valve cusp; *PPC,* posterior pulmonic valve cusp; *RACC,* right anterior coronary cusp; *LACC,* left anterior coronary cusp; *NCC,* noncoronary cusp; *PA,* pulmonary artery; *PV,* pulmonic valve; *IVS,* interventricular septum; *RVFW,* right ventricular free wall; *R,* right; *L,* left; *A,* anterior; *P,* posterior.

tween the posterior right and left pulmonic valve leaflets; the separation of the left intercalated and the dextrosuperior truncal swellings forms the commissure between the anterior and posterior right pulmonic valve cusps; the separation of the left intercalated and the sinistroinferior truncal swellings makes up the commissure between the left posterior and the anterior leaflets.

The morphogenetic mechanism that causes valve pulmonic stenosis is not well known. Two morphogenetic processes have been suggested to explain the absence of one or more of the commissures of the semilunar valves: (a) complete deletion of the separation between two or more of the embryologic structures of the truncus that give rise to the semilunar valves during an early stage of development, and (b) fusion of two or more of these structures during a later stage of development, with a resulting connective tissue band or raphe (34,35) (Fig. 18-1B,C). Van Mierop suggests that the pure form, which lacks a raphe, could be due to the complete absence of the primordium of a cusp (36). An inflammatory process or ''fetal endocarditis'' has also been proposed as a morphogenetic mechanism (23,37,38).

ANATOMIC AND ECHOCARDIOGRAPHIC CONSIDERATIONS

The echocardiographic study of valvular pulmonic stenosis should include the following: (a) the morphology of the stenotic pulmonic valve; (b) the diameter of the ''pulmonary annulus''; (c) the size of the right ventricle; (d) the degree of dilatation of the pulmonary artery; (e) the severity of the obstruction; and (f) associated anomalies.

Morphology of the Stenotic Pulmonic Valve

The congenital anomalies of the pulmonic valve comprise a spectrum that includes an increase or decrease in the number of cusps as well as variations in their shape and size.

Unicuspid Pulmonic Valve. The valve is composed of a single cusp, which can be acommissural or unicommissural (Fig. 18-1B,C). An acommissural valve is made of one single cusp in the shape of a dome, with a central orifice that is circular, lacking any commissure (Fig. 18-1B). The presence of a single cusp is due to fusion of the commissures, and three raphes may be observed adjacent to the pulmonary arterial wall that do not reach the free edge of the valve cusp. The valve is thickened, and its mobility is reduced. This type of unicuspid valve is more commonly seen in the pulmonic than in the aortic position and is the usual type of valve found in isolated pulmonic valve stenosis (9,10,39–43). The most severe form of a domed acommissural unicuspid pulmonic valve is that seen in critical pulmonic stenosis of the newborn. The unicommissural unicuspid pulmonic valve is seen much less frequently; it has only one cusp and one commissure, which reaches the pulmonary arterial wall and results in an eccentric orifice of variable size (Fig. 18-1C). Normally, one or two raphes can be seen adjacent to the arterial wall that do not reach the free edge of the leaflet. Rarely, four raphes can be seen as a result of fusion of the commissures of a quadricuspid valve (9,27,39).

Bicuspid Pulmonic Valve. Contrary to the aortic valve, a bicuspid pulmonic valve is rare as an isolated lesion, being found usually in association with tetralogy of Fallot (10,31,44,45). Initially, the bicuspid valve is either not stenotic or only mildly so. Different from a bicuspid aortic valve, the cusps are commonly similar in size (Fig. 18-1D,E). The valve is slightly thickened, and usually there is a raphe that does not reach the valve orifice, being more a depression than a hole.

Tricuspid and Quadricuspid Valves. Rarely, there may

be a tricuspid stenotic pulmonic valve, having an incidence of 6% of all stenotic pulmonic valves (42). The valve is usually dysplastic; the leaflets are thickened and redundant and are composed of myxomatous dysplastic tissue of nodular appearance. The commissures are not fused, and the obstruction is due to thickening of the leaflets with a usually hypoplastic "pulmonary annulus" (9,10,43,44,46). This type of valve is most commonly seen in Noonan's syndrome and in multiple lentigenes syndrome (9,10,40,43,47,48). A quadricuspid valve is seen more frequently in the pulmonary than the aortic position (10,34,49,50). In the majority of cases, the valve functions normally; only 4% are functionally abnormal, with two-thirds being regurgitant and one-third being stenotic (49). The morphologic characteristics of the pulmonic valve are best seen echocardiographically from the parasternal short-axis view, the parasternal long-axis view tilted towards the right ventricular outflow and from the subcostal short-axis view. In these views, the thickened and redundant dysplastic leaflets are evident, and their motion during the cardiac cycle, particularly in systole when the valve appears to dome, is apparent (Echo. 18-1). Also from these views the presence of a unicuspid acommissural or unicommissural valve can be established; however, due to the spatial plane of the pulmonic leaflets, it is not always possible to determine the number of cusps with certainty.

Size of the "Pulmonary Annulus"

In the normal heart, the pulmonary valve lacks a fibrous annulus. The site of insertion of the pulmonary leaflets, which is classically called the "pulmonary annulus," is totally muscular and corresponds to the union or junction between the right ventricular infundibulum and the pulmonary trunk (51) (Fig. 18-1B). The site of insertion of the pulmonary valve leaflets, similar to the aortic valve (see Fig. 19-3), is semicircular; the portion of the leaflets that forms the commissures inserts into the arterial wall, while the body of the leaflets inserts in the infundibular myocardium (42). In isolated pulmonic valve stenosis, the "pulmonary annulus" is usually normal in size but can also be hypoplastic such as in critical pulmonary stenosis of the neonate and in the presence of a dysplastic valve (9,10,43,44,46).

The echocardiographic views used to evaluate the morphology of the leaflets can also be used to assess the size of the "annulus" or right ventricular-pulmonary trunk junction (Echo. 18-1). The measurements should be made at the lowest point of insertion of the valve leaflets.

Size of the Right Ventricle

The right ventricle is usually concentrically hypertrophied. Infundibular hypertrophy, characterized by a diffuse narrowing of the right ventricular infundibulum, can result in subvalve obstruction, which has been seen in up to 37.5% of cases of valvular pulmonic stenosis (53) (Fig. 18-2A). It can regress after surgical valvotomy (52–54) or balloon valvuloplasty (55).

The size of the right ventricle can range from normal in the presence of mild valvular stenosis to severely hypoplastic, as seen in critical pulmonic stenosis of the newborn. In these latter cases, the right ventricle can be diminutive (56,57). The function of the left ventricle can be altered either due to changes in the left ventricular geometry secondary to the right ventricular hypertrophy or due to myocardial alterations, which can be seen in severe pulmonary stenosis (58,59). In rare instances, the elevated right ventricular pressure can cause bowing of the infundibular septum towards the left with secondary obstruction of the left ventricular outflow.

The size of the right ventricle can be assessed echocardiographically from the parasternal long-axis view tilted towards the inflow of the right ventricle, from the short-axis view, and from the apical four-chamber and subcostal four-chamber and short-axis view. The infundibulum of the right ventricle can be studied from the parasternal long axis aimed towards the right ventricular outflow and from the subcostal short-axis views.

Degree of Dilatation of the Pulmonary Arteries

Isolated valvular pulmonic stenosis is almost always associated with poststenotic dilatation of the pulmonary artery, which can extend to the proximal portion of the left branch. This is a result of the high-velocity flow across the stenotic valve impacting on the arterial wall (60,61). The degree of poststenotic dilatation is not related to the severity of obstruction, as it is not seen in critical

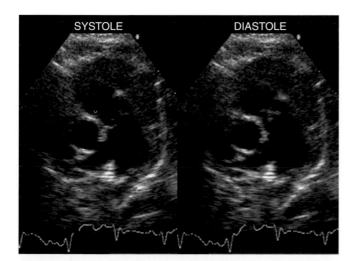

ECHO. 18-1. Parasternal short-axis view of a stenotic pulmonic valve. Note the doming of the valve in systole and the thickened, redundant tissue in diastole. The annular size can be measured from this view.

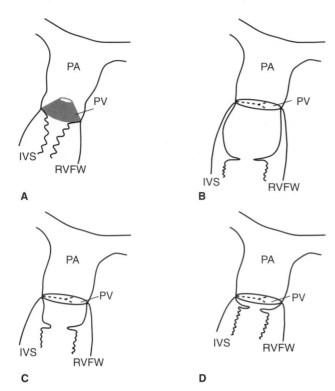

FIG. 18-2. Schematic drawings showing the various types of obstruction of the right ventricular outflow tract. **A:** Subvalvular pulmonary obstruction secondary to infundibular hypertrophy in the presence of valvular pulmonic stenosis. **B:** Discrete fibromuscular obstruction in the lower portion of the pulmonary infundibulum. **C:** Discrete fibromuscular obstruction in the mid portion of the pulmonary infundibulum. **D:** Discrete fibromuscular obstruction immediately below the pulmonary valve. *PA,* pulmonary artery; *PV,* pulmonary valve; *IVS,* interventricular septum; *RVFW,* right ventricular free wall.

pulmonary stenosis of the neonate or in the presence of a dysplastic valve.

The dilatation of the main and left branches of the pulmonary artery can be seen best from the parasternal long-axis view of the outflow tract of the right ventricle and from the short-axis views obtained from the parasternal and subcostal windows (Echos. 18-1, 18-2; see color plate 51 following p. 364).

Severity of the Obstruction

The severity of the pulmonary valve stenosis is assessed by recording of the maximal velocities across the valve with continuous-wave Doppler techniques and converting these to peak and mean gradients through the application of the simplified Bernoulli equation (gradient = 4 velocity^2). Because the stenotic jet is frequently eccentric, color Doppler flow mapping of the area is very useful as an aid in positioning the sampling line along the direction of the jet (Echo. 18-2). The outflow tract of the right ventricle should be interrogated with pulsed and/or high pulse rate frequency (PRF) Doppler to establish the pres-

ence of any infundibular obstruction. Ideally, the sample volumes in high PRF mode should be carefully positioned along the length of the outflow tract, across the pulmonic valve and along the main pulmonary artery to map the velocities and establish the level(s) and relative severity of the obstruction(s). In isolated valvular stenosis without infundibular obstruction, there is a dramatic increase in the peak flow velocity within the main pulmonary artery, just above the level of the pulmonic valve (62). In the presence of infundibular obstruction, on the other hand, high velocities are recorded in the outflow tract, below the level of the valve. Once the level(s) of obstruction is established and the severity estimated, the peak velocity should be confirmed with the Pedof Doppler probe, guided by the audio and spectral signal.

In the presence of left-to-right shunts, the velocity in the pulmonary artery is increased due to the increased flow (63). This should not be confused with true valvular pulmonic stenosis. In these cases, a careful analysis of the anatomy of the valve using two-dimensional imaging should reveal normal leaflet morphology and mobility.

In neonates with critical pulmonic stenosis, the gradient may be underestimated due to a variety of factors. Some of the important ones to keep in mind are (a) the relatively high pulmonary artery pressure found in the newborn; (b) the presence of a patent ductus arteriosus augmenting the pulmonary pressure distally; (c) the presence of significant tricuspid valve regurgitation and/or right-to-left atrial shunting, which would diminish the forward pulmonary blood flow; and (d) right ventricular dysfunction. In the presence of severe tricuspid valve regurgitation and right-to-left atrial shunting, critical pulmonic stenosis can be erroneously diagnosed as pulmonary valve atresia because of the virtual lack of forward pulmonary blood flow; however, identification of even trivial pulmonary regurgitation with color Doppler flow mapping estab-

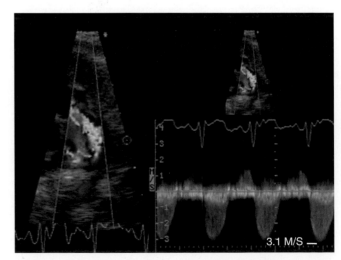

ECHO. 18-2. Color Doppler flow map and spectral velocity recording across a stenotic pulmonic valve. Note the color aliasing and high velocity as well as the poststenotic dilatation extending to the left pulmonary artery branch.

lishes the fact that the valve is patent and therefore more amenable to balloon valvuloplasty (Echo. 18-3; see color plate 52 following p. 364). In the presence of a significant patent ductus arteriosus or pulmonary hypertension, the true gradient across the stenotic valve may not be revealed until the ductus closes or the pulmonary arterial pressure drops. In these instances, however, the morphology of the valve aids in the assessment of the severity of the lesion. Further, the gradient between the aorta and pulmonary artery estimated from the velocity across the patent ductus provides an approximation of the pulmonary pressure.

Associated Anomalies

It is unusual to find other anomalies in association with pulmonic stenosis with intact ventricular septum (9,39). The most common one is patent foramen ovale or atrial septal defect of the ostium secundum type (1,2,7–9,26, 27,39,46,53). Others include patent ductus arteriosus (1,2, 7–9,39,53), valve aortic stenosis (9,39), bicuspid aortic valve (8,9,39), dynamic subvalve aortic stenosis (2), subvalve pulmonic stenosis (1,9,46), right ventricular anomalous muscle bundles (39), supravalve pulmonic stenosis (9,46), peripheral pulmonary stenosis (39), partial anomalous pulmonary venous drainage (8,9,53), anomalous left superior vena cava draining into the coronary sinus (8,53), right aortic arch (9,39), aortopulmonary window (8), tricuspid stenosis (53), and single coronary artery (26).

SUBVALVULAR PULMONARY STENOSIS

Subvalvular pulmonary stenosis includes infundibular stenosis and double-chamber right ventricle.

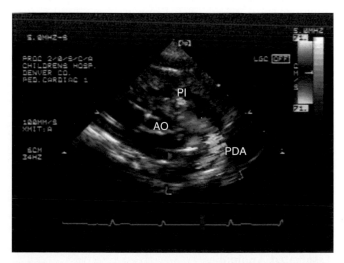

ECHO. 18-3. Color Doppler flow map of mild pulmonary insufficiency associated with a patent ductus arteriosus in the presence of critical pulmonic valve stenosis. Note the small and hypertrophied right ventricle. The identification of even trace pulmonic insufficiency documents the valve is patent. *PI*, pulmonic insufficiency jet; *PDA*, patent ductus arteriosus; *AO*, aorta.

INFUNDIBULAR PULMONARY STENOSIS

Infundibular pulmonary stenosis with intact ventricular septum can be primary or secondary (64). In the primary form, there are two types, that seen with idiopathic hypertrophic cardiomyopathy, which is not discussed in this chapter, and discrete fibromuscular obstruction or isolated infundibular pulmonary stenosis. The secondary form occurs as a result of an aneurysm of the membranous septum, an aneurysm of the right sinus of Valsalva, ectopic tricuspid valve tissue, and cardiac tumors, and right ventricular hypertrophy from valvular pulmonic stenosis (64).

Isolated infundibular pulmonary stenosis was originally described by Elliotson in 1830 (65) and later by Peacock in 1858, who called it "supernumerary septum in the right ventricle" (66). Keith termed it "sub-division of the right ventricle" in 1909 (67). Its incidence varies between 0.2% and 8% of all cases of pulmonary stenosis (10,11,25,30,53,68).

EMBRYOLOGIC CONSIDERATIONS

The conus or primordium of the infundibulum of both ventricles appears in the loop stage, at the extreme cephalic end of the heart and is continuous with the primordium of the trabecular portion of the morphologic right ventricle (69) (see Fig. 1-5). The conus is divided by the conal crests into an anterolateral and a posteromedial conus (see Figs. 1-12 and 1-14A). The anterolateral conus remains connected to the primordium of the trabecular portion of the right ventricle and makes up its outlet portion or pulmonary infundibulum. The union between the trabecular portion and the outlet portion of the right ventricle is called the "ostium infundibuli" (66) or "ostium bulbi." The incorporation of the posteromedial conus into the left ventricle and later total absorption results in the mitral-aortic continuity (70,71).

A defect in the process of absorption of the anterolateral conus or pulmonary infundibulum has been proposed as the embryologic mechanism resulting in discrete fibromuscular obstruction or isolated pulmonary infundibular stenosis (67,71,72).

ANATOMIC AND ECHOCARDIOGRAPHIC CONSIDERATIONS

The echocardiographic study of infundibular stenoses should comprise the following: (a) the morphologic characteristics of the obstruction; (b) the severity of the obstruction; and (c) associated anomalies.

Morphologic Characteristics of the Obstruction

In discrete fibromuscular obstruction, there is a ring or fibromuscular diaphragm with a central orifice of variable size that can be located at different levels within the right ventricular infundibulum (Fig. 18-2B–D). The location of the fibromuscular ring is most commonly at the lower portion of the pulmonary infundibulum, at the union with the trabecular portion of the right ventricle or ostium infundibuli (1,2,9,31,53,68,73) (Fig. 18-2B). The infundibular chamber is dilated and its walls are thin, the pulmonary valve and "pulmonary annulus" are normal and there is no dilatation of the pulmonary arterial trunk. Rarely the obstruction is at the mid portion of the infundibulum (74,75) (Fig. 18-2C) or immediately below the pulmonic valve (3,68,73–75) (Fig. 18-2D). Similarly, there is no dilatation of the pulmonary trunk in these types either.

There have been various causes identified in the genesis of secondary infundibular obstruction. Some of these are aneurysm of the right sinus of Valsalva (10,64), aneurysm of the membranous septum (76–78), incomplete fibrous membrane immediately below the pulmonic valve associated with fibrous tissue of tricuspid valve origin (79), mobile fibrous tissue attached to a normal papillary muscle (80), accessory tricuspid valve tissue (10,81), and cardiac tumors such as rhabdomyoma, myxoma, and sarcoma (10,82–87).

The morphologic characteristics of the right ventricular infundibulum can be studied echocardiographically by using the parasternal long-axis view tilted towards the outflow tract of the right ventricle, the parasternal short-axis view positioned slightly lower on the chest so as to "elongate" the outflow tract and from the subcostal short-axis view. These views allow determination of the site of obstruction, its characteristics, the size of the infundibular chamber, and the morphology of the valve and of the "pulmonary annulus" and of the main and proximal branches of the pulmonary artery. A fibromuscular membrane located immediately below the pulmonic valve may be difficult to image as a separate structure so in all instances the morphology and mobility of the valve leaflets throughout the cardiac cycle should be studied carefully. These would be typically normal in isolated infundibular stenosis but can exhibit some fluttering and early closure due to the high-velocity infundibular jet striking it in mid systole.

Severity of the Obstruction

The gradient across the right ventricular outflow tract can be estimated by measuring the velocity from parasternal long-axis and short-axis and subcostal short-axis views. The velocities across the entire right ventricular outflow tract should be recorded using high PRF Doppler techniques with careful placement of the sample volumes to accurately estimate the relative gradients at the various sites. Color flow mapping can serve as an indicator of the site(s) of obstruction by demonstrating serial color aliasing (Echos. 18-4, 18-5; see color plates 53 and 54 following p. 364). Even though the valve and "annulus"

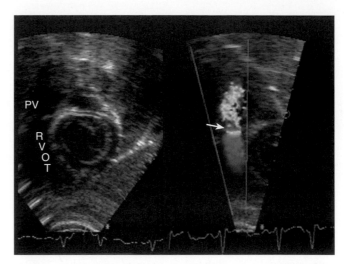

ECHO. 18-4. Subcostal short-axis view demonstrating the length of the right ventricular outflow tract and the pulmonic valve in subvalvular pulmonic stenosis. Note the sudden aliasing of the color Doppler flow map *(arrow)*, indicating the site of stenosis immediately below the valve. *PV,* pulmonic valve; *RVOT,* right ventricular outflow tract.

are usually normal in the presence of infundibular obstruction, it is important to continue the mapping of velocities with high PRF Doppler through the valve to assure no further significant stenoses.

The peak and mean gradients are calculated using the simplified Bernoulli equation. It is important to realize, however, that, in cases where the most significant obstruction is at the ostium infundibuli, the maximal velocity will be obtained immediately distal to this site and not beyond the valve. In the presence of obstruction at the mid portion of the infundibulum, the highest velocity will occur between the stenosis and the valve. In these two situations, use of high PRF Doppler is essential as the only method that can accurately resolve the velocities with some degree of range gating. Continuous wave Doppler can be used to confirm the highest velocities across the entire outflow tract but without definition of the actual site(s) of the gradients. Finally, if the obstruction is very close to the valve, the highest velocities can occur immediately distal to the valve, so in these cases continuous wave Doppler can be an acceptable method to record them. Doppler-estimated gradients will usually be higher than those measured by catheters due to pressure recovery effects that take place beyond the point of maximal flow constriction (see Chapter 6).

Associated Anomalies

In the majority of cases infundibular pulmonary stenosis is an isolated lesion. The presence of small ventricular septal defects (53,75) and subaortic stenosis (88) have been reported.

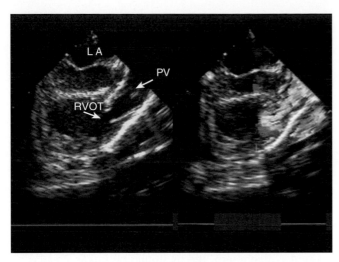

ECHO. 18-5. Left: Transesophageal longitudinal view of the right ventricular outflow tract showing the presence of a subpulmonic membrane *(arrow)*. **Right:** Color Doppler flow map across the outflow tract. Note the acceleration of flow with narrowing of the flow stream at the point of maximal obstruction. *LA,* left atrium; *PV,* pulmonic valve; *RVOT,* right ventricular outflow tract.

DOUBLE-CHAMBER RIGHT VENTRICLE

Double-chamber right ventricle is a malformation characterized by the presence of one or more anomalous muscle bundles that divide the right ventricular cavity into a proximal and a distal chamber. In the literature, it has been called "two-chambered right ventricle" (89,90), "cor triventriculare" (91), "anomalous muscle bundle of the right ventricle" (92), "double-chambered right ventricle" (93), "right ventricular obstruction by aberrant muscle bands" (94), "anomalous right ventricular muscles" (95), "double-chamber right ventricle" (96), and "divided right ventricle" (97).

In 1858, Peacock (66) described a group of hearts with what he called "supernumerary septum in the right ventricle," which included one heart with a thick muscular septum separating the sinus from the infundibular portions of the right ventricle. In 1909, Keith (67) reported a series of hearts with subdivided right ventricles in which he mentioned two hearts with a completely muscular separation, one of which had the infundibular chamber reaching the cardiac apex. However, it was not until the 1960s that the morphology of this malformation was clearly defined as different from infundibular stenosis at the level of the ostium infundibuli (89–95,98).

The actual incidence of double-chamber right ventricle, either relative to all congenital cardiac malformations or within the groups of pulmonary stenoses, has not been established.

EMBRYOLOGIC CONSIDERATIONS

The embryologic origin of double-chamber right ventricle has not yet been well defined. Some authors consider it to be due to a high takeoff of the septomarginal trabecula or to hypertrophy of the moderator band (96,99). Others suggest that it is an acquired lesion due to hypertrophy of an abnormally implanted moderator band in patients with ventricular septal defects (94,100,101) and that it regresses after spontaneous closure of the defects (100). Finally, others propose that it is due to persistence of septoparietal bands that are prominent in the embryonic heart (92,95,102,103).

ANATOMIC AND ECHOCARDIOGRAPHIC CONSIDERATIONS

The echocardiographic study in double-chamber right ventricle includes definition of the following features: (a) the anatomical characteristics of the obstruction; (b) presence of a ventricular septal defect; (c) degree of obstruction; and (d) associated anomalies.

Anatomical Characteristics of the Obstruction

Double-chamber right ventricle is characterized by the presence of one or several anomalous muscular bands located in the body of the right ventricle and which divide it into a proximal and a distal chamber. Usually, the anomalous muscle band is due to a hypertrophied moderator band that has a higher than normal origin on the septomarginal trabecula (Fig. 18-3). It is a thick muscular band

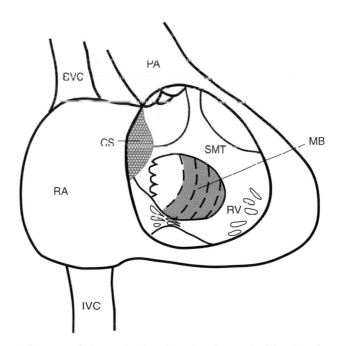

FIG. 18-3. Schematic drawing showing a double-chamber right ventricle. Note the higher than normal origins of the moderator band on the septomarginal trabecula. *RA,* right atrium; *RV,* right ventricle; *MB,* moderator band; *SMT,* septomarginal trabecula; *CS,* crista supraventricularis; *PA,* pulmonary artery; *SVC,* superior vena cava; *IVC,* inferior vena cava.

that is perpendicular to the interventricular septum and is oriented from the septum towards the free wall of the ventricle, immediately below the union of the right ventricular inlet and outlet portions. Occasionally, the anomalous muscle band divides the right ventricular cavity in two but without causing intraventricular obstruction. In the more severe forms, the anomalous muscle band is found adjacent to the crista supraventricularis and hypertrophy of the crista can aggravate the obstruction. The proximal or entry chamber is found between the tricuspid valve and the anomalous muscle band; it is separated from the outlet chamber, which is distal to the muscle band, by one or more totally muscular orifices (Echo. 18-6; see color plate 55 following p. 364). There can also be several septoapical muscle bands.

The double-chamber right ventricle is differentiated from low infundibular stenosis (Figs. 18-2B, 18-3) in that in double-chamber right ventricle the obstruction is lower within the body of the ventricle, the orifice(s) which communicates both chambers is totally muscular and the infundibular portion of the right ventricle is normal in size and characteristics and does not form part of the obstruction.

Recently, Restivo et al. (97) described various anatomic types of divided right ventricle: (a) anomalous septoparietal band dividing the entrance of the ventricular outlet into two pathways; (b) high takeoff of a prominent septoparietal band or anomalous apical shelf and hypertrophy of the apical trabeculations; (c) anomalous apical shelf with Ebstein's anomaly of the tricuspid valve; (d) high takeoff of a prominent septoparietal band with hypertrophy of the ventricular trabeculae forming a muscular shelf extending from the outlet septum to the apex; (e) sequestered ventricular inlet portion with a muscular shelf separating the inlet from the apical trabecular components of the ventricle; (f) sequestered trabecular component with endocardial fibroelastosis of the right ventricle associated with a horizontal extension of the trabecula septomarginalis forming a smooth plate across the ventricle allowing a direct pathway from the inlet to the outlet portions of the ventricle, thereby sequestering the apical trabecular septum from the rest of the ventricular cavity; the associated endocardial fibroelastosis of the left ventricle did not result in sequestration of its apical trabecular component; and (g) sequestration of the outlet portion in a heart with tetralogy of Fallot in which a circumferential muscular diaphragm, the os infundibuli, was created by a deviation of the infundibular septum and a prominent septoparietal trabeculation. This latter case could be considered a low infundibular stenosis and not a true double-chamber right ventricle. The case in which the muscular shelf extended from the outlet septum to the ventricular apex (see list above) had been previously reported by Beitzke et al. (104) as a case of two-chambered right ventricle simulating two-chambered left ventricle.

The morphologic characteristics of the double-chamber right ventricle can be evaluated from the apical four-chamber view and from the subcostal coronal or long-axis view and the subcostal short-axis or sagittal view (105,106). From the subcostal long-axis view, rotating the transducer slightly towards a short axis, the muscular band can be seen within the cavity of the right ventricle as well as the presence of a proximal and a distal chamber (Echo. 18-6). In the subcostal short-axis view, the anomalous muscle band is seen crossing from the ventricular septum to the free wall of the ventricle. The parasternal short-axis view also serves to demonstrate the presence of the anomalous muscle band (106).

Based on the hypothesis that there is a superior displacement of the moderator band in double-chamber right ventricle (96), Wong et al. (99) quantified the degree of displacement echocardiographically by measuring the distance between the pulmonary valve "annulus" and the septal insertion of the moderator band normalized against the diameter of the tricuspid annulus. The authors performed the measurements at end diastole in the subcostal short-axis view from the mid point of the insertion of the moderator band to the pulmonary valve annulus. The tricuspid annulus was measured at its largest dimension, in mid-diastole from the apical four-chamber view. In patients with double-chamber right ventricle, the displacement index was less than 1.0, with a mean index of 0.78 ± 0.19, whereas normal controls had a displacement index of greater than 1.15, with a mean index of 1.4 ± 0.14 (99).

The use color Doppler flow mapping from the subcostal long-axis and short-axis views and the parasternal short-axis view can aid in the demonstration of the site(s) of

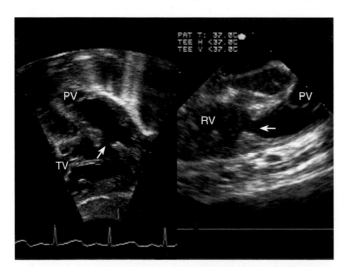

ECHO. 18-6. Left: Subcostal view with the transducer tilted superiorly to deomonstrate the presence of a double-chamber right ventricle. Note the hypertrophied muscle band with a completely muscular orifice (*arrow*) separating the proximal and distal right ventricular chambers. **Right:** Transesophageal longitudinal view of a patient with infundibular pulmonary stenosis. Note the fibromuscular ring located at the lower portion of the infundibulum or ostium infundibuli (*arrow*) separating the trabecular portion of the right ventricle from the pulmonary infundibulum. *PV,* pulmonic valve; *RV,* right ventricle; *TV,* tricuspid valve.

obstruction and of the orifice(s) communicating the proximal and distal chambers. These are represented by flow acceleration proximal to the obstruction and velocity variance distally (Echo. 18-6).

Presence of a Ventricular Septal Defect

In 64% to 96% of reported cases of double-chamber right ventricle there has been a ventricular septal defect present (90,92,94–96,99,102,105,107,108). It is usually perimembranous, of variable size, and located below the crista supraventricularis, covered by the septal leaflet of the tricuspid valve. It is connected with the proximal, high-pressured chamber. In one series, the septal defects had extensions towards the inlet in 69% of cases and towards the outlet in the remaining 31% (105).

The echocardiographic views that would reveal the presence of a ventricular septal defect would be the parasternal long-axis and short-axis views, the apical four-chamber view and the subcostal long- and short-axis views. Its anatomical location, size and direction of flow should be determined from a combination of two-dimensional imaging and color flow mapping. Since the ventricular septal defect is related to the proximal or high-pressure chamber, the direction of flow is dependent on the relative pressures of that chamber and the systemic ventricle. It can be completely left to right, bidirectional, or mostly right to left. Spectral Doppler recording of velocities and the color M-mode traces of the flow through the defect can best demonstrate the dynamics of the flow across it as well as the pressure drop from the left ventricle to the proximal chamber.

Degree of Obstruction

The degree of obstruction can be determined by measuring the velocities across the stenotic orifice separating the two chambers with high PRF Doppler techniques. Similar to that described above for infundibular obstructions, the high PRF method allows resolution of high velocities with range-gating capabilities. Color Doppler is helpful in visually demonstrating the site(s) of obstruction and thereby in positioning the sample volumes for recording the velocities. The views most suited for visualizing the two chambers within the right ventricular cavity and outflow tract are the parasternal long-axis view tilting the transducer slightly towards the pulmonary valve, the apical four-chamber view aiming superiorly, and the subcostal long- and short-axis views also aiming superiorly towards the right ventricular outflow tract.

Associated Anomalies

A number of associated anomalies have been reported with double-chamber right ventricle. These include valve pulmonic stenosis (92,93,95,96,105,107), tetralogy of Fallot (105), pulmonary atresia (93), valve aortic stenosis (95), subvalve aortic stenosis (95,96,105,107–109), prolapse of the aortic valve with regurgitation (96,107,108), atrial septal defect (95,96,107,108), patent ductus arteriosus (95), complete transposition of the great arteries (95), double outlet right ventricle (95,107,108), mitral atresia (95), hypoplastic left ventricle (95), cor triatriatum (95), partial anomalous pulmonary venous drainage, scimitar syndrome (107), total anomalous pulmonary venous drainage (95,96), bilateral inferior vena cava (95), peripheral pulmonary branch stenosis (96), and right aortic arch (105,110), which can be seen in up to 15% of patients with double-chamber right ventricle (110).

PULMONARY VALVULAR INSUFFICIENCY

Pulmonary valvular insufficiency can be physiologic, as seen in up to 92% of normal individuals (111,112). It can also be secondary to a number of conditions such as a morphologically abnormal valve like a quadricuspid (49) or a dysplastic valve, due to pulmonary hypertension, after balloon valvuloplasty or surgical valvotomy for valvular pulmonic stenosis, after reconstruction of the outflow tract in the surgery for tetralogy of Fallot, in the absence of the pulmonary valve, etc. We will specifically consider isolated absence of the pulmonary valve in this section. Pulmonary regurgitation occurring after therapeutic interventions is discussed below in "Intra- and Postoperative Evaluation." Other types are discussed in the corresponding chapters.

The first report of isolated absence of the pulmonary valve was by Chevers in 1847 (113), who described a syndrome characterized by absence of the leaflets of the pulmonary valve, ventricular septal defect, pulmonary annular stenosis and dilation of the pulmonary trunk and of one or both branches. Since then most cases reported have been in association with tetralogy of Fallot, having an incidence of 2.1% to 6.3% of cases of tetralogy (114–116). The first case of isolated absence of the pulmonary valve was described by Ehrenhaft (117) in a youth 14 years of age and the first case in a premature infant was reported by Smith et al. in 1959 (118). Very few additional cases have been reported in the literature (119–125). Only 2.4% of published cases of agenesis of the pulmonic valve are isolated (114); its incidence corresponds to 0.13% of all congenital heart disease (12).

EMBRYOLOGIC CONSIDERATIONS

The morphogenetic process that causes isolated agenesis of the pulmonic valve is unknown. In the first described case, Ehrenhaft considered it secondary to destruction of the valve from an acquired process (117). Smith et al. (118), on the other hand, suggested that it was congenital since there was absence of an inflammatory process or of destruction of valvular tissue. Probably failure of development of the truncal swellings would explain those cases in which there is absence of all valve tissue, while an abnormal development of the truncal swellings could be the cause in cases where there are leaflet remnants or dysplastic leaflets.

ANATOMIC AND ECHOCARDIOGRAPHIC CONSIDERATIONS

The echocardiographic study of isolated agenesis of the pulmonic valve would include the following: (a) morphology of the pulmonic valve remnants; (b) the size of the right ventricular-pulmonary trunk junction or "pulmonary annulus"; (c) the size of the main and branch pulmonary arteries; (d) presence and severity of pulmonary insufficiency; and (e) associated anomalies.

Morphology of the Pulmonic Valve, Size of the "Pulmonary Annulus" and of the Main and Branch Pulmonary Arteries

The term absent pulmonary valve has been used in the literature to describe a condition in which there is a rudimentary or dysplastic pulmonic valve (120–122,124). In the majority of cases, there is rudimentary valvular tissue having a nodular appearance or remnants of dysplastic leaflets that are thickened and gelatinous. Histologically, they are composed of young and avascular connective tissue (118). There have been only two cases in which no valve tissue remnants were seen (117,123). The right ventricular-pulmonary trunk junction or "pulmonary annulus" is almost always diminished in size, and only rarely is it normal or dilated. Gross dilatation of the main pulmonary artery, extending either to the left or to both branches, is the norm. These can be aneurysmatically dilated, causing bronchial compression. The adventitia of the pulmonary artery has fibrous thickening, and there are alterations in the elastic medial layer, with histologic characteristics similar to those seen in cystic medial necrosis (118). The right ventricle is usually dilated and hypertrophic.

Absence of the pulmonary valve can be detected echocardiographically from the parasternal long-axis view tilted towards the pulmonary outflow, from the parasternal short-axis view aimed at the level of the great arteries and from the subcostal long- and short-axis views. These views would also reveal any remnant of fibrous tissue or dysplastic leaflets (Echo. 18-7). The size of the right ventricular-pulmonary trunk junction ("pulmonary annulus") can be measured from these views as well. The main and branch pulmonary arteries can be seen best from the short-axis views; in the parasternal position the transducer should be placed slightly lower or higher than the usual site to image as much as possible of the length of the pulmonary branches. The peripheral pulmonary

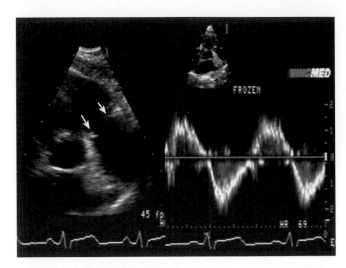

ECHO. 18-7. Left: Short-axis view of the right ventricular outflow tract demonstrating the remnants of the pulmonic leaflets *(arrows)* in isolated absence of the pulmonary valve. **Right:** Spectral Doppler recording of velocities across the pulmonary annulus. The traces exhibit low velocity forward and reverse flow, indicating wide-open regurgitation.

arteries can also be seen from the suprasternal views (see Figs. 4-20C, 4-21C, 4-22, and 4-23) and from the left subclavicular view (see Figs. 4-24A and 4-25A). If the "pulmonary annulus" is stenotic, the velocities across it should be measured with continuous wave Doppler to establish the presence and severity of the gradient. This will also reveal the pulmonary regurgitation (Echo. 18-7).

Presence and Severity of Pulmonary Insufficiency

Absence of the pulmonary valve or presence of only dysplastic leaflet remnants causes severe pulmonary regurgitation. This is readily seen on color Doppler flow mapping of the right ventricular outflow (Echo. 18-8; see color plate 56 following p. 364). Spectral Doppler recording of the regurgitant jet velocities permits estimation of its severity by the intensity of the signal itself as well as by the slope of the deceleration curve (Echo. 18-7). The more severe the regurgitation, the sharper the deceleration slope since the diastolic pressure in the pulmonary artery approaches the right ventricular end diastolic pressure faster.

If there is a patent ductus arteriosus with pulmonary hypertension, the ductal flow is bidirectional; during systole, the flow is from the pulmonary artery to the aorta, whereas in diastole it is from the aorta to the pulmonary artery and into the right ventricular cavity.

Associated Anomalies

Contrary to what is seen in tetralogy of Fallot with absent pulmonary valve, in isolated absence of the valve the ductus arteriosus is usually patent (118–125). Other

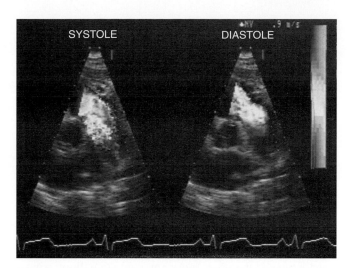

ECHO. 18-8. Color Doppler maps of the systolic and diastolic flows across the right ventricular outflow tract in the presence of isolated absence of the pulmonic valve. Note the aliasing of velocities, in both directions, at the narrowest point along the outflow tract.

associated anomalies include patent foramen ovale (118,119,122), atrial septal defect (120), and anomalous origin of the right subclavian artery from the descending aorta (124).

PULMONARY ATRESIA WITH INTACT VENTRICULAR SEPTUM

Pulmonary atresia with intact ventricular septum or pulmonary atresia with normal aortic root are part of the spectrum of right ventricular outflow tract anomalies and are characterized by the absence of a connection between the right ventricle and the pulmonary artery, intact ventricular septum, perforated tricuspid valve and two ventricles clearly differentiated (see Fig. 2-8G). The first case of this malformation was published by Hunter in 1783 (126) who described it as "The pulmonary artery, which, at its beginning from the right ventricle, was contracted into a solid substance or chord, and absolutely and completely impervious; so that the lungs had not received one drop of blood from the heart by the trunk of the pulmonary artery." Later, Peacock (127) published three cases in 1858 in which the orifice or trunk of the pulmonary artery was totally impervious and the ventricular septum was intact.

The first classification of this malformation was suggested by Greenwold et al. (128), who recognized two types, one with small right ventricle (type 1) and one with normal or dilated right ventricle (type 2). More recently, Bull et al. (129) proposed a new classification based on the presence or absence of inlet, trabecular or outlet portions of the right ventricular cavity.

Pulmonary atresia with intact ventricular septum carries an incidence of 43.9% of all pulmonary atresias (130)

and varies between 0.71% and 3.1% of all congenital cardiac anomalies (12,25,131).

EMBRYOLOGIC CONSIDERATIONS

The morphogenetic process that causes pulmonary atresia with intact septum is not well defined. The presence of raphes in the membrane that forms the plane of the valve has led investigators to propose that this malformation occurs late in cardiac development, after cardiac septation is complete, due to fusion of the pulmonary leaflets, similar to that in valvular pulmonary stenosis (36,103,132). This is different from that proposed for tetralogy of Fallot with pulmonary atresia.

ANATOMIC AND ECHOCARDIOGRAPHIC CONSIDERATIONS

The echocardiographic study of pulmonary atresia with intact ventricular septum should include, in addition to determination of the visceroatrial situs and the type of atrioventricular and ventriculoarterial connection, the following features: (a) the morphologic characteristics of the atretic segment; (b) the size and anatomical characteristics of the right ventricle and the tricuspid valve; (c) the presence of anomalies of the coronary arteries; (d) the presence of atrial shunting; (e) the presence of a patent ductus arteriosus; (f) anatomical characteristics of the main and branch pulmonary arteries; and (g) associated anomalies.

Visceroatrial Situs and Type of Atrioventricular and Ventriculoarterial Connection

In the vast majority of cases of pulmonary atresia with intact ventricular septum, the heart is in levocardia, the visceroatrial situs is solitus and the atrioventricular and ventriculoarterial connections are concordant (130,131,133–136). Only one case of dextrocardia and situs inversus (133) and three cases with atrioventricular and ventriculoarterial discordance (congenitally corrected transposition) have been reported (136–138).

Morphologic Characteristics of the Atretic Segment

In the majority of cases the atresia is at the valvular level and is represented by a fibrous diaphragm with three raphes corresponding to the three fused leaflets, which are more or less developed. Zuberbuhler et al. (139,140) described two types of atresia, one in which the raphes are located exclusively in the periphery with a smooth central dome that protrudes into the main pulmonary trunk and another in which prominent raphes are seen corresponding to the fused commissures and that converge in the middle of the fibrous diaphragm. The first type is seen in cases where the infundibulum is permeable and not severely stenotic, and the tricuspid valve is neither severely stenotic nor markedly regurgitant so that there is a high right ventricular pressure pressing against the infundibular surface of the pulmonary membrane. The second type is seen in cases of severe stenosis or atresia of the infundibulum and severe tricuspid regurgitation resulting in a low right ventricular pressure (139,140). These same authors have found one case in which there was only one raphe and two cases having four raphes (139,140). In rare instances, there can be no valvular tissue present along with a small pulmonary arterial trunk (139,140) or a fibrous chord extending to the branch pulmonary arteries (133,141) or an infundibular atresia without recognizable valve tissue in its dimple (132,142). One case of a bicuspid, perforated pulmonic valve associated with infundibular atresia and intact ventricular septum was reported by Freedom and Keith (133). Infundibular and valvular pulmonary atresia can be seen with an intact ventricular septum (130,136,139,140); in these instances there is a variable sized bar of muscular tissue that separates the atretic pulmonic valve from the right ventricular cavity. The two cases published by Van Praagh et al. (130) also had congenital absence of the tricuspid valve similar to what had been previously denominated congenital unguarded tricuspid orifice associated with pulmonary atresia by Kanjuh et al. (143).

The echocardiographic views that allow analysis of the atretic segment are the parasternal long-axis view of the outflow tract, the parasternal short-axis view with the transducer positioned slightly lower on the chest to allow a somewhat elongated projection of the outflow tract, and the subcostal long-axis and short-axis views (Echo. 18-9). From the subcostal approach, Marino et al. (144) suggest a view intermediate between the coronal and sagittal ones, a right oblique equivalent view, as the most adequate for evaluation of this anatomy. Color Doppler is quite useful for the confirmation of the absence of flow from the right ventricle to the pulmonary artery. As mentioned previously, it is important to differentiate true pulmonic valve atresia from functional atresia, which can occur in the presence of tricuspid regurgitation and high pulmonary vascular resistance, particularly in the newborn period (145–147). Frame-by-frame analysis of the color Doppler images usually reveals even small amounts of forward flow through the valve; however, the relatively poor temporal resolution of this technique can lead to errors in diagnosis. Nonetheless, a useful parameter on color Doppler flow mapping is the presence of pulmonary valvular regurgitation, which implies that the valve is permeable and therefore more amenable to balloon valvuloplasty (148) (Echo. 18-3).

Size and Anatomical Characteristics of the Right Ventricle and Tricuspid Valve

Classically, pulmonary atresia with intact ventricular septum was classified according to the size of the right ventricle, namely those with small, normal, or large right ventricular cavities (128). However, since the size of the right ventricle comprises a large spectrum from diminutive to severely dilated, classification according to this parameter is difficult (130,134–136,139,140,149,150). As such, a new classification has been proposed according to the presence of inlet, trabecular, and outlet portions of the ventricular cavity: (a) right ventricle having identifiable inlet, trabecular and outlet portions; (b) right ventricle with absence of trabecular portion; and (c) right ventricle having only an inlet portion, with absent trabecular and outlet portions (129). In a morphologic study of 60 cases of pulmonary atresia with intact ventricular septum, Freedom et al. (134) noted a dilated right ventricular cavity in 13% of cases, a normal cavity in 6.5%, a mildly underdeveloped cavity in 10%, a moderately hypoplastic one in 30%, and a markedly underdeveloped cavity in 40% of cases. The degree of development of the right ventricle is related to the size of the tricuspid orifice and to the presence of incompetence of the valve. In the presence of a stenotic and competent tricuspid valve, the right ventricle is small and hypertrophied, whereas in the presence of tricuspid regurgitation, the right ventricle is dilated (130,134–136,140,149,150). Endocardial fibroelastosis is usual in the presence of a small right ventricular cavity with a hypoplastic or atretic infundibulum.

The tricuspid valve is usually abnormal in pulmonary atresia with intact ventricular septum (129,134,136,139, 140,151). The size of the right ventricular cavity is related to the degree of stenosis and regurgitation of the tricuspid valve so that when the right ventricle is markedly or moderately hypoplastic, the tricuspid orifice is usually stenotic and the valve competent. In these cases, the

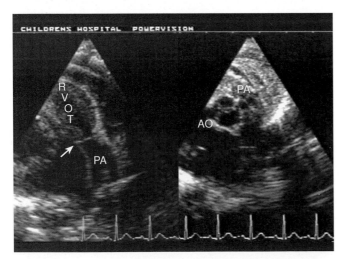

ECHO. 18-9. Left: Parasternal view tilted towards the right ventricular outflow tract demonstrating an atretic pulmonic valve *(arrow)* and a small and severely hypertrophied right ventricular outflow tract. **Right:** A high short-axis view shows the atretic pulmonic valve in cross section. *RVOT*, right ventricular outflow tract; *PA*, pulmonary artery; *AO*, aorta.

leaflets of the tricuspid valve are generally thickened and dysplastic, the tendinous chords are short and deficient and the papillary muscles are rudimentary. Occasionally, the leaflets insert directly into the papillary muscles without intervening tendinous chords (134). When the right ventricle is normal or dilated, the tricuspid valve orifice is usually dilated and the tricuspid valve regurgitant with dysplastic, redundant leaflets, and deficient tendinous chords and papillary muscles (134,150). The tricuspid valve leaflets can present variable grades of downward displacement or Ebstein's malformation.

The echocardiographic views that best demonstrate the anatomical characteristics of the right ventricular cavity and tricuspid valve are the parasternal long-axis view tilted towards the inflow of the right ventricle, the parasternal short-axis view, the apical four-chamber view, the subcostal four-chamber and short-axis views and the right oblique equivalent view. The morphology of the tricuspid valve and the size of the orifice can be evaluated from these views, particularly the four-chamber apical and the parasternal short-axis views. Measurement of the right ventricular size and volume and the diameter of the tricuspid valve annulus are best performed from the subcostal long-axis and short-axis views. These measurements have been found to be predictive of the postoperative outcome and useful in the preoperative planning for these patients, according to the recommendations of the Congenital Heart Surgeons Society (152). The Z-score of the tricuspid valve is obtained using the following formula:

Z value

$$= \frac{\text{Measured diameter} - \text{Mean normal diameter}}{\text{Standard deviation of the mean normal diameter}}$$

The measured diameter is the tricuspid orifice diameter measured echocardiographically and the mean normal diameter is that found in normal individuals of comparable body surface area (152). Analysis of the Z value in relation to the predicted prevalence of the initial surgical approach demonstrated that pulmonary valvulotomy without a systemic to pulmonary shunt was optimal for neonates with a Z value for the tricuspid valve of greater than −0.15. For patients with Z values between −1.5 and −4, the best initial intervention was the placement of a transannular patch along with a shunt (152). The predicted prevalence with respect to the definitive surgical procedure demonstrated that the Z value was lower in patients 5 years after univentricular repair (Fontan type of operation) while it was higher in patients after a biventricular repair (152). Color Doppler flow mapping is helpful in defining the forward flow across the tricuspid valve and the presence of regurgitation. Spectral Doppler recording of the forward and regurgitant velocities aids in the estimation of any gradient across the tricuspid valve and of the severity of the regurgitation. The severity of the valvular stenosis can be assessed by measuring the pressure half time of the forward Doppler velocity curve as well

as the peak pressure drop from the simplified Bernoulli equation. The regurgitant jet velocity allows for the estimation of the pressure drop between the right ventricle and the right atrium and therefore of the right ventricular systolic pressure. In the presence of wide-open tricuspid regurgitation, however, the right ventricular and right atrial cavities function as a single unit physiologically without a pressure difference between them, so the Doppler velocity of the regurgitant jet is low. This should not be erroneously interpreted as lack of right ventricular outflow obstruction.

Presence of Anomalies of the Coronary Arteries

Since the first report by Grant in 1926 of an anomalous communication between the right ventricular cavity and the coronary arteries (153), a series of other publications have documented their presence in pulmonary atresia with intact ventricular septum (130,134,136,140,149, 154–163). These include ventriculocoronary communications, intramyocardial sinusoids, coronary obstructive lesions occurring proximally or distally to the ventriculocoronary communications, absence of connection between a coronary artery and the aorta, anomalies in the origin of the coronary arteries and presence of a single coronary artery.

Ventriculocoronary Communications and Intramyocardial Sinusoids. Between 47% and 60% of cases of pulmonary atresia with intact ventricular septum, small right ventricle, and competent tricuspid valve have ventriculocoronary communications and intramyocardial sinusoids (140,159,163). During early stages of development, the ventricular walls are nourished through imbibition of the circulating blood and later through intramyocardial sinusoids that establish contact with the subepicardial vascular network, which will give rise to the coronary circulation. When the subepicardial vascular network comes in contact with the aorta, the intramyocardial sinusoids disappear (see Fig. 1-15). In pulmonary atresia with intact ventricular septum, competent tricuspid valve and small right ventricular cavity, the pressure within the right ventricle is high, thereby preventing the disappearance of the intramyocardial sinusoids. These persist as channels in the right ventricular myocardium originating from the ventricular cavity and either ending as blind sacs in the myocardium itself or establishing connections with the coronary arteries or coronary veins, giving rise to the ventriculocoronary communications that link the right ventricular cavity with the coronary circulation.

The ventriculocoronary communications can be single or multiple and can establish connections between the right ventricular cavity and either the right coronary artery, the anterior descending coronary artery or both. Rarely is there a communication between the right ventricular cavity and the left main coronary artery (158,160). Normally, coronary arterial flow occurs in diastole; however, in these patients, coronary flow occurs during right ventricular systole so that the normal diastolic flow is impaired by the retrograde systolic flow through the ventriculocoronary communications, which can result in ischemia and myocardial dysfunction. In the presence of obstructive coronary lesions, the coronary circulation perfusing the major part of the left ventricular myocardium may be dependent on the right ventricle in which case decompression of the right ventricle during blade/balloon valvuloplasty or surgical valvotomy can have devastating consequences.

Obstructive Coronary Lesions. Presence of ventriculocoronary communications may result in coronary obstructive lesions proximal or distal to the communications. The pattern of abnormal coronary flow with systolic coronary perfusion under suprasystemic pressures would give rise to lesions characterized by variable degrees of thickening of the media and intima (158,159). This results in luminal narrowing or even complete obstruction. Cases with lack of connection between the main and branches of one or both coronary arteries have been reported (131,136,161).

Anomalous Origin of the Coronary Arteries. In 20% of cases studied by Calder et al. (159), there was only a single coronary artery. In one case, the left coronary artery emerged from the right coronary and in four cases the right coronary artery originated from the left coronary artery; in three of these cases, it arose from the anterior descending coronary and in the fourth from the trunk of the left coronary artery. In all instances, the right coronary artery crossed in front of the right ventricular outflow tract (159). Anomalous origin of a coronary from the pulmonary arterial trunk has also been reported (157).

Echocardiographically the ventriculocoronary communications can be seen with color Doppler flow mapping within the right ventricular myocardium from the parasternal long- and short-axis views, and the apical and the subcostal views (Echo. 18-10; see color plate 57 following p. 364). If prominent, the velocities can be recorded with pulsed wave Doppler and the systolic timing of the flow documented (Echo. 18-10). Obstructive coronary lesions cannot be detected by echocardiography at present. The origin and proximal course of the coronary arteries can be seen from a low parasternal short-axis view angled slightly superior to the plane of the aortic root. Normally, the right coronary can be seen coursing along the right atrioventricular groove and if there are significant branches crossing in front of the outflow tract, these can usually be seen within the right ventricular anterior wall. The left anterior descending and circumflex branches are normally observed coursing leftward, anterior to the pulmonary outflow, by angling the transducer superiorly from a standard parasternal short-axis view.

Presence of Atrial Level Shunting

An atrial level shunt allowing blood flow from the right atrium to the left atrium is mandatory for survival of

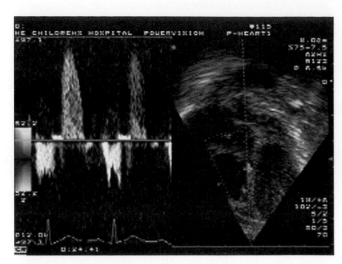

ECHO 18-10. Right: Apical view of ventriculocoronary communications demonstrated on color Doppler flow map. **Left:** Spectral Doppler recording of the systolic velocity obtained at the site of the ventriculocoronary communication.

patients with this lesion. Almost always there is a patent foramen ovale of adequate size but in the presence of a restrictive atrial communication, the atrial septum bulges to the left. An ostium secundum atrial septal defect is seen in only 20% to 23% of cases (131,134). Only rarely is the atrial septum intact, and then the left atrium communicates with an unroofed coronary sinus, allowing a right-to-left shunt; unfortunately, in these cases, the coronary sinus is stenotic (136). The right atrium is always dilated and its size is related to the severity of the tricuspid valve regurgitation.

The atrial level shunt can be demonstrated echocardiographically from the subcostal long-axis view using color Doppler flow mapping. Recording of the velocity of the shunt flow with pulsed wave Doppler can aid in the determination of the physiologic adequacy of the communication and can supplement the anatomic information derived from the two-dimensional images of the atrial septum.

Presence of a Patent Ductus Arteriosus

The presence of a patent ductus arteriosus allowing blood flow into the pulmonary circulation is the rule and survival depends on its permeability. Different from pulmonary atresia with ventricular septal defect, in which the ductal union with the aorta has an acute angle, in pulmonary atresia with intact ventricular septum, the ductal angle is obtuse, similar to that seen in normal newborns (164). The ductal size can be quite variable, but usually it is small and tortuous. Bilateral ducti can also be the only origin of flow into separate pulmonary arteries that are not confluent (Echo. 18-11; see color plates 58 and 59 following p. 364). Rarely there may be systemic to pulmonary collaterals supplying the pulmonary blood flow (131).

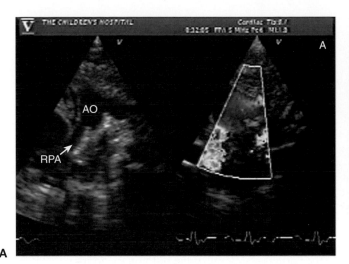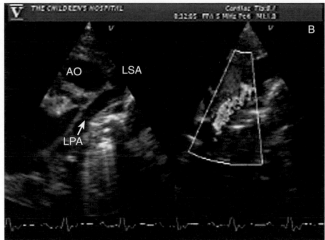

ECHO. 18-11. Example of separate origins of nonconfluent pulmonary arteries from bilateral ducti in pulmonary atresia. **A:** Anatomical image and color Doppler flow map of the right pulmonary artery originating from a right-sided ductus. **B:** Anatomical image and color Doppler flow map of the left pulmonary artery originating from a left-sided ductus. *AO,* aorta; *LSA,* left subclavian artery; *LPA,* left pulmonary artery; *RPA,* right pulmonary artery.

The presence of a patent ductus can be seen echocardiographically from the parasternal long-axis view tilted towards the right ventricular outflow, from the parasternal short-axis view and from the suprasternal long- and short-axis views. The presence and direction of the shunt can be easily appreciated with color Doppler flow mapping which can also aid in determining the anatomical size of the ductus. The spectral Doppler velocity traces permit a better analysis of the timing of the shunting and can help determine the degree of constriction of the ductus by estimating the pressure drop from aorta to pulmonary artery. These techniques are essential in the early management of these infants when maintaining a patent ductus of adequate size with prostaglandin infusion is critical for survival.

Anatomical Characteristics of the Main and Branch Pulmonary Arteries

The main and branch pulmonary arteries are almost always present, but the main trunk is usually smaller than normal (130,140,149) and absent in 3.8% to 5% of cases (130,131). The branches of the pulmonary artery are variably hypoplastic. In the 52 necropsy cases studied by Van Praagh et al. (130), 84% had moderately or severely hypoplastic branches; however, in a study of 171 neonates, Hanley et al. (163) found only 3.5% of patients with significant hypoplasia of the branches. Most likely this discrepancy can be explained by the fact that Van Praagh's study included only necropsy cases, perhaps representing the worst in the spectrum.

The size of the main and branch pulmonary arteries can be best appreciated echocardiographically from the parasternal and subcostal short-axis views and from the suprasternal and left subclavicular views (Echo. 18-12).

Associated Anomalies

Persistence of the right sinus venosus valve has been found in 20.4% of cases in a published series (130). Other reported associated lesions are bicuspid aortic valve (130), aortic valvular stenosis (131,136,165), subvalvular aortic stenosis due to bulging of the ventricular septum

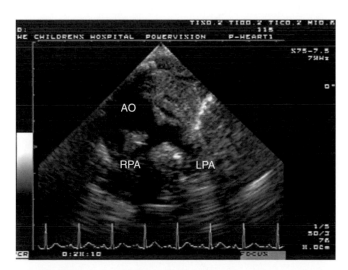

ECHO. 18-12. Left subclavicular view showing the confluence and proximal branches of the right and left pulmonary arteries in atresia of the pulmonary valve and main pulmonary segment. *AO,* aorta; *RPA,* right pulmonary artery; *LPA,* left pulmonary artery.

(139), dysplastic mitral valve (131,136), mitral valve arcade (140), right aortic arch (131), parachute tricuspid valve (139), persistence of the right sinus venosus valve, and Uhl's anomaly (130,131,166).

ANOMALIES OF THE PULMONARY ARTERY AND ITS BRANCHES

This section will include stenosis of the main and branches of the pulmonary arteries and anomalous origin of a pulmonary artery from the ascending aorta. Anomalous origin of the left pulmonary branch from the right pulmonary artery or pulmonary arterial sling is discussed in Chapter 31.

STENOSIS OF THE MAIN AND BRANCH PULMONARY ARTERIES

Stenosis of the trunk and branches of the pulmonary artery form the complex known as supravalve pulmonary stenosis. The obstruction can be found in the trunk, immediately above the valve (Fig. 18-4), near the bifurcation and at the origin or the periphery of the pulmonary branches. The first publication of a case of supravalve pulmonary stenosis at the level of the arterial trunk was made by Chevers in 1847 (113) and the first report of bilateral stenosis of the branches was written by Oppenheimer in 1938 (167). The incidence of this lesion ranges between 2% and 4.2% of all congenital heart disease (168–170).

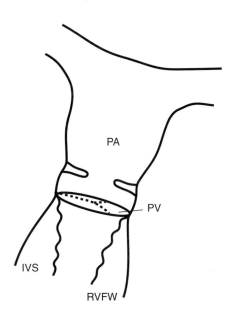

FIG. 18-4. Schematic drawing of supravalve pulmonary stenosis. *PA*, pulmonary artery; *PV*, pulmonic valve; *IVS*, interventricular septum; *RVFW*, right ventricular free wall.

EMBRYOLOGIC CONSIDERATIONS

The main and branch pulmonary arteries have different embryologic origins and the structures that form them appear at different stages in cardiac development. The aortopulmonary septum divides the aortic sac into ascending aorta and main pulmonary trunk. The proximal portion of the right and left pulmonary arteries originates from the proximal portion of the right and left sixth aortic arch, respectively. The distal or intrahilar branches of the right and left pulmonary arteries arise from the right and left primitive pulmonary arteries, respectively. The morphogenetic mechanisms that give rise to supravalve pulmonary stenoses are not known. Any alteration in the development of the embryologic structures that give rise to the various segments of the pulmonary artery will cause stenosis at that level. The rubella virus has been recognized as a teratogenic agent causing peripheral pulmonary artery stenosis (171–173). The syndrome of supravalve aortic stenosis, peripheral pulmonary artery stenosis, mental retardation and characteristic elfin facies, described by Williams et al. (174) and Beuren et al. (175,176) has been associated with idiopathic familial hypercalcemia (177,178).

ANATOMIC AND ECHOCARDIOGRAPHIC CONSIDERATIONS

The echocardiographic study of supravalve pulmonary stenoses should be directed towards determining the anatomical characteristics and location of the obstruction and any associated anomalies.

Morphology and Location of the Obstruction

Franch and Gay proposed a classification of supravalve pulmonary stenosis that was based on the various classifications previously suggested by Gyllensward et al. (179), Smith (180), and Arvidsson et al. (181). The classification of Franch and Gay (182) included four types of stenoses of the pulmonary arteries: Type I, isolated central stenosis; Type II, stenosis at the bifurcation; Type III, multiple peripheral stenoses; and Type IV, combined central and peripheral stenoses.

Type I was observed by these authors in 38% of their cases. The stenosis can be at the level of the trunk of the pulmonary artery, subtype IA, and be formed either by a membranous diaphragm or by a diffuse segment. The membranous diaphragm can be located immediately above the valve, at the mid third of the main trunk or close to the bifurcation; the diffuse segment is close to the bifurcation. When the stenotic segment is located in the right pulmonary branch it is classified as subtype 1B and when it is in the left pulmonary branch it is named subtype 1C. Type II was seen in 20% of cases. The stenosis is found at the level of the bifurcation and encompasses the distal portion of the main pulmonary trunk and the origin of both branch pulmonary arteries. It can be a short segment, subtype IIA, or a long one, subtype IIB. Type III was seen in 18% of cases. This type has multiple peripheral stenoses that involve only the segmental pulmonary arterial branches and are usually accompanied by poststenotic dilatation; the main trunk and branches are normal. Type IV was found in 24% of cases. These present with multiple peripheral stenoses at the level of the segmental branches similar to type III but associated with stenosis of the main trunk and branches as well (182).

Stenosis of the main trunk and/or branches of the pulmonary arteries can be visualized by echocardiography from the parasternal and subcostal short-axis views, from the suprasternal long- and short-axis views and from the left subclavicular view (Echos. 18-13, 18-14; see color plates 60 and 61 following p. 364). The presence of a discrete diaphragm or of a diffuse type of stenosis can be appreciated as well as the size of the branches distal to the stenotic site(s). The suprasternal short-axis views (see Figs. 4-20C, 4-21C, 4-22, and 4-23) allows visualization of the peripheral branches up to the hilum in some patients; beyond, they cannot be studied with echocardiography. Color Doppler can help assess the size of the branches beyond the stenoses, particularly when these are very small and cannot be defined with two-dimensional imaging alone.

Associated Anomalies

Stenosis of the pulmonary arteries exists as an isolated malformation in up to 40% of cases (182). In addition to the supravalve aortic stenosis already mentioned above, other associations have been valvular pulmonic stenosis

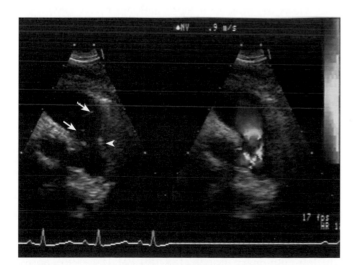

ECHO. 18-13. Parasternal view tilted towards the right ventricular outflow tract in the presence of supravalve pulmonary stenosis. Note the valve leaflets *(arrows)*, the area of narrowing above the valve *(arrowhead)*, and the aliasing of velocities at that site on color Doppler flow mapping.

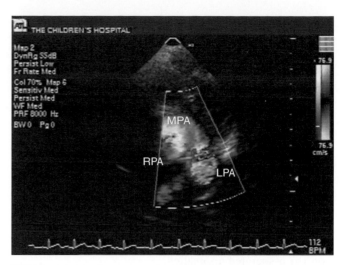

ECHO. 18-14. Parasternal short-axis view demonstrating stenosis of the left pulmonary arterial branch at its bifurcation. Note the velocity aliasing on the color Doppler map. *MPA*, main pulmonary artery; *RPA*, right pulmonary artery; *LPA*, left pulmonary artery.

(168,179,181–186), tetralogy of Fallot (168,182–184), patent foramen ovale (167), atrial septal defect (182,185), ventricular septal defect (168,181–183,185), patent ductus arteriosus (168,181–183), valvular aortic stenosis (181,182), persistent left superior vena cava (179), partial anomalous pulmonary venous drainage (168,179), and coarctation of the aorta (184).

ANOMALOUS ORIGIN OF A PULMONARY ARTERY FROM THE ASCENDING AORTA

Origin of a pulmonary artery from the ascending aorta or "hemitruncus" is a rare congenital malformation characterized by one pulmonary artery emerging from the ascending aorta and the other one emerging normally from the main pulmonary trunk. The first case was published by Fraentzel in 1868 and described a case of anomalous origin of the right pulmonary artery from the ascending aorta and aortopulmonary window (187). The incidence of this malformation is very low, between 0.05% and 0.09% of all congenital heart disease (188,189).

EMBRYOLOGIC CONSIDERATIONS

There is no consensus regarding the morphogenesis of anomalous origin of a pulmonary artery from the ascending aorta. Cucci et al. (190) postulated that this is a partial form of truncus arteriosus and is a consequence of abnormal truncal septation. Penkoske et al. (191) consider the cause to be failure of leftward migration of the right sixth aortic arch. Kutsche and Van Mierop (189) attribute the cause of anomalous origin near the aortic valve to an incomplete leftward migration of the right pulmonary artery while that in which the origin is close to the innominate artery would be due to development of the fifth right aortic arch and failure of development of the sixth right arch. The same would be assumed for anomalous origin of the left pulmonary artery from a site close to the innominate artery (189).

ANATOMIC AND ECHOCARDIOGRAPHIC CONSIDERATIONS

The echocardiographic study of this malformation should include (a) which pulmonary arterial branch is anomalous and its site of origin in the ascending aorta; and (b) associated anomalies.

Anomalous Origin of the Right Pulmonary Artery

This type is seen in 83% to 87% of all cases of anomalous pulmonary arterial origin from the ascending aorta (189,191). The right pulmonary artery emerges from the posterior or left posterior wall of the ascending aorta, near the aortic valve in 85% of cases (Echo. 18-15; see color plate 62 following p. 364) and near the innominate artery in 15% (189). In the latter cases, the right pulmonary artery can originate directly from the ascending aorta, from the innominate artery or receive blood flow through a patent ductus arteriosus or aortopulmonary collateral. In 54% of cases of origin close to the innominate artery, the right pulmonary branch is stenotic at its origin or close to it (189).

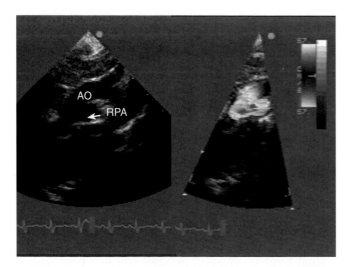

ECHO. 18-15. Left: Suprasternal long-axis view demonstrating an anomalous origin of the right pulmonary artery from the posterior wall of the ascending aorta. **Right:** Color Doppler color map showing the flow entering the right pulmonary artery from the ascending aorta. *AO,* aorta; *RPA,* right pulmonary artery.

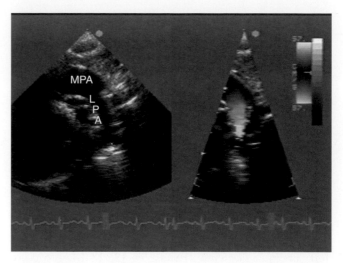

ECHO. 18-16. Anatomical and color Doppler image of the normal origin of the left pulmonary artery from the main pulmonary artery in the same patient illustrated on Echo 18-15. *MPA,* main pulmonary artery; *LPA,* left pulmonary artery.

Anomalous Origin of the Left Pulmonary Artery

Usually, the left pulmonary artery emerges from the left lateral wall, the anterior wall or the posterior wall of the ascending aorta, near the aortic valve. Rarely its origin is close to the innominate artery (189,191–193). In this latter type, the left pulmonary branch can emerge directly from the aorta or receive the blood flow from a ductus arteriosus or a systemic to pulmonary collateral (191). Occasionally, the left pulmonary branch can have a slight kink at its origin (194).

Echocardiographically the best views to visualize an anomalous pulmonary origin are the parasternal long-axis view tilted towards the pulmonary trunk, the apical long-axis view, the subcostal long- and short-axis views and the suprasternal long-axis view. One branch can be seen emerging from the ascending aorta while the contralateral branch is seen to be normal (Echos. 18-15, 18-16; see color plate 63 following p. 364). Color and pulsed wave Doppler can serve to confirm the systolic arterial flow pattern in the anomalous branch.

Associated Anomalies

In 85% of cases, there are associated anomalies present (195). The most common is patent ductus arteriosus, which can be seen in 38% to 76% of cases (188,189, 191,195,196). Others include tetralogy of Fallot, most commonly seen in association with anomalous origin of the left pulmonary branch (188,189,191,194–196), aortopulmonary window (189,191,195), atrial septal defect (189,191,195), patent foramen ovale (195), persistent left superior vena cava (189), coarctation of the aorta (188,189,191,195), interrupted aortic arch (189,195), right aortic arch (188,189,196,197), bicuspid aortic valve (188), bicuspid pulmonic valve (188), ventricular septal defect (188,191,195), and tricuspid atresia (195).

INTRAOPERATIVE AND POSTOPERATIVE EVALUATION

Valvular Pulmonary Stenosis

Balloon valvuloplasty is the therapy of choice in the treatment of valvular pulmonary stenosis. The procedure was originally described by Semb et al. (198) in 1979 in a newborn and by Kan et al. (199) in 1982 in a child 8 years old as an alternative to surgical valvotomy. At present, it is used in all forms of valvular stenosis but is least effective in dysplastic valves (200–204). In our center, the gradient is estimated by Doppler velocities obtained transthoracically, in the cardiac catheterization laboratory simultaneously with hemodynamic recordings. Usually, the window employed is the parasternal short-axis view. After the balloon valvuloplasty, the same procedure is used so that the residual Doppler gradient serves as a baseline relative to the residual catheter-measured gradient, for the continued follow-up of the patient. In this study also, presence of valvular regurgitation is assessed carefully and its severity estimated through the intensity of the spectral Doppler signal and the deceleration slope of the regurgitant velocity curve.

In the presence of dysplastic valves or a small "pulmonary annulus" requiring surgical intervention, the transesophageal approach is used intraoperatively. Pre-bypass the ventricular function is assessed from the transgastric short-axis view (see Fig. 4-27A,B). The gradient across the right ventricular outflow tract is best measured from the longitudinal transgastric views, which afford the best angle of incidence for the Doppler beam (see Fig. 4-27E). The size of the right ventricle and the competence of the tricuspid valve are best evaluated from the transverse four-chamber view (see Fig. 4-28A,B) and also from the longitudinal inflow view of the tricuspid valve. The morphology of the right ventricular outflow tract and "pulmonary annulus" is seen from the longitudinal view of the outflow tracts, although the gradient cannot usually be recorded from this approach due to an unfavorable angle of interrogation (see Fig. 4-29D,E).

Post-bypass, the same views as described for the pre-bypass study are utilized. In this study, however, the reconstructed right ventricular outflow tract should be carefully reviewed from the longitudinal view of the outflows, and any regurgitation of the valve should be noted and estimated with the use of spectral Doppler. The longitudinal transgastric view is used to measure the transannular velocities and also to record the spectral signals from the regurgitant curves (see Fig. 4-27E). The gradient across the valve can also be recorded from the transverse view of the main and branch pulmonary arteries obtained with

extreme anteflexion and slight withdrawal of the transducer from the short-axis view of the aortic valve (see Fig. 4-31A,B).

Subvalvular Pulmonary Stenosis

The treatment for infundibular obstruction and for double-chamber right ventricle is surgical resection of the stenotic area. The pre-bypass study is similar to that described above. Post-bypass, the ventricular function is assessed transgastrically. Further, the velocity across the outflow tract is measured from the longitudinal transgastric view to detect any area of significant residual gradient (see Fig. 4-27E). Regurgitation of the pulmonary valve can be produced after resection of subvalvular areas of stenosis and this should be evaluated carefully from the transgastric longitudinal views and from the longitudinal views of the outflow tracts. The transverse view of the main and proximal branches of the pulmonary artery obtained by extreme anteflexion of the transducer at the level of the aortic valve also permits good alignment of the Doppler beam for velocity measurements (see Fig. 4-31A,B).

Isolated Absence of the Pulmonary Valve

The surgical treatment of this malformation varies from banding of the pulmonary artery, plication of the aneurysmally dilated artery, and resection of the pulmonary trunk with placement of a valved conduit between the right ventricular outflow tract and the distal pulmonary artery (123). The post-bypass study should be directed at estimating any residual regurgitation and assessing the size of the plicated pulmonary trunk. Evaluation of the valved conduit intraoperatively should include an attempt at estimating forward velocities and detecting any regurgitation that is usually present, particularly when using homografts. This study would serve as a baseline for the long-term follow-up of the patient.

Pulmonary Atresia with Intact Ventricular Septum

The type of surgical approach for this lesion varies according to the size of the right ventricle, the morphology and competence of the tricuspid valve and the presence of ventriculocoronary communications. It can consist of surgical perforation or resection of the atretic segment with or without placement of a shunt in cases where the right ventricle is considered adequate and there are no significant ventriculocoronary communications. This would eventually be followed by takedown of the shunt and placement of a patch across the "pulmonary annulus" to widen it if necessary. In these instances, the post-bypass study is directed towards documenting any residual gradient and establishing the severity of regurgitation. A careful analysis of the tricuspid valve for its size and competence should be undertaken as well.

In patients in whom the right ventricle is not adequate in size and/or there are significant ventriculocoronary communications making the decompression of the right ventricle dangerous, the first procedure would be a systemic to pulmonary shunt followed by a right heart bypass operation (Fontan type). The intraoperative and late postoperative follow-up after the Fontan type of operation has been discussed in detail in Chapter 17.

Supravalvular Pulmonary Stenosis and Anomalous Origin of a Pulmonary Branch from the Ascending Aorta

The surgical treatment of supravalvular pulmonary stenosis consists of widening of the area(s) of obstruction with a Dacron patch. The intraoperative evaluation in these cases would be limited to the ventricular function and any associated anomalies because it is usually difficult to visualize the peripheral pulmonary arteries in detail from the transesophageal approach.

Anomalous origin of a pulmonary artery from the ascending aorta is repaired by transecting the anomalous branch from the aorta and reimplanting it into the main pulmonary trunk. As in supravalve stenosis, the intraoperative study is mostly limited to the evaluation of ventricular function and associated lesions. It may be possible to visualize the site of anastomosis of the anomalous branch to the pulmonary trunk but this depends on the location of the anastomosis.

The long-term follow-up of patients with anomalies of the right ventricular outflow tract and pulmonary arteries emphasizes the evaluation of right ventricular size and function. The tricuspid valve also needs serial examination since it is commonly abnormal so that an initially competent valve can become regurgitant with time. The gradient across the right ventricular outflow tract and the presence and severity of pulmonary valve regurgitation should be estimated with Doppler techniques to detect any significant increase. If a valved conduit has been implanted, the velocities across the conduit should be obtained, ideally with resolution of the specific site(s) of obstruction using high PRF Doppler if possible, as well as an estimate of the presence and degree of regurgitation, which can be progressive. The long-term follow-up of patients after a right heart bypass operation has been discussed in Chapter 17.

REFERENCES

1. Wood P. Pulmonary stenosis. In: Wood P, ed. *Diseases of the heart and circulation.* 2nd ed. Philadelphia: JB Lippincott Co, 1956:407–424.
2. Malo Concepcion P, Caffarena Raggio JM. Estenosis pulmonar. In: Sanchez PA, ed. *Cardiologia pediatrica. Clinica y cirugia. Vol. I.* Barcelona: Salvat Editores, S.A., 1986:429–452.
3. Cheatham JP. Pulmonary stenosis. In: Garson A Jr, Bricker JT, McNamara DG, eds. *The science and practice of pediatric cardiology. Vol. II.* Philadelphia: Lea & Febiger, 1990:1382–1420.
4. Fyler DC. Pulmonary stenosis. In: Fyler DC, ed. *Nadas' pediatric cardiology.* Philadelphia: Hanley & Belfus, 1992:459–470.
5. Rocchini AP, Emmanouilides GC. Pulmonary stenosis. In: Emmanouilides GC, Riemenschneider TA, Allen HD, Gutgesell HP, eds. *Moss and Adams' heart disease in infants, children, and adolescents. Including the fetus and young adult. Vol. II.* 5th ed. Baltimore: Williams & Wilkins, 1995:930–962.
6. Abrahams DG, Wood P. Pulmonary stenosis with normal aortic root. *Br Heart J* 1951;13:519–548.
7. Adams FH, Veasy LG, Jorgens J, et al. Congenital valvular pulmonary stenosis with or without an interatrial communication: physiologic studies as diagnostic aids. *J Pediatr* 1951;38:431–441.
8. Campbell M. Simple pulmonary stenosis. Pulmonary valvular stenosis with a closed ventricular septum. *Br Heart J* 1954;16:273–300.
9. Lucas RV Jr, Moller JH. Pulmonary valvular stenosis. *Cardiovasc Clin* 1970;2:155–184.
10. Castaneda-Zuniga WR, Formanek A, Amplatz K. Radiologic diagnosis of different types of pulmonary stenoses. *Cardiovasc Radiol* 1978;1:45–57.
11. Rowe RD. Pulmonary stenosis with normal aortic root. In: Keith JD, Rowe RD, Vlad P, eds. *Heart disease in infancy and childhood.* 3rd ed. New York: Macmillan, 1978:761–788.
12. Fyler DC, Buckley LP, Hellenbrand WE, Cohn HE. Report of the New England Regional Infant Cardiac Program. *Pediatrics* 1980;65[Suppl]:375–461.
13. Hoffman JIE. Incidence of congenital heart disease: I. Postnatal incidence. *Pediatr Cardiol* 1995;16:103–113.
14. Morgagni JB. *De sedibus et causis morborum per anatomen indagatis. Libri quince (Epist. 17, art. 12). Vol. 1.* Venice: Remondini, 1761.
15. Ogle JW. Abnormal condition of the valve at the root of the pulmonary artery, with consequent hypertrophy of the parietes of the right ventricle of the heart. *Trans Pathol Soc Lond* 1854;5:69–71.
16. Peacock TB. Contraction of the orifice of the pulmonary artery; communication between the cavities of the auricles by the foramen ovale; septum of ventricles entire. In: Peacock TB, ed. *On malformations, and C., of the human heart. With original cases* [1858]. Boston: Mildford House, 1973:83–92.
17. Peacock TB. Contraction of the orifice of the pulmonary artery from fusion of the valves. *Trans Pathol Soc Lond* 1859;10:107–108.
18. Andrew J. Congenital malformation of pulmonary valves. *Trans Pathol Soc Lond* 1865;16:81–82.
19. Peacock TB. Case of stenosis of the pulmonary artery from disease of the valves, probably of congenital origin. *Trans Pathol Soc Lond* 1879;30:258–262.
20. Barlow T. Congenital heart disease; pulmonary stenosis, with dilated pulmonary artery above the stenosis. *Trans Pathol Soc Lond* 1879;30: 272–273.
21. Finlay DW. Malformation of the heart; stenosis of the pulmonary valve, with dilatation of the pulmonary artery and hypertrophy of the right ventricle; patency of the foramen ovale, with a cribriform opening in the septum of the auricles (ductus arteriosus closed). *Trans Pathol Soc Lond* 1879;30:262–265.
22. Fallot A. Contribution a l'anatomie pathologique de la maladie bleue (cyanose cardiaque). *Marseille Med* 1888;25:77,138,207,270,341,403.
23. Abbott ME, Lewis DS, Beattie WW. Differential study of a case of pulmonary stenosis of inflammatory origin (ventricular septum closed) and two cases of (a) pulmonary stenosis and (b) pulmonary atresia of developmental origin with associated ventricular septal defect and death from paradoxical cerebral embolism. In three cases, aged respectively, fourteen, ten, and eleven years. *Am J Med Sci* 1923;165:636–659.
24. Abbott ME. Congenital cardiac disease. In: Osler W, ed. *Modern medicine. Its theory and practice. In original contributions by American and foreign authors. Vol. 4.* 3rd ed. Philadelphia: Lea & Febiger, 1927:612–812.
25. Abbott ME. A. Pulmonary and tricuspid stenosis with closed ventricular septum. In: Abbott ME, ed. *Atlas of congenital cardiac disease.* New York: American Heart Association, 1936:44–45.

26. Currens JH, Kinney TD, White PD. Pulmonary stenosis with intact interventricular septum. Report of eleven cases. *Am Heart J* 1945; 30:491–510.

27. Selzer A, Carnes WH, Noble CA Jr, Higgins WH, Holmes RO. The syndrome of pulmonary stenosis with patent foramen ovale. *Am J Med* 1949;6:3–23.

28. Greene DG, Baldwin ED, Baldwin JS, Himmelstein A, Roh CE, Cournand A. Pure congenital pulmonary stenosis and idiopathic congenital dilatation of the pulmonary artery. *Am J Med* 1949;6: 24–40.

29. Allanby KD, Campbell M. Congenital pulmonary stenosis with closed ventricular septum. *Guy's Hosp Rep* 1949;98:18– 53.

30. Wood P. Congenital heart disease. A review of its clinical aspects in the light of experience gained by means of modern techniques. Part II. *BMJ* 1950;2:693–698.

31. Brock R. *The anatomy of congenital pulmonary stenosis.* New York: Paul B. Hoeber Inc., 1957.

32. Kramer TC. The partitioning of the truncus and conus and the formation of the membranous portion of the interventricular septum in the human heart. *Am J Anat* 1942;71:343–370.

33. Netter FH, Van Mierop LHS. Embryology. In: Netter FH, Yonkman FF, eds. *Heart.* Summit, NJ: Ciba Publications Department, 1969:112–130 *(The Ciba collection of medical illustrations, vol. 5).*

34. Peacock TB. Malformations which do not interfere with the functions of the heart, but may lay the foundations of disease in after life. Irregularities of the valves. In: Peacock TB, ed. *On malformations, and C., of the human heart. With original cases* [1858]. Boston: Mildford House, 1973:93–102.

35. Moore GW, Hutchins GM, Brito JC, Kang H. Congenital malformations of the semilunar valves. *Hum Pathol* 1980;11:367–372.

36. Van Mierop LHS. Pathology and pathogenesis of the common cardiac malformations. *Cardiovasc Clin* 1970;2:27–59.

37. Farber S, Hubbard J. Fetal endomyocarditis: intrauterine infection as the cause of congenital cardiac anomalies. *Am J Med Sci* 1933; 186:705–713.

38. Oka M, Angrist A. Mechanism of cardiac valvular fusion and stenosis. *Am Heart J* 1967;74:37–47.

39. Edwards JE. Congenital malformations of the heart and great vessels. C. Malformations of the valves. In: Gould SE, ed. *Pathology of the heart and blood vessels.* 3rd ed. Springfield, IL: Charles C. Thomas Publisher, 1968:312–351.

40. Becker AE, Anderson RH. Ventricular outflow abnormalities. In: Becker AE, Anderson RH, eds. *Pathology of congenital heart disease.* London: Butterworths, 1981:165–190.

41. Becker AE, Anderson RH. Ventricular outflow tract malformations. In: Becker AE, Anderson RH, eds. *Cardiac pathology. An integrated text and colour atlas.* New York: Raven Press, 1982: 13.15–13.22.

42. Gikonyo BM, Lucas RV, Edwards JE. Anatomic features of congenital pulmonary valvar stenosis. *Pediatr Cardiol* 1987;8:109– 115.

43. Milo S, Fiegel A, Shem-Tov A, Neufeld HN, Goor DA. Hourglass deformity of the pulmonary valve: a third type of pulmonary valve stenosis. *Br Heart J* 1988;60:128–133.

44. Jeffery RF, Moller JH, Amplatz K. The dysplastic pulmonary valve: a new roentgenographic entity. With a discussion of the anatomy and radiology of other types of valvular pulmonary stenosis. *Am J Roentgenol* 1972;114:322–339.

45. Roberts WC, Dangel JC, Bulkley BH. Nonrheumatic valvular cardiac disease: a clinicopathologic survey of 27 different conditions causing valvular dysfunction. *Cardiovasc Clin* 1973;5:334–446.

46. Koretzky ED, Moller JH, Korns ME, Schwartz CJ, Edwards JE. Congenital pulmonary stenosis resulting from dysplasia of valve. *Circulation* 1969;40:43–53.

47. Noonan JA, Ehmke DA. Associated noncardiac malformations in children with congenital heart disease. *J Pediatr* 1963;63:468–470.

48. Gorlin RJ, Anderson RC, Blaw M. Multiple lentigenes syndrome. Complex comprising multiple lentigenes, electrocardiographic conduction abnormalities, ocular hypertelorism, pulmonary stenosis, abnormalities of genitalia, retardation of growth, sensorineural deafness, and autosomal dominant hereditary pattern. *Am J Dis Child* 1969;117:652–662.

49. Hurwitz LE, Roberts WC. Quadricuspid semilunar valve. *Am J Cardiol* 1973;31:623–626.

50. Davia JE, Fenoglio JJ, DeCastro CM, McAllister HA, Cheitlin MD. Quadricuspid semilunar valves. *Chest* 1977;2:186–189.

51. Anderson RH, Becker AE. The morphologically right ventricle. In: Anderson RH, Becker AE, eds. *Cardiac anatomy. An integrated text and color atlas.* London: Gower Medical Publishing, 1980:3.12–3.24.

52. Engle MA, Holswade GR, Goldberg HP, Lukas DS, Glenn F. Regression after open valvotomy of infundibular stenosis accompanying severe valvular pulmonic stenosis. *Circulation* 1958;17: 862–873.

53. Brock R. The surgical treatment of pulmonary stenosis. *Br Heart J* 1961;23:337–356.

54. Gilbert JW, Morrow AG, Talbert JL. The surgical significance of hypertrophic infundibular obstruction accompanying valvular pulmonic stenosis. *J Thorac Cardiovasc Surg* 1963;46:457–467.

55. Fontes VF, Sousa JEMR, Esteves CA, Dias da Silva MV. Regression of the infundibular hypertrophy after pulmonary valvuloplasty in patients with suprasystemic pressure of the right ventricle. *J Am Coll Cardiol* 1987;9:75A(abst).

56. Williams JCP, Barrat-Boyes BG, Lowe LB. Underdeveloped right ventricle and pulmonary stenosis. *Am J Cardiol* 1963;11:458–468.

57. Freed MD, Rosenthal A, Bernhard WF, Litwin SB, Nadas AS. Critical pulmonary stenosis with a diminutive right ventricle in neonates. *Circulation* 1973;48:875–881.

58. Becu L, Somerville J, Gallo A. Isolated pulmonary valve stenosis as part of more widespread cardiovascular disease. *Br Heart J* 1976;38:472–482.

59. Harinck E, Becker AE, Gittenberger-De Groot AC, Oppenheimer-Dekker A, Versprille A. The left ventricle in congenital isolated pulmonary valve stenosis. A morphological study. *Br Heart J* 1977;39:429–435.

60. Holman E. The obscure physiology of poststenotic dilatation: its relation to the development of aneurysms. *J Thorac Surg* 1954; 28:109–133.

61. Rodbard S, Ikeda K, Montes M. Mechanisms of poststenotic dilatation. *Circulation* 1963;28:791.

62. Hatle L, Angelsen B. Pulsed and continuous wave Doppler in diagnosis and assessment of various heart lesions. In: Hatle L, Angelsen B, eds. *Doppler ultrasound in cardiology. Physical principles and clinical applications.* 2nd ed. Philadelphia: Lea & Febiger, 1985:97–292.

63. Rao PS, Awa S, Linde LM. Role of kinetic energy in pulmonary valvar pressure gradients. *Circulation* 1973;48:65–73.

64. Zaret BL, Conti CR. Infundibular pulmonic stenosis with intact ventricular septum in the adult. *Hopkins Med J* 1973,132:30–60.

65. Elliotson J. *The recent improvements in the art of distinguishing the various diseases of the heart.* London: Longmans and Co, 1830; cited in Blount SG, Vigoda PS, Swan H. Isolated infundibular stenosis. *Am Heart J* 1959;57:684–700..

66. Peacock TB. Supernumerary septum in the right ventricle; heart otherwise well formed. In: Peacock TB, ed. *On malformations, and C., of the human heart. With original cases* [1858]. Boston: Mildford House, 1973:68–71.

67. Keith A. The Hunterian Lectures on malformations of the heart. Lecture I. *Lancet* 1909;2:359–363.

68. Blount SG, Vigoda PS, Swan H. Isolated infundibular stenosis. *Am Heart J* 1959;57:684–700.

69. De la Cruz MV, Sanchez Gomez C, Arteaga MM, Arguello C. Experimental study of the development of the truncus and the conus in the chick embryo. *J Anat* 1977;123:661–686.

70. Goor DA, Dische R, Lillehei CW. The conotruncus. I. Its normal inversion and conus absorption. *Circulation* 1972;46:375–384.

71. Goor DA, Lillehei CW. The embryology of the heart. In: Goor DA, Lillehei CW, eds. *Congenital malformations of the heart. Embryology, anatomy and operative considerations.* New York: Grune & Stratton, 1975:38–102.

72. Swan H, Hederman WP, Vigoda PS, Blount SG Jr. The surgical treatment of isolated infundibular stenosis. *J Thorac Cardiovasc Surg* 1959;38:319–335.

73. Glover RP, O'Neill TJE, Gontigo H, McAuliffe TC, Wells CRE. The surgery of infundibular pulmonic stenosis with intact ventricular septum (a type of "pure" pulmonic stenosis). *J Thorac Surg* 1954;28:481–503.

74. Heim de Balsac R, Escalle JE. Anomalies de l'orifice pulmonaire.

In: Donzelot E, D'Allaines F, eds. *Traite des cardiopathies congenitales*. Paris: Masson et Cie, Editeurs, 1954:357–386.

75. Slade PR. Isolated infundibular stenosis. *J Thorac Cardiovasc Surg* 1963;45:775–788.

76. Varghese PJ, Izukawa T, Celermajer J, Simon A, Rowe RD. Aneurysm of the membranous ventricular septum. A method of spontaneous closure of small ventricular septal defect. *Am J Cardiol* 1969;24:531–536.

77. Falsetti HL, Andersen MN. Aneurysm of the membranous ventricular septum producing right ventricular outflow tract obstruction and left ventricular failure. *Chest* 1971;59:578–580.

78. Bonvicini M, Piovaccari G, Picchio FM. Severe subpulmonary obstruction caused by an aneurysmal tissue tag complicating an infundibular perimembranous ventricular septal defect. *Br Heart J* 1982;48:189–191.

79. Cosio FG, Wang Y, Nicoloff DM. Membranous right ventricular outflow obstruction. *Am J Cardiol* 1973;32:1000–1003.

80. Pate JW, Richardson RL, Giles HH. Accessory tricuspid leaflet producing right ventricular outflow tract obstruction. *N Engl J Med* 1968;279:867–868.

81. Pate JW, Ainger LE, Butterick OD. A new form of right ventricular outflow obstruction. *Am Heart J* 1964;68:249–251.

82. Pund EE Jr, Collier TM, Cunningham JE Jr, Hayes JR. Primary cardiac rhabdomyosarcoma presenting as pulmonary stenosis. *Am J Cardiol* 1963;12:249–253.

83. Hallermann FJ, Kincaid OW, Brown AL Jr, Daugherty GW. Rhabdomyosarcoma of the heart producing right ventricular outflow obstruction. *JAMA* 1963;184:939–942.

84. Gottsegen G, Wessely J, Arvay A, Temesvari A. Right ventricular myxoma simulating pulmonic stenosis. *Circulation* 1963;27:95–97.

85. Goldstein S, Mahoney EB. Right ventricular fibrosarcoma causing pulmonic stenosis. *Am J Cardiol* 1966;17:570–578.

86. Nanda NC, Barold SS, Gramiak R, Ong LS, Heinle RA. Echocardiographic features of right ventricular outflow tumor prolapsing into the pulmonary artery. *Am J Cardiol* 1977;40:272–276.

87. Chandraratna PAN, San Pedro S, Elkins RC, Grantham N. Echocardiographic, angiocardiographic, and surgical correlations in right ventricular myxoma simulating valvar pulmonic stenosis. *Circulation* 1977;55:619–622.

88. Neufeld HN, Ongley PA, Edwards JE. Combined congenital subaortic stenosis and infundibular pulmonary stenosis. *Br Heart J* 1960;22:686–690.

89. Tsifutis AA, Hartmann AF Jr, Arvidsson H. Two-chambered right ventricle: report on seven patients. *Circulation* 1961;24:1058(abst).

90. Hartmann AF Jr, Tsifutis AA, Arvidsson H, Goldring D. The two-chambered right ventricle. Report of nine cases. *Circulation* 1962;26:279–287.

91. Watler DC, Wynter L. Cor triventriculare: infundibular stenosis with subdivision of the right ventricle. *Br Heart J* 1961;23:599–602.

92. Lucas RV Jr, Varco RL, Lillehei CW, Adams P Jr, Anderson RC, Edwards JE. Anomalous muscle bundle of the right ventricle. Hemodynamic consequences and surgical considerations. *Circulation* 1962;25:443–455.

93. Coates JR, McClenathan JE, Scott LP. The double-chambered right ventricle. A diagnostic and operative pitfall. *Am J Cardiol* 1964;14:561–567.

94. Hartmann AF Jr, Goldring D, Carlsson E. Development of right ventricular obstruction by aberrant muscular bands. *Circulation* 1964;30:679–685.

95. Hindle WV Jr, Engle MA, Hagstrom JWC. Anomalous right ventricular muscles. A clinicopathologic study. *Am J Cardiol* 1968;21:487–495.

96. Rowland TW, Rosenthal A, Castaneda AR. Double-chamber right ventricle: experience with 17 cases. *Am Heart J* 1975;89:455–462.

97. Restivo A, Cameron AH, Anderson RH, Allwork SP. Divided right ventricle: a review of its anatomical varieties. *Pediatr Cardiol* 1984;5:197–204.

98. Warden HE, Lucas RV Jr, Varco RL. Right ventricular obstruction resulting from anomalous muscle bundles. *J Thorac Cardiovasc Surg* 1966;51:53–65.

99. Wong PC, Sanders SP, Jonas RA, et al. Pulmonary valve-moderator band distance and association with development of double-chambered right ventricle. *Am J Cardiol* 1991;68:1681–1686.

100. Lintermans JP, Roberts DB, Guntheroth WG, Figley MM. Two-chambered right ventricle without outflow obstruction in ventricular septal defect. A case of spontaneous correction. *Am J Cardiol* 1968;21:582–587.

101. Pongiglione G, Freedom RM, Cook D, Rowe RD. Mechanism of acquired right ventricular outflow tract obstruction in patients with ventricular septal defect: an angiocardiographic study. *Am J Cardiol* 1982;50:776–780.

102. Forster JW, Humphries JO. Right ventricular anomalous muscle bundle. Clinical and laboratory presentation and natural history. *Circulation* 1971;43:115–127.

103. Goor DA, Lillehei CW. Obstruction of the pulmonary arterial pathways. In: Goor DA, Lillehei CW, eds. *Congenital malformations of the heart. Embryology, anatomy and operative considerations*. New York: Grune & Stratton, 1975:312–339.

104. Beitzke A, Anderson RH, Wilkinson JL, Shinebourne EA. Two-chambered right ventricle: simulating two-chambered left ventricle. *Br Heart J* 1979;42:22–26.

105. Matina D, Van Doesburg NH, Fouron JC, Guerin R, Davignon A. Subxiphoid two-dimensional echocardiographic diagnosis of double-chambered right ventricle. *Circulation* 1983;67:885–888.

106. Von Doenhoff LJ, Nanda NC. Obstruction within the right ventricular body: two-dimensional echocardiographic features. *Am J Cardiol* 1983;51:1498–1501.

107. Cazzaniga M, Dietl C, Gamboa R, et al. Ventriculo derecho bicameral. Una obstruccion intraventricular singular. *Rev Arg Cardiol* 1992;60:477–482.

108. Dietl CA, Torres AR, Cazzaniga ME, Favaloro RG. Double-chambered right ventricle. In: Crupi G, Parenzan L, Anderson RH, eds. *Perspectives in pediatric cardiology. Vol. 2. Pediatric cardiac surgery. Part 3*. Mount Kisco, NY: Futura Publishing, 1990:284–288.

109. Baumstark A, Fellows KE, Rosenthal A. Combined double chambered right ventricle and discrete subaortic stenosis. *Circulation* 1978;57:299–303.

110. Freedom RM, Culham JAG, Moes CAF. Anomalous right ventricular muscle bundle (so-called double-chambered right ventricle). In: Freedom RM, Culham JAG, Moes CAF, eds. *Angiocardiography of congenital heart disease*. New York: Macmillan, 1984:161–168.

111. Kostucki W, Vandenbossche J-L, Friart A, Englert M. Pulsed Doppler regurgitant flow patterns of normal valves. *Am J Cardiol* 1986;58:309–313.

112. Yoshida K, Yoshikawa J, Shakudo M, et al. Color Doppler evaluation of valvular regurgitation in normal subjects. *Circulation* 1988;78:840–847.

113. Chevers N. Recherches sur les maladies de l'artere pulmonaire. *Arch Gen Med* 1847;15:488–508.

114. Calder AL, Brandt PWT, Barrat-Boyes BG, Neutze JM. Variant of tetralogy of Fallot with absent pulmonary valve leaflets and origin of one pulmonary artery from the ascending aorta. *Am J Cardiol* 1980;46:106–116.

115. Anderson RH, Allwork SP, Ho SY, Lenox CC, Zuberbuhler JR. Surgical anatomy of tetralogy of Fallot. *J Thorac Cardiovasc Surg* 1981;81:887–896.

116. Karczenski K. The syndrome of congenital absence of pulmonary valve. In: Rosenberg, HS, Bernstein J, eds. *Perspectives in Pediatric Pathology. Vol 12. Cardiovasular diseases*. Basel, Germany: Karger: 1988:128–138.

117. Ehrenhaft JL. Discussion. *J Thorac Surg* 1955;30:641.

118. Smith RD, DuShane JW, Edwards JE. Congenital insufficiency of the pulmonary valve including a case of fetal cardiac failure. *Circulation* 1959;20:554–560.

119. Ito T, Engle MA, Holswade GR. Congenital insufficiency of the pulmonic valve. A rare cause of neonatal heart failure. *Pediatrics* 1961;28:712–718.

120. Alpert BS, Moore HV. "Absent" pulmonary valve with atrial septal defect and patent ductus arteriosus. *Pediatr Cardiol* 1985;6:107–112.

121. Thanapoulos BD, Fisher EA, Hastreiter AR. Large ductus arteriosus and intact ventricular septum associated with congenital absence of the pulmonary valve. *Br Heart J* 1986;55:602–604.

122. Sethia B, Jamieson MPG, Houston AB. "Absent" pulmonary

valve with ASD and PDA [Letter]. *Pediatr Cardiol* 1986;7:119–120.

123. Kron IL, Johnson AM, Carpenter MA, Gutgesell HP Jr, Overholt ED, Rheuban KS. Treatment of absent pulmonary valve syndrome with homograft. *Ann Thorac Surg* 1988;46:579–581.

124. Lau K, Cheung HH, Mok C. Congenital absence of the pulmonary valve, intact interventricular septum, and patent ductus arteriosus: management in a newborn infant. *Am Heart J* 1990;120:711–714.

125. Berman W Jr, Fripp RR, Rowe SA, Yabek SM. Congenital isolated pulmonary valve incompetence: neonatal presentation and early natural history. *Am Heart J* 1992;124:248–251.

126. Hunter W. Three cases of mal-conformation in the heart. *Med Observations Inquiries* 1783;6:291–299.

127. Peacock TB. Obliteration of the pulmonary orifice. In: Peacock TB, ed. *On malformations, and C., of the human heart. With original cases* [1858]. Boston: Mildford House, 1973:51–57.

128. Greenwold WE, DuShane JW, Burchell HB, Bruwer A, Edwards JE. Congenital pulmonary atresia with intact ventricular septum: two anatomic types. *Circulation* 1956;14:945–946(abst).

129. Bull C, De Leval MR, Mercanti C, Macartney FJ, Anderson RH. Pulmonary atresia and intact ventricular septum: a revised classification. *Circulation* 1982;66:266–272.

130. Van Praagh R, Ando M, Van Praagh S, et al. Pulmonary atresia: anatomic considerations. In: Kidd BSL, Rowe RD, eds. *The child with congenital heart disease after surgery.* Mount Kisco, NY: Futura Publishing, 1976:103–134.

131. Freedom RM. *Pulmonary atresia with intact ventricular septum.* Mount Kisco, NY: Futura Publishing, 1989.

132. Samanek M, Slavik Z, Zborilova B, Hrobonova V, Voriskova M, Skovranek J. Prevalence, treatment, and outcome of heart disease in live-born children: a prospective analysis of 91,823 live-born children. *Pediatr Cardiol* 1989;10:205–211.

133. Freedom RM, Keith JD. Pulmonary atresia with normal aortic root. In: Keith JD, Rowe RD, Vlad P, eds. *Heart disease in infancy and childhood.* 3rd ed. New York: Macmillan, 1978:506–517.

134. Freedom R, Dische MR, Rowe RD. The tricuspid valve in pulmonary atresia and intact ventricular septum. A morphological study of 60 cases. *Arch Pathol Lab Med* 1978;102:28–31.

135. Freedom RM. The morphologic variations of pulmonary atresia with intact ventricular septum: guidelines for surgical intervention. *Pediatr Cardiol* 1983;4:183–188.

136. Freedom RM, Wilson G, Trusler GA, Williams WG, Rowe RD. Pulmonary atresia and intact ventricular septum. A review of the anatomy, myocardium, and factors influencing right ventricular growth and guidelines for surgical intervention. *Scand J Thorac Cardiovasc Surg* 1983;17:1–28.

137. Steeg CN, Ellis K, Bransilver B, Gersony WM. Pulmonary atresia and intact ventricular septum complicating corrected transposition of the great arteries. *Am Heart J* 1971;82:382–386.

138. Shimizu T, Ando M, Takao A. Pulmonary atresia with intact ventricular septum and corrected transposition of the great arteries. *Br Heart J* 1981;45:471–474.

139. Zuberbuhler JR, Anderson RH. Morphological variations in pulmonary atresia with intact ventricular septum. *Br Heart J* 1979;41:281–288.

140. Zuberbuhler JR, Fricker FJ, Park SC, et al. Pulmonary atresia with intact ventricular septum: morbid anatomy. In: Godman MJ, Marquis RM, eds. *Paediatric cardiology. Vol. 2. Heart disease in newborn.* Edinburgh: Churchill Livingstone, 1979:285–296.

141. Kugel MA. Congenital heart disease. A clinical and pathological study of two cases of truncus solitarius aorticus (pulmonary atresia). *Am Heart J* 1932;7:262–273.

142. Becker AE, Anderson RH. Hypoplasia of the right ventricle. In: Becker AE, Anderson RH, eds. *Pathology of congenital heart disease.* London: Butterworths, 1981:119–127.

143. Kanjuh VI, Stevenson JE, Amplatz K, Edwards JE. Congenitally unguarded tricuspid orifice with coexistent pulmonary atresia. *Circulation* 1964;30:911–917.

144. Marino B, Franceschini E, Ballerini L, Marcelletti C, Thiene G. Anatomical-echocardiographic correlations in pulmonary atresia with intact ventricular septum. Use of subcostal cross-sectional views. *Int J Cardiol* 1986;11:103–109.

145. Schrire V, Sutin GJ, Barnard CN. Organic and functional pulmonary atresia with intact ventricular septum. *Am J Cardiol* 1961;8:100–108.

146. Neufeld EA, Cole RB, Paul MH. Ebstein's malformation of the tricuspid valve in the neonate. Functional and anatomic pulmonary outflow tract obstruction. *Am J Cardiol* 1967;19:727–732.

147. Freedom RM, Culham G, Moes F, Olley PM, Rowe RD. Differentiation of functional and structural pulmonary atresia: role of aortography. *Am J Cardiol* 1978;41:914–920.

148. Smallhorn JF, Izukawa T, Benson L, Freedom RM. Noninvasive recognition of functional pulmonary atresia by echocardiography. *Am J Cardiol* 1984;54:925–926.

149. Edwards JE, Carey LS, Neufeld HN, Lester RG. Pulmonary atresia with intact ventricular septum. In: Edwards JE, Carey LS, Neufeld HN, Lester RG, eds. *Congenital heart disease. Correlation of pathologic anatomy and angiocardiography. Vol. II.* Philadelphia: WB Saunders, 1965:575–598.

150. Bharati S, McAllister HA, Chiemmongkoltip P, Lev M. Congenital pulmonary atresia with tricuspid insufficiency: morphologic study. *Am J Cardiol* 1977;40:70–75.

151. Soto B, Pacifico AD. Pulmonary atresia with intact ventricular septum. In: Soto B, Pacifico AD, eds. *Angiocardiography in congenital heart malformations.* Mount Kisco, NY: Futura Publishing, 1990:493–516.

152. Hanley FL, Sade RM, Blackstone EH, Kirklin JW, Freedom RM, Nanda NC. Outcomes in neonatal pulmonary atresia with intact ventricular septum. A multiinstitutional study. *J Thorac Cardiovasc Surg* 1993;105:406–427.

153. Grant RT. An unusual anomaly of the coronary vessels in the malformed heart of a child. *Heart* 1926;13:273–283.

154. Lauer RM, Fink HP, Petry EL, Dunn MI, Diehl AM. Angiographic demonstration of intramyocardial sinusoids in pulmonary-valve atresia with intact ventricular septum and hypoplastic right ventricle. *N Engl J Med* 1964;271:68–72.

155. Cornell SH. Myocardial sinusoids in pulmonary valvular atresia. *Radiology* 1966;86:421–424.

156. Freedom RM, Harrington DP. Contributions of intramyocardial sinusoids in pulmonary atresia and intact ventricular septum to a right-sided circular shunt. *Br Heart J* 1974;36:1061–1065.

157. Dusek J, Ostadal B, Duskova M. Postnatal persistence of spongy myocardium with embryonic blood supply. *Arch Pathol* 1975;99:312–317.

158. O'Connor WN, Cottrill CM, Johnson GL, Noonan JA, Todd EP. Pulmonary atresia with intact ventricular septum and ventriculo-coronary communications: surgical significance. *Circulation* 1982;65:805–809.

159. Calder AL, Co EE, Sage MD. Coronary arterial abnormalities in pulmonary atresia with intact ventricular septum. *Am J Cardiol* 1987;59:436–442.

160. O'Connor WN, Stahr BJ, Cottrill CM, Todd EP, Noonan JA. Ventriculocoronary connections in hypoplastic right heart syndrome: autopsy serial section study of six cases. *J Am Coll Cardiol* 1988;11:1061–1072.

161. Gittenberger–De Groot AC, Sauer U, Bindl L, Babic R, Essed CE, Buhlmeyer K. Competition of coronary arteries and ventriculo-coronary arterial communications in pulmonary atresia with intact ventricular septum. *Int J Cardiol* 1988;18:243–258.

162. Mainwaring RD, Lamberti JJ. Pulmonary atresia with intact ventricular septum. Surgical approach based on ventricular size and coronary anatomy. *J Thorac Cardiovasc Surg* 1993;106:733–738.

163. Hanley FL, Sade RM, Blackstone EH, Kirklin JW, Freedom RM, Nanda NC. Outcomes in neonatal pulmonary atresia with intact ventricular septum. A multiinstitutional study. *J Thorac Cardiovasc Surg* 1993;105:406–427.

164. Santos MA, Moll JN, Drumond C, Araujo WB, Romao N, Reis NB. Development of the ductus arteriosus in right ventricular outflow tract obstruction. *Circulation* 1980;62:818–822.

165. Patel RG, Freedom RM, Bloom KR, Rowe RD. Truncal or aortic valve stenosis in functionally single arterial trunk. *Am J Cardiol* 1978;42:800–809.

166. Cote M, Davignon A, Fouron JC. Congenital hypoplasia of right ventricular myocardium (Uhl's anomaly) associated with pulmonary atresia in a newborn. *Am J Cardiol* 1973;31:658–661.

167. Oppenheimer EH. Partial atresia of the main branches of the pulmonary artery occurring in infancy and accompanied by calcification of the pulmonary artery and aorta. *Bull Johns Hopkins Hosp* 1938;63:261–277.

168. D'Cruz IA, Agustsson MH, Bicoff JP, Weinberg M Jr, Arcilla RA. Stenotic lesions of the pulmonary arteries. Clinical and hemodynamic findings in 84 cases. *Am J Cardiol* 1964;13:441–450.

169. Mudd JG, Walter KE, Willman VL. Pulmonary artery stenosis: diagnostic and therapeutic considerations. *Am J Med Sci* 1965; 249:125–134.

170. Fouron JC, Favreau-Ethier M, Marion P, Davignon A. Les stenoses pulmonaires peripheriques congenitales: presentation de 16 observations et revue de la litterature. *Can Med Assoc J* 1967;96:1084–1094.

171. Emmanouilides GC, Linde LM, Crittenden IH. Pulmonary artery stenosis associated with ductus arteriosus following maternal rubella. *Circulation* 1964;29:514–522.

172. Campbell PE. Vascular abnormalities following maternal rubella. *Br Heart J* 1965;27:134–138.

173. Rowe RD. Cardiovascular disease in the rubella syndrome. *Cardiol Clin* 1973;4:61–80.

174. Williams JCP, Barrat-Boyes BG, Lowe JB. Supravalvular aortic stenosis. *Circulation* 1961;24:1311–1318.

175. Beuren AJ, Apitz J, Harmjanz D. Supravalvular aortic stenosis in association with mental retardation and a certain facial appearance. *Circulation* 1962;26:1235–1240.

176. Beuren AJ, Schulze C, Eberle P, Harmjanz D, Apitz J. The syndrome of supravalvular aortic stenosis, peripheral pulmonary stenosis, mental retardation and similar facial appearance. *Am J Cardiol* 1964;13:471–483.

177. Black JA, Bonham-Carter RE. Association between aortic stenosis and facies of severe infantile hypercalcemia. *Lancet* 1963;2:745–749.

178. Garcia RE, Friedman WF, Kaback MM, Rowe RD. Idiopathic hypercalcemia and supravalvular aortic stenosis. Documentation of a new syndrome. *N Engl J Med* 1964;271:117–120.

179. Gyllensward A, Lodin H, Lundberg A, Moller T. Congenital, multiple peripheral stenoses of the pulmonary artery. *Pediatrics* 1957; 19:399–410.

180. Smith WG. Pulmonary hypertension and a continuous murmur due to multiple peripheral stenoses of the pulmonary arteries. *Thorax* 1958;13:194–200.

181. Arvidsson H, Carlsson E, Hartmann A Jr, Tsifutis A, Crawford C. Supravalvular stenoses of the pulmonary arteries. Report of eleven cases. *Acta Radiol* 1961;56:466–480.

182. Franch RH, Gay BB Jr. Congenital stenosis of the pulmonary artery branches. A classification, with postmortem findings in two cases. *Am J Med* 1963;35: 512–529.

183. Luan LL, D'Silva JL, Gasul BM, Dillon RF. Stenosis of the right main pulmonary artery. Clinical, angiocardiographic, and catheterization findings in ten patients. *Circulation* 1960;21:1116–1125.

184. Delaney TB, Nadas AS. Peripheral pulmonic stenosis. *Am J Cardiol* 1964;13:451–461.

185. Agustsson MH, Arcilla RA, Gasul BM, Bicoff JP, Nassif SI, Lendrum BL. The diagnosis of bilateral stenosis of the primary pulmonary artery branches based on characteristic pulmonary trunk pressure curves. A hemodynamic and angiocardiographic study. *Circulation* 1962;26:421–427.

186. Edwards JE, Carey LS, Neufeld HN, Lester RG. Peripheral pulmonary arterial stenosis. In: Edwards JE, Carey LS, Neufeld HN, Lester RG, eds. *Congenital heart disease. Correlation of pathologic anatomy and angiocardiography. Vol. 2.* Philadelphia: WB Saunders, 1965:673–675.

187. Fraentzel O. Ein fall von abnormer communication der aorta mit der arteria pulmonalis. *Virchows Arch* 1868;43:420–426.

188. Keane JF, Maltz D, Bernhard WF, Corwin RD, Nadas AS. Anomalous origin of one pulmonary artery from the ascending aorta: diagnostic, physiological, and surgical considerations. *Circulation* 1974;50:588–594.

189. Kutsche LM, Van Mierop LHS. Anomalous origin of a pulmonary artery from the ascending aorta: associated anomalies and pathogenesis. *Am J Cardiol* 1988;61:850–856.

190. Cucci CE, Doyle EF, Lewis EW. Absence of a primary division of the pulmonary trunk, an ontogenetic theory. *Circulation* 1964; 29:124–131.

191. Penkoske PA, Castaneda AR, Fyler DC, Van Praagh R. Origin of pulmonary artery branch from ascending aorta. Primary surgical repair in infancy. *J Thorac Cardiovasc Surg* 1983;85:537–545.

192. Sotomora RF, Edwards JE. Anatomic identification of so-called absent pulmonary artery. *Circulation* 1978;57:624–633.

193. Smallhorn JF, Anderson RH, Macartney FJ. Two-dimensional echocardiography assessment of communications between ascending aorta and pulmonary trunk or individual pulmonary arteries. *Br Heart J* 1982;47:563–572.

194. Morgan JR. Left pulmonary artery from ascending aorta in tetralogy of Fallot. *Circulation* 1972; 45: 653–657.

195. Fontana GP, Spach MS, Effmann EL, Sabiston DC Jr. Origin of the right pulmonary artery from the ascending aorta. *Ann Surg* 1987;206:102–113.

196. Fong LV, Anderson RH, Siewers RD, Trento A, Park SC. Anomalous origin of one pulmonary artery from the ascending aorta: a review of echocardiographic, catheter, and morphological features. *Br Heart J* 1989;62:389–395.

197. Stewart JR, Kincaid OW, Edwards JE. Other and rare malformations of the aortic arch system. In: Stewart JR, Kincaid OW, Edwards JE, eds. *An atlas of vascular rings and related malformations of the aortic arch system.* Springfield, IL: Charles C. Thomas Publisher, 1964:130–155.

198. Semb BKH, Tjonneland S, Stake G, Aabyholm G. ''Balloon valvulotomy'' of congenital pulmonary valve stenosis with tricuspid valve insufficiency. *Cardiovasc Radiol* 1979;2:239–241.

199. Kan JS, White RI Jr, Mitchell SE, Gardner TJ. Percutaneous balloon valvuloplasty: a new method for treating congenital pulmonary-valve stenosis. *N Engl J Med* 1982;307:540–542.

200. Sullivan ID, Robinson PJ, Macartney FJ, et al. Percutaneous balloon valvuloplasty for pulmonary valve stenosis in infants and children. *Br Heart J* 1985;54:435–441.

201. Musewe NN, Robertson MA, Benson LN, et al. The dysplastic pulmonary valve: echocardiographic features and results of balloon dilatation. *Br Heart J* 1987;57:364–370.

202. Marantz PM, Huhta JC, Mullins CE, et al. Results of balloon valvuloplasty in typical and dysplastic pulmonary valve stenosis: Doppler echocardiographic follow-up. *J Am Coll Cardiol* 1988; 12:476–479.

203. Stanger P, Cassidy SC, Girod DA, Kan JS, Lababidi Z, Shapiro SR. Balloon pulmonary valvuloplasty: results of the valvuloplasty and angioplasty of congenital anomalies registry. *Am J Cardiol* 1990;65:775–783.

204. Cazzaniga M, Vagnola O, Alday L, et al. Balloon pulmonary valvuloplasty in infants: a quantitative analysis of pulmonary valve-anulus-trunk structure. *J Am Coll Cardiol* 1992;20:345–349.

CHAPTER 19

Anomalies of the Left Ventricular Outflow Tract

Lilliam M. Valdes-Cruz and Raul O. Cayre

The obstructions to left ventricular outflow, classically denominated aortic stenosis, comprise a spectrum of malformations that include valvular, subvalvular, and supravalvular aortic stenosis. Their incidence varies between 1.9% and 7.6% of all cases of congenital cardiac anomalies (1–7). Aortic atresia with normal or dilated left ventricle is also included within the left ventricular outflow obstructions. Obstructions due to leftward and posterior displacement of the infundibular septum or due to the presence of an anterolateral muscular band seen in complete interruption of the aortic arch, those seen in atrioventricular univentricular connection caused by a restrictive intercameral or bulboventricular foramen, those presenting in ventriculoarterial discordance, those caused by anomalous insertions of the mitral valve, and aortic atresia as an integral part of the syndrome of hypoplastic left ventricle are not included in this chapter; they are discussed in their respective chapters.

Aortic valvular insufficiency can be associated with any type of aortic stenosis and therefore will be considered in each of the subsequent sections.

VALVULAR AORTIC STENOSIS

Valvular aortic stenosis accounts for 70% to 91% of aortic obstructions (1,3,7), with an incidence of 2% in neonates and 11% in young adults with congenital heart disease (8). The first description of a calcified aortic valve is attributed to Carolus Rayger in 1672, cited by T. Bonetus in 1679 (9). The first reference to an aortic orifice "contracted at birth" was by N. Chevers in 1842 (10).

EMBRYOLOGIC CONSIDERATIONS

The semilunar valves of the great vessels originate from the truncal valve swellings and from the intercalated cush-

ions. The dextrosuperior and the sinistroinferior truncal swellings give rise to the posterior pulmonary leaflets and to the anterior aortic leaflets; the anterior pulmonary leaflet arises from the left intercalated truncal swelling and the posterior noncoronary aortic cusp from the right intercalated truncal swelling (11) (see Fig. 1-14B). The separation of the truncal swellings gives origin to the aortic and pulmonic valve commissures. The separation between the dextrosuperior and the sinistroinferior truncal swellings gives rise to the commissure between the anterior right and the anterior left aortic cusps and the posterior right and left pulmonary cusps. The separation between the right intercalated and the sinistroinferior truncal swellings results in the commissure between the left anterior and the posterior noncoronary cusps. The separation between the right intercalated and the dextrosuperior truncal swellings gives rise to the commissure between the posterior noncoronary and the right anterior coronary cusps (see Fig. 1-14B).

The morphogenetic mechanism that results in valvular aortic stenosis is not well known. Absence of one or more commissures would be due to either a complete lack of separation between the embryologic structures, which give rise to the semilunar valves early in development, or to the fusion of these structures at a later stage so that a band of connective tissue or raphe remain in place of the commissure (12,13). According to Van Mierop (14), the pure form with absence of a raphe would be due to the complete lack of primordium of one of the cusps. An inflammatory process or "fetal endocarditis" has been proposed as the morphogenetic factor in the production of these types of malformations (15–17).

ANATOMIC AND ECHOCARDIOGRAPHIC CONSIDERATIONS

The echocardiographic study of valvular aortic stenosis should include the following features: (a) the morphology of the stenotic valve; (b) the diameter of the "aortic annulus"; (c) the size and function of the left ventricle; (d) the degree of obstruction; and (e) associated anomalies. The intra- and postinterventional evaluation is discussed at the end for all types of left ventricular outflow obstructions.

Morphology of the Stenotic Valve

Aortic valve stenosis can be congenital or acquired; this latter can occur on a valve that is congenitally malformed but that functions well during early life or on a normal valve (7,18). The congenital anomalies of the aortic valve comprise a spectrum of deformities, which includes a decrease or an increase in the number of valve cusps, their form and size.

Unicuspid aortic valve is the most common form found in critical aortic stenosis in the neonate (19,20). The valve has only one cusp and can be of two types, unicommissural or acommissural (7,21) (Fig. 19-1A,B), the unicommissural type being the most common (20,21) (Fig. 19-1A). There is only one commissure, which extends to the aortic wall, resulting in the presence of an eccentric orifice whose diameter determines the severity of stenosis (Echo. 19-1). The valve is thickened and of poor mobility, which may cause insufficiency. Usually, one or two raphes can be seen adjacent to the aortic wall, but these do

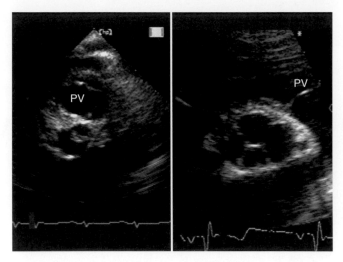

ECHO. 19-1. Parasternal short-axis views of a unicommissural aortic valve (**left**) and a quadricuspid valve (**right**). *PV*, pulmonic valve.

not reach the free border of the valve cusp (7,13,22,23) (Fig. 19-1A). These raphes are found in the locations that would correspond to the true commissures, and their presence indicates that the existence of only one cusp is due to fusion of two commissures during fetal development. An acommissural valve is seen much less frequently. It has the shape of a dome, with only one cusp, no commissure, and only one central orifice (7,21) (Fig. 19-1B). Similar to the unicommissural valve, raphes can be seen along the sites corresponding to the true commissures.

Bicuspid aortic valve and mitral valve prolapse are considered the most common forms of congenital cardiac anomalies (24). This is the most common congenital malformation of the aortic valve (7,13,18) and is found in association with coarctation of the aorta in 46% to 85% of cases (25,26).

The leaflets are usually unequal in size, and two types can be recognized: one with cusps located to the right and left, and one with anterior and posterior cusps (Fig. 19-1C,D). Frequently, in cases with right and left cusps, the raphe is in the right cusp and with anterior and posterior cusps, the raphe is in the anterior cusp (7,13,27). The raphe can be of variable size and extends from the aortic wall to the free border of the cusp dividing it in two portions, so it can be confused with a tricuspid leaflet. The height of the raphe has been related to the moment in development when the fusion occurs; a low raphe can indicate early fusion, while a higher raphe is the result of later fusion (13). In 16% of cases, no raphe can be found (27).

A bicuspid aortic valve is not stenotic at birth except if it has dysplastic tissue, in which case the cusps are thickened and redundant, with myxomatous tissue, which appears nodular (1,28). In adulthood, stenosis can develop due to fusion of the commissures, fibrosis of the leaflets,

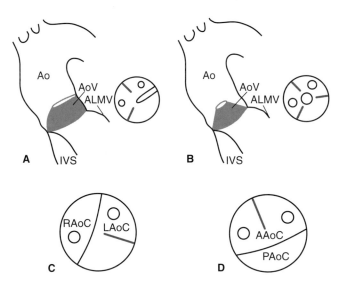

FIG. 19-1. Schematic drawings showing the various anatomical types of abnormal aortic valves. **A:** Unicommissural aortic valve. Note that the raphes are located at the line of fusion of the commissures. **B:** Acommissural aortic valve. As in A, raphes are along the line of fusion of the commissures. **C:** Bicuspid aortic valve with one right and one left cusp. **D:** Bicuspid aortic valve with one anterior and one posterior cusp. *Ao*, aorta; *AoV*, aortic valve; *ALMV*, anterior leaflet of the mitral valve; *IVS*, interventricular septum; *RAoC*, right aortic cusp; *LAoC*, left aortic cusp; *AAoC*, anterior aortic cusp; *PAoC*, posterior aortic cusp.

and sometimes later calcification. Presence of a bicuspid valve in adulthood can be due to a congenitally bicuspid valve or to an acquired deformity due to fusion of two adjacent cusps (29,30). Morphologically, it is not always possible to establish the difference between them; however, it is generally thought that a raphe that does not extend to the free border of the leaflet indicates a congenitally malformed valve (31). Histologically, it is also possible to differentiate them since the raphe in a congenitally bicuspid valve is composed of elastic fibers, which are similar to the media of the aortic wall, whereas fused cusps contain only fibrous tissue similar to that found in the leaflets (29).

The coronary arteries emerge from the anterior leaflet in cases with anterior and posterior cusps (Fig. 19-1D) or from the posterior leaflet when there is complete transposition of the great vessels in association with a bicuspid aortic valve. In the presence of right and left cusps, the left coronary artery emerges from the anterior portion of the left sinus and the right coronary from the anterior part of the right sinus in front of the raphe when it is present (7,27) (Fig. 19-1C). In 44% of cases, a high origin of the left coronary above the sinus of Valsalva has been found (32). A high left coronary origin is seen in 30% of normal subjects (33).

Tricuspid aortic valves are usually not stenotic at birth, and if there is obstruction, it is usually caused by a small "aortic annulus" (7). Stenosis of a tricuspid aortic valve is common in adults due to fusion of the commissures. Rarely, there can be three cusps, with one being so small that the valve is functionally bicuspid (12).

Quadricuspid aortic valves usually have three normal-sized leaflets and one very small leaflet and are rarely stenotic (34,35) (Echo. 19-1). In the majority of cases, a quadricuspid valve functions normally, but a large percentage is insufficient (34,36,37).

The morphologic characteristics of a stenotic aortic valve can be accurately observed with two-dimensional echocardiography. The parasternal short-axis view demonstrates the number of cusps. Presence of an eccentric orifice with one commissure or of a unicuspid valve establishes the differential diagnosis between a unicommissural and an acommissural valve, respectively (Fig. 19-1A,B) (Echo. 19-1). This view also allows observation of thickened leaflets and their degree of mobility during the cardiac cycle. In the presence of a bicuspid valve, the parasternal short-axis view also illustrates the location of the cusps (Echo. 19-2). It is not possible to always differentiate a raphe from a real commissure of a tricuspid valve; however, the fact that a raphe does not extend to the free border of the leaflet and that the systolic opening of a bicuspid valve is circular or somewhat oval in shape (Echo. 19-2), while it is more or less triangular in a tricuspid valve, can help establish the difference. The size of the leaflets can also be seen from this view.

Color Doppler flow mapping is of great utility in dem-

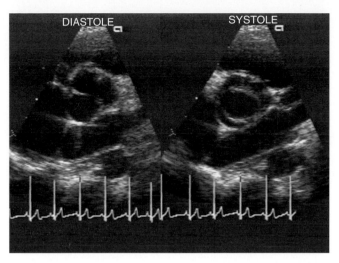

ECHO. 19-2. Short-axis view of a bicuspid valve with one anterior and one posterior cusp. The raphe is in the anterior cusp.

onstrating the direction of a central or eccentric jet as well as its point of origin. There can be dilation of the aortic wall at the site where the jet is directed. The location of this poststenotic dilatation can be useful in selecting the most appropriate view for recording of the highest spectral Doppler velocity (38), which is obtained within the ascending aorta (39) (Echo. 19-3; see color plate 64 following p. 364).

Regurgitation of the aortic valve can be easily detected with color Doppler flow mapping from the parasternal long- and short-axis views and from the apical and subcostal long-axis and outflow views. It can be found in association with any type of congenitally stenotic valve (4,21); however, it is seen in 36% to 43% of quadricuspid valves (34,35) and in 20% to 25% of bicuspid valves (29,31). It is less common in the presence of a unicuspid or a tricuspid valve.

Diameter of the "Aortic Annulus"

Despite several published studies that undertake a detailed analysis of the anatomy and histology of the aortic valvular apparatus (20,27,40–45), there is still confusion about the nomenclature applied to its different portions particularly in reference to the aortic valve "annulus." Consequently, we will define the terminology that will be used to identify the different anatomic structures that compose the aortic valvular apparatus.

Ascending aorta is composed in its proximal portion by the aortic sinus or the sinuses of Valsalva and distally by the tubular portion (46) (Fig. 19-2).

Sinotubular junction is the point of union of the aortic sinuses and the tubular portion of the ascending aorta. At this level, there is a small crest in the internal aortic wall called the "sinotubular ridge" (47) (Fig. 19-2). The apex

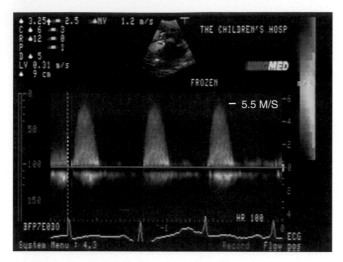

ECHO. 19-3. Spectral Doppler velocity through a severely stenotic aortic valve derived from a right parasternal color Doppler guided image.

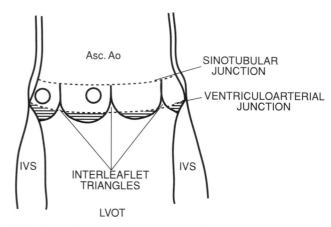

FIG. 19-3. Schematic drawing showing the sinotubular junction and the ventriculoarterial union between the aorta and the left ventricle. Note the portion of the wall of the aorta or interleaflet triangles that forms part of the outflow tract of the left ventricle and the portion of the left ventricular wall located within the sinuses of Valsalva *(shaded areas). Asc Ao,* ascending aorta; *IVS,* interventricular septum; *LVOT,* left ventricular outflow tract.

of the aortic valve commissures or point of union of the leaflets is found at the sinotubular junction (45) and corresponds to the highest point of insertion of the aortic cusps on the lateral wall of the aorta (Fig. 19-2). There has been no circular connective tissue structure or "fibrous annulus" demonstrated to support these insertions (44,45).

Ventriculoarterial junction anatomically corresponds to the insertion of the arterial trunk into the ventricular structures that support it (44,45) (Fig. 19-3). In the left ventricle, this insertion acquires the shape of a fibromuscular ring, which can be described as an annulus. The muscular portion corresponds to the left ventricular myocardium, which supports the valve, and the fibrous portion corresponds to the insertion at the level of the fibrous

continuity between the aortic and mitral valve leaflets (44,45).

The insertion of the leaflets of the aortic valve into the wall of the aortic sinus is semilunar or similar to a hyperbola in shape (44,45,48) and makes up its hinge point (20) (Fig. 19-3). Its free border is the coapting surface (20). The highest level corresponds to the point of insertion of the commissure into the lateral wall of the aorta and the lowest level to the point of insertion into the ventricular wall adjacent to the anatomic ventriculoarterial junction (20,27,44,45) (Fig. 19-3). This type of insertion determines that there is a portion of the aortic wall below the commissures called the "interleaflet triangle," which hemodynamically forms part of the outflow tract of the left ventricle and which is the hemodynamic ventriculoarterial junction (44,45) (Fig. 19-3). Likewise, there is a portion of the ventricular wall, above the basal insertion, which is included in the sinuses of Valsalva and which from the hemodynamic standpoint is arterial (44,45) (Fig. 19-3).

Valvular orifice corresponds to the circular or oval-shaped orifice limited by the coapting surfaces of the valve leaflets and whose area is related to the degree of fusion of the adjacent leaflets that starts at the level of the commissures. The valve orifice is usually found more or less at the level of the insertion of the commissures into the aortic wall (44) (Fig. 19-3). The plane of this orifice does not correspond to the anatomic plane of the ventriculoarterial junction, generally considered the "aortic annulus" (Fig. 19-2).

The echocardiographic parasternal long-axis view permits determination of the plane of the anatomic ventriculoarterial junction or "aortic annulus," the basal insertion of the leaflets or lowest hinge point, the thickness and

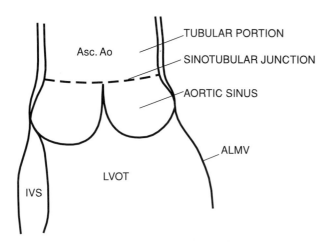

FIG. 19-2. Schematic drawing showing the various portions of the ascending aorta. The *dotted line* indicates the sinotubular junction. *Asc Ao,* ascending aorta; *IVS,* interventricular septum; *LVOT,* left ventricular outflow tract; *ALMV,* anterior leaflet of the mitral valve.

mobility of the leaflets, the plane of the valvular orifice, the sinuses of Valsalva, the sinotubular junction, and the proximal part of the tubular portion of the ascending aorta. This is the view commonly used to measure the various parameters that enter into the evaluation of aortic stenosis, particularly critical stenosis (49,50).

The aortic root is that portion of the aorta that contains the semilunar valve leaflets (51). It includes the sinuses of Valsalva or aortic sinus, the leaflets and the interleaflet triangles of the subaortic outflow tract (27). Due to the configuration of the aortic valve, all these various elements that make up the aortic valvular apparatus are not at the same level. This has resulted in confusion when measurements are made of the aortic root from the parasternal long-axis view, be it at the point of maximum dimension of the sinuses of Valsalva (50), at the site of insertion of the aortic valve cusps at end diastole (52) or at the lowest hinge point of the aortic leaflets (53). The point of insertion of the aortic cusps into the wall of the aorta, which corresponds more or less to the plane of the valvular orifice, and the basal insertion of the leaflets into the ventricular wall or lowest hinge point of the leaflets have the narrowest diameters of the aortic valve complex (27). We consider the latter to be the level where the aortic root should be measured. It is the point of the anatomic ventriculoarterial junction and where the "aortic annulus" is usually found (Echo. 19-4).

Size and Function of the Left Ventricle

The left ventricle is usually hypertrophied with increased contractility and a small cavity. A large percentage of cases, particularly of critical aortic stenosis of the neonate, have endocardial fibroelastosis (8,19,49,54,55).

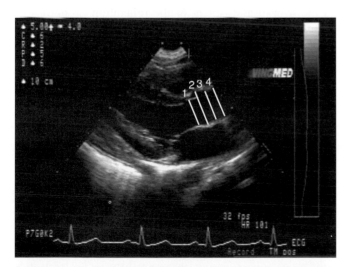

ECHO. 19-4. Parasternal long-axis view demonstrating the sites for anatomical measurements of the aortic root and ascending aorta. *1,* aortic root; *2,* aortic sinuses; *3,* sinotubular junction; *4,* ascending aorta.

The size of the left ventricular cavity in critical aortic stenosis can be markedly hypoplastic, normal or even dilated.

The left ventricular size determines the clinical course of the patient and is one of the predictive factors in the outcome following balloon valvuloplasty or surgical valvotomy in the neonate (8,19,49,50,53,54–56). Its size can be assessed echocardiographically from a parasternal long-axis view measured at end diastole using the simultaneous EKG as a reference signal or from a derived M-mode obtained from a short-axis parasternal view. The long-axis views (parasternal, apical and subcostal) are also used to measure other structures such as the aortic root in early systole and the mitral valve annular diameter in early diastole. This latter structure can also be measured from the apical four-chamber view (49,53,56).

Leung et al. (49) utilized the long-axis and the apical four-chamber views to measure the inflow of the left ventricle from the insertion of the posterior mitral valve leaflet to the apex at end diastole, the diameter of the ventriculoarterial junction, and the mitral valve annulus. These authors found that infants with a left ventricular inflow measuring less than 25 mm, a ventriculoarterial junction under 5 mm and a mitral annulus less than 9 mm did not have acceptable results following valvotomy and therefore should be considered for heart transplantation or a Norwood type of operation. Parsons et al. (57) found that in infants with critical aortic stenosis, a mitral valve annulus under 6 mm measured from the apical four-chamber view, an end diastolic left ventricular dimension less than 13 mm obtained from a derived M-mode and a left ventricular cross-sectional area at end diastole of less than 2 cm² measured from the long-axis parasternal view all predicted a poor outcome following surgical valvotomy.

Rhodes et al. (50) developed a detailed scoring system to evaluate the adequacy of left heart structures as predictors of survival after balloon or surgical valvotomy (two ventricle repair) by retrospectively evaluating the echocardiograms of a series of neonates with critical aortic stenosis. Their approach was based on the hypothesis that the functional consequences of hypoplasia of several left heart structures is additive and that left ventricular size alone is not fully predictive of survival. As such, an adequate systemic ventricle must have an adequately sized inflow, chamber, and outflow. They obtained measurements from two-dimensional echocardiographic images. The aortic root dimension was measured as the maximal dimension at the level of the sinuses of Valsalva from a parasternal long-axis view. The mitral valve area was obtained from the anteroposterior and lateral dimensions of the mitral annulus in diastole measured from the parasternal long-axis and the apical four-chamber views, respectively, and applied to the formula for an ellipse (area= $\pi[D_1 \times D_2]/4$). The long-axis length of the left ventricle was measured as the distance from the apex of the ventricle to the mitral valve plane obtained from the subcostal long-axis view. The long axis of the heart was measured as the distance from the crux cordis to the apical endocardium (of the right or left ventricle, whichever forms the cardiac apex) from an apical four-chamber view. The left ventricular mass was calculated as the difference between epicardial and endocardial volumes multiplied by the specific gravity of the myocardium (1.04 gm/ml). The critical levels of the four anatomic factors found to be most predictive of outcome after valvotomy were (a) left ventricular long-axis to heart long-axis ratio of less than or equal to 0.8; (b) indexed aortic root diameter of less than or equal to 3.5 cm/m^2; (c) indexed mitral valve area of less than or equal to 4.75 cm^2/m^2; and (d) left ventricular mass index of less than or equal to 35 g/m^2. All patients with two or more risk factors died, whereas 92% of those with no or one risk factors survived valvotomy. Exclusion of the left ventricular mass index reduced the predictive accuracy of nonsurvival from 100% to 79%. The authors proposed a predictive survival score based on these anatomical measurements as follows:

$$\text{Score} = 14.0 \, (\text{BSA}) + 0.943 \, (\text{ROOT}_i) + 4.78 \, (\text{LAR})$$
$$+ 0.157 \, (\text{MVA}_i) - 12.03$$

where BSA = body surface area in m^2; ROOT$_i$ = indexed aortic root dimension; LAR = ratio of long-axis dimension of the left ventricle to long-axis dimension of the heart; and MVA$_i$ = indexed mitral valve area. A score under -0.35 was predictive of death after valvotomy.

Mitral valve regurgitation is found frequently and can be due to anomalies of the valvular and/or subvalvular apparatus, to ischemia or infarct of the papillary muscles, or to endocardial fibroelastosis (8,18,29,54,55,58,59). In a study of the clinical and anatomical findings of patients with endocardial fibroelastosis, Moller et al. (60) described a group of patients with aortic stenosis, dilated left ventricle and endocardial fibroelastosis who, despite pathologic evidence of an abnormal mitral valve apparatus, did not have auscultatory findings of mitral regurgitation. Further, their findings of endocardial fibroelastosis in all the morphologic types of congenital anomalies of the aortic valve led these authors to postulate that the valvular abnormality and the endocardial process could be either separate abnormalities having the same etiology or that the primary process could be the valvular stenosis causing the endocardial fibroelastosis secondarily. Endocardial fibroelastosis can be suspected echocardiographically by the presence of a highly echo-dense and bright endocardium (Echo. 19-5).

Ventricular function is assessed through a combination of views and techniques. Systolic function is estimated from a derived M-mode trace recorded from either a parasternal short-axis or from a long-axis view. Parameters such as end diastolic dimension, end systolic dimension, shortening fraction and ejection fraction, percent thick-

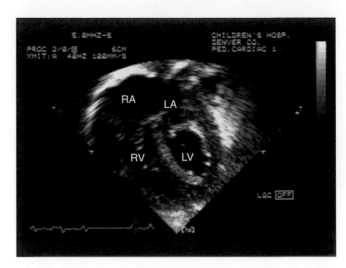

ECHO. 19-5. Apical view of the left ventricular cavity in the presence of bright, highly dense echoes along its endocardium, suggesting endocardial fibroelastosis. *RA,* right atrium; *RV,* right ventricle; *LA,* left atrium; *LV,* left ventricle.

ening of the septum and of the posterior wall can all be measured from these traces. An estimate of the rate of pressure rise (dP/dT) in the left ventricle can be derived from the continuous wave Doppler recording of the mitral regurgitant curve by measuring the time between two arbitrarily selected points on the spectral curve (usually at 1 m/s and 3 m/s) at which the pressures are derived using the Bernoulli equation. In addition, diastolic ventricular function is estimated from the Doppler inflow velocities of the left ventricle recorded at the tip of the mitral leaflets. Measurements of the velocity, duration and velocity time integrals (VTI) of the filling during early diastole (E wave) and atrial systole (A wave) as absolute measurements and in ratios (E/A) and of the isovolumic relaxation time of the left ventricle are helpful in the overall assessment of the relaxation properties of the ventricle. In addition, the pulmonary venous wave forms, their velocity and VTI measured in systole and diastole, and particularly the duration of the pulmonary venous A wave reversal in comparison to the duration of the mitral valve A wave are important in estimating the left atrial and pulmonary venous pressures. Segmental wall motion abnormalities should be assessed globally since there can be ischemia and/or infarcts of the papillary muscles and ventricular walls that would impact on the short- and long-term clinical outcomes. Wall motion is studied utilizing a segmental approach encompassing all echocardiographic views.

It is important to take into consideration the left ventricular function in assessing the severity of the gradient across the obstruction. In the presence of diminished systolic ventricular function, the gradient may be "falsely" low and misleading as to the true degree of stenosis. Likewise in the presence of valve regurgitation, the left ventricular systolic function should be hyperdynamic. If the fractional shortening or ejection fraction are normal or slightly diminished, this implies ventricular dysfunction and would indicate the need for surgical replacement of the regurgitant valve.

Assessment of left ventricular systolic and diastolic function is discussed in detail in Chapters 5 and 6.

Degree of Obstruction

It is important to obtain a clean continuous wave Doppler spectral signal of the highest transvalvular velocity (Echo. 19-3). This requires recording it from all transducer locations, namely the apical and subcostal outflow and long-axis views, the suprasternal long-axis view, and the high subclavicular views. It is recommended that the velocities also be obtained using the stand-alone Pedof transducer due to its greater sensitivity. Commonly, the highest velocity is obtained from the high right subclavicular position with the stand-alone transducer due to the direction of the jet within the ascending aorta. The peak and mean gradients across the valve can be estimated using the simplified Bernoulli equation (39). It is not unusual to find discrepancies between the Doppler-calculated gradients and those recorded at cardiac catheterization. There are various reasons that account for this. The ones most commonly implicated are (a) the difference between peak instantaneous gradients recorded by Doppler and the peak-to-peak gradients usually used in catheterization data and (b) the fact that catheters measure the distal pressures at a location beyond that of the vena contracta, which is defined as the point of maximal contraction of flow and therefore of highest velocity and highest gradient. Doppler, on the other hand, records the velocity at the vena contracta, leading to a higher gradient estimation. Other factors such as inertial and viscous forces as demonstrated by the Reynolds number have been implicated (61). In general, these discrepancies are less obvious when calculating and comparing mean Doppler and catheterization gradients, probably due to the inclusion of lower and higher velocities in the calculations. For these reasons the use of mean gradients rather than peak gradients is becoming more common.

Skjaerpe et al. (62) first described the use of the Doppler continuity equation to estimate the effective aortic valve area. It includes measurement of the diameter and velocity of the left ventricular outflow tract and the velocity across the stenotic aortic valve according to the equation:

Aortic valve area

$$= \frac{\text{Velocity} \times \text{Area of the LV outflow tract}}{\text{Velocity across the aortic valve}}$$

The variability in results obtained by Myreng et al. (63) was attributed to errors in the measurement of the left ventricular outflow tract dimensions. However, there appears to be a dependence of the continuity equation on flow so that at lower outputs, the Doppler-calculated effective orifice area is smaller than that calculated at higher outputs for the same valve in the same subject. This has been attributed to a failure of complete opening of the valve leaflets at low flow rates (64). Recently, however, *in vitro* studies using precise laser Doppler techniques visualizing the vena contracta have suggested that the errors may be due to an underestimation of effective flow areas by the Doppler continuity equation secondary to a departure from a flat flow profile at low flow states and that the actual effective orifice area or vena contracta area remains moderately constant through a wide range of flows (65).

The Doppler methods for assessing the degree of aortic valve obstruction are discussed in detail in Chapter 6.

Associated Anomalies

A patent ductus arteriosus is seen in 20% to 65% of cases of valvular aortic stenosis (8,13,19,29,49,55,59,66). Coarctation of the aorta is found in 11% to 53% of cases (8,13,29,49,51,67) and stenosis of the mitral valve in 25% of patients (8,55,59). Other associated anomalies are patent foramen ovale (18,19,66), atrial septal defect (19,49), Ebstein's anomaly of the tricuspid valve (19), tricuspid valve atresia (13), bicuspid pulmonic valve (29), pulmonary valve atresia with ventricular septal defect (55) or with intact ventricular septum (55), supravalvular mitral ring (55,59), mitral arcade (49), mitral atresia (13), atrioventricular septal defect (49,55), ventricular septal defect (13,49), subvalve aortic stenosis (67), supravalve aortic stenosis (67), hypoplastic ascending aorta (8,66), interrupted aortic arch (8), right aortic arch (29), and anomalous origin of the right coronary artery from the left ventricular outflow tract (68).

SUBVALVE AORTIC STENOSIS

In 1842, Norman Chevers wrote in the *Guy's Hospital Reports:* "The part of the orifice immediately below the valves is probably less frequently the seat of marked organic lesions than any other portion of the aortic outlet: still it is liable to become generally rigid and contracted from inflammatory change; and one portion of its compass—the upper part of the larger mitral curtain, which is attached to the bases of two of the aortic valves—is occasionally found coated with masses of fibrinous and other deposit: this layer of fibrous structure is also apt to become hardened, and rather contracted, after attacks of endocarditis and in cases of disease affecting the left auriculo-ventricular orifice; in this way forming the cause of narrowing of the lower part of the aortic ostium, which I believe to be frequently overlooked" (10). This is the first reference to this type of pathology. In 1882, Moore described the existence of a thickened ring of fibrous tissue just below the aortic valve (69). In 1904 (70) and 1905 (71), two cases were published under the denomination of stenosis of the aortic orifice. Keith in 1909 (72) and Thursfield and Scott in 1913 (73) used the term "subaortic stenosis." The "phrase discrete subaortic stenosis" was proposed by Reis et al. in 1971 (74).

This type of malformation is found in 8% to 30% of cases of aortic stenosis (7,75–80) and corresponds to 1.2% of all congenital cardiac anomalies (81).

EMBRYOLOGIC CONSIDERATIONS

The embryologic origin of subaortic stenosis has not been completely elucidated. The association with an inflammatory process, initially proposed by Chevers (10) was discarded after the histologic studies of Moore (68). Its congenital origin was suggested by Keith (72,82), who proposed that it could be due to failure of reabsorption of the bulbus cordis, which would remain within the left ventricular outflow tract. For Van Mierop (14), it could be due to a malformation of the proximal portion of the truncal septum where it joins the conal septum. Van Praagh (83) considered that probably the majority, if not all cases, of subaortic stenosis due to a fibrous annulus would be the result of an abnormal development of endocardial tissue of the atrioventricular canal, which normally forms the anterior mitral leaflet. The theory proposed by Rosenquist et al. (84,85) states that persistence of the bulboventricular flange would cause an increase in the separation between the anterior mitral leaflet and the aorta or mitral-aortic discontinuity; this would alter the angle at which the blood is ejected from the left ventricle with later differentiation of cells of the crest of the ventricular septum into a fibroelastic band or ring.

The existence of discrete subaortic stenosis in Newfoundland dogs led Pyle et al. (86) to consider that it is not truly a congenital defect but rather that it develops later; the fibrous ring would originate from persistence of embryonic endocardial tissue, which retains its proliferative capabilities after birth. This anomaly would be inherited as a polygenic trait or as an autosomal dominant trait with modifiers (86). These findings as well as the fact that only rarely is discrete subaortic stenosis seen in the newborn period, that it usually develops later in life, and that it recurs after surgical resection or appears after surgery for other associated cardiac malformations have led some authors to conclude that it should be considered an acquired lesion on a preexistent anatomical substrate. With abnormal turbulent flows within the left ventricular outflow tract, connective tissue would be stimulated and progressive obstruction would result (4,87–96). The occurrence of discrete subaortic stenosis in identical twins (80) and in several members of the same family (95) have been reported.

ANATOMIC AND ECHOCARDIOGRAPHIC CONSIDERATIONS

The echocardiographic study of subvalve aortic stenosis should include (a) the morphology of the subvalve stenosis; (b) the presence of aortic valvular insufficiency; and (c) associated anomalies.

Morphology of the Subvalve Stenosis

Classically, subvalve aortic stenosis has been divided into fixed and dynamic types. The fixed obstructions, membranous or fibromuscular, include the various types of discrete subaortic stenoses as well as the obstructions caused by other mechanisms within a variety of malformations listed above, in the introduction to this chapter. These latter types are discussed in the respective chapters. The dynamic or muscular obstructions are found within the spectrum of the hypertrophic cardiomyopathies and will not be included since there is no general agreement as to the congenital or acquired nature of these pathologies.

There are three types of fixed subaortic obstructions that have been recognized (80) (Fig. 19-4): membranous type, in which there is a thin fibrous membrane underneath the aortic valve or up to 2.5 cm below it (Fig. 19-4A); fibromuscular type, in which there is a thick ridge or diaphragm of fibroelastic or fibromuscular tissue that can be found in the same locations within the left ventricular outflow tract (Fig. 19-4B); and fibromuscular tunnel type, in which the obstruction extends for several centimeters below the valve (Fig. 19-4C). By definition, this last one is not considered a discrete form of subaortic stenosis.

Reis et al. (74) used the term "discrete subaortic stenosis" to indicate obstruction caused by a discrete fibrous membrane and called "subaortic tunnel" that in which there is a segment of the left ventricular outflow tract with a diffuse obstruction. Anderson and Becker also recognized two types of subaortic obstructions, one due to a fibrous diaphragm and one due to a fibromuscular tunnel (29,97). Somerville (4,91) and Somerville et al. (88)

FIG. 19-4. Schematic drawings showing the various types of fixed subvalve aortic stenosis. **A:** Membranous type. **B:** Fibromuscular type. **C:** Fibromuscular tunnel type. Note the septal hypertrophy and thickened anterior mitral leaflet. *Asc Ao,* ascending aorta; *IVS,* interventricular septum; *ALMV,* anterior leaflet of the mitral valve; *LVOT,* left ventricular outflow tract.

stated that a true thin membrane cannot be demonstrated by pathologists at necropsy so that the tissue resected by the surgeons is truly a ridge of fibroelastic tissue that protrudes into the left ventricular outflow tract.

Echocardiographically, it is not possible to differentiate between a fibrous and a fibromuscular discrete membrane; therefore, for our purposes, the fixed subaortic obstructions will be divided into discrete type and fibromuscular tunnel type.

Discrete subaortic stenosis is caused by a ridge or diaphragm of fibroelastic or fibromuscular tissue that can be located immediately below or up to 2.5 cm below the aortic valve (74,78–80,96,98) (Fig. 19-4A,B). The diaphragm extends from the interventricular septum to the anterior leaflet of the mitral valve and in those cases in which it abuts the valve, mitral regurgitation can occur. In the majority of instances it has the shape of a horseshoe and rarely it is a complete ring. In cases where the diaphragm is immediately below the valve, it can abut or be joined to one of the aortic cusps by a strand of tissue (71,75). The aortic valve is usually normal but it can also be stenotic with thickened cusps. In children over 5 years of age, damage to the aortic cusps can be found due to the high-velocity jet across the membrane (4).

Fibromuscular tunnel can be considered to be a more severe case of a fibrous diaphragm (23,97). The left ventricular outflow tract is deformed and has a diffuse obstruction that can extend from the aortic valve to the free border of the mitral valve (Fig. 19-4C). Usually the anterior mitral leaflet and the aortic cusps have a degree of thickening (71).

In both forms of subvalve aortic stenosis, the left ventricle is hypertrophied if the obstruction is at least of moderate severity and the ascending aorta is usually not dilated.

It is important to point out that this type of cardiac malformation is progressive. This is evidenced by the fact that in many patients these lesions are not detected on initial exam (92,93) as well as by the fact that they frequently recur after surgical resection. Recurrence has been reported in 11% to 86% of clinical series (80,88,93,99). In the majority of cases reported by Firpo et al. (93), trivial residual discrete subaortic stenosis was seen on echo; the authors attributed these findings to the sensitivity and precision of the echocardiographic methods used.

Echocardiographically, discrete and tunnel subaortic stenoses can be studied from the parasternal long-axis, the apical long-axis and outflow views and the subcostal outflow view.

A discrete membrane is seen from these views as a shelf adhered to the interventricular septum. Since the membranous diaphragm is directed posteriorly towards the left ventricular posterior wall and mitral valve, it is not possible to appreciate its true extent from the parasternal long-axis view since the ultrasound beam is parallel to it. The apical and subcostal long-axis and outflow views

are more likely to demonstrate the entire ridge since the ultrasound beam is perpendicular to it (Echo. 19-6). It is important to measure the distance between the diaphragm and the aortic valve since damage to the valve from a jet lesion is more likely if it is a distance away from the valve. Likewise, if a membrane is very close to the valve it can be confused with valvar stenosis. M-mode traces of the aortic valve leaflet motion demonstrate a slight flutter and early systolic closure of the leaflets in the presence of a fixed subaortic obstruction that is not seen in valve stenosis (100).

A fibromuscular tunnel is easily diagnosed from these same views by the appearance of a long and diffusely narrowed outflow tract (Echo. 19-7; see color plate 65 following p. 364). No evidence of a discrete shelf can be appreciated in these cases.

Doppler serves to demonstrate the sites of obstruction along the length of the outflow tract. Color Doppler illustrates the flow acceleration at the site(s) of stenosis by color aliasing and the deceleration beyond the stenosis by velocity variance (Echo. 19-7). The relative severities of the stenoses can be evaluated by the use of high pulse rate frequency (PRF) Doppler with careful positioning of the sample volumes along the various sites of the outflow tract. This is best accomplished from the apical long-axis and outflow views and in smaller children also from the subcostal views. Continuous wave Doppler should be used to measure the total gradient (101); in order to assure a true recording of maximal velocity, this should be attempted from all views using the stand-alone Pedof probe as well as the combined imaging and Doppler probes. The right infraclavicular view with the patient turned towards the right usually results in the highest velocity recording.

The discrepancies between Doppler- and catheter-

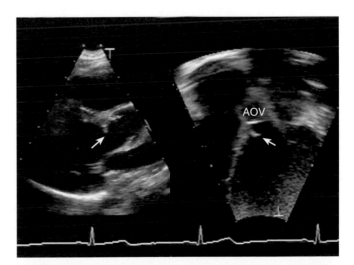

ECHO. 19-6. Left: Parasternal long-axis view demonstrating the presence of a discrete subaortic membrane *(arrow).* **Right:** Apical outflow view of the subaortic membrane *(arrow). AOV,* aortic valve.

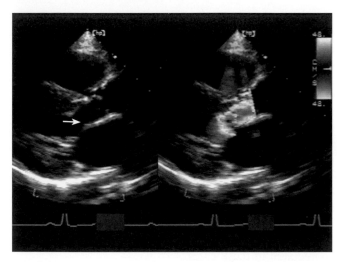

ECHO. 19-7. Parasternal long-axis views of fibromuscular subaortic tunnel. Note the narrowest point along the subaortic area *(arrow)*. The color Doppler flow map **(right)** exhibits flow acceleration towards this point and aliasing of the velocities beyond it.

measured gradients become more of a problem in the presence of subvalve obstructions than in isolated valvar stenosis (102,103). With a discrete membrane located at a distance from an essentially normal aortic valve, the highest velocity is recorded between the membrane and the valve, with pressure recovery effects already seen in the proximal aortic root just beyond the valve leaflets. This is very difficult to document in the cardiac catheterization laboratory even with the use of end-hole catheters and slow pull-backs. If the membrane is close to the aortic valve, the highest velocities will be recorded beyond the valve itself and it will be difficult to assess whether the valve contributes to the overall gradient. In these cases, two-dimensional imaging can be helpful in establishing the differential diagnosis. In the hemodynamic laboratory, this would be almost impossible to assess by simple catheter pull-back due to the proximity of the membrane and valve. In diffuse tunnel obstruction, the maximal velocity is produced inside the tunnel and this can be missed altogether by catheter measurement and sometimes even by Doppler techniques if the tunnel is very long and narrowed (102). In these latter cases, the pressure drop caused by viscous friction along the tunnel may cause a lower Doppler velocity to be recorded, resulting in an underestimation of the true gradient (38).

Presence of Aortic Regurgitation

Aortic valve regurgitation in the presence of subvalve obstruction is seen in 28% to 55% of pediatric patients with a discrete type of stenosis (78,80,93). Flow disturbances produced by the subvalve jet cause a progressive alteration in the closing mechanism of the valve with resulting regurgitation (79,104). Regurgitation can be seen even in patients after resection of a discrete membrane (93).

Associated Anomalies

The valve lesions caused by the high-velocity stenotic jet predispose towards the occurrence of bacterial endocarditis, which has a greater incidence in patients with discrete subaortic stenosis and which increases with age (104). For these reasons, it is important to maintain a high degree of suspicion when studying these patients echocardiographically if the clinical presentation involves febrile episodes.

The incidence of associated anomalies in the presence of subaortic obstructions is high, varying between 57% and 72% of reported cases (74,80,88,91,93,99). The most frequent ones include coarctation of the aorta, patent ductus arteriosus and ventricular septal defect (7,74,78–80,88,90,92,93,99). Others found with less frequency are valve pulmonic stenosis (74,79,92,93), bicuspid aortic valve (74,79,88), mitral regurgitation (78,88,99), valvar aortic stenosis (80,98), abnormal aortic valve (88,99), supravalve aortic stenosis (79,88), mitral valve stenosis (80,99), anomalies of the mitral valve (90,93), aortopulmonary window (80,92), atrial septal defect (92,99), persistent left superior vena cava (74,88), aberrant subclavian artery (93,99), atrioventricular septal defect (92), tetralogy of Fallot (92), absent pulmonary valve (92), double outlet right ventricle (74), anomalous coronary ostia (99), infundibular pulmonic stenosis (105), double orifice mitral valve (106), and aortic arch interruption (107).

SUPRAVALVE AORTIC STENOSIS

Supravalve aortic stenosis is a complex form of left ventricular outflow tract obstruction characterized by obstruction of the aorta above the sinuses. The first description of this type of pathology was by Chevers in 1842 (10) and the term ''supravalve aortic stenosis'' was first proposed by Mencarelli in 1930 (108). The association of supravalve stenosis, elfin facies, and mental retardation was described by Williams et al. in 1961 (109) and by Beuren et al. in 1962 (110). The association of this syndrome with familial idiopathic hypercalcemia was suggested by Black and Bonham-Carter in 1963 (111) and confirmed by Garcia et al. in 1964 (112). Presence of central or peripheral pulmonary arterial stenosis in association with supravalve aortic stenosis was pointed out by Bourassa and Campeau in 1963 (113) and by Beuren et al. in 1964 (114). Stenosis of systemic arteries in patients with supravalve aortic stenosis was studied by Ottesen et al. (115).

The incidence of supravalve aortic stenosis varies between 2% and 11% of all cases of aortic stenosis (3,4,7,

76,77,116,117) and corresponds to 0.11% of all congenital cardiac anomalies (118).

EMBRYOLOGIC CONSIDERATIONS

Knowledge of the morphogenetic processes responsible for the various types of supravalve aortic stenosis continues to be in the realm of speculation. Goor and Lillehei (117) recognize a similarity between coarctation of the aorta and supravalve stenosis and attribute them to a stricture at the point of union of two developing aortic segments. In cases where the supravalve stenosis is located immediately above the aortic valve cusps, the stricture could be due to an abnormal development between the truncus arteriosus or extreme cephalic end of the heart and the aortic sac. When the stenosis encompasses the entire length of the tubular portion of the ascending aorta, the lesion could represent a hypoplasia of the embryonic aortic sac (117).

In cases related to familial idiopathic hypercalcemia, the lesion could be related to an abnormality of vitamin D metabolism (111,112,119,120), and as such some cases have been produced experimentally (119). In patients without the stigmata of Williams' syndrome, the anomaly would be familial and transmitted as an autosomal dominant trait (7,121). Recent studies appear to indicate that the gene for supravalve aortic stenosis could be located in the same chromosomal subunit as that for elastin and a mutation in that gene could cause the malformation (122).

The association of supravalve aortic stenosis with rubella syndrome has also been mentioned (123).

ANATOMIC AND ECHOCARDIOGRAPHIC CONSIDERATIONS

The echocardiographic study of supravalve aortic stenosis should include the following: (a) morphology of the supravalve stenotic area; (b) anomalies of the aortic valve; (c) presence of stenosis of the central or branch pulmonary arteries; (d) presence of coronary lesions; and (e) associated anomalies.

Morphology of the Supravalve Stenotic Area

Classically, it is considered that there are three types of supravalve aortic stenosis: membranous, hourglass-shaped, and hypoplastic. The first two are localized, and the third type is diffuse (18,23,97,116,124,125) (Fig. 19-5).

The membranous type of lesion is located immediately above the aortic valve and consists of a thin membrane or fibrous diaphragm with a central orifice. There is no constriction on the external aortic wall corresponding to the site of the diaphragm internally. This type of stenosis

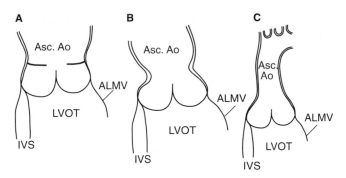

FIG. 19-5. Schematic drawings of the various types of supravalvular aortic stenosis. **A:** Membranous type. **B:** Hourglass type. **C:** Tubular or diffuse type. *Asc Ao,* ascending aorta; *LVOT,* left ventricular outflow tract; *IVS,* interventricular septum; *ALMV,* anterior leaflet of the mitral valve.

is found in 13.2% to 17% of all cases of supravalve stenosis (7,116,126) (Fig. 19-5A).

The hourglass type of deformities is the most common form of supravalve aortic stenosis, with an incidence of 66% of all cases (7,116,126). There is dysplasia of the wall of the aorta with disorganization and thickening of the medial fibers immediately above the aortic cusps and fibrosis and thickening of the intima at the same site, resulting in narrowing of the aortic lumen (116,126). Along the external wall of the aorta at the same level there is an hourglass-shaped narrowing (Fig. 19-5B).

In both types of localized stenoses, the Venturi effect of the jet can cause a dilation of the distal portion of the ascending aorta (23,97).

The tubular or diffuse type of supravalve stenosis involves a uniform and diffuse hypoplasia of the tubular portion of the ascending aorta, beginning immediately above the sinuses of Valsalva and extending to the origin of the innominate artery (Fig. 19-5C). This is the most severe form and sometimes includes the arterial branches of the aortic arch (23,97). The incidence varies between 13% and 24% of all cases of supravalve aortic stenosis (7,116,121,125–127).

According to the facial characteristics and the presence of mental retardation, patients with supravalve aortic stenosis have been classified into three groups; any of the morphologic types described above can be found in any of the clinical groups (115,121,127). Group 1 includes patients with a sporadic, nonfamilial form who have normal facies and normal intelligence; these comprise 37% to 52% of cases (115,120,125,127). Group 2 are patients with a nonfamilial form, elfin facies characteristic of Williams' syndrome, and mental retardation; the incidence varies between 28% and 50% of cases (77,115,120,126,127). Group 3 includes patients with a familial autosomal dominant form with normal facies and intelligence, which comprise 19% to 27% of all cases (115,125,127).

The association of supravalve aortic stenosis with Marfan's syndrome was reported by Burry (128) and has been observed in 4.4% of cases (116).

The echocardiographic study of the different anatomic types of supravalve stenosis can be performed from the parasternal, apical, and subcostal long-axis views and from the high right parasternal long-axis view of the ascending aorta. These views allow determination of the site and extent of the stenosis and the high right parasternal view demonstrates any involvement of the aortic arch branches in the diffuse form (Echo. 19-8; see color plate 66 following p. 364). Spectral Doppler techniques (pulsed and high PRF) manifest the site(s) and severity of the stenosis. The accuracy of the Bernoulli equation for calculation of the gradients would be acceptable in cases of localized stenosis. However, in diffuse narrowing, Doppler is not accurate in the absolute determination of the gradient. As in all instances of long, narrowed obstructions, the maximal velocities occur within the tunnel itself and losses due to viscous friction are not accounted for by the distal velocity alone (102). Color Doppler aids in the detection of the site(s) of stenosis and of any valvular regurgitation.

Left ventricular hypertrophy may be present depending on the severity of the stenosis. This is usually evaluated on M-mode traces derived from parasternal short-axis and/or long-axis views.

Anomalies of the Aortic Valve

These have been reported in 25% to 45% of cases of supravalve aortic stenosis (18,116,125,129). These include valve dysplasia, thickening and fibrosis of the free borders, commissural fusion, attachment of the cusps to

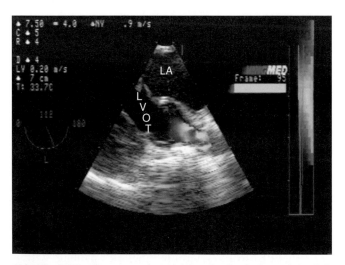

ECHO. 19-8. Transesophageal longitudinal view of the left ventricular outflow tract and ascending aorta in the presence of diffuse supravalve aortic stenosis. Note the narrowing and aliasing of color velocities above the valve. *LA,* left atrium; *LVOT,* left ventricular outflow tract.

the wall of the aorta, fusion of aortic cusps to the membrane or diaphragm causing the obstruction, and bicuspid aortic valve (7,18,76,77,109,116,125,127–129). Occasionally, fusion of the cusps with the supravalve tissue is represented by a band of fibrous tissue or cusp-tuck and is generally found between the right and left coronary cusps (127). Anomalies of the aortic valve can cause valvular regurgitation, which has been reported in 13% to 66% of cases of supravalve stenosis (115,125).

Anomalies of the aortic valve can be seen echocardiographically from the same views as described for valvar stenosis—namely, from the parasternal long- and short-axis views, and from the apical and subcostal outflow views. It is important to point out the need for assessing the dynamics of the aortic valve motion throughout the cardiac cycle. In diastole, the valve may function normally; however, in systole, its motion can be limited and its opening incomplete due to spatial restriction; this has been called "pseudo-valvar stenosis" (130).

Presence of Stenosis of the Central or Branch Pulmonary Arteries

Stenosis of the pulmonary arteries at the bifurcation or at the branches is associated with supravalve aortic stenosis, particularly in Williams' syndrome (114–116,120, 126,131,132). The stenosis can occur in the region of the proximal pulmonary artery, at the bifurcation, at the origin of the right or left branch or peripherally, in which case it can be at multiple sites along the branches or be a generalized hypoplasia (7,97,113,115,116,120,133). Usually, it is diffuse and tubular rather than discrete and at the sites of the lesions there is a thickening of the media with an increase in the elastic fibers that can be in a mosaic orientation (23,134).

Supravalve aortic stenosis is a progressive lesion, with an increasing degree of severity of obstruction with time, while the stenosis of the branch pulmonary arteries tends to improve with time (131,132).

The echocardiographic views that facilitate the study of the pulmonary artery and its branches are the parasternal short-axis view and the suprasternal short-axis view. From these views the site(s) of stenosis can be seen, particularly if these are located in the main pulmonary artery or at the bifurcation. Obstructions along the branches can also be seen from these views, particularly from the suprasternal short-axis, which demonstrates the area almost up to the hilum. Stenoses beyond the hilum cannot be seen echocardiographically. Color Doppler aids in the visual demonstration of the main sites of narrowing and also in the placement of the spectral Doppler sample volume for measurement of velocities. The gradient can be estimated through the Bernoulli equation mostly at a discrete, proximal site but may not be accurate in cases of long, tubular narrowing or in the presence of multiple discrete sites along the length of the branches.

Presence of Anomalies of the Coronary Arteries

Different from what occurs in subvalve and valve aortic stenosis, in which the coronary arteries are distal to the obstruction, in supravalve stenosis the coronary arteries are located proximally and so are subjected to higher pressures. This results in dilated and tortuous arteries with thickened media and intimal fibrosis, which can bring about premature arteriosclerosis (7,18,23,97,109,113,115, 116,121,125,129,134). Partial or total occlusion of a coronary ostium due to fusion of a cusp to the aortic wall has been mentioned (7,116). The incidence of coronary anomalies in supravalve aortic stenosis varies between 45% and 61% of cases (105,116,125). These coronary anomalies and the left ventricular hypertrophy, which is the result of the supravalve obstruction, can explain the angina and syncope as well as the sudden death that has been seen in these patients (23,97,125,135). Presence of collateral circulation between the coronary arteries and the mediastinal arteries has been reported (110).

The origin and proximal portion of the coronary arteries can be seen by echocardiography from the parasternal short-axis view, particularly by positioning the transducer slightly higher or lower on the chest to visualize the branching. The apical four-chamber view demonstrates the right coronary artery coursing along the right atrioventricular groove, and aiming the transducer superiorly towards the outflow of the left ventricle, the branching of the left anterior descending and the circumflex may be seen. The posterior descending branch is observed coursing along the posterior interventricular groove from the parasternal long-axis view tilted medially and posteriorly.

Associated Anomalies

Anomalies that have been described in association with supravalve aortic stenosis are ventricular septal defects, atrial septal defects, patent ductus arteriosus, coarctation of the aorta, subvalve pulmonic stenosis, anomalies of the mitral valve, mitral regurgitation, and subvalve aortic stenosis (4,113,120,125,127,136,137).

AORTIC ATRESIA WITH NORMAL OR DILATED LEFT VENTRICLE

An unusual form of left ventricular outflow tract obstruction is aortic valve atresia, with normal or dilated left ventricle. Aortic atresia was considered an integral component of the hypoplastic left heart syndrome (138–142); however, in 1974 Rosenquist et al. (142) reported a case of aortic atresia, aortopulmonary window, interrupted aortic arch, ventricular septal defect, and patent ductus arteriosus with a left ventricle measuring 2.7 cm. Later in 1976, Pellegrino and Thiene, Freedom et al., and Roberts et al. published seven cases with aortic atresia

and ventricular septal defect with a normal or dilated left ventricle; five cases had a normal-sized mitral valve, one had an atrioventricular septal defect, and one had mitral atresia (143–145). The incidence of this type of aortic atresia ranges from 5% to 7% of cases of aortic valve atresia (145–147).

EMBRYOLOGIC CONSIDERATION

The morphogenetic mechanism that would give rise to atresia of the aortic valve with normal or dilated left ventricle would be the same as that causing valvar aortic stenosis—that is, fusion of the commissures of the valve during a late stage in development (14,148,149). This would result in a membranous type of atresia. In cases where there is aortic valve atresia with "virtual" muscular subaortic atresia, this would be the result of a leftward and superior displacement of the infundibular septum (146,150). In cases associated with an atrioventricular septal defect, the mechanism would be an abnormal attachment of undifferentiated tissue of the endocardial cushions to the interventricular septum (150).

ANATOMIC AND ECHOCARDIOGRAPHIC CONSIDERATIONS

The echocardiographic study of aortic atresia with normal or dilated left ventricle should determine the following features: (a) the morphologic characteristics of the atretic segment, the size of the cardiac cavities, and the morphology of the atrioventricular valves and of the great vessels; (b) the location of the interventricular septal defect; (c) the presence of a patent ductus arteriosus; and (d) associated anomalies.

Morphologic Characteristics of the Atretic Segment, Size of the Cardiac Cavities, Morphology of the Atrioventricular Valves and of the Great Vessels

The left ventricular infundibulum is a blind-ending sac. In the majority of cases, there is an atretic aortic valve at the blind end of the infundibulum represented by an imperforate membrane in which two or three fused cusps can be identified (144,146–149). In situations where there is superior and leftward displacement of the infundibular septum, there is a portion of muscular tissue below the atretic valve that virtually obliterates the subaortic vestibule (146).

In the majority of cases, the right atrium is dilated, the right ventricle is dilated and hypertrophied, the left atrium is of normal size, and the left ventricle is either normal or moderately dilated (142–149).

The tricuspid valve is normal except in cases associated with atrioventricular septal defects (144,146,149,150).

The mitral valve is usually of normal size; however, it can have a variable degree of hypoplasia, with thickening of the leaflets (147,148), or can even be atretic (145).

In all cases reported in the literature, the spatial relationship of the great arteries was normal, with a dilated pulmonary artery and a moderately hypoplastic ascending aorta (142–149).

The morphologic characteristics of the atretic segment can be evaluated echocardiographically through the parasternal long-axis, the apical outflow view, the apical two-chamber and long-axis views, and the subcostal outflow view (Echo. 19-9). In the membranous type of aortic atresia, an imperforate membrane is seen at the level of the aortic valve with variable movement during the cardiac cycle. In the muscular type of atresia, the tissue underneath the plane of the aortic valve is thick and echodense. Color flow Doppler demonstrates the lack of flow from the left ventricle to the ascending aorta. The size of the cardiac chambers and the anatomic characteristics of the atrioventricular valves can also be evaluated from these views, as well as from the short-axis parasternal and the four-chamber apical and subcostal views. The velocity across the mitral valve should be recorded with pulsed and/or continuous wave Doppler from the four-chamber view to assess the presence of stenosis. Color Doppler will aid in demonstrating any regurgitation of the mitral or tricuspid valves. This should be evaluated from various positions on the chest to assure that an eccentrically located jet is not missed. The severity of the regurgitation can be estimated semiquantitatively from the intensity of the spectral signal and the width of the jet at the base.

The spatial relationship of the great vessels can be determined best from a parasternal short-axis view and complemented through the parasternal long-axis sweeping the

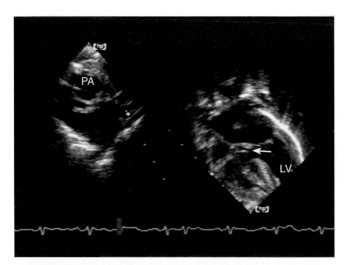

ECHO. 19-9. Left: Parasternal short-axis view of the great vessels in the presence of aortic atresia with diminutive aortic root. **Right:** Apical outflow view demonstrating the diminutive aortic root *(arrow)*. *PA,* pulmonary artery; *LV,* left ventricle.

transducer from a standard position slightly towards the outflow of the right ventricle. The size of the ascending aorta can be evaluated simultaneously from these views and from the suprasternal long-axis, the high right parasternal and the apical outflow and long-axis views (Echo. 19-9).

Location of the Ventricular Septal Defect

Presence of a ventricular septal defect is the rule in this malformation. Absence of a ventricular septal defect is extremely rare (148,149). The defect is of the infundibular type and in a large percentage of cases is due to malalignment between the interventricular and infundibular septa, the latter being displaced superiorly and leftward (146,147,150). Seen from the right side, the defect is located between the limbs of the septomarginal trabecula and, in the presence of displacement of the infundibular septum, the pulmonary artery overrides the interventricular septum (97,146,147). The posterior border of the defect is constituted by the fusion of the infundibular septum and the ventriculoinfundibular fold, which is the structure that separates the pulmonary valve from the atrioventricular valve(s) (143,146,147). In the absence of displacement of the infundibular septum, the defect can be membranous with infundibular or trabecular extensions (144,146,147).

The echocardiographic views that would best demonstrate the defect are the parasternal long-axis and short-axis views, apical four-chamber and outflow views, and subcostal four-chamber view (Echo 19-9). The posterior displacement of the infundibular septum and the subpulmonary location of the defect are particularly evident from the parasternal long-axis view, tilting the transducer slightly towards the pulmonary outflow to demonstrate the infundibular septum and also from the apical and subcostal outflow views. Color Doppler flow mapping would show the passage of blood from the left ventricle through the defect into the pulmonary artery. Spectral Doppler recordings of the flow through the defect would best demonstrate its timing and dynamics.

Presence of a Patent Ductus Arteriosus

In all reported cases, there has been a patent ductus arteriosus allowing blood to flow from the descending aorta to the ascending aorta in a retrograde fashion, thereby perfusing the coronary arteries (142–149). In a report by Thiene et al. (147), there were bilateral ducti; the right ductus connected the right pulmonary artery with the right subclavian artery in one case and with the brachiocephalic artery in the other.

Presence of a patent ductus can be seen echocardiographically with the use of color Doppler from the parasternal short-axis view aiming towards the pulmonary artery and from the suprasternal long- and short-axis views. This demonstrates the passage of blood from the pulmonary artery to the descending aorta through the ductus as well as the retrograde flow within the ascending aorta.

Associated Anomalies

Some of the anomalies reported in association with aortic atresia with normal or dilated left ventricle include atrial septal defect or patent foramen ovale, which are almost always present and are mandatory for the survival of the patients when there is mitral valve atresia; aortic coarctation; bicuspid pulmonic valve; anomalous origin of the right subclavian artery; and double aortic arch (142,145,147–149).

INTRAOPERATIVE AND POSTOPERATIVE EVALUATION (INCLUDING POSTINTERVENTIONAL CATHETERIZATION)

Valve Aortic Stenosis

Balloon dilation of a stenotic aortic valve was originally reported by Lababidi in 1983 (151) and by Lababidi et al. in 1984 (152). It was first used in children by Rupprath and Neuhaus (153) and by Sanchez et al. (154) and in critical aortic stenosis of the newborn by Lababidi and Weinhaus in 1986 (155). Since then it has become a therapeutic alternative in the presence of aortic valve stenosis with results that are comparable to those of surgery but with less morbidity and mortality (53,56,156–164). This technique is also used in recurrent aortic stenosis (165).

In our institution, the gradient is assessed by transthoracic Doppler simultaneously with measurement by catheters immediately prior to balloon valvuloplasty. The valve area is also estimated using the continuity equation (62). These are performed from a combination of a parasternal long-axis and apical outflow views. The velocity across the valve is confirmed with the use of a stand-alone Pedof probe from the suprasternal and right or left subclavicular area. These studies are repeated after the balloon valvuloplasty and compared with the catheter measurements in order to establish a new baseline after intervention. After the balloon study, a careful examination is performed for the presence of regurgitation.

Regurgitation of the aortic valve is one of the complications of therapeutic interventions on the aortic valve. It has been observed in 10% to 70% of cases after balloon valvuloplasty in various published series (53,56,156–158,160–163,165). The mechanism causing the regurgitation has not been clearly defined; however, rupture of the commissures of a rigid valve is the most likely cause, although leaflet perforation and evulsion of cusp tissue from the annulus have been reported (162). Presence of

aortic regurgitation is easily detected by color Doppler flow mapping (Echo. 19-10; see color plate 67 following p. 364). Additionally, various echocardiographic and Doppler methods that have been proposed for estimating the severity of aortic regurgitation. All have limitations; however, their combined use can provide a fairly accurate assessment of severity (166,182). One indirect sign of severe aortic regurgitation is early closure of the mitral valve by the regurgitant jet and consequent mitral valve regurgitation. Both of these phenomena can be documented echocardiographically (Echo. 19-11). Doppler techniques are specifically discussed in detail in Chapter 6.

Subvalve and Supravalve Aortic Stenosis

In these lesions, the treatment of choice is surgery. There has been one case reported of balloon angioplasty in subvalve aortic stenosis (183).

The pre-bypass study is directed towards defining the anatomical characteristics of the ventricular obstruction. The aortic valve can be seen from the transverse retrocardiac views at the base, which also allows determination of the presence of regurgitation (see Fig. 4-29). The transverse four-chamber view, withdrawing the transducer slightly to visualize the left ventricular outflow tract, aids in the diagnosis of a subvalve membrane or diffuse obstruction (see Fig. 4-29A). The longitudinal views are helpful in imaging the left ventricular outflow tract, aortic valve and ascending aorta (184–187) (see Fig. 4-29E,F) (Echo. 19-8). The presence of ventricular hypertrophy and the overall ventricular function can be evaluated from the transgastric short-axis views.

Post-bypass, the transesophageal intraoperative study begins by assessing ventricular function from the trans-

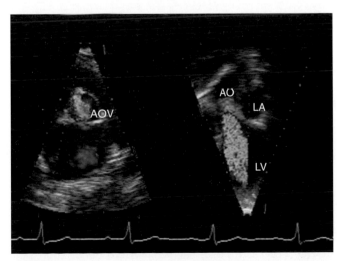

ECHO. 19-10. Color Doppler flow maps of an aortic regurgitant jet obtained from the parasternal short-axis view **(left)** and from an apical outflow view **(right)**. *AOV*, aortic valve; *AO*, aorta; *LA*, left atrium; *LV*, left ventricle.

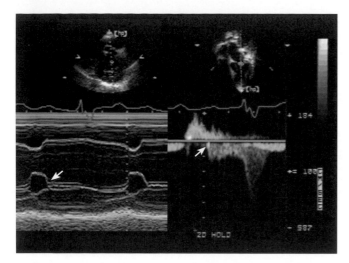

ECHO. 19-11. Left: M-mode trace demonstrating early closure of the mitral valve due to severe aortic regurgitation *(arrow)*. **Right:** Spectral Doppler recording of the mitral valve. Arrow points to the beginning of diastolic mitral regurgitant flow corresponding to the same time point *(arrow)* in the M-mode trace.

gastric views (see Fig. 4-27A,B). In cases where the aortic annulus is hypoplastic, an extended aortic root replacement may need to be performed using cryopreserved allografts (188) (Echo. 19-12). In severe aortic valve regurgitation, the valve may either be replaced with a prosthetic valve or the patient's own pulmonary valve may be used in the aortic position and a homograft would be implanted from the right ventricle to the pulmonary artery (Ross operation) (189). In any of these procedures, the postbypass study should include recording of the velocities across the replaced valve and assessment of any regurgita-

tion particularly if a homograft has been implanted (Echo. 19-13; see color plate 68 following this page).

In subvalve stenosis (membranous or fibromuscular type), the surgical procedure entails resection of the subaortic diaphragm and additional myectomy when there is important septal hypertrophy. In diffuse or tubular stenosis with a small aortic annulus and valve, a ventricular aortoplasty or Konno operation (190) or alternatively an extended aortic root replacement with cryopreserved allograft may be performed. Rarely, a conduit from the left ventricular apex to the descending aorta may be considered (191,192).

Supravalve aortic stenosis of the discrete, localized type is treated surgically with resection of the ring or fibrous diaphragm and enlargement of the site of obstruction with a diamond-shaped pericardial or Dacron patch (193) or with a pantaloon-shaped synthetic patch (130). In diffuse supravalve stenosis, the stenotic area is resected and the aortotomy is closed with a Dacron patch (194). The postbypass study should include measurement of the velocity across the resected site and assessment of any residual regurgitation of the valve.

The late postoperative follow-up in all types of left ventricular outflow tract obstructions must emphasize the fact that these lesions usually recur and that aortic regurgitation is progressive. As such, continued long-term echocardiographic assessments are recommended which would include serial measurements of the gradients and evaluation of the aortic regurgitation by the methods outlined above. In addition, the degree of left ventricular

(text continues)

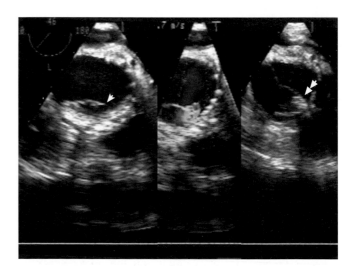

ECHO. 19-13. Transesophageal short-axis views obtained intraoperatively in a patient with a perforated right coronary cusp after an earlier Ross procedure. **Left:** Open aortic valve leaflets with the perforation of the right coronary cusp *(arrow)*. **Middle:** Color Doppler flow map of the regurgitant jet through the perforation. **Right:** Repaired cusp immediately post-bypass *(double arrows)*.

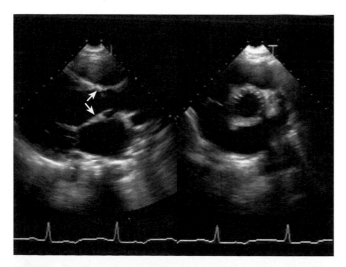

ECHO. 19-12. Parasternal long- **(left)** and short-axis **(right)** views in a patient after extended aortic root replacement. The arrows point to the suture line on the long-axis view. The sutures are easily seen on the short axis, below the aortic valve.

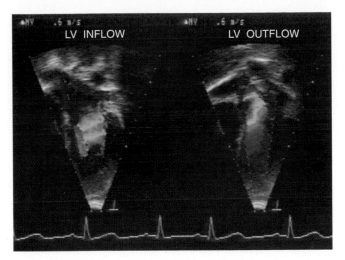

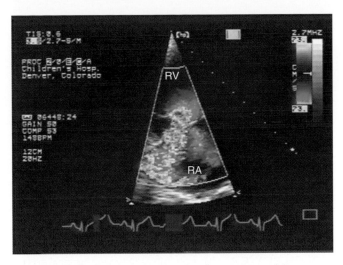

COLOR PLATE 1. Color Doppler aliasing can be seen in normal physiologic flow situations as shown here in the color Doppler flow images of the left ventricular inflow **(left)** and the left ventricular outflow **(right)**. The maximum pulse repetition frequency (PRF), which can be utilized in most color flow imaging systems is relatively low, which leads to such aliasing. *LV,* left ventricle.

COLOR PLATE 3. Color Doppler flow image of flow convergence region with isovelocity surfaces visualized as aliasing hemicircular concentric rings shown here on the right ventricular side of the tricuspid valve. *RV,* right ventricle; *RA,* right atrium.

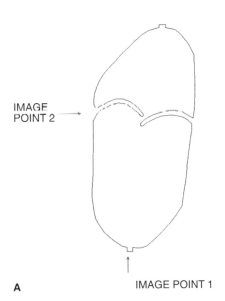

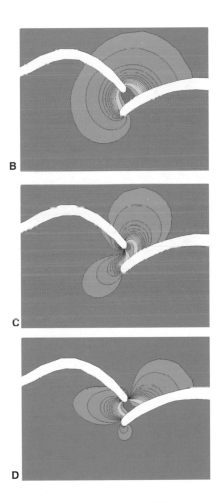

COLOR PLATE 2. Numerical simulation of regurgitant flow through a prolapsed mitral valve demonstrating the angle dependence of Doppler color imaging. "Echo" Doppler color images were simulated from two transducer sites in the numerical model **(A).** True isovelocity contours are shown **(B),** along with "echo" Doppler isovelocity contours imaging from point 1 **(C)** and point 2 **(D).** Note how the image changes depending on where the "transducer" is placed.

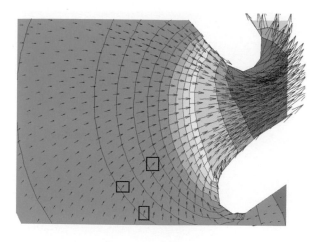

COLOR PLATE 4. Example of velocity vectors and an isovelocity surface in the flow convergence region of a finitely sized orifice. Note the velocity vectors *(boxes)* are not normal to the isovelocity surface. Only the component of the velocity vector normal to the isovelocity surface should be used in the control volume calculation of flow rate.

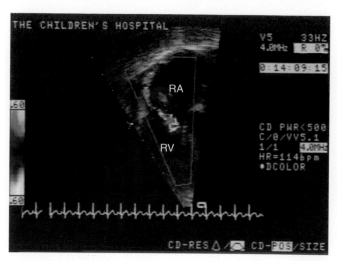

COLOR PLATE 5. Example of a jet spreading out over a wall. Two-dimensional color Doppler flow images of such a jet may not show full extent of regurgitant flow area. *RA,* right atrium; *RV,* right ventricle.

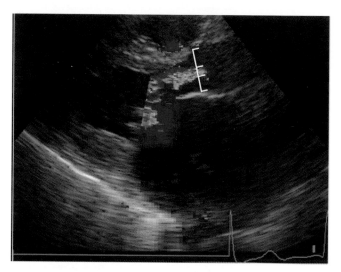

COLOR PLATE 6. Example of proximal flow jet width measurement *(inner bars)* taken from the color Doppler velocity parasternal long-axis image of aortic regurgitation.

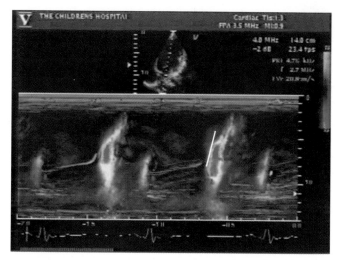

COLOR PLATE 7. Color Doppler M-mode tracings of mitral valve inflow demonstrating how propagation velocity is measured. A line is drawn from the leading edge of the early diastolic inflow wave on the color Doppler M-mode signal, and the slope of this line represents the propagation velocity (a measure of diastolic function). A diminished propagation slope occurs with worsening ventricular diastolic function.

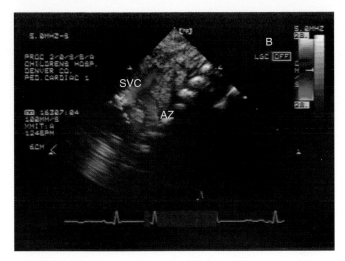

COLOR PLATE 8. Drainage of the azygous vein into the posterior aspect of the right-sided superior vena cava. Color Doppler flow image. *SVC*, superior vena cava; *AZ*, azygous vein.

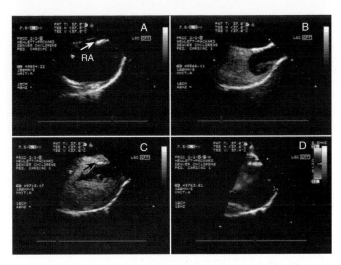

COLOR PLATE 9. Transesophageal longitudinal view of the atria, emphasizing the atrial septum and right superior vena cava. **A:** Anatomic view. The *arrow* points to the flap of the foramen ovale. **B:** Peripheral venous contrast injection performed with the patient on room air. The right atrium is filled completely. Note the negative contrast of the superior vena caval inflow. No right-to-left shunting is seen. **C:** Peripheral venous contrast injection with the patient breathing 17% oxygen. The right atrium fills and there is right-to-left interatrial shunting. **D:** Color Doppler flow mapping of the right-to-left shunt. *RA*, right atrium.

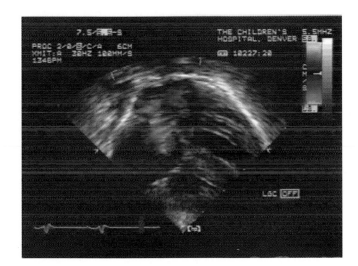

COLOR PLATE 10. Color Doppler flow image from a subcostal long-axis view illustrating left-to-right shunting across an ostium secundum atrial septal defect.

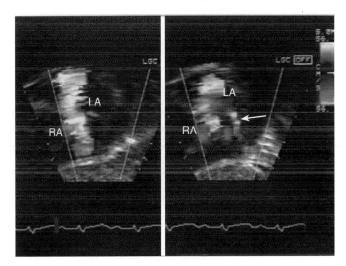

COLOR PLATE 11. Color Doppler flow images of a fenestrated atrial septum with left-to-right shunting through several defects. The *arrow* points to one of the smaller defects. *RA*, right atrium; *LA*, left atrium.

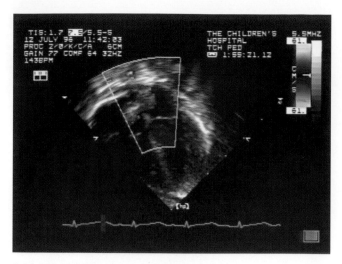

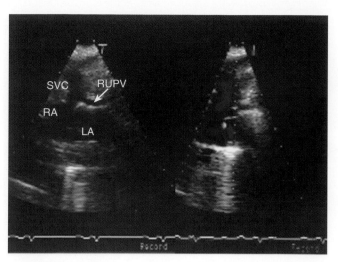

COLOR PLATE 12. Apical four-chamber view demonstrating left-to-right shunting through an ostium secundum atrial septal defect. Note that the defect is far from the insertion of the tricuspid and mitral valves.

COLOR PLATE 13. Suprasternal view tilted toward the superior vena cava demonstrating anomalous drainage of the right upper pulmonary vein at the junction of the right superior vena cava and right atrium. The color Doppler image also shows the superior vena caval inflow (*blue*) and the left-to-right atrial shunt (*red*). *SVC*, superior vena cava; *RA*, right atrium; *LA*, left atrium; *RUPV*, right upper pulmonary vein.

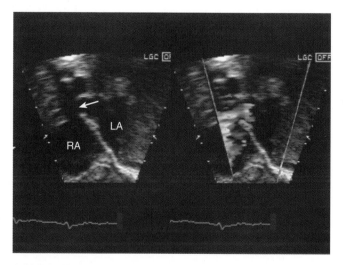

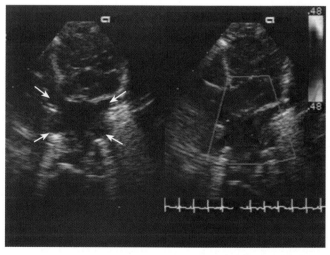

COLOR PLATE 14. Anatomic and color flow image from the subcostal sagittal projection of the atrial septum demonstrating left-to-right shunting across a sinus venosus defect of the superior vena caval type (*arrow*). *RA*, right atrium; *LA*, left atrium.

COLOR PLATE 15. Suprasternal short-axis view of the four pulmonary veins connecting to the left atrium (*arrows*).

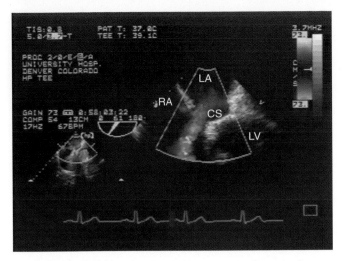

COLOR PLATE 16. Transesophageal color Doppler image of the left-to-right flow across an atrial septal defect of the coronary sinus type. The endoscope must be retroflexed to image this portion of the atrial septum clearly. *LA*, left atrium; *RA*, right atrium; *CS*, coronary sinus; *LV*, left ventricle.

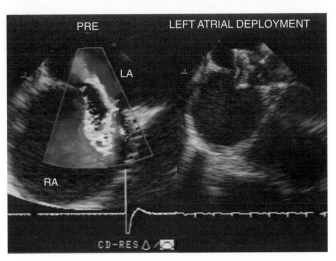

COLOR PLATE 17. Left: Transesophageal view of the left-to-right shunt across an atrial septal defect immediately before deployment of a closure device under echocardiographic guidance. **Right:** View of the closure device as it is deployed through the left atrium. *RA*, right atrium; *LA*, left atrium.

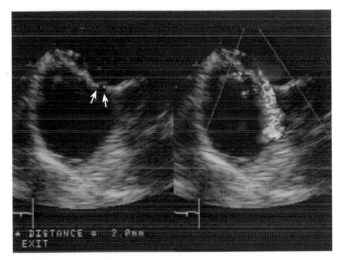

COLOR PLATE 18. Transesophageal view of a tiny residual left-to-right shunt at the bottom edge of the closure device. *Arrows* point to the edges of the residual defect, which measured 2 mm.

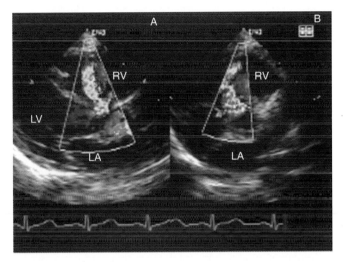

COLOR PLATE 19. Echocardiograms demonstrating shunting through a perimembranous ventricular septal defect. **A:** Parasternal long-axis view with the transducer tilted toward the right ventricular inflow. **B:** Parasternal short-axis view. *RV*, right ventricle; *LV*, left ventricle; *LA*, left atrium.

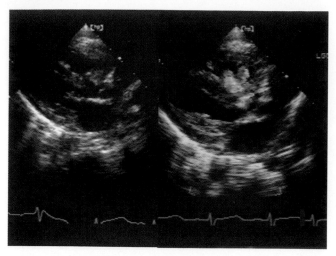

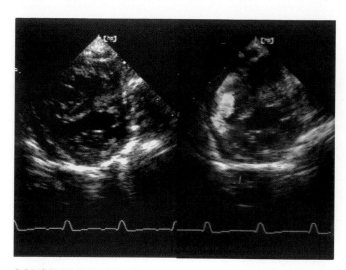

COLOR PLATE 20. Parasternal long-axis view demonstrating a perimembranous defect with extension toward the trabecular septum.

COLOR PLATE 21. Short-axis view of the ventricles demonstrating the presence of a large ventricular septal defect in the muscular inlet septum. *RV,* right ventricle; *LV,* left ventricle.

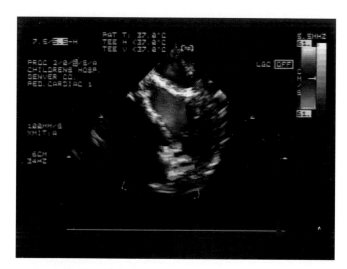

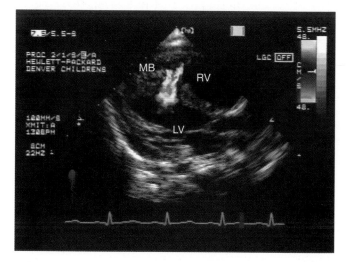

COLOR PLATE 22. Color Doppler flow map obtained from a transesophageal horizontal view demonstrating left-to-right shunting across multiple small ventricular septal defects of the apical portion of the trabecular septum.

COLOR PLATE 23. Parasternal long-axis view demonstrating the left-to-right shunt across a defect of the muscular trabecular ventricular septum adjacent to the moderator band. *RV,* right ventricle; *LV,* left ventricle; *MB,* moderator band.

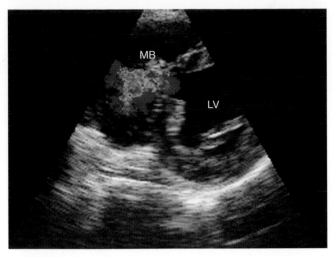

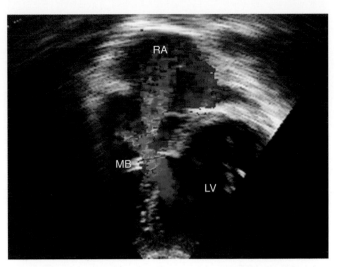

COLOR PLATE 24. Parasternal short-axis view of the ventricles demonstrating left-to-right shunting across a defect of the muscular trabecular septum, adjacent to the moderator band. *LV,* left ventricle; *MB,* moderator band.

COLOR PLATE 25. Apical four-chamber view modified to emphasize the shunt across a defect of the trabecular muscular ventricular septum, adjacent to the moderator band. *RA,* right atrium; *MB,* moderator band; *LV,* left ventricle.

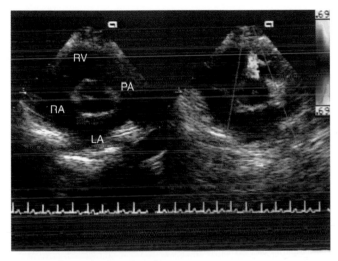

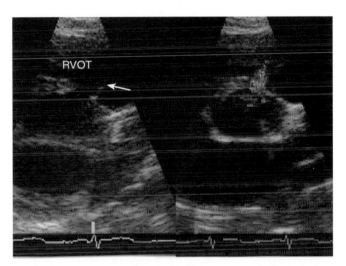

COLOR PLATE 26. Parasternal short-axis view illustrating the presence of a defect of the outlet ventricular septum. There is muscular tissue separating the defect from both the tricuspid and pulmonic valves. *RV,* right ventricle; *RA,* right atrium; *LA,* left atrium; *PA,* pulmonary artery.

COLOR PLATE 27. Parasternal long- and short-axis views tilted toward the right ventricular outflow showing a subarterial ventricular septal defect of moderate size immediately below the pulmonic valve, with absence of the infundibular septum. The *arrow* points to the pulmonic valve leaflets. *RVOT,* right ventricular outflow tract.

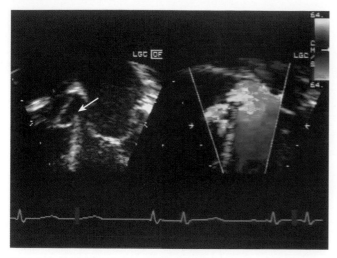

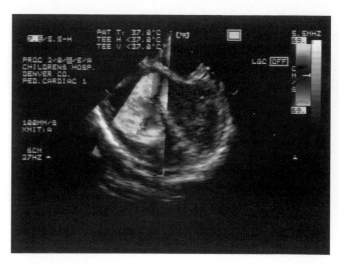

COLOR PLATE 28. Magnified view of a perimembranous ventricular septal defect undergoing spontaneous closure. The *arrow* points to the defect partially covered by tricuspid valve tissue.

COLOR PLATE 29. Transesophageal view of the ventricular septum from the horizontal plane. The endoscope is withdrawn slightly toward the left ventricular outflow, revealing the presence of a perimembranous defect immediately below the aortic valve.

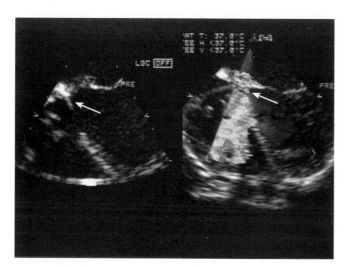

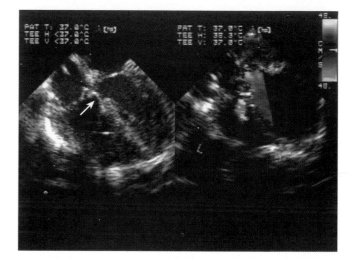

COLOR PLATE 30. Transesophageal view of the ventricular septum from the horizontal plane demonstrating a ventricular septal defect of the inlet muscular septum. The *arrows* point to muscular tissue on the superior edge of the defect.

COLOR PLATE 31. Transesophageal view of the ventricular septum from the horizontal plane demonstrating the surgical patch used to close a perimembranous ventricular septal defect (*arrow*). The color Doppler flow image reveals a tiny residual shunt detected immediately postoperatively, most likely through the patch itself.

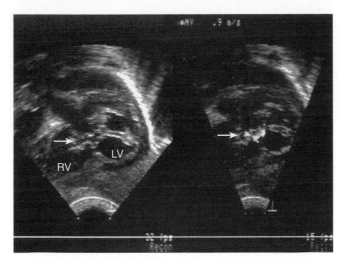

COLOR PLATE 32. Left: Subcostal view illustrating the commissure between the bridging leaflets (*arrow*). **Right:** The color Doppler flow map of the regurgitation through the commissural space is shown (*arrow*). *RV*, right ventricle; *LV*, left ventricle.

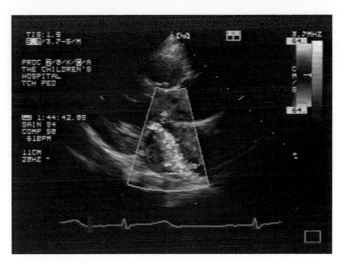

COLOR PLATE 33. Color Doppler flow map from a parasternal long-axis view demonstrating a central regurgitant jet most likely originating around the inferior bridging and left mural leaflets.

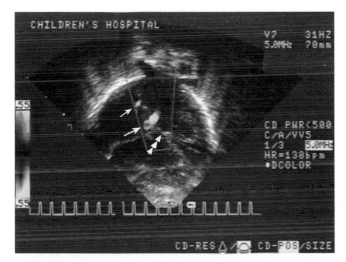

COLOR PLATE 34. Color Doppler flow map of the left-to-right shunt across an ostium primum atrial septal defect (*large arrow*). Note the presence of a smaller shunt across a patent foramen ovale (*small arrow*). The ventricular septum, through which there is no shunt, is shown (*triple arrows*).

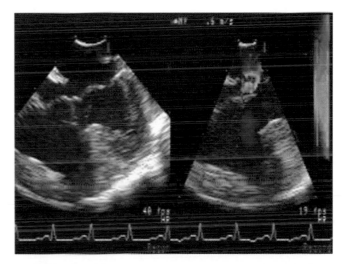

COLOR PLATE 35. Transesophageal horizontal four-chamber view of a complete atrioventricular septal defect with atrial and ventricular defects. There is mild bridging of the superior leaflet and left-to-right shunting across both defects.

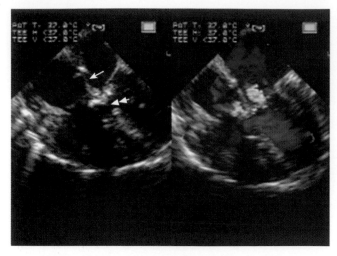

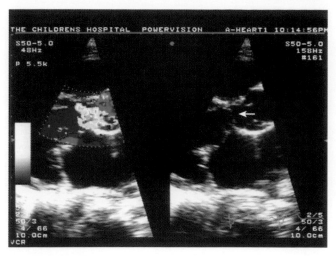

COLOR PLATE 36. Transesophageal four-chamber views obtained immediately post repair of complete atrioventricular septal defect. **Left:** The atrial patch (*single arrow*) and the presence of a small residual ventricular septal defect (*double arrow*). **Right:** The color Doppler flow map of mild atrioventricular valve regurgitation.

COLOR PLATE 37. Parasternal long-axis view of residual left ventricular outflow tract obstruction following repair of a complete atrioventricular septal defect. **Right:** The site of encroachment of the left-sided valve into the outflow tract is shown (*arrow*). **Left:** Color aliasing due to flow velocity acceleration at that same site is shown.

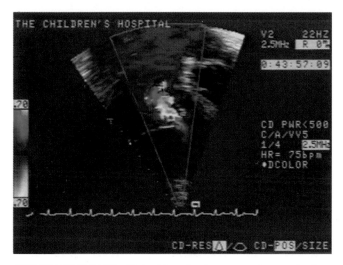

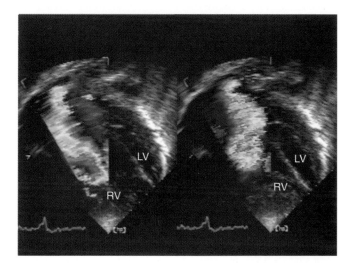

COLOR PLATE 38. Color Doppler flow map demonstrating the jet of tricuspid valve regurgitation in Ebstein's anomaly. Note the point of origin of the regurgitant jet.

COLOR PLATE 39. Color Doppler flow map of the free flow between the right atrium and right ventricle in diastole **(left)** and systole **(right)** in the presence of an unguarded tricuspid orifice. *RV,* right ventricle; *LV,* left ventricle.

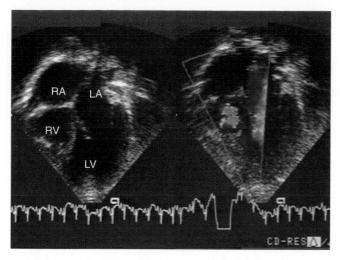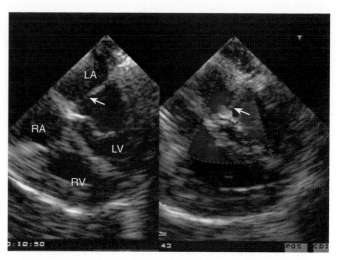

COLOR PLATE 40. Left: Apical four-chamber view demonstrating the presence of tricuspid atresia due to an imperforate valve; the right ventricle is hypoplastic. **Right:** Normal inflow through the mitral valve; the blue color Doppler signal in the right ventricle represents low velocity swirling flow within the right ventricle from a small ventricular septal defect. *RA,* right atrium; *RV,* right ventricle; *LA,* left atrium; *LV,* left ventricle.

COLOR PLATE 41. Left: Transesophageal four-chamber view of cor triatriatum sinister. The membrane is perpendicular to the atrial septum and more or less parallel to the plane of the mitral valve, dividing the left atrium into a proximal or accessory chamber, which receives the pulmonary veins, and a distal or true chamber. **Right:** The color Doppler map of the flow between the two chambers through an orifice in the membrane (*arrow*). *RA,* right atrium; *RV,* right ventricle; *LA,* left atrium; *LV,* left ventricle.

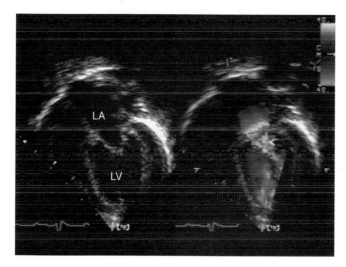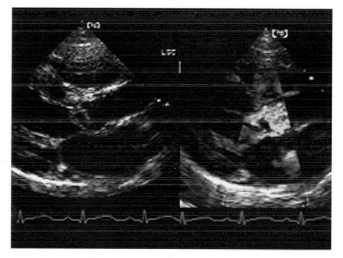

COLOR PLATE 42. Apical views showing a dysplastic, stenotic mitral valve that is domed in the open position **(left)** and showing flow acceleration through it in diastole **(right).** *LA,* left atrium; *LV,* left ventricle.

COLOR PLATE 43. Parasternal long-axis view of accessory mitral valve tissue, causing left ventricular outflow tract obstruction.

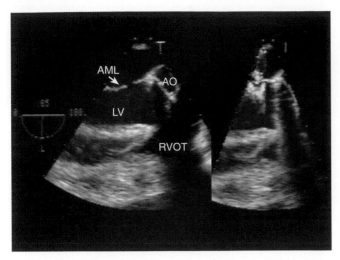

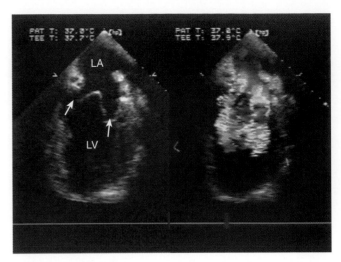

COLOR PLATE 44. Transesophageal longitudinal view of the left ventricle demonstrating the presence of a perforation of the anterior mitral leaflet (**left,** *arrow*) and regurgitation through the defect in the leaflet tissue (**right**). *AML,* anterior mitral leaflet; *LV,* left ventricle; *AO,* aorta; *RVOT,* right ventricular outflow tract.

COLOR PLATE 45. Transesophageal longitudinal view of a double orifice mitral valve. **Left:** Anatomic image of the two orifices. The major and minor orifices are indicated (*arrows*). **Right:** Color Doppler flow map demonstrating the flow through the two orifices. *LA,* left atrium; *LV,* left ventricle.

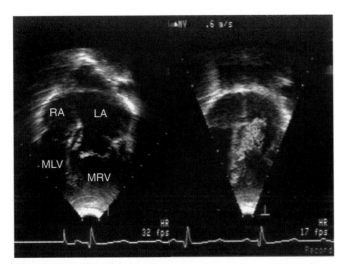

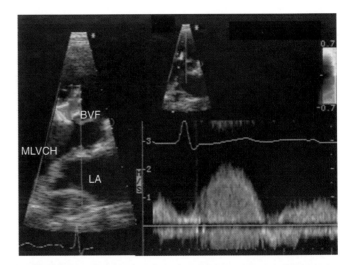

COLOR PLATE 46. Apical four-chamber view of Ebstein's malformation of the left-sided tricuspid valve. The **right** panel shows tricuspid regurgitation originating from the inferiorly displaced septal and posterior leaflets. *RA,* right atrium; *MLV,* morphologic left ventricle; *LA,* left atrium; *MRV,* morphologic right ventricle.

COLOR PLATE 47. Color Doppler flow map and spectral recording of velocities across a restrictive bulboventricular foramen connecting a main left ventricular chamber to an anterior rudimentary right ventricular chamber. *BVF,* bulboventricular foramen; *MLVCH,* main left ventricular chamber; *LA,* left atrium.

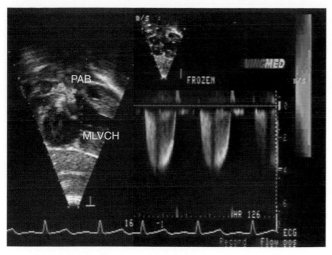

COLOR PLATE 48. Subcostal view tilted superiorly to image the banded pulmonary artery emerging from a main left ventricular chamber. Note the aliasing of the color Doppler flow and the high velocity spectral signal across the band. *PAB*, pulmonary artery band; *MLVCH*, main left ventricular chamber.

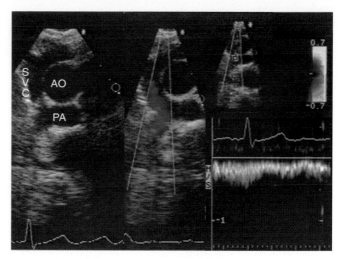

COLOR PLATE 49. Right subclavicular view of a bidirectional Glenn connection between the superior vena cava and the right pulmonary artery. **Left:** Anatomic view of the superior vena cava-pulmonary artery connection. **Middle:** Color Doppler map of the unrestricted superior vena cava-to-pulmonary artery flow. **Right:** Spectral Doppler velocity recording of the low-velocity flow with accentuation in inspiration. *SVC*, superior vena cava; *AO*, aorta; *PA*, pulmonary artery.

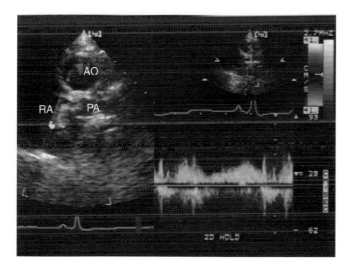

COLOR PLATE 50. Right subclavicular view demonstrating the Fontan connection between the right atrium and pulmonary artery. **Left:** Color Doppler flow map. **Right:** Spectral Doppler recording of velocities through the Fontan connection. Note the biphasic velocity curves with peaks in middle-late systole and diastole. *AO*, aorta; *RA*, right atrium; *PA*, pulmonary artery.

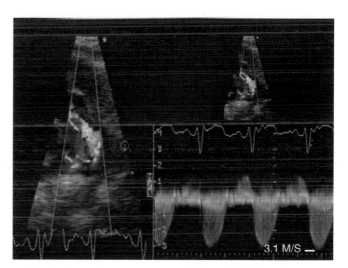

COLOR PLATE 51. Color Doppler flow map and spectral velocity recording across a stenotic pulmonic valve. Note the color aliasing and high velocity as well as the poststenotic dilatation extending to the left pulmonary artery branch.

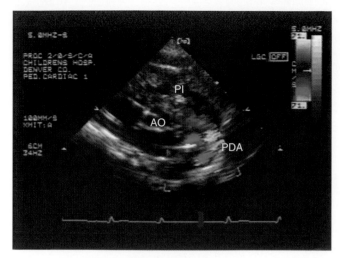

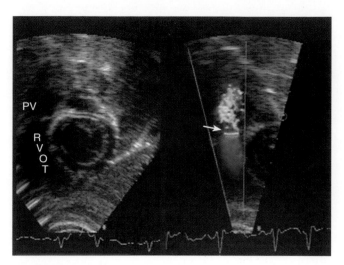

COLOR PLATE 52. Color Doppler flow map of mild pulmonary insufficiency associated with a patent ductus arteriosus in the presence of critical pulmonic valve stenosis. Note the small and hypertrophied right ventricle. The identification of even trace pulmonic insufficiency documents the valve is patent. *PI,* pulmonic insufficiency jet; *PDA,* patent ductus arteriosus; *AO,* aorta.

COLOR PLATE 53. Subcostal short-axis view demonstrating the length of the right ventricular outflow tract and the pulmonic valve in subvalve pulmonic stenosis. Note the sudden aliasing of the color Doppler flow map (*arrow*) indicating the site of stenosis immediately below the valve. *PV,* pulmonic valve; *RVOT,* right ventricular outflow tract.

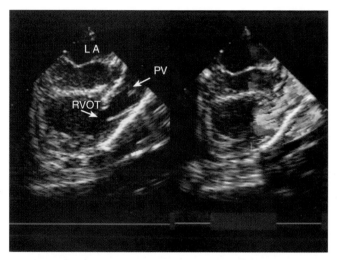

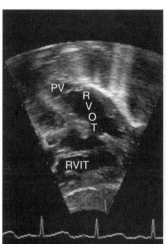
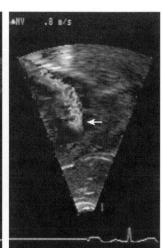
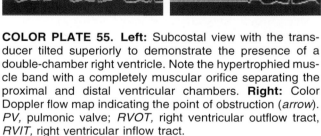

COLOR PLATE 54. Left: Transesophageal longitudinal view of the right ventricular outflow tract showing the presence of a subpulmonic membrane (*arrow*). **Right:** Color Doppler flow map across the outflow tract. Note the acceleration of flow with narrowing of the flow stream at the point of maximal obstruction. *LA,* left atrium; *PV,* pulmonic valve; *RVOT,* right ventricular outflow tract.

COLOR PLATE 55. Left: Subcostal view with the transducer tilted superiorly to demonstrate the presence of a double-chamber right ventricle. Note the hypertrophied muscle band with a completely muscular orifice separating the proximal and distal ventricular chambers. **Right:** Color Doppler flow map indicating the point of obstruction (*arrow*). *PV,* pulmonic valve; *RVOT,* right ventricular outflow tract, *RVIT,* right ventricular inflow tract.

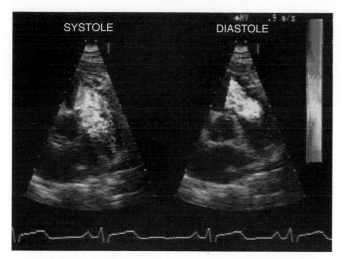

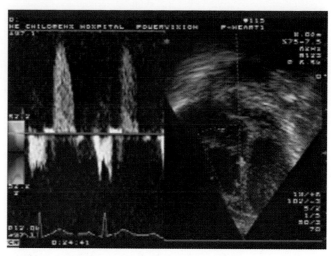

COLOR PLATE 56. Color Doppler maps of the systolic and diastolic flows across the right ventricular outflow tract in the presence of isolated absence of the pulmonic valve. Note the aliasing of velocities, in both directions, at the narrowest point along the outflow tract.

COLOR PLATE 57. Right: Apical view of ventriculo-coronary communications demonstrated on color Doppler flow map. **Left:** Spectral Doppler recording of the systolic velocity obtained at the site of the ventriculocoronary communication.

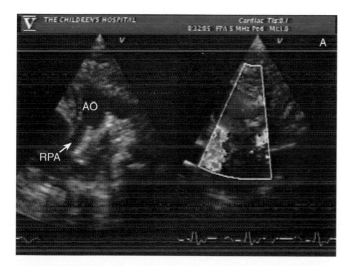

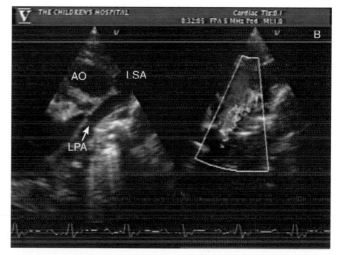

COLOR PLATE 58. Example of separate origins of non-confluent pulmonary arteries from bilateral ducti in pulmonary atresia. (*with color plate 59*). Anatomic image and color Doppler flow map of the right pulmonary artery originating from a right-sided ductus. *AO,* aorta; *RPA,* right pulmonary artery.

COLOR PLATE 59. Example of separate origins of non-confluent pulmonary arteries from bilateral ducti in pulmonary atresia (*with color plate 58*). Anatomic image and color Doppler flow map of the left pulmonary artery originating from a left-sided ductus. *AO,* aorta; *LSA,* left subclavian artery; *LPA,* left pulmonary artery.

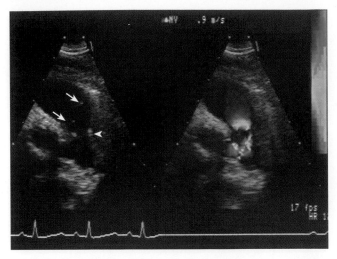

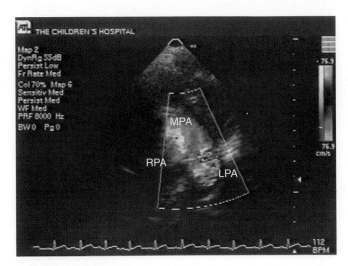

COLOR PLATE 60. Parasternal view tilted towards the right ventricular outflow tract in the presence of supravalve pulmonary stenosis. Note the valve leaflets (*arrows*), the area of narrowing above the valve (*arrowhead*), and the aliasing of velocities at that site on color Doppler flow mapping.

COLOR PLATE 61. Parasternal short-axis view demonstrating stenosis of the left pulmonary arterial branch at its bifurcation. Note the velocity aliasing on the color Doppler map. *MPA*, main pulmonary artery; *RPA*, right pulmonary artery; *LPA*, left pulmonary artery.

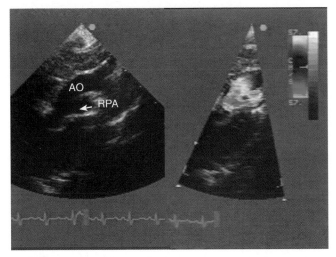

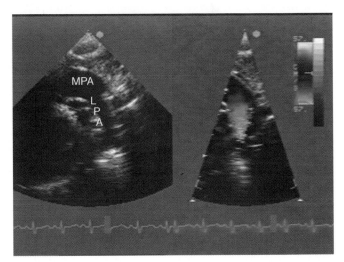

COLOR PLATE 62. Left: Suprasternal long-axis view demonstrating an anomalous origin of the right pulmonary artery from the posterior wall of the ascending aorta. **Right:** Color Doppler color map showing the flow entering the right pulmonary artery from the ascending aorta. *AO*, aorta; *RPA*, right pulmonary artery.

COLOR PLATE 63. Anatomical and color Doppler image of the normal origin of the left pulmonary artery from the main pulmonary artery in the same patient illustrated on color plate 62. *MPA*, main pulmonary artery; *LPA*, left pulmonary artery.

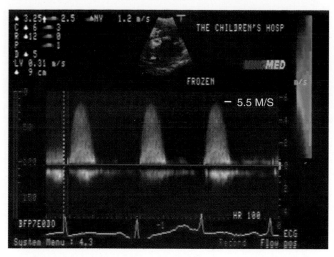

COLOR PLATE 64. Spectral Doppler velocity through a severely stenotic aortic valve derived from a right parasternal color Doppler guided image.

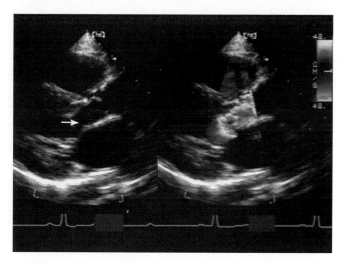

COLOR PLATE 65. Parasternal long-axis views of fibromuscular subaortic tunnel. Note the narrowest point along the subaortic area (*arrow*). The color Doppler flow map **(right)** exhibits flow acceleration towards this point and aliasing of the velocities beyond it.

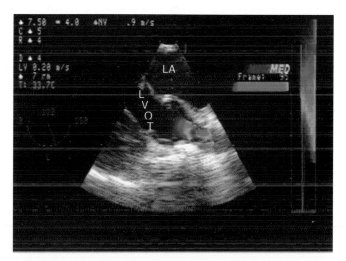

COLOR PLATE 66. Transesophageal longitudinal view of the left ventricular outflow tract and ascending aorta in the presence of diffuse supravalve aortic stenosis. Note the narrowing and aliasing of color velocities above the valve. *LA,* left atrium; *LVOT,* left ventricular outflow tract.

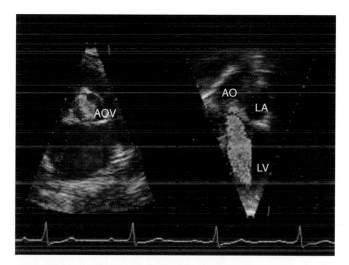

COLOR PLATE 67. Color Doppler flow maps of an aortic regurgitant jet obtained from the parasternal short-axis view **(left)** and from an apical outflow view **(right).** *AOV,* aortic valve; *AO,* aorta; *LA,* left atrium; *LV,* left ventricle.

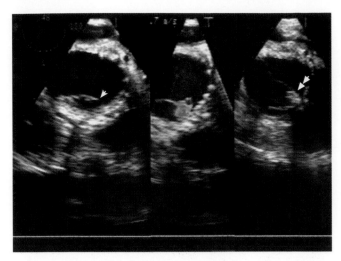 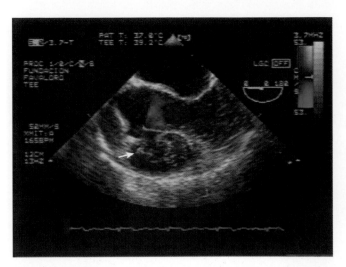

COLOR PLATE 68. Transesophageal short-axis views obtained intraoperatively in a patient with a perforated right coronary cusp after an earlier Ross procedure. **Left:** Open aortic valve leaflets with the perforation of the right coronary cusp (*arrow*). **Middle:** Color Doppler flow map of the regurgitant jet through the perforation. **Right:** Repaired cusp immediately post-bypass (*double arrows*).

COLOR PLATE 69. Color Doppler flow map from the same patient as in Echo. 20-1. The *arrow* indicates the point of rupture of the aneurysm into the right ventricle. Note the jet of flow entering the right ventricle. (*Echocardiogram courtesy of Drs. Ana Maria de Dios and Pedro Weisberg, Fundacion Favaloro, Buenos Aires, Argentina*)

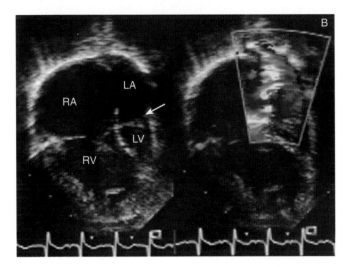 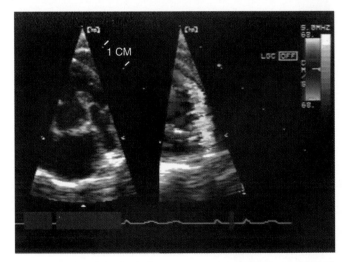

COLOR PLATE 70. Apical four-chamber view of the hypoplastic left ventricle, dilated right ventricle, and large atrial communication with left-to-right shunting. Note the lack of flow across the atretic mitral valve (*arrow*). *RV*, right ventricle; *LV*, left ventricle; *ASC AO*, ascending aorta; *LA*, left atrium; *RA*, right atrium.

COLOR PLATE 71. Left: Parasternal short-axis view of the right ventricular infundibulum in tetralogy of Fallot. Note the hypertrophied and anteriorly displaced infundibular septum, and the small pulmonary annulus and main pulmonary artery. The *1-cm marks* are highlighted at the right side of the image. **Right:** Color Doppler flow map across the right ventricular outflow tract and main pulmonary artery. Note the aliasing of velocities at the site corresponding to the infundibular septum.

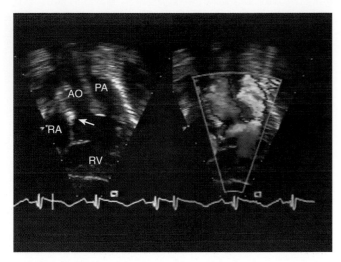

COLOR PLATE 72. Apical view with the transducer tilted anteriorly toward the outflow tracts. The *arrow* points to the muscular ventriculoinfundibular fold separating the tricuspid and aortic valves. The color Doppler flow map illustrates the aliasing of the color velocities at the point of maximum obstruction resulting from hypertrophy and anterior displacement of the infundibular septum. *RA*, right atrium; *RV*, right ventricle; *AO*, aorta; *PA*, pulmonary artery.

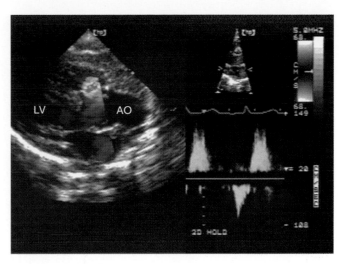

COLOR PLATE 73. **Left:** Parasternal long-axis view of the malalignment ventricular septal defect, with this frame demonstrating the color Doppler flow map of the left-to-right shunting. **Right:** The spectral velocity recording shows the bidirectional shunting across the defect. *LV*, left ventricle; *AO*, aorta.

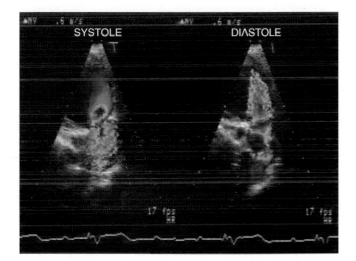

COLOR PLATE 74. Color Doppler flow maps of the systolic and diastolic flows across the pulmonary outflow in tetralogy of Fallot with absent pulmonary valve. The restriction occurs at the annulus itself. Note the acceleration of the forward flow toward the annulus in systole and of the regurgitant flow in diastole.

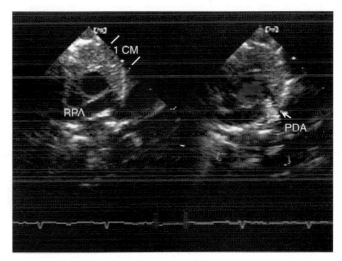

COLOR PLATE 75. **Left:** Suprasternal view of the confluence and branch pulmonary arteries, which are supplied only by a patent ductus arteriosus. Note the *1-cm marks* at the right of the image. **Right:** Shunt from the ductus into the left pulmonary artery (*arrow*). *RPA*, right pulmonary artery; *PDA*, patent ductus arteriosus.

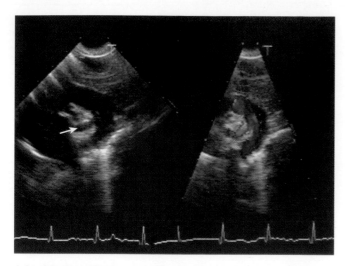

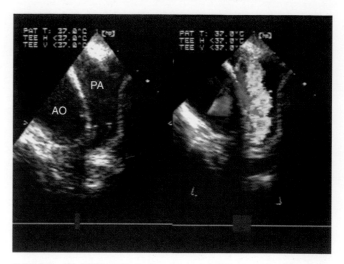

COLOR PLATE 76. Suprasternal notch view of a large collateral supplying the pulmonary arteries. **Left:** Anatomic view of the collateral (*arrow*). **Right:** Color Doppler image of the flow from the aorta through the collateral vessel.

COLOR PLATE 77. Left: Transesophageal transverse short-axis view of the pulmonary annulus, main pulmonary artery, and branches. **Right:** Color Doppler flow map of the forward flow into the pulmonary arteries. Note the color aliasing, implying high velocities. *AO*, aorta; *PA*, pulmonary artery.

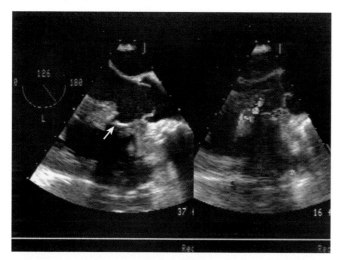

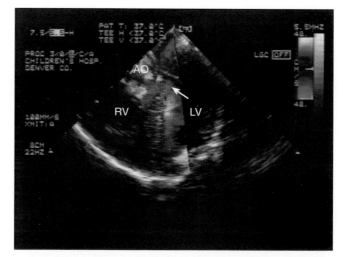

COLOR PLATE 78. Left: Transesophageal longitudinal view of the left ventricular outflow tract immediately after bypass. The patch closing the ventricular septal defect is seen committing the aorta to the left ventricle. *Arrow* points to the site of a small residual ventricular septal defect. **Right:** Color Doppler flow map of the left-to-right shunting across the small residual ventricular septal defect.

COLOR PLATE 79. Transesophageal transverse view with the endoscope slightly withdrawn to demonstrate the ventricular septal defect and aorta. The *arrow* points to the large ventricular septal defect. *RV*, right ventricle; *LV*, left ventricle; *AO*, aorta.

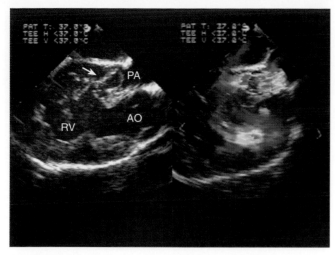

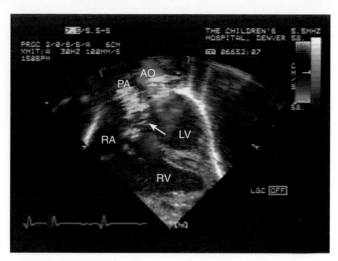

COLOR PLATE 80. Transesophageal longitudinal view of the outflow tracts. **Left:** The anatomic view reveals an anteroposterior infundibular relationship, with the aorta anterior to the pulmonary artery. Posterior displacement of the infundibular septum and accessory tricuspid valve tissue (*arrow*) is causing subpulmonary obstruction. **Right:** Color Doppler flow map demonstrates the flow from the right ventricle to both great arteries and the aliasing of the color flow across the pulmonary infundibulum resulting from obstruction. *PA,* pulmonary artery; *AO,* aorta; *RV,* right ventricle.

COLOR PLATE 81. Color Doppler flow map of the patient in Echo. 23-12. The *arrow* points to the area of subpulmonic obstruction. Note the color aliasing beyond the obstruction. There is streaming of right ventricular blood into the pulmonary artery and of left ventricular blood into the left ventricle. *RA,* right atrium; *RV,* right ventricle; *LV,* left ventricle; *AO,* aorta; *PA,* pulmonary artery.

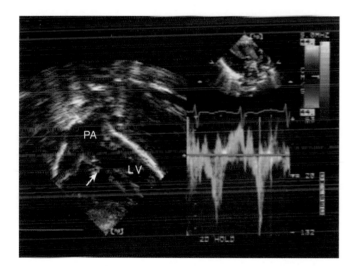

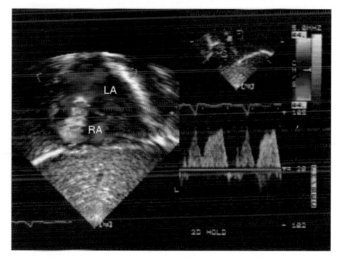

COLOR PLATE 82. Left: Subcostal view aimed towards the outflow tracts demonstrating a subpulmonary ventricular septal defect (*arrow*). **Right:** Spectral Doppler recording of the low velocity bidirectional shunt across the ventricular septal defect. *PA,* pulmonary artery; *LV,* left ventricle.

COLOR PLATE 83. Subcostal view of the atrial septum demonstrating color and spectral Doppler velocity recordings of the left to right flow across an atrial defect. *LA,* left atrium; *RA,* right atrium.

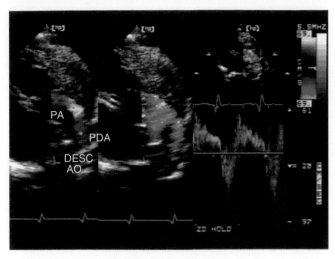

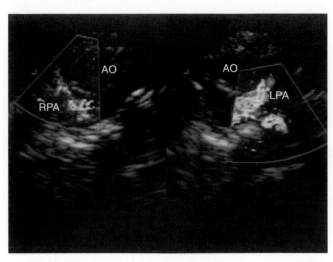

COLOR PLATE 84. Parasternal short-axis views of the color and spectral Doppler recordings of flow across a bidirectional patent ductus arteriosus. **Left:** Left-to-right shunting from descending aorta to pulmonary artery. **Middle:** Right-to-left shunting from the pulmonary artery to the aorta. **Right:** Spectral Doppler recording of the low velocity bidirectional shunt. *PA,* pulmonary artery; *DESC AO,* descending aorta; *PDA,* patent ductus arteriosus.

COLOR PLATE 85. Transesophageal horizontal view of the color Doppler map of the flow into the branch pulmonary arteries obtained from the same patient as in Echo 24-13. *AO,* neoaorta; *RPA,* right pulmonary artery; *LPA,* left pulmonary artery.

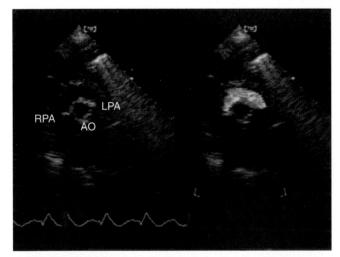

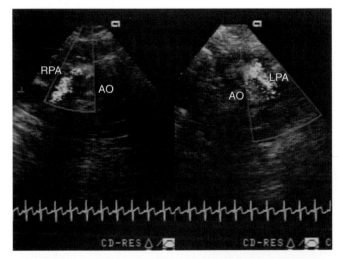

COLOR PLATE 86. Transthoracic high parasternal view imaging the relationship between the pulmonary arteries and the neoaorta after arterial switch operation for transposition of the great arteries. Note the laminar flow into both pulmonary arteries without evidence of obstruction. *AO,* neoaorta; *RPA,* right pulmonary artery; *LPA,* left pulmonary artery.

COLOR PLATE 87. Transthoracic high parasternal view of the pulmonary arteries after arterial switch operation. Note the narrow jets and color aliasing of the flow into both branches of the pulmonary arteries, implying stenosis at these sites. *AO,* neoaorta; *RPA,* right pulmonary artery; *LPA,* left pulmonary artery.

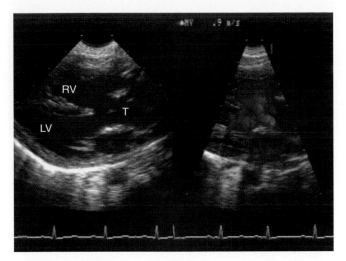

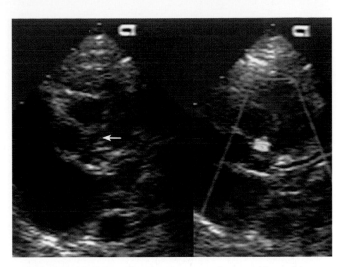

COLOR PLATE 88. Parasternal long-axis views of truncus arteriosus demonstrating the large-outlet ventricular septal defect and overriding of the truncus over the interventricular septum. Note that the truncal valve forms the roof of the ventricular defect. The **right** panel is the color Doppler flow map of the shunt across the ventricular defect. There is direct flow from the right ventricle to the truncus (*blue*) as well as flow from the left ventricle to the truncus (*red*). *RV,* right ventricle; *LV,* left ventricle; *T,* truncus.

COLOR PLATE 89. Short-axis view of a quadricuspid truncal valve. The *arrow* points to the regurgitant orifice in the middle of the valve. **Right:** Cross-section of the regurgitant jet occupying the orifice.

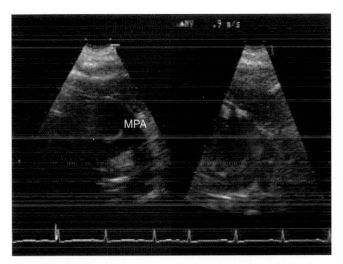

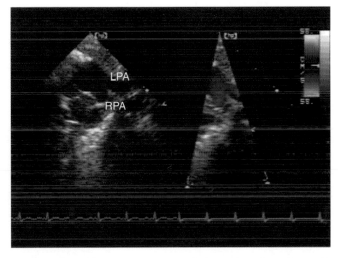

COLOR PLATE 90. Left: Parasternal short-axis view of type I truncus showing the origin of the main pulmonary trunk and branches. **Right:** Color Doppler flow map demonstrating the flow from the truncus to the pulmonary arteries. A coronary artery is seen emerging from the truncus anteriorly. *MPA,* main pumonary artery.

COLOR PLATE 91. Left: Left subclavicular view of type II truncus with the origin of the right and left pulmonary arteries directly from the truncus without a common pulmonary trunk. **Right:** Color Doppler map of the flow from the truncus into the branch pulmonary arteries. *LPA,* left pulmonary artery; *RPA,* right pulmonary artery.

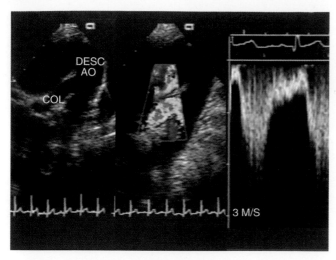

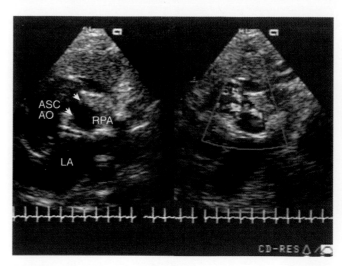

COLOR PLATE 92. Left: Suprasternal long-axis view demonstrating the truncus and descending aorta. A large systemic-to-pulmonary collateral vessel is seen emerging from the underside of the transverse arch supplying the pulmonary circulation. This is an example of type IV truncus, which should instead be considered a form of pulmonary atresia with ventricular communication. **Middle:** The color Doppler flow map demonstrates the flow into the collateral vessel. **Right:** Spectral Doppler recording of the flow into the collateral vessel. It is exclusively left to right. *DESC AO,* descending aorta; *COL,* collateral vessel.

COLOR PLATE 93. Left: Suprasternal long-axis view demonstrating the aortopulmonary window (*arrows*). **Right:** Color Doppler flow map of the shunting across the communication. *ASC AO,* ascending aorta; *RPA,* right pulmonary artery; *LA,* left atrium.

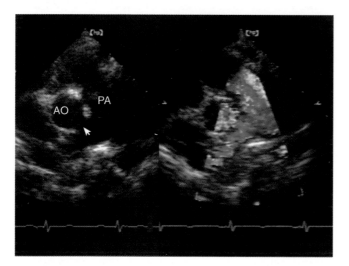

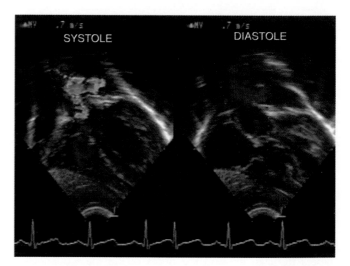

COLOR PLATE 94. Parasternal short-axis view in a normal heart demonstrating a false echo dropout (*arrow*), which should not be confused with a true aortopulmonary window. *AO,* aorta; *PA,* pulmonary artery.

COLOR PLATE 95. Subcostal view aimed superiorly towards the outflow tracts in the presence of an aortopulmonary window. The systolic frame demonstrates high-velocity aortic outflow and aliased shunting into the pulmonary artery through the window. The diastolic frame shows the lower velocity retrograde flow into the pulmonary artery.

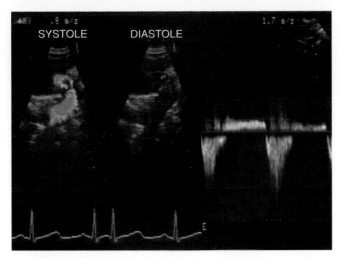

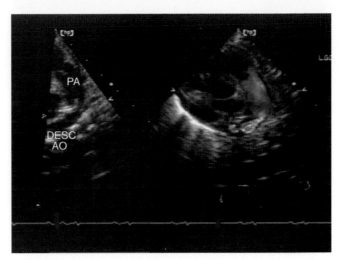

COLOR PLATE 96. Color Doppler map of the flow in the descending aorta in the presence of an aortopulmonary window. Note the reversal of flow in the descending aorta during diastole due to the run-off into the pulmonary circulation. The spectral Doppler velocity recording demonstrates the slightly disturbed forward systolic flow and the reversed diastolic flow.

COLOR PLATE 97. High parasternal short-axis view demonstrating the pulmonary artery, patent ductus arteriosus, and adjacent coarctation of the aorta. Note the normal forward flow in the main pulmonary artery. The pulmonary flow aliases at the site of the coarctation and supplies the descending aorta. *PA*, pulmonary artery; *DESC AO*, descending aorta.

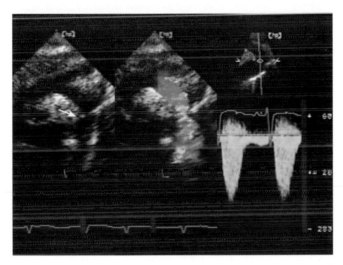

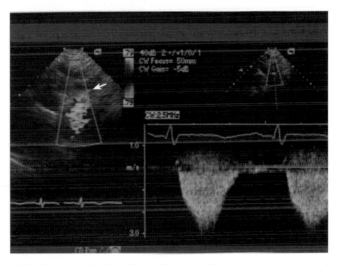

COLOR PLATE 98. Left: Suprasternal long-axis view of the aorta in a neonate. There is a shelf at the site of the ductal junction (*arrow*) with slight narrowing at that site. **Middle:** Color Doppler flow map through the descending aorta. There is slight narrowing of the color flow and aliasing at the site of the shelf. **Right:** Spectral Doppler velocity recording through the descending aorta demonstrating low velocity, without the typical diastolic high-velocity flow.

COLOR PLATE 99. Color Doppler flow map and spectral velocity recording across a mild coarctation of the aorta. The *arrow* indicates the point of velocity aliasing. Note the high velocity is recorded only in systole, without high-velocity diastolic flows.

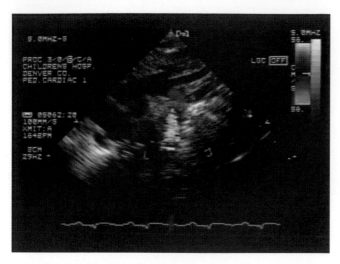

COLOR PLATE 100. Suprasternal long-axis view of type A interruption of the aortic arch (between the left subclavian artery and the ductus arteriosus). The aliased flow seen in the descending aorta originates from the pulmonary artery through a patent ductus arteriosus.

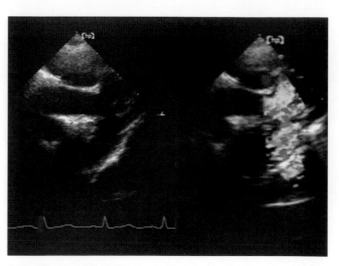

COLOR PLATE 101. Suprasternal long-axis view of repaired interruption of the aortic arch. **Left:** Anatomic view demonstrating an apparently unobstructed arch. **Right:** Color Doppler flow map of the area of repair with aliasing of velocities indicating mild flow disturbance. This is usually of no clinical significance.

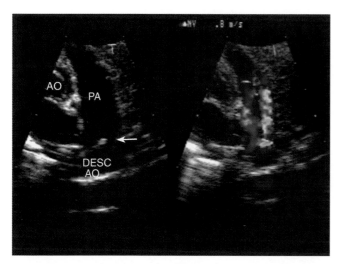

COLOR PLATE 102. Parasternal short-axis view in the presence of a patent ductus arteriosus. **Left:** Anatomic image of the ductus (*arrow*) connecting the pulmonary artery and descending aorta. **Right:** Color Doppler flow map of a left-to-right shunt across a patent ductus arteriosus. Note the trace pulmonary insufficiency caused by the ductal jet striking the pulmonic valve. *AO*, aorta; *PA*, pulmonary artery; *DESC AO*, descending aorta.

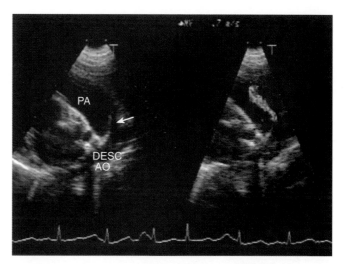

COLOR PLATE 103. Left: High left sagittal view of the pulmonary artery and ductus arteriosus (*arrow*). **Right:** Color Doppler flow map of the left-to-right shunt across the patent ductus arteriosus. *PA*, pulmonary artery; *DESC AO*, descending aorta.

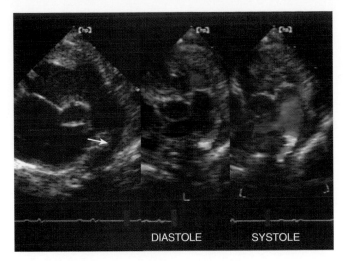

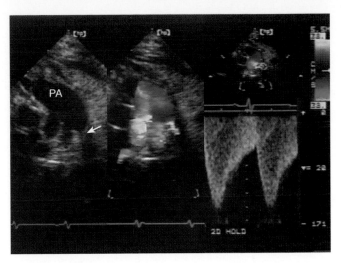

COLOR PLATE 104. Parasternal short-axis view of a ductus arteriosus in the presence of pulmonary hypertension. **Left:** Anatomic view of the large ductus (*arrow*). Note the dilated pulmonary artery. **Middle:** Color Doppler flow map of the left-to-right shunt across the ductus during diastole. **Right:** Color Doppler flow map of the right-to-left shunt across the ductus in systole.

COLOR PLATE 105. Patent ductus arteriosus in severe pulmonary hypertension. **Left:** *Arrow* points to the ductus. Note the very dilated main pulmonary artery. **Middle:** Color Doppler map of the flow in the main and proximal pulmonary arterial branches and in the ductus arteriosus. The ductal shunt is from right to left. **Right:** Spectral Doppler recording of the flow across the ductus. Note the continuous right-to-left flow persisting throughout the cardiac cycle. *PA,* pulmonary artery.

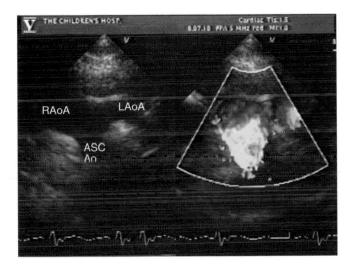

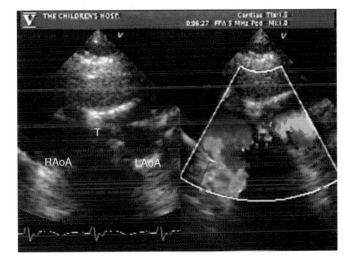

COLOR PLATE 106. Short-axis suprasternal view aimed anteriorly demonstrating a double aortic arch. A segment of the ascending aorta is seen with the two arches emerging from it. The right arch is larger than the left. *ASC AO,* ascending aorta; *RAOA,* right aortic arch; *LAOA,* left aortic arch.

COLOR PLATE 107. Suprasternal short-axis view demonstrating the two arches bifurcating from the aorta. *RAoA,* right aortic arch; *LAoA,* left aortic arch; *T,* trachea.

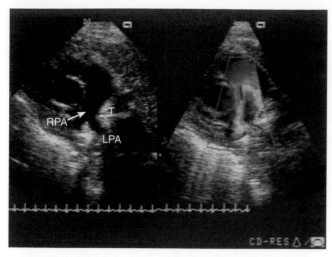

COLOR PLATE 108. Short-axis view of a pulmonary sling (same patient as in Echo. 31-5). **Left:** Anatomic image of anomalous origin of the left pulmonary artery from the right pulmonary artery. **Right:** Color Doppler map of the flow in the pulmonary arteries. *RPA*, right pulmonary artery; *LPA*, left pulmonary artery.

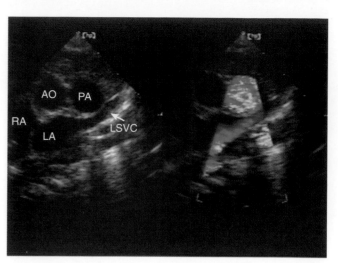

COLOR PLATE 109. Suprasternal short-axis view with the transducer tilted to the left to demonstrate the persistence of a left superior vena cava draining into the roof of the left atrium. **Left:** Anatomic image of the connection between the left superior vena cava (*arrow*) and the left atrium. The left-sided pulmonary veins are also seen in this view connecting normally to the left atrium. **Right:** Color Doppler image of the flow of the left superior vena cava into the left atrium. The flow within the pulmonary artery is also seen in this frame. *AO*, aorta; *PA*, pulmonary artery; *RA*, right atrium; *LA*, left atrium; *LSVC*, left superior vena cava.

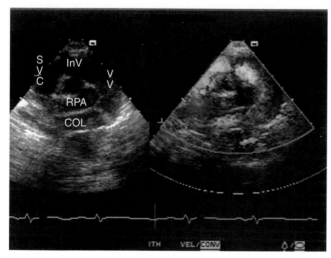

COLOR PLATE 110. Suprasternal view of total anomalous venous connection to a vertical vein. The common venous collector is seen connecting with the vertical vein, which in turn joins a dilated innominate vein and the right superior vena cava. Anatomic image **(left)** and color Doppler image **(right)** of the drainage of the common venous collector into the vertical vein, innominate vein, and superior vena cava. *SVC*, superior vena cava; *InV*, innominate vein; *VV*, vertical vein; *RPA*, right pulmonary artery; *COL*, common venous collector.

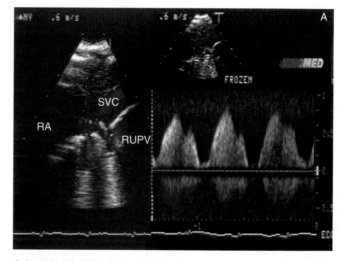

COLOR PLATE 111. Color Doppler and spectral Doppler recordings in a case of total anomalous pulmonary venous connection, mixed type (*with color plate 112*). Right subclavicular view **(left)** demonstrating the connection of the right upper pulmonary vein to the superior vena cava directly, and the spectral Doppler recording **(right)** of the velocities at the site of connection of the pulmonary vein to the superior vena cava. *RA*, right atrium; *SVC*, superior vena cava; *RUPV*, right upper pulmonary vein.

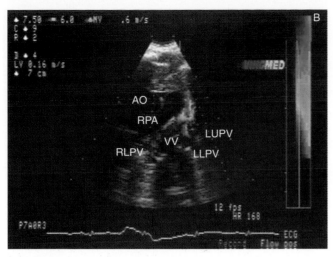

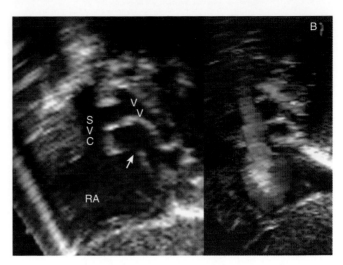

COLOR PLATE 112: Color Doppler and spectral Doppler recordings in a case of total anomalous pulmonary venous connection, mixed type (*with color plate 111*). Color Doppler flow image identifying the three remaining pulmonary veins draining into a vertical vein. *AO*, aorta; *RPA*, right pulmonary artery *RLPV*, right lower pulmonary vein; *LUPV*, left upper pulmonary vein; *LLPV*, left lower pulmonary vein; *VV,* vertical vein.

COLOR PLATE 113. Images from a case with total anomalous pulmonary venous connection to a vertical vein. Anatomic image **(left)** and color Doppler image **(right)** from the subcostal sagittal position of the connection of the vertical vein to the right superior vena cava through an innominate vein. *RA*, right atrium; *SVC*, superior vena cava; *VV*, vertical vein.

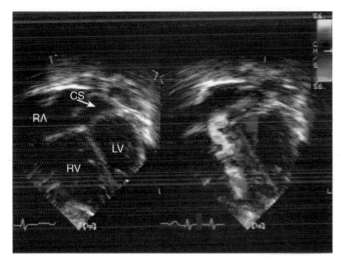

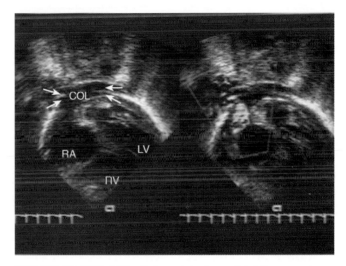

COLOR PLATE 114. Images from a case with total anomalous pulmonary venous connection to the coronary sinus. Apical four-chamber view **(left)** of the dilated coronary sinus opening into the right atrium (*arrow*). Color Doppler image **(right)** of the flow from the coronary sinus into the right atrium. *RA*, right atrium; *RV*, right ventricle; *LV*, left ventricle; *CS*, coronary sinus.

COLOR PLATE 115. Subcostal view of total anomalous venous connection directly to the right atrium. **Left:** Anatomic image demonstrating the four pulmonary veins (*arrows*) connecting to a common venous collector, which in turn connects to the right atrium. **Right:** Color Doppler image of the flow from the collector into the right atrium. *COL*, common venous collector; *RA*, right atrium; *RV*, right ventricle; *LV*, left ventricle.

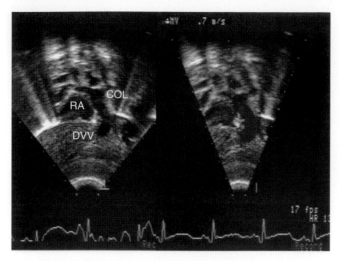

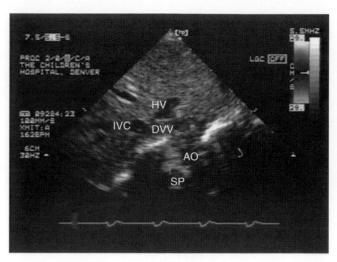

COLOR PLATE 116. Images from a case with total anomalous venous connection, infradiaphragmatic type. **Left:** Anatomic image of the pulmonary veins joining a common collector, which connects to a descending vertical vein directed toward the liver. **Right:** Color Doppler image of the flow in the descending vertical vein. *RA*, right atrium; *COL*, common venous collector; *DVV*, descending vertical vein.

COLOR PLATE 117. Abdominal short-axis view of total anomalous pulmonary venous connection, infradiaphragmatic type, showing the descending vertical vein in cross section. *HV*, hepatic vein; *IVC*, inferior vena cava; *DVV*, descending vertical vein; *AO*, aorta; *SP*, spine.

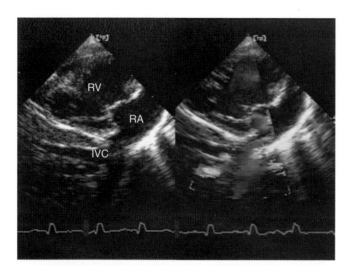

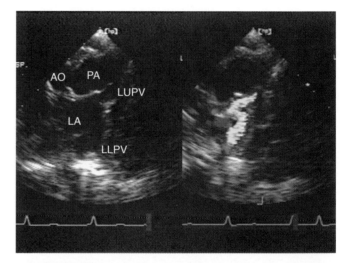

COLOR PLATE 118. Parasternal long-axis view with the transducer tilted toward the right ventricular inflow in total anomalous pulmonary venous connection, infradiaphragmatic type. **Left:** The view demonstrates the connection of the inferior vena cava and the returning venous channel to the right atrium. **Right:** The color Doppler image illustrates the flow of the pulmonary venous channel at the inferior vena caval-right atrial-hepatic junction. *RV*, right ventricle; *RA*, right atrium, *IVC*, inferior vena cava.

COLOR PLATE 119. Suprasternal short-axis view demonstrating stenosis of the left-sided pulmonary veins. **Left:** The anatomic image suggests narrowing at the junction of the left pulmonary veins to the left atrium. **Right:** The color Doppler image demonstrates aliasing of the velocities at the sites of obstruction. *AO*, aorta; *PA*, pulmonary artery; *LUPV*, left upper pulmonary vein; *LLPV*, left lower pulmonary vein.

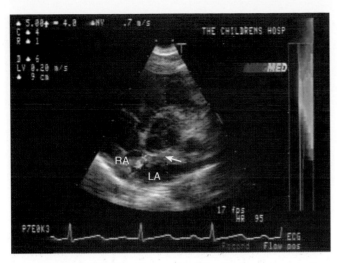

COLOR PLATE 120. Short axis of the aorta demonstrating the color Doppler flow image of the fistulous drainage of a left coronary artery into the right atrium (*arrow*). RA, right atrium; *LA,* left atrium.

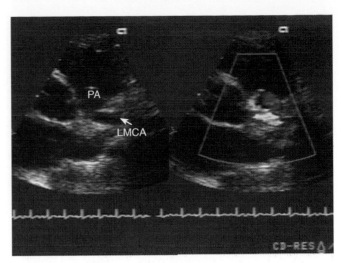

COLOR PLATE 121. Parasternal short-axis view demonstrating anomalous origin of the left coronary artery from the pulmonary artery. **Left:** Anatomical image indicating the anomalous coronary artery (*arrow*). **Right:** Color Doppler image of the flow of the left coronary artery into the pulmonary artery. *PA,* pulmonary artery; *LMCA,* left main coronary artery.

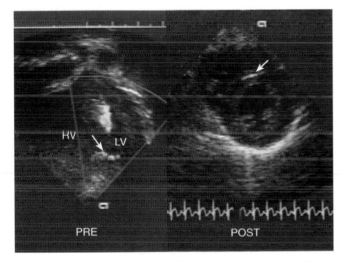

COLOR PLATE 122. Images from a case of coronary fistulae. **Left:** Apical view of a coronary fistula draining into the right ventricle (*arrow*). **Right:** Short-axis view demonstrating the coil used to close the fistulous connection (*arrow*). RV, right ventricle; *LV,* left ventricle.

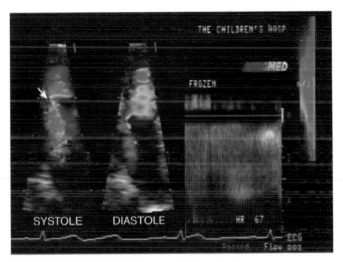

COLOR PLATE 123. Color Doppler and spectral velocity recording of a fistula between the left coronary artery and the pulmonary artery (*arrow*) after tunnel repair of anomalous origin of the left coronary artery from the pulmonary artery. Images were obtained from the same patient as in Echos. 34-6 and 34-7. The recordings demonstrate continuous, high-velocity flow from the left coronary artery to the pulmonary artery.

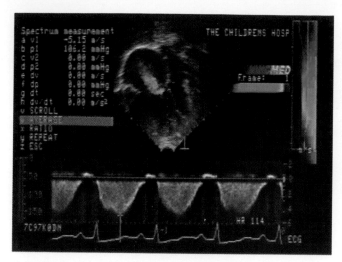

COLOR PLATE 124. Spectral Doppler velocity traces from a tricuspid regurgitant jet. Note the high velocity and the slow acceleration seen in pulmonary hypertension.

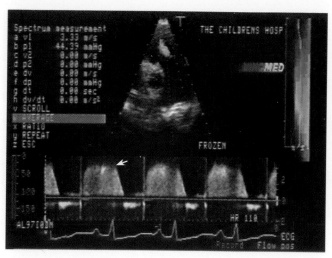

COLOR PLATE 125. Spectral Doppler recording of a pulmonary insufficiency curve. The velocity at the "shoulder" of the waveform is high (*arrow*), indicating the presence of elevated pulmonary end diastolic pressures.

hypertrophy, the size of the left ventricular cavity and the systolic and diastolic function of the left ventricle must be evaluated serially as well, particularly if there is significant residual aortic regurgitation. In the pediatric population, the postoperative follow-up is performed transthoracically and only rarely is a transesophageal study required.

In cases where the aortic valve has been replaced with a mechanical prosthetic valve, usually of the St. Jude type, the valve motion should be studied qualitatively to evaluate restricted motion secondary to clots (rarely) or panus formation (usually) (Echo. 19-14). The metallic cage of the valve causes artifacts that impede the ultrasound beam from penetrating the leaflet structure itself. Consequently, the valve motion should be evaluated for several cardiac cycles for the presence of abnormal delay, and/or intermittent and uneven motion from all available acoustic windows and transducer positions. Ideally, the ultrasound beam should be directed parallel to the direction of motion of the discs to ensure appropriate evaluation. The valve should remain open throughout systole and there should be no delay in the onset of valve opening. In a normally functioning St. Jude valve, color Doppler flow mapping demonstrates three thin jets ejecting from the valve itself and directed somewhat eccentrically into the aortic root. Pulsed and continuous waves are useful in the assessment of prosthetic valve function. Because the velocities through normally functioning prosthetic valves are almost always higher than those found in native valves, it is important to obtain baseline velocity measurements prior to discharge from the hospital. Gradients can be calculated using the Bernoulli equation in conjunction with the continuity equation. Measurement of the mean pressure gradients are preferable in most instances since

usually these correlate better with transcatheter pressure gradients than do the peak instantaneous gradients. Pressure half-time is also useful in assessing valve function and in calculating valve areas in the absence of significant regurgitation. Prosthetic valves are usually minimally regurgitant and this is usually evident on color Doppler flow mapping examination. Guided by these images, the spectral Doppler sampling line can be positioned along the direction of the jet to obtain the velocity wave form for evaluation of signal intensity (195,196).

Following extended aortic root replacement, the major concern in long-term follow-up is the development of stenosis and/or regurgitation of the cryopreserved homograft. Mild degrees of regurgitation are detected immediately postoperatively in most instances. Late stenosis and regurgitation are common, leading to a high percentage of late replacements (197).

The possibility of endocarditis affecting the aortic valve postoperatively must always be kept in mind. This applies whether the valve is the patient's own or whether it has been replaced with a bioprosthetic valve, a mechanical prosthesis, or the patient's pulmonic valve as in a Ross procedure.

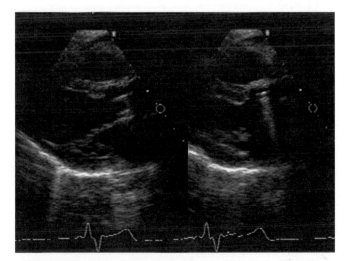

ECHO. 19-14. Parasternal long-axis view of a St. Jude prosthetic valve in the aortic position. **Left:** Valve in systole with the two leaflets and three orifices clearly demonstrated. **Right:** Valve in diastole with the reflection from the metallic structures shadowing posteriorly.

REFERENCES

1. Cheitlin MD, Fenoglio JJ, McAllister HA, Davia JE, DeCastro CM. Congenital aortic stenosis secondary to dysplasia of congenital bicuspid aortic valves without commissural fusion. *Am J Cardiol* 1978;42:102–107.
2. Hoffman JIE, Christianson R. Congenital heart disease in a cohort of 19,502 births with long-term follow-up. *Am J Cardiol* 1978; 42:641–647.
3. Fyler DC, Buckley LP, Hellenbrand WE, Cohn HE. Report of the New England Regional Infant Cardiac Program. *Pediatrics* 1980; 65[Suppl]:375–461.
4. Somerville J. Aortic stenosis and incompetence. In: Anderson RH, Macartney FJ, Shinebourne EA, Tynan M, eds. *Paediatric cardiology. Vol. 1.* Edinburgh: Churchill Livingstone, 1987:977–999.
5. Samanek M, Slavik Z, Zborilova B, Hrobonova V, Voriskova M, Skovranek J. Prevalence, treatment, and outcome of heart disease in live-born children: a prospective analysis of 91,823 live-born children. *Pediatr Cardiol* 1989;10:205–211.
6. Hoffman JIE. Incidence of congenital heart disease: I. Postnatal incidence. *Pediatr Cardiol* 1995;16:103–113.
7. Roberts WC. Valvular, subvalvular, and supravalvular aortic stenosis: morphologic features. *Cardiovasc Clin* 1973;5:98–126.
8. Jarmakani JM. Valvar aortic stenosis. *Prog Pediatr Cardiol* 1994; 3:115–131.
9. Bonetus T. *Sepulchretum sive anatomia practica ex cadaveribus morbo denatis. Vol. 1, book 2* [1679]. Geneva: Observatio XXVI, 1700:891.
10. Chevers N. Observations on the diseases of the orifice and valves of the aorta. *Guy's Hosp Rep* 1842;7:387–452.
11. Kramer TC. The partitioning of the truncus and conus and the formation of the membranous portion of the interventricular septum in the human heart. *Am J Anat* 1942;71:343–370.
12. Peacock TB. Malformations which do not interfere with the functions of the heart, but may lay the foundation of disease in after life. Irregularities of the valves. In: Peacock TB, ed. *On malformations, and C., of the human heart. With original cases* [1858]. Boston: Mildford House, 1973:93–102.
13. Moore GW, Hutchins GM, Brito JC, Kang H. Congenital malformations of the semilunar valves. *Hum Pathol* 1980;11:367–372.

14. Van Mierop LHS. Pathology and pathogenesis of the common cardiac malformations. *Cardiovasc Clin* 1970;2:28–59.

15. Osler W. The bicuspid condition of the aortic valves. *Trans Assoc Am Physicians* 1886;1:185–192.

16. Farber S, Hubbard J. Fetal endomyocarditis: intrauterine infection as the cause of congenital cardiac anomalies. *Am J Med Sci* 1933;186:705–713.

17. Oka M, Angrist A. Mechanism of cardiac valvular fusion and stenosis. *Am Heart J* 1967;74:37–47.

18. Edwards JE. Pathology of left ventricular outflow tract obstruction. *Circulation* 1965;31:586–599.

19. Lakier JB, Lewis AB, Heymann MA, Stanger P, Hoffman JIE, Rudolph AM. Isolated aortic stenosis in the neonate: natural history and hemodynamic considerations. *Circulation* 1974;50:801–808.

20. McKay R, Smith A, Leung MP, Arnold R, Anderson RH. Morphology of ventriculoaortic junction in critical aortic stenosis. Implications for hemodynamic function and clinical management. *J Thorac Cardiovasc Surg* 1992;104:434–442.

21. Edwards JE. Pathologic aspects of cardiac valvular insufficiencies. *Arch Surg* 1958;77:634–649.

22. Roberts WC, Morrow AG. Congenital aortic stenosis produced by a unicommissural valve. *Br Heart J* 1965;27:505–510.

23. Becker AE, Anderson RH. Ventricular outflow abnormalities. In: Becker AE, Anderson RH, eds. *Pathology of congenital heart disease.* London: Butterworths, 1981:165–190.

24. Roberts WC. The two most common congenital heart diseases [Editorial]. *Am J Cardiol* 1984;53:1198.

25. Edwards JE. The congenital bicuspid aortic valve. *Circulation* 1961;23:485–488.

26. Becker AE, Becker MJ, Edwards JE. Anomalies associated with coarctation of the aorta. Particular reference to infancy. *Circulation* 1970;41:1067–1075.

27. Angelini A, Ho SY, Anderson RH, Devine WA, Zuberbuhler JR, Becker AE. The morphology of the normal aortic valve as compared with the aortic valve having two leaflets. *J Thorac Cardiovasc Surg* 1989;98:362–367.

28. Davis GL, McAlister WH, Friedenberg MJ. Congenital aortic stenosis due to failure of histogenesis of the aortic valve (myxoid dysplasia). *Am J Roentgenol* 1965;95:621–628.

29. Roberts WC. The congenitally bicuspid aortic valve: a study of 85 autopsy cases. *Am J Cardiol* 1970;26:72–83.

30. Waller BF, Carter JB, Williams HJ Jr, Wang K, Edwards JE. Bicuspid aortic valve. Comparison of congenital and acquired types. *Circulation* 1973;48:1140–1150.

31. Thubrikar M. Diseases of the aortic valve. In: Thubrikar M, ed. *The aortic valve.* Boca Raton, FL: CRC Press, 1990:157–174.

32. Lerer PK, Edwards WD. Coronary arterial anatomy in bicuspid aortic valve. Necropsy study of 100 hearts. *Br Heart J* 1981;45:142–147.

33. Vlodaver Z, Neufeld HN, Edwards JE. Positions of coronary ostia. In: Vlodaver Z, Neufeld HN, Edwards JE, eds. *Coronary arterial variations in the normal heart and in congenital heart disease.* New York: Academic Press, 1975:19–22.

34. Hurwitz LE, Roberts WC. Quadricuspid semilunar valve. *Am J Cardiol* 1973;31:623–626.

35. Davia JE, Fenoglio JJ, DeCastro CM, McAllister HA, Cheitlin MD. Quadricuspid semilunar valves. *Chest* 1977;72:186–189.

36. Fernicola DJ, Mann JM, Roberts WC. Congenitally quadricuspid aortic valve: analysis of six necropsy patients. *Am J Cardiol* 1989;63:136–138.

37. Titus JL, Edwards JE. The aortic root and valve. Development, anatomy, and congenital anomalies. In: Emery RW, Arom KV, eds. *The aortic valve.* Philadelphia: Hanley & Belfus, 1991:1–8.

38. Snider AR, Serwer GA. Abnormalities of the left ventricular outflow. Valvular aortic stenosis. In: Snider AR, Serwer GA, eds. *Echocardiography in pediatric heart disease.* Chicago: Year Book Medical Publisher, 1990:242–263.

39. Hatle L, Angelsen B. Pulsed and continuous wave Doppler in diagnosis and assessment of various heart lesions. In: Hatle L, Angelsen B, eds. *Doppler ultrasound in cardiology. Physical principles and clinical applications.* 2nd ed. Philadelphia: Lea & Febiger, 1985:97–292.

40. Lewis T, Grant RT. Observations relating to subacute infective endocarditis. *Heart* 1923;10:21–99.

41. Gross L, Kugel MA. Topographic anatomy and histology of the valves in the human heart. *Am J Pathol* 1932;7:445–473.

42. Brewer RJ, Deck JD, Capati B, Nolan SP. The dynamic aortic root. Its role in aortic valve function. *J Thorac Cardiovasc Surg* 1976;72:413–417.

43. Thubrikar M, Piepgrass WC, Shaner TW, Nolan SP. The design of the normal aortic valve. *J Am Physiol* 1981;241:H795–H801.

44. Anderson RH. Editorial note: the anatomy of arterial valvar stenosis. *Int J Cardiol* 1990;26:355–359.

45. Anderson RH, Devine WA, Ho SY, Smith A, McKay R. The myth of the aortic annulus: the anatomy of subaortic outflow tract. *Ann Thorac Surg* 1991;52:640–646.

46. Edwards JE. Manifestations of acquired and congenital diseases of the aorta. *Curr Prob Cardiol* 1979;3:1–62.

47. Tveter KJ, Edwards JE. Calcified aortic sinotubular ridge: a source of coronary ostial stenosis or embolism. *J Am Coll Cardiol* 1988;12:1510–1514.

48. Mercer JL, Benedicty M, Bahnson HT. The geometry and construction of the aortic leaflet. *J Thorac Cardiovasc Surg* 1973;65:511–518.

49. Leung MP, McKay R, Smith A, Anderson RH, Arnold R. Critical aortic stenosis in early infancy. Anatomic and echocardiographic substrates of successful open valvotomy. *J Thorac Cardiovasc Surg* 1991;101:526–535.

50. Rhodes LA, Colan SD, Perry SB, Jonas RA, Sanders SP. Predictors of survival in neonates with critical aortic stenosis. *Circulation* 1991;84:2325–2335.

51. Anderson RH, Becker AE. The morphologically left ventricle. In: Anderson RH, Becker AE, eds. *Cardiac anatomy. An integrated text and color atlas.* London: Gower Medical Publishing, 1980:4.2–4.19.

52. El Habbal M, Somerville J. Size of the normal aortic root in normal subjects and in those with left ventricular outflow obstruction. *Am J Cardiol* 1989;63:322–326.

53. Donti A, Bonvicini M, Gargiulo G, Frascaroli G, Picchio FM. Criteria for selection of balloon valvoplasty for treatment of aortic stenosis in neonates. *Cardiol Young* 1995;5:31–35.

54. Moller JH, Nakib A, Eliot RS, Edwards JE. Symptomatic congenital aortic stenosis in the first year of life. *J Pediatr* 1966;69:728–734.

55. Pelech AN, Dyck JD, Trusler GA, et al. Critical aortic stenosis. Survival and management. *J Thorac Cardiovasc Surg* 1987;94:510–517.

56. Cazzaniga M, Faella H, Gamboa R, et al. Valvotomia percutanea con balon en la cardiopatia obstructiva neonatal. Parte II. Estenosis valvular aortica critica. *An Esp Pediatr* 1993;38:407–412.

57. Parsons MK, Moreau GA, Graham TP Jr, Johns JA, Boucek RJ Jr. Echocardiographic estimation of critical left ventricular size in infants with isolated aortic valve stenosis. *J Am Coll Cardiol* 1991;18:1049–1055.

58. Moller JH, Nakib A, Edwards JE. Infarction of papillary muscles and mitral insufficiency associated with congenital aortic stenosis. *Circulation* 1966;34:87–91.

59. Dick JD, Freedom RM. Aortic stenosis. In: Freedom RM, Benson LN, Smallhorn JF, eds. *Neonatal heart disease.* London: Springer-Verlag, 1992:357–373.

60. Moller JH, Lucas RV, Adams P Jr, Anderson RC, Jorgens J, Edwards JE. Endocardial fibroelastosis. A clinical and anatomic study of 47 patients with emphasis on its relationship to mitral insufficiency. *Circulation* 1964;30:759–781.

61. Cape ED, Jones M, Yamada I, VanAuker MD, Valdes-Cruz LM. Turbulent/viscous interactions control Doppler/catheter pressure discrepancies in aortic stenosis: the role of the Reynolds number. *Circulation* 1996;94:2975–2981.

62. Skjaerpe T, Hegrenaes L, Hatle L. Noninvasive estimation of valve area in patients with aortic stenosis by Doppler ultrasound and two-dimensional echocardiography. *Circulation* 1985;72:810–818.

63. Myreng Y, Molstad P, Endresen K, Ihlen H. Reproducibility of echocardiographic estimates of the area of stenosed aortic valves using the continuity equation. *Int J Cardiol* 1990;26:349–354.

64. Pascoe RD, Roger VL, Pellikka PA, Seward JB, Tajik AJ. Use of

Dobutamine stress echocardiography in patients with aortic stenosis, reduced left ventricular ejection fraction and low mean transvalvular gradient: preliminary experience. *J Am Soc Echocardiogr* 1994;7[Suppl]:S8(abst).

65. Shandas R, Trujillo N, Kwon J, Gill EA, Valdes-Cruz L. A new method to measure actual vena contracta areas for regurgitant and stenotic jets: in vitro studies on steady and pulsatile flows. Presented at the American Heart Association Scientific Sessions, 1996. *Circulation* 1996;94:I442 (abst).

66. Quero Jimenez M, Casanova Gomez M. Left ventricular outflow tract obstruction—pathology. In: Godman M, Marquis RM, eds. *Paediatric cardiology. Vol. 2. Heart disease in the newborn.* Edinburgh: Churchill Livingstone, 1979:196–209.

67. Hastreiter AR, Oshima M, Miller RA, Lev M, Paul MH. Congenital aortic stenosis syndrome in infancy. *Circulation* 1963;28: 1084–1095.

68. Culbertson C, De Campli W, Williams R, Helton G, Young N, Hardy C. Congenital valvar aortic stenosis and abnormal origin of the right coronary artery: rare combination with important clinical implications. *Pediatr Cardiol* 1995;16:73–75.

69. Moore N. III. Diseases, etc., of the organs of circulation. 1. Abnormal heart. *Trans Pathol Soc Lond* 1882;34:29–31.

70. Smart A. A case of double stenosis of the aortic orifice. *Lancet* 1904;2:1417–1418.

71. Shennan T. Note on a case of double stenosis of the aortic orifice. *Lancet* 1905;1:21.

72. Keith A. The Hunterian Lectures on malformations of the heart. Lecture I. *Lancet* 1909;2:359–363.

73. Thursfield H, Scott HW. Sub-aortic stenosis. *Br J Child Dis* 1913; 10:104–109.

74. Reis RL, Peterson LM, Mason DT, Simon AL, Morrow AG. Congenital fixed subvalvular aortic stenosis. An anatomical classification and correlations with operative results. *Circulation* 1971; 43[Suppl 1]:I-11–I-18.

75. Taussig HB. Anomalies of aortic valve and of the ascending aorta. In: Taussig HB, ed. *Congenital malformations of the heart. Vol. II.* Cambridge, MA: Commonwealth Fund, Harvard University Press, 1960:835–865.

76. Gordon AS. The surgical management of congenital supravalvular, valvular, and subvalvular aortic stenosis using deep hypothermia. *J Thorac Cardiovasc Surg* 1962;43:141–156.

77. Cooley DA, Beall AC Jr, Hallman GL, Bricker DL. Obstructive lesions of the left ventricular outflow tract. Surgical treatment. *Circulation* 1965;31:612–621.

78. Kelly DT, Wulfsberg E, Rowe RD. Discrete subaortic stenosis. *Circulation* 1972;46:309–322.

79. Champsaur G, Trusler GA, Mustard WT. Congenital discrete subvalvular aortic stenosis. Surgical experience and long-term follow-up in 20 paediatric patients. *Br Heart J* 1973;35:443–446.

80. Newfeld EA, Muster AJ, Paul MH, Idriss FS, Riker WL. Discrete subvalvular aortic stenosis in childhood. *Am J Cardiol* 1976;38: 53–61.

81. Abbott ME. Subaortic stenosis. In: Abbott ME, ed. *Atlas of congenital cardiac disease.* New York: American Heart Association, 1936:60–61.

82. Keith A. Schorstein Lecture on the fate of the bulbus cordis in the human heart. Schorstein Lecture. *Lancet* 1924;2:1267–1273.

83. Van Praagh R, Corwin RD, Dahlquist EH Jr, Freedom RM, Mattioli L, Nebesar RA. Tetralogy of Fallot with severe left ventricular outflow tract obstruction due to anomalous attachment of the mitral valve to the ventricular septum. *Am J Cardiol* 1970;26:93–101.

84. Rosenquist GC, Clark EB, Sweeney LJ, McAllister HA. The normal spectrum of mitral and aortic valve discontinuity. *Circulation* 1976;54:298–301.

85. Rosenquist GC, Clark EB, McAllister HA, Bharati S, Edwards JE. Increased mitral-aortic separation in discrete subaortic stenosis. *Circulation* 1979;60:70–74.

86. Pyle RL, Patterson DF, Chacko S. The genetics and pathology of discrete subaortic stenosis in the Newfoundland dog. *Am Heart J* 1976;92:324–334.

87. Somerville J. Congenital heart disease changes in form and function. *Br Heart J* 1979;41:1–22.

88. Somerville J, Stone S, Ross D. Fate of patients with fixed subaortic stenosis after surgical removal. *Br Heart J* 1980;43:629–647.

89. Freedom RM, Fowler RS, Duncan WJ. Rapid evolution from "normal" left ventricular outflow tract to fatal subaortic stenosis in infancy. *Br Heart J* 1981;45:605–609.

90. Freedom RM, Pelech A, Brand A, et al. The progressive nature of subaortic stenosis in congenital heart disease. *Int J Cardiol* 1985;8:137–143.

91. Somerville J. Fixed subaortic stenosis—a frequently misunderstood lesion. *Int J Cardiol* 1985;8:145–148.

92. Leichter DA, Sullivan I, Gersony WM. "Acquired" discrete subvalvular aortic stenosis: natural history and hemodynamics. *J Am Coll Cardiol* 1989;14:1539–1544.

93. Firpo C, Maitre Azcarate MJ, Quero Jimenez M, Saravalli O. Discrete subaortic stenosis (DSS) in chilhood: a congenital or acquired disease? Follow-up in 65 patients. *Eur Heart J* 1990;11: 1033–1040.

94. DeLeon SY, Ilbawi MN, Roberson DA, et al. Conal enlargement for diffuse subaortic stenosis. *J Thorac Cardiovasc Surg* 1991; 102:814–820.

95. Richardson ME, Menahem S, Wilkinson JL. Familial fixed subaortic stenosis. *Int J Cardiol* 1991;30:351–353.

96. Maginot KR, Williams RG. Fixed subaortic stenosis. *Prog Pediatr Cardiol* 1994;3:141–149.

97. Becker AE, Anderson RH. *Cardiac pathology. An integrated text and color atlas.* New York: Raven Press, 1982:13.1–13.22.

98. Brock R, Fleming PR. Aortic subvalvular stenosis. A report of 5 cases diagnosed during life. *Guy's Hosp Rep* 1956;105:391–408.

99. Chaikhouni A, Crawford FA Jr, Sade RM, Taylor AB, Riopel DA, Hohn AR. Discrete subaortic stenosis. *Clin Cardiol* 1984;7:289–293.

100. Ten Cate FJ, Van Dorp WG, Hugenholtz PG, Roelandt J. Fixed subaortic stenosis. Value of echocardiography for diagnosis and differentiation between various types. *Br Heart J* 1979;41:159–166.

101. Hatle L. Noninvasive assessment and differentiation of left ventricular outflow obstruction with Doppler ultrasound. *Circulation* 1981;64:381–387.

102. Yoganathan AP, Valdes-Cruz LM, Schmidt-Dohna J, et al. Continuous wave Doppler velocities and gradients across fixed tunnel obstructions: studies in vitro and in vivo. *Circulation* 1987;76: 657–666.

103. Simpson IA, Valdes-Cruz LM, Yoganathan AP, Sung HW, Jimoh A, Sahn DJ. Spatial velocity distribution and acceleration in serial subvalve tunnel and valvular obstructions: an in vitro study using Doppler color flow mapping. *J Am Coll Cardiol* 1989;13:241–248.

104. Sung C, Price EC, Cooley DA. Discrete subaortic stenosis in adults. *Am J Cardiol* 1978;42:283–290.

105. Zuberbuhler JR, Bauersfeld SR, Bahnson HT. Ventricular septal defect associated with combined subvalvular aortic and pulmonic stenosis. *J Thorac Cardiovasc Surg* 1965;50:721–725.

106. Johnson TB, Fyfe DA, Swanger SJ. Double orifice mitral valve associated with subaortic stenosis—echocardiographic and anatomic findings. *Cardiol Young* 1994;4:168–171.

107. Pinto RJ, Sharma S, Shah N. Interruption of the aortic arch with patency of the arterial duct, discrete subaortic stenosis, resctrictive ventricular septal defect and severe pulmonary hypertension survival to adulthood and successful correction by balloon dilatation and surgery. *Cardiol Young* 1995;5:367–369.

108. Mencarelli L. Stenosi sopravalvolare aortica ad anello. *Arch Ital Anat Istol Patol* 1930;1:829–841.

109. Williams JCP, Barrat-Boyes BG, Lowe JB. Supravalvular aortic stenosis. *Circulation* 1961;24:1311–1318.

110. Beuren AJ, Apitz J, Harmjanz D. Supravalvular aortic stenosis in association with mental retardation and a certain facial appearance. *Circulation* 1962;26:1235–1240.

111. Black JA, Bonham-Carter RE. Association between aortic stenosis and facies of severe infantile hypercalcemia. *Lancet* 1963;2:745–749.

112. Garcia RE, Friedman WF, Kaback MM, Rowe RD. Idiopathic hypercalcemia and supravalvular aortic stenosis. Documentation of a new syndrome. *N Engl J Med* 1964;271:117–120.

113. Bourassa MG, Campeau L. Combined supravalvular aortic and pulmonic stenosis. *Circulation* 1963;28:572–581.

114. Beuren AJ, Schulze C, Eberle P, Harmjanz D, Apitz J. The syn-

drome of supravalvular aortic stenosis, peripheral pulmonary stenosis, mental retardation and similar facial appearance. *Am J Cardiol* 1964;13:471–483.

115. Ottesen OE, Antia AU, Rowe RD. Peripheral vascular anomalies associated with the supravalvular aortic stenosis syndrome. *Radiology* 1966;86:430–435.

116. Peterson TA, Todd DB, Edwards JE. Supravalvular aortic stenosis. *J Thorac Cardiovasc Surg* 1965;50:734–741.

117. Goor DA, Lillehei CW. Malformations of the aortic pathway. In: Goor DA, Lillehei CW, eds. *Congenital malformations of the heart. Embryology, anatomy, and operative considerations.* New York: Grune & Stratton, 1975:237–263.

118. Attie F, Ovseyevitz J, Buendia A, De Rossi RL. Estenosis aorticas. In: Sanchez PA, ed. *Cardiologia pediatrica. Clinica y cirugia. Vol. I.* Barcelona: Salvat Editores S.A., 1986:652–668.

119. Friedman WF, Roberts WC. Vitamin D and the supravalvular aortic stenosis syndrome. The transplacental effects of vitamin D on the aorta of the rabbit. *Circulation* 1966;34:77–86.

120. Antia AU, Wiltse HE, Rowe RD, et al. Pathogenesis of the supravalvular aortic stenosis syndrome. *J Pediatr* 1967;71:431–441.

121. Friedman WF. Supravalvular aortic stenosis. *Prog Pediatr Cardiol* 1994;3:133–139.

122. Curran ME, Atkinson DL, Ewart AK, Morris CA, Leppert MF, Keating MT. The elastin gene is disrupted by a translocation associated with supravalvular aortic stenosis. *Cell* 1993;73:159–168.

123. Varghese PJ, Izukawa T, Rowe RD. Supravalvular aortic stenosis as part of rubella syndrome, with discussion of pathogenesis. *Br Heart J* 1969;31:59–62.

124. Sissman NJ, Neill CA, Spencer FC, Taussig HB. Congenital aortic stenosis. *Circulation* 1959;19:458–468.

125. Rastelli GC, McGoon DC, Ongley PA, Mankin HT, Kirklin JW. Surgical treatment of supravalvular aortic stenosis. Report of 16 cases and review of literature. *J Thorac Cardiovasc Surg* 1966; 51:873–882.

126. O'Connor WN, Davis JB Jr, Geissler R, Cottrill CM, Noonan JA, Todd EP. Supravalvular aortic stenosis. Clinical and pathologic observations in six patients. *Arch Pathol Lab Med* 1985;109:179–185.

127. Flaker G, Teske D, Kilman J, Hosier D, Wooley C. Supravalvular aortic stenosis. A 20-year clinical perspective and experience with patch aortoplasty. *Am J Cardiol* 1983;51:256–260.

128. Burry AF. Supra-aortic stenosis associated with Marfan's syndrome. *Br Heart J* 1958;20:143–146.

129. Soto B, Pacifico AD. Congenital aortic stenosis. In: Soto B, Pacifico AD, eds. *Angiocardiography in congenital heart malformations.* Mount Kisco, NY: Futura Publishing, 1990:545–563.

130. Doty DB, Polansky DB, Jenson CB. Supravalvular aortic stenosis. Repair by extended aortoplasty. *J Thorac Cardiovasc Surg* 1977; 74:362–371.

131. Giddins NG, Finley JP, Nanton MA, Roy DL. The natural course of supravalvular aortic stenosis and peripheral pulmonary artery stenosis in William's syndrome. *Br Heart J* 1989;62:315–319.

132. Wren C, Oslizlok P, Bull C. Natural history of supravalvular aortic stenosis and pulmonary artery stenosis. *J Am Coll Cardiol* 1990; 15:1625–1630.

133. Rowe RD. Pulmonary arterial stenosis. In: Keith JD, Rowe RD, Vlad P, eds. *Heart disease in infancy and childhood.* 3rd ed. New York: Macmillan, 1978:789–801.

134. Blieden LC, Lucas RV Jr, Carter JB, Miller K, Edwards JE. A developmental complex including supravalvular stenosis of the aorta and pulmonary trunk. *Circulation* 1974;49:585–590.

135. Bristow JD. Recognition of left ventricular outflow obstruction. *Circulation* 1965;31:600–611.

136. Becker AE, Becker MJ, Edwards JE. Mitral valvular abnormalities associated with supravalvular aortic stenosis. Observations in three cases. *Am J Cardiol* 1972;29:90–94.

137. Kirklin JW, Barrat-Boyes BG. Congenital aortic stenosis. In: Kirklin JW, Barrat-Boyes BG, eds. *Cardiac surgery. Morphology, diagnostic criteria, natural history, techniques, results, and indications. Vol. 2.* 2nd ed. New York: Churchill Livingstone, 1994: 1195–1237.

138. Lev M. Pathologic anatomy and interrelationship of hypoplasia of the aortic tract complexes. *Lab Invest* 1952;1:61–70.

139. Noonan JA, Nadas AS. The hypoplastic left heart syndrome. An analysis of 101 cases. *Pediatr Clin North Am* 1958;5:1029–1056.

140. Watson DG, Rowe RD. Aortic-valve atresia. Report of 43 cases. *JAMA* 1962;179:112–116.

141. Kanjuh VI, Eliot RS, Edwards JE. Coexistent mitral and aortic valvular atresia. A pathologic study of 14 cases. *Am J Cardiol* 1965;15:611–621.

142. Rosenquist GC, Taylor JFN, Stark J. Aortopulmonary fenestration and aortic atresia. Report of an infant with ventricular septal defect, persistent ductus arteriosus, and interrupted aortic arch. *Br Heart J* 1974;36:1146–1148.

143. Pellegrino PA, Thiene G. Aortic valve atresia with a normally developed left ventricle. *Chest* 1976;69:121–122.

144. Freedom RM, Williams WG, Dische MR, Rowe RD. Anatomical variants in aortic atresia. Potential candidates for ventriculoaortic reconstitution. *Br Heart J* 1976;38:821–826.

145. Roberts WC, Perry LW, Chandra RS, Myers GE, Shapiro SR, Scott LP. Aortic valve atresia: a new classification based on necropsy study of 73 cases. *Am J Cardiol* 1976;37:753–756.

146. Freedom RM, Dische MR, Rowe RD. Conal anatomy in aortic atresia, ventricular septal defect, and normally developed left ventricle. *Am Heart J* 1977;94:689–698.

147. Thiene G, Gallucci V, Macartney FJ, Del Torso S, Pellegrino PA, Anderson RH. Anatomy of aortic atresia. Cases presenting with a ventricular septal defect. *Circulation* 1979;59:173–178.

148. Esteban I, Cabrera A. Aortic atresia with normal left ventricle and intact ventricular septum. *Chest* 1978;73:883–884.

149. Houyel L, Zupan V, Roset F. Aortic atresia with normal left ventricle and intact ventricular septum—a major form of subaortic stenosis complicating an atrioventricular septal defect with intact septal structures. *Cardiol Young* 1995;5:282–285.

150. Freedom RM, Dische MR, Rowe RD. Pathologic anatomy of subaortic stenosis and atresia in the first year of life. *Am J Cardiol* 1977;39:1035–1044.

151. Lababidi Z. Aortic balloon valvuloplasty. *Am Heart J* 1983;106: 751–752.

152. Lababidi Z, Wu JR, Walls JT. Percutaneous balloon aortic valvuloplasty: results in 23 patients. *Am J Cardiol* 1984;53:194–197.

153. Rupprath G, Neuhaus KL. Percutaneous balloon valvuloplasty for aortic valve stenosis in infancy. *Am J Cardiol* 1985;55:1655–1656.

154. Sanchez GR, Metha AV, Ewing LL, Brickley SE, Anderson TM, Black IFS. Successful percutaneous balloon valvuloplasty of the aortic valve in an infant. *Pediatr Cardiol* 1985;6:103–106.

155. Lababidi Z, Weinhaus L. Successful balloon valvuloplasty for neonatal critical aortic stenosis. *Am Heart J* 1986;112:913–916.

156. Wren C, Sullivan I, Bull C, Deanfield J. Percutaneous balloon dilatation of aortic valve stenosis in neonates and infants. *Br Heart J* 1987;58:608–612.

157. Sholler GF, Keane JF, Perry SB, Sanders SP, Lock JE. Balloon dilatation of congenital aortic valve stenosis. Results and influence of technical and morphological features on outcome. *Circulation* 1988;78:351–360.

158. Zeevi B, Keane JF, Castaneda AR, Perry SB, Lock JE. Neonatal critical valvar aortic stenosis. A comparison of surgical and balloon dilatation therapy. *Circulation* 1989;80:831–839.

159. Freedom RM. Balloon therapy of critical aortic stenosis in the neonate. The therapeutic conundrum resolved? *Circulation* 1989; 80:1087–1088.

160. Vogel M, Benson LN, Burrows P, Smallhorn JF, Freedom RM. Balloon dilatation of congenital aortic stenosis in infants and children: short-term and intermediate results. *Br Heart J* 1989;62: 148–153.

161. Kasten-Sportes CH, Piechaud JF, Sidi D, Kachaner J. Percutaneous balloon valvuloplasty in neonates with critical aortic stenosis. *J Am Coll Cardiol* 1989;13:1101–1105.

162. Rocchini AP, Beekman RH, Shachar GB, Benson L, Schwartz D, Kan JS. Balloon aortic valvuloplasty: results of the valvuloplasty and angioplasty of congenital anomalies registry. *Am J Cardiol* 1990;65:784–789.

163. Beekman RH, Rocchini AP, Andes A. Balloon valvuloplasty for critical aortic stenosis in the newborn: influence of new catheter technology. *J Am Coll Cardiol* 1991;17:1172–1176.

164. Tometzki AJP, Gibbs JL, Weil J. Balloon valvoplasty of critical

aortic and pulmonary stenosis in the premature neonate. *Int J Cardiol* 1991;30:248–249.

165. Meliones JN, Beekman RH, Rocchini AP, Lacina SJ. Balloon valvuloplasty for recurrent aortic stenosis after surgical valvotomy in childhood: immediate and follow-up studies. *J Am Coll Cardiol* 1989;13:1106–1110.

166. Galassi AR, Nihoyannopoulus P, Pupita G, Odawara H, Crea F, McKenna WJ. Assessment of colour flow imaging in the grading of valvular regurgitation. *Eur Heart J* 1990;11:1101–1108.

167. Klein AL, Davison MB, Vonk G, Tajik AJ. Doppler echocardiographic assessment of aortic regurgitation: uses and limitations. *Cleve Clin J Med* 1992;59:359–368.

168. Ciobanu M, Abbasi AS, Allen M, Hermer A, Spellberg R. Pulsed Doppler echocardiography in the diagnosis and estimation of severity of aortic insufficiency. *Am J Cardiol* 1982;49:339–343.

169. Veyrat C, Ameur A, Gourtchiglouian C, Lessana A, Abitbol G, Kalmanson D. Calculation of pulsed Doppler left ventricular outflow tract regurgitant index for grading the severity of aortic regurgitation. *Am Heart J* 1984;108:507–516.

170. Kandath D, Nanda NC. Part I. Assessment of aortic regurgitation by noninvasive techniques. *Curr Probl Cardiol* 1990;15:45–58.

171. Perry GJ, Helmcke F, Nanda NC, Byard C, Soto B. Evaluation of aortic insufficiency by Doppler color flow mapping. *J Am Coll Cardiol* 1987;9:952–959.

172. Masuyama T, Kodama K, Kitabatake A, et al. Noninvasive evaluation of aortic regurgitation by continuous-wave Doppler echocardiography. *Circulation* 1986;73:460–466.

173. Labovitz AJ, Ferrara RP, Kern MJ, Bryg RJ, Mrosek DG, Williams GA. Quantitative evaluation of aortic insufficiency by continuous wave Doppler echocardiography. *J Am Coll Cardiol* 1986;8:1341–1347.

174. Samstad SO, Hegrenaes L, Skjaerpe T, Hatle L. Half time of the diastolic aortoventricular pressure difference by continuous wave Doppler ultrasound: a measure of the severity of aortic regurgitation? *Br Heart J* 1989;61:336–343.

175. Teague SM, Heinsimer JA, Anderson JL, et al. Quantification of aortic regurgitation utilizing continuous wave Doppler ultrasound. *J Am Coll Cardiol* 1986;8:592–599.

176. Grayburn PA, Handshoe R, Smith MD, Harrison MR, DeMaria AN. Quantitative assessment of the hemodynamic consequences of aortic regurgitation by means of continuous wave Doppler recordings. *J Am Coll Cardiol* 1987;10:135–141.

177. Beyer RW, Ramirez M, Josephson MA, Shah PM. Correlation of continuous-wave Doppler assessment of chronic aortic regurgitation with hemodynamics and angiography. *Am J Cardiol* 1987;60:852–856.

178. Touche T, Prasquier R, Nitenberg A, De Zuttere D, Gourgon R. Assessment and follow-up of patients with aortic regurgitation by an updated Doppler echocardiographic measurement of the regurgitant fraction in the aortic arch. *Circulation* 1985;72:819–824.

179. Rokey R, Sterling LL, Zoghbi WA, et al. Determination of regurgitant fraction in isolated mitral or aortic regurgitation by pulsed Doppler two-dimensional echocardiography. *J Am Coll Cardiol* 1986;7:1273–1278.

180. Shandas R, Yamata I, Solowiejcyk D, Manduley R, Jones M, Valdes-Cruz L. A modified flow convergence equation for calculation of aortic regurgitant volume: studies in a quantified animal model. *J Am Coll Cardiol* 1996;27[Suppl A]:396A(abst).

181. Shiota T, Jones M, Yamada I, et al. Effective regurgitant orifice area by the color Doppler flow convergence method for evaluating the severity of chronic aortic regurgitation. An animal study. *Circulation* 1996;93:594–602.

182. Reimold SC, Maier SE, Fleischmann KE, et al. Dynamic nature of the aortic regurgitant orifice area during diastole in patients with chronic aortic regurgitation. *Circulation* 1994;89:2085–2092.

183. Lababidi Z, Weinhaus L, Stoeckle H Jr, Walls JT. Transluminal balloon dilatation for discrete subaortic stenosis. *Am J Cardiol* 1987;59:423–425.

184. Seward JB, Khandheria BK, Edwards WD, Oh J, Freeman WK, Tajik AJ. Biplanar transesophageal echocardiography: anatomic correlations, image orientation, and clinical applications. *Mayo Clin Proc* 1990;65:1193–1213.

185. Lam J, Neirotti RA, Lubbers WJ, et al. Usefulness of biplane transesophageal echocardiography in neonates, infants and children with congenital heart disease. *Am J Cardiol* 1993;72:699–706.

186. Benheim A, Karr SS, Sell JE, Midgley FM, Holley D, Martin GR. Routine use of transesophageal echocardiography and color flow imaging in the evaluation and treatment of children with congenital heart disease. *Echocardiography* 1993;10:583–593.

187. Leung MP, Yung TC, Chan B, Chiu C, Lee J, Mok CK. The role of transesophageal echocardiography in the diagnosis and management of children and young adults with valvar diseases of the left heart. *Cardiol Young* 1994;4:373–380.

188. Clarke DR. Extended aortic root replacement with cryopreserved allografts: do they hold up? *Ann Thorac Surg* 1991;52:669–675.

189. Ross DN. Replacement of aortic and mitral valves with a pulmonary autograft. *Lancet* 1967;2:956–958.

190. Konno S, Imai Y, Iida Y, Nakajima M, Tatsuno K. A new method for prosthetic valve replacement in congenital aortic stenosis associated with hypoplasia of the aortic valve ring. *J Thorac Cardiovasc Surg* 1975;70:909–917.

191. Castaneda AR, Jonas RA, Mayer JE Jr, Hanley FL. Obstruction of the left ventricular outflow tract. In: Castaneda AR, Jonas RA, Mayer JE Jr, Hanley FL, eds. *Cardiac surgery of the neonate and infant.* Philadelphia: WB Saunders, 1994:315–332.

192. Drinkwater DC Jr, Laks H. Surgery for subvalvular aortic stenosis. *Prog Pediatr Cardiol* 1994;3:189–201.

193. McGoon DC, Mankin HT, Vlad P, Kirklin JW. The surgical treatment of supravalvular aortic stenosis. *J Thorac Cardiovasc Surg* 1961;41:125–133.

194. Van Son JAM, Danielson GK, Puga FJ, et al. Supravalvular aortic stenosis. Long-term results of surgical treatment. *J Thorac Cardiovasc Surg* 1994;107:103–115.

195. Nanda NC, Cooper JW, Mahan EF III, Fan PH. Echocardiographic assessment of prosthetic valves. *Circulation* 1991[Suppl I]:84:I-228–I-239.

196. Reisner SA, Meltzer RS. Normal values of prosthetic valve Doppler echocardiographic parameters: a review. *J Am Soc Echocardiogr* 1988;1:201–210.

197. Cripe LH, Clarke DR, Campbell DN, Fullerton DA, Shaffer EM, Valdes-Cruz LM. Performance of cryopreserved pulmonary homografts in the right ventricular outflow tract in children: an echocardiographic study. *Pediatr Res* 1995;37:24A(abst).

CHAPTER 20

Miscellaneous Anomalies of the Left Ventricular Outflow Tract

Lilliam M. Valdes-Cruz and Raul O. Cayre

AORTICO-LEFT VENTRICULAR TUNNEL

Aortico-left ventricular tunnel is a rare cardiac malformation characterized by the presence of an abnormal communication that originates in the ascending aorta and terminates in the left ventricle, bypassing the aortic valve (1). In 1961, Edwards (2) described the anatomy of this malformation for the first time; the term aortico-left ventricular tunnel was proposed by Levy et al. in 1963 (1). The incidence is 0.1% of all congenital cardiac malformations (3). Cook et al. (4) noted four cases of aortico-left ventricular tunnel in 872 cases of congenital anomalies diagnosed by fetal echocardiography.

EMBRYOLOGIC CONSIDERATIONS

The embryologic origin of aortico-left ventricular tunnel is not known. Nonetheless, several theories have been advanced: (a) an anomalous coronary artery connected with the left ventricular cavity through an intramyocardial sinusoid (1); (b) an anomalous coronary artery connected to the left ventricle via a persistent mesocardial cyst (5); (c) an anomaly of the aortic wall similar to that of Marfan syndrome, with increased deposit of acid mucopolysaccharides in the media of the aorta (6); (d) rupture of a supravalvar aortic aneurysm caused by mural tension generated by turbulence as a result of an intercommissural fibrous crest (7); (e) abnormal development and incorporation of the distal bulbus cordis (8).

ANATOMIC AND ECHOCARDIOGRAPHIC CONSIDERATIONS

The echocardiographic study of aortico-left ventricular tunnel should include the following: (a) anatomic definition of the malformation; and (b) evaluation of associated anomalies.

Anatomic Definition of the Malformation

In all cases reviewed by us in the literature, the tunnel originated in the anterolateral wall of the aorta, directly above or above and to the left of the right coronary ostium (1–23). The tunnel orifice was separated from the right coronary ostium by a crest of fibrous tissue. The tunnel coursed downward along the superior aspect of the interventricular septum, crossed behind the posterior wall of the right ventricular outflow tract, and opened into the left ventricular cavity immediately below either the right coronary cusp or the posterior, noncoronary cusp (Fig. 20-1). In some cases, the intraventricular portion of the tunnel, located behind the right ventricular outflow tract, was dilated, resulting in some obstruction of the right ventricular outflow (1,7,9,12,16).

The tunnel has two portions: an aortic portion, which is generally dilated or even aneurysmatic, and an intraventricular portion, which is narrower or tubular. The presence of an aneurysmatic aortic portion can be confused with an aneurysm of the right sinus of Valsalva opening into the left ventricle. Levy et al. (1) postulate that in aortico-left ventricular tunnel, the tunnel orifice is located above the coronary ostia, whereas in aneurysms of the sinus of Valsalva opening into the left ventricle, the aneurysm is found below the coronary ostia. Histologically, the aortic or extracardiac portion has elastic fibers similar to those of the media of the aorta. As the tunnel progresses into the interventricular septum, the elastic fibers diminish, and a fibrous tissue rich in collagen appears surrounded by striated muscle fibers (1,3,4,6,12). In three published cases, accessory valvular tissue was present in the tunnel orifice (4,7,19).

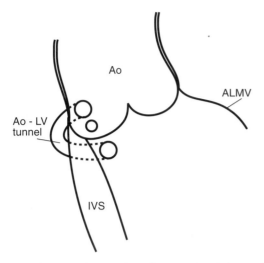

FIG. 20-1. Schematic drawing of an aortico-left ventricular tunnel. *Ao,* aorta; *IVS,* interventricular septum; *ALMV,* anterior leaflet of the mitral valve; *Ao-LV tunnel,* aortico-left ventricular tunnel.

The coronary arteries usually originate normally and are not included in the malformation. The right coronary artery emerged from the tunnel in only one reported case (16). The aortic valve is abnormal in a large percentage of cases. The leaflets are thickened, and the aortic-left ventricular junction is frequently dilated, with resulting aortic valvular regurgitation (13,21,22,24). The ascending aorta is always dilated, and the left ventricle is dilated and hypertrophied.

Two-dimensional echocardiography has been found to be useful in the diagnosis of aortico-left ventricular tunnel (16,18–20). The views utilized are the parasternal long- and short-axis, apical long-axis, and apical and subcostal four-chamber views, with the transducer angled superiorly or anteriorly to image the left ventricular outflow tract. In the parasternal long-axis, apical long-axis, and subcostal long-axis views, two left ventricular outflows are seen, a posterior one corresponding to the aorta and an anterior one that corresponds to the tunnel and terminates in the anterior aortic wall. The parasternal short-axis view at the level of the aortic valve demonstrates the tunnel orifice located in front of the anterior right coronary cusp. With the transducer aimed posteriorly or inferiorly, the tunnel can be visualized in front of the left ventricular outflow tract. Color Doppler flow mapping demonstrates systolic and retrograde diastolic flow at the level of the tunnel. The aortic regurgitant jet can also be seen from this view. The anatomic characteristics of the aortic valve should be evaluated carefully because a severe gradient across the aortic valve can be underestimated owing to the flow through the tunnel, only to be revealed after surgical closure of the tunnel.

Associated Anomalies

Anomalies that have been found in association with aortico-left ventricular tunnel include bicuspid aortic valve (1,2,7,9,16), critical aortic stenosis (23), pulmonic valve stenosis (1,16), patent foramen ovale (7,16,21), patent ductus arteriosus (6,7,16,21), aneurysm of the right sinus of Valsalva (14), absence of the right coronary artery (8), and ventricular septal defect (19).

ANEURYSMS OF THE SINUSES OF VALSALVA

Congenital aneurysms of the sinuses of Valsalva are a very rare cardiac malformation, found in fewer than 0.1% of patients with congenital heart disease (25) and in 0.05% of all autopsies (26). The incidence is much higher in Orientals: 2% to 3.5% of all congenital cardiac malformations (27,28). The first case of a ruptured aneurysm of the sinus of Valsalva into the right ventricle was observed by Hope in 1837 in a 25-year-old man; this was reported in the third English edition of his book entitled *A Treatise on the Diseases of the Heart and Great Vessels,* published in 1839, and in the first American edition, published in 1842 (29). Aneurysms of the sinuses of Valsalva without rupture are asymptomatic in the first decades of life and cause symptoms only when they obstruct neighboring structures or rupture. Of the 255 cases reviewed by us in the literature, 187 stated the age of the patient, and 83 of these were under the age of 20 (44%) (26–78).

EMBRYOLOGIC CONSIDERATIONS

The embryologic origin of aneurysms of the sinuses of Valsalva is not known. Several theories have been proposed regarding morphogenesis: (a) a defect at the point of fusion of the distal bulbar septum with the aorticopulmonary septum, resulting in thinning of the tissue in that region (39); (b) a local deficiency in the elastic tissue at the base of the aorta (40); (c) failure of continuity between the media of the aorta and the aortic valve annulus (48,49); and (d) a defect in the fibrous annulus of the aorta (63).

ANATOMIC AND ECHOCARDIOGRAPHIC CONSIDERATIONS

The echocardiographic study of aneurysms of the sinuses of Valsalva includes the following: (a) definition of the sinus(es) involved and anatomic characteristics of the aneurysm; (b) determination of the presence of obstruction or rupture and the cavity or structure involved; and (c) evaluation of associated anomalies.

Sinus(es) Involved and Anatomic Characteristics of the Aneurysm

In 99.1% of cases reviewed, only one sinus was involved (26–32,35,67–78). Rarely, two sinuses were dilated (66), and only exceptionally were all three sinuses affected (33). The fundamental pathology of this type of anomaly is the separation between the media of the aorta and the attachment of the leaflets of the aortic valve. The aortic medial layer retracts and does not form part of the dilated sinus of Valsalva, which is made up of dense collagenous fibers without smooth muscular fibers or elastic tissue (48,49,63).

The anterior right coronary sinus was involved in 73% of cases reviewed (Echo. 20-1). The posterior, noncoronary cusp was involved in 20% and the anterior left coronary cusp in 6%. Two sinuses were affected in 0.6% of cases: the anterior right and posterior, noncoronary sinus in 0.3%, and the anterior right and anterior left in 0.3%. The three sinuses were involved in 0.3% of cases reviewed (26–78).

Presence of Obstruction or Rupture and Cavity or Structure Involved

Because of the central anatomic position of the aorta, the four cardiac cavities, pulmonary artery, and pericardial space can be affected by an aneurysm of the sinus of Valsalva (Fig. 20-2). An aneurysm of the anterior right sinus can involve the right ventricle, right atrium, left ventricle, pulmonary artery, and pericardium (Fig. 20-2A). An aneurysm of the posterior, noncoronary sinus can extend to the right atrium and ventricle, left atrium and ventricle, and pericardial space (Fig. 20-2B). An aneurysm of the anterior left coronary sinus can affect the right and left atria, right and left ventricles, pulmonary artery, and pericardial space (Fig. 20-2C).

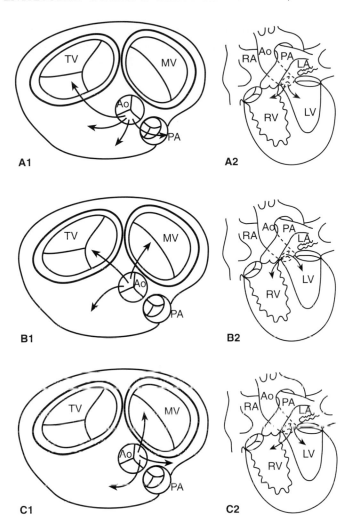

FIG. 20-2. Schematic drawings demonstrating the various locations of aneurysms of the sinuses of Valsalva and the sites of probable rupture into the cardiac chambers, pulmonary artery, or pericardial space (*arrows*). **A1,2:** Aneurysm of the right anterior sinus of Valsalva. **B1,2:** Aneurysm of the posterior, noncoronary sinus of Valsalva. **C1,2:** Aneurysm of the left anterior sinus of Valsalva. *TV*, tricuspid valve; *MV*, mitral valve; *Ao*, aorta; *PA*, pulmonary artery; *RA*, right atrium; *LA*, left atrium; *RV*, right ventricle; *LV*, left ventricle.

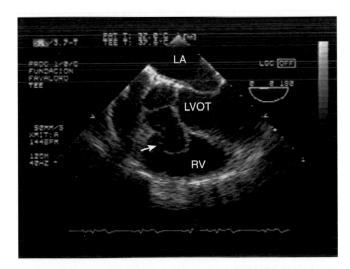

ECHO. 20-1. Transesophageal horizontal view of the aortic valve demonstrating an aneurysm of the right sinus of Valsalva. The *arrow* indicates the point of rupture into the right ventricle. *LA*, left atrium; *LVOT*, left ventricular outflow tract; *RV*, right ventricle. (*Echocardiogram courtesy of Drs. Ana Maria de Dios and Pedro Weisberg, Fundacion Favaloro, Buenos Aires, Argentina*)

Of the 255 cases reviewed in the literature, rupture was present in 222 (87%). In almost all cases, there was only one perforation of the aneurysm, but cases with two or more perforations have been reported (29,42,48,49). Rupture of the anterior right coronary sinus was seen in 161 cases (72.5%); of the posterior, noncoronary sinus in 50 cases (22.7%); of the anterior left sinus in 10 cases (4.4%); and of the anterior right sinus and posterior, noncoronary sinus in one case (0.4%). Of the 161 cases of ruptured aneurysm of the anterior right coronary sinus (Fig. 20-2A), rupture was into the right ventricle in 132 cases (82%) (27,28,30,39,41,42,44,45,47,50,51,56,60,63, 65,66,72,74,77). These cases should not be confused with aortico-right ventricular tunnel, in which the communication with the right ventricle originates in the lateral wall of the aorta, above the anterior right sinus of Valsalva (57,79,80). Rupture into the right atrium was seen in 20 cases (12.5%) (27,28,40,44,51,64,74), and these cases should not be confused with the extremely rare aortico-right atrial tunnel, in which the origin of the communication is found in the lateral wall of the aorta, above the right sinus of Valsalva (81). Rupture into the left ventricle was found in seven cases (4.3%) (38,39,51,55,62,70), into the right atrium and right ventricle in one case (0.6%) (51), and into the pulmonary artery in one case (0.6%) (51).

Of the 50 cases of rupture of an aneurysm of the posterior, noncoronary sinus (Fig. 20-2B), 41 drained into the right atrium (82%) (31,35–37,44,48–51,54,56,60,65, 66,72,74,78) and nine into the right ventricle (18%) (60,64–66). We did not find any cases with rupture into the left atrium or left ventricle; however, Nowicki et al. (67) make reference to one case draining into the left atrium and one into the left ventricle.

Of the 10 cases of rupture of the anterior left coronary sinus (Fig. 20-2C), there was drainage into the left atrium in four cases (40%) (53,58,60,67). In one case of aortico-left ventricular tunnel reported by Yu et al. (82), in which the tunnel communicated with the left atrium at the base of the appendage, it originated in the lateral wall of the aorta, above the anterior left sinus of Valsalva, unlike what is seen in aneurysms. Rupture into the right atrium was found in three cases (30%) (32,69), into the pulmonary artery in two cases (20%) (73,76), and into the left ventricle in one case (10%) (67). Nowicki et al. (67) reported three cases of rupture into the right ventricle in their review of the literature.

Unruptured aneurysms of the sinuses of Valsalva can obstruct the cardiac cavities or adjacent vascular structures or can enter the pericardial space. Cases with obstruction of the right ventricular outflow tract (72,75), dissection of the interventricular septum (70), coronary obstruction (34,61), and protrusion into the pericardial cavity have all been reported (51,61).

The ascending aorta is generally dilated. Anomalies of the aortic valve, such as thickened leaflets, are common, as well as aortic regurgitation resulting from prolapse of a cusp, distortion of the valvular apparatus, or the presence of an interventricular defect (26–28,59,60,64–67,72,83). Cases in which the aneurysm ruptures into the right-sided cavities have a left-to-right shunt with dilatation of the right side of the heart. When the rupture is into the left side of the heart, volume overload of these cavities occurs.

The transthoracic echocardiographic study of congenital aneurysms of the sinuses of Valsalva is performed with the parasternal long- and short-axis views, the apical four-chamber and long-axis views, and the subcostal long- and short-axis views, with the transducer aimed toward the outflows. The parasternal long-axis view allows visualization of the anterior right and posterior, noncoronary sinuses, whereas the short-axis view demonstrates all three sinuses.

An aneurysm of the right anterior sinus of Valsalva can be seen from the standard parasternal long-axis view and from the long-axis view with the transducer tilted toward the right ventricular inflow or outflow, depending on the direction of the aneurysm (Fig. 20-2A). The size of the aneurysm varies during the cardiac cycle, usually being larger in diastole. This type of aneurysm can also be observed from the parasternal short-axis view protruding into the right atrium or the right ventricular inflow or outflow. The apical and subcostal four-chamber views, with anterior or superior angulation of the transducer to visualize the right ventricular outflow tract, also demonstrate the extent of the aneurysm.

Aneurysms of the posterior, noncoronary sinus of Valsalva can be visualized from the parasternal long- and short-axis views (Fig. 20-2B). Those involving the anterior left coronary sinus can be evaluated from the parasternal short-axis and apical four-chamber and long-axis views (Fig. 20-2C).

Color Doppler flow mapping allows demonstration of rupture of an aneurysm and the cavity into which it drains. Rupture into the right or left atrium, right ventricle, or pulmonary artery results in continuous flow throughout systole and diastole (Echo. 20-2). Rupture into the left ventricle causes only diastolic flow. Aortic regurgitation is also seen.

Associated Anomalies

The most common associated anomaly is an interventricular septal defect (27,28,30,39,42,49,56,60,64,66, 72,74,76,83). Others are bicuspid aortic valve (27,31, 39,60,61,67), valvar aortic stenosis (39,46), subvalvar aortic stenosis (39,66), unicommissural aortic valve (66), valvar pulmonic stenosis (64,67), infundibular pulmonic stenosis (39,66), bicuspid pulmonic valve (60), tetralogy of Fallot (66,67), pulmonary atresia with ventricular septal defect (76), atrial septal defect (27,58,66,67,76), patent foramen ovale (39,58,67,72,74), coarctation of the aorta (27,39,43,46,52,66), patent ductus arteriosus (27,66,67), persistent left superior vena cava (27,66), tricuspid regurgitation (31,67), mitral stenosis (46), and single coronary artery (39).

INTRAOPERATIVE AND POSTOPERATIVE EVALUATION

The treatment of aortico-left ventricular tunnel is surgical and should be undertaken at the moment of diagnosis to avoid left ventricular dysfunction. Several techniques have been proposed: (a) direct closure of the aortic end of the tunnel with interrupted or continuous sutures, which causes distortion of the aortic cusp coaptation with severe aortic regurgitation in the late postoperative period; (b) closure of the aortic end of the tunnel with a Dacron or pericardial patch; and (c) closure of the aortic and ventricular ends of the tunnel with a Dacron or pericardial patch. In cases in which there is aneurysmal dilatation of the intracardiac portion of the tunnel, a reinforcing patch technique is recommended involving the subvalvular septum and aortic annulus. Some patients require aortic valve replacement during the late postoperative period when aortic regurgitation occurs secondary to distortion of the aortic valve.

Intraoperative study from the transesophageal approach demonstrates the aortic and ventricular ends of the tunnel and the diastolic flow through the tunnel into the left ventricular cavity, similar to that of aortic valve regurgitation.

The treatment of aneurysms of the sinuses of Valsalva is also surgical whether they are ruptured or not, as long as they cause hemodynamic compromise. The surgical treatment of small, unruptured aneurysms that do not produce hemodynamic compromise, with the sole purpose of preventing later complications, is controversial. The surgical treatment consists of closure of the orifice of the aneurysm in the sinus of Valsalva with a Dacron patch and resection of the windsock in the chamber into which it ruptured. In cases associated with aortic regurgitation, this should be dealt with at the time of surgery, either with a plastic repair or valve replacement.

The transesophageal study demonstrates the dilatation of the aortic sinuses associated with aneurysms, the typical windsock, and the presence of aortic regurgitation

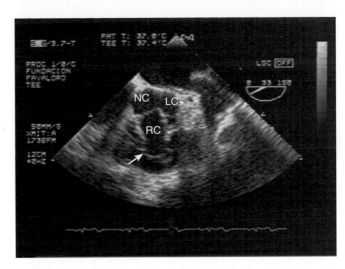

ECHO 20-3. Transesophageal short-axis view of the aortic valve, showing the aneurysm of the right sinus of Valsalva. *Arrow* indicates the point of rupture. *RC*, right coronary cusp; *LC*, left coronary cusp; *NC*, noncoronary cusp. (*Echocardiogram courtesy of Drs. Ana Maria de Dios and Pedro Weisberg, Fundacion Favaloro, Buenos Aires, Argentina*)

(Echos. 20-1–20-3; see also color plate 69 following p. 364).

REFERENCES

1. Levy MJ, Lillehei CW, Anderson RC, Amplatz K, Edwards JE. Aortico-left ventricular tunnel. *Circulation* 1963;27:841–853.
2. Edwards JE. Aneurysm of lower part of ascending aorta rupturing into left ventricle. In: Edwards JE, ed. *Diseases of the great vessels*. Philadelphia: WB Saunders, 1961:1142–1143 (*Atlas of acquired diseases of the heart and great vessels*, Vol. 3).
3. Okorama EO, Perry LW, Scott III LP, McClenathan JE. Aortico-left ventricular tunnel. Clinical profile, diagnostic features, and surgical considerations. *J Thorac Cardiovasc Surg* 1976;71:238–244.
4. Cook AC, Fagg NLK, Ho SY, et al. Echocardiographic-anatomical correlations in aorto-left ventricular tunnel. *Br Heart J* 1995;74:443–448.
5. Goor DA, Lillehei CW. Malformation of the aortic pathway. In: Goor DA, Lillehei CW, eds. *Congenital malformations of the heart*. New York: Grune & Stratton, 1975:237–311.
6. Cooley RN, Harris LC, Rodin AE. Abnormal communication between the aorta and left ventricle. Aortico-left ventricular tunnel. *Circulation* 1965;31:564–571.
7. Bove KE, Schwartz DC. Aortico-left ventricular tunnel. A new concept. *Am J Cardiol* 1967;19:696–709.
8. Somerville J, English T, Ross DN. Aorto-left ventricular tunnel. Clinical features and surgical management. *Br Heart J* 1974;36:321–328.
9. Roberts WC, Morrow AG. Aortico-left ventricular tunnel. A cause of massive aortic regurgitation and of intracardiac aneurysm. *Am J Med* 1965;39:662–667.
10. Bernhard WF, Plauth W, Fyler D. Unusual abnormalities of the aortic root or valve necessitating surgical correction in early childhood. *N Engl J Med* 1970;282:68–71.
11. Fishbone G, DeLeuchtenberg N, Stansel HC Jr. Aortico-left ventricular tunnel. *Radiology* 1971;98:579–580.
12. Perez-Martinez V, Quero M, Castro C, Moreno F, Brito JM, Merino G. Aortico-left ventricular tunnel. A clinical and pathologic review of this uncommon entity. *Am Heart J* 1973;85:237–245.
13. Nichols GM, Lees MH, Henken DP, Sunderland CO, Starr A.

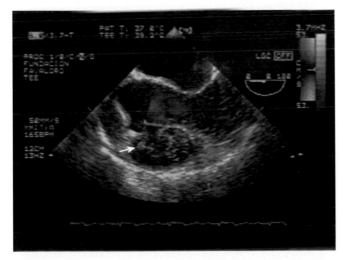

ECHO. 20-2. Color Doppler flow map from the same patient as in Echo. 20-1. The *arrow* indicates the point of rupture of the aneurysm into the right ventricle. Note the jet of flow entering the right ventricle. (*Echocardiogram courtesy of Drs. Ana Maria de Dios and Pedro Weisberg, Fundacion Favaloro, Buenos Aires, Argentina*)

Aortico-left ventricular tunnel. Recognition and repair in infancy. *Chest* 1976;70:74–76.

14. Spooner EW, Dunn JM, Behrendt DM. Aortico-left ventricular tunnel and sinus of Valsalva aneurysm. Case report with operative repair. *J Thorac Cardiovasc Surg* 1978;75:232–236.

15. Sung CS, Leachman RD, Zerpa F, Angelini P, Lufschanowski R. Aortico-left ventricular tunnel. *Am Heart J* 1979;98:87–93.

16. Turley K, Silverman NH, Teitel D, Mavroudis C, Snider R, Rudolph A. Repair of aortico-left ventricular tunnel in the neonate: surgical, anatomic and echocardiographic considerations. *Circulation* 1982; 65:1015–1020.

17. Levy MJ, Schachner A, Blieden LC. Aortico-left ventricular tunnel. Collective review. *J Thorac Cardiovasc Surg* 1982;84:102–109.

18. Perry JC, Nanda NC, Hicks DG, Harris JP. Two-dimensional echocardiographic identification of aortico-left ventricular tunnel. *Am J Cardiol* 1983;52:913–914.

19. Bash SE, Huhta JC, Nihill MR, Vargo TA, Hallman GL. Aortico-left ventricular tunnel with ventricular septal defect: two-dimensional/Doppler echocardiographic diagnosis. *J Am Coll Cardiol* 1985;5:757–760.

20. Humes RA, Hagler DJ, Julsrud PR, Levy JM, Feldt RH, Schaff HV. Aortico-left ventricular tunnel: diagnosis based on two-dimensional echocardiography, color flow Doppler imaging, and magnetic resonance imaging. *Mayo Clin Proc* 1986;61:901–907.

21. Hovaguimian H, Cobanoglu A, Starr A. Aortico-left ventricular tunnel: a clinical review and new surgical classification. *Ann Thorac Surg* 1988;45:106–112.

22. Sreeram N, Franks R, Walsh K. Aortic-ventricular tunnel in a neonate: diagnosis and management based on cross sectional and colour Doppler ultrasonography. *Br Heart J* 1991;65:161–162.

23. Webber S, Johnston B, LeBlanc J, Patterson M. Aortico-left ventricular tunnel associated with critical aortic stenosis in the newborn. *Pediatr Cardiol* 1991;12:237–240.

24. Edwards JE. Aortico-left ventricular tunnel. The case for early treatment [Editorial]. *Chest* 1976;70:5–6.

25. Anderson RH, Macartney FJ, Shinebourne EA, Tynan M, Bush A. The child with a continuous murmur. In: Anderson RH, Macartney FJ, Shinebourne EA, Tynan M, eds. *Paediatric cardiology*, Vol. 2. Edinburgh: Churchill Livingstone, 1987:1001–1022.

26. Falholt W, Thomsen G. Congenital aneurysm of the right sinus of Valsalva, diagnosed by aortography. *Circulation* 1953;8:549–553.

27. Taguchi K, Sasaki N, Matsuura Y, Uemura R. Surgical correction of aneurysm of the sinus of Valsalva. A report of forty-five consecutive patients including eight with total replacement of the aortic valve. *Am J Cardiol* 1969;23:180–191.

28. Tanabe T, Yokota A, Sugie S. Surgical treatment of aneurysms of the sinus of Valsalva. *Ann Thorac Surg* 1979;27:133–136.

29. Hope J. Case of an aneurismal pouch of the aorta bursting into the right ventricle. In: Hope J, ed. *A treatise on the diseases of the heart and great vessels*, 1st American ed. Philadelphia: Lea & Blanchard, 1842:437–439.

30. Hart K. Uber das aneurysma des rechten sinus valsalvae der aorta und seine beziehungen zum oberen ventrikelseptum. *Virchows Arch* 1905;182:167–178.

31. Goehring C. Congenital aneurysm of the aortic sinus of Valsalva. *J Med Res* 1920/1921;42:49–59.

32. Higgins AR. Aneurysm of sinus of Valsalva with rupture into right auricle and death. *U S Naval Bull* 1934;32:47–49.

33. Micks RH. Congenital aneurysms of all three sinuses of Valsalva. *Br Heart J* 1940;2:63–78.

34. Chipps HD. Aneurysm of the sinus of Valsalva causing coronary occlusion. *Arch Pathol* 1941;31:627–630.

35. Kawasaki IA, Benenson AS. Rupture of an aneurysm of a sinus of Valsalva into the right auricle. *Ann Intern Med* 1946;25:150–153.

36. Herrmann GR, Schofield ND. The syndrome of rupture of aortic root or sinus of Valsalva aneurysm into the right atrium. *Am Heart J* 1947;34:87–99.

37. Maynard RM, Thompson CW. Congenital aneurysm of an aortic sinus. *Arch Pathol* 1948;45:65–71.

38. Warthen RO. Congenital aneurysm of the right anterior sinus of Valsalva (interventricular aneurysm) with spontaneous rupture into the left ventricle. *Am Heart J* 1949;37:975–981.

39. Morgan Jones A, Langley FA. Aortic sinus aneurysms. *Br Heart J* 1949;11:325–341.

40. Venning GR. Aneurysms of the sinuses of Valsalva. *Am Heart J* 1951;42:57–69.

41. Fowler REL, Bevil HH. Aneurysms of the sinuses of Valsalva. With report of a case. *Pediatrics* 1951;8:340–348.

42. Burchell HB, Edwards JE. Aortic sinus aneurysm with communications into the right ventricle and associated ventricular septal defect. *Proc Staff Meet Mayo Clin* 1951;26:336–340.

43. Steinberg I, Finby N. Congenital aneurysm of the right aortic sinus associated with coarctation of the aorta and subacute bacterial endocarditis. Ante-mortem report of a case. *N Engl J Med* 1955;253: 549–552.

44. Oram S, East T. Rupture of aneurysm of aortic sinus (of Valsalva) into the right side of the heart. *Br Heart J* 1955;17:541–551.

45. Brown JW, Heath D, Whitaker W. Cardioaortic fistula. A case diagnosed in life and treated surgically. *Circulation* 1955;12:819–826.

46. Steinberg I, Finby N. Clinical manifestations of the unperforated aortic sinus aneurysm. *Circulation* 1956;14:115–124.

47. Harris EJ. Aneurysms of the sinus of Valsalva. *Am J Roentgenol* 1956;76:767–772.

48. Edwards JE, Burchell HB. Specimen exhibiting the essential lesion in aneurysm of the aortic sinus. *Proc Staff Meet Mayo Clin* 1956; 31:407–412.

49. Edwards JE, Burchell HB. The pathological anatomy of deficiencies between the aortic root and the heart, including aortic sinus aneurysms. *Thorax* 1957;12:125–139.

50. Lillehei CW, Stanley P, Varco RL. Surgical treatment of ruptured aneurysms of the sinus of Valsalva. *Ann Surg* 1957;146:459–472.

51. Sawyers JL, Adams JE, Scott HW Jr. Surgical treatment for aneurysms of the aortic sinuses with aorticoatrial fistula. Experimental and clinical study. *Surgery* 1957;41:26–42.

52. Steinberg I, Sammons BP. Aneurysmal dilatation of the aortic sinuses in coarctation of the aorta: report of two new cases and review of the literature. *Ann Intern Med* 1958;49:922–934.

53. Kay JH, Anderson RM, Lewis RR, Reinberg M. Successful repair of sinus of Valsalva-left atrial fistula. *Circulation* 1959;20:427–429.

54. Winfield ME. Rupture of an aneurysm of the posterior sinus of Valsalva into the right atrium. *Am J Cardiol* 1959;3:688–691.

55. Tasaka S, Yoshitoshi Y, Seki K, Koide K, Ogata E, Nakamura K. Congenital aneurysm of the right coronary sinus of Valsalva with rupture into the left ventricle. *Jpn Heart J* 1960;1:106–112.

56. Sakakibara S, Konno S. Congenital aneurysm of the sinus of Valsalva. Anatomy and classification. *Am Heart J* 1962;63:405–424.

57. Houel J, Raynaud R, Morand P, Pinet F. Communication aorte-ventricule droit (à propos de 3 observations). *Arch Mal Coeur Vaiss* 1961;54:1346–1356.

58. Heiner DC, Hara M, White HJ. Cardioaortic fistulas and aneurysms of sinus of Valsalva in infancy. A report of an aortic-left atrial communication indistinguishable from a ruptured aneurysm of the aortic sinus. *Pediatrics* 1961;27:415–426.

59. London SB, London RE. Production of aortic regurgitation by unperforated aneurysm of the sinus of Valsalva. *Circulation* 1961;24: 1403–1406.

60. Magidson O, Kay JH. Ruptured aortic sinus aneurysms. Clinical and surgical aspects of seven cases. *Am Heart J* 1963;65:597–606.

61. Eliot RS, Wolbrink A, Edwards JE. Congenital aneurysm of the left aortic sinus. A rare lesion and a rare cause of coronary insufficiency. *Circulation* 1963;28:951–956.

62. Morgan RI, Mazur JH. Congenital aneurysm of aortic root with fistula to left ventricle. A case report with autopsy findings. *Circulation* 1963;28:589–594.

63. Kwittken J, Christopoulus P, Dua NK, Bruno MS. Congenital and acquired aortic sinus aneurysm. A case report of each with histologic study. *Arch Intern Med* 1965;115:684–691.

64. Morch JE, Greenwood WF. Rupture of the sinus of Valsalva. A study of eight cases with discussion on the differential diagnosis of continuous murmurs. *Am J Cardiol* 1966;18:827–836.

65. Morgan JR, Rogers AK, Fosburg RG. Ruptured aneurysms of the sinus of Valsalva. *Chest* 1972;61:640–643.

66. Howard RJ, Moller J, Castaneda AR, Varco RL, Nicoloff DM. Surgical correction of sinus of Valsalva aneurysm. *J Thorac Cardiovasc Surg* 1973;66:420–427.

67. Nowicki ER, Aberdeen E, Friedman S, Rashkind WJ. Congenital

left aortic sinus-left ventricle fistula and review of aortocardiac fistulas. *Ann Thorac Surg* 1977;23:378–388.

68. Spooner EW, Dunn JM, Behrendt DM. Aortico-left ventricular tunnel and sinus of Valsalva aneurysm. Case report with operative repair. *J Thorac Cardiovasc Surg* 1978;75:232–236.

69. Oberhansli I, Friedli B. Aneurysm of the left sinus of Valsalva draining into the right atrium. *Chest* 1979;76:322–324.

70. Engel PJ, Held JS, Van der Bel-Kahn J, Spitz H. Echocardiographic diagnosis of congenital sinus of Valsalva aneurysm with dissection of the interventricular septum. *Circulation* 1981;63:705–711.

71. Lewis BS, Agathangelou NE. Echocardiographic diagnosis of unruptured sinus of Valsalva aneurysm. *Am Heart J* 1984;107:1025–1027.

72. Terdjman M, Bourdarias JP, Farcot JC, et al. Aneurysms of sinus of Valsalva: two-dimensional echocardiographic diagnosis and recognition of rupture into the right heart cavities. *J Am Coll Cardiol* 1984;3:1227–1235.

73. Heilman KJ III, Groves BM, Campbell D, Blount SG Jr. Rupture of left sinus of Valsalva aneurysm into the pulmonary artery. *J Am Coll Cardiol* 1985;5:1005–1007.

74. Mayer ED, Ruffmann K, Saggau W, et al. Ruptured aneurysms of the sinus of Valsalva. *Ann Thorac Surg* 1986;42:81–85.

75. Kiefaber RW, Tabakin BS, Coffin LH, Gibson TC. Unruptured sinus of Valsalva aneurysm with right ventricular outflow obstruc-

tion diagnosed by two-dimensional and Doppler echocardiography. *J Am Coll Cardiol* 1986;7:438–442.

76. Scagliotti D, Fisher EA, Deal BJ, Gordon D, Chomka EV, Brundage BH. Congenital aneurysm of the left sinus of Valsalva with an aortopulmonary tunnel. *J Am Coll Cardiol* 1986;7:443–445.

77. Chia BL, Ee BK, Choo MH, Yan PC. Ruptured aneurysm of sinus of Valsalva: recognition by Doppler color flow mapping. *Am Heart J* 1988;115:686–688.

78. Peters P, Juziuk E, Gunther S. Doppler color flow mapping detection of ruptured sinus of Valsalva aneurysm. *J Am Soc Echocardiogr* 1989;2:195–197.

79. Bharati S, Lev M, Cassels DE. Aortico-right ventricular tunnel. *Chest* 1973;63:198–202.

80. Saylam A, Tuncali T, Ikizler C, Aytac A. Aorto-right ventricular tunnel. A new concept in congenital cardiac malformations. *Ann Thorac Surg* 1974;18:634–637.

81. Otero Coto E, Caffarena JM, Such M, Marques JL. Aorta-right atrial communication. Report of an unusual case. *J Thorac Cardiovasc Surg* 1980;80:941–944.

82. Yu LC, Bharati S, Thilenius O, Lamberti J, Lev M, Arcilla RA. Congenital aortico-left atrial tunnel. *Pediatr Cardiol* 1979/80;1:153–158.

83. Sakakibara S, Konno S. Congenital aneurysm of the sinus of Valsalva associated with ventricular septal defect. Anatomical aspects. *Am Heart J* 1968;75:595–603.

CHAPTER 21

Hypoplastic Left-Heart Syndrome

Lilliam M. Valdes-Cruz and Raul O. Cayre

The hypoplastic left-heart syndrome comprises a complex of malformations characterized by aortic atresia, hypoplasia of the ascending aorta, left ventricular hypoplasia, and stenosis or atresia of the mitral valve. The first case of aortic atresia was reported by Canton in 1850 (1). Several cases of aortic atresia and hypoplastic left ventricle associated with ascending aortic hypoplasia and mitral stenosis or atresia were later published under the denomination of aortic atresia (2–9). Mueller (10) was the first to use the term congenital left-sided stenosis of the cavity of the heart. Friedman et al. in 1951 (11) reported four cases of aortic atresia or severe stenosis with hypoplasia of the left atrium, mitral valve, left ventricle, and aortic arch under the name of aortic atresia with hypoplasia of the left heart and aortic arch. Lev in 1952 (12) included cases of hypoplasia of the aorta with stenosis or atresia of the valve in a group of cases demonstrating what he called hypoplasia of the aortic tract complex. The term hypoplastic left-heart syndrome, the most commonly used in reference to this type of cardiac malformation, was first proposed by Noonan and Nadas in 1958 (13).

The incidence of hypoplastic left-heart syndrome varies between 1.3% and 7.5% of all cases of congenital heart disease (14–18).

EMBRYOLOGIC CONSIDERATIONS

The morphogenetic processes that result in hypoplastic left-heart syndrome are not completely known. Some authors suggest that narrowing or premature closure of the foramen ovale during an early developmental stage causes a reduction in blood flow to the left-sided cardiac cavities of the embryo, resulting in failure of development of the left-sided structures (19–22). Observations by Hawkins et al. (23) of hearts with aortic atresia support the theory of blood flow as one of the factors contributing to cardiac development. Harh et al. (24) demonstrated experimentally that obstruction of mitral blood flow results in vari-

able degrees of hypoplasia of the mitral valve, left ventricle, and aorta. Van der Linde-Sipman and Wensing (25) have proposed that the primary anomaly resulting in aortic atresia occurs at the level of the atrioventricular junction. According to these authors, an abnormal development of the cushions of the atrioventricular canal is principally responsible for a reduction in blood flow to the left-sided cavities, with resultant failure of development

ANATOMIC AND ECHOCARDIOGRAPHIC CONSIDERATIONS

The echocardiographic study of hypoplastic left-heart syndrome should assess the following: (a) visceroatrial situs, (b) anatomic characteristics of the malformation, (c) any shunting at atrial and/or ductal levels, (d) any ventriculocoronary communications, and (e) any associated anomalies. Intraoperative and postoperative evaluation should be included.

Visceroatrial Situs

The vast majority of cases of hypoplastic left-heart syndrome present with levocardia and situs solitus, and atrioventricular and ventriculoarterial concordance (6–9,11–13,19–21,23,26–35). Few cases present with situs solitus and dextrocardia (36) or situs inversus (37), and rarely is this syndrome associated with bilateral right-sidedness or left-sidedness syndromes (38–42).

Anatomic Characteristics of the Malformation

The right atrium is always dilated, with variable grades of hypertrophy of its walls (Fig. 21-1). In the majority of cases, the venae cavae and coronary sinus drain normally into the right atrium. The right atrial appendage is larger than the left atrial appendage. The annulus of the tricuspid

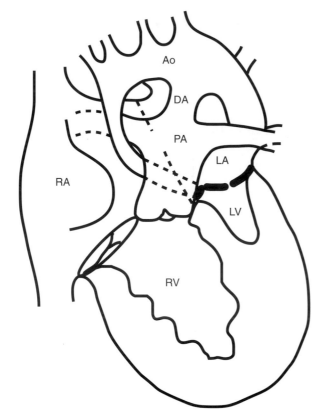

FIG. 21-1. Schematic drawing of a heart with hypoplastic left-heart syndrome with valvular mitral stenosis and aortic valve atresia. Note the *dotted line* indicating the plane of the atrial septum and presence of a defect. *RA*, right atrium; *LA*, left atrium; *RV*, right ventricle; *LV*, left ventricle; *Ao*, aorta; *PA*, pulmonary artery; *DA*, ductus arteriosus.

valve is always dilated, and the valve can be morphologically normal or dysplastic, with thickened leaflets, fused commissures, rolled cusps, shortened chordae, and thickened and small papillary muscles (6,7,9,11,19). The right ventricle is dilated and hypertrophied and forms the cardiac apex; on rare occasions it is only dilated (8,9). The pulmonic valve is almost always normal, and the pulmonary arterial trunk and its branches are dilated. Hypoplasia of the pulmonary arteries has been seen in aortic atresia associated with corrected transposition of the great arteries and severe regurgitation of the systemic atrioventricular valve (35,43,44).

The left atrium is hypoplastic and sometimes very small, and its walls are thin (11,19). Usually, the pulmonary veins drain normally into the left atrium. The left atrial appendage is small. The mitral valve is stenotic in 64% to 66% of cases and atretic in the rest (31,42). In cases with mitral atresia, the valve is represented by an imperforate membrane separating the left atrium and ventricle. If stenotic, the valve can be severely dysplastic, with a small annulus, thickened leaflets, short chordae inserting directly into the ventricular wall, and poorly developed or rudimentary papillary muscles (6,7,

11,19,21). The valve can also be hypoplastic and competent (23).

The left ventricle is extremely hypoplastic and can be reduced to a slit covered with endothelium within the right ventricular wall in cases with mitral valve atresia. If the mitral valve is patent, the left ventricle can be a small, moderately hypertrophied cavity with thickened endocardium and endocardial fibroelastosis.

The aortic valve is atretic. Frequently, three fused cusps are present with three raphes representing the points of fusion of the leaflets. More rarely, there may be a membrane without vestiges of commissural fusion (7,19). The ventriculoaortic junction or aortic annulus, as well as the aortic root and ascending aorta, are hypoplastic. Coarctation of the aorta is seen in 70% to 80% of cases (32,35,42,44–46) and is considered an integral component of the syndrome (35).

The echocardiographic views used to define the anatomic characteristics of all structures involved in the hypoplastic left-heart syndrome are the standard parasternal long-axis view and long-axis view of the right ventricular inflow; the parasternal short-axis view; the apical four-chamber, two-chamber, and long-axis views; the subcostal long- and short-axis views; and the suprasternal long- and short-axis views (Echo. 21-1). These views allow evaluation of the size of the cardiac cavities and the characteristics of the atrioventricular and semilunar valves, pulmonary artery and its branches, and ascending, transverse, and descending aorta.

Presence of Shunting at Atrial and/or Ductal Levels

The atrial septum is usually thickened, and a patent foramen ovale or a small ostium secundum type of atrial septal defect is frequently present. Mahowald et al. (42) reported three cases with a sinus venosus type of atrial defect. In some cases, the floor of the fossa ovalis is fenestrated (19,29,42). Cases with an intact atrial septum have been reported (8,11,13,20,21,23,28,42). In the presence of mitral valve atresia and either an intact atrial septum or a restrictive defect, the outflow from the left atrium is a venous channel, called the levoatriocardinal vein, connecting a pulmonary vein with a systemic vein (35,47–49), the left atrium with the superior vena cava (42), or the left atrium with the coronary sinus (unroofed coronary sinus) (26,50,51). In 25% of cases, a redundant atrial septum can cause a degree of obstruction to tricuspid inflow (52). Watson and Rowe (26) and Kanjuh et al. (27) published cases with totally absent interatrial septum or common atrium.

A large patent ductus arteriosus is present in most cases of hypoplastic left-heart syndrome. The ductus allows retrograde flow into the ascending aorta and is the only source of blood flow into the coronary arteries.

The echocardiographic study of the atrial septum is

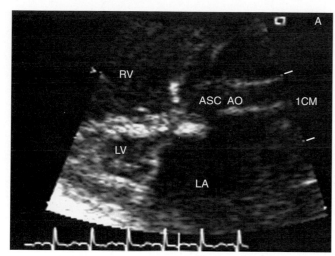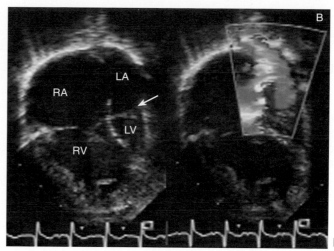

A
B

ECHO. 21-1. **A:** Parasternal long-axis view, magnified to demonstrate the atretic aortic valve and hypoplastic left ventricle and ascending aorta. Note the *1-cm mark* at the right edge of the image. **B:** Apical four-chamber view of the hypoplastic left ventricle, dilated right ventricle, and large atrial communication with left-to-right shunting. Note the lack of flow across the atretic mitral valve (*arrow*). *RV*, right ventricle; *LV*, left ventricle; *ASC AO*, ascending aorta; *LA*, left atrium; *RA*, right atrium.

accomplished from the parasternal short-axis view, the apical four-chamber view, and the subcostal long- and short-axis views (Echos. 21-1B, 21-2; see also color plate 70 following p. 364). Color Doppler flow mapping demonstrates the presence and direction of shunting across the atrial septum. Spectral Doppler allows recording of the velocity of flow across the defect and confirmation of the direction and timing of the shunting, which is mostly from left to right. This is important to determine if the communication is restrictive or not (Echo. 21-2).

The ductus arteriosus can be seen echocardiographically from the parasternal long-axis view of the right ventricular outflow tract, the parasternal short-axis view, the subcostal four-chamber view with superior or anterior angulation of the transducer, the high left parasternal or subclavicular view, and the suprasternal long-axis view. From these views, Doppler color flow mapping and spectral Doppler traces confirm the presence, direction, and velocity of the flow at ductal level (Echo. 21-3). The pulmonary arterial flow is continuous with that of the

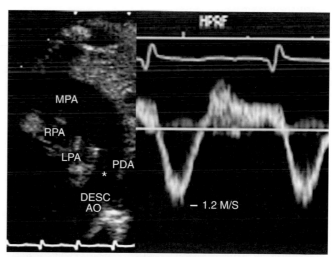

ECHO. 21-3. **Left:** Short-axis view of the pulmonary arteries and a large patent ductus arteriosus (*asterisk*) connecting the descending aorta and main pulmonary artery. Note that the descending aorta is of normal size because of the blood flow from the pulmonary artery through the ductus. **Right:** Spectral Doppler recording of the velocities at the asterisk. Note that the flow is predominantly from right to left (pulmonary artery to aorta), although there is also some left-to-right shunting in diastole. *MPA*, main pulmonary artery; *RPA*, right pulmonary artery; *LPA*, left pulmonary artery; *PDA*, patent ductus arteriosus; *DESC AO*, descending aorta.

ECHO. 21-2. **Left:** Subcostal view in hypoplastic left-heart syndrome demonstrating the interatrial communication. **Right:** Spectral Doppler recording of the velocity across the atrial communication. Note the low velocity and predominant left-to-right shunt. *LA*, left atrium; *RA*, right atrium; *RV*, right ventricle; *LV,* left ventricle.

descending aorta, and the ascending aorta is filled in retrograde fashion (Echo. 21-4).

Presence of Ventriculocoronary Communications

Almost always, the origin and distribution of the coronary arteries are normal in cases of hypoplastic left-heart syndrome (Echo. 21-5). Bharati et al. (53) published one case with anomalous origin of both coronary arteries from the pulmonary artery. The presence of single right and single left coronary arteries has been reported by Baffa et al. (54). In patients with a competent mitral valve, ventriculocoronary communications can be seen between the left ventricular cavity and the coronary arteries (21,32,54–56). These communications are similar to those seen in pulmonary atresia with intact ventricular septum and a competent tricuspid valve and can be found between the left ventricle and any of the coronary arteries. Raghib et al. (21) reported one case with communications between the left ventricle and right coronary artery and between the left ventricle and circumflex coronary artery, and an arteriovenous fistula between the circumflex artery and coronary sinus.

Color Doppler flow mapping demonstrates the presence of these communications. From the apical and subcostal four-chamber views, color Doppler identifies them as systolic flows at the level of the interventricular septum or the right ventricular free wall. The origin and distribution of the proximal coronary arteries can be seen from the parasternal short-axis view with the transducer aimed toward the aortic valve level.

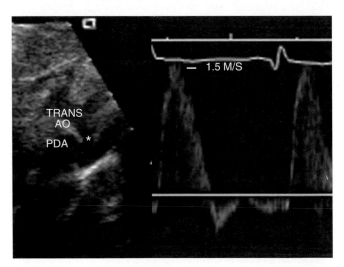

ECHO. 21-4. Left: Suprasternal notch view of the hypoplastic transverse aortic arch and patent ductus arteriosus in hypoplastic left-heart syndrome. **Right:** The spectral Doppler velocity obtained at the asterisk demonstrates the retrograde flow into the transverse aortic arch through the patent ductus arteriosus supplying the ascending aorta and coronary circulation. *TRANS AO,* transverse aortic arch; *PDA,* patent ductus arteriosus.

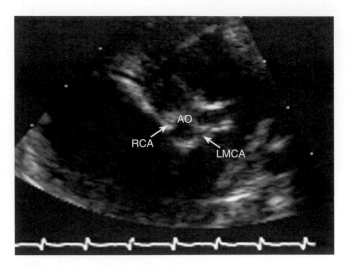

ECHO. 21-5. Parasternal short-axis view of the hypoplastic aortic root showing the normal origins of the right and left coronary arteries. *AO,* aorta; *RCA,* right coronary artery; *LMCA,* left main coronary artery.

Associated Anomalies

The following anomalies have been found in association with the hypoplastic left-heart syndrome: bicuspid pulmonic valve (32,42), dysplastic pulmonic valve (19,33), stenosis of the pulmonic valve (11), tricuspid stenosis (32), Ebstein's anomaly of the tricuspid valve (42), double tricuspid orifice (32,55), double-outlet right ventricle (55,57), complete transposition of the great vessels (42,55,57), corrected transposition of the great vessels (58), partial or complete atrioventricular septal defect (26,42,55), unbalanced atrioventricular septal defect (57), pulmonary vein hypoplasia (32), partial or total anomalous pulmonary venous connection (19,42,59–63), persistent left superior vena cava draining into the coronary sinus (19,32,52), persistent left superior vena cava draining directly into the left atrium with absence of the coronary sinus (42), bilateral inferior vena cava (42), cor triatriatum sinister (42,59,62), absent coronary sinus (29), atresia of the coronary sinus orifice (29), juxtaposed atrial appendages (55), interrupted aortic arch (55), superoinferior ventricles (36), and right aortic arch (32).

INTRAOPERATIVE AND POSTOPERATIVE EVALUATION

Two options are available for the surgical treatment of hypoplastic left-heart syndrome: cardiac transplantation and staged reconstructive techniques.

The staged reconstructive technique was first proposed and accomplished by Norwood et al. in 1980 (64); since then, it has undergone various modifications (55,65–69). At present, it comprises three stages: stage I or Norwood operation in the neonatal period, stage II or bidirectional cavopulmonary shunt (Glenn) or hemi-Fontan procedure undertaken at 4 to 10 months of age, and stage III or

Fontan procedure carried out at 12 to 24 months of age (65–69).

The objectives of the stage I or Norwood operation are (a) prevention of pulmonary venous obstruction, (b) unobstructed flow from the right ventricle to the aorta and coronary arteries, (c) preservation of right ventricular function, and (d) pulmonary blood flow adequate to permit growth of the pulmonary arteries without resulting in right ventricular volume overload (55,64–69). To accomplish these goals, the ductus arteriosus is ligated at a point distal to its aortic end, the pulmonary artery is sectioned near its bifurcation, and the distal portion is closed. The ascending aorta and aortic arch are opened to the juxtaductal area of the isthmus, and an anastomosis is created between the ascending aorta and divided main pulmonary artery with a supplementary cuff of homograft arterial wall to create a neoaorta. The procedure is completed with an atrial septectomy and implantation of a systemic-to-pulmonary arterial shunt. The echocardiographic evaluation following the stage I procedure should focus on assessing the presence of stenosis at any of the anastomotic sites, the patency of the aorticopulmonary shunt, and the presence of any obstruction to the pulmonary venous flow. The most common site of stenosis is at the aortic anastomosis, where narrowing similar to a "coarctation" is commonly seen. The spectral Doppler flow pattern in these cases exhibits the diastolic runoff typically seen in coarctation. In addition, because of the presence of an anastomosis between the main pulmonary artery and ascending aorta, the pulmonary branches are directed around both sides of the neoaorta. Consequently, the classic short-axis view of the great vessels with the right ventricular outflow tract around a central aortic root is not usually obtained.

The objective of stage II is to diminish the volume and pressure overload of the right ventricle. As such, this stage involves ligation of the aorticopulmonary shunt and implantation of a cavopulmonary anastomosis. This can be an end-to-side anastomosis of the superior vena cava to the superior aspect of the right pulmonary artery with ligation of the cardiac end of the sectioned superior vena cava (bidirectional Glenn). The hemi-Fontan is similar, but the superior vena cava is anastomosed to the inferior wall of the right pulmonary artery. The echocardiographic evaluation after stage II includes imaging and Doppler interrogation of the superior vena cava-to-pulmonary artery anastomosis. This is best accomplished from the right subclavicular view, the long-axis suprasternal view with the transducer tilted to the right to reveal the superior vena cava, and the subcostal short-axis sagittal view of the atria. Color Doppler is helpful in visualizing the flow into the right pulmonary artery. The spectral Doppler pattern is characteristic, with low velocity, continuous flow, and accentuation during inspiration.

Stage III is the completion of the Fontan procedure, or total cavopulmonary connection. This involves creation

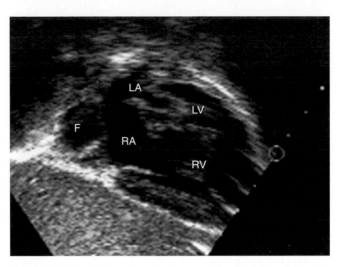

ECHO. 21-6. Subcostal view in a patient with hypoplastic left-heart syndrome who underwent the three stages of the Norwood operation. Note the small left ventricle and the Fontan connection in the right atrium. *RA*, right atrium; *F*, Fontan connection; *LA*, left atrium; *RV*, right ventricle; *LV*, left ventricle.

of a lateral tunnel to channel blood return from the inferior vena cava into the pulmonary artery. Frequently, the intraatrial baffle is fenestrated, thus allowing decompression of the right side of the heart during the early postoperative period. This communication is closed later, either surgically or with a transcatheter device. Echocardiographic study includes evaluation of the right ventricular size and function, the permeability of the cavopulmonary anastomoses, and the shunting across the fenestrated intraatrial baffle. Eventually, as the right ventricular function improves, the right-to-left shunting across the baffle diminishes and may revert to left-to-right shunting. At this time, the fenestration can be closed safely.

The late postoperative echocardiographic evaluation following the three stages would be very similar to that after a Fontan procedure for atrioventricular univentricular connection (Echo. 21-6). The most important features to be considered are size and function of the right ventricle, which is sustaining the systemic circulation; competence of the tricuspid valve; flow across the neoaorta; and flow through the cavopulmonary anastomosis. This is discussed in detail in Chapter 17 (see "Intraoperative and Postoperative Evaluation").

REFERENCES

1. Canton M. Congenital obliteration of origin of the aorta. *Trans Pathol Soc London* 1850;2:38.
2. Martens G. Zwei falle von aortenatresie. *Virchows Arch* 1890;121:322–335.
3. Dudzus M. Uber "Cor triloculare biatriatum" mit atresie des linken venosen ostiums. *Virchows Arch* 1922;237:32–43.
4. Abbott M. Congenital cardiac disease. In: Osler W, ed. *Modern*

medicine. Its theory and practice, Vol 4, 3rd ed. Philadephia: Lea & Febiger, 1927:612–812.

5. Philpott N. Congenital atresia of aortic ring. *Ann Intern Med* 1928; 2:422–427.

6. Roberts JT. A case of congenital aortic atresia. With hypoplasia of ascending aorta, normal origin of coronary arteries, left ventricular hypoplasia and mitral stenosis. *Am Heart J* 1936;12:448–457.

7. Lippincott S. Congenital atresia of the aortic valve without septal defect. Report of case. *Am Heart J* 1939;17:502–506.

8. Anderson NA, Sano ME. Aortic atresia with hypoplasia of the left ventricle. *Am J Dis Child* 1941;62:629–633.

9. Newerla GJ. Associated mitral and aortic atresia or hypoplasia. Case report and review of the literature. *Arch Pediatr* 1944;61:68–74.

10. Mueller B. Ein beitrag zur kenntnis der angeborenen linksseitingen konusverengerungen des herzens. *Virchows Arch* 1924;249:368–373.

11. Friedman S, Murphy L, Ash R. Aortic atresia with hypoplasia of the left heart and aortic arch. *J Pediatr* 1951;38:354–368.

12. Lev M. Pathologic anatomy and interrelationship of hypoplasia of the aortic tract complexes. *Lab Invest* 1952;1:61–70.

13. Noonan JA, Nadas AS. The hypoplastic left heart syndrome. An analysis of 101 cases. *Pediatr Clin North Am* 1958;5:1029–1056.

14. Mitchell SC, Korones SB, Berendes HW. Congenital heart disease in 56,109 births. Incidence and natural history. *Circulation* 1971; 43:323–332.

15. Hoffman JIE, Christianson R. Congenital heart disease in a cohort of 19,502 births with long-term follow-up. *Am J Cardiol* 1978;42: 641–647.

16. Fyler DC, Buckley LP, Hellenbrand WE, Cohn HE. Report of the New England Regional Infant Cardiac Program. *Pediatrics* 1980; 65[Suppl]:375–461.

17. Samanek M, Slavik Z, Zborilova B, Hrobonova V, Voriskova M, Skovranek J. Prevalence, treatment, and outcome of heart disease in live-born children: a prospective analysis of 91,823 live-born children. *Pediatr Cardiol* 1989;10:205–211.

18. Hoffman JIE. Incidence of congenital heart disease: I. Postnatal incidence. *Pediatr Cardiol* 1995;16:103–113.

19. Friedman S, Murphy L, Ash R. Congenital mitral atresia with hypoplastic nonfunctioning left heart. *Am J Dis Child* 1955;90:176–188.

20. Lev M, Arcilla R, Rimoldi HJA, Licata RH, Gasul BM. Premature narrowing or closure of the foramen ovale. *Am Heart J* 1963;65: 638–647.

21. Raghib G, Bloemendaal RD, Kanjuh VI, Edwards JE. Aortic atresia and premature closure of foramen ovale. Myocardial sinusoids and coronary arteriovenous fistula serving as outflow channel. *Am Heart J* 1965;70:476–480.

22. Schall SA, Dalldorf FG. Premature closure of the foramen ovale and hypoplasia of the left heart. *Int J Cardiol* 1984;5:103–107.

23. Hawkins JA, Clark EB, Doty DB. Morphologic characteristics of aortic atresia: implications for fetal hemodynamics. *Int J Cardiol* 1986;10:127–132.

24. Harh JY, Paul MH, Gallen WJ, Friedberg DZ, Kaplan S. Experimental production of hypoplastic left heart syndrome in chick embryo. *Am J Cardiol* 1973;31:51–56.

25. Van der Linde-Sipman JS, Wensing CJG. The left hypoplastic heart syndrome in the minipig. In *Birth defects: original article series*, Vol 14. Baltimore: Williams & Wilkins, 1978:295–314.

26. Watson DG, Rowe RD. Aortic-valve atresia. Report of 43 cases. *JAMA* 1962;179:14–18.

27. Kanjuh VI, Eliot RS, Edwards JE. Coexistent mitral and aortic valvular atresia. A pathologic study of 14 cases. *Am J Cardiol* 1965; 15:611–621.

28. Sinha SN, Rusnak SL, Sommers HM, Cole RB, Muster AJ, Paul MH. Hypoplastic left ventricle syndrome. Analysis of thirty autopsy cases in infants with surgical considerations. *Am J Cardiol* 1968; 21:166–173.

29. Saied A, Folger GM Jr. Hypoplastic left heart syndrome. Clinico-pathologic and hemodynamic correlation. *Am J Cardiol* 1972;29: 190–196.

30. Freedom RM, Williams WG, Dische MR, Rowe RD. Anatomical variants in aortic atresia. Potential candidates for ventriculoaortic reconstitution. *Br Heart J* 1976;38:821–826.

31. Roberts WC, Perry LW, Chandra RS, Myers GE, Shapiro SR, Scott LP. Aortic valve atresia: a new classification based on necropsy study of 73 cases. *Am J Cardiol* 1976;37:753–756.

32. Bharati S, Lev M. The surgical anatomy of hypoplasia of aortic tract complex. *J Thorac Cardiovasc Surg* 1984;88:97–101.

33. Bharati S, Nordenberg A, Brock RR, Lev M. Hypoplastic left heart syndrome with dysplastic pulmonary valve with stenosis. *Pediatr Cardiol* 1984;5:127–130.

34. Lloyd TR, Evans TC, Marvin WJ Jr. Morphologic determinants of coronary blood flow in the hypoplastic left heart syndrome. *Am Heart J* 1986;112:666–671.

35. Freedom RM, Nykanen D. Hypoplastic left heart syndrome: pathologic considerations of aortic atresia and variations on the theme. *Prog Pediatr Cardiol* 1996;5:3–18.

36. Thilenius OG, Bharati S, Lev M, Karp RB, Arcilla RA. Horizontal ventricular septum with dextroversion: hearts with and without aortic atresia. *Pediatr Cardiol* 1987;8:187–193.

37. Raines KH, Armstrong BE. Aortic atresia with visceral situs inversus with mirror-image dextrocardia. *Pediatr Cardiol* 1989;10:232–235.

38. Jue KL. Edwards JE. Anomalous attachments of mitral valve causing subaortic atresia. Observations in a case with other cardiac anomalies and multiple spleens. *Circulation* 1967;35:928–932.

39. Friedberg DZ, Gallen WJ, Oechler HW, Glicklich M. Ivemark syndrome with aortic atresia. *Am J Dis Child* 1973;126:106–108.

40. Freedom RM. Aortic valve and arch anomalies in the congenital asplenia syndrome. Case report, literature review and re-examination of the embryology of the congenital asplenia syndrome. *Johns Hopkins Med J* 1974;135:124–135.

41. Salazar J, Martinez F, Valero MI, Casado de Frias E. Polysplenia with left ventricular hypoplasia and partial anomalous pulmonary venous connection. *Acta Cardiol* 1976;31:483–490.

42. Mahowald JM, Lucas RV Jr, Edwards JE. Aortic valvular atresia. Associated cardiovascular anomalies. *Pediatr Cardiol* 1982;2:99–105.

43. Freedom RM, Benson LN. Hypoplastic left heart syndrome. In: Emmanouilides GC, Allen HD, Riemenschneider TA, Gutgesell HP, eds. *Moss and Adams heart disease in infants, children, and adolescents. Including the fetus and young adult*, Vol. 2, 5th ed. Baltimore: Williams & Wilkins, 1995:1133–1153.

44. Freedom RM, Benson LN, Smallhorn JF. Hypoplastic left heart syndrome. In: Freedom RM, Benson LN, Smallhorn JF, eds. *Neonatal heart disease*. London: Springer-Verlag, 1992:333–356.

45. Von Rueden TJ, Knight L, Moller JH, Edwards JE. Coarctation of aorta associated with aortic valvular atresia. *Circulation* 1975;52: 951–954.

46. Lang P, Jonas RA, Norwood WI, Mayer JE Jr, Castaneda AR. The surgical anatomy of hypoplasia of aortic tract complex [Letter to the Editor]. *J Thorac Cardiovasc Surg* 1985;89:149.

47. Lucas RV Jr, Lester RG, Lillehei CW, Edwards JE. Mitral atresia with levoatriocardinal vein. A form of congenital pulmonary venous obstruction. *Am J Cardiol* 1962;9:607–613.

48. Edwards JE. Malformations of the thoracic veins. In Gould SE, ed. *Pathology of the heart and blood vessels*, 3rd ed. Springfield, IL: Charles C Thomas Publisher, 1968:463–478.

49. Moreira Pinto CA, Ho SY, Redington A, Shinebourne EA, Anderson RH. Morphological features of the levoatriocardinal (or pulmonary-to-systemic collateral) vein. *Pediatr Pathol* 1993;13: 751–761.

50. Rose AG, Beckman CB, Edwards JE. Communications between coronary sinus and left atrium. *Br Heart J* 1974;36:182–185.

51. Freedom RM, Culhman JAG, Rowe RD. Left atrial to coronary sinus fenestration (partially unroofed coronary sinus). Morphological and angiocardiographic observations. *Br Heart J* 1981;46:63–68.

52. Sade RM, Crawford FA Jr, Fyfe DA. Symposium on hypoplastic left heart syndrome [Letter to the Editor]. *J Thorac Cardiovasc Surg* 1986;91:937–939.

53. Bharati S, Szarnicki RJ, Popper R, Fryer A, Lev M. Origin of both coronary arteries from the pulmonary trunk associated with hypoplasia of the aortic tract complex: a new entity. *J Am Coll Cardiol* 1984;3:437–441.

54. Baffa JM, Chen SL, Guttenberg ME, Norwood WI, Weinberg PM. Coronary artery abnormalities and right ventricular histology in

hypoplastic left heart syndrome. *J Am Coll Cardiol* 1992;20:350–358.

55. Norwood WI, Lang P, Castaneda AR, Campbell DN. Experience with operations for hypoplastic left heart syndrome. *J Thorac Cardiovasc Surg* 1981;82:511–519.

56. O'Connor WN, Cash JB, Cottrill CM, Johnson GL, Noonan JA. Ventriculocoronary connections in hypoplastic left hearts: an autopsy microscopic study. *Circulation* 1982;66:1078–1086.

57. Rychik J, Gullquist SD, Jacobs ML, Norwood WI. Doppler echocardiographic analysis of flow in the ductus arteriosus of infants with hypoplastic left heart syndrome: relationship of flow patterns to systemic oxygenation and size of interatrial communication. *J Am Soc Echocardiogr* 1996;9:166–173.

58. Deanfield JE, Anderson RH, Macartney FJ. Aortic atresia with "corrected transposition of the great arteries" (atrioventricular and ventriculoarterial discordance). *Br Heart J* 1981;46:683–686.

59. Gerlis LM, Dickinson DF, Fagan DG. An unusual type of anomalous pulmonary venous drainage associated with a complex left heart hypoplasia and a variety of divided left atrium (cor triatriatum). *Int J Cardiol* 1985;7:245–250.

60. Seliem MA, Chin AJ, Norwood WI. Patterns of anomalous pulmonary venous connection/drainage in hypoplastic left heart syndrome: diagnostic role of Doppler color flow mapping and surgical implications. *J Am Coll Cardiol* 1992;19:135–141.

61. Lucas RV Jr, Anderson RC, Amplatz K, Adams P Jr, Edwards JE. Congenital causes of pulmonary venous obstruction. *Pediatr Clin North Am* 1963;10:781–836.

62. Al-Fadley F, Galal O, Wilson N, Aloufi S. Cor triatriatum associated with total anomalous pulmonary venous drainage in the setting of mitral atresia and a restrictive interatrial communication. *Pediatr Cardiol* 1992;13:125–126.

63. Shone JD, Edwards JE. Mitral atresia associated with pulmonary venous anomalies. *Br Heart J* 1964;26:241–249.

64. Norwood WI, Kirklin JK, Sanders SP. Hypoplastic left heart syndrome: experience with palliative surgery. *Am J Cardiol* 1980;45:87–91.

65. Norwood WI. Hypoplastic left heart syndrome. *Ann Thorac Surg* 1991;52:688–695.

66. Castaneda AR, Jonas RA, Mayer JE Jr, Hanley FL. Hypoplastic left heart syndrome. In: Castaneda AR, Jonas RA, Mayer JE Jr, Hanley FL, eds. *Cardiac surgery of the neonate and infant*. Philadelphia: WB Saunders, 1994:363–385.

67. Norwood WI, Jacobs ML. Hypoplastic left heart syndrome. In: Stark J, De Leval M. *Surgery for congenital heart defects*, 2nd ed. Philadelphia: WB Saunders, 1994:587–598.

68. Backer CL, Bove EL, Zales VR, Mavroudis C. Hypoplastic left heart syndrome. In: Mavroudis C, Backer CL, eds. *Pediatric cardiac surgery*, 2nd ed. St. Louis: Mosby–Year Book, 1994:442–453.

69. Bove EL, Mosca RS. Surgical repair of the hypoplastic left heart syndrome. *Prog Pediatr Cardiol* 1996;5:23–35.

PART IX

Conotruncal Anomalies

CHAPTER 22

Tetralogy of Fallot

Lilliam M. Valdes-Cruz and Raul O. Cayre

Tetralogy of Fallot is a malformation characterized by infundibular pulmonary stenosis, dextroposition of the aorta so that it overrides the ventricular septum, interventricular communication, and hypertrophy of the right ventricle. The first anatomic report, by Niels Stensen, dates from 1671–1672 (1). A detailed anatomic description and discussion of some clinical aspects was authored by Edouard Sandifort in 1777 (2). The first clinical report of a crisis of paroxysmal dyspnea was written by Hunter in 1784 (3), and the most complete description of the four components of the syndrome and its clinical manifestations was made by Arthur Fallot in 1888 (4). Its incidence varies between 3.5% and 10% of all congenital cardiac malformations (5–10).

EMBRYOLOGIC CONSIDERATIONS

The processes of conal, truncal, and aorticopulmonary septation contribute to the morphogenesis of tetralogy of Fallot. An unequal partition of the conus and truncus occurs at the expense of the right ventricular outflow tract, pulmonary valve, and pulmonary artery as a result of an anomalous origin of the conal and truncal crests (11–13) and of the aorticopulmonary septum.

The dextrodorsal and sinistroventral conal crests fuse and give origin to the conal septum, which divides the conus into an anterolateral and a posteromedial conus (see Figs. 1-12, 1-14A). The conal or infundibular septum makes up the septal portion of the crista supraventricularis, which corresponds to the septal surface of the right ventricle located between the limbs of the septomarginal trabecula, and it is normally aligned with the interventricular septum (Fig. 22-1A). The parietal portion of the crista extends from the interventricular septum to the free wall of the right ventricle (Fig. 22-1B). The crista supraventricularis is the fibrous or muscular structure that in hearts with normal outflow tracts separates the pulmonic valve from the tricuspid valve (14) (Fig. 22-1). The dextrodorsal

conal crest and the right lateral cushion of the atrioventricular canal as well as the posterior wall of the conus or conoventricular flange contribute to its embryologic development (15) (see Fig. 1-13).

In tetralogy of Fallot, the conal crests develop abnormally (Fig. 22-2A) and give rise to a conal or infundibular septum that is displaced anteriorly, rightward, and superiorly, causing obstruction of the subpulmonary outflow tract (11,12,16–18) (Fig. 22-2B). Because of the anterior and rightward displacement of the conal septum, the conal or infundibular septum and the interventricular septum are malaligned, which produces the malalignment type of interventricular communication (9,18) and the overriding aorta (18) (Fig. 22-2C).

The anterior and rightward displacement of the infundibular septum, also called the septal portion of the crista supraventricularis, results in a separation between it and the parietal portion of the crista, which in this case is called the ventriculoinfundibular fold (Fig. 22-2B). The ventriculoinfundibular fold is the muscular or fibrous structure that in hearts with pathology of the outflow tracts separates one or both semilunar valves from the atrioventricular orifices (14,18). In tetralogy of Fallot, attenuation of the posterior wall of the conus or conoventricular flange will produce a fibrous ventriculoinfundibular fold, with resulting aortic-tricuspid continuity (Fig. 22-3A,C). Failure of attenuation will be expressed as a muscular ventriculoinfundibular fold, resulting in discontinuity between the aortic and tricuspid valves (Fig. 22-3B).

Van Praagh et al. (19) consider that tetralogy of Fallot is caused by an incomplete development of the subpulmonary conus, which as a consequence would be short, narrow, and shallow. However, the subpulmonary infundibulum in tetralogy is significantly longer than that in normal hearts (20). Therefore, this theory would be valid only in cases of tetralogy with hypoplasia or agenesis of the infundibular septum (Fig. 22-3C).

Several mechanisms have been proposed to explain the

morphogenesis of dextroposition of the aorta. These include rightward displacement and clockwise rotation of the aortic valve (17), retention of the aortic valve in its embryologic position (17), anterior displacement of the conal septum (13,17,21), and failure of normal incorporation of the posterior conus into the left ventricle (13,22,23). We consider these latter two mechanisms most likely to be the ones involved in the morphogenesis of the dextroposed aorta.

Pulmonic valve stenosis, as well as the varying degrees of hypoplasia of the main and branch pulmonary arteries commonly seen in tetralogy of Fallot, are caused by an anomalous partition of the truncus at the expense of the pulmonary artery (11). The truncal swellings develop abnormally, so that the dextrosuperior truncal swelling adopts a more dorsal position and the sinistroinferior truncal swelling acquires a more ventral position (12) (Fig. 22-2A). The aorticopulmonary septum also develops abnormally, resulting in an uneven partition of the truncus, with a pulmonary artery that is smaller than usual (Fig. 22-2A,C).

Tetralogy of Fallot with Pulmonary Atresia

Pulmonary atresia with ventricular septal defect is an extreme form of tetralogy of Fallot (17,24–27). Because of atresia of the infundibulum and/or pulmonic valve, blood enters the pulmonary circulation through a patent

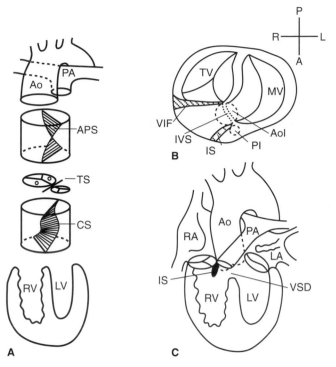

FIG. 22-2. Schematic drawings of the morphogenesis and anatomic characteristics of tetralogy of Fallot. **A:** Schema of the morphogenesis. **B:** View of a transverse cut at the base of the heart. The *dotted lines* indicate the spatial position of the ventricular infundibula and interventricular septum; **C:** Schematic representation of a heart showing the anatomic components of tetralogy of Fallot. *RA*, right atrium; *LA*, left atrium; *RV*, right ventricle; *LV*, left ventricle; *CS*, conal septum; *TS*, truncal septum; *APS*, aorticopulmonary septum; *TV*, tricuspid valve; *MV*, mitral valve; *AoI*, aortic infundibulum; *PI*, pulmonic infundibulum; *IS*, infundibular septum; *IVS*, interventricular septum; *VSD*, ventricular septal defect; *VIF*, ventriculoinfundibular fold; *Ao*, aorta; *PA*, pulmonary artery. *A*, anterior; *P*, posterior; *R*, right; *L*, left.

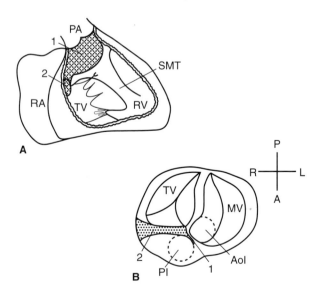

FIG. 22-1. Schematic representation of the anatomic characteristics of the crista supraventricularis. **A:** View of the right septal surface. **B:** View of a transverse cut at the base of the heart. *1*, septal portion of the crista supraventricularis; *2*, parietal portion of the crista supraventricularis; *TV*, tricuspid valve; *MV*, mitral valve; *SMT*, septomarginal trabecula; *PI*, pulmonary infundibulum; *AoI*, aortic infundibulum; *PA*, pulmonary artery; *RA*, right atrium; *RV*, right ventricle. *A*, anterior; *P*, posterior; *R*, right; *L*, left.

ductus arteriosus, systemic arterial collaterals, or bronchial arteries (28). The morphogenesis, although similar to that of tetralogy with pulmonic stenosis, differs in two respects: (a) the infundibular septum, which is displaced anteriorly and rightward, is fused with the free wall of the right ventricle (26), and (b) systemic-to-pulmonary collaterals are present.

The morphogenesis of these collaterals is related to the development of the intersegmentary arteries, which in turn is related to the formation of the respiratory apparatus. The respiratory apparatus originates from an evagination of the anterior wall of the foregut. This evagination is surrounded by a pulmonary vascular plexus, which is connected to the dorsal aortas by the intersegmentary arteries (29,30) (Fig. 22-4A). The sixth aortic arch, which will give rise to the right and left pulmonary arterial branches and to the ductus arteriosus, appears later in development. When the sixth aortic arch connects with the pulmonary plexus, blood flow to the arch through the intersegmentary arteries ceases, and the intersegmentary arteries subsequently involute and disappear (Fig. 22-4B). The bronchial arteries appear later in development, after the intersegmentary arteries have been resorbed (31). In pulmonary atresia with interventricular communication, failure of connection between the sixth aortic arch and the pulmonary vascular plexus determines that the intersegmentary arteries will persist as systemic arterial collaterals providing blood flow to the pulmonary circulation. If the pulmonary branches and ductus arteriosus (sixth arch) fail to develop at an early stage, the intersegmentary arteries will persist as large systemic-to-pulmonary collaterals (28). If the ductus is present, no systemic collateral branches will supply the same lung as the duct (28,32–34), as the presence of a ductus and the presence of systemic-to-pulmonary collaterals are mutually exclusive (28,33). If pulmonary atresia occurs later in development, the pulmonary circulation will be supported by bronchial arteries (35).

Tetralogy of Fallot with Absent Pulmonary Valve

This is a rare variant of tetralogy of Fallot characterized by, in addition to the anatomic characteristics of

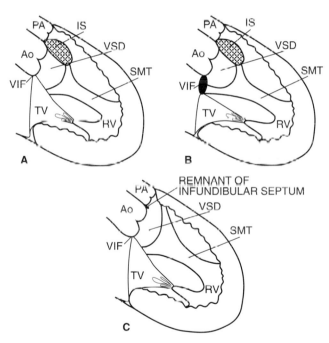

FIG. 22-3. Schematic drawings of the anatomic characteristics of the right ventricle and the relationship of the atrioventricular and semilunar valves with the ventricular septal defect in the variants of tetralogy of Fallot. **A:** With fibrous ventriculoinfundibular fold and aortic-tricuspid continuity. **B:** With muscular ventriculoinfundibular fold and aortic-tricuspid discontinuity. **C:** With absence of the infundibular septum, doubly committed ventricular septal defect, and aortic-tricuspid continuity. *IS*, infundibular septum; *VIF*, ventriculoinfundibular fold; *VSD*, ventricular septal defect; *SMT*, septomarginal trabecula; *RV*, right ventricle; *Ao*, aorta; *PA*, pulmonary artery; *TV*, tricuspid valve.

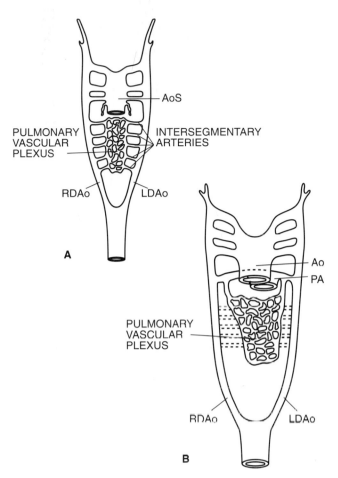

FIG. 22-4. Schematic representation of the development of the pulmonary vascular plexus, the intersegmentary arteries, and the connection between the pulmonary arteries and the pulmonary vascular plexus. **A:** Development of the intersegmentary arteries between the pulmonary vascular plexus and the dorsal aortas. **B:** Connection of the pulmonary arteries with the pulmonary vascular plexus. The *dotted lines* indicate the intersegmentary arteries, which disappear. *AoS*, aortic sac; *RDAo*, right dorsal aorta; *LDAo*, left dorsal aorta; *Ao*, aorta; *PA*, pulmonary artery.

tetralogy, a hypoplastic pulmonary annulus, rudimentary or absent pulmonic valve cusps, aneurysmal dilatation of the pulmonary arterial branches, and absence of the ductus arteriosus (25,36). The morphogenetic mechanism is similar to that of tetralogy. The embryologic origin of the absence or rudimentary development of the pulmonic valve and of the aneurysmal dilatation of the branches is unknown; however, an alteration in the cells of the neural crest has been mentioned as a possible mechanism interfering with the normal development of the pulmonic valve (37,38). Absence of the ductus arteriosus and the resulting failure of the pulmonary circulation to decompress through the ductus have been proposed to explain the intrauterine dilatation of the pulmonary branches (39). Other mechanisms that have been proposed to explain such dilatation are stenosis of the pulmonary annulus (39); histologic abnormalities of the pulmonary arterial wall, such as cystic medial necrosis similar to that seen in Marfan syndrome (40); and the orientation of the infundibular septum (41).

ANATOMIC AND ECHOCARDIOGRAPHIC CONSIDERATIONS

The echocardiographic study of tetralogy of Fallot, in addition to a determination of visceroatrial situs, atrioventricular concordance, and systemic and pulmonary venous drainages, should comprise an analysis of (a) the subpulmonary infundibular obstruction, (b) the location and anatomic characteristics of the interventricular communication, (c) the degree of dextroposition and overriding of the aorta, (d) the size of the right ventricle-pulmonary trunk junction (pulmonary annulus) and characteristics of the valve, (e) the size of the main and branch pulmonary arteries and sources of the pulmonary blood flow, (f) the origin and distribution of the coronary arteries, and (g) any associated anomalies. Intraoperative and postoperative echocardiographic evaluation should be included.

Subpulmonary Infundibular Obstruction

The fundamental morphologic characteristic of tetralogy of Fallot is the anterior, rightward, and superior displacement of the infundibular septum (42–44) (Figs. 22-2; 22-3A,B). In the normal heart, the infundibular septum or septal portion of the crista supraventricularis is a small structure located between the two limbs of the septomarginal trabecula (Fig. 22-1A). It is aligned with the interventricular septum and occupies an oblique spatial position with respect to the frontal plane (Fig. 22-1B). The infundibular septum forms a unit with the parietal portion of the crista supraventricularis, which extends from the interventricular septum to the free wall of the right ventricle and separates the pulmonic from the tricuspid valve (Fig. 22-1B). In tetralogy of Fallot, the infundibular septum (septal portion of the crista) is displaced anteriorly, rightward, and superiorly, thereby losing its alignment with the interventricular septum, forming a structure located completely within the right ventricle, and adopting a spatial position almost parallel to the frontal plane (Fig. 22-2). It inserts into the anterior limb of the septomarginal trabecula or immediately in front of it (19,42) (Fig. 22-3A,B) and is separated from the ventriculoinfundibular fold, which is the fibrous or muscular structure that separates the aortic and tricuspid valves (Figs. 22-2B, 22-3B).

The displaced infundibular septum obstructs the subpulmonary outflow and plays a fundamental role in the development of the pulmonary stenosis present in tetralogy (Fig. 22-3A,B). Additional mechanisms of obstruction include hypertrophy of the infundibular septum and right ventricular free wall as well as of the body of the septomarginal trabecula (42,45). Anomalous muscle bands described between the region of the septomarginal trabecula and the anterior right ventricular free wall may also contribute to the obstruction of the subpulmonary infundibulum (46).

The infundibular stenosis can be either localized or diffuse, depending on the characteristics of the obstruction. If the obstruction is low, at the level of the os infundibuli, it is produced by displacement of the infundibular septum and hypertrophy of the body of the septomarginal trabecula and/or free wall of the infundibulum. Generally, the infundibular chamber and main and branch pulmonary arteries are well developed. When the obstruction is diffuse, the entire pulmonary infundibulum is narrowed; in these cases, obstruction is caused by displacement and hypertrophy of the infundibular septum and by hypertrophy of the free wall of the infundibulum. The length of the subpulmonary infundibulum depends on the development of the infundibular septum. In tetralogy of Fallot, the pulmonary infundibulum is generally as long as or longer than that found in the normal heart (23); however, sometimes it is shorter than normal or even totally absent (42,47,48). When the infundibular septum is absent, stenosis is caused by deviation of the aorticopulmonary septum at the expense of the pulmonary arterial trunk (42) and by hypertrophy of the free wall of the infundibulum (49) (Fig. 22-3C).

In tetralogy of Fallot with pulmonary atresia, there is no continuity between the body of the right ventricle and the lumen of the main and branch pulmonary arteries (50). The extreme displacement of the infundibular septum causes it to fuse with the free wall of the infundibulum, resulting in either a blind-ending or absent right ventricular infundibulum. Rarely, atresia is caused by an imperforate pulmonic valve (51); in such cases, the infundibulum is present but narrow because of hypertrophy and displacement of the infundibular septum and free wall, and a fibrous membrane is present at the level of the pulmonic valve. These two types of tetralogy with congenital pulmonary atresia have to be differentiated from tetralogy with acquired atresia that develops after birth as a consequence of severe pulmonic stenosis or after palliative surgery (52).

The echocardiographic views used to study the right ventricular infundibulum, type and characteristics of the subpulmonary obstruction, and hemodynamic effects on the right ventricle are the parasternal long-axis view with the transducer tilted to visualize the right ventricular outflow tract, the parasternal short-axis view at the base, and the subcostal long- and short-axis views, from which the right ventricular outflow tract can be best seen in its entirety (Echo. 22-1; see color plate 71 following p. 364). These views permit a detailed observation of the length and width of the right ventricular outflow tract; the size, degree of displacement, and location of the infundibular septum within the right ventricular outflow tract; and the

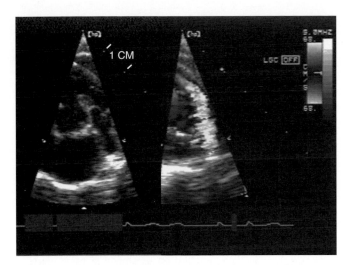

ECHO. 22-1. **Left:** Parasternal short-axis view of the right ventricular infundibulum in tetralogy of Fallot. Note the hypertrophied and anteriorly displaced infundibular septum, and the small pulmonary annulus and main pulmonary artery. The *1-cm marks* are highlighted at the right side of the image. **Right:** Color Doppler flow map across the right ventricular outflow tract and main pulmonary artery. Note the aliasing of velocities at the site corresponding to the infundibular septum.

grade of hypertrophy of the septum and of other components of the subpulmonary infundibulum. These same echocardiographic cuts will reveal the size and severity of right ventricular hypertrophy resulting from the outflow tract obstruction. The apical four-chamber view can complement the other views in regard to size of the right ventricular cavity. Spectral Doppler can help define the site(s) of obstruction with high PRF (pulsed repetition frequency) and the severity of the gradient with continuous-wave sampling. The presence of dynamic infundibular obstruction can be appreciated from the shape of the spectral waveform, which peaks later in systole, giving the appearance of a "reverse dagger" (Echo. 22-2). Color flow mapping will demonstrate the flow from the right ventricle to the main and branch pulmonary arteries, as well as the right-to-left shunt from the right ventricle to the aorta.

Interventricular Communication

The ventricular septal defect in tetralogy of Fallot is subaortic and is caused by malalignment between the infundibular and interventricular septa (43) secondary to the anterior, rightward, and superior displacement of the infundibular septum. The ventricular septal defect is usually perimembranous (42,50,53) and located between the limbs of the septomarginal trabecula (Fig. 22-3). Its anterosuperior edge is constituted by the infundibular septum, its anteroinferior and inferior borders by the bifurcation of the limbs of the septomarginal trabecula, and its posterior

border by the central fibrous body. If the ventriculoinfundibular fold is fibrous, which is the most common situation, there is mitral-aortic-tricuspid continuity (Fig. 22-3A). In more than a third of cases, a fibrous remnant of the membranous septum is present, which is of considerable importance in the surgical closure of the defect (54). When the ventriculoinfundibular fold is present and fused with the posterior limb of the septomarginal trabecula (Fig. 22-3B), there is aortic-tricuspid discontinuity (53,54) and the defect is separated from the tricuspid annulus by a bar of muscular tissue, which is the ventriculoinfundibular fold; therefore, the defect is classified as being of the muscular infundibular type (53). In the absence of the infundibular septum, the defect is subarterial or doubly committed (53–55) (Fig. 22-3C) and is related to both semilunar valves, which are located at the same level and separated by a fibrous remnant of the infundibular septum, and which form the roof of the defect. The other borders of the defect consist of the free edge of the trabecular septum and are completely muscular.

The ventricular septal defect in tetralogy can be studied echocardiographically from the parasternal long- and short-axis views, the apical four-chamber and outflow views, and the subcostal long- and short-axis views. The malalignment defect can be easily seen in the long-axis views immediately below the aortic valve, as well as from the parasternal short-axis view at the level of the aortic valve (Echo. 22-3). The defect is located immediately below the tricuspid valve in the usual position of the membranous septum. From the apical four-chamber view, the septal defect can be visualized below the aortic valve by sweeping the transducer posteroanteriorly toward the left ventricular outflow tract. From this sweep, the mitral-aortic-tricuspid continuity can be seen when the ventriculoinfundibular fold is fibrous, or the aortic-tricuspid dis-

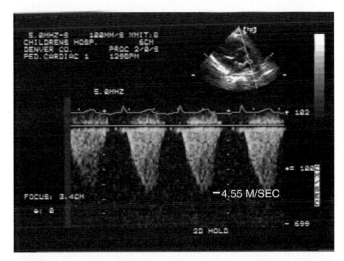

ECHO. 22-2. Spectral continuous-wave Doppler recording of the velocities across the right ventricular outflow tract and pulmonic valve. The waveform suggests dynamic infundibular obstruction.

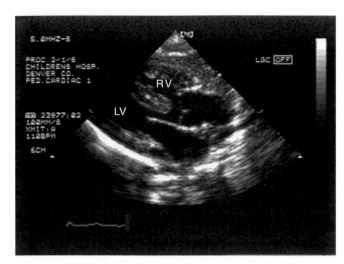

ECHO. 22-3. Parasternal long-axis view demonstrating the overriding aorta and malalignment type of ventricular septal defect. *RV*, right ventricle; *LV*, left ventricle.

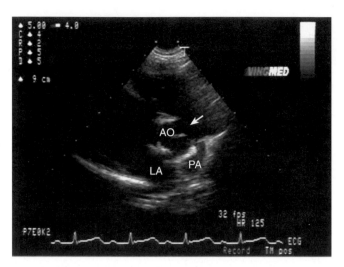

ECHO. 22-5. Parasternal short-axis view at the level of the great vessels. The *arrow* points to the absent infundibular septum, which results in a ventricular septal defect that is subarterial or doubly committed. Note the hypoplastic pulmonary annulus and main pulmonary artery. *AO*, aorta; *PA*, pulmonary artery; *LA*, left atrium.

continuity when it is muscular (Echo. 22-4; see color plate 72 following p. 364). The same features can be seen from the subcostal four-chamber view, with superior angulation of the transducer, and from the subcostal short-axis view of the right ventricular outflow tract.

Doubly committed or subarterial defects can be seen from the standard parasternal long-axis view immediately below the aortic valve (Echo. 22-5). From the long-axis view of the right ventricular outflow tract and the short-axis view at the level of the great vessels, the defect can be seen just below the pulmonic valve. The membranous septum is intact. A sweep from the standard long-axis view toward the right ventricular outflow tract will reveal the relationship of the defect with both semilunar valves, the absence of the infundibular septum, and the pulmonic and aortic valves at the same level and in fibrous continuity.

Color Doppler will demonstrate the direction of the shunt, which is usually bidirectional and directed in its right-to-left phase from right ventricle to aorta rather than into the left ventricular cavity (Echo. 22-6; see color plate 73 following p. 364). Flow mapping can also help identify

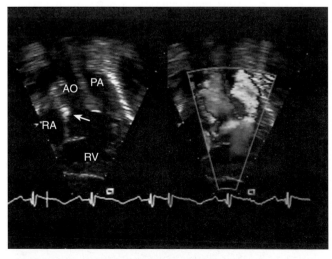

ECHO. 22-4. Apical view with the transducer tilted anteriorly toward the outflow tracts. The *arrow* points to the muscular ventriculoinfundibular fold separating the tricuspid and aortic valves. The color Doppler flow map illustrates the aliasing of the color velocities at the point of maximum obstruction resulting from hypertrophy and anterior displacement of the infundibular septum. *RA*, right atrium; *RV*, right ventricle; *AO*, aorta; *PA*, pulmonary artery.

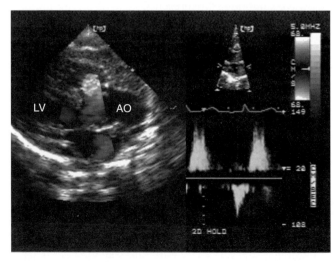

ECHO. 22-6. Left: Parasternal long-axis view of the malalignment ventricular septal defect, with this frame demonstrating the color Doppler flow map of the left-to-right shunting. **Right:** The spectral velocity recording shows the bidirectional shunting across the defect. *LV*, left ventricle; *AO*, aorta.

any other defects present. From the long-axis parasternal view, the color Doppler signal can help position the continuous- or pulsed-wave sample volume to measure the velocity across the defect, which is usually low because both ventricles are at the same pressure. Spectral velocity recordings and color M-mode traces of the shunt flow will demonstrate the phasic changes in the direction of shunting better than the two-dimensional color flow mapping because of the better time resolution (Echo. 22-6).

Aortic Dextroposition and Overriding

In the normal heart, the aortic valve overrides the interventricular septum (19,20). Therefore, there has always been a question as to whether the overriding of the aorta seen in tetralogy is truly an anomaly specific to this syndrome (19) and whether the aorta in tetralogy is truly dextroposed (56). Van Praagh et al. (19) state that the increase in overriding seen in tetralogy as a result of dilatation of the aorta is not a true malformation, even if it is secondary to abnormal hemodynamics; they also consider that an abnormal degree of overriding occurs only in cases of extremely severe pulmonary stenosis or infundibular atresia. The echocardiographic findings reported by Isaaz et al. (56) demonstrate an increase in the degree of aortic override resulting from dilation of the aorta, leftward movement of the interventricular septum caused by abnormal hemodynamics, an anterior displacement of the infundibular septum, and dextroposition of the aorta. These findings confirm those postulated by Goor and Lillehei (17) and Becker et al. (20), who state that in tetralogy there is true dextroposition of the aorta as a result of a rightward displacement of the aortic root. The aortic valve is also displaced anteriorly relative to the atrioventricular valves and so is not wedged between them, as in the normal heart (20) (Figs. 22-1B, 22-2B).

In double-outlet right ventricle with an anterior pulmonary artery, a posterior aorta, and pulmonary stenosis (called double-outlet right ventricle of the tetralogy type, tetralogy of Fallot with double-outlet right ventricle, or double-outlet right ventricle with pulmonic stenosis), dextroposition of the aorta is also seen. Originally, it was felt that the aorta had to override the ventricular septum by at least 50% to differentiate these hearts from those with tetralogy of Fallot (57). Later, cases with as much as 95% overriding were considered to be tetralogy of Fallot; it was pointed out that there can be tetralogy with double outlet of the right ventricle (42). Piccoli et al. (58) consider double outlet to be present when there is more than 90% overriding of the aorta. We consider double-outlet right ventricle to be a type of ventriculoarterial connection, and, as suggested by Lev and co-workers (59), we use the term double-outlet right ventricle to include hearts in which both great arteries emerge completely or almost completely from the morphologic right ventricle, or in

which one great artery emerges from the right ventricle and the other one overrides the ventricular septum by at least 50% in the direction of the right ventricle.

The dextroposition and overriding of the aorta can be seen well from the parasternal long-axis view in its standard projection, from the apical views with the transducer swept from a four-chamber to an outflow view, and from the subcostal long-axis view with the transducer tilted anteriorly or superiorly toward the aortic outflow (Echo. 22-3).

Size of the Right Ventricle-Pulmonary Trunk Junction (Pulmonary Annulus) and Characteristics of the Pulmonic Valve

In the normal heart, the pulmonic valve lacks a fibrous annulus at the site of insertion of its leaflets—that is, the union of the right ventricle and the pulmonary trunk (the valvular annulus) is always muscular. In tetralogy of Fallot, this union is almost always smaller than the aortic annulus and is rarely of normal size (25,50). The diameter of the "pulmonic valve annulus" is of great importance to the cardiologist and surgeon because placement of a transannular patch to augment the union always results in pulmonary regurgitation and hemodynamic effects on the right ventricle. In tetralogy with absent pulmonary valve, the right ventricle-pulmonary trunk union is always hypoplastic (8,36,37,41).

The pulmonic valve in tetralogy is usually abnormal, and a degree of valvar stenosis is almost always present. In cases without valvar stenosis, the area of the pulmonic valve is smaller than that of the aorta, contrary to what is found in the normal heart (50). The leaflets are thickened; in 55% to 70% of cases the valve is bicuspid (8,17,25,42,43,50), and sometimes the leaflets adhere to the pulmonary arterial wall (43). The valve is tricuspid in a third of cases of tetralogy. A unicuspid valve has been described in 1.6% to 10% of hearts with tetralogy (17,42). In tetralogy with absent pulmonic valve, the valve can be either totally absent or consist only of fibrous tissue remnants.

Echocardiographically, the views that allow study of the right ventricle-pulmonary trunk union and of the pulmonic valve itself are the same as those described above for the right ventricular outflow tract. These are the long-axis parasternal view of the right ventricular outflow tract, the parasternal short-axis view at the level of the great vessels, and the subcostal long- and short-axis views with the transducer aimed superiorly toward the right ventricular outflow (Echo. 22-1). From these views, it is important to measure the "valve annulus" for surgical planning. Mapping of the velocities across the pulmonic valve from the right ventricular infundibulum with the careful use of high PRF Doppler will permit an assessment of the relative severity of stenosis at sites throughout this area.

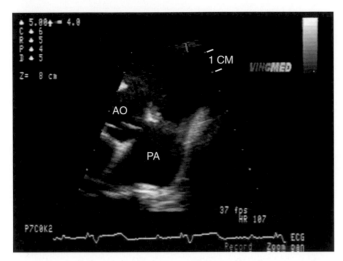

ECHO. 22-7. Short-axis parasternal view of the pulmonary annulus, main pulmonary artery, and bifurcation in tetralogy of Fallot with absent pulmonary valve. Note the very dilated pulmonary arteries. *AO*, aorta; *PA*, pulmonary artery.

In absent pulmonic valve syndrome, these same views allow evaluation of the degree of annular hypoplasia and determination of the presence of residual valve tissue or a fibrous annular ring (60) (Echo. 22-7). In these cases, valvar regurgitation can be demonstrated with color Doppler flow mapping and its severity estimated from the intensity of the spectral Doppler signal and slope of the regurgitant jet (Echos. 22-8, 22-9; see color plate 74 following p. 364). Pulmonary regurgitation causes a volume overload of the right ventricle with resultant dilatation of the right ventricular cavity and abnormal septal motion (61). These can be best evaluated from M-mode traces,

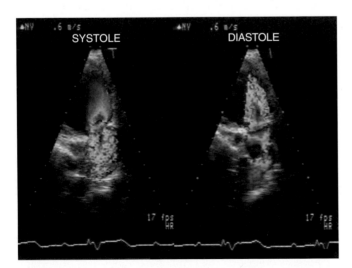

ECHO. 22-8. Color Doppler flow maps of the systolic and diastolic flows across the pulmonary outflow in tetralogy of Fallot with absent pulmonary valve. The restriction occurs at the annulus itself. Note the acceleration of the forward flow toward the annulus in systole and of the regurgitant flow in diastole.

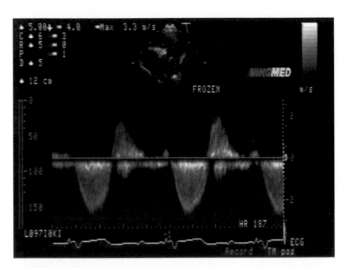

ECHO. 22-9. Spectral Doppler recording of the velocities across the pulmonary outflow in tetralogy of Fallot with absent pulmonary valve. Note the increased forward velocities in systole and the rapidly decelerating flows in diastole. The rapid return to baseline of the diastolic flow implies wide open pulmonary regurgitation.

derived ideally from a parasternal short-axis view to ensure correct alignment of the M-mode line. In adults or patients with difficult short-axis windows, the M-mode can be recorded from a long-axis parasternal view as well.

Size of the Main and Branch Pulmonary Arteries and Source(s) of Pulmonary Blood Flow

The anatomic characteristics of the main pulmonary trunk and its branches and the blood flow to them vary in the different types of tetralogy of Fallot, depending on whether the valve is stenotic, atretic, or absent.

In stenosis, the main and branch arteries are hypoplastic to some degree, which in the report of Rao et al. (62) was mild to moderate in 53% of cases and severe in 29%. The main pulmonary trunk is always smaller than the aorta and can exhibit supravalvar stenosis associated with a fibrous ring or narrowing at the junction of the leaflet cusps to the arterial wall. At the bifurcation, narrowing is frequently present, which can include the origin of both branches or of only one, more commonly the left branch (63,64). The peripheral and intrahilar branches can also be stenotic. Nonconfluent pulmonary arteries have been reported in association with tetralogy of Fallot and pulmonic stenosis. An atretic proximal left pulmonary artery may be continuous distally with the ductus arteriosus (63,65) or branch directly from the ascending aorta (66), or a right pulmonary artery can branch directly from the ascending aorta (65). Systemic-pulmonary collaterals are rare in tetralogy with pulmonic stenosis (67), and because the body of the right ventricle is connected with the pulmonary artery, these are bronchial collaterals when they are present (35) (see "Embryologic Considerations").

In tetralogy with pulmonary atresia, the anatomy of the pulmonary arterial tree and the source(s) of pulmonary blood flow must be elucidated. According to the type of branching, there are four types of pulmonary atresia (68): type I denotes the presence of both a main trunk and confluent branches; in type II, the main trunk is absent but branches are present, whether confluent or not; in type III, the trunk and one branch are absent, but hilar arteries are present in that lung; type IV indicates absence of the trunk and both pulmonary branches. Usually, stenosis is present at the origin of one or both pulmonary arteries, at their midsegment, and even in the intraparenchymal branches (69). Pulmonary blood flow can be through a patent ductus, from major systemic-to-pulmonary collaterals originating directly from the descending aorta or indirectly from branches other than the bronchials (persistent intersegmentary arteries), from major collaterals coming off the bronchial arteries, or from minor acquired collaterals originating from the bronchial or intercostal arteries (27,28,32–35,70,71). As previously mentioned (see "Embryologic Considerations"), when pulmonary atresia occurs early in development, there is no connection between the sixth aortic arch and the pulmonary vascular plexus, and the intersegmentary arteries therefore persist as major systemic-to-pulmonary collateral vessels. If pulmonary atresia occurs later in development, after the disappearance of the intersegmentary arteries, the pulmonary blood flow is supplied by the bronchial arteries.

Macartney et al. (72,73) have proposed classifying pulmonary blood flow in tetralogy with pulmonary atresia as unifocal or multifocal, based on the definition of a focus as a common pressure head providing effective pulmonary blood flow to one, some, or all lung segments. They consider that the denomination of pulmonary arteries as confluent indicates anatomic continuity of the pulmonary branches but offers no information regarding hemodynamic status. Therefore, the term should not be used synonymously with unifocal or multifocal blood flow. Unifocal pulmonary blood flow requires the presence of confluent pulmonary arteries. On the other hand, pulmonary arteries may or may not be confluent, and their central portions can even be absent when the pulmonary blood flow is multifocal—that is, having various sources from the aorta. In the presence of confluent pulmonary arteries that are normal or minimally diminished in size, the ductus is usually present and no systemic-to-pulmonary arterial collaterals supply the same lung as the duct, there being a mutually exclusive relationship between the presence of a ductus and of systemic-to-pulmonary collaterals (28,32–34). Bilateral ducti can be seen when the pulmonary arteries are not confluent. If the ductus is small or absent, the pulmonary arteries are diminutive and major systemic-to-pulmonary collaterals are present. In the absence of central pulmonary arterial branches, major systemic-to-pulmonary collaterals are also present, supplying blood to the intrahilar branches.

In tetralogy with absent pulmonary valve, severe and sometimes aneurysmal dilatation of the main and branch arteries occurs. The right branch is usually more dilated than the left, and it has been suggested that the orientation of the right ventricular outflow tract has a role in the greater dilatation of this branch (41). The extremely dilated pulmonary arteries can cause compression of the bronchial tree, with respiratory compromise commonly seen in these patients (74). The ductus is always absent (25,36,39). Generally, the pulmonary arteries are confluent; however, three cases have been reported with associated nonconfluent branches, two in which the left branch and one in which the right branch originated from the ascending aorta, with stenosis at its origin in two of the cases (75).

The echocardiographic evaluation of the main and branch pulmonary arteries—their size and source of the pulmonary blood flow—is very important in the clinical and surgical management of patients with tetralogy of Fallot. The best views to see the pulmonary arteries are the parasternal short-axis view at the level of the great vessels, the subcostal four-chamber view with superior angulation of the transducer to see the outflow tract and main and branch pulmonary arteries, the subcostal short axis view of the right ventricular outflow tract, and the suprasternal short axis view, from which confluence and branching can be visualized. These views can be used in tetralogy with pulmonary stenosis (Echo. 22-10), with pulmonary atresia (Echo. 22-11; see color plate 75 following p. 364), or with absence of the pulmonary valve (Echo. 22-7) Measurement of the size of the arteries is best performed from the parasternal short-axis as well as from the suprasternal short-axis views (76). In cases with severe dilatation of the right pulmonary branch, the indentation in the left atrial wall caused by the dilatation can give the false impression of a membrane within the left

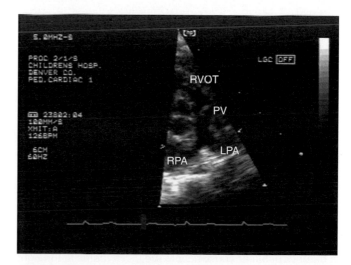

ECHO. 22-10. Parasternal short-axis view demonstrating the main and proximal branches of the pulmonary arteries. Note the *1-cm marks* on the right of the image.

atrial cavity, similar to a cor triatriatum, when it is imaged from a subcostal four-chamber view (60).

Color Doppler flow mapping in all these views is invaluable to demonstrate the source of flow into the main and branch pulmonary arteries (Echos. 22-11, 22-12; see color plate 76 following p. 364). It can help reveal the presence or absence of confluence as well as flow acceleration in cases of stenosis of the branches. In the parasternal and suprasternal short-axis views, color Doppler can aid in the positioning of the spectral sample volume to record the velocity of blood flow at various locations and thereby confirm the site(s) of stenosis. Color Doppler is also extremely helpful in confirming the presence of a ductus arteriosus and estimating its size and shunt direction, which is of particular importance in cases of pulmonary atresia.

It is possible to determine the presence of systemic-to-pulmonary collaterals with color Doppler flow mapping, particularly from the suprasternal long-axis and short-axis views, by imaging both the aorta and pulmonary arteries (Echo. 22-12). However, this technique does not allow precise determination of the location and number of all collaterals, particularly in cases of multifocal pulmonary blood flow with nonconfluent arteries (77,78).

Origin and Distribution of the Coronary Arteries

Anomalies in the origin and distribution of the coronary arteries have been reported in 2.5% to 9% of cases of tetralogy of Fallot (10,54,63,79). They are of importance at the time of surgery, particularly when a branch follows an epicardial course along the anterior wall of the right

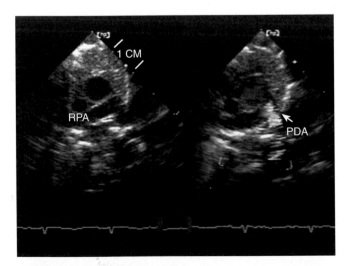

ECHO. 22-11. Left: Suprasternal view of the confluence and branch pulmonary arteries, which are supplied only by a patent ductus arteriosus. Note the *1-cm marks* at the right of the image. **Right:** Shunt from the ductus into the left pulmonary artery (*arrow*). *RPA*, right pulmonary artery; *PDA*, patent ductus arteriosus.

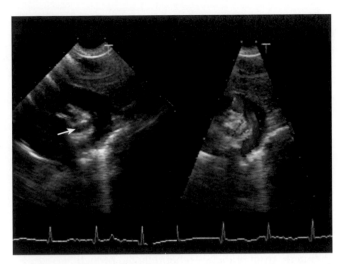

ECHO. 22-12. Suprasternal notch view of a large collateral supplying the pulmonary arteries. **Left:** Anatomic view of the collateral (*arrow*). **Right:** Color Doppler image of the flow from the aorta through the collateral vessel.

ventricular infundibulum. This can occur in cases with origin of the anterior descending from the right coronary artery, origin of the left coronary artery from a single coronary that emerges from the right anterior aortic cusp, origin of the right coronary artery from a single coronary emerging from the left anterior aortic cusp, and origin of the right coronary artery from the anterior right aortic cusp (which is rotated leftward), and in the presence of a large conal branch that branches normally from the right coronary artery.

The echocardiographic views that permit definition of the origin and distribution of the coronaries as well as of branches that may cross in front of the free wall of the right ventricular infundibulum have been described by Berry et al. (80) and Jureidini et al. (81). The origin and proximal distribution of the left and right coronary arteries can be studied from the parasternal short-axis views with left or right angulation, respectively, just above the short axis of the aortic valve. These views can be recorded from standard transducer positions or from a modified position on the first or second intercostal space (80,81). The high parasternal long-axis view of the right ventricular outflow tract demonstrates the position of the anterior descending coronary either in front of or behind the outflow tract (80). The proximal course of the coronaries can be seen also from the apical outflow views, with the transducer positioned 2 to 3 cm lateral to the left parasternal border (81). From an apical four-chamber view, with posterior and lateral angulation and slight rotation of the transducer, the longitudinal course of the anterior descending branch can be seen (81).

Associated Anomalies

The most common associated anomaly in tetralogy of Fallot is an interatrial communication, which is present in 9% to 40% of reported cases (10,25,50,62). Other, less frequent anomalies are a patent ductus arteriosus, atrioventricular septal defects, drainage of a left superior vena cava into the coronary sinus, multiple ventricular septal defects, tricuspid stenosis, aberrant right subclavian artery, aberrant left subclavian artery, total or partial anomalous pulmonary venous drainage, mitral stenosis, parachute deformity of the mitral valve, aorticopulmonary window, pulmonary vein stenosis, cor triatriatum, anomalous origin of the left coronary artery from the pulmonary artery, subaortic stenosis, unroofed coronary sinus, vascular rings, Ebstein's anomaly, tricuspid valve straddling, and juxtaposition of the atrial appendages (9,10,25, 50,62,82–87).

Anomalies of the aortic valve are rare in tetralogy; however, aortic regurgitation can be seen, particularly after the first decade of life and in adulthood (84,88). Aortic regurgitation has been reported in the presence of doubly committed ventricular septal defects (49,89), in prolapse of the right coronary cusp (25,62) or of the right and noncoronary cusps (90), with bicuspid aortic valve (90,91), with dilation of the aortic root in patients having large ventricular septal defects and volume overload caused by surgical aorticopulmonary shunts or collaterals (88), or secondary to bacterial endocarditis (88,92). A right aortic arch is present in 20% to 30% of cases with tetralogy of Fallot (10,19,44,62,82).

INTRAOPERATIVE AND POSTOPERATIVE EVALUATION

Intraoperative assessment is usually performed from a transesophageal approach, with either a biplane or multiplane probe (93–101). The pre-bypass study should include a confirmation of the anatomic details seen transthoracically before surgery and an evaluation of ventricular function.

Ventricular function is best evaluated from the transgastric transverse views with anteflexion of the transducer, which provides a short-axis view of the ventricle (see Fig. 4-27A,B). If necessary, M-mode traces can be derived from this view. Segmental wall motion can be assessed from this view and from the four-chamber and two-chamber transverse and longitudinal views, respectively (see Fig. 4-28A,C).

The transverse four-chamber views with slight withdrawal of the transducer permit examination of the ventricular septal defect resulting from malalignment, the degree of dextroposition and overriding of the aorta, and the origin and proximal distribution of the coronary arteries (see Fig. 4-29A) (Echo. 22-13). These views also allow determination of the continuity between the aorta and atrioventricular valves, degree of right ventricular hypertrophy, and size of the left ventricle, as well as anomalies of the atrioventricular valves. Rotation of the

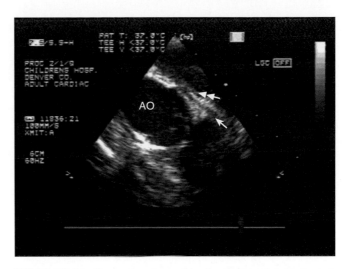

ECHO. 22-13. Transesophageal horizontal short-axis view of the aorta demonstrating the origin of the left coronary artery. *Single arrow* points to the left anterior descending artery. *Double arrow* points to the circumflex artery. *AO*, aorta.

transducer permits evaluation of the atrial septum for the presence of a defect or patent foramen ovale, which should always be closed surgically (see Fig. 4-29B). Color and spectral Doppler from these positions permits evaluation of the ventricular inflows and any regurgitation of the atrioventricular valves, the direction of shunting across the ventricular septal defect, and any aortic valve regurgitation, and it may reveal the presence of additional ventricular defects, although the apical trabecular septum is difficult to image from the transesophageal approach. It is useful to routinely record the velocity across the atrioventricular valves and aortic valve with pulsed Doppler. From a transverse short-axis view at the level of the aortic valve, slow withdrawal of the transducer will reveal a segment of the main pulmonary artery, the branches, and their confluence (see Fig. 4-31A,B). This is the best view from which to record the velocity in the pulmonary artery because it allows alignment of the Doppler sampling line along the direction of flow (Echo. 22-14; see color plate 77 following p. 364).

The longitudinal views permit evaluation of the segmental wall motion from the two-chamber (see Fig. 4-28C) and long-axis equivalent views (see Fig. 4-27D). These views of the left ventricular inflow also allow imaging of the mitral valve, the left atrium and its appendage, and the drainage of the left upper pulmonary vein. Slow rotation of the transducer rightward reveals the outflow tract of the right ventricle, which is of prime importance in tetralogy of Fallot (see Fig. 4-29D,E) (Echo. 22-15). The right ventricular cavity, outflow tract, pulmonic valve, and main and proximal branches, particularly the left, come into view. The infundibular septum can also be seen, and its anterior and superior displacement and hypertrophy can be evaluated. The size of the right ventricle-pulmonary trunk junction can also be mea-

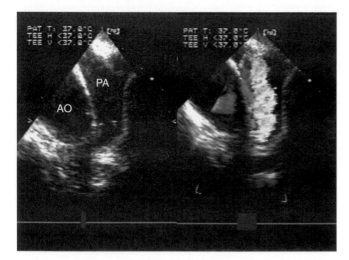

ECHO. 22-14. **Left:** Transesophageal transverse short-axis view of the pulmonary annulus, main pulmonary artery, and branches. **Right:** Color Doppler flow map of the forward flow into the pulmonary arteries. Note the color aliasing, implying high velocities. *AO,* aorta; *PA,* pulmonary artery.

sured. The anatomic characteristics in cases of valve atresia and of absent pulmonary valve can be confirmed from these views as well. Color Doppler will demonstrate the high-velocity forward flow across the outflow tract in cases of stenosis, the lack of antegrade flow in atresia, any flow resulting from the presence of collaterals or a ductus, and pulmonary regurgitation in cases of absent valve syndrome. Further rightward rotation of the transducer (see Fig. 4-29E,F) reveals the left ventricular outflow tract with the overriding aorta, the malalignment

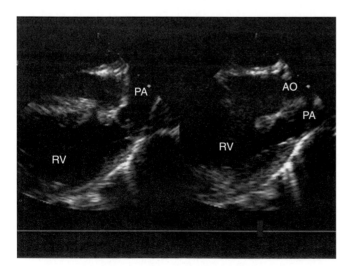

ECHO. 22-15. **Left:** Transesophageal longitudinal view of the right ventricular outflow tract and main pulmonary artery. The hypertrophied and anteriorly displaced infundibular septum is seen clearly. **Right:** The endoscope has been moved slightly to reveal the overriding aorta. The infundibular septum is also prominent in this view, in which less of the distal pulmonary artery is evident. *RV,* right ventricle; *PA,* pulmonary artery; *AO,* aorta.

ventricular septal defect, and any aortic regurgitation (Echos. 22-15, 22-16). Additionally, the coronaries can be evaluated from this position, which can provide information complementary to that obtained from the transverse views. With additional rotation to the right, the atrial septal view can be obtained, which permits further confirmation of an atrial defect or patent foramen ovale (see Fig. 4-30B).

The post-bypass study should be tailored to the specific type of repair performed.

In tetralogy with pulmonic stenosis, the surgical technique varies in different centers because presently there is no clear consensus regarding the best type of repair, particularly in infants and neonates. In some centers, early total repair is advocated, irrespective of age or weight, in an attempt to preserve the ventricular myocardium, protect ventricular function in the short and long term, and reduce the incidence of arrhythmias in the late postoperative period (102–108). Complete correction consists of closure of the ventricular defect and enlargement of the right ventricular outflow tract with a patch along with resection of parietal and/or septal infundibular muscle. If the right ventricle-pulmonary artery junction is small, the patch must be transannular and may need to be extended to the branches. This results in obligatory pulmonary regurgitation, which may affect the short- and long-term function of the right ventricle (104,109). At altitude, pulmonary regurgitation has been very detrimental, leading to the frequent implantation of cryopreserved pulmonary homografts when extensive reconstruction is needed across the pulmonary annulus (110).

Other centers propose a two-stage repair of tetralogy (44,64,111–114), either in infants under 3 months (112) or under 6 months of age (9). The initial palliation is performed with a systemic-to-pulmonary shunt, usually

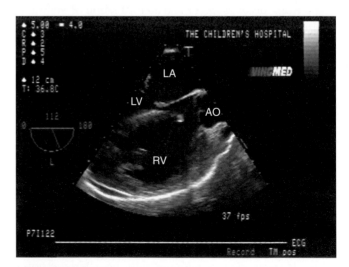

ECHO. 22-16. Transesophageal longitudinal view of the left ventricular outflow tract revealing the overriding aorta and malalignment type of ventricular septal defect. *LA,* left atrium; *LV,* left ventricle; *AO,* aorta; *RV,* right ventricle.

of the Blalock-Taussig type (115), modified by using a presized Gore-Tex tube between the subclavian and pulmonary arteries. The Waterston shunt is rarely performed between the ascending aorta and right pulmonary artery (9,64,114,116). This shunt permits greater pulmonary blood flow and may contribute to enhanced growth of the peripheral pulmonary arteries, allowing later complete repair. In the presence of a major coronary artery coursing in front of the right ventricular outflow tract, a conduit is needed from the right ventricle to the pulmonary artery. Therefore, in these cases a shunt may be used as a first-stage palliation (108). When shunts are placed, the intraoperative evaluation is of limited utility and is not routinely performed in our center.

With the advent of interventional catheterization procedures, a balloon valvuloplasty of the pulmonary valve has been used in the palliation of tetralogy of Fallot (117). When successful, this procedure permits growth of the pulmonary "annulus" and branch pulmonary arteries (117). However, some authors suggest that this should be attempted only after a systemic-to-pulmonary shunt has been performed (118). In any event, transesophageal monitoring during the valvuloplasty can aid in positioning of the balloon as well as in immediate assessment of the success of the procedure.

The surgical correction of tetralogy with pulmonary atresia has as its objective closure of the ventricular septal defect and the establishment of continuity between the right ventricle and pulmonary artery. Various techniques have been proposed, depending on the presence of pulmonary arteries, their confluence and size, and the characteristics of the systemic-to-pulmonary collaterals (50,108,119–124). Usually, when confluent pulmonary arteries are present, a Blalock-Taussig type of shunt is performed first in the neonatal period, followed by complete repair with closure of the septal defect and placement of a conduit between the right ventricle and pulmonary artery. When the central pulmonary branches are not confluent and are small, a shunt is required to allow growth, followed by repair with a conduit if their size is eventually considered adequate. When the central pulmonary arteries are absent and systemic collaterals are providing the pulmonary flow, various techniques of unifocalization are utilized in which the collateral arteries are progressively connected to the hilar branches, either directly or through Gore-Tex tubes. The objective is to eventually to establish antegrade flow by placing a conduit between the right ventricle and unifocalized arteries (108,121–124).

In tetralogy with absent pulmonary valve, the surgery is aimed at resection and plication of the aneurysmally dilated pulmonary arteries, particularly if they are causing respiratory symptoms. In addition, the ventricular septal defect is closed, and a valve is usually placed between the right ventricle and pulmonary artery (50,125,126).

The intraoperative post-bypass study should begin with a global assessment of ventricular function from the transgastric transverse short-axis view (see Fig. 4-27A). Withdrawal of the transducer into a transverse four-chamber view (see Fig. 4-28A) will permit evaluation of residual ventricular defects and of the functional status of the atrioventricular valves. Further rotation of the transducer will permit assessment of the atrial septum and any shunting at this site (see Fig. 4-29B). From the short axis of the aortic root, further slow withdrawal of the transducer will reveal the main pulmonary artery and the bifurcation with the reconstruction performed at these sites (see Fig. 4-31A,B). Pulsed- and/or continuous-wave Doppler sampling along the direction of flow from this view is utilized for the estimation of residual gradients at these sites. The longitudinal views will reveal the ventricular septal patch and the presence of any residual pulmonary stenosis and regurgitation, providing an overall assessment of their severity (see Fig. 4-29D,E) (Echo. 22-17; see color plate 78 following p. 364). Conduits from the right ventricle to the pulmonary artery are difficult to view from conventional transesophageal views because their placement varies widely depending on the size of the patient and anatomy of the pulmonary arteries. However, it is useful to attempt to document forward velocities through the conduit as well as the presence and degree of regurgitation, which is quite commonly seen immediately after implantation. These studies will serve as a baseline for the follow-up of these conduits in the late postoperative period.

The late postoperative evaluation of tetralogy of Fallot following palliative shunting is directed toward assessment of the patency of the shunt, progression of stenosis of the right ventricular outflow tract, hypertrophy of the

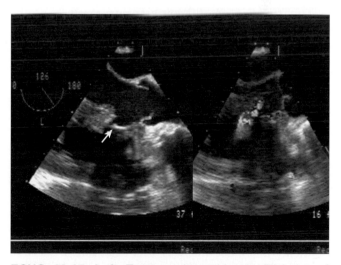

ECHO. 22-17. Left: Transesophageal longitudinal view of the left ventricular outflow tract immediately after bypass. The patch closing the ventricular septal defect is seen committing the aorta to the left ventricle. *Arrow* points to the site of a small residual ventricular septal defect. **Right:** Color Doppler flow map of the left-to-right shunting across the small residual ventricular septal defect.

right ventricle and size of the cavity, and growth of the peripheral pulmonary arteries to optimize the timing of complete repair. This is best accomplished through the transthoracic approach from the parasternal and suprasternal short-axis views.

Following complete repair without a transannular patch, the main objective of continued echocardiographic evaluation is to assess ventricular function and hypertrophy and to determine the presence and severity of residual pulmonary stenosis and/or regurgitation. This is best performed from a parasternal short-axis view with derived M-mode traces for measurement of global systolic ventricular function, size, and hypertrophy. Pulmonary stenosis and regurgitation are also best evaluated from the long- and short-axis views of the right ventricular outflow tract. Color Doppler can help guide placement of the continuous-wave Doppler sample line to measure forward velocities and calculate the degree of stenosis, if present. With regurgitation, the intensity of the pulsed-wave signal and slope of the regurgitant velocity trace can aid in the estimation of severity.

If the repair has involved a transannular patch, the echocardiogram will reveal pulmonary regurgitation, and its severity can be assessed as explained above. In these cases, the size and function of the right ventricle must be carefully evaluated serially because the right ventricle will be under ongoing volume overload. Evaluation is best performed quantitatively from the parasternal short-axis view with a derived M mode. The values obtained are followed serially.

In repairs involving the placement of conduits, the objectives of the follow-up studies should be the serial quantitation of ventricular size and function and the detection and quantitation of stenosis and/or regurgitation of the conduit. Conduits are difficult to image transthoracically because of their unusual positions within the chest. Attempts to image them should be made from the standard parasternal long- and short-axis views of the right ventricular outflow tract as well as from high right and left subclavicular positions. The suprasternal long- and short-axis views are also sometimes helpful in imaging the peripheral pulmonary arteries and the distal portion of the conduit. Doppler measurement of the forward conduit velocities should be attempted from all views. Stenosis of the conduit can occur at the proximal or distal anastomotic sites as well as at the valve through calcification. If the different sites cannot be viewed and sampled individually, at least a total velocity should be measured if possible with the stand-alone Pedof probe. Regurgitation is equally important to assess with color and/or spectral Doppler. The intensity of the Doppler signal and slope of the velocity curve will serve as an estimate of the severity of regurgitation along with the size of the right ventricle, degree of dilation and/or hypertrophy, and septal motion.

Patients with tetralogy of Fallot and doubly committed or subarterial ventricular defects are particularly prone to residual obstruction of the pulmonary valve annulus, and this should be specifically looked for in the late postoperative follow-up of these patients (127).

Balloon valvuloplasty has been very successful in our center as palliation for severe tetralogy of Fallot and for tetralogy with short-segment atresia. In these cases, often the right ventricular cavity and the pulmonary annulus and branches grow with time, so that complete repairs can be performed successfully.

REFERENCES

1. Stensen Niels. *Acta medica et philosophica hafniencia* 1671–1672;1:202–203. Cited by Goldstein HI in discussion of Jarcho S: Giovanni Battista Morgagni. *Bull Hist Med* 1948;22:503–527.
2. Sandifort E; Bennett LR, trans. *Anatomicopathologic observations 1777*. Chapter I, Concerning a very rare disease of the heart. I. Tetralogy of Fallot or Sandifort? *Bull Hist Med* 1946;20:539–570.
3. Hunter W. Three cases of mal-conformation in the heart. *Medical observations and inquiries by a society of physicians in London* 1784;6:291–303.
4. Fallot A. Contribution à l'anatomie pathologique de la maladie bleue (cyanose cardiaque). *Marseille Med* 1888;25:77,138,207, 270,341,403.
5. Mitchel SC, Korones SB, Berendes HW. Congenital heart disease in 56,109 births. Incidence and natural history. *Circulation* 1971; 43:323–332.
6. Campbell M. Incidence of cardiac malformations at birth and later, and neonatal mortality. *Br Heart J* 1973;35:189–200.
7. Hoffman JIE, Christianson R. Congenital heart disease in a cohort of 19,502 births with long-term follow-up. *Am J Cardiol* 1978; 42:641–647.
8. Rowe RD. Tetralogy of Fallot. In: Keith JD, Rowe RD, Vlad P, eds. *Heart disease in infancy and childhood*, 3rd ed. New York: Macmillan, 1978:470–505.
9. Arque Gibernau JM, Quero Jimenez M, Alvarez Diaz F, Cabo Salvador FJ, Sanchez PA. Tetralogia de Fallot. In: Sanchez PA, ed. *Cardiologia pediatrica, clinica y cirugia*, Vol. 1. Barcelona: Salvat Editores SA, 1986:365–403.
10. Fyler DC. Tetralogy of Fallot. In: Fyler DC, ed. *Nadas' pediatric cardiology*. Philadelphia: Hanley & Belfus, 1992:471–491.
11. Patten BM. Developmental disturbances of cardiovascular system. In: Patten BM, ed. *Human embryology*, 2nd ed. New York: McGraw-Hill, 1953:673–691.
12. De la Cruz MV, DaRocha JP. An ontogenetic theory for the explanation of congenital malformations involving the truncus and the conus. *Am Heart J* 1956;51:782–805.
13. Van Mierop LHS, Patterson DF, Schnarr WR. Hereditary conotruncal septal defects in Keeshond dogs: embryologic studies. *Am J Cardiol* 1977;40:936–950.
14. Anderson RH, Becker AE, Van Mierop LHS. What shall we call the crista? *Br Heart J* 1977;39:856–859.
15. De la Cruz MV, Quero-Jimenez M, Arteaga Martinez M, Cayre R. Morphogenèse du septum interventriculaire. *Coeur* 1982;13: 443–448.
16. Van Mierop LHS. Pathology and pathogenesis of the common cardiac malformations. *Cardiovasc Clin* 1970;2:27–59.
17. Goor DA, Lillehei CW. Dextroposition of the aorta. In: Goor DA, Lillehei CW, eds. *Congenital malformations of the heart. Embryology, anatomy, and operative considerations*. New York: Grune & Stratton, 1975:169–202.
18. Becker AE, Anderson RH. Fallot's tetralogy—developmental aspects, anatomy and conducting tissues. In: Anderson RH, Shinebourne EA, eds. *Paediatric Cardiology 1977*. Edinburgh: Churchill Livingstone, 1978:245–257.
19. Van Praagh R, Van Praagh S, Nebesar RA, Muster AJ, Sinha SN, Paul MH. Tetralogy of Fallot: underdevelopment of the pulmonary infundibulum and its sequelae. *Am J Cardiol* 1970;26:25–33.

20. Becker AE, Connor M, Anderson RH. Tetralogy of Fallot: a morphometric and geometric study. *Am J Cardiol* 1975;35:402–412.
21. Van Mierop LHS, Wiglesworth FW. Pathogenesis of transposition complexes. II. Anomalies due to faulty transfer of the posterior great artery. *Am J Cardiol* 1963;12:226–232.
22. Van Mierop LHS, Patterson DF. Pathogenesis of conotruncal defects and some other cardiovascular anomalies in the Keeshond dog. In: Van Praagh R, Takao A, eds. *Etiology and morphogenesis of congenital heart disease*. Mount Kisco, NY: Futura Publishing, 1980:177–193.
23. Anderson RH, Wilkinson JL, Arnold R, Becker AE, Lubkiewicz K. Morphogenesis of bulboventricular malformations. II. Observations on malformed hearts. *Br Heart J* 1974;36:948–970.
24. Taussig HB. The tetralogy of Fallot. Pulmonary stenosis or atresia combined with dextroposition of the aorta. In: Taussig HB, ed. *Congenital malformations of the heart*, Vol. II. Cambridge, MA: Harvard University Press, 1960:3–61.
25. Lev M, Eckner FAO. The pathologic anatomy of tetralogy of Fallot and its variations. *Dis Chest* 1964;45:251–261.
26. Van Praagh R, Ando M, Van Praagh S, et al. Pulmonary atresia: anatomic considerations. In: Kidd BSL, Rowe RD, eds. *The child with congenital heart disease after surgery*. Mount Kisco, NY: Futura Publishing, 1976:103–134.
27. Becker AE, Anderson RH. Ventricular outflow tract atresia. In: Becker AE, Anderson RH, eds. *Pathology of congenital heart disease. Postgraduate pathology series*. London: Butterworth-Heineman, 1981:199–208.
28. Thiene G, Bortolotti U, Gallucci V, Valente ML, Dalla Volta S. Pulmonary atresia with ventricular septal defect. Further anatomical observations. *Br Heart J* 1977;39:1223–1233.
29. Huntington GS. The morphology of the pulmonary artery in the mammalia. *Anat Rec* 1919–1920;17:165–201.
30. Congdon ED. Transformation of the aortic arch system during the development of the human embryo. *Carnegie Inst Contrib Embryol* 1922;14:47–110.
31. Boyden EA. The time lag in the development of bronchial arteries. *Anat Rec* 1970;166:611–614.
32. Liao PK, Edwards WD, Julsrud PR, Puga FJ, Danielson GK, Feldt RH. Pulmonary blood supply in patients with pulmonary atresia and ventricular septal defect. *J Am Coll Cardiol* 1985;6:1343–1350.
33. Bharati S, Paul MH, Idriss FS, Potkin RT, Lev M. The surgical anatomy of pulmonary atresia with ventricular septal defect: pseudotruncus. *J Thorac Cardiovasc Surg* 1975;69:713–721.
34. Thiene G, Frescura C, Bortolotti U, Del Maschio A, Valente M. The systemic pulmonary circulation in pulmonary atresia with ventricular septal defect: concept of reciprocal development of the fourth and sixth aortic arches. *Am Heart J* 1981;101:339–344.
35. Rabinovitch M, Herrera-De Leon V, Castaneda AR, Reid L. Growth and development of the pulmonary vascular bed in patients with tetralogy of Fallot with or without pulmonary atresia. *Circulation* 1981;64:1234–1249.
36. Freedom RM, Rabinovitch M. Tetralogy of Fallot with absent pulmonary valve. In: Freedom RM, Benson LN, Smallhorn JF, eds. *Neonatal heart disease*. London: Springer-Verlag, 1992:257–267.
37. Momma K, Ando M, Takao A. Fetal cardiac morphology of tetralogy of Fallot with absent pulmonary valve in the rat. *Circulation* 1990;82:1343–1351.
38. Fouron JC. Tetralogy of Fallot with absent pulmonary valve. Clarification of a complex malformation and of its therapeutic challenge. *Circulation* 1990;82:1531–1532.
39. Emmanouilides GC, Thanopoulus B, Siassi B, Fishbein M. Agenesis of ductus arteriosus associated with the syndrome of tetralogy of Fallot and absent pulmonary valve. *Am J Cardiol* 1976;37:403–409.
40. Childers RW, McCrea PC. Absence of the pulmonary valve: a case occurring in the Marfan syndrome. *Circulation* 1964;29:598–603.
41. Lakier JB, Stanger P, Heymann MA, Hoffman JIE, Rudolph AM. Tetralogy of Fallot with absent pulmonary valve. Natural history and hemodynamic considerations. *Circulation* 1974;50:167–175.
42. Anderson RH, Allwork SP, Ho SY, Lenox CC, Zuberbuhler JR. Surgical anatomy of tetralogy of Fallot. *J Thorac Cardiovasc Surg* 1981;81:887–896.
43. Anderson RH, Tynan M. Tetralogy of Fallot—a centennial review. *Int J Cardiol* 1988;21:219–232.
44. Freedom RM, Benson LN. Tetralogy of Fallot. In: Freedom RM, Benson LN, Smallhorn JF, eds. *Neonatal heart disease*. London: Springer-Verlag, 1992:213–228.
45. Soto B, Pacifico AD, Ceballos R, Bargeron LM. Tetralogy of Fallot: an angiographic-pathologic correlative study. *Circulation* 1981;64:558–566.
46. Acerete Guillen F, Quero Jimenez M. Las otras obstrucciones del ventriculo derecho. *Rev Esp Cardiol* 1981;34:255–257.
47. Ando M. Subpulmonary ventricular septal defect with pulmonary stenosis [Letters to the Editor]. *Circulation* 1974;50:412.
48. Neirotti R, Galindez E, Kreutzer G, Coronel AR, Pedrini M, Becu L. Tetralogy of Fallot with sub-pulmonary ventricular septal defects. *Ann Thorac Surg* 1978;25:51–56.
49. Rodriguez-Lopez Domingo AM. *Tetralogia de Fallot con ausencia o hipoplasia del septum infundibular* [Tesina de Licenciatura]. Santa Cruz de Tenerife, Spain: Universidad de La Laguna, 1986:28–31.
50. Kirklin JW, Barrat-Boyes BG. Ventricular septal defect and pulmonary stenosis or atresia. In: Kirklin JW, Barrat-Boyes BG, eds. *Cardiac surgery. Morphology, diagnostic criteria, natural history, techniques, results and indications*, Vol. 2, 2nd ed. New York: Churchill Livingstone, 1993:861–1012.
51. Thiene G, Anderson RH. Anatomy. In: Anderson RH, Macartney FJ, Shinebourne EA, Tynan M, eds. *Paediatric cardiology 5*. Edinburgh: Churchill Livingstone, 1983:80–101.
52. Fabricius J, Hansen PF, Lindeneg O. Pulmonary atresia developing after a shunt operation for Fallot's tetralogy. *Br Heart J* 1961;23:556–560.
53. Soto B, Pacifico AD. Tetralogy of Fallot. In: Soto B, Pacifico AD, eds. *Angiocardiography in congenital heart malformations*. Mount Kisco, NY: Futura Publishing, 1990:353–376.
54. Suzuki A, Ho SY, Anderson RH, Deanfield JE. Further morphologic studies on tetralogy of Fallot, with particular emphasis on the prevalence and structure of the membranous flap. *J Thorac Cardiovasc Surg* 1990;99:528–535.
55. Capelli H, Somerville J. Atypical Fallot's tetralogy with doubly committed subarterial ventricular septal defect. Diagnostic value of 2-dimensional echocardiography. *Am J Cardiol* 1983;51:282–285.
56. Isaaz K, Cloez JL, Marcon F, Worms AM, Pernot C. Is the aorta truly dextroposed in tetralogy of Fallot? A two-dimensional echocardiographic answer. *Circulation* 1986;73:892–899.
57. Kirklin JW, Pacifico AD, Bargeron LM, Soto B. Cardiac repair in anatomically corrected malposition of the great arteries. *Circulation* 1973;48:153–159.
58. Piccoli G, Pacifico AD, Kirklin JW, Blackstone EH, Kirklin JK, Bargeron LM. Changing results and concepts in the surgical treatment of double-outlet right ventricle: analysis of 137 operations in 126 patients. *Am J Cardiol* 1983;52:549–554.
59. Lev M, Bharati S, Meng CCL, Liberthson RR, Paul MH, Idriss F. A concept of double-outlet right ventricle. *J Thorac Cardiovasc Surg* 1972;64:271–281.
60. Di Segni E, Einzig S, Bass JL, Edwards JE. Congenital absence of pulmonary valve associated with tetralogy of Fallot: diagnosis by 2-dimensional echocardiography. *Am J Cardiol* 1983;51:1798–1800.
61. Cheatham JP, Latson LA, Gutgesell HP. Echocardiographic pulsed Doppler features of absent pulmonary valve syndrome in the neonate. *Am J Cardiol* 1982;49:1773–1777.
62. Rao BNS, Anderson RC, Edwards JE. Anatomic variations in the tetralogy of Fallot. *Am Heart J* 1971;81:361–371.
63. Fellows KE, Smith J, Keane JF. Preoperative angiocardiography in infants with tetrad of Fallot. Review of 36 cases. *Am J Cardiol* 1981;47:1279–1285.
64. Arciniegas E. Tetralogy of Fallot. In: Arciniegas E, ed. *Pediatric cardiac surgery*. Chicago: Year Book, 1985:203–217.
65. Anderson RH, Macartney FJ, Shinebourne EA, Tynan M. Fallot's tetralogy. In: Anderson RH, Macartney FJ, Shinebourne EA, Tynan M, eds. *Paediatric cardiology*, Vol. 2. Edinburgh: Churchill Livingstone, 1987:765–798.

66. Morgan JR. Left pulmonary artery from ascending aorta in tetralogy of Fallot. *Circulation* 1972;45:653–657.

67. Ramsay JM, Macartney FJ, Haworth SG. Tetralogy of Fallot with major aortopulmonary collateral arteries. *Br Heart J* 1985;53:167–172.

68. Jefferson K, Rees S, Somerville J. Systemic arterial supply to the lungs in pulmonary atresia and its relation to pulmonary artery development. *Br Heart J* 1972;34:418–427.

69. Soto B, Pacifico AD. Pulmonary atresia with ventricular septal defect. In: Soto B, Pacifico AD, eds. *Angiocardiography in congenital heart malformations.* Mount Kisco, NY: Futura Publishing, 1990:449–491.

70. Anderson RH, Macartney FJ, Shinebourne EA, Tynan M. Pulmonary atresia with ventricular septal defect. In: Anderson RH, Macartney FJ, Shinebourne EA, Tynan M, eds. *Paediatric cardiology,* Vol. 2. Edinburgh: Churchill Livingstone, 1987:799–827.

71. Thiene G, Frescura C. Pathological anatomy of pulmonary atresia with ventricular septal defect. In: Crupi G, Parenzan L, Anderson RH, eds. *Pediatric cardiac surgery,* Part 1. Mount Kisco, NY: Futura Publishing, 1989:222–225 (*Perspectives in pediatric cardiology,* Vol. 2).

72. Macartney FJ, Scott O, Deverall PB. Haemodynamic and anatomical characteristics of pulmonary blood supply in pulmonary atresia with ventricular septal defect—including a case of persistent fifth aortic arch. *Br Heart J* 1974;36:1049–1060.

73. Macartney FJ, Haworth SG. The pulmonary blood supply in pulmonary atresia with ventricular septal defect. In: Godman MJ, Marquis RM, eds. *Paediatric cardiology,* Vol. 2. Edinburgh: Churchill Livingstone, 1979:314–338.

74. Rabinovitch M, Grady S, David I, et al. Compression of intrapulmonary bronchi by abnormally branching pulmonary arteries associated with absent pulmonary valves. *Am J Cardiol* 1982;50:804–813.

75. Calder AL, Brandt PWT, Barrat-Boyes BG, Neutze JM. Variant of tetralogy of Fallot with absent pulmonary valve leaflets and origin of one pulmonary artery from the ascending aorta. *Am J Cardiol* 1980;46:106–116.

76. Huhta JC, Piehler JM, Tajik AJ, et al. Two dimensional echocardiographic detection and measurement of the right pulmonary artery in pulmonary atresia-ventricular septal defect: angiographic and surgical correlation. *Am J Cardiol* 1982;49:1235–1240.

77. Hagler DJ. Doppler color flow imaging and determination of pulmonary blood supply in infants with pulmonary atresia with ventricular septal defect. *J Am Coll Cardiol* 1989;14:1766–1767.

78. Smyllie JH, Sutherland GR, Keeton BR. The value of Doppler color flow mapping in determining pulmonary blood supply in infants with pulmonary atresia with ventricular septal defect. *J Am Coll Cardiol* 1989;14:1759–1765.

79. Dabizzi RP, Teodori G, Barletta GA, Caprioli G, Baldrighi G, Baldrighi V. Associated coronary and cardiac anomalies in the tetralogy of Fallot. An angiographic study. *Eur Heart J* 1990;11:692–704.

80. Berry JM, Einzig S, Krabill KA, Bass JL. Evaluation of coronary artery anatomy in patients with tetralogy of Fallot by two-dimensional echocardiography. *Circulation* 1988;78:149–156.

81. Jureidini SB, Appleton RS, Nouri S, Crawford CJ. Detection of coronary artery abnormalities in tetralogy of Fallot by two-dimensional echocardiography. *J Am Coll Cardiol* 1989;14:960–967.

82. Nagao GI, Daoud GI, McAdams AJ, Schwartz DC, Kaplan S. Cardiovascular anomalies associated with tetralogy of Fallot. *Am J Cardiol* 1967;20:206–215.

83. Hohn AR, Jain KK, Tamer DM. Supravalvular mitral stenosis in a patient with tetralogy of Fallot. *Am J Cardiol* 1968;22:733–737.

84. Higgins CB, Mulder DG. Tetralogy of Fallot in the adult. *Am J Cardiol* 1972;29:837–846.

85. Perez-Martinez VM, Burgueros M, Quero M, Perez Leon J, Hafer G. Aorticopulmonary window associated with tetralogy of Fallot. Report of one case and review of the literature. *Angiology* 1976;27:526–534.

86. Akasaka T, Itoh K, Ohkawa Y, et al. Surgical treatment of anomalous origin of the left coronary artery from the pulmonary artery associated with tetralogy of Fallot. *Ann Thorac Surg* 1981;31:469–474.

87. Gutierrez J, Perez de Leon J, De Marco E, et al. Tetralogy of Fallot associated with total anomalous pulmonary venous drainage. *Pediatr Cardiol* 1983;4:293–296.

88. Capelli H, Ross D, Somerville J. Aortic regurgitation in tetrat of Fallot and pulmonary atresia. *Am J Cardiol* 1979;49:1979–1983.

89. Matsuda H, Ihara K, Mori T, Kitamura S, Kawashima Y. Tetralogy of Fallot associated with aortic insufficiency. *Ann Thorac Surg* 1980;29:529–533.

90. Van Praagh R, McNamara JJ. Anatomic types of ventricular septal defect with aortic insufficiency. Diagnostic and surgical considerations. *Am Heart J* 1968;75:604–619.

91. Glancy DL, Morrow AG, Roberts WC. Malformations of the aortic valve in patients with tetralogy of Fallot. *Am Heart J* 1968;76:755–759.

92. Emanuel R, Somerville J, Prusty S, Ross DN. Aortic regurgitation from infective endocarditis in Fallot's tetralogy and pulmonary atresia. *Br Heart J* 1975;37:365–370.

93. Cyran SE, Kimball TR, Meyer RA, et al. Efficacy of intraoperative transesophageal echocardiography in children with congenital heart disease. *Am J Cardiol* 1989;63:594–598.

94. Stumpfer OFW, Elzenga NJ, Hess J, Sutherland GR. Transesophageal echocardiography in children with congenital heart disease: an initial experience. *J Am Coll Cardiol* 1990;16:433–441.

95. Ritter SB. Transesophageal echocardiography in children: new peephole to the heart. *J Am Coll Cardiol* 1990;16:447–450.

96. Muhiudeen IA, Roberson DA, Silverman NH, Hass G, Turley K, Cahalan MK. Intraoperative echocardiography in infants and children with congenital cardiac shunt lesions: transesophageal versus epicardial echocardiography. *J Am Coll Cardiol* 1990;16:1687–1695.

97. Ritter SB. Transesophageal real-time echocardiography in infants and children with congenital heart disease. *J Am Coll Cardiol* 1991;18:569–580.

98. Lam J, Neirotti RA, Lubbers WJ, et al. Usefulness of biplane transesophageal echocardiography in neonates, infants and children with congenital heart disease. *Am J Cardiol* 1993;72:699–706.

99. Seward JB, Khandheria BK, Oh JK, et al. Transesophageal echocardiography: technique, anatomic correlations, implementation, and clinical applications. *Mayo Clin Proc* 1988;63:649–680.

100. Seward JB, Khandheria BK, Edwards WD, Oh JK, Freeman WK, Tajik AJ. Biplanar transesophageal echocardiography: anatomic correlations, image orientation, and clinical applications. *Mayo Clin Proc* 1990;65:1193–1213.

101. Seward JB, Khandheria BK, Freeman WK, et al. Multiplane transesophageal echocardiography: image orientation, examination technique, anatomic correlations, and clinical applications. *Mayo Clin Proc* 1993;68:523–551.

102. Walsh EP, Rockenmacher S, Keane JF, Houghen TJ, Lock JE, Castaneda AR. Late results in patients with tetralogy of Fallot repaired during infancy. *Circulation* 1988;77:1062–1067.

103. Castaneda A, Mayer J, Jonas R, Walsh EP, Lang P. Repair of tetralogy of Fallot in infancy. In: Crupi G, Parenzan L, Anderson RH, eds. *Pediatric cardiac surgery,* Part 1. Mount Kisco, NY: Futura Publishing, 1989:155–158 (*Perspectives in pediatric cardiology,* Vol. 2).

104. Raudkivi PJ, Balaji S, Thomas D, Sutherland GR, Keeton BR, Monro JL. Primary correction of tetralogy of Fallot in the first year of life. In: Crupi G, Parenzan L, Anderson RH, eds. *Pediatric cardiac surgery,* Part 1. Mount Kisco, NY: Futura Publishing, 1989:159–162 (*Perspectives in pediatric cardiology,* Vol. 2).

105. Deanfield JE. Late ventricular arrhythmias occurring after repair of tetralogy of Fallot: do they matter? *Int J Cardiol* 1991;30:143–150.

106. Mitsuno M, Nakano S, Shimazaki Y, et al. Fate of right ventricular hypertrophy in tetralogy of Fallot after corrective surgery. *Am J Cardiol* 1993;72:694–698.

107. Castaneda AR, Mayer J. Tetralogy of Fallot. In: Stark J, De Leval M, eds. *Surgery for congenital heart defects,* 2nd ed. Philadelphia: WB Saunders, 1994:405–416.

108. Castaneda AR, Jonas RA, Mayer JE Jr, Hanley FL. Tetralogy of Fallot. In: Castaneda AR, Jonas RA, Mayer JE Jr, Hanley FL, eds. *Cardiac surgery of the neonate and infant.* Philadelphia: WB Saunders, 1994:215–234.

109. Kirklin JK, Kirklin JW, Blackstone EH, et al. Sudden death and arrhythmic events after repair of tetralogy of Fallot. In: Crupi G, Parenzan L, Anderson RH, eds. *Pediatric cardiac surgery*, Part 1. Mount Kisco, NY: Futura Publishing, 1989:204–208 (*Pespectives in pediatric cardiology*, Vol. 2).

110. Cripe LH, Clarke DR, Campbell DN, Fullerton DA, Shaffer EM, Valdes-Cruz LM. Performance of cryopreserved pulmonary homografts in the right ventricular outflow tract in children: an echocardiographic study. *Pediatr Res* 1995;37[Part 2]:24A(abst).

111. Parenzan L, Annecchino FP, Gamba A. The impact of initial palliation in the first two years of life upon the result of later total repair for tetralogy of Fallot. In: Crupi G, Parenzan L, Anderson RH, eds. *Pediatric cardiac surgery*, Part 1. Mount Kisco, NY: Futura Publishing, 1989:169–172 (*Perspectives in pediatric cardiology*, Vol. 2).

112. Kirklin JW, Blackstone EH, Pacifico AD, Kirklin JK, Bargeron LM Jr. Tetralogy of Fallot with and without pulmonary atresia. In: Anderson RH, Neches WH, Park SC, Zuberbuhler JR, eds. Mount Kisco, NY: Futura Publishing, 1988:199–211 (*Perspectives in pediatric cardiology*, Vol. 1).

113. Arciniegas E, Farooki ZK, Hakimi M, Green EW. Results of two-stage surgical treatment of tetralogy of Fallot. *J Thorac Cardiovasc Surg* 1980;79:876–883.

114. Alvarez Diaz F, Sanz E, Sanchez PA, et al. Fallot's tetralogy—palliation and repair with a previous shunt. In: Anderson RH, Shinebourne EA, eds. *Paediatric cardiology 1977*. Edinburgh: Churchill Livingstone, 1978;273–282.

115. Blalock A, Taussig HB. The surgical treatment of malformations of the heart in which there is pulmonary stenosis or pulmonary atresia. *JAMA* 1945;128:189–202.

116. Rammos S, Krian A, Kramer HH, Kozlik R, Bircks W, Bourgeois M. Growth of the ventriculo-pulmonary junction (the "annulus") and the pulmonary arteries following construction of a Waterston shunt as palliation in patients with tetralogy of Fallot. In: Crupi G, Parenzan L, Anderson RH, eds. *Pediatric cardiac surgery*, Part 1. Mount Kisco, NY: Futura Publishing, 1989:196–200 (*Perspectives in pediatric cardiology*, Vol. 2).

117. Sreeram N, Saleem M, Jackson M, et al. Results of balloon pulmonary valvuloplasty as a palliative procedure in tetralogy of Fallot. *J Am Coll Cardiol* 1991;18:159–165.

118. Sommer RJ, Golinko RJ. Is there a choice of palliation for tetralogy of Fallot? [Editorial Comment]. *J Am Coll Cardiol* 1991;18:166–167.

119. Livi U, Kay P, Ross D. The pulmonary homograft: an improved conduit for right ventricular outflow tract reconstruction. *Circulation* 1986;74:II-250(abst).

120. Matsuda H, Shimazaki Y, Nakano S, Iio N, Miura T, Kawashima Y. The indications for and results of corrective surgery for pulmonary atresia with ventricular septal defect. In: Crupi G, Parenzan L, Anderson RH, eds. *Pediatric cardiac surgery*, Part 1. Mount Kisco, NY: Futura Publishing, 1989:239–243 (*Perspectives in pediatric cardiology*, Vol. 2).

121. Mee RBB, Brawn W. The Melbourne approach to multistaged repair of pulmonary atresia with ventricular septal defect in the presence of hypoplastic pulmonary arteries, arborization defects, and major aortopulmonary collateral arteries. In: Crupi G, Parenzan L, Anderson RH, eds. *Pediatric cardiac surgery*, Part 1. Mount Kisco, NY: Futura Publishing, 1989:244–248 (*Perspectives in pediatric cardiology*, Vol. 2).

122. Barbero-Marcial M, Rizzo A, Jatene AD. New techniques for correction of pulmonary atresia with ventricular septal defect and severe vascular anomalies. In: Crupi G, Parenzan L, Anderson RH, eds. *Pediatric cardiac surgery*, Part 1. Mount Kisco, NY: Futura Publishing, 1989;249–251 (*Perspectives in pediatric cardiology*, Vol. 2).

123. Sawatari K, Imai Y, Kurosawa H, Momma K. Staged operation for pulmonary atresia and ventricular septal defect with major aortopulmonary collateral arteries. Remodeling of the pulmonary arteries by complete unifocalization. In: Crupi G, Parenzan L, Anderson RH, eds. *Pediatric cardiac surgery*, Part 1. Mount Kisco, NY: Futura Publishing, 1989:252–255 (*Perspectives in pediatric cardiology*, Vol. 2).

124. De Leval M. Pulmonary atresia and ventricular septal defect. In: Stark J, De Leval M, eds. *Surgery for congenital heart defects*, 2nd ed. Philadelphia: WB Saunders, 1994;417–428.

125. Snir E, De Leval MR, Elliot MJ, Stark J. Current surgical technique to repair Fallot's tetralogy with absent pulmonary valve syndrome. *Ann Thorac Cardiovasc Surg* 1991;51:979–982.

126. Elliot MJ. Absent pulmonary valve syndrome. In: Stark J, De Leval M, eds. *Surgery for congenital heart defects*, 2nd ed. Philadelphia: WB Saunders, 1994;429–435.

127. Okita Y, Miki S, Ueda Y, et al. Early and late results of repair of tetralogy of Fallot with subarterial ventricular septal defect. A comparative evaluation of tetralogy with perimembranous ventricular septal defect. *J Thorac Cardiovasc Surg* 1995;110:180–185.

CHAPTER 23

Double-outlet Ventricle

Lilliam M. Valdes-Cruz and Raul O. Cayre

The term double-outlet ventricle refers to a specific type of ventriculoarterial connection in which both great arteries emerge completely or almost completely from the same ventricle, or one great artery emerges completely from one ventricle and the other overrides the interventricular septum by more than 50% over the same ventricle, or more than half the circumference of both semilunar valves is connected to the same ventricle (1–7). Within the context of segmental analysis of congenital cardiac anomalies, the double-outlet ventriculoarterial connection includes the connection of both great arteries to a right ventricle, left ventricle, main chamber, or outlet chamber (3,8,9). For the purposes of this chapter, however, we use the term double-outlet ventricle only for cases in which two ventricles are present, and not for cases with a double outlet from either a single ventricle or an outlet chamber (3,8,9) (see Chapter 17).

Either a right or a left ventricle can have a double outlet, and either situation can present in situs solitus, situs inversus, or situs ambiguus. For each type of double-outlet ventricle there are several subtypes, according to the spatial relationship of the infundibula (10–12) and great arteries (4,5,13,14) and the relationship of the ventricular septal defect to the semilunar valves and atrioventricular valves (1,4,5,13–17). It is important to point out that these pathologies exist as a spectrum, with double-outlet right ventricle at one extreme and double-outlet left ventricle at the other.

DOUBLE-OUTLET RIGHT VENTRICLE

Double-outlet right ventricle refers to a ventriculoarterial connection in which either both great arteries emerge completely or almost completely from the anatomic right ventricle, or one great artery emerges completely from the anatomic right ventricle and the other overrides the ventricular septum so that more than 50% emerges from the anatomic right ventricle (Fig. 23-1). The term double-

outlet right ventricle was first used by Witham in 1957 (18); however, hearts with this same malformation had been previously described as partial or complete transpositions or as dextroposition of the aorta (19–22). The incidence ranges between 0.5% and 1.5% of all congenital cardiac malformations (6,23–27) and varies according to the application of a 50% (2) or 90% (14) override rule.

EMBRYOLOGIC CONSIDERATIONS

Double-outlet right ventricle includes a spectrum of conotruncal malformations, ranging from tetralogy of Fallot to complete transposition of the great arteries (1,28). The visceroatrial situs, type of ventricular looping, conal septation, incorporation of the medial conus, and truncal and aorticopulmonary septation should all be considered in the morphogenesis.

Visceroatrial Situs and Bulboventricular Looping

The vast majority of cases of double-outlet right ventricle occur in situs solitus, although this malformation can also occur in situs inversus or situs ambiguus. In situs solitus, there will be atrioventricular concordance with D bulboventricular looping (Fig. 23-1A) and atrioventricular discordance with L looping (Fig. 23-1B). Hearts in situs inversus will be a mirror image of those in situs solitus. In situs ambiguus, the atrioventricular connection will be ambiguous and can present with right or left isomerism and with D or L ventricular looping. Double-outlet right ventricle with superoinferior ventricles is discussed in Chapter 16.

Conal Septation, Incorporation of the Medial Conus into the Left Ventricle, Truncal and Aorticopulmonary Septation

The conus appears in the loop stage in the cephalic end of the heart and is continuous caudally with the primordium

409

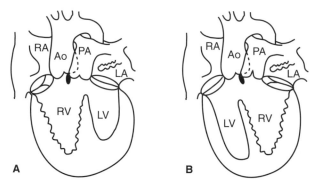

FIG. 23-1. Schematic drawings of hearts with double-outlet right ventricle and situs solitus. **A:** Atrioventricular concordance. **B:** Atrioventricular discordance. *RA*, right atrium; *LA*, left atrium; *RV*, right ventricle; *LV*, left ventricle; *Ao*, aorta; *PA*, pulmonary artery.

of the trabecular portion of the right ventricle (see Fig. 1-5B). The dextrodorsal and sinistroventral conal crests normally divide the conus into two coni, one anterolateral and one posteromedial, and both are connected with the primordium of the trabecular portion of the right ventricle (see Fig. 1-12). The medially positioned conus is eventually incorporated into the left ventricle and becomes its outflow tract (see Fig. 1-5D,E). The interinfundibular relationship depends on the conal septation, whereas the spatial relationship between the great arteries and between the semilunar valves depends on aorticopulmonary and truncal septation, respectively (see Fig. 1-14).

Several embryologic theories have been proposed to explain the morphogenesis of the various types of double-outlet right ventricle, and this topic is still controversial today. Some of these theories include (a) failure of conal inversion (28,29), (b) failure of absorption of the so-called bulboventricular flange or ventriculoinfundibular fold (1,6,20,25,30–34), (c) failure of incorporation of the posterior conus (6,10,11,25,28,30,32), (d) malalignment between the conal and interventricular septum (32), (e) failure of incorporation of the anterior conus (28), and (f) anomalous development of the conal, truncal, and aorticopulmonary septa (11,25,32,34). Because various embryologic structures contribute to the formation of double-outlet right ventricle, none of the theories mentioned can explain by itself all the various anatomic types of double-outlet right ventricle. In each case, the specific developmental alterations should be analyzed in relation to the spatial relationship of the great arteries, interinfundibular relationship, location of the ventricular septal defect, and presence or absence of infundibular stenosis. All these anatomic factors have been used to classify double-outlet right ventricle because all are important to the cardiologist and surgeon (1,4,5,10–17). We analyze these factors without attempting any particular classification (Table 23-1).

Double-outlet Right Ventricle, Anterior and Posterior Infundibula, Normally Related Great Arteries, Subaortic Ventricular Septal Defect, and Absence of Pulmonic Stenosis (Fig. 23-2A). In this type of double-outlet right ventricle, the conal, truncal, and aorticopulmonary septa

TABLE 23-1. *Double-outlet right ventricle[a]*

Interinfundibular relationship		Spatial relationship of the great arteries	Ventricular septal defect[b]				Figure
			Subaortic	Subpulmonic	Noncommitted	Doubly committed	
Anterior and posterior Anterolateral and posteromedial	⊘	Normally related	X	—	?	—	23-2A, B
		Side by side with aorta to the right	—	?	X	—	23-2C
		Aorta anterior and to the right	—	X	?	—	23-2D
Anterior and posterior	⊖	Aorta anterior and to the right	—	?	X	—	23-2E
Anteromedial and posterolateral	⊘	Aorta anterior and to the left	X	—	X	—	23-2F, G
Side by side	⊕	Normally related	—	?	X	—	23-3A
		Side by side with aorta to the right	—	X	?	—	23-3B
		Side by side with aorta to the left	X	—	?	—	23-3C
		Aorta anterior and to the right	—	X	X	—	23-3D
Absent infundibular septum	○	Normally related	—	—	—	X	23-4

[a] Table shows the various anatomic types of double-outlet right ventricle according to the spatial relationship of the infundibula, spatial relationship of the great vessels, and location of the ventricular septal defect. Figure numbers refer to the schematic drawings illustrating the specific anatomic type.

[b] X, known cases; ?, possible cases, not described in the literature.

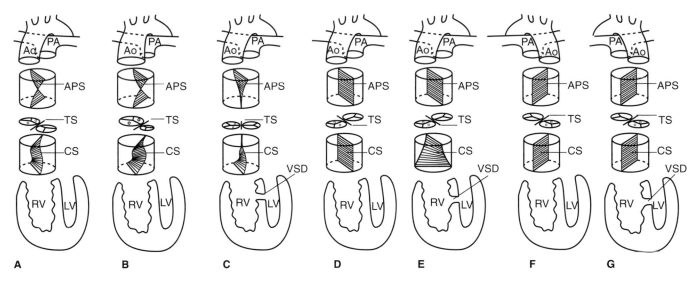

FIG. 23-2. Schematic drawings demonstrating the probable morphogenesis of the different types of double-outlet right ventricle with anterior and posterior infundibula. **A:** Normally related great arteries, no pulmonic stenosis, and subaortic ventricular septal defect. **B:** Normally related great arteries, pulmonic stenosis, and subaortic ventricular septal defect. **C:** Side-by-side great arteries with aorta to the right and noncommitted ventricular septal defect. **D:** Aorta anterior and to the right and subpulmonic ventricular septal defect. **E:** Aorta anterior and to the right and noncommitted ventricular septal defect. **F:** Aorta anterior and to the left and subaortic ventricular septal defect. **G:** Aorta anterior and to the left and noncommitted ventricular septal defect. *RV,* right ventricle; *LV,* left ventricle; *CS,* conal septum; *TS,* truncal septum; *APS,* aorticopulmonary septum; *VSD,* ventricular septal defect; *Ao,* aorta; *PA,* pulmonary artery.

all develop normally. The aorta, which is anterior and to the right cephalically, occupies a posterior and rightward position at the valvular level and connects with the posterior infundibulum. Failure of incorporation of the posterior conus into the left ventricle causes the aorta, which is connected to that conus, to override the ventricular septum, so that more than 50% emerges from the right ventricle. The infundibular septum remains totally within the right ventricle, so a subaortic ventricular septal defect is formed as a result of malalignment between the infundibular and interventricular septa.

Double-outlet Right Ventricle, Anterior and Posterior Infundibula, Normally Related Great Arteries, Subaortic Ventricular Septal Defect, and Pulmonary Stenosis (Fallot Type) (Fig. 23-2B). The morphogenesis of this type of double-outlet right ventricle is similar to that described for tetralogy of Fallot. An abnormal development of the conal crests gives rise to an infundibular septum that is displaced anteriorly, to the right, and superiorly, causing obstruction of the right ventricular outflow tract. The displacement of the infundibular septum also results in the formation of a subaortic ventricular septal defect resulting from malalignment of the infundibular and ventricular septa. Failure of incorporation of the posterior conus into the left ventricle determines the more than 50% aortic override of the right ventricle. Abnormal development of the truncal and aorticopulmonary septa results in an uneven partition of the truncus at the expense of the pulmonary artery; however, the spatial position of the truncal

septum and the spiral shape of the aorticopulmonary septum are normal.

Double-outlet Right Ventricle, Anterior and Posterior Infundibula, Great Arteries Side by Side with Aorta to the Right, Noncommitted Muscular Ventricular Septal Defect (Fig. 23-2C). The direction of the aorticopulmonary septum is normal at its cephalic end, posterior to anterior and right to left, but the septum fails to adopt a spiral shape as it proceeds caudally so that it maintains an anteroposterior direction, with the aorta situated to the right and the pulmonary artery to the left. The truncal septum develops abnormally because of the presence of an anterior or superior truncal swelling and a posterior or inferior truncal swelling, which give rise to a truncal septum directed anteroposteriorly; the aortic valve then develops on the right and the pulmonary valve on the left. The conal septum is also abnormal. The dextrodorsal conal crest becomes continuous with the superior truncal swelling and the sinistroventral conal crest with the inferior truncal swelling. The result is that the infundibular septum maintains a normal spatial position caudally—that is, its direction is posterior to anterior and right to left; however, cephalically it is anteroposterior. The noncommitted muscular ventricular septal defect is a consequence of abnormal development of the interventricular septum at this location.

Double-outlet Right Ventricle, Anterior and Posterior Infundibula, Aorta to the Right and Anterior, Subpulmonary Ventricular Septal Defect (Transposition Type) (Fig.

23-2D). In these cases (Fig. 23-2D), the development of the aorticopulmonary and truncal septa is abnormal, similar to that seen in complete transposition of the great arteries, with the aorta anterior and to the right. The aorticopulmonary septum is normal at its cephalic end, with a direction that is posterior to anterior and right to left, but it fails to acquire a spiral shape, so that caudally its direction is also posterior to anterior and right to left, with a straight shape. The truncal septum is also abnormal because of the development of a sinistrosuperior and a dextroinferior truncal swelling, so that its direction is posterior to anterior and right to left. The conal crests are normal, so that the direction of the infundibular septum is normal, posterior to anterior and right to left. The failure of incorporation of the posteromedial conus into the left ventricle causes the pulmonary artery, which is connected to that conus, to override the septum so that more than 50% emerges from the right ventricle. The ventricular septal defect is the result of malalignment between the infundibular and interventricular septa.

Double-outlet Right Ventricle, Anterior and Posterior Infundibula, Aorta Anterior and to the Right, Noncommitted Muscular Ventricular Septal Defect (Fig. 23-2E). The aorticopulmonary and truncal septa develop abnormally, as in complete transposition of the great arteries and in double-outlet right ventricle of the transposition type (see immediately above). However, in these cases, there is also an abnormal development of the conal septum because of the presence of a right and a left conal crest, resulting in a spatial position of the infundibular septum that is right to left—namely, parallel to the frontal plane. The aorta, located anteriorly and to the right, connects with the anterior infundibulum, and the pulmonary artery emerges from the posterior infundibulum. Failure of incorporation of the conus into the left ventricle results in both coni remaining connected to the anatomic right ventricle. The noncommitted muscular ventricular septal defect is the result of abnormal development of the ventricular septum in this location.

Double-outlet Right Ventricle, Anterior and Posterior Infundibula, Aorta Anterior and to the Left, Subaortic Ventricular Septal Defect or Noncommitted Muscular Ventricular Septal Defect (Fig. 23-2F, 23-2G). This type of double-outlet right ventricle is within the spectrum of anatomically corrected malposition of the great arteries. In these cases of double-outlet right ventricle, the development of the aorticopulmonary, truncal, and conal septa is abnormal, similar to that occurring in anatomically corrected malposition of the great arteries with aorta anterior and to the left. The aorticopulmonary septum is straight rather than spiral, maintaining a spatial position that is posterior to anterior and left to right. The truncal and infundibular septa also have the same direction, posterior to anterior and left to right. The difference between this type of double-outlet right ventricle and anatomically corrected

malposition is in the degree of overriding of the aorta over the anatomic right ventricle resulting from the failure of incorporation of the anteromedial conus into the left ventricle. In double-outlet right ventricle, the anterior and leftward aorta, which is connected to the anteromedial infundibulum, overrides the septum by more than 50% over the anatomic right ventricle, and a subaortic ventricular septal defect is caused by malalignment of the infundibular and ventricular septa. The muscular ventricular septal defect is caused by abnormal development of the ventricular septum in that location.

Double-outlet Right Ventricle, Infundibula Side by Side, Normally Related Great Arteries, Noncommitted Muscular Ventricular Septal Defect (Fig. 23-3A). The aorticopulmonary and truncal septa are normally developed, so the great arteries have a normal spatial relationship, with the aortic valve located posteriorly and to the right of the pulmonary valve. The conal crests are abnormally positioned, with one located dorsally or posteriorly and one located ventrally or anteriorly, so that the infundibular septum has an anteroposterior spatial position, resulting in side-by-side infundibula. The failure of incorporation of the medial conus into the left ventricle results in both infundibula being connected to the right ventricle. The noncommitted muscular ventricular septal defect is the result of abnormal development of the septum in this region.

Double-outlet Right Ventricle, Infundibula Side by Side, Great Arteries Side by Side with Aorta to the Right, Subpulmonary Ventricular Septal Defect (Fig. 23-3B). The aorticopulmonary and truncal septa develop abnormally in a manner similar to that described immediately above, so that both great arteries are side by side, with the aorta to the right and the pulmonary artery to the left. The development of the infundibular septum, however, is different in this case. The conal crests are abnormal in that one is located anteriorly and one posteriorly, resulting in an infundibular septum directed anteroposteriorly—that is, perpendicular to the frontal plane. The abnormal incorporation of the medial conus into the left ventricle results in a subpulmonary ventricular septal defect caused by malalignment between the infundibular and ventricular septa.

Double-outlet Right Ventricle, Infundibula Side by Side, Great Arteries Side by Side with Aorta to the Left, Subaortic Ventricular Septal Defect (Fig. 23-3C). The aorticopulmonary septum is developed abnormally. At its cephalic end it has a posterior-to-anterior and a left-to-right direction, whereas at its caudal end it is strictly anteroposterior. It is continuous with the truncal septum, which is also anteroposterior. This results in a side-by-side relationship of the great arteries, with the aorta to the left and the pulmonary artery to the right. The conal crests also develop abnormally in that there is one anterior or ventral crest and one posterior or dorsal crest, dividing the conus into a lateral conus and a medial conus. The

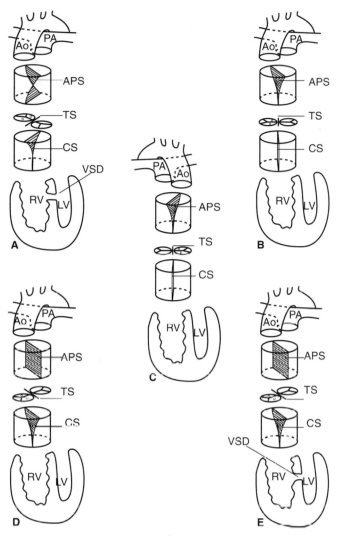

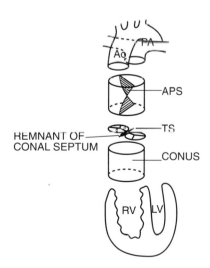

tricular Septal Defect or Noncommitted Muscular Ventricular Septal Defect (Fig. 23-2D, 23-2E). The aorticopulmonary and truncal septa develop abnormally in a manner similar to that described above for double-outlet right ventricle of the transposition type and to that for anterior and posterior infundibula and noncommitted muscular ventricular septal defect. In these cases, however, the conal septum develops differently. The conal crests are located anteriorly and posteriorly; therefore, the spatial location of the infundibular septum is posterior to anterior, perpendicular to the frontal plane. The abnormal incorporation of the medial conus into the left ventricle results in a greater than 50% override of the pulmonary artery, which is connected to that conus, over the right ventricle. The subpulmonary ventricular septal defect is caused by malalignment between the infundibular and ventricular septa (Fig. 23-3D). The muscular ventricular septal defect is caused by abnormal development of the ventricular septum in that location (Fig. 23-3E).

Double-outlet Right Ventricle, Hypoplasia or Absence of the Infundibular Septum, Normally Related Great Arteries, Doubly Committed Ventricular Septal Defect (Fig. 23-4). The aorticopulmonary and truncal septa are normally developed; therefore, the relationship of the great arteries is normal and the spatial position of the semilunar valves is also normal. Failure of development of the conal crests results in hypoplasia or absence of the infundibular septum, so that the semilunar valves are separated by a remnant of fibrous tissue. Failure of incorporation of the conus into the left ventricle results in overriding of the semilunar valves by more than 50% over the right ventricle.

In all anatomic types of double-outlet right ventricle,

FIG. 23-3. Schematic drawings demonstrating the probable morphogenesis of the various types of double-outlet right ventricle with side-by-side infundibula. **A:** Normally related great arteries and noncommitted ventricular septal defect. **B:** Side by side great arteries with aorta to the right and subpulmonic ventricular septal defect. **C:** Side-by-side great arteries with aorta to the left and subaortic ventricular septal defect. **D:** Aorta anterior and to the right and subpulmonic ventricular septal defect. **E:** Aorta anterior and to the right and noncommitted ventricular septal defect. *RV,* right ventricle; *LV,* left ventricle; *CS,* conal septum; *TS,* truncal septum; *APS,* aorticopulmonary septum; *VSD,* ventricular septal defect; *Ao,* aorta; *PA,* pulmonary artery.

infundibular septum, which develops from them, also has an abnormal spatial position, being perpendicular to the frontal plane. An abnormal incorporation of the medial conus into the left ventricle causes the aorta, which is connected to that conus, to override the septum by more than 50% over the right ventricle. The subaortic ventricular septal defect is a result of the malalignment between the infundibular and ventricular septa.

Double-outlet Right Ventricle, Infundibula Side by Side, Aorta Anterior and to the Right, Subpulmonary Ven-

FIG. 23-4. Schematic drawing representing the probable morphogenesis of double-outlet right ventricle with absence of the infundibular septum, normally related great arteries, and doubly committed ventricular septal defect. *RV,* right ventricle; *LV,* left ventricle; *TS,* truncal septum; *APS,* aorticopulmonary septum; *Ao,* aorta; *PA,* pulmonary artery.

the continuity or discontinuity between the great arteries and atrioventricular valves depends on the degree of absorption of the so-called bulboventricular flange or ventriculoinfundibular fold (1,6,20,25,30–34).

ANATOMIC AND ECHOCARDIOGRAPHIC CONSIDERATIONS

The echocardiographic study of double-outlet right ventricle should address the situs, atrioventricular connection, and sites of pulmonary and systemic venous drainage. Specific to this spectrum of malformations, the following should be determined: (a) infundibular morphology and interinfundibular relationship, (b) location and anatomic characteristics of the ventricular communication, (c) spatial relationship of the great arteries, (d) relationship of the semilunar valves with the atrioventricular valves, (e) infundibular connections to the great vessels and relationship of the great vessels to the ventricular communication, (f) presence of stenosis of the outflow tracts, (g) origin and distribution of the coronary arteries, and (h) presence of associated anomalies. Intraoperative and postoperative evaluation should be included.

Infundibular Morphology and Interinfundibular Relationship

Double-outlet right ventricle is essentially an infundibular malformation (10,11). In this lesion, the infundibular or outlet septum is located completely within the morphologic right ventricle and therefore does not form part of the outlet portion of the interventricular septum (4,5,12). The interventricular septum in double-outlet right ventricle has exclusively membranous, inlet, and trabecular portions. The infundibular or outlet septum separates both outflow tracts and, according to its insertion, determines the interinfundibular relationship (10–12). It can insert into the anterior limb of the septomarginal trabecula (12,35) (Fig. 23-5A), at the point of fusion of the posterior limb of the septomarginal trabecula with the ventriculoinfundibular fold (Fig. 23-5B1), in the proximity of the anterior limb of the septomarginal trabecula (Fig. 23-5B2) (*personal observation of author R.O.C.*), or into the ventriculoinfundibular fold itself (12,35) (Fig. 23-6). When the infundibular septum inserts into the anterior limb of the septomarginal trabecula, the interinfundibular relationship is anterior-posterior (12) (Fig. 23-5A). This can include different spatial positions of the infundibula, such that there can be one anterolateral and one posteromedial (Fig. 23-2A–D), one strictly anterior and the other strictly posterior (Fig. 23-2E), or one anteromedial and one posterolateral (Fig. 23-2F,G). This latter type of relationship can also be seen when the infundibular septum inserts at the point of fusion of the posterior limb of the septomarginal trabecula with the ventriculoinfundibular

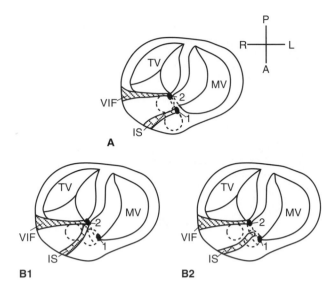

FIG. 23-5. Schematic drawings of a transverse cut at the base of the heart demonstrating the sites of insertion of the infundibular septum in the various types of double-outlet right ventricle with anterior and posterior infundibula. The *dotted lines* indicate the spatial position of the semilunar valves and the ventricular septal defect. **A:** Infundibular septum inserting in the anterior limb of the septomarginal trabecula. **B1:** Infundibular septum inserting at the point of union of the posterior limb of the septomarginal trabecula and the ventriculoinfundibular fold. **B2:** Infundibular septum inserting in the proximity of the anterior limb of the septomarginal trabecula. *IS*, infundibular septum; *VIF*, ventriculoinfundibular fold; *1*, anterior limb of the septomarginal trabecula; *2*, posterior limb of the septomarginal trabecula; *TV*, tricuspid valve; *MV*, mitral valve. *A*, anterior; *P*, posterior; *R*, right; *L*, left.

fold (Fig. 23-5B1). If the infundibular septum inserts into the ventriculoinfundibular fold itself (Fig. 23-6), the infundibular relationship will be side by side (12,35) (Fig. 23-3A–E).

In an anterolateral and posteromedial infundibular relationship, the infundibular septum occupies an oblique spatial position with respect to the frontal plane and is more or less parallel to the interventricular septum (Fig. 23-2A–D). The walls of the anterolateral infundibulum comprise the free wall of the right ventricle, the infundibular septum, and the right surface of the outflow portion of the ventricular septum, which is also the free right ventricular wall (12). The walls of the posteromedial infundibulum are formed by the free right ventricular wall, the infundibular septum, and the portion of the interventricular septum comprising the limbs of the septomarginal trabecula and the ventriculoinfundibular fold, which can be fibrous or muscular (12) (Fig. 23-5A). Only the posteromedial infundibulum has a wall to which the interventricular septum contributes, so only the great vessel connected to this infundibulum can be related to the ventricular septal defect (Fig. 23-2A,B,D).

In a strictly anterior-to-posterior infundibular relationship, the infundibular septum has an oblique position rela-

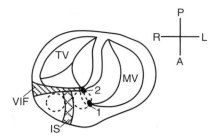

FIG. 23-6. Schematic drawing of a transverse cut of the heart at the level of the base showing the point of insertion of the infundibular septum in double-outlet right ventricle with side-by-side infundibula. The *dotted lines* indicate the spatial position of the semilunar valves and the ventricular septal defect. *IS*, infundibular septum; *VIF*, ventriculoinfundibular fold; *1*, anterior limb of the septomarginal trabecula; *2*, posterior limb of the septomarginal trabecula; *TV*, tricuspid valve; *MV*, mitral valve. *A*, anterior; *P*, posterior; *R*, right; *L*, left.

tive to the interventricular septum and is more or less parallel to the frontal plane (Fig. 23-2E). The anatomic components of the infundibular walls are the same as those described immediately above for posteromedial and anterolateral infundibula. Only the great vessel connected to the posterior infundibulum can be related to the ventricular septal defect.

With an anteromedial and a posterolateral infundibular relationship, the infundibular septum has a spatial position that is perpendicular to the interventricular septum and more or less oblique to the frontal plane (Fig. 23-5B1). The anatomic components of the infundibular walls vary according to the site of insertion of the infundibular septum. If the septum inserts at the point of fusion of the posterior limb of the septomarginal trabecula and the ventriculoinfundibular fold (Fig. 23-5B1), the walls of the posterolateral infundibulum are the infundibular septum, the free wall of the right ventricle, and the ventriculoinfundibular fold. The walls of the anteromedial infundibulum are the infundibular septum, the free wall of the right ventricle, and the portion of the interventricular septum comprising the limbs of the septomarginal trabecula. The artery connected to the anteromedial infundibulum will be the only one related to the ventricular septal defect (Fig. 23-2F). If the infundibular septum inserts in the proximity of the anterior limb of the septomarginal trabecula (Fig. 23-5B2), the walls of the anteromedial infundibulum will be the free wall of the right ventricle, the infundibular septum, and the outflow portion of the right side of the ventricular septum. The walls of the posterolateral infundibulum will be the infundibular septum, the free wall of the right ventricle, the ventriculoinfundibular fold, fibrous or muscular, and the portion of the ventricular septum comprising the limbs of the septomarginal trabecula. Only the artery connected with the posterolateral infundibulum will have a relationship to the ventricular septal defect (5).

If the infundibular septum inserts into the ventriculoinfundibular fold (12–35) (Fig. 23-6), the infundibular rela-

tionship will be side by side, and there will be a medial and a lateral infundibulum (12). The infundibular septum will have an oblique spatial position with respect to the interventricular septum and will be more or less perpendicular to the frontal plane (Fig. 23-3A–E). The walls of the lateral infundibulum will be the ventriculoinfundibular fold, the free wall of the right ventricle, and the infundibular septum (12). The walls of the medial infundibulum will be the free wall of the right ventricle, the infundibular septum, the ventriculoinfundibular fold, fibrous or muscular, and the portion of the ventricular septum located between the limbs of the septomarginal trabecula (12) (Fig. 23-6). Only the artery connected with the medial infundibulum will be related to the defect located in this portion of the ventricular septum (12) (Fig. 23-3B–D).

The echocardiographic views that permit elucidation of the interinfundibular relationship, site of insertion of the infundibular septum, and anatomic characteristics of the infundibula are the parasternal long-axis view of the outflow tract of the right ventricle, the apical views with slow rotation of the transducer between the four-chamber and outflow views, and the subcostal long- and short-axis views of the outflow tract (36). The insertion of the infundibular septum, either to the anterior limb of the septomarginal trabecula, which determines the anterior-posterior interinfundibular relationship (Echo. 23-1), or to the ventriculoinfundibular fold, which determines a side-by-side infundibular relationship, can be seen in these views (Echo. 23-2). The malalignment between the interventricular and the infundibular septa can be seen from the parasternal long-axis view (Echo. 23-1) and from the apical and subcostal four-chamber views, with the

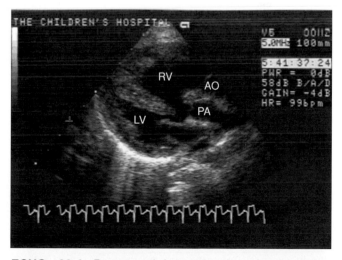

ECHO. 23-1. Parasternal long-axis view demonstrating double-outlet right ventricle with anteroposterior infundibular relationship resulting from insertion of the infundibular septum into the anterior limb of the septomarginal trabeculation. The ventricular septal defect is perimembranous with extensions toward the trabecular septum. Note the malalignment between the infundibular and interventricular septa. *RV*, right ventricle; *LV*, left ventricle; *AO*, aorta; *PA*, pulmonary artery.

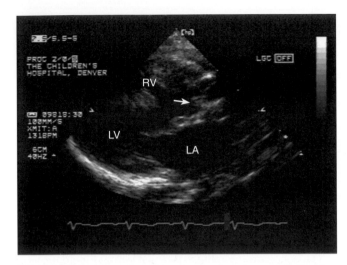

ECHO. 23-2. Parasternal long-axis view demonstrating insertion of the infundibular septum into the ventriculoinfundibular fold (*arrow*), determining a side-by-side infundibular relationship. *RV*, right ventricle; *LV*, left ventricle; *LA*, left atrium.

transducer swept from the crux cordis to the outflow tracts (Echo. 23-3). These views will also establish the relationship between the infundibula and the anatomic right ventricle.

Location and Anatomic Characteristics of the Ventricular Communication

Although rare cases of double-outlet right ventricle without a ventricular septal defect have been published (1,4,34,37–44), generally the rule is that a septal defect is present. The defect is usually large and can be perimembranous or muscular. The latter type can be located in the portion of the ventricular septum between the limbs of the septomarginal trabecula or in the inlet or trabecular portion of the interventricular septum (4,5,12).

In 80% of cases with anterior and posterior infundibula (Fig. 23-5), the defect is located between the limbs of the septomarginal trabecula (12). Depending on the site of insertion of the infundibular septum, the ventricular septal defect can be related to the posteromedial infundibulum (Fig. 23-2A,B,D), posterior infundibulum, anteromedial infundibulum (Fig. 23-2F), or posterolateral infundibulum, as only these infundibula have the ventricular septum as one of the walls (12) (see above). In 79% of these cases, the semilunar valve connected to the particular infundibulum is in continuity with the defect and forms its roof. The borders of the ventricular septal defect are the infundibular septum, the septomarginal trabecula, and the ventriculoinfundibular fold, which can be fibrous, fibromuscular, or muscular (12) (Echo. 23-3A). In the remaining 21% of cases, there is discontinuity between the defect and the corresponding semilunar valve, which are separated by muscular tissue of the ventriculoinfundibular fold. In these cases, the borders of the defect are completely muscular and are made up of the ventriculoinfundibular fold, infundibular septum, and limbs of the septomarginal trabecula (12) (Echo. 23-3B). Because the outflow tracts are abnormal, the ventricular communications are named according to their relationship to the great arteries as subaortic, subpulmonary, or noncommitted (12). When the ventricular septal defect is located in the inlet or trabecular portion of the septum, the defects are considered noncommitted, according to the classification

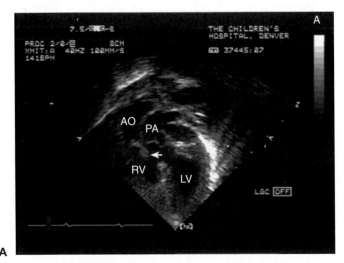
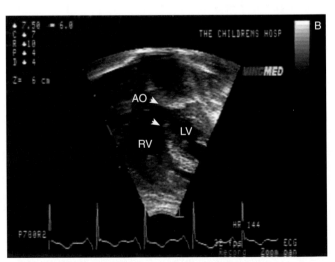

ECHO. 23-3. Apical view with the transducer tilted anteriorly toward the outflows. **A:** The *arrow* points to the malalignment between the infundibular and interventricular septa, which results in a malalignment type of ventricular septal defect. The pulmonary valve forms the roof of the ventricular septal defect. **B:** The *arrow* points to the limits of the ventricular septal defect. In this case there is discontinuity between the aortic valve and the ventricular septal defect, caused by the presence of a muscular ventriculoinfundibular fold. *AO*, aorta; *PA*, pulmonary artery; *RV*, right ventricle; *LV*, left ventricle.

originally established by Lev et al. (1) (Fig. 23-2C,E,G). When the infundibular septum is hypoplastic or absent, the ventricular communication is doubly committed (Fig. 23-4).

In 92% of cases in which the infundibular relationship is side by side (Fig. 23-6), the ventricular septal defect is located between the limbs of the septomarginal trabecula (12). The artery connected to the medial infundibulum is the only one that can be related to the defect, and there is continuity between it and the defect in most cases. The great artery makes up the roof of the defect (Fig. 23-3B–D). The borders of the defect are the limbs of the septomarginal trabecula and the ventriculoinfundibular fold, which can be fibrous or muscular (12). Muscular defects in the trabecular portion of the septum have been described in 8% of cases with side-by-side infundibular relationships (12) (Fig. 23-3A,E).

Anatomic specimens with multiple ventricular septal defects have been reported (7,14,43,45), as have atrioventricular septal defects with common atrioventricular valve (1,4,6,7,12,46) and perimembranous defects with extensions into the inlet, trabecular, or outlet septum (Echos. 23-1, 23-4).

The perimembranous or muscular defects located between the limbs of the septomarginal trabecula can be seen echocardiographically from the parasternal long-axis and short-axis views, from the apical views, and from the subcostal long- and short-axis views. When the defect is perimembranous, the relationship between it and the atrioventricular valves can be seen, particularly from the parasternal long-axis view with the transducer tilted toward the right ventricular inflow and from the apical views with the transducer swept from the plane of the atrioventricular valves to that of the semilunar valves.

When the defect is muscular, a muscular rim is present between the defect and the atrioventricular valves. However, it is sometimes difficult to differentiate these two types of defects echocardiographically, particularly when the muscular ring below the defect is under 1 mm in thickness (47). The malalignment between the infundibular septum and the muscular portion of the ventricular septum can be seen from the parasternal long-axis view and from the apical four-chamber to outflow sweeps (Echos. 23-1, 23-3A).

The muscular inlet defects can be seen best from the apical four-chamber views and the subcostal long-axis view, with the transducer swept posteriorly. The defect is separated from the tricuspid valve by a rim of muscular tissue. These can also be seen from the parasternal short-axis view, with the transducer swept from apex to base.

The muscular trabecular defects can be seen echocardiographically from the parasternal long-axis and short-axis views, the apical four-chamber view, and the subcostal long-axis view. Color Doppler flow mapping aids in demonstrating the defect in these various transducer projections and also helps define their relationship to the infundibulum.

Spectral Doppler is used to determine the velocity across the ventricular septal defects and estimate the gradient between the ventricles. Usually, the defects are large and the velocities consequently are low; however, a velocity greater than 2.5 m/s can imply that the defect is restrictive, and the surgeon may be required to augment it depending on the surgical procedure undertaken. Color Doppler can also ascertain the presence of small and/or multiple defects, which can be missed with two-dimensional echocardiography alone.

Spatial Relationship of the Great Arteries

The spatial relationship of the great arteries is defined based on the position of the aorta and pulmonary artery relative to each other (5,12,14,17,25,43,46–50) (Fig. 23-7). The spatial relationship of the great vessels can be more or less normal (aorta located posteriorly and to the right of the pulmonary artery), the vessels can be side by side (aorta to the right or left), or the aorta can be anterior and to the right, strictly anterior, or anterior and to the left. One case (No. 70-422P) has been reported in the literature by Cameron et al. (46) with an aorta located posteriorly and to the left, and Anderson et al. (5) refer to a patient with spiral great vessels but with the aorta located posteriorly and to the left of the pulmonary artery. The spatial relationship of the great arteries does not always agree with the interinfundibular relationship (12,36), and rarely, it may not correspond with the spatial position of the semilunar valves, as in the case reported by Otero Coto et al. (49), in which the aorta was located anteriorly and to the left but the valves were in a side-

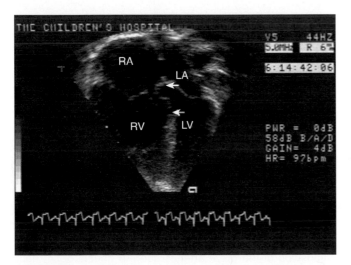

ECHO. 23-4. Apical four-chamber view demonstrating the inlet extensions of this perimembranous defect in double-outlet right ventricle. The *arrows* point to the limits of the defect. *RA*, right atrium; *LA*, left atrium; *RV*, right ventricle; *LV*, left ventricle.

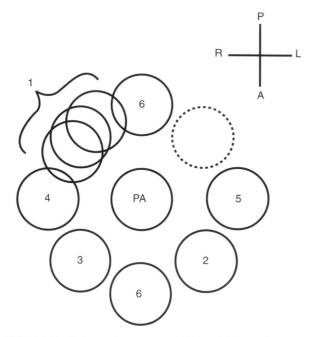

FIG. 23-7. Schematic representation of the various types of spatial relationship of the great vessels in double-outlet right ventricle. *1*, more or less normally related; *2*, aorta anterior and to the left; *3*, aorta anterior and to the right; *4*, side-by-side great arteries with aorta to the right; *5*, side-by-side great arteries with aorta to the left; *6*, aorta strictly anterior or posterior. The *dotted lines* indicate the probable location of the aorta posterior and to the left. *PA*, pulmonary artery. *A*, anterior; *P*, posterior; *R*, right; *L*, left.

by-side relationship. This can occur because different embryologic processes are involved in their formation. The spatial relationship of the great vessels depends on the shape of the aorticopulmonary septum, whereas the relationship of the semilunar valves depends on the development of the truncal septum. The interinfundibular relationship is determined by the shape and site of insertion of the infundibular septum.

The parasternal short-axis view at the level of the valve leaflets will demonstrate the spatial relationship of the great arteries (Echo. 23-5). This can also be seen from the parasternal, apical, and subcostal outflow and long-axis views with the transducer angled superiorly to visualize the great vessels.

Relationship of the Semilunar and Atrioventricular Valves

The ventriculoinfundibular fold is the muscular or fibrous structure separating one or both semilunar valves from the atrioventricular orifices in all hearts with malformations of the outflow tracts (51). The continuity or discontinuity between the aortic and/or pulmonic valves and the atrioventricular valves depends on the presence of a either a fibrous or a muscular ventriculoinfundibular fold,

respectively, as well as on the interinfundibular relationship. In the presence of anterior-posterior infundibula, only the vessel connected to the posterior infundibulum can have a relationship to the atrioventricular valves (Fig. 23-5A,B). In side-by-side infundibula, both arteries have a relationship to the atrioventricular valves (12,36) (Fig. 23-6).

Discontinuity between the semilunar and atrioventricular valves has been considered a criterion in the definition of double-outlet right ventricle by some authors (33,40,42,52–55). However, cases of double-outlet right ventricle have been reported with mitral-aortic continuity, mitral-pulmonary continuity, and bilateral absence of a muscular ventriculoinfundibular fold, and resulting fibrous continuity of the aorta and pulmonary artery with both atrioventricular valves (1,4,5,12,34,36,44). In fact, fibrous continuity has sometimes been found more frequently (12), so that this parameter should not be considered a defining characteristic of double-outlet right ventricle.

The presence or absence of continuity between the semilunar and atrioventricular valves can be assessed echocardiographically through the parasternal long-axis, apical four-chamber, and subcostal long-axis views, with the transducer angled superiorly slowly toward the outflow tracts (Echos. 23-1, 23-2, 23-6).

Infundibular Connections to the Great Vessels and Relationship of the Great Vessels to the Ventricular Communication

Because the relationship between the infundibula is not always the same as that of the great vessels (12,36), a

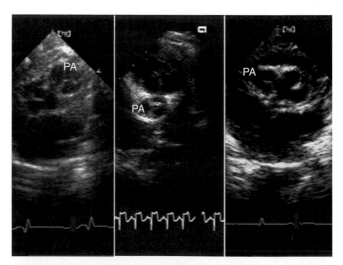

ECHO. 23-5. Parasternal short-axis views of the spatial relationships of the great arteries seen in double-outlet right ventricle. **Left:** The location of the pulmonary artery is to the left of and slightly anterior to the aorta. **Middle:** The aorta is strictly anterior to the pulmonary artery, which is stenotic. **Right:** The aorta is to the left in a strictly side-by-side relationship with the pulmonary artery. *PA*, pulmonary artery.

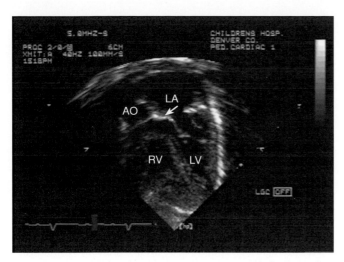

ECHO. 23-6. Apical view with the transducer tilted anteriorly. Discontinuity between the mitral and aortic valves is caused by the presence of a muscular ventriculoinfundibular fold (*arrow*). *AO*, aorta; *LA*, left atrium; *RV*, right ventricle; *LV*, left ventricle.

wide variety of types of double-outlet right ventricle can be seen. The variations in the infundibular-arterial connection depend on the interinfundibular relationship and the shape of the aorticopulmonary and truncal septa. The interinfundibular relationship and location of the ventricular septal defect determine the relationship between the ventricular communication and great vessels.

Muscular defects of the inlet or trabecular type have no relationship to the semilunar valves and therefore are considered noncommitted (1). Defects located between the limbs of the septomarginal trabecula can be related only to the artery connected to the medial infundibulum, in which case they are subaortic or subpulmonary, and they can be continuous with the semilunar valves if they are perimembranous or discontinuous if they are muscular. The types of double-outlet right ventricle with subpulmonary ventricular septal defects have been considered within the spectrum of Taussig-Bing malformations (1,21,31,43,44). When the infundibular septum is hypoplastic or absent, the defect is related to both great arteries and is referred to as doubly committed.

Echocardiography can demonstrate the interinfundibular relationship, location of the ventricular septal defect, spatial relationship of the great vessels and relationship between the semilunar and atrioventricular valves, and the connection between the great vessels and infundibula and therefore to the ventricular septal defect (see specific sections above). This latter point is of extreme surgical importance because it will determine the type of correction to be used.

Stenosis of the Outflow Tracts

Infundibular, valvular, or mixed stenosis is common in double-outlet right ventricle (1,7,25,39–41,43,44,46,47,

50,56,57). In general, it occurs in the infundibulum connected to the artery that is not related to a large ventricular septal defect. Rarely, if the defect is small or restrictive, the obstruction can develop in the infundibulum connected to the artery related to the defect, as a result of connective tissue growths from the fibrous trigone of the heart (25). In the presence of noncommitted, small ventricular septal defects, the obstruction can be present in either infundibulum. The mechanism of obstruction in any of these instances can be displacement of the infundibular septum or hypertrophy of the infundibular septum, infundibular wall, or ventriculoinfundibular fold (Echo. 23-7).

In double-outlet right ventricle of the tetralogy type (normally related great arteries, subaortic ventricular septal defect, and pulmonic stenosis) (Fig. 23-8A), the infundibular morphology is similar to that in tetralogy, the only difference being the greater degree of aortic override in double-outlet right ventricle. The infundibular obstruction can be associated with valvular stenosis as well. Rarely, there can also be stenosis of the subaortic infundibulum (1,25,27).

In double-outlet right ventricle with the aorta located anteriorly and to the left, the ventricular communication is subaortic or noncommitted, and infundibular and/or valvular pulmonic stenosis is frequently present (48).

In double-outlet right ventricle with side-by-side great arteries, aorta to the right, and a subpulmonary ventricular septal defect (Fig. 23-9A), as well as in double-outlet right ventricle with the aorta anterior and to the right and a subpulmonary ventricular septal defect (transposition

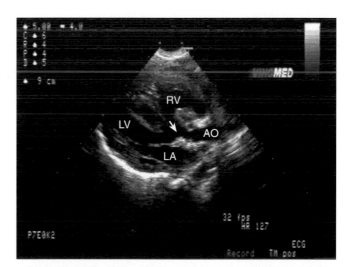

ECHO. 23-7. Parasternal long-axis view in double-outlet right ventricle with an anteroposterior infundibular relationship resulting from anterior displacement of the infundibular septum, which inserts into the anterior limb of the septomarginal trabeculation. Obstruction of the right ventricular outflow is caused by hypertrophy of the infundibular septum. Obstruction of the left ventricular outflow is caused by additional hypertrophy of the muscular ventriculoinfundibular fold (*arrow*). *RV*, right ventricle; *LV*, left ventricle; *LA*, left atrium; *AO*, aorta.

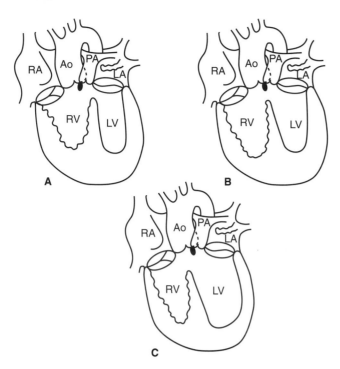

FIG. 23-8. Schematic demonstration of the anatomic spectrum of double-outlet ventricle around tetralogy of Fallot. See text for details. **A:** Double-outlet right ventricle. **B:** Tetralogy of Fallot. **C:** Double-outlet left ventricle. *RA*, right atrium; *LA*, left atrium; *RV*, right ventricle; *LV*, left ventricle; *Ao*, aorta; *PA*, pulmonary artery.

type) (Fig. 23-10A), associated infundibular or valvular stenosis is frequently present in the infundibulum connected to the aorta (1,25,39,41,43,44,47,50,57). The obstruction is caused by the rightward displacement and hypertrophy of the infundibular septum and hypertrophy of the free wall of the ventricle and/or ventriculoinfundibular fold. Much less frequently, there can be stenosis of the infundibulum connected to the pulmonary artery (25,43,58). In these cases, the stenosis is caused by an anomalous origin of the infundibular septum at the expense of the pulmonary infundibulum or by hypertrophy of the infundibular septum and infundibular walls. Frequently, a small ventricular septal defect with various degrees of hypoplasia of the left ventricle and pulmonary valve annulus is present (25).

Echocardiographically, the obstructions to the outflow tracts should be evaluated from the standard parasternal long-axis view as well as with the transducer tilted toward the right ventricular outflow tract, from the parasternal short-axis view at the level of the semilunar valves, from the apical views with the transducer tilted superiorly toward the outflows, and from the subcostal long-axis and short-axis views (Echos. 23-7, 23-8). These views allow localization of the site(s) of obstruction, whether infundibular, valvular, or both. Spectral Doppler, both with high PRF (pulsed repetition frequency) interrogation for better confirmation of the level and relative severity of

the stenoses and with continuous-wave sampling for total velocity recording, need to be performed from these views for an accurate estimation of the gradients. This becomes important in presurgical planning.

Origin and Distribution of the Coronary Arteries

Most commonly, the origin and distribution of the coronary arteries in double-outlet right ventricle are those found in the normal heart (1,4,50,59). Anomalous patterns have been described in 2% to 30% of reported series (1,4,25,40,43,44,48,50,58,60). These can be important in surgical planning and can vary based on the spatial relationship of the great arteries. Because double-outlet ventricle falls within a spectrum of malformations from tetralogy of Fallot through complete transposition of the great arteries to corrected malposition of the great arteries, the coronary patterns are similar to those associated with these defects and are covered in detail in the corresponding chapters.

Associated Anomalies

In double-outlet right ventricle, the great artery that is not related to the ventricular septal defect can show vary-

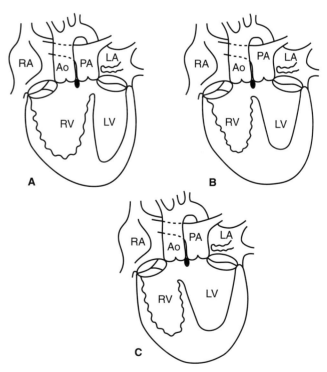

FIG. 23-9. Schematic demonstration of the anatomic spectrum of double-outlet ventricle around transposition of the great arteries with side-by-side great vessels and aorta to the right. See text for details. **A:** Double-outlet right ventricle. **B:** Ventriculoarterial discordance. **C:** Double-outlet left ventricle. *RA*, right atrium; *LA*, left atrium; *RV*, right ventricle; *LV*, left ventricle; *Ao*, aorta; *PA*, pulmonary artery.

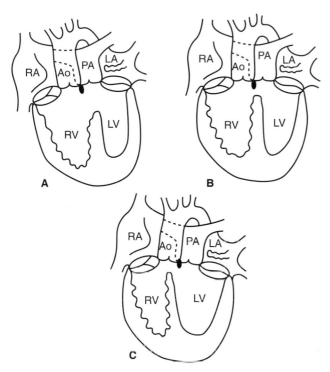

FIG. 23-10. Schematic demonstration of the anatomic spectrum of double-outlet ventricle around classic transposition of the great arteries (aorta anterior and to the right). See text for details. **A:** Double-outlet right ventricle. **B:** Ventriculoarterial discordance (classic complete transposition). **C:** Double-outlet left ventricle. *RA,* right atrium; *LA,* left atrium; *RV,* right ventricle; *LV,* left ventricle; *Ao,* aorta; *PA,* pulmonary artery.

ing degrees of hypoplasia, in addition to infundibular and/or valvular stenosis. As such, in cases with normally related great arteries, subaortic defect, and pulmonic stenosis (tetralogy type), some degree of hypoplasia of the main and branch pulmonary arteries is commonly seen. Pulmonary branch hypoplasia has also been reported in the presence of small subpulmonary ventricular defects and hypoplastic left ventricle (25), and in cases with an anterior and leftward aorta and subaortic ventricular communication (48). In cases of a subpulmonary ventricular septal defect and subaortic infundibular or valvular stenosis, coarctation of the aorta with aortic arch hypoplasia (1,4,6,7,14,27,39,41,43,47,50,52,56,60,61) or interrupted aortic arch (4,6,7,39,41,43,47,60) is frequently present.

Other associated malformations that have been seen with double-outlet right ventricle are ostium secundum atrial septal defects (4,6,39,40,46,50,60), patent foramen ovale (22,44), atrioventricular septal defects (4,6,40, 41,43,46,56,61), straddling or overriding of the mitral valve (4,6,7,27,41,43,44,46,50,61–63), mitral stenosis (4,6,14,41,43,46,50), mitral atresia (4,6,39,41,43,46), left ventricular hypoplasia (14,25,43,46,50,61), parachute deformity of the mitral valve (39,40,43), mitral regurgitation (1,50), supravalve mitral ring (39), overriding or straddling of the tricuspid valve (7,50,61), tricuspid valve ste-

nosis (4,61), tricuspid insufficiency (14,50,61), Ebstein's malformation (61), tricuspid valve cleft (4), tricuspid atresia (6,43), total anomalous pulmonary venous drainage (4,6,39,41,43,60), partial anomalous pulmonary venous drainage (7,39,46), patent ductus arteriosus (4,14,40,44, 46,50,60,61), juxtaposition of the atrial appendages (4,6,7,43,50,56), persistent left superior vena cava (1,4,39,46,50,60), unroofed coronary sinus (14,50), right aortic arch (1,41,50), and absence of the left pulmonary artery (48).

INTRAOPERATIVE AND POSTOPERATIVE EVALUATION

The intraoperative evaluation is conducted through the transesophageal approach. Before bypass, the objectives are to confirm the anatomic characteristics determined in the preoperative transthoracic studies. The ventricular function is best evaluated from the transgastric transverse short-axis view (see Fig. 4-27). Withdrawing the transducer to the four-chamber view (see Fig. 4-28A,B) permits localization of the ventricular communication and determination of its relationship to the great arteries and its size, which are of great surgical importance (Echo. 23-9; see color plate 79 following p. 364). From this view, by tilting the transducer, the atrial septum can be imaged for the presence of a defect or a patent foramen ovale, which should always be closed at surgery (see Fig. 4-29B). The origins and proximal distribution of the coronary arteries can be also seen in these views with anteflexion of the transducer. The atrioventricular valves can be studied from the transverse and longitudinal views (see

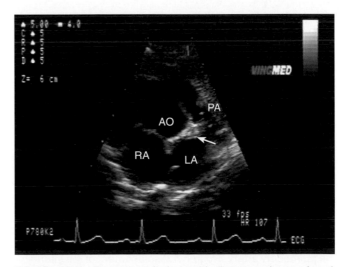

ECHO. 23-8. Parasternal view with the transducer aimed toward the right ventricular outflow. There is narrowing of the right ventricular outflow tract with stenosis at the level of the pulmonic valve and hypertrophy of a muscular ventriculoinfundibular fold (*arrow*). *AO,* aorta; *PA,* pulmonary artery; *RA,* right atrium; *LA,* left atrium.

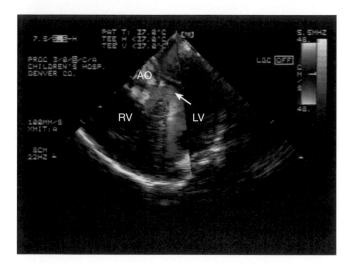

ECHO. 23-9. Transesophageal transverse view with the endoscope slightly withdrawn to demonstrate the ventricular septal defect and aorta. The *arrow* points to the large ventricular septal defect. *RV*, right ventricle; *LV*, left ventricle; *AO*, aorta.

Fig. 4-28). Progressive rightward rotation of the transducer from a longitudinal position allows examination of the aortic and pulmonary outflow tracts to determine the presence of any obstruction and the relationship of the infundibula to each other and to the ventricular septal defect (Fig. 4-29D,E) (Echo. 23-10; see color plate 80 following p. 364). The best views to measure velocity across the outflow tracts by spectral Doppler are the trans-

gastric longitudinal views, in which both outflows are displayed in parallel (see Fig. 4-27E), and the transverse short-axis view of the aorta, with the transducer withdrawn superiorly to bring the pulmonary arteries into view (see Fig. 4-31A,B).

The post-bypass study should begin with evaluation of the ventricular function from the transverse transgastric approach, as in the pre-bypass study. The rest of the examination should be directed to the type of repair performed.

In the presence of subaortic ventricular septal defects with no pulmonic stenosis, the repair will consist of connecting the aorta to the left ventricle through the septal defect by constructing an intraventricular tunnel with a patch (64,65). To avoid obstruction, Sakata et al. (66) consider the distance between the tricuspid and pulmonic valves critical. If the distance is equal to or greater than the aortic diameter, subaortic obstruction is unlikely to occur either early or late postoperatively; if the distance is less than the aortic diameter, subaortic stenosis is likely. When the pulmonic valve is very close to the tricuspid valve, the Rastelli operation is recommended (67). A small ventricular communication is not necessarily a contraindication for placement of a tunnel as long as the defect can be enlarged. Banding of the pulmonary artery can be performed in newborns or small infants with intractable heart failure (68) (Echo. 23-11).

In the presence of pulmonic stenosis and subaortic ventricular septal defect, the surgery is very similar to that performed in tetralogy of Fallot with or without placement of an extracardiac conduit (65) (see Chapter 22).

In the presence of associated hypoplasia or atresia of one of the atrioventricular valves, a staged single ventric-

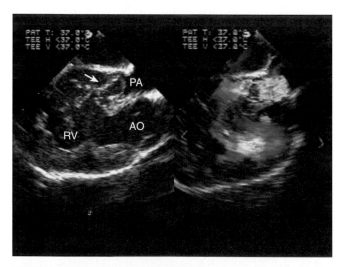

ECHO. 23-10. Transesophageal longitudinal view of the outflow tracts. **Left:** The anatomic view reveals an anteroposterior infundibular relationship, with the aorta anterior to the pulmonary artery. Posterior displacement of the infundibular septum and accessory tricuspid valve tissue (*arrow*) is causing subpulmonary obstruction. **Right:** Color Doppler flow map demonstrates the flow from the right ventricle to both great arteries and the aliasing of the color flow across the pulmonary infundibulum resulting from obstruction. *PA*, pulmonary artery; *AO*, aorta; *RV*, right ventricle.

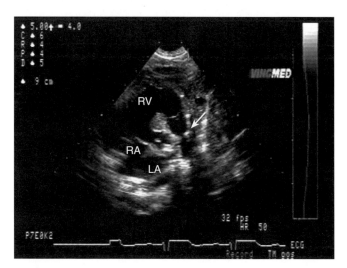

ECHO. 23-11. Parasternal short-axis view at the base of the heart. Note the commitment of both great arteries to the right ventricle. The ventricular septal defect is perimembranous and subaortic. There is hypertrophy and slight posterior displacement of the infundibular septum, causing subaortic narrowing. The *arrow* points to the pulmonary artery band positioned in the midportion of the main pulmonary artery. *RV*, right ventricle; *RA*, right atrium; *LA*, left atrium.

ular repair of the Fontan type is recommended, depending on the status and competence of the existing atrioventricular valve (65,69,70) (see Chapter 17).

When the interventricular communication is subpulmonary and there is minimal or no subpulmonary stenosis, the initial surgery may have to be a palliative banding of the pulmonary artery to prevent pulmonary vascular disease. The definitive surgery can consist of placement of an intraventricular tunnel connecting the pulmonary artery to the left ventricle, followed by an arterial switch or an atrial switch or the Damus-Kaye-Stansel procedure (see Chapter 24). In some cases, the aorta can be connected to the left ventricle via a tunnel without causing subpulmonary obstruction and without the need for an extracardiac conduit (71–73). If pulmonic stenosis is present, the Rastelli type of repair can be performed along with placement of an extracardiac conduit. If a tunnel cannot be implanted without causing obstruction, the ventricular septal defect can be closed and an atrial switch performed with placement of an extracardiac conduit (65).

In the presence of noncommitted ventricular septal defects with pulmonic stenosis, several surgical alternatives have been considered. An intraventricular tunnel can be created between the aorta and left ventricle along with placement of an extracardiac conduit. Closure of the ventricular septal defect, which creates ventriculoarterial discordance, is followed by an atrial switch and placement of an extracardiac conduit between the pulmonary artery and left ventricle. Alternatively, a Fontan type of procedure can be considered (65,67,74).

When the ventricular communication is doubly committed, surgery consists of augmenting the ventricular septal defect anteriorly and creating an intraventricular tunnel to connect the left ventricle to the aorta (50).

The immediate and late postoperative evaluation should be directed to detection of residual ventricular septal defects and any obstruction of the intraventricular tunnel and outflow tracts. If an extracardiac conduit was placed, attempts should be made to measure velocities at the proximal and distal ends of the conduit as well as across the valve and to record and grade the severity of regurgitation. As mentioned previously, regurgitation of conduit valves is very common immediately after implantation and may progress with time.

If an arterial switch operation was performed, the postsurgical evaluation should include specific interrogation of the supravalve neoaortic and neopulmonary anastomotic sites, which are prone to become restrictive. If an atrial switch was required, the late follow-up should include examination of the systemic and pulmonary venous conduits for obstructions or leaks. These concerns are considered in detail in Chapter 24.

DOUBLE-OUTLET LEFT VENTRICLE

Double-outlet left ventricle is a type of ventriculoarterial connection in which more than half of both great arteries emerge from the anatomic left ventricle (16,75), both great arteries emerge completely or almost completely from the left ventricle (13,76), or one great vessel emerges completely from the left ventricle and the other overrides the ventricular septum by more than 50% over the left ventricle (2) (see Fig. 2-8D). In the context of this chapter, we require the presence of two ventricles, so that we exclude double-outlet left ventricle with atrioventricular univentricular connection, considered by some as a subtype of double-outlet left ventricle (16).

Double-outlet left ventricle is a rare malformation, occurring in 0.1% to 0.23% of all congenital cardiac anomalies (77,78) and in fewer than 5% of all hearts with atrioventricular biventricular connection and a double outlet. Its incidence is less than 1 in 200,000 live births (6).

EMBRYOLOGIC CONSIDERATIONS

The fact that the first case, described by Maréchal in 1819 (79), was actually a single ventricle with outlet chamber, and that the case described by Fragoyannis and Kardalinos (80) was a double-outlet right ventricle with atrioventricular discordance and situs solitus and that its existence was considered embryologically improbable or impossible (30,81) all contributed to a general doubt about the existence of this malformation. However, the first successful surgical repair of double-outlet left ventricle, reported by Sakakibara et al. in 1967 (82), and the description of a case of double-outlet left ventricle with intact ventricular septum by Paul et al. in 1970 (83) removed all doubts.

Morphogenetically, double-outlet left ventricle is caused by an exaggerated displacement of the conus to the left (29,75,78), which results in both infundibula connecting with the morphologic left ventricle. In addition, anomalies in the origin or shape of the conal or infundibular septum, and of the truncal and aorticopulmonary septa, result in the various types of double-outlet left ventricle (Figs. 23-8C, 23-9C, 23-10C, 23-11C, 23-12C, 23-13C; see color plate 81 following p. 364). The theory of differential conal growth (84), which considers bilateral absence of the conus an integral component in the morphogenesis of double-outlet left ventricle and a differential characteristic for its diagnosis (83,85), is erroneous because there are cases of double-outlet left ventricle with subpulmonary, subaortic, or double conus (6,15,16, 75,78,86,87). Like double-outlet right ventricle, it can present in situs solitus, situs inversus, or situs ambiguus and, according to the ventricular loop, can have atrioventricular concordance or discordance (Fig. 23-14).

Double-outlet right and left ventricles can be considered to occupy the extremes of a variety of anatomic spectra depending on the spatial relationship of the great arteries and the ventriculoarterial connection. With Fig. 23-7 used as a reference, the spectra can be classified as follows: (a)

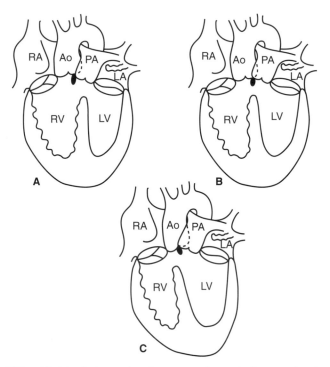

FIG. 23-11. Schematic demonstration of the anatomic spectrum of double-outlet ventricle with normally related great arteries without pulmonic stenosis. See text for details. **A:** Double-outlet right ventricle. **B:** Ventriculoarterial discordance with posterior aorta. **C:** Double-outlet left ventricle. *RA*, right atrium; *LA*, left atrium; *RV*, right ventricle; *LV*, left ventricle; *Ao*, aorta; *PA*, pulmonary artery.

double-outlet right ventricle with normally related arteries and subaortic ventricular septal defect, ventriculoarterial discordance with posterior aorta and double-outlet left ventricle with posterior and rightward aorta (Fig. 23-11); (b) double-outlet right ventricle with aorta to the left and anterior, anatomically corrected malposition of the great arteries and double-outlet left ventricle with aorta to the left and anterior (Fig. 23-13); (c) double-outlet right ventricle with aorta anterior and to the right and subpulmonary ventricular septal defect, ventriculoarterial discordance with aorta anterior and to the right (classic complete transposition of the great arteries) and double-outlet left ventricle with aorta anterior and to the right (Fig. 23-10); (d) double-outlet right ventricle with side-by-side great vessels and aorta on the right, ventriculoarterial discordance with side-by-side great arteries and rightward aorta and double-outlet left ventricle with side-by-side great vessels and aorta on the right (Fig. 23-9); and (e) double-outlet right ventricle with side-by-side great vessels and aorta to the left of the pulmonary artery, anatomically corrected malposition with side-by-side great arteries and leftward aorta and double-outlet left ventricle with side-by-side great vessels and aorta to the left (Fig. 23-12).

ANATOMIC AND ECHOCARDIOGRAPHIC CONSIDERATIONS

The echocardiographic study in double-outlet left ventricle should consider the visceroatrial situs, atrioventricu-

lar connection, and systemic and pulmonary venous drainage. In addition, the specific details pertaining to this malformation are (a) location of the ventricular septal defect and its relation to the great vessels and atrioventricular valves, (b) the spatial relationship of the great vessels, (c) presence of stenosis of the outflow tracts, (d) origin and distribution of the coronary arteries, and (e) presence of associated anomalies. Intraoperative and postoperative evaluation should be included.

Location of the Ventricular Septal Defect and Its Relation to the Great Vessels and Atrioventricular Valves

With the exception of the case reported by Paul et al. (83), a ventricular septal defect is always present in this malformation. Generally, it is located between the limbs of the septomarginal trabecula, and its roof is the semilunar valve of the great artery that overrides the ventricular septum (Fig. 23-15). Sometimes, the defect is in continuity with the tricuspid valve (Fig. 23-15A,E) or may be separated by a muscular band, the ventriculoinfundibular fold (Fig. 23-15B,D). Its inferior and anterior borders are the limbs of the septomarginal trabecula. The infundibular

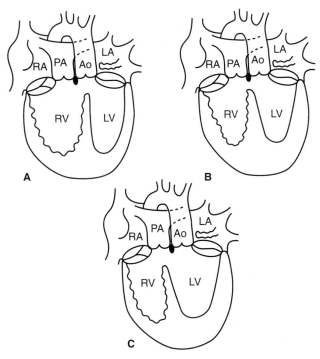

FIG. 23-12. Schematic demonstration of the anatomic spectrum of double-outlet ventricle around anatomically corrected malposition of the great arteries with side-by-side great vessels and aorta to the left. See text for details. **A:** Double-outlet right ventricle. **B:** Anatomically corrected malposition of the great arteries. **C:** Double-outlet left ventricle. *RA*, right atrium; *LA*, left atrium; *RV*, right ventricle; *LV*, left ventricle; *Ao*, aorta; *PA*, pulmonary artery.

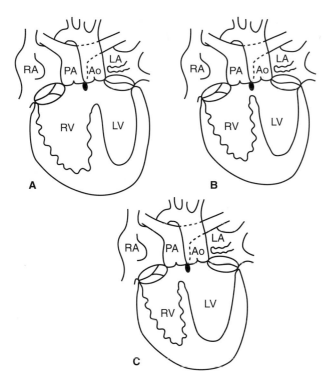

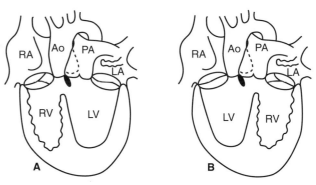

FIG. 23-14. Schematic drawings of hearts with double-outlet left ventricle and situs solitus. **A:** With atrioventricular concordance. **B:** With atrioventricular discordance. *RA,* right atrium; *LA,* left atrium; *RV,* right ventricle; *LV,* ventricle; *Ao,* aorta; *PA,* pulmonary artery.

FIG. 23-13. Schematic demonstration of the anatomic spectrum of double-outlet ventricle around anatomically corrected malposition of the great arteries with aorta anterior and to the left. **A:** Double-outlet right ventricle. **B:** Anatomically corrected malposition of the great arteries. **C:** Double-outlet left ventricle. *RA,* right atrium; *LA,* left atrium; *RV,* right ventricle; *LV,* left ventricle; *Ao,* aorta; *PA,* pulmonary artery.

septum is displaced to the left and located completely within the left ventricle; therefore, the ventricular septal defect is caused by a malalignment between the infundibular and ventricular septa (78,87–89).

The relationship of the defect to the great vessels has

been used to classify double-outlet left ventricle (13,15,16). In the majority of cases, the semilunar valve that is related to the defect is the aortic valve (Figs. 23-8C, 23-9C, 23-10C, 23-11C). The incidence of subaortic defects is between 68% and 77.5% of all cases of double-outlet left ventricle (16,89,90). The second type of ventricular defect is related to the pulmonic valve and is found in 13.7% to 17% of cases (16,89) (Figs. 23-12C, 23-13C). In 10% of cases, the infundibular septum is hypoplastic or absent and the defect is doubly committed, being related to both semilunar valves (16,89,90) (Fig. 23-15C). The incidence of noncommitted interventricular communications is very small, and these are usually associated with multiple defects (16,86). Continuity or discontinuity between the semilunar valves and atrioventricular valves depends on the spatial position of the great vessel valves and the presence of the ventriculoinfundibular fold (Fig. 23-15).

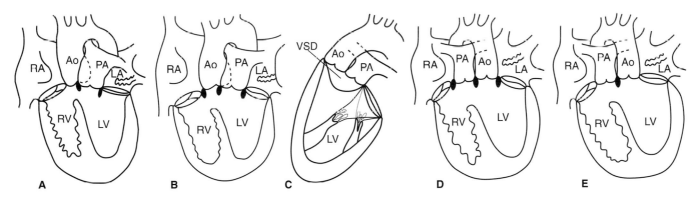

FIG. 23-15. Schematic drawings of hearts with double-outlet left ventricle demonstrating the relationship of the atrioventricular valves, the ventricular septal defect, and the semilunar valves. **A:** Subaortic ventricular septal defect, aortic-tricuspid continuity, and pulmonic-mitral discontinuity. **B:** Subaortic ventricular septal defect, aortic-tricuspid discontinuity, and pulmonic-mitral discontinuity. **C:** Doubly committed ventricular septal defect and pulmonic-mitral continuity. **D:** Side-by-side great arteries with the aorta to the left, subpulmonic ventricular septal defect, and pulmonic-tricuspid and aortic-mitral discontinuity. **E:** Side-by-side great arteries with the aorta to the left, subpulmonic ventricular septal defect, and pulmonic-tricuspid and aortic-mitral continuity. *RA,* right atrium; *LA,* left atrium; *RV,* right ventricle; *LV,* left ventricle; *Ao,* aorta; *PA,* pulmonary artery; *VSD,* ventricular septal defect.

The echocardiographic views that are best to determine the location of the ventricular defect and its relationship to the semilunar valves are the parasternal long- and short-axis views at the level of the valve leaflets as well as the apical four-chamber and subcostal long-axis views, with the transducer tilted toward the outflows (91) (Echo. 23-12). Specific details to note in these views are the degree of override and relation of the left ventricle to both great vessels, relationship of the defect with the valve of the artery that overrides the septum, and continuity or lack thereof between the semilunar and atrioventricular valves. The malalignment between the infundibular and ventricular septa can be seen from the parasternal long-axis view, from the apical four-chamber view with the transducer swept from a posterior to an anterior orientation to view the outflow tracts, and similarly from the subcostal four-chamber view (Echo. 23-12). The pattern of blood flow across the defect can be visualized on color Doppler flow mapping from any of these views and will reveal the streaming that may occur favoring one or the other great vessel depending on the location of the defect, the spatial position of the vessels, and the degree of override (Echo. 23-13).

The presence of a bilateral muscular infundibulum (double conus) or a muscular subaortic or subpulmonary infundibulum or the bilateral absence of a muscular infundibulum can be determined from the same views. This will determine the continuity or discontinuity between the semilunar and atrioventricular valves (Echo. 23-12).

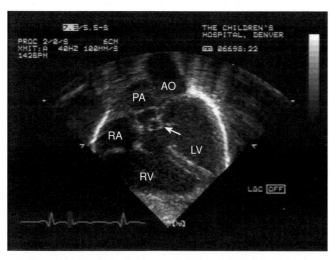

ECHO. 23-12. Subcostal view with the transducer tilted toward the outflow tracts in a patient with double-outlet left ventricle. There is override of the pulmonary artery over the interventricular septum so that it is almost completely committed to the left ventricle. The ventricular septal defect is subpulmonic. There is discontinuity between the tricupid and pulmonic valves and between the mitral and aortic valves. The *arrow* points to a subpulmonic obstruction caused by accessory mitral valve tissue below the pulmonic valve. *RA*, right atrium; *RV*, right ventricle; *LV*, left ventricle; *PA*, pulmonary artery; *AO*, aorta.

Spatial Relationship of the Great Vessels

When the relative spatial positions of the great arteries are defined, the range is similar to that described for double-outlet right ventricle (Fig. 23-7). They can be more or less normally related, with the aorta posterior and to the right and the pulmonary artery anterior and to the left. They can be side by side, with the aorta to the right or left, or the aorta can be anterior and to the right, strictly anterior, or anterior and to the left.

The spatial relationship of the great vessels can be determined by echocardiography from the parasternal short-axis view at the level of the great vessels, from the long-axis parasternal and subcostal views, and from the apical outflow views (Echo. 23-5).

Stenosis of the Outflow Tracts

As in double-outlet right ventricle, infundibular and/or valvular stenosis can be seen in the artery that is not related to the ventricular septal defect (6,13,16,75,76,89–92). Obstruction can be caused by hypertrophy of the muscular infundibulum (ventriculoinfundibular fold), displacement and hypertrophy of the infundibular septum, and/or hypertrophy of the free wall of the infundibulum.

With a subaortic defect, stenosis of the pulmonary infundibulum and valve is usually present, which can be associated with some degree of right ventricular hypoplasia. When the defect is subpulmonary, there is some degree of subaortic obstruction in 50% of cases (75). Obstruction of the outflow tract of the great artery that overrides the septum can occur but is very rare (16,75) (Echos. 23-12, 23-13). Echocardiographically, the obstructions can be demonstrated in the parasternal long-axis view, the apical and subcostal four-chamber to outflow sweep, and the apical long-axis view. Gradients can be estimated from the velocity recorded across the outflows with continuous-wave Doppler. If several sites of stenosis (e.g., subvalvular as well as valvular) are present, high PRF should be used to estimate their relative severity.

Origin and Distribution of the Coronary Arteries

Anomalies of the origin and distribution of the coronaries can be seen in 20% of cases (75). These include single coronary artery and origin of the anterior descending from the right coronary artery (16,75,78,87,93). This information is important at the time of surgical repair, particularly in the presence of infundibular stenosis. The views to study the coronary arteries include the parasternal short-axis view, from which both the left main coronary artery and its branches can be seen as well as the right main coronary artery coursing along the right atrioventricular groove. From this view especially, large conal branches

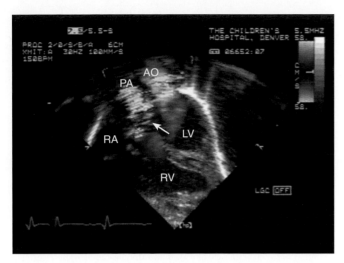

ECHO. 23-13. Color Doppler flow map of the patient in Echo. 23-12. The *arrow* points to the area of subpulmonic obstruction. Note the color aliasing beyond the obstruction. There is streaming of right ventricular blood into the pulmonary artery and of left ventricular blood into the left ventricle. *RA*, right atrium; *RV*, right ventricle; *LV*, left ventricle; *AO*, aorta; *PA*, pulmonary artery.

can be identified as well as anomalous origins of the anterior descending branch. The posterior descending artery can be identified from the parasternal long-axis view of the inflow, coursing along the ventricular septum posteriorly.

Associated Anomalies

Some of the associated anomalies reported include malformations of the tricuspid valve, such as stenosis, Ebstein's anomaly, and straddling and atresia (13,15, 16,47,75,78,87,89,90,94,95); malformations of the mitral valve, including cleft, stenosis, and atresia (13,15,47,95); coarctation of the aorta (13,15,47,89); patent ductus arteriosus (13,78); juxtaposition of the atrial appendages (13,47); atrial septal defect (13,78); and persistent left superior vena cava draining into the coronary sinus (13).

INTRAOPERATIVE AND POSTOPERATIVE EVALUATION

The intraoperative studies are usually conducted from the transesophageal approach. The pre-bypass study should start with an evaluation of ventricular size and function, best performed from the transverse transgastric view (see Fig. 4-27A). Withdrawal of the transducer to the four-chamber view (see Fig. 4-28A,B) will permit recording of the ventricular septal defect and its relationship to the great arteries. It will also afford another view of the two ventricular cavities and their size and allow examination of the atrioventricular

valves for any anatomic abnormalities, such as straddling or overriding. The forward velocities and any regurgitation should be documented by color and spectral Doppler from these views. The coronary arterial origin and proximal distribution can be seen by anteflexing the transducer to a short axis of the aortic root along with slight right and left rotation (see Fig. 4-29B). This view also permits examination of the atrial septum for the presence of shunts, which should always be closed at the time of surgery (see Figs. 4-29B, 4-30A). The longitudinal views will provide another perspective of the atrioventricular valves and ventricular cavities (see Fig. 4-28C,D). More importantly, the two outflow tracts and the relationship of the great vessels to the ventricles and to the septal defect can be determined (see Fig. 4-29E). Extreme rightward rotation of the transducer will reveal the atrial septum and the systemic and some of the pulmonary venous connections (see Fig. 4-30D).

After bypass, the study should begin with a global assessment of ventricular function from the transverse transgastric approach. This should be supplemented with an assessment of wall motion from the various transverse and longitudinal views. The study should proceed to analyze those factors specific to the repair performed.

The aim of the surgical repair is to close the ventricular septal defect, connect the left ventricle to the aorta and the right ventricle to the pulmonary artery, and if needed place an extracardiac conduit (86,92,96). If the ventricular defect is subpulmonary and there is no stenosis, the defect can be closed so as to connect the pulmonary artery to the right ventricle directly (82,97). In cases with atresia or stenosis of the tricuspid valve and/or hypoplasia of the right ventricle, a single ventricle repair of the Fontan type is recommended (92,94,98).

Postoperatively, the features that should be specifically assessed are the presence and amount of any residual shunting at the ventricular or atrial level, possible stenosis of either outflow tract, atrioventricular valve regurgitation and stenosis, and/or regurgitation of the extracardiac conduits if these were implanted. It is important to recall that regurgitation of the conduits immediately after implantation is common, and it is useful to obtain an estimate intraoperatively that can be used as a baseline for the late follow-up.

REFERENCES

1. Lev M, Bharati S, Meng CCL, Liberthson RR, Paul MH, Idriss F. A concept of double-outlet right ventricle. *J Thorac Cardiovasc Surg* 1972;64:271–281.
2. Kirklin JW, Pacifico AD, Bargeron LM Jr, Soto B. Cardiac repair in anatomically corrected malposition of the great arteries. *Circulation* 1973;48:153–159.
3. Tynan MJ, Anderson RH, Macartney FJ, Shinebourne EA. The ventricular origin of the great arteries. In: Anderson RH, Shine-

bourne EA, eds. *Paediatric cardiology 1977*. Edinburgh: Churchill Livingstone, 1978:36–42.

4. Wilcox BR, Ho SY, Macartney FJ, Becker AE, Gerlis LM, Anderson RH. Surgical anatomy of double-outlet right ventricle with situs solitus and atrioventricular concordance. *J Thorac Cardiovasc Surg* 1981;82:405–417.

5. Anderson RH, Becker AE, Wilcox BR, Macartney FJ, Wilkinson JL. Surgical anatomy of double-outlet right ventricle—a reappraisal. *Am J Cardiol* 1983;52:555–559.

6. Wilkinson JL. Double outlet ventricle. In: Anderson RH, Macartney FJ, Shinebourne EA, Tynan M, eds. *Paediatric cardiology*, Vol. 2. Edinburgh: Churchill Livingstone, 1987:889–911.

7. Musumeci F, Shumway S, Lincoln C, Anderson RH. Surgical treatment for double-outlet right ventricle at the Brompton Hospital, 1973 to 1986. *J Thorac Cardiovasc Surg* 1988;96:278–287.

8. Tynan MJ, Becker AE, Macartney FJ, Quero Jimenez M, Shinebourne EA, Anderson RH. Nomenclature and classification of congenital heart disease. *Br Heart J* 1979;41:544–553.

9. Anderson RH, Ho SY. Tomographic anatomy of the normal and congenitally malformed heart. In: Higgins CB, Silverman NH, Kersting-Sommerhoff B, Schmidt KG, eds. *Congenital heart disease: echocardiography and magnetic resonance imaging*. New York: Raven Press, 1990:1–35.

10. Arteaga M, De la Cruz MV, Sanchez C, Diaz GF. Double outlet right ventricle: experimental morphogenesis in the chick embryo heart. *Pediatr Cardiol* 1982;3:219–227.

11. De la Cruz MV, Cayre R. Doble salida ventricular derecha. Embriogenesis, tipos anatomicos e implicaciones quirurgicas. *Rev Lat Cardiol y Cir Cardiovasc Inf* 1985;1:18–24.

12. De la Cruz MV, Cayre R, Arista-Salado Martinez O, Sadowinski S, Serrano A. The infundibular interrelationships and the ventriculoarterial connection in double outlet right ventricle. Clinical and surgical implications. *Int J Cardiol* 1992;35:153–164.

13. Bharati S, Lev M, Stewart R, McAllister HA, Kirklin JW. The morphologic spectrum of double outlet left ventricle and its surgical significance. *Circulation* 1978;58:558–565.

14. Piccoli G, Pacifico AD, Kirklin JW, Blackstone EH, Kirklin JK, Bargeron LM Jr. Changing results and concepts in the surgical treatment of double-outlet right ventricle: analysis of 137 operations in 126 patients. *Am J Cardiol* 1983;52:549–554.

15. Van Praagh R, Weinberg PM. Double-outlet left ventricle. In: Adams FH, Emmanouilides GC, eds. *Moss heart disease in infants, children, and adolescents*, 3rd ed. Baltimore: Williams & Wilkins, 1983:370–385.

16. Otero Coto E, Quero Jimenez M, Anderson RH, et al. Double outlet left ventricle. In: Anderson RH, Macartney FJ, Shinebourne EA, Tynan M, eds. *Paediatric cardiology 5*. Edinburgh: Churchill Livingstone, 1983:451–465.

17. Howell CE, Ho SY, Anderson RH, Elliott MJ. Fibrous skeleton and ventricular outflow tracts in double-outlet right ventricle. *Ann Thorac Surg* 1991;51:394–400.

18. Witham AC. Double outlet right ventricle: a partial transposition complex. *Am Heart J* 1957;53:928–939.

19. Abbott ME. *Atlas of congenital cardiac disease*. New York: American Heart Association, 1936.

20. Saphir O, Lev M. The tetralogy of Eisenmenger. *Am Heart J* 1941;21:31–46.

21. Taussig HB, Bing RJ. Complete transposition of the aorta and a levoposition of the pulmonary artery. *Am Heart J* 1949;37:551–559.

22. Braun K, De Vries A, Feingold DS, Ehrenfeld NE, Feldman J, Schorr S. Complete dextroposition of the aorta, pulmonary stenosis, interventricular septal defect, and patent foramen ovale. *Am Heart J* 1952;43:773–780.

23. Mitchell SC, Korones SB, Berendes HN. Congenital heart disease in 56,109 births. *Circulation* 1971;43:323–332.

24. Hoffman JIE, Christianson R. Congenital heart disease in a cohort of 19,502 births with long-term follow up. *Am J Cardiol* 1978;42:641–647.

25. Herraiz Sarachaga I, Quero Jimenez M, Santalla Rando A, Sanchez PA. Ventriculo derecho de doble salida. In: Sanchez PA, ed. *Cardiologia pediatrica, clinica y cirugia*, Vol 1. Barcelona: Salvat Editores SA, 1986:567–592.

26. Fyler DC. Prevalence. Trends. In: Fyler DC, ed. *Nadas' pediatric cardiology*. Philadelphia: Hanley & Belfus, 1992:273–280.

27. Freedom RM, Smallhorn JF. Double-outlet right ventricle. In: Freedom RM, Benson LN, Smallhorn JF, eds. *Neonatal heart disease*. London: Springer-Verlag, 1992:453–470.

28. Anderson RH, Wilkinson JL, Arnold R, Becker AE, Lubkiewicz K. Morphogenesis of bulboventricular malformations II. Observations on malformed hearts. *Br Heart J* 1974;36:948–970.

29. Goor DA, Edwards JE. The spectrum of transposition of the great arteries with specific reference to developmental anatomy of the conus. *Circulation* 1973;48:406–415.

30. Van Mierop LHS, Wiglesworth FW. Pathogenesis of transposition complexes II. Anomalies due to faulty transfer of the posterior great artery. *Am J Cardiol* 1963;12:226–232.

31. Van Praagh R. What is the Taussig-Bing malformation? *Circulation* 1968;38:445–449.

32. Gessner IH, Van Mierop LHS. Experimental production of cardiac defects: the spectrum of dextroposition of the aorta. *Am J Cardiol* 1970;25:272–278.

33. Baron MG. Radiologic notes in cardiology. Angiographic differentiation between tetralogy of Fallot and double-outlet right ventricle. Relationship of the mitral and aortic valves. *Circulation* 1971;43:451–455.

34. Angelini P, Leachman RD. The spectrum of double-outlet right ventricle: an embryologic interpretation. *Cardiovasc Dis* 1976;3:127–149.

35. Anderson RH. The morphogenesis of ventriculo-arterial discordance. In: Van Mierop LHS, Oppenheimer-Deker A, Bruins CLDC. *Embryology and teratology of the heart and the great arteries*. Leiden, Germany: Leiden University Press, 1978:93–111.

36. Arista-Salado Martinez O, Arango Casado J, De la Cruz MV, Diaz F, Cubero O. Double outlet right ventricle—an echocardiographic study. *Cardiol Young* 1993;3:124–131.

37. MacMahon HE, Lipa M. Double-outlet right ventricle with intact interventricular septum. *Circulation* 1964;30:745–748.

38. Ainger LE. Double-outlet right ventricle: intact ventricular septum, mitral stenosis and blind left ventricle. *Am Heart J* 1965;70:521–525.

39. Zamora R, Moller JH, Edwards JE. Double-outlet right ventricle. Anatomic types and associated anomalies. *Chest* 1975;68:672–677.

40. Sridaromont S, Feldt RH, Ritter DG, Davis GD, Edwards JE. Double outlet right ventricle: hemodynamic and anatomic correlations. *Am J Cardiol* 1976;38:85–94.

41. Sondheimer HM, Freedom RM, Olley PM. Double outlet right ventricle: clinical spectrum and prognosis. *Am J Cardiol* 1977;39:709–714.

42. Sridaromont S, Ritter DG, Feldt RH, Davis GD, Edwards JE. Double-outlet right ventricle. Anatomic and angiocardiographic correlations. *Mayo Clin Proc* 1978;53:555–577.

43. Wilkinson JL, Wilcox BR, Anderson RH. Anatomy of double outlet right ventricle. In: Anderson RH, Macartney FJ, Shinebourne EA, Tynan M, eds. *Paediatric cardiology*, Vol. 5. Edinburgh: Churchill Livingstone, 1983:397–407.

44. Stellin G, Zuberbuhler JR, Anderson RH, Siewers RD. The surgical anatomy of the Taussig-Bing malformation. *J Thorac Cardiovasc Surg* 1987;93:560–569.

45. De Oliveira e Silva ER, Snyder MS, O'Loughlin JE, et al. Unique variant of Taussig-Bing heart: double-outlet right ventricle with double ventricular septal defects and double overriding of great arteries. *Pediatr Cardiol* 1991;12:123–125.

46. Cameron AH, Acerete F, Quero M, Castro MC. Double outlet right ventricle. Study of 27 cases. *Br Heart J* 1976;38:1124–1132.

47. Roberson DA, Silverman NH. Malaligned outlet septum with subpulmonary ventricular septal defect and abnormal ventriculoarterial connection: a morphologic spectrum defined echocardiographically. *J Am Coll Cardiol* 1990;16:459–468.

48. Lincoln C, Anderson RH, Shinebourne EA, English TAH, Wilkinson JL. Double outlet right ventricle with l-malposition of the aorta. *Br Heart J* 1975;37:453–463.

49. Otero Coto E, Castaneda AR, Caffarena JM, Deverall PB, Cabrera A, Quero Jimenez M. L-malposed great arteries with situs solitus and concordant atrioventricular connection. *J Cardiovasc Surg* 1982;23:277–286.

50. Kirklin JW, Barrat-Boyes BG. Double outlet right ventricle. In:

Kirklin JW, Barrat-Boyes BG, eds. *Cardiac surgery. morphology, diagnostic criteria, natural history, techniques, results, and indications*, Vol 2, 2nd ed. New York: Churchill Livingstone, 1993:1469–1500.

51. Anderson RH, Becker AE, Van Mierop LHS. What should we call the crista? *Br Heart J* 1977;39:856–859.
52. Neufeld HN, DuShane JW, Wood EH, Kirklin JW, Edwards JE. Origin of both great vessels from the right ventricle. I. Without pulmonary stenosis. *Circulation* 1961;23:399–412.
53. Neufeld HN, DuShane JW, Edwards JE. Origin of both great vessels from the right ventricle. II. With pulmonary stenosis. *Circulation* 1961;23:603–612.
54. Carey LS, Edwards JE. Roentgenographic features in cases with origin of both great vessels from the right ventricle without pulmonary stenosis. *Am J Roentgenol* 1965;93:269–297.
55. Hallermann FJ, Kincaid OW, Ritter DG, Titus JL. Mitral-semilunar valve relationships in the angiography of cardiac malformations. *Radiology* 1970;94:63–68.
56. Hagler DJ, Tajik AJ, Seward JB, Mair DD, Ritter DG. Double-outlet right ventricle: wide-angle two dimensional echocardiographic observations. *Circulation* 1981;63:419–428.
57. Anderson RH, Becker AE, Lucchese FA, Meier MA, Rigby ML, Soto B. Double outlet right ventricle. In: Anderson RH, Becker AE, Lucchese FA, Meier MA, Rigby ML, Soto B. *Morphology of congenital heart disease. angiocardiographic, echocardiographic and surgical correlates.* Baltimore: University Park Press, 1983:51–64.
58. Navarro Lopez F, Dobben GG, Rabinowitz M, et al. Taussig Bing complex with pulmonary stenosis. *Dis Chest* 1966;50:1–12.
59. Neufeld HN, Schneeweiss A. Origin of both great vessels from the right ventricle. In: Neufeld HN, Schneeweiss A, eds. *Coronary artery disease in infants and children.* Philadelphia: Lea & Febiger, 1983:102–106.
60. Luber JM, Castaneda AR, Lang P, Norwood WI. Repair of double-outlet right ventricle: early and late results. *Circulation* 1983;68[Suppl II].II-144–II-147.
61. Battistessa S, Soto B. Double outlet right ventricle with discordant atrioventricular connexion: an angiographic analysis of 19 cases. *Int J Cardiol* 1990;27:253–263.
62. Kitamura N, Takao A, Ando M, Imai Y, Konno S. Taussig-Bing heart with mitral valve straddling: case report and post-mortem study. *Circulation* 1974;49:761–767.
63. Muster AJ, Bharati S, Aziz KU, et al. Taussig Bing anomaly with straddling mitral valve. *J Thorac Cardiovasc Surg* 1979;77:832–842.
64. Kirklin JW, Harp RA, McGoon DC. Surgical treatment of origin of both vessels from right ventricle, including cases of pulmonary stenosis. *J Thorac Cardiovasc Surg* 1964;48:1026–1036.
65. Kirklin JW, Pacifico AD, Blackstone EH, Kirklin JK, Bargeron LM. Current risks and protocols for operations for double-outlet right ventricle. *J Thorac Cardiovasc Surg* 1986;92:913–930.
66. Sakata R, Lecompte Y, Battise A, Borromee L, Durandy Y. Anatomic repair of anomalies of ventriculoarterial connection associated with ventricular septal defect. I. Criteria of surgical decision. *J Thorac Cardiovasc Surg* 1988;95:90–95.
67. Castaneda AR, Jonas RA, Mayer JE, Hanley FL. Double-outlet right ventricle. In: Castaneda AR, Jonas RA, Mayer JE, Hanley FL, eds. *Cardiac surgery of the neonate and infant.* Philadelphia: WB Saunders, 1994:445–459.
68. Harvey JC, Sondheimer HM, Williams WG, Olley PM, Trusler GA. Repair of double-outlet right ventricle. *J Thorac Cardiovasc Surg* 1977;73:611–615.
69. DeLeon SY, Ilbawi MN, Idriss FS, et al. Fontan type operation for complex lesions. Surgical considerations to improve survival. *J Thorac Cardiovasc Surg* 1986;92:1029–1037.
70. Kirklin JW, Blackstone EH, Kirklin JK, Pacifico AD, Bargeron LM. The Fontan operation. Ventricular hypertrophy, age, and date of operation as risk factors. *J Thorac Cardiovasc Surg* 1986;92:1049–1064.
71. Patrick DL, McGoon DC. An operation for double-outlet right ventricle with transposition of the great arteries. *J Cardiovasc Surg* 1968;9:537–542.
72. Kawashima Y, Fujita T, Miyamoto T, Manabe H. Intraventricular

rerouting of blood for the correction of Taussig-Bing malformation. *J Thorac Cardiovasc Surg* 1971;62:825–829.
73. Pacifico AD, Kirklin JK, Colvin EV, Bargeron LM Jr. Intraventricular tunnel repair for Taussig-Bing heart and related cardiac anomalies. *Circulation* 1986;74[Suppl I]:I-53–I-60.
74. Russo P, Danielson GK, Puga FJ, McGoon DC, Humes R. Modified Fontan procedure for biventricular hearts with complex forms of double-outlet right ventricle. *Circulation* 1988;78[Suppl III]:III-20–III-25.
75. Arque Gibernau JM, Quero Jimenez M, Otero Coto E. Ventriculo izquierdo de doble salida. In: Sanchez PA, ed. *Cardiologia pediatrica, clinica y cirugia*, Vol 1. Barcelona: Editorial Salvat, 1986:593–599.
76. Soto B, Pacifico AD. Double-outlet left ventricle. In: Soto B, Pacifico AD, eds. *Angiocardiography in congenital heart malformations.* Mount Kisco, NY: Futura Publishing, 1990:395–404.
77. Ferencz C. A case-control study of cardiovascular malformations in liveborn infants: the morphogenetic relevance of epidemiologic findings. In: Clark EB, Takao A, eds. *Developmental cardiology. Morphogenesis and function.* Mount Kisco, NY: Futura Publishing, 1990:523–539.
78. Otero Coto E, Quero Jimenez M, Castaneda AR, Rufilanchas JJ, Deverall PB. Double outlet from chambers of left ventricular morphology. *Br Heart J* 1979;42:15–21.
79. Maréchal. Conformation vicieuse du coeur d'un enfant affecté de la maladie bleue. *J Gen Med* 1819;69:354.
80. Fragoyannis S, Kardalinos A. Transposition of the great vessels, both arising from the left ventricle (juxtaposition of pulmonary artery). Tricuspid atresia, atrial septal defect and ventricular septal defect. *Am J Cardiol* 1962;10:601–604.
81. Grant RP. The morphogenesis of transposition of the great vessels. *Circulation* 1962;26:819–840.
82. Sakakibara S, Takao A, Arai T, Hashimoto A, Nogi M. Both great vessels arising from the left ventricle. *Bull Heart Inst Jpn* 1967:66–86.
83. Paul MH, Muster AJ, Sinha SN, Cole RB, Van Praagh R. Double outlet left ventricle with intact ventricular septum: clinical and autopsy diagnosis and developmental implications. *Circulation* 1970;41:129–139.
84. Van Praagh R, Van Praagh S. Isolated ventricular inversion. A consideration of the morphogenesis, definition and diagnosis of nontransposed and transposed great arteries. *Am J Cardiol* 1966;17:395–406.
85. Stegmann T, Oster H, Bissenden J, Kallfelz HC, Oelert H. Surgical treatment of double-outlet left ventricle in 2 patients with D-position and L-position of the aorta. *Ann Thorac Surg* 1979;27:121–129.
86. Pacifico AD, Kirklin JW, Bargeron LM Jr, Soto B. Surgical treatment of double-outlet left ventricle. Report of four cases. *Circulation* 1973;48[Suppl III]:III-19–III-23.
87. Quero Jimenez M, Maitre Azcarate MJ. Ventriculo izquierdo de doble salida: estudio de un caso y revision de la literatura. *Rev Esp Cardiol* 1975;28:587–596.
88. Otero Coto E, Quero Jimenez M, Cabrera A, Deverall PB, Caffarena JM. Aortic levopositions without ventricular inversion. *Eur J Cardiol* 1978;8:523–541.
89. Van Praagh R, Weinberg PM, Srebro JP. Double-outlet left ventricle. In: Adams FH, Emmanouilides GC, Riemenschneider TA, eds. *Moss heart disease in infants, children, and adolescents*, 4th ed. Baltimore: Williams & Wilkins, 1989:461–485.
90. Hagler DJ, Edwards WD. Double-outlet left ventricle. In: Emmanouilides GC, Reimenscheider TA, Allen HD, Gutgesell, HP, eds. *Moss and Adams' heart disease in infants, children, and adolescents. Including the fetus and young adult*, Vol. II, 5th ed. Baltimore: Williams & Wilkins, 1995:1270–1278.
91. Bengur AR, Snider AR, Peters J, Merida-Asmus L. Two-dimensional echocardiographic features of double outlet left ventricle. *J Am Soc Echocardiogr* 1990;3:320–325.
92. Kirklin JW, Barrat-Boyes BG. Double outlet left ventricle. In: Kirklin JW, Barrat-Boyes BG, eds. *Cardiac surgery. Morphology, diagnostic criteria, natural history, techniques, results, and indications*, Vol. 2, 2nd ed. New York: Churchill Livingstone, 1993:1501–1509.
93. Neufeld HN, Schneeweiss A. Origin of both great vessels from the left ventricle. In: Neufeld HN, Schneeweiss A, eds. *Coronary artery*

disease in infants and children. Philadelphia: Lea & Febiger, 1983:106–109.

94. Sharrat GP, Sbokos CG, Johnson AM, Anderson RH, Monro JL. Surgical correction of solitus-concordant, double-oulet left ventricle with L-malposition and tricuspid stenosis with hypoplastic right ventricle. *J Thorac Cardiovasc Surg* 1976;71:853–858.

95. Freedom RM. Double-outlet left ventricle. In: Freedom RM, Benson LN, Smallhorn JF, eds. *Neonatal heart disease*. London: Springer-Verlag, 1992:561–562.

96. Stark J. Double-outlet ventricles. In: De Leval M, Stark J, eds. *Surgery for congenital heart defects*, 2nd ed. Philadelphia: WB Saunders, 1994:437–446.

97. Planche C, Pernot C, Battise A, et al. Traitement chirurgical du ventricule gauche à double issue. *Arch Mal Coeur Vaiss* 1979;72: 503–514.

98. Replogle RL, Campbell DJ, Campbell CD, Arcilla RA. Double outlet ventricles. In: Arciniegas E, ed. *Pediatric cardiac surgery*. Chicago: Year Book, 1985:231–245.

CHAPTER 24

Complete Transposition of the Great Arteries

Lilliam M. Valdes-Cruz and Raul O. Cayre

Complete transposition of the great arteries is a congenital cardiac malformation characterized by atrioventricular concordance and ventriculoarterial discordance. It has an incidence of 5% to 10% of all congenital heart disease (1–6).

EMBRYOLOGIC CONSIDERATIONS

The morphogenesis of complete transposition of the great arteries involves conal and truncal septation. The conus appears during the loop stage (7); it makes up the cephalic end of the heart and is continuous with the primordium of the trabeculated portion of the right ventricle caudally (see Fig. 1-5B). During the early post-loop stage, the truncus appears. It is continuous with the conus caudally and with the aortic sac cephalically (8) (see Fig. 1-5C).

Cardiac septation begins during the early post loop stage (8). The conal crests appear in the conus or primordium of the infundibulum of both ventricles; there is a dextrodorsal and a sinistroventral conal crest that will give origin to the conal septum, dividing the conus in two, an anterolateral and a posteromedial conus (see Figs. 1-12 and 1-14A). Simultaneously, two truncal swellings appear in the proximal end of the truncus, one sinistroinferior and one dextrosuperior (9), which will fuse to form the truncal septum (see Figs. 1-12B and 1-14B). Eventually, the dextrodorsal conal crest becomes continuous with the dextrosuperior truncal swelling and the sinistroventral conal crest with the sinistroinferior truncal swelling (9) (see Fig. 1-14).

The aortopulmonary septum appears between the fourth and sixth aortic arches and is composed of cells originating from the neural crest (10). This septum is spiral and becomes continuous with the truncal septum, thereby dividing the truncus into the ascending aorta and the main pulmonary artery (see Fig. 1-14). The spiral shape of the aortopulmonary, truncal and conal septa causes the aorta, which occupies an anterior position in the aortic sac, to connect with the posteromedial conus, which will eventually become incorporated into the anatomic left ventricle and give rise to its outflow tract. Similarly, the pulmonary artery, which occupies a posterior position in the aortic sac, connects with the anterolateral conus, which will become the infundibulum of the anatomic right ventricle (see Fig. 1-14).

An abnormal development of the aortopulmonary, truncal, and conal septa will give origin to the different types of complete transposition of the great arteries. Usually, complete transposition occurs in the presence of visceroatrial situs solitus and normal bulboventricular looping (D loop), i.e., atrioventricular concordance.

In *complete transposition with an anterior and rightward aorta and a posterior and leftward pulmonary artery* (Fig. 24-1A), there is an abnormal development of the aortopulmonary and truncal septa and normal development of the dextrodorsal and sinistroventral conal crests. At the proximal end of the truncus, the truncal swellings develop abnormally in a sinistrosuperior and a dextroinferior orientation (11). As a result the normally situated dextrodorsal conal crest becomes continuous with the dextroinferior truncal swelling and the normally positioned sinistroventral conal crest with the sinistrosuperior truncal swelling (11–13). The conal septum is therefore straight, losing the semispiral shape it normally has. The aortopulmonary septum becomes continuous with the malposed truncal swellings and also assumes a straight rather than spiral shape (14). Consequently, the anterior and rightward aorta becomes continuous with the anterolateral infundibulum connected to the anatomic right ventricle and the posterior and leftward pulmonary artery becomes continuous with the posteromedial infundibulum connected to the anatomic left ventricle (15).

In *transposition of the great arteries with side-by-side great vessels* (Fig. 24-1B), the conal septum develops abnormally with conal crests positioned dorsally and ven-

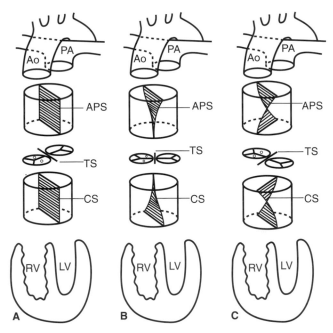

FIG. 24-1. Schematic representation of the probable morphogenesis of the various types of complete transposition of the great arteries. **A:** Anterior and rightward aorta and posterior and leftward pulmonary artery. **B:** Side-by-side great arteries. **C:** Posterior and rightward aorta and anterior and leftward pulmonary artery. *RV*, right ventricle; *LV*, left ventricle; *CS*, conal septum; *TS*, truncal septum; *APS*, aorticopulmonary septum; *Ao*, aorta; *PA*, pulmonary artery.

trally (14,16). The crests divide the conus into one lateral and one medial conus (14) with the conal septum having an anteroposterior direction perpendicular to the frontal plane. The truncal septum also acquires an abnormal orientation perpendicular to the frontal plane. The aortopulmonary septum loses its normal spiral shape. Distally, it starts normally, having an axis that is posterior to anterior and right to left; however, proximally, it becomes continuous with the truncal septum and therefore adopts an anteroposterior direction. The aorta will connect with the lateral infundibulum related to the anatomic right ventricle while the pulmonary artery will connect with the medial infundibulum related to the anatomic left ventricle.

In *complete transposition of the great arteries with posterior aorta* (Fig. 24-1C), the conal crests develop abnormally in a dextroventral and sinistrodorsal position (14). When they fuse, the resulting conal septum assumes a directional axis from posterior to anterior and left to right that divides the conus into an anteromedial and a posterolateral conus (15). The truncal crests develop normally and therefore the truncal septum has a direction from posterior to anterior and left to right. The aortopulmonary septum also develops normally. In its cephalic end it is oriented from posterior to anterior and right to left while caudally it is directed from posterior to anterior and left to right. The aorta connects with the posterolateral conus related to the anatomic right ventricle and the pul-

monary artery connects with the anteromedial conus, which is related to the anatomic left ventricle.

ANATOMIC AND ECHOCARDIOGRAPHIC CONSIDERATIONS

The definition of transposition of the great arteries has been a source of much controversy in the pediatric cardiac literature. In general, there are two schools: those who define transposition in terms of the relations of the great arteries and those who define it based on the ventriculoarterial connections. The original anatomic description by Baillie in 1797 was that of a heart in which the aorta arose from the right ventricle and the pulmonary artery from the left ventricle (17). In 1814, Farre first utilized the term "transposition of the aorta and pulmonary artery," thereby defining the term based on ventriculoarterial connections (18). Nevertheless, subsequent publications advocated the arterial relations and conal anatomy as the core of the malformation, i.e., an anterior aorta with a subaortic infundibulum (11,19–26). Additional controversy emerged when proponents of the connection approach qualified their definition in terms of great vessel relations, resulting in the commonly used "D-transposition" and "L-transposition" as synonymous with complete and congenitally corrected transpositions, respectively (26–28), which is not universally the case (29). Most recently, another source of confusion has been introduced by defining ventriculoarterial connection as "the manner in which the great arteries are connected to the ventricles, with emphasis on the semilunar-atrioventricular anatomic relations" and ventriculoarterial alignment as "the spatial relation between the great arteries and the ventricles, or which ventricle ejects into which great artery"(30).

Without implying any fundamental criticism towards one or another school of thought, we have elected to use a simplified definition of complete transposition as the presence of concordant atrioventricular connection with discordant ventriculoarterial connection and qualifying it with the particular great artery relation, infundibular morphology, and associated malformations found in the specific case discussed. We feel this approach will be clear to all individuals including those involved in the ongoing care of adult patients with congenital heart disease. Therefore, complete transposition of the great arteries will define a group of malformations in which the morphologic right atrium is connected to the morphologic right ventricle, which gives rise to the aorta, and the morphologic left atrium is connected with the morphologic left ventricle, which gives rise to the pulmonary artery (see Fig. 2-8B). In this arrangement, there can be situs solitus or situs inversus, but by definition it cannot exist with atrial isomerism, univentricular hearts of indeterminate type, double-inlet or double-outlet ventricles, or single arterial trunk (31). The resultant physiology is that of two circulations in parallel rather than in series.

The echocardiographic study of patients with complete transposition should include (a) characteristic anatomic features and connections within the context of a segmental approach; (b) great artery relationships; (c) infundibular morphology; (d) origin and distribution of the coronary arteries; (e) associated anomalies; and (f) intra- and post-operative evaluation.

Characteristic Anatomic Features and Connections Within the Context of a Segmental Approach

The essential anatomic characteristic of complete transposition of the great arteries is that of a discordant ventriculoarterial connection with a concordant atrioventricular connection. This results in changes in the morphology of the outflow tracts, which in turn cause slight differences in the atrioventricular junction and intraventricular anatomy. In the majority of cases of uncomplicated complete transposition, the right and left ventricular outflow tracts run parallel to each other so that the ventricular septum is a straight structure, i.e., the inlet, trabecular, and outlet septa are aligned (32–35). Seen from a short-axis view of the heart, the pulmonic valve is not as wedged between the tricuspid and mitral valves as is the normal aorta (32,34–37), resulting in an underdeveloped central fibrous body, atrioventricular septum and membranous septum. The latter is absent in most cases of complete transposition with intact ventricular septum (38). Because of the deficiency in the atrioventricular septum, the tricuspid and mitral valves insert closer to the same level so the inlet septum separates the right and left ventricles only (37). Further, the left ventricular outlet is disproportionately longer than its inlet although not to the degree observed in atrioventricular septal defects (34).

The parasternal long-axis view demonstrates the parallel arrangement of the outflow tracts of the ventricles with the pulmonary artery coursing sharply posteriorly and bifurcating into a right and left branch (Echo. 24-1). In this view, the relatively elongated outlet resulting from an unwedging of the posterior great vessel can also be seen. At this point determination of the atrial and ventricular arrangement is important. This can be accomplished with a combination of apical and subcostal views.

Examination of the inferior vena cava, aorta, and hepatic venous connections to the atria from a subcostal approach is most commonly the starting point. Beginning at the level of the diaphragm, cross-sectional views of the abdominal great vessels reveal an inferior vena cava positioned to the right and slightly anterior to the aorta in normal situs with a mirror image arrangement in situs inversus. Occasionally, atrial isomerism can be found in the presence of ventriculoarterial discordance; however, these cases would not be included in the definition of

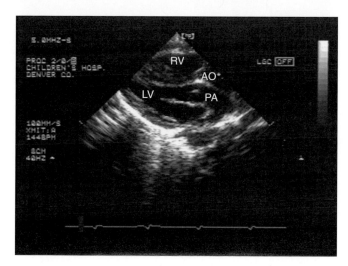

ECHO. 24-1. Parasternal long-axis view in complete transposition of the great arteries demonstrating the parallel outflow tracts and posterior course of the pulmonary artery. *RV*, right ventricle; *AO*, aorta; *LV*, left ventricle; *PA*, pulmonary artery.

complete transposition of the great vessels (see above). The presence of a finger-like appendage on the left-sided atrium seen from a parasternal short-axis view and of a broad-based appendage on the right-sided atrium imaged from the parasternal right ventricular inflow view further confirms the presence of situs solitus (or situs inversus if appearance is in mirror image).

The apical and subcostal four-chamber views demonstrate the atrioventricular connections and ventricular morphology. The presence of a tricuspid valve and a moderator band in the anterior (right) ventricle and of a bileaflet mitral valve, an anterolateral and a posteromedial papillary muscle, and smoother trabeculations in the posterior (left) ventricle establishes the echocardiographic diagnosis of concordant atrioventricular connection. Additional cranial angulation of the transducer from a four-chamber view demonstrates the main pulmonary artery arising from the left ventricle and bifurcating immediately while the aorta arises from the right ventricle and does not branch until the transverse arch (Echo. 24-2). A four-chamber apical sweep from posterior to anterior further confirms the underdevelopment of the atrioventricular septum with the resultant closer than usual insertion levels of the tricuspid and mitral valves (Echo. 24-3).

The cavity size, wall thickness of the ventricular chambers, and the motion of the interventricular septum are all of importance in the assessment of the capability of the left ventricle to sustain systemic circulation in infants considered for the arterial switch operation. Due to the relative pulmonary hypertension present in newborns, the left ventricle usually maintains its ventricular mass until the normal fall in pulmonary resistance occurs, approximately three weeks in the absence of a ventricular septal defect and/or a patent ductus arteriosus. This elevated

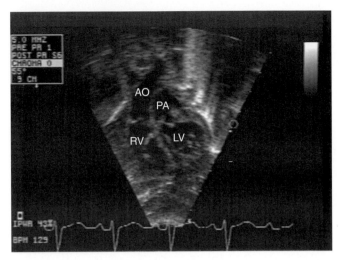

ECHO. 24-2. Apical view with extreme cranial angulation demonstrating the outflow tracts in complete transposition. The aorta emerges from the right ventricle and the pulmonary artery from the left ventricle. *RV*, right ventricle; *AO*, aorta; *LV*, left ventricle; *PA*, pulmonary artery.

left ventricular pressure is manifested by a rounded or elliptical left ventricular cavity, wall thickness at least equal to that of the right ventricle and an interventricular septal motion that does not bow towards the left ventricle in systole. These features can be accurately evaluated from the parasternal and subcostal long- and short-axis views (Echo. 24-4).

Great Artery Relationships

By far the most common relationship of the great arteries in complete transposition is with the aorta anterior

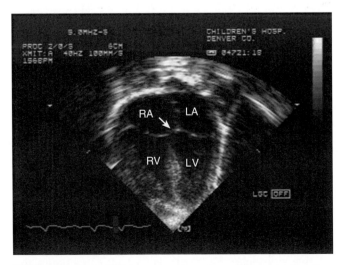

ECHO. 24-3. Apical four-chamber view demonstrating the smaller than usual atrioventricular septum seen in complete transposition *(arrow)*. As a result, the points of insertion of the atrioventricular valves are closer to each other. *RA*, right atrium; *LA*, left atrium; *RV*, right ventricle; *LV*, left ventricle.

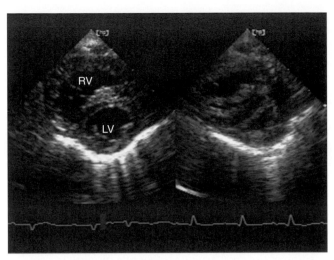

ECHO. 24-4. Left: Parasternal short-axis view of the ventricles showing a round left ventricle without systolic bowing of the interventricular septum. **Right:** Short-axis view demonstrating compression of the left ventricle with systolic bowing of the septum towards the left ventricle in systole as a result of a drop in pulmonary arterial resistance. *RV*, right ventricle; *LV*, left ventricle.

and to the right of the pulmonary artery (29,34,35,39) (see Fig. 2-9). However, the aorta can be directly anterior or anterior and to the left of the pulmonary artery. In the presence of an anterior aorta, there is usually a subaortic muscular infundibulum and the pulmonary valve is in fibrous continuity with the mitral valve (35). The interventricular septum is straight due to alignment of the inlet, trabecular and outlet septa and the right and left ventricular outflow tracts run parallel to each other, as do the arterial trunks. The axis of the outlet septum is directed posterior to anterior and right to left.

Less commonly, the great vessels are side by side, and the aorta can be either to the right or to the left of the pulmonary artery. In these cases, it is more common to find abnormal coronary arterial patterns (36) and bilateral infundibula (35). The outlet septum is semispiral in shape, with its major axis directed posterior to anterior and perpendicular to the frontal plane.

The least common relationship is with the aorta positioned posteriorly and to the right of the pulmonary artery (26,35,36,40–43). In these cases, the arteries appear normally related; however, the right ventricle is connected to the aorta and the left ventricle to the pulmonary artery. These cases also have aortic-mitral fibrous continuity and pulmonary-mitral discontinuity (35). The outlet septum is posterior to anterior and left to right.

The echocardiographic demonstration of the great artery relationships is best accomplished from the parasternal short-axis views, where the anteroposterior and right-left coordinates can be defined (Echo. 24-5). The presence of semilunar-atrioventricular valve continuity and infundibular orientation are best shown from the parasternal

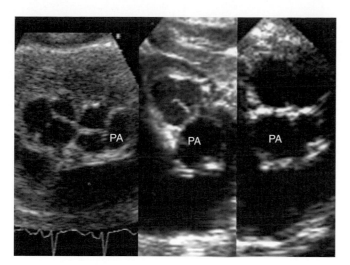

ECHO. 24-5. Parasternal short-axis views of the various spatial relationships of the great vessels seen in complete transposition of the great arteries. **Left:** Side-by-side relationship with aorta to the right of the pulmonary artery. **Middle:** Aorta positioned to the right and anterior to the pulmonary artery. **Right:** Aorta situated strictly anterior to the pulmonary artery. *PA, pulmonary artery.*

long-axis view and the subcostal four-chamber views with anterior angulation to expose the outflow tracts of both ventricles and their connections with the great arteries (Echos. 24-1, 24-2).

Infundibular Morphology

The echocardiographic examination of the infundibular anatomy is best accomplished from the parasternal long-axis and subcostal long- and short-axis views, with anterior angulation of the transducer towards the outflow tracts. In the presence of a muscular subarterial infundibulum, there is discontinuity between the corresponding atrioventricular and semilunar valves seen on the echocardiogram as muscle tissue. In the presence of a fibrous infundibulum, there is continuity between the respective atrioventricular and semilunar valves.

The most frequent infundibular morphology is that of a subaortic muscular infundibulum, with aortic-tricuspid discontinuity and pulmonary-mitral continuity. In these instances, the aorta is most likely anterior, to the right and superior to the pulmonary artery. This infundibular arrangement is seen best from the parasternal long-axis views, rotating the transducer slowly between both ventricular outflows to demonstrate the relative positions of the great arteries (Echo. 24-1). The relationship between the semilunar and atrioventricular valves is best evaluated from the apical and subcostal four-chamber views, sweeping the transducer between the inflows and the outflows to define the presence of thicker muscular tissue echocardiographically in the presence of discontinuity (Echo. 24-2).

The next most common type of infundibular morphology is that of a muscular infundibulum below both the aorta and pulmonary arteries (bilateral infundibula), resulting in discontinuity between the aortic and tricuspid valves and also between the pulmonic and mitral valves. The pulmonary root in these cases would have a more superior and anterior location than would normally be expected in complete transposition but would be clearly related to the left ventricle. This latter feature would differentiate it from double-outlet right ventricle transposition type. Commonly the subpulmonary infundibulum is narrowed due to leftward displacement of the infundibular or outlet septum, leading to obstruction. If the outlet septum is displaced to the right, the result would be subaortic obstruction. These are best demonstrated from a parasternal long-axis, apical outflow and long-axis views as well as from the subcostal outflow and short-axis views (Echo. 24-6).

Presence of a subpulmonary infundibulum only with absent subaortic infundibulum is rare. The pulmonary trunk is superior and anterior to the aorta due to the presence of the infundibular muscle and could give the appearance of a normal great artery relationship from subcostal views with extreme anterior and superior angulation of the transducer. Sweeping slowly posteriorly, however, would reveal the discordant ventriculoarterial connection. There is usually a subaortic ventricular septal defect, with aortic-mitral fibrous continuity through the defect. Occasionally the aorta may override the septal defect, suggesting a double-outlet left ventricle. The aorta is usually posterior and to the right of the pulmonary trunk but can also be anterior and to the left. This fact demonstrates once again that the spatial relationship of the

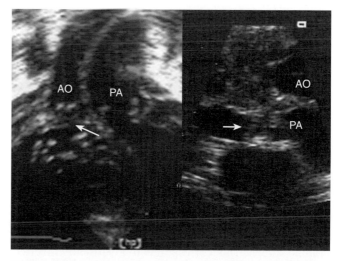

ECHO. 24-6. **Left:** Apical view tilted superiorly demonstrating the parallel outflow tracts. *Arrow* points to the subaortic stenosis. **Right:** Parasternal long-axis view demonstrating an anterior aorta and a posterior pulmonary artery. There is subpulmonic stenosis (*arrow*). *AO, aorta; PA, pulmonary artery.*

great arteries is not solely dependent on the infundibular anatomy. Pulmonary obstruction is common and can be valvular or subvalvular (30).

The absence of an infundibulum below both great arteries results in fibrous continuity between the aorta and tricuspid valves and between the pulmonic and mitral valves. These are evident echocardiographically from parasternal long-axis and subcostal long- and short-axis views with angulation towards the outflows. In the two cases reported by Pasquini et al. (30), the aorta was located slightly posterior to the pulmonary trunk in one case and side by side in the other. In both instances, there was a prominent infundibulum present anterior to both semilunar valves but ending blindly since neither great vessel arose from it. A ventricular septal defect was present in both cases, allowing communication between both ventricular outflow tracts through the infundibular chamber. The authors demonstrated these features from parasternal short-axis scans.

Origin and Distribution of the Coronary Arteries

The coronary arteries in complete transposition of the great arteries originate from the aortic sinuses that face the pulmonary trunk (35,36,39,44–49); therefore, the spatial variability in their origin can be accounted for by the variations in great artery relationships. There are various nomenclatures that have been advanced for naming the coronary sinuses in complete transposition; however, the system advocated by the Leiden group seems easiest (46). The sinuses that face the pulmonary trunk are called the "facing" sinuses, and the third sinus, which is not related to the pulmonary, is called the "nonfacing" or noncoronary sinus. Since sinusal position varies with great artery relationship, their position is best described as if the surgeon were standing within the nonfacing (noncoronary) sinus looking towards the pulmonary trunk (Fig. 24-2B): the sinus to the right of the observer would be sinus no. 1 (right-hand sinus) and that to the left would be sinus no. 2 (left-hand sinus). Morphologically, the left coronary artery is identified by having a short pedicle that branches into the anterior descending and circumflex arteries while the right coronary artery is that which surrounds the tricuspid orifice.

The right-hand sinus (sinus no. 1) is the left coronary sinus, which in the conventional echocardiographic display (Fig. 24-2A) is on the right side of the screen. The left-hand sinus (sinus no. 2), which is the right coronary sinus, is displayed on the left side of the echocardiographic screen. This corresponds to a vertically inverted and mirror image of the anatomic orientation of the aortic cusps seen in complete transposition. As such, following the Leiden convention, the surgeon would be standing upside down within the nonfacing aortic cusp (Fig. 24-2).

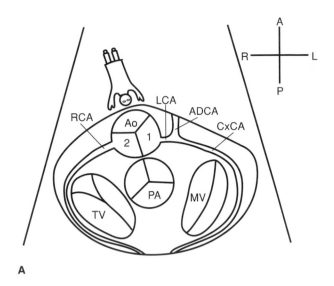

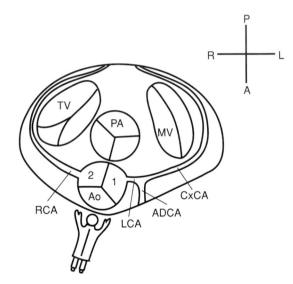

FIG. 24-2. Schematic drawings of a transverse cut of the heart at the base demonstrating the Leiden convention (46) for naming the coronary sinuses in complete transposition of the great arteries. See text for details. **A:** Conventional echocardiographic display. **B:** Anatomical position (surgeon's view). *TV*, tricuspid valve; *MV*, mitral valve; *Ao*, aorta; *PA*, pulmonary artery; *1*, right-hand sinus; *2*, left-hand sinus; *RCA*, right coronary artery; *LCA*, left coronary artery; *ADCA*, anterior descending coronary artery; *CxCA*, circumflex coronary artery; *A*, anterior; *P*, posterior; *R*, right; *L*, left.

In the vast majority of cases with anterior aorta (Figs. 24-3–24-5), the left coronary artery originates from sinus no. 1 and divides into left anterior descending and circumflex; the right coronary artery originates from sinus no. 2 and supplies the posterior descending (34–36,45,48) (Figs. 24-3B, 24-4B, 24-5B) (Echo. 24-7). The next most common pattern is that in which the circumflex and the right coronary artery originate from sinus no. 2 and the left anterior descending originates from sinus no. 1 (34–36,45,48) (Figs. 24-3C, 24-4C) (Echo. 24-8). In these

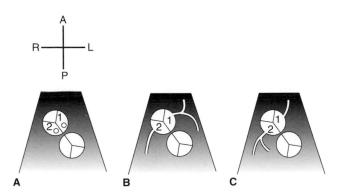

FIG. 24-3. Schematic drawings of the echocardiographic views of the spatial relationship of the semilunar valves and the most common coronary patterns found in complete transposition of the great arteries with aorta anterior and to the right. See text for details. **A:** Spatial relationship of the great arteries. **B,C:** Coronary patterns. *1,* right-hand sinus; *2,* left-hand sinus; *A,* anterior; *P,* posterior; *R,* right; *L,* left.

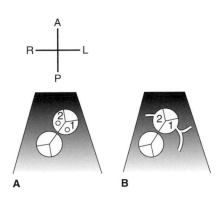

FIG. 24-5. Schematic drawings of the echocardiographic views of the spatial relationship of the semilunar valves and the most common coronary artery pattern found in complete transposition of the great arteries with aorta anterior and leftward. See text for details. **A:** Spatial relationship of the semilunar valves. **B:** Coronary pattern. *1,* right-hand sinus; *2,* left-hand sinus; *A,* anterior; *P,* posterior; *R,* right; *L,* left.

cases, the circumflex usually takes a retropulmonary course towards the left atrioventricular groove. Although these two relatively simple patterns account for most observations, it is important to keep in mind that any of the three main coronary branches (right, left anterior descending and circumflex) can arise from any of the two facing sinuses via one, two or three orifices; therefore, the echocardiographer must account for the origin, branching and proximal distribution of the three major arteries separately. This is best accomplished through a low parasternal short-axis view with the transducer aiming superiorly and anteriorly to display the aortic root and proximal ascending aorta. Rotating the transducer slowly counterclockwise and to the right permits visualization of the trajectory of the right coronary artery within the right atrioventricular groove (50). Angling the transducer left-

ward, one can observe the origin and distribution of the left coronary artery (50). From the subcostal approach, rotation of the transducer to a short-axis view with superior and anterior angulation from the standard four-chamber projection also permits demonstration of the coronary arteries arising from the aorta.

Side-by-side great artery relationship is more frequently associated with unusual coronary patterns (34,48) (Fig. 24-6). These include the circumflex arising from sinus no. 2 and following a retropulmonary course and the right coronary and anterior descending arising from sinus no. 1 (Fig. 24-6B). Other unusual patterns observed are illustrated in Fig. 24-6C–E (34).

Coronary patterns observed in the rare cases of com-

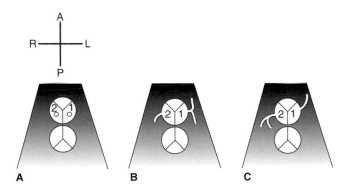

FIG. 24-4. Schematic drawings of the echocardiographic views of the spatial relationship of the semilunar valves and the most common coronary artery patterns found in complete transposition of the great arteries with aorta strictly anterior to the pulmonary artery. See text for details. **A:** Spatial relationship of the semilunar valves. **B,C:** Coronary patterns. *1,* right-hand sinus; *2,* left-hand sinus; *A,* anterior; *P,* posterior; *R,* right; *L,* left.

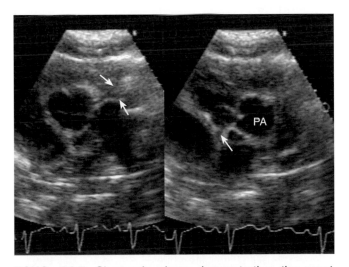

ECHO. 24-7. Short-axis views demonstrating the most common coronary arterial pattern seen in complete transposition. **Left:** (*arrow*) The left coronary artery originates from sinus no. 1 and gives rise to the left anterior descending and circumflex branches. **Right:** (*arrow*) The right coronary artery originates from sinus no. 2.

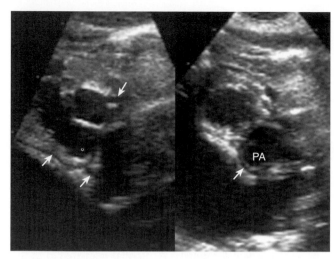

ECHO. 24-8. Short-axis view demonstrating the second most common pattern of coronary arterial distribution in complete transposition. **Left:** Origin of the left anterior descending from sinus no. 1 *(top arrow)* and of the right coronary artery and circumflex from sinus no. 2 *(bottom arrows, respectively)*. **Right:** The circumflex branch is seen coursing leftward behind the pulmonary artery *(arrow)*. *PA*, pulmonary artery.

plete transposition with posterior aorta are also unusual (Fig. 24-7). These include the anterior descending and circumflex originating from sinus no. 2 and the right coronary from sinus no. 1 (Fig. 24-7B); or the anterior descending and right coronary from sinus no. 1 and the circumflex from sinus no. 2 (Fig. 24-7C) (34).

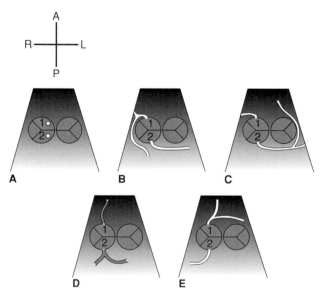

FIG. 24-6. Schematic drawings of the echocardiographic views of the spatial relationship of the semilunar valves and the common coronary patterns found in complete transposition of the great arteries with side-by-side great arteries. See text for details. **A:** Spatial relationship of the semilunar valves. **B–E:** Coronary patterns. *1*, right-hand sinus; *2*, left-hand sinus; *A*, anterior; *P*, posterior; *R*, right; *L*, left.

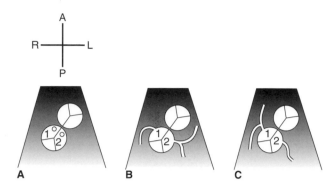

FIG. 24-7. Schematic drawings of the echocardiographic view of the spatial relationship of the semilunar valves and the common coronary patterns found in complete transposition of the great arteries with posterior aorta. See text for details. **A:** Spatial relationship of the semilunar valves. **B,C:** Coronary patterns. *1*, right-hand sinus; *2*, left-hand sinus; *A*, anterior; *P*, posterior; *R*, right; *L*, left.

Intramural coronary arteries occur in 3% to 7% of cases of complete transposition (51,52). This can cause technical difficulties during the arterial switch operation and can also result in higher mortality following this operation (48,53–55) particularly if the left coronary originates from sinus no. 2 (or left-hand sinus) and follows an intramural course between the aortic and pulmonary trunks (48,54,55). Recently, Pasquini et al. (52) reported certain diagnostic characteristics evident on the parasternal short-axis view that aid in the detection of intramural coronary arteries. According to these authors, the most reliable criterion is the identification of a coronary artery originating from the contralateral sinus of Valsalva, which then courses between both arterial roots, giving the appearance of a "double border" to the posterior wall of the aortic root. This double border appearance is caused by the intramural course of the coronary artery within the aortic wall. They also point out that origin of a coronary artery higher than normal above a sinus of Valsalva, close to the supravalvar annular ring, is suggestive although not diagnostic of an intramural coronary artery. Another variation that presents difficulties for the arterial switch operation is when the arteries appear to arise from separate sinuses but instead one tunnels along the aortic wall and crosses a valve commissure, resulting in all three coronaries arising from the same sinus.

An origin of all three coronaries from a single sinus separately or through a common stem was found in 6% of cases in the series reported by Mayer et al. (54). This has been associated with anterior displacement of the infundibular septum within the right ventricle (48). Difficulties can also result if the pulmonary and aortic trunks are rotated relative to one another, so there is a greater distance between the facing sinuses (36).

Associated Anomalies

Ventricular septal defect is the most common associated anomaly found with complete transposition of the great arteries; it is present in 30% to 45% of cases (2,44,56,57). These can be outlet, perimembranous with outlet or inlet extensions, muscular, or doubly committed (3,31,32,34,35,56,58).

Outlet defects or perimembranous defects with outlet extensions can be due to hypoplasia or abnormal development of the outlet septum or due to malalignment between the outlet and trabecular septa. In these latter cases, the outlet septum is displaced rightward, into the right ventricle, permitting an override of the pulmonary valve over the ventricular septum therefore the septal defect is subpulmonary. The degree of overriding of the pulmonary valve over the ventricular septum presents a spectrum that ranges from minimal to extreme overriding, in which case the pulmonary artery emerges almost completely from the right ventricle and should be considered double-outlet right ventricle, transposition type. The ventricular communication and the degree of overriding of the pulmonary artery, if present, can be seen from a parasternal long-axis view and from an apical and subcostal four-chamber view, angling the transducer into a superior or anterior plane (Echo. 24-9; see color plate 82 following p. 364). Greater detail can be observed from subcostal long-axis and oblique right and left views (30,59–62). A right oblique subcostal view is obtained by rotating the transducer from a standard long-axis subcostal plane approximately 45° to 55° until the right atrium, right ventricular body, outflow tract and aorta are seen. The left oblique subcostal view allows examination of both ventricles, the outflow tracts and the trabecular and infundibular septa as well as the pulmonary artery and aorta. This view can be obtained by rotating the transducer approximately 70° from the standard subcostal long-axis position. The shunt flow is best visualized by color Doppler from parasternal

long- and short-axis views by tilting the transducer towards the outlet portions of the septum. It is usually directed from the right (systemic) to the left (pulmonary) ventricle immediately below the pulmonic valve. Because the jet is parallel to the Doppler beam, it is possible to obtain the velocity gradient between both ventricles for pressure estimation (Echo. 24-9).

Perimembranous defects with inlet extensions can be evaluated from an apical four-chamber view by sweeping the transducer from the crux cordis posteriorly to the level of the outflow of the ventricles anteriorly/superiorly. This view allows imaging of the interventricular communication underneath the septal leaflet of the tricuspid valve, extending from the region of the membranous septum posteriorly towards the septum that separates the two ventricular inflows. It is also important to note in these views the presence of tendinous chords from the tricuspid valve, which may be crossing in front of the defect. This type of defect can be accompanied by a malalignment between the atrial septum and trabecular septum with overriding or straddling of the tricuspid valve (32,34,36,63). This type of septal malalignment can be best seen from the four-chamber views. Color Doppler flow mapping from these views will clearly demonstrate the direction of shunting across the defect, usually from right to left ventricle as well as the presence of tricuspid regurgitation. Flow mapping will also define any preferential streaming of blood into either ventricle in cases with straddling and/or overriding of the tricuspid valve.

Muscular ventricular septal defects are not common in complete transposition. When present, these can be single or multiple and located in the muscular portion of the inlet septum, in the outlet septum, or in the medial or apical portion of the trabecular septum. The parasternal long-axis and short-axis views and the apical and subcostal four-chamber views can be used to detect the presence of muscular defects, particularly with the use of color Doppler flow mapping, by sweeping the transducer from the cardiac apex to the base. The gradient between both ventricles can be measured with continuous wave (CW) Doppler by aligning the beam as parallel as possible to the direction of flow. Perimembranous defects can be present in association with muscular ones.

It is important to point out that, in addition to locating a defect of the interventricular septum, there is a need to define its relationship with the great arteries. When the aorta is either right and anterior or right in a side-by-side great vessel relationship, the defect is usually related with the pulmonary artery since this is the great vessel adjacent to the ventricular septum. However, if there is a posterior and leftward displacement of the outlet septum, resulting in its incorporation into the left ventricle, the defect is due to malalignment between the outlet and trabecular septa and there would be mild overriding of the aortic valve (64).

When the aorta is located either to the left and anterior

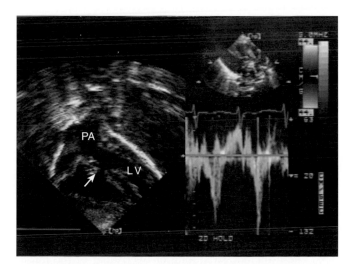

ECHO. 24-9. Left: Subcostal view aimed towards the outflow tracts demonstrating a subpulmonary ventricular septal defect *(arrow).* **Right:** Spectral Doppler recording of the low velocity bidirectional shunt across the ventricular septal defect. *PA,* pulmonary artery; *LV,* left ventricle.

or to the right and posterior of the pulmonary artery, the septal defect can be either subpulmonary or subaortic because both great arteries are adjacent to the ventricular septum and therefore either one can be related to the defect. Usually, however, when the aorta is to the right and posterior, the defect is subaortic (3,42,65), although it can also be doubly committed or juxtaarterial (3). The parasternal short-axis view permits definition of the spatial position of the great arteries and a combination of the parasternal long-axis view, apical four-chamber view, and subcostal long-axis and oblique views helps define the relationship of the septal defect to the great arteries.

Obstruction of the ventricular outflow tracts. In 25% of cases of complete transposition with ventricular septal defect, there is obstruction of the right ventricular outflow tract (64). The obstruction can be caused by an anterior and rightward displacement of the outlet septum, by hypertrophy of anomalous muscle bands within the right ventricular outflow tract, by hypertrophy of the ventriculoinfundibular fold or secondary to aortic valve stenosis. Obstruction to the right ventricular outflow tract can be accompanied by hypoplasia or interruption of the aortic arch or aortic coarctation (64,67,68). Echocardiographically, the parasternal long-axis view tilted towards the right ventricular outflow and the apical four-chamber position with superior-anterior transducer angulation allow examination of the right ventricular outflow tract. The subcostal long-axis and right oblique echocardiographic views are also important to demonstrate this anatomy (Echo. 24-6). From any of these views, spectral Doppler interrogation of velocities can be performed using either high pulse rate frequency (PRF) or CW techniques for localization of the site(s) of stenosis, estimation of their relative severity and calculation of the pressure gradient(s). Color Doppler flow mapping will aid in the localization of the areas of stenosis and in the positioning of the Doppler interrogating beam, particularly in the presence of eccentric jets. The aortic arch can be examined from the suprasternal and high left infraclavicular positions. From these views, Doppler velocities of the descending aorta can also be recorded for evaluation of possible coarctation or interruption of the aortic arch.

Obstruction to the left ventricular outflow tract can be basically of two types—dynamic or fixed. Dynamic obstruction is most commonly present with intact ventricular septum. The higher right ventricular pressure causes bulging of the interventricular septum into the left ventricular outflow tract during systole with or without anterior motion of the mitral valve, thereby causing obstruction (69–72). This dynamic obstruction can be seen at birth and either increase or diminish in severity depending on the relative pressures of the right and left ventricle. It usually disappears completely after anatomical repair (arterial switch operation) (72).

Fixed left ventricular outflow tract obstruction can have various underlying mechanisms: leftward deviation of the outlet septum (70,71); subvalve diaphragm or fibrous ring (70,73), muscular ring (74), or tunnel (35); hypertrophy of the anterolateral muscular band or muscle of Moulaert (75); accessory mitral valve tissue (73); anomalous insertion of anterior mitral leaflet chords (56,73,74,76–78); valve pulmonic stenosis (56,70,73); tricuspid valve pouch protruding though the ventricular septal defect (56,70); and aneurysm of the membranous septum (79).

Left ventricular outflow tract obstruction should be carefully evaluated by echocardiography with specific attention to differentiating dynamic from fixed obstruction and, within the latter, what type is involved and which are the possible surgical approaches. This has particular relevance in deciding what surgical procedure will be used for correction of transposition. In the presence of ventricular septal defects, particularly, the left ventricular outflow tract requires special attention for the presence of a potential subvalvular obstruction, which may reveal itself only after surgical closure of the ventricular defect. Echocardiographically, obstructions to the left ventricular outflow tract can be evaluated from the standard parasternal long-axis view, the apical outflow and long-axis views and the oblique subcostal views (30,59–62,80) (Echo. 24-6). Velocity traces using high PRF and CW Doppler spectral signals can be recorded for localization of the site and extent of the stenosis and estimation of total gradient by the simplified Bernoulli equation. M-mode recordings of the mitral valve aid in the detection of systolic anterior motion of the anterior mitral leaflet and its possible role in creating dynamic outflow obstruction. The relative sizes of the aorta and main pulmonary artery become important when planning for the arterial switch operation. As such, measurements of the valve annuli, sinotubular junction, ascending aorta, and main pulmonary artery should be routinely performed and compared (Echo. 24-10).

Anomalies of the tricuspid and mitral valves. In addition to overriding or straddling of the tricuspid valve over the interventricular septum and obstruction of the left ventricular outflow tract due to protrusion of tricuspid valve tissue through a ventricular septal defect mentioned previously, there are other described anomalies of the tricuspid valve in complete transposition (3,44,81,82). These include dysplastic or redundant valve tissue, anomalous insertions of tendinous chords onto the edges of the ventricular septal defect, hypoplasia of the valve and tissue gap between the septal and anterosuperior leaflets. This could be a cause of tricuspid regurgitation, often seen in complete transposition.

Anomalies of the mitral valve have also been reported in association with complete transposition (3,76–78,83–85). These include straddling or overriding of the mitral valve with malalignment between the atrial and ventricular septa, cleft of the anterior mitral leaflet, tissue gap at the anterior commissure, abnormal insertions of the tendinous chords to the edge of the ventricular defect,

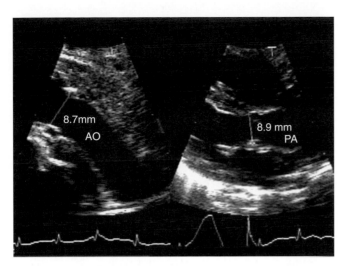

ECHO. 24-10. Parasternal views of the great vessels demonstrating the anatomical measurements of importance in planning an arterial switch operation. *AO*, aorta; *PA*, pulmonary artery.

parachute mitral valve and a forme fruste of parachute valve due to hypoplasia of the papillary muscles and short tendinous chords.

Detection of anomalies of the atrioventricular valves by echocardiography has obvious surgical importance, not only in selecting the type of surgical correction to be used, but also in the long-term clinical outcome since both hemodynamic and anatomical corrections require integrity of either the tricuspid or mitral valves, respectively, to support systemic resistance. The best echocardiographic views to visualize the atrioventricular valves are the parasternal long- and short-axis views, the four and two-chamber views obtained from the apex, and the subcostal four-chamber and short-axis views. Color and spectral Doppler are essential for a thorough evaluation of the atrioventricular valves. Color Doppler will reveal the presence of regurgitation and the direction of the jet. The intensity of the spectral Doppler signal will provide an indirect estimate of the severity of the insufficiency. Further, forward velocities recorded with pulsed and/or CW Doppler will reveal any tricuspid or mitral valve gradients.

Atrial septal defect or patent foramen ovale. Either a patent foramen ovale or an interatrial communication of the ostium secundum or fossa ovalis type is almost always present. Other types of atrial defects are extremely rare in complete transposition (31). Communications at the atrial level play an important physiologic role in complete transposition, particularly in cases with intact interventricular septum since they allow mixing of the two parallel circulations.

The size and location of the atrial communication and the results of a balloon or a blade septostomy can be accurately evaluated with two-dimensional echocardiography, particularly in association with spectral and color

Doppler mapping, through the parasternal short-axis and the apical and subcostal four-chamber views (Echo. 24-11; see color plate 83 following p. 364). Blood flow through the atrial communication is bidirectional in complete transposition thereby permitting the physiologic mixing of the two circulations. During ventricular diastole, flows are from right atrium to left atrium due to the lower pressure in the left atrium as a result of the greater compliance of the left (pulmonary) ventricle (86). During ventricular systole, shunting is from left atrium to right atrium due to a higher left atrial pressure during this portion of the cardiac cycle, resulting from lower distensibility of the left atrium (87). If the atrial communication is anatomically very small, only right to left shunting is seen. The timing and flow characteristics of atrial level shunting can be evaluated best with spectral Doppler and color M-mode traces, which provide better time resolution than two-dimensional color flow mapping (Echo. 24-11).

The use of two-dimensional echocardiography from either a transthoracic (especially subcostal views) or a transesophageal approach during atrial septostomy is particularly helpful because it allows a clear view of the atrial septum, the atrioventricular valves, and the pulmonary veins as well as of the position of the balloon or blade in relationship to these structures.

Patent ductus arteriosus. A patent ductus arteriosus also allows mixing of blood between the venous and systemic circulations and frequently survival in the newborn period depends on its patency. Echocardiographically, the ductus can be visualized from a parasternal short-axis view at the level of the great vessels, from a parasternal long-axis view of the right ventricular outflow, from suprasternal long- and short-axis views and from a subcostal short-axis view. Spectral Doppler, either pulsed wave or CW, and color flow mapping are essential for the accurate

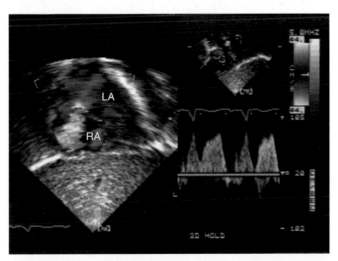

ECHO. 24-11. Subcostal view of the atrial septum demonstrating color and spectral Doppler velocity recordings of the left to right flow across an atrial defect. *LA*, left atrium; *RA*, right atrium.

evaluation of the direction and estimation of the amount of ductal shunt. In the immediate neonatal period, shunting can be from the pulmonary artery to the aorta (88) during ventricular systole while during ventricular diastole it reverses and goes from the aorta to the pulmonary artery due to the higher systemic vascular resistance (86). Pulmonary arterial pressure can be estimated from the spectral velocity recorded across the ductus when the systemic pressure is measured simultaneously. This can be a useful parameter to follow in planning the timing of anatomic repair before the pulmonary pressures drop to a level where the left ventricle loses its ability to sustain systemic pressures and resistances (Echo. 24-12; see color plate 84 following p. 364).

Juxtaposition of the atrial appendages. Left juxtaposition of the atrial appendages occurs in 1% to 2.5% of cases of complete transposition of the great arteries, particularly in those with the aorta located anterior and to the left (3,31,89–91). The right atrial appendage crosses behind the great vessels and comes to be located anteriorly and inferiorly to the left atrial appendage. In these cases the atrial septum adopts an abnormal spatial orientation: posteriorly, it is normally positioned or slightly oblique while anteriorly it take a horizontal position parallel to the frontal plane. Left juxtaposition of the atrial appendages can be observed echocardiographically in a parasternal short-axis view and from a four-chamber apical or subcostal view.

INTRAOPERATIVE AND POSTOPERATIVE EVALUATION

The intraoperative and postoperative evaluation in complete transposition of the great arteries varies with the type of surgical procedure utilized.

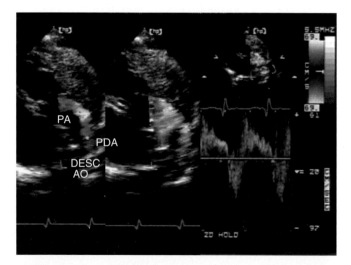

ECHO. 24-12. Parasternal short-axis views of the color and spectral Doppler recordings of flow across a bidirectional patent ductus arteriosus. **Left:** Left-to-right shunting from descending aorta to pulmonary artery. **Middle:** Right-to-left shunting from the pulmonary artery to the aorta. **Right:** Spectral Doppler recording of the low velocity bidirectional shunt. *PA,* pulmonary artery; *DESC AO,* descending aorta; *PDA,* patent ductus arteriosus.

The surgical techniques can be palliative or corrective. The *Blalock-Hanlon operation,* rarely used today, consists of the surgical creation of an atrial septal defect by performing an atrial septectomy (92). The *Senning operation* or atrial switch consists of placing an intraatrial baffle utilizing the atrial wall and a portion of the atrial septum in order to direct blood from the superior and inferior vena cavae towards the mitral valve and from the pulmonary veins towards the tricuspid valve (93). The *Mustard operation* uses the same physiologic principle of atrial switch as the Senning but the surgical technique involves resection of the atrial septum and the use of pericardium for the baffle (94). The *Jatene operation* or anatomic correction is performed by switching the great arteries with reimplantation of the coronary arteries; it is currently the preferred surgical procedure (95). In those cases with a large ventricular septal defect and stenosis of the left ventricular outflow tract not amenable to surgical resection, the *Rastelli operation* is used, during which the left ventricle is connected to the aorta via a Dacron patch through the ventricular defect (96,97). The pulmonary artery is then connected to the right ventricle through an extracardiac valved conduit or a homograft. The *Damus-Kaye-Stansel* operation is rarely used in complete transposition (79). In this procedure, the main pulmonary artery is sectioned at the bifurcation and anastomosed to the lateral wall of the ascending aorta, the aortic valve is oversewn and the distal pulmonary arteries are attached to the right ventricle via an extracardiac valved conduit. The coronary arteries are perfused by retrograde flow from the ascending aorta.

The intraoperative pre-bypass evaluation should serve to complement and clarify the transthoracic study. Ventricular function is evaluated through the transgastric transverse view (see Fig. 4-27A); this is particularly important when the arterial switch operation is being performed in order to compare it to the post-bypass study. The presence and location of ventricular and atrial defect(s) should be confirmed from transverse four-chamber and short-axis views (see Figs. 4-27A,B and 4-28A,B). Defects extending to the outlet septum are best visualized from the longitudinal views (see Fig. 4-29E). Competence of the atrioventricular valves should also be evaluated from the four-chamber views. The right and left ventricular outflow tracts must be specifically studied from the longitudinal views for the presence of obstruction (see Fig. 4-29D–F). Spectral Doppler velocities should be recorded as baseline values from these views and from the transgastric longitudinal views (see Fig. 4-27E), which usually provide for better positioning of the Doppler sampling line. The coronary anatomy can be confirmed from short-axis transverse views with slight anteflexion and retroflexion of the transducer to visualize their proximal course (see Fig. 4-29B,C).

The intraoperative post-bypass evaluation should include the same factors as in the pre-bypass study. First, ventricular function should be assessed from the transgastric short-axis views, particularly in the arterial switch operation. Second, this should be followed by examination of the ventricular and atrial septa for residual defects, of the atrioventricular valves for regurgitation and of the outflow tracts, particularly the left, for possible residual obstruction.

In *atrial switch repairs*, the systemic and pulmonary venous baffles should be assessed echocardiographically by spectral and color flow mapping to assure no significant leaks or obstruction. In these cases, the tricuspid valve, which remains as the systemic atrioventricular valve, should be studied carefully with Doppler for the presence of regurgitation, which would affect the short- and long-term prognosis.

In arterial switch repairs, the mitral valve should be carefully studied with Doppler for regurgitation, since this is the systemic atrioventricular valve. Further, an attempt should be made to visualize the coronary arteries and the sites of implantation. Also the suture lines of the neoaorta and neopulmonary anastomosis should be examined with two-dimensional imaging and Doppler to rule out stenosis, a common complication of this type of repair (Echos. 24-13, 24-14; see color plate 85 following p. 364).

In patients in whom a *Rastelli type repair* was performed, the post-bypass study should specifically evaluate for presence of residual shunts across the ventricular septal patch and for obstruction of the subaortic outflow due to the intracardiac baffle directing the flow from the left ventricle to the aorta. Frequently there is a mild degree of insufficiency of the pulmonary extracardiac conduit valve immediately postimplantation (98) so it is important to establish a baseline study with a combination of spectral and color Doppler for comparison during the long-term follow-up.

The late postoperative studies should address the complications that may occur in the specific surgical technique utilized.

In the *atrial switch operations* (Senning and Mustard), the right ventricle is kept as the systemic ventricle with late dysfunction seen commonly (99–105). The right ventricle is usually hypertrophied with the septum convex to the left, opposite the normal heart (Echo. 24-15). This is seen in the long-axis, short-axis, and four-chamber views, parasternally, apically, and subcostally. Schmidt et al. (106) have proposed a Doppler method to assess right ventricular performance using the acceleration variables of the aortic flow curve measured with pulsed Doppler. Insufficiency of the tricuspid valve, which is seen frequently in these patients and which can further aggravate the right (systemic) ventricular dysfunction (28,99,100,102,105), can be detected and its severity estimated from parasternal long-axis inflow views and from four-chamber apical and subcostal views using a combination of spectral and color Doppler methods. The left ventricular outflow tract should be assessed

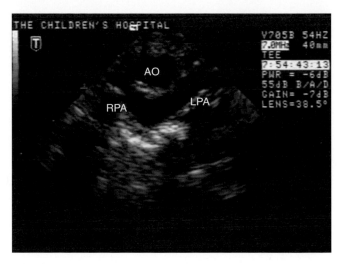

ECHO. 24-13. Transesophageal horizontal view of the relationship between the pulmonary arteries and neoaorta after arterial switch operation for complete transposition of the great arteries. Note the disposition of the pulmonary arteries around the neoaorta. *AO,* neoaorta; *RPA,* right pulmonary artery; *LPA,* left pulmonary artery.

for the presence of obstruction from the parasternal long-axis and the apical outflow views and its severity can be estimated using CW Doppler. The dynamic type of left ventricular outflow tract obstruction, which is commonly seen in complete transposition with intact ventricular septum, rarely progresses after atrial switch operations (107). Following the Mustard repair and less frequently after the Senning, there can be obstruction of the systemic venous baffle, particularly at the union of the superior vena cava to the superior end of the baffle (28,99,102,105,108,109). Attempts should be made to visualize the systemic venous baffle in its entirety from views that allow observation of the systemic venous atrium such as the apical four-chamber view and the subcostal four-chamber sagittal and oblique views (Echo. 24-16). The presence of obstructions can be demonstrated with color flow mapping and the severity estimated from spectral Doppler velocities using the simplified Bernoulli equation. The pulmonary venous baffle and atrium can be evaluated from apical four-chamber views (28). Angling the transducer anteriorly or superiorly one can see the pulmonary venous flows into the right atrium and the tricuspid valve (Echo. 24-17). It is important to note that in this view the systemic venous atrium occupies an anterior and medial plane with respect to the pulmonary venous atrium, which is posterior and lateral. In the standard parasternal long-axis view, the systemic venous atrium is located anteriorly and inferiorly to the pulmonary atrium. A baffle leak, which can occur from a dehiscence of the baffle patch, results in an atrial level shunt, which can be best seen with color Doppler from an apical four-chamber view.

The late postoperative follow-up of *arterial switch re-*

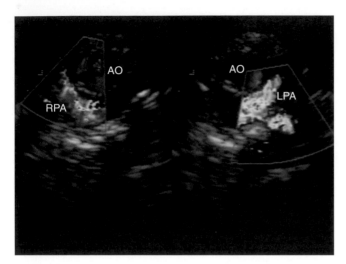

ECHO. 24-14. Transesophageal horizontal view of the color Doppler map of the flow into the branch pulmonary arteries obtained from the same patient as in Echo 24-13. *AO,* neo-aorta; *RPA,* right pulmonary artery; *LPA,* left pulmonary artery.

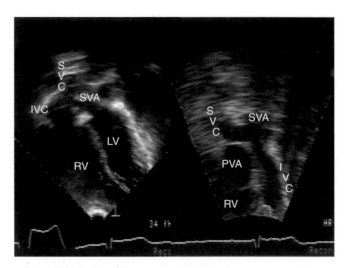

ECHO. 24-16. Apical views demonstrating the systemic venous atrium directing blood from the vena cavae to the left ventricle. *SVC,* superior vena cava; *IVC,* inferior vena cava; *SVA,* systemic venous atrium; *RV,* right ventricle; *LV,* left ventricle.

pairs usually presents few complications. Some that have been described include left ventricular outflow tract stenosis, dynamic and/or fixed subpulmonary stenosis, valve pulmonic stenosis, supravalve pulmonic stenosis, and supravalve aortic stenosis (110,111). Aortic valve regurgitation has also been described (112,113). The postoperative echocardiographic evaluation in these patients should include an examination of the coronary neoanastomoses, which are visible from a parasternal short-axis and apical and subcostal four-chamber views angling the transducer towards the outflow tracts. Ventricular function should be evaluated carefully including overall systolic function

from a short-axis view, segmental wall motion from a combination of four-chamber, two-chamber, and long-axis views imaged from all windows (parasternal, apical, and subcostal) and diastolic function by pulsed wave Doppler recording of velocities across the atrioventricular valves, systemic veins and pulmonary veins. The presence of stenosis of the outflow tracts can be revealed in the parasternal long-axis, apical outflow and subcostal outflow views. The actual gradients can be estimated from the spectral Doppler velocities recorded from the above views. The supravalve pulmonic and aortic areas, at the site of anastomosis, should be studied carefully since obstructions at these sites are common late sequelae of this

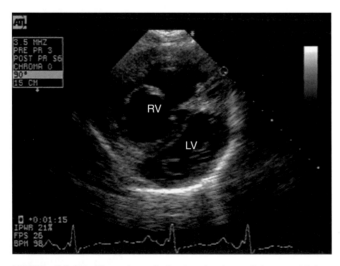

ECHO. 24-15. Parasternal short-axis view of the ventricles after atrial switch repair for transposition of the great arteries. Note the dilated and hypertrophied right ventricle and the convex septum compressing the left ventricle. *RV,* right ventricle; *LV,* left ventricle.

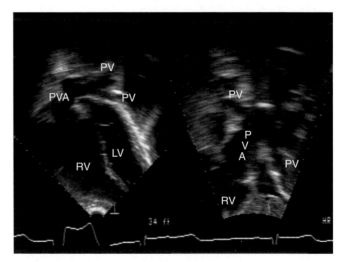

ECHO. 24-17. Apical view demonstrating the pulmonary venous atrium directing pulmonary venous blood into the right ventricle. *PV,* pulmonary veins; *PVA,* pulmonary venous atrium; *RV,* right ventricle; *LV,* left ventricle.

operation (Echo. 24-18; see color plate 86 following p. 364). The peripheral pulmonary arteries are best imaged from a short-axis suprasternal or high left subclavicular area (Echo. 24-19; see color plate 87 following p. 364). Regurgitation of the aortic valve can be seen from a parasternal long-axis view and from the apical and subcostal outflow views. Its degree of severity can be estimated from the spectral Doppler signal intensity, the slope of the regurgitant jet, and from the degree of flow reversal present in the descending aorta seen from a suprasternal long-axis view. Atrioventricular valves should also be examined specifically for the presence of regurgitation. This is best accomplished from the long-axis and the four- and two-chamber views obtained from the parasternal, apical, and subcostal windows.

Patients after the *Rastelli type of operation* can have residual shunts at the ventricular level, usually detected in the perioperative period. In the late follow-up, the most common sequelae are calcification of the pulmonary valved conduit with various degrees of stenosis and/or regurgitation of the conduit valve, and stenosis of the proximal and/or distal conduit anastomotic sites (114–119). Conduits are sometimes difficult to image in their full length, depending on their position; however, the usual approach includes the parasternal long-axis view with slight clockwise transducer rotation, the subcostal short-axis view with angulation of the transducer superiorly towards the right ventricular outflow tract, and the suprasternal long-axis view with slight clockwise rotation to achieve a longitudinal view of the conduit (120). Doppler flow mapping by color and pulsed (or high PRF) sampling of the length of the conduit can reveal the site(s) of obstruction and the presence and severity of regurgitation.

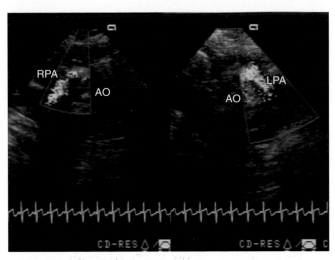

ECHO. 24-19. Transthoracic high parasternal view of the pulmonary arteries after arterial switch operation. Note the narrow jets and color aliasing of the flow into both branches of the pulmonary arteries, implying stenosis at these sites. *AO*, neoaorta; *RPA*, right pulmonary artery; *LPA*, left pulmonary artery.

The presence of tricuspid valve regurgitation can aid in the estimation of right ventricular pressure and therefore serve as an indirect measure of the severity of conduit malfunction. Meliones et al. (121) failed to detect conduit regurgitation in 35% of cases in the immediate postoperative period and in 26% of cases in the late follow-up period using transthoracic Doppler. However, using transesophageal echo, color Doppler is very sensitive in detecting conduit regurgitation, which is usually observed to a mild degree immediately postimplantation (98). In our experience, there is almost always some degree of conduit regurgitation in the late postoperative period, which increases progressively. Spectral Doppler sampling of the regurgitant jet can provide a good estimate of the severity of insufficiency from the intensity of the Doppler signal as well as from the slope of the decelerating regurgitant curve, which is in direct relationship to how fast the pulmonary arterial and right ventricular pressures approximate each other. Sometimes at sea level and in the presence of low pulmonary resistances a nonvalved conduit can be used to avoid reoperation due to conduit valve calcification; in these cases conduit regurgitation is present from implantation and should be evaluated similarly to the approaches used for valved conduits.

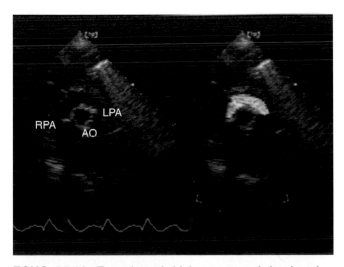

ECHO. 24-18. Transthoracic high parasternal view imaging the relationship between the pulmonary arteries and the neoaorta after arterial switch operation for transposition of the great arteries. Note the laminar flow into both pulmonary arteries without evidence of obstruction. *AO*, neoaorta; *RPA*, right pulmonary artery; *LPA*, left pulmonary artery.

REFERENCES

1. MacMahon B, McKeown T, Record RG. The incidence and life expectation of children with congenital heart disease. *Br Heart J* 1953;15:121–129.
2. Langford Kidd BS. Complete transposition of the great arteries. In: Keith JD, Rowe RD, Vlad P, eds. *Heart disease in infancy and childhood.* 3rd ed. New York: Macmillan, 1978:590–611.
3. Quero Jimenez M, Arque Gibernau JM, Maitre Azcarate MJ, Go-

mez Gonzalez R, Sanchez PA. Transposicion completa de las grandes arterias. In: Sanchez PA, ed. *Cardiologia pediatrica. Clinica y cirugia. Vol. 1.* Barcelona: Salvat Editores S.A., 1986:487–546.

4. Fyler DC. Prevalence. Trends. In: Fyler DC, ed. *Nadas pediatric cardiology.* Philadelphia: Hanley & Belfus, 1992:273–280.

5. Neches WH, Park SC, Ettedgui JA. Transposition of the great arteries. In: Garson A Jr, Bricker JT, Mcnamara DG, eds. *The science and practice of pediatric cardiology. Vol. II.* Philadelphia: Lea & Febiger, 1990:1175–1212.

6. Paul MH. Complete transposition of the great arteries. In: Adams FH, Emmanouilides GC, Riemenschneider TA, eds. *Moss heart disease in infants, children and adolescents.* 4th ed. Baltimore: Williams & Wilkins, 1989:371–423.

7. De la Cruz MV, Sanchez Gomez C, Arteaga MM, Arguello C. Experimental study of the development of the truncus and the conus in the chick embryo. *J Anat* 1977;123:661–686.

8. De la Cruz MV, Cayre R. Desarrollo embriologico del corazon y las grandes arterias. In: Sanchez PA, ed. *Cardiologia pediatrica. Clinica y cirugia.* Barcelona: Salvat Editores S.A., 1986:10–18.

9. Netter FH, Van Mierop LHS. Embryology. In: Netter FH, Yonkman FF, eds. *Heart.* Summit, NJ: Ciba Publications Department, 1969:111–130 *(The Ciba collection of medical illustrations, vol. 5).*

10. Kirby ML, Gale TF, Steward DE. Neural crest cells contribute to aorticopulmonary septation. *Science* 1983;220:1059–1061.

11. Van Mierop LHS, Wiglesworth FW. Pathogenesis of transposition complexes. III. True transposition of the great vessels. *Am J Cardiol* 1963;12:233–239.

12. Dor X, Corone P. Migration et cloisonnement du cono-truncus. Etude experimentale sur le coeur d'embryon de poulet. *Coeur* 1982;13:453–460.

13. Toussaint M, Lemoine G, Planche CL, Ribierre M. Transposition des gros vaisseaux avec aorta posterieure. Aspects anatomiques et embryologiques a propos d'une observation. *Coeur* 1982;13:461–465.

14. De la Cruz MV, Arteaga M, Quero Jimenez M. Conexiones y relaciones ventriculo-arteriales. Clasificacion anatomica y embriogenesis. *Rev Lat Cardiol* 1981;2:66–75.

15. De la Cruz MV, Arteaga M, Espino-Vela J, Quero Jimenez M, Anderson RH, Diaz GF. Complete transposition of the great arteries: types and morphogenesis of ventriculoarterial discordance. *Am Heart J* 1981;102:271–281.

16. Anselmi G, Munoz OH, Espino Vela J, Arguello C. Side-by-side great arteries. Embryologic considerations. In: Mendez Oteo F, ed. *Side-by-side great arteries.* Caracas, Venezuela: Instituto Venezolano de Cardiologia, 1984:2–21.

17. Baillie M. *The morbid anatomy of some of the most important parts of the humman body.* 2nd ed. London: Johnson & Nicol, 1797:38–40.

18. Farre JR. *Pathological researches. Essay 1: on malformation of the human heart.* London: Longman, Hurst, Rees, Orme, Brown, 1814:1–46.

19. Geipel P. Weitere beitrage zum situs transversus und zur hehre von den transpositionen der grossen gefasse des herzens. *Arch Kinderheilkunde* 1903;35:112–161.

20. Keith A. Hunterian lectures on malformations of the heart. *Lancet* 1909;2:433–435.

21. Monckeberg JG. Die missbildungen des herzens. In: Henke F, Lubarsh J, eds. *Handbuch der speciellen pathologischen anatomie und histologie. Vol. 2.* Berlin: Springer, 1924.

22. De la Cruz MV, Da Rocha JP. An ontogenetic theory for the explanation of congenital malformations involving the truncus and conus. *Am Heart J* 1956;51:782–805.

23. Grant RP. The morphogenesis of transposition of the great vessels. *Circulation* 1962;26:819–840.

24. Shaher RM. Complete and inverted transposition of the great vessels. *Br Heart J* 1964;26:51–66.

25. Van Mierop LHS. Transposition of the great arteries. I. Clarification or further confusion? *Am J Cardiol* 1971;28:735–738.

26. Van Praagh RV. Transposition of the great arteries. II. Transposition clarified. *Am J Cardiol* 1971;28:739–741.

27. Bourlon F, Fouron JC, Battle-Diaz J, Ducharme G, Davingnon A. Relation between isovolumic relaxation period of left ventricle and pulmonary artery pressure in d-transposition of the great arteries. *Br Heart J* 1980;43:226–231.

28. Aziz KU, Paul MH, Bharati S, et al. Two-dimensional echocardiographic evaluation of Mustard operation for d-transposition of the great arteries. *Am J Cardiol* 1981;47:654–664.

29. Carr I, Tynan MJ, Aberdeen E, Bonham-Carter RE, Graham G, Waterston DJ. Predictive accuracy of the loop-rule in 109 children with classical complete transposition of the great arteries. *Circulation* 1968;38[Suppl VI]:52(abst).

30. Pasquini L, Sanders SP, Parness IA, et al. Conal anatomy in 119 patients with d-loop transposition of the great arteries and ventricular septal defect: an echocardiographic and pathologic study. *J Am Coll Cardiol* 1993;21:1712–1721.

31. Anderson RH, Ho SY. Morphology of complete transposition. In: Anderson RH, Neches WH, Park SC, Zuberbuhler JR, eds. *Perspectives in pediatric cardiology. Vol. 1.* Mount Kisco, NY: Futura Publishing, 1988:217–227.

32. Anderson RH, Becker AE, Lucchese FA, Meier MA, Rigby ML, Soto B. Complete transposition. In: Anderson RH, Becker AE, Lucchese FA, Meier MA, Rigby ML, Soto B, eds. *Morphology of congenital heart disease. Angiocardiographic, echocardiographic and surgical correlates.* Kent, U.K.: Castle House Publications, 1983:84–100.

33. Goor DA, Edwards JE. The spectrum of transposition of the great arteries with specific reference to developmental anatomy of the conus. *Circulation* 1973;48:406–415.

34. Anderson RH, Macartney FJ, Shinebourne EA, Tynan M. Complete transposition. In: Anderson RH, Macartney FJ, Shinebourne EA, Tynan M, eds. *Paediatric cardiology. Vol. 2.* Edinburgh: Churchill Livingstone, 1987:829–865.

35. Soto B, Pacifico AD. Transposition of the great arteries. In: Soto B, Pacifico AD, eds. *Angiocardiography in congenital heart malformations.* Mount Kisco, NY: Futura Publishing, 1990:405–432.

36. Anderson RH, Henry GW, Becker AE. Morphologic aspects of complete transposition. *Cardiol Young* 1991;1:41–53.

37. Chiu IS, Anderson RH, Macartney FJ, De Leval MR, Stark J. Morphologic features of an intact ventricular septum susceptible to subpulmonary obstruction in complete transposition. *Am J Cardiol* 1984;53:1633–1638.

38. Smith A, Wilkinson JL, Anderson RH, Arnold R, Dickinson DF. Architecture of the ventricular mass and atrioventricular valves in complete transposition with intact septum compared with the normal. II. The right ventricle and tricuspid valve. *Pediatr Cardiol* 1986;6:299–305.

39. Elliott LP, Neufeld HN, Anderson RC, Adams P Jr, Edwards JE. Complete transposition of the great vessels. I. An anatomic study of sixty cases. *Circulation* 1963;27:1105–1117.

40. Van Praagh R, Perez-Trevino C, Lopez-Cuellar M, et al. Transposition of the great arteries with posterior aorta, anterior pulmonary artery, subpulmonary conus and fibrous continuity between aortic and atrioventricular valves. *Am J Cardiol* 1971;28:621–631.

41. Wilkinson JL, Arnold R, Anderson RH, Acerete F. Posterior transposition reconsidered. *Br Heart J* 1975;37:757–766.

42. Arteaga Martinez M, Fernandez-Espino R, Quero-Jimenez M, Noriega N, De la Cruz MV. Discordancia ventriculo-arterial con aorta posterior. Estudio anatomico de nueve casos. *Rev Lat Cardiol* 1981;4:277–286.

43. Miyake T, Yokoyama T, Shitorani H. Transposition of the great arteries with posterior aorta: detection by two-dimensional echocardiography. *Pediatr Cardiol* 1990;11:102–105.

44. Kirklin JW, Barrat-Boyes BG. Complete transposition of the great arteries. In: Kirklin JW, Barrat-Boyes BG, ed. *Cardiac surgery. Morphology, diagnostic criteria, natural history, techniques, results, and indications. Vol. 2.* 2nd ed. New York: Churchill Livingstone, 1993:1383–1467.

45. Shaher RM, Puddu GC. Coronary arterial anatomy in complete transposition of the great vessels. *Am J Cardiol* 1966;17:355–361.

46. Gittenberg-De Groot AC, Sauer U, Oppenheimer-Dekker A, Quaegebeur J. Coronary arterial anatomy in transposition of the great arteries. A morphologic study. *Pediatr Cardiol* 1983;4[Suppl I]:15–24.

47. Yacoub MH, Radley-Smith R. Anatomy of the coronary arteries

in transposition of the great arteries and methods for their transfer in anatomical correction. *Thorax* 1978;33:418–428.

48. Kurosawa H, Imai Y, Kawada M. Coronary arterial anatomy in regard to the arterial switch procedure. *Cardiol Young* 1991;1:54–62.

49. Smith A, Arnold R, Wilkinson JL, Hamilton DI, McKay R, Anderson RH. An anatomical study of the patterns of the coronary arteries and sinus nodal artery in complete transposition. *Int J Cardiol* 1986;12:295–304.

50. Pasquini L, Sanders SP, Parness IA, Colan SD. Diagnosis of coronary artery anatomy by two-dimensional echocardiography in patients with transposition of the great arteries. *Circulation* 1987;75:557–564.

51. Gittenberger-De Groot AC, Sauer U, Quaegebeur J. Aortic intramural coronary artery in three hearts with transposition of the great arteries. *J Thorac Cardiovasc Surg* 1986;91:566–571.

52. Pasquini L, Parness IA, Colan SD, Wernovsky G, Mayer JE, Sanders SP. Diagnosis of intramural coronary artery in transposition of the great arteries using two-dimensional echocardiography. *Circulation* 1993;88:1136–1141.

53. Ebels T, Meuzelaar K, Gallandat Huet RCG, et al. Neonatal arterial switch operation complicated by intramural left coronary artery and treated by left internal mammary bypass graft. *J Thorac Cardiovasc Surg* 1989;97:473–475.

54. Mayer JE, Sanders SP, Jonas RA, Castaneda AR, Wernovsky G. Coronary artery pattern and outcome of arterial switch operation for transposition of the great arteries. *Circulation* 1990;82[Suppl IV]:IV-139–IV-145.

55. Day RW, Laks H, Drinkwater DC. The influence of coronary anatomy on the arterial switch operation in neonates. *J Thorac Cardiovasc Surg* 1992;104:706–712.

56. Silberbach M, Castro WL, Goldstein MA, Lucas RV Jr, Edwards JE. Comparison of types of pulmonary stenosis with the state of the ventricular septum in complete transposition of the great arteries. *Pediatr Cardiol* 1989;10:11–15.

57. Idriss FS, Aubert J, Paul M, Nikaidoh H, Lev M, Newfeld EA. Transposition of the great vessels with ventricular septal defect. Surgical and anatomic considerations. *J Thorac Cardiovasc Surg* 1974;68:732–741.

58. Kurosawa H, Van Mierop LHS. Surgical anatomy of the infundibular septum in transposition of the great arteries with ventricular septal defect. *J Thorac Cardiovasc Surg* 1986;91:123–132.

59. Bierman FZ, Williams RG. Prospective diagnosis of d-transposition of the great arteries in neonates by subxiphoid, two-dimensional echocardiography. *Circulation* 1979;60:1496–1502.

60. Sanders SP, Bierman FZ, Williams RG. Conotruncal malformations: diagnosis in infancy using subxiphoid two-dimensional echocardiography. *Am J Cardiol* 1982;50:1361–1367.

61. Marino B, De Simone G, Pasquini L, et al. Complete transposition of the great arteries: visualization of left and right outflow tract obstruction by oblique subcostal two-dimensional echocardiography. *Am J Cardiol* 1985;55:1140–1145.

62. Roberson DA, Silverman NH. Malaligned outlet septum with subpulmonary ventricular septal defect and abnormal ventriculoarterial connection: a morphologic spectrum defined echocardiographically. *J Am Coll Cardiol* 1990;16:459–468.

63. Aziz KU, Paul MH, Muster AJ, Idriss FS. Positional abnormalities of atrioventricular valves in transposition of the great arteries including double outlet right ventricle, atrioventricular valve straddling and malattachment. *Am J Cardiol* 1979;44:1135–1145.

64. Milanesi O, Ho SY, Thiene G, Frescura C, Anderson RH. The ventricular septal defect in complete transposition of the great arteries: pathologic anatomy in 57 cases with emphasis on subaortic, subpulmonary, and aortic arch obstruction. *Hum Pathol* 1987;18:392–396.

65. Benatar A, Antunes MJ, Levin SE. Posterior d-transposition of the great arteries with an unusual form of aortic obstruction. *Pediatr Cardiol* 1990;11:170–172.

66. Lincoln C, Hasse J, Anderson RH, Shinebourne EA. Surgical correction in complete levotransposition of the great arteries with an unusual subaortic ventricular septal defect. *Am J Cardiol* 1976;38:344–351.

67. Milanesi O, Thiene G, Bini RM, Pellegrino PA. Complete transpo-sition of great arteries with coarctation of aorta. *Br Heart J* 1982;48:566–571.

68. Schneeweiss A, Motro M, Shem-Tov A, Neufeld HN. Subaortic stenosis: an unrecognized problem in transposition of the great arteries. *Am J Cardiol* 1981;48:336–339.

69. Nanda NC, Gramiak R, Manning JA, Lipchik EO. Echocardiographic features of subpulmonic obstruction in dextro-position of the great vessels. *Circulation* 1975;51:515–521.

70. Sansa M, Tonkin IL, Bargeron LM Jr, Elliot LP. Left ventricular outflow tract obstruction in transposition of the great arteries: an angiographic study of 74 cases. *Am J Cardiol* 1979;44:88–95.

71. Aziz KU, Paul MH, Idriss FS, Wilson AD, Muster AJ. Clinical manifestations of dynamic left ventricular outflow tract stenosis in infants with d-transposition of the great arteries with intact ventricular septum. *Am J Cardiol* 1979;44:290–297.

72. Yacoub MH, Arensman FW, Bernhard A, Heintzen PH, Lange PE, Radley-Smith R. Preparation of the left ventricle for anatomical correction of transposition of the great arteries. *Pediatr Cardiol* 1983;4:83–92.

73. Shrivastava S, Tadavarthy M, Fukuda T, Edwards JE. Anatomic causes of pulmonary stenosis in complete transposition. *Circulation* 1976;54:154–159.

74. Tonkin IL, Sansa M, Elliot LP, Bargeron LM. Recognition of developing left ventricular outflow tract obstruction in complete transposition of the great arteries. *Radiology* 1980;134:53–59.

75. Quero Jimenez M, Perez Martinez V. Uncommon conal pathology in complete dextrotransposition of the great arteries with ventricular septal defect. *Chest* 1974;66:411–417.

76. Rosenquist GC, Stark J, Taylor JFN. Congenital mitral valve disease in transposition of the great arteries. *Circulation* 1975;51:731–737.

77. Moene RJ, Oppenheimer-Dekker A. Congenital mitral valve anomalies in transposition of the great arteries. *Am J Cardiol* 1982;49:1972–1977.

78. Ammirati A, Arteaga M, Garcia-Pelaez I, et al. Congenital mitral valve anomalies in transposition of the great arteries. *Jpn Heart J* 1989;30:187–195.

79. Freedom RM, Smallhorn JF, Trusler GA. Transposition of the great arteries. In: Freedom RM, Benson LN, Smallhorn JF, eds. *Neonatal heart disease.* London: Springer-Verlag, 1992:179–212.

80. Chin AJ, Yeager SB, Sanders SP, et al. Accuracy of prospective two-dimensional echocardiographic evaluation of left ventricular outflow tract in complete transposition of the great arteries. *Am J Cardiol* 1985;55:759–764.

81. Huhta JC, Edwards WD, Danielson GK, Feldt RH. Abnormalities of the tricuspid valve in complete transposition of the great arteries with ventricular septal defect. *J Thorac Cardiovasc Surg* 1982;83:569–576.

82. Daskalopoulos DA, Edwards WD, Driscoll DJ, Seward JB, Tajik AJ, Hagler DJ. Correlation of two-dimensional echocardiographic and autopsy findings in complete transposition of the great arteries. *J Am Coll Cardiol* 1983;2:1151–1157.

83. Layman TE, Edwards JE. Anomalies of the cardiac valves associated with complete transposition of the great vessels. *Am J Cardiol* 1967;19:247–255.

84. Otero Coto E, Quero Jimenez M, Deverall PB, Bain H. Anomalous mitral cleft with abnormal ventriculo-arterial connection: anatomical findings and surgical implications. *Pediatr Cardiol* 1984;5:1–5.

85. Deal BJ, Chin AJ, Sanders SP, Norwood WI, Castaneda AR. Subxiphoid two-dimensional echocardiographic identification of tricuspid valve abnormalities in transposition of the great arteries with ventricular septal defect. *Am J Cardiol* 1985;55:1146–1151.

86. Hoffman JIE, Heymann MA, Rudolph AM. Complete transposition: physiological considerations on the neonatal transition. In: Anderson RH, Neches WH, Park SC, Zuberbuhler JR, eds. *Perspectives in pediatric cardiology. Vol. 1.* Mount Kisco, NY: Futura Publishing, 1988:229–232.

87. Carr I. Timing of bidirectional atrial shunts in transposition of the great arteries and atrial septal defect. *Circulation* 1971;44[Suppl II]:II-70.

88. Rudolph AM. Aortopulmonary (complete) transposition—medical and surgical treatment during the first week of life. In: Marcelletti C, Anderson RH, Becker AE, Corno A, Di Carlo D, Mazzera E,

eds. *Paediatric cardiology 6.* Edinburgh: Churchill Livingstone, 1986:298–306.

89. Melhuish BPP, Van Praagh R. Juxtaposition of the atrial appendages. A sign of severe cyanotic congenital heart disease. *Br Heart J* 1968;30:269–284.

90. Urban AE, Stark J, Waterston DJ. Mustard's operation for transposition of the great arteries complicated by juxtaposition of the atrial appendages. *Ann Thorac Surg* 1976;21:304–310.

91. Wood AE, Freedom RM, Williams WG, Trusler GA. The Mustard procedure in transposition of the great arteries associated with juxtaposition of the atrial appendages with and without dextrocardia. *J Thorac Cardiovasc Surg* 1983;85:451–456.

92. Blalock A, Hanlon CR. The surgical treatment of complete transposition of the aorta and the pulmonary artery. *Surg Gynecol Obstet* 1950;90:1–15.

93. Senning A. Surgical correction of transposition of the great vessels. *Surgery* 1959;45:966–980.

94. Mustard WT. Successful two-stage correction of transposition of the great vessels. *Surgery* 1964;55:469–472.

95. Jatene A, Fontes VF, Paulista PP, et al. Anatomic correction of transposition of the great vessels. *J Thorac Cardiovasc Surg* 1976; 72:364–370.

96. Rastelli GC. A new approach to anatomic repair of transposition of the great arteries. *Mayo Clin Proc* 1969;44:1–12.

97. Rastelli GC, Wallace RB, Ongley PA. Complete repair of transposition of the great arteries with pulmonary stenosis. A review and report of a case corrected by using a new surgical technique. *Circulation* 1969;39:83–95.

98. Golebiovski P, Elkadi T, Moises V, Valdes-Cruz LM, Sahn DJ. Biplane transesophageal imaging provides complete visualization of human allograft conduits placed for reconstruction of the right ventricular outflow tract. *J Am Coll Cardiol* 1993;21:390A(abst).

99. Warnes CA, Somerville J. Transposition of the great arteries: late results in adolescents and adults after the Mustard procedure. *Br Heart J* 1987;58:148–155.

100. Rees S, Somerville J, Warnes C, et al. Assessing cardiac function and anatomy following Mustard's operation for transposition of the great arteries. *Am J Cardiol* 1988;61:1316–1322.

101. Kato H, Nakano S, Matsuda H, Hirose H, Shimazaki Y, Kawashima Y. Right ventricular myocardial function after atrial switch operation for transposition of the great arteries. *Am J Cardiol* 1989;63:226–230.

102. Bender HW Jr, Stewart JR, Merrill WH, Hammon JW Jr, Graham TP. Ten years experience with the Senning operation for transposition of the great arteries: physiological results and late follow-up. *Ann Thorac Surg* 1989;47:218–223.

103. Martin RP, Qureshi SA, Ettedegui JA, et al. An evaluation of right and left ventricular function after anatomical correction and intraatrial repair operations for complete transposition of the great arteries. *Circulation* 1990;82:808–816.

104. Redington AN. Functional assessment of the heart after corrective surgery for complete transposition. *Cardiol Young* 1991;1:84–90.

105. Merrill WH, Stewart JR, Hammon JW Jr, Johns JA, Bender HW. The Senning operation for complete transposition: mid-term physiologic, electrophysiologic, and functional results. *Cardiol Young* 1991;1:80–83.

106. Schmidt KG, Cloez JL, Silverman NH. Assessment of right ventricular performance by pulsed Doppler echocardiography in patients after intraatrial repair of aortopulmonary transposition in infancy or childhood. *J Am Coll Cardiol* 1989;13:1578–1585.

107. Park SC, Neches WH, Mathews RA, et al. Hemodynamic function after the Mustard operation for transposition of the great arteries. *Am J Cardiol* 1983;51:1514–1519.

108. Campbell RM, Moreau GA, Johns JA, et al. Detection of caval obstruction by magnetic resonance imaging after intraatrial repair of transposition of the great arteries. *Am J Cardiol* 1987;60:688–691.

109. Kaulitz R, Stumper OFW, Geuskens R, et al. Comparative values of the precordial and transesophageal approaches in the echocardiographic evaluation of atrial baffle function after an atrial correction procedure. *J Am Coll Cardiol* 1990;16:686–694.

110. Wernovsky G, Jonas RA, Colan SD, et al. Results of the arterial switch operation in patients with transposition of the great arteries and abnormalities of the mitral valve or left ventricular outflow tract. *J Am Coll Cardiol* 1990;16:1446–1454.

111. Castaneda AR, Mayer JE Jr. Neonatal repair of transposition of the great arteries. In: Long WA, ed. *Fetal and neonatal cardiology.* Philadelphia: WB Saunders, 1990:789–795.

112. Planche C, Serraf A, Lacour-Gayet F, Bruniaux J, Bouchart F. Anatomic correction of complete transposition with ventricular septal defect in neonates: experience with 42 consecutive cases. *Cardiol Young* 1991;1:101–103.

113. Martin RP, Ettedgui JA, Qureshi SA, et al. A quantitative evaluation of aortic regurgitation after anatomic correction of transposition of the great arteries. *J Am Coll Cardiol* 1988;12:1281–1284.

114. Heck HA, Schieken RM, Lauer RM, Doty DB. Conduit repair for complex congenital heart disease. Late follow-up. *J Thorac Cardiovasc Surg* 1978;75:806–814.

115. Mair DD, Fulton RE, Danielson GK. Thrombotic occlusion of Hancock conduit due to severe dehydration after Fontan operation. *Mayo Clin Proc* 1978;53:397–402.

116. Geha AS, Laks H, Stansel HC, et al. Late failure of porcine valve heterografts in children. *J Thorac Cardiovasc Surg* 1979;78:351–364.

117. McGoon DC, Danielson GK, Puga FJ, Ritter DG, Mair DD, Ilstrup DM. Late results after extracardiac conduit repair for congenital cardiac defects. *Am J Cardiol* 1982;49:1741–1749.

118. Vergesslich KA, Gersony WM, Steeg CN, et al. Postoperative assessment of porcine-valved right ventricular-pulmonary artery conduits. *Am J Cardiol* 1984;53:202–205.

119. Jonas RA, Freed MD, Mayer JE Jr, Castaneda AR. Long-term follow-up of patients with synthetic right heart conduits. *Circulation* 1985;72[Suppl II]:II-77–II-83.

120. Canale JM, Sahn DJ, Copeland JG, et al. Two-dimensional Doppler echocardiographic/M mode echocardiographic and phonocardiographic method for study of extracardiac heterograft valved conduits in the right ventricular outflow tract position. *Am J Cardiol* 1982;49:100–107.

121. Meliones JN, Snider AR, Bove EL, et al. Doppler evaluation of homograft valved conduits in children. *Am J Cardiol* 1989;64:354–358.

CHAPTER 25

Truncus Arteriosus

Lilliam M. Valdes-Cruz and Raul O. Cayre

Truncus arteriosus is a congenital cardiac malformation characterized by the presence of one arterial trunk emerging from the heart that gives origin to the coronary, pulmonary, and systemic arteries (1–6). The requirement for the presence of only one arterial valve in the definition of truncus is important in order to differentiate it from aortopulmonary window, in which there are two separate arterial valves (7–9).

The first anatomical case was reported by Wilson in 1798 (10). In 1864, Buchanan (11) described the clinical symptoms and autopsy findings in one case and called it "undivided truncus arteriosus." Since then, different names have been used to label this malformation: truncus arteriosus communis persistents (1), persistent truncus arteriosus (2,7–9,12), common aorticopulmonary trunk (3), truncus arteriosus communis (4–6), single arterial trunk (13), and single outlet heart via a persistent truncus arteriosus (14). Its incidence varies between 0.7% and 2.5% of all congenital cardiac malformations (15–19) and between 1% and 4% in necropsy series (18,20).

EMBRYOLOGIC CONSIDERATIONS

The structures and mechanisms that contribute to the morphogenesis of truncus arteriosus are the conal, truncal, and aortopulmonary septa and the incorporation of the conus into the left ventricle.

Conal Septation

The conus, primordium of the infundibula of both ventricles, appears in the loop stage (21) and makes up the cephalic end of the heart (22) (see Fig. 1-5B). During the early loop stage, two mesenchymal tissue masses appear in the internal wall of the conus, which are the dextrodorsal and sinistroventral conal crests (23) (see Fig. 1-12). The fusion of the conal crests gives origin to the conal

or infundibular septum, which separates the conus in two: one anterolateral conus and one posteromedial conus (see Fig. 1-14A).

Truncal Septation

The truncus appears in the early post-loop stage in the extreme cephalic end of the heart (21); distally it is continuous with the aortic sac and proximally with the conus (see Fig. 1-5C). Simultaneously with the appearance of the conal crests, two mesenchymal tissue masses also appear in the proximal end of the truncus and are called the "dextrosuperior" and "sinistroinferior truncal swellings" (24) (see Fig. 1-12B). The fusion of the truncal swellings gives rise to the truncal septum, which separates the semilunar valves (see Fig. 1-14B).

Aortopulmonary Septation

Truncal septation is also contributed to by the aortopulmonary septum. This septum has an extracardiac origin between the fourth and sixth aortic arches, from cells of the neural crest (25). The aortopulmonary septum is spiral, grows in a cephalocaudal direction, and fuses with the truncal septum, thereby separating the ascending aorta from the main pulmonary trunk (see Fig. 1-14C).

Incorporation of the Conus into the Left Ventricle

As the ventriculoinfundibular fold diminishes in size, the conus migrates (26) from a rightward position related to the primordium of the trabeculated portion of the right ventricle, to an anteromedial position. In this manner, the left ventricle acquires its outflow tract (see Fig. 1-5D,E).

Truncus arteriosus is caused by a failure of conal septation, a complete absence of the truncal septum, and an incomplete development or absence of the aortopulmo-

449

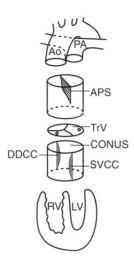

FIG. 25-1. Schematic drawing demonstrating the probable morphogenesis of truncus arteriosus. Note the underdevelopment of the conal crests, the absence of the truncal septum and the failure in development of the aortopulmonary septum. *RV,* right ventricle; *LV,* left ventricle; *DDCC,* dextrodorsal conal crest; *SVCC,* sinistroventral conal crest; *TrV,* truncal valve; *Ao,* aorta; *PA,* pulmonary artery.

nary septum (20,27–29) (Fig. 25-1). Failure of fusion of the conal crests will determine the presence of a ventricular septal defect, which will be the result of absence of the infundibular septum (20,30). The truncal septum is always absent; therefore, there is only one arterial valve (Fig. 25-1). Cases with two arterial valves should be considered aortopulmonary windows (7,8,28). The degree of development of the aortopulmonary septum forms the basis for the classification of truncus arteriosus proposed by Collet and Edwards (2) (Fig. 25-2). Type I truncus (Fig. 25-2A) is caused by an incomplete development of the aortopulmonary septum, whereas type II (Fig. 25-2B) and type III (Fig. 25-2C) are the result of a complete absence of aortopulmonary septation. Truncus type IV (Fig.

25-2D) should be considered a form of pulmonary atresia with ventricular septal defect rather than a type of truncus arteriosus (8,31). The theory proposed by Van Praagh and Van Praagh (3), which emphasizes the similarities between tetralogy of Fallot with pulmonary atresia and truncus arteriosus, lacks sustaining embryologic and anatomic evidence, as has been demonstrated by various authors (8,28,32).

Generally, the truncus overrides the ventricular septum and is related to both ventricles in a balanced manner (Fig. 25-3A). If there is failure of conal incorporation into the left ventricle, the truncus arteriosus can be predominantly related with the right ventricle, called "right predominance" (Fig. 25-3B). If there is excessive incorporation of the conus into the left ventricle, there can be left predominance (Fig. 25-3C).

ANATOMIC AND ECHOCARDIOGRAPHIC CONSIDERATIONS

The echocardiographic study of truncus arteriosus should establish the visceroatrial situs, the atrioventricular concordance, and the pulmonary and systemic venous drainages. Specifically related to the truncus arteriosus, the following should be studied: (a) the ventricular septal defect; (b) the truncal valve; (c) the relationship of the truncal valve to the atrioventricular valves and to the ventricles; (d) the type of truncus arteriosus; (e) origin and distribution of the coronary arteries; (f) associated anomalies; and (g) intra- and postoperative evaluation.

Ventricular Septal Defect

Except in extremely rare cases (33), there is always a large ventricular septal defect present in truncus arteriosus. Rarely, it is small and restrictive (34), particularly

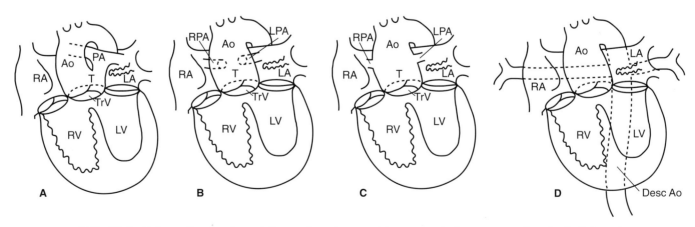

FIG. 25-2. Schematic drawing of the various types of truncus arteriosus according to Collet and Edwards (2). **A:** Type I. **B:** Type II. **C:** Type III. **D:** Type IV. *RA,* right atrium; *LA,* left atrium; *RV,* right ventricle; *LV,* left ventricle; *TrV,* truncal valve; *T,* truncus; *Ao,* aorta; *PA,* pulmonary artery; *RPA,* right pulmonary artery; *LPA,* left pulmonary artery; *Desc Ao,* descending aorta.

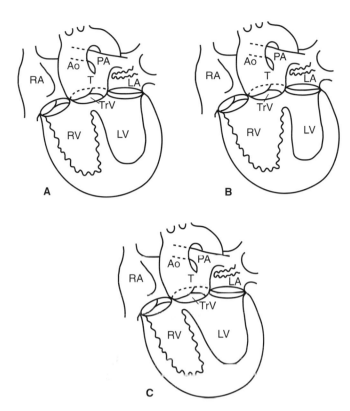

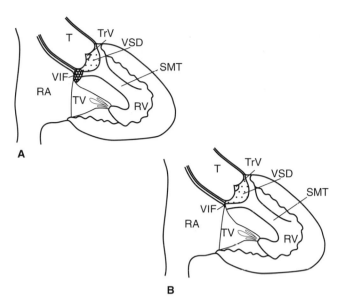

FIG. 25-3. Schematic drawings demonstrating the different types of overriding of the truncus arteriosus over the ventricular septum. **A:** Balanced manner. **B:** Right predominance. **C:** Left predominance. *RA*, right atrium; *LA*, left atrium; *RV*, right ventricle; *LV*, left ventricle; *TrV*, truncal valve; *T*, truncus; *Ao*, aorta; *PA*, pulmonary artery.

FIG. 25-4. Schematic drawings of the right ventricle showing the relationship between the tricuspid valve, the truncal valve, and the ventricular septal defect. **A:** Truncal valve-tricuspid valve discontinuity. **B:** Truncal valve-tricuspid valve continuity. *RA*, right atrium; *RV*, right ventricle; *TV*, tricuspid valve; *TrV*, truncal valve; *SMT*, septomarginal trabecula; *T*, truncus; *VSD*, ventricular septal defect; *VIF*, ventriculoinfundibular fold.

in cases of marked right predominance. Absence of the infundibular septum determines the presence of the ventricular septal defect, located between the limbs of the septomarginal trabecula; the anterior limb makes the anterior border and the posterior limb the posterior border of the defect (Fig. 25-4). The truncal valve forms the roof and the superior border of the defect, which is separated from the tricuspid valve by the muscular ventriculoinfundibular fold (Fig. 25-4A). Occasionally, the ventriculoinfundibular fold is fibrous, resulting in continuity between the tricuspid valve and the defect, in which case it has perimembranous extensions (35) (Fig. 25-4B). In this case, the truncal valve makes the superior border of the defect, the anterior and posterior limbs of the septomarginal trabecula form the superior and inferior borders of the defect, respectively, and the fibrous ventriculoinfundibular fold forms its posterior border.

The echocardiographic views that allow a study of the ventricular septal defect are the parasternal long-axis, the apical four-chamber, and the subcostal four-chamber views, aiming superiorly towards the outflow tract. The defect is seen in the region corresponding to the outlet septum and roofed by the truncal valve (Echo. 25-1; see color plate 88 following p. 364). Differentiation from

tetralogy of Fallot with pulmonary atresia should be made from these views since in both lesions there is one great vessel overriding the ventricular septum, which is roofed by one arterial valve, and the other arterial valve is absent. In tetralogy with pulmonary atresia, the ventricular septal

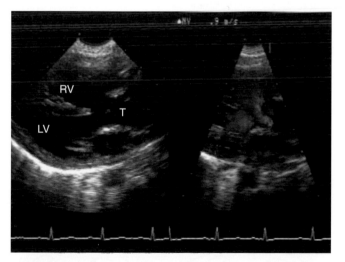

ECHO. 25-1. Parasternal long-axis views of truncus arteriosus demonstrating the large-outlet ventricular septal defect and overriding of the truncus over the interventricular septum. Note that the truncal valve forms the roof of the ventricular defect. The **right** panel is the color Doppler flow map of the shunt across the ventricular defect. There is direct flow from the right ventricle to the truncus *(blue)* as well as flow from the left ventricle to the truncus *(red)*. *RV*, right ventricle; *LV*, left ventricle; *T*, truncus.

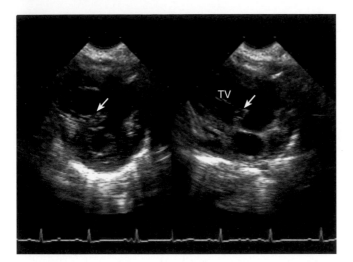

ECHO. 25-2. Parasternal short-axis views in truncus arteriosus. **Left:** The short axis at the ventricular level demonstrates the presence of a ventricular defect in the outlet septum. The *arrow* points to the muscular septum separating the tricuspid valve from the defect. **Right:** The *arrow* points to the intact membranous septum. The ventricular defect is in the outlet septum and there is discontinuity between the defect and the tricuspid valve. *TV,* tricuspid valve.

defect is perimembranous and usually there is mitral-aortic-tricuspid continuity, and the outlet septum is present and attached to the right ventricular infundibular free wall, whereas in truncus the defect is in the outlet septum, which is underdeveloped, and rarely extends to the perimembranous septum; therefore, there is discontinuity between the defect and the tricuspid valve (Echo. 25-2). Doppler color flow mapping clearly demonstrates the defect under the truncal valve and the bidirectional shunting that is present, as there are balanced pressures between the ventricles. Spectral Doppler velocities can be recorded with pulsed wave and are usually low due to the low gradient across the defect.

Truncal Valve

The single truncal valve present in truncus arteriosus serves to differentiate it from the aortopulmonary window. It can have a variable number of cusps. The truncal cusps can be classified according to two characteristics: the spatial position and the number of cusps (36) (Fig. 25-5). The position of each cusp is defined in relation to the atrioventricular valve orifices in the coronal plane: those adjacent to the atrioventricular orifices are called "posterior cusps," and those that are not are named "anterior cusps" (36). The cusps located to the right or the left of the anteroposterior axis of the heart are called "right" and "left," respectively (36).

Three cusps are found in 49% to 70% of cases of truncus (2–6,8,9,35–37) (Figs. 25-5A–C). Most commonly, there is one anterior and to the right, one anterior and to the left, and one posterior (Fig. 25-5A). The second most common situation seen is that of four cusps, found in 11.3% to 26.5% of cases (2–6,8,9,35,37), with two anterior and two posterior cusps (Fig. 25-5D), or one anterior, one right, one left, and one posterior (Fig. 25-5E). A bicuspid truncal valve has been seen in 1.2% to 32% of reports (2–6,8,9,35,37), with one located on the right and one on the left (Fig. 25-5F), or one anterior and one posterior (Fig. 25-5G). More rarely, the valve can have five leaflets (0.5% to 2% of cases) (4,8,37), six leaflets (1.2%), (2) or one leaflet (4%) (9).

The truncal valve cusps are abnormal in a high percentage of cases. Anomalies that have been reported include different sized cusps, variable degrees of myxomatous dysplasia with thickening, nodular fibrosis on the free borders of the cusps, and imperfections of the commissures (4,6,8,9,34,37–41). These anomalies result in truncal valve insufficiency, which is reported in 2.2% to 58.3% of cases of truncus arteriosus (4,5,8,20,38,39). More rarely, in 3.7% to 18% of cases, there can also be

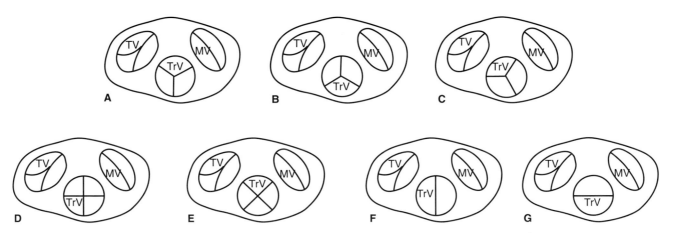

FIG. 25-5. Schematic drawings demonstrating the various anatomic variants of the truncal valve. **A–C:** Tricuspid. **D,E:** Quadricuspid. **F,G:** Bicuspid. *TV,* tricuspid valve; *MV,* mitral valve; *TrV,* truncal valve.

stenosis of the truncal valve, either as an isolated or as a mixed lesion with insufficiency (4,5,9,40–42).

Echocardiographically, the truncal valve should be studied both anatomically and functionally from all available windows. The short-axis view at the level of the valve itself offers the best cross-sectional cut to determine the number, size, and location of the cusps (Echo. 25-3; see color plate 89 following p. 364). Its relationship to the ventricular septal defect can be appreciated from the parasternal long-axis and the four-chamber views (both apical and subcostal) aiming the transducer superiorly towards the truncal valve. The long-axis view of the right ventricular outflow reveals the absence of an outlet septum and the fact that the roof of the defect is formed by the truncal valve.

The functional anatomy of the valve involves assessment of possible stenosis and/or insufficiency with color and spectral Doppler. The parasternal long-axis view reveals the presence of regurgitation of the valve and the cusp(s) from which the regurgitant jet mostly originates. Depending on the direction of the jet on color flow mapping, the continuous wave Doppler interrogation line may be aligned with the regurgitant jet from this view to record the velocities and thereby estimate the severity of regurgitation based on the intensity of the spectral signal and on the slope of the diastolic velocity curve. The parasternal short-axis view reveals the cross-sectional size of the jet at its origin and also the cusp(s) involved. The four-chamber views tilted superiorly towards the truncal valve and the two-chamber views (apical and subcostal) also permit assessment of the regurgitant jet and its direction, and estimation of its severity by Doppler interrogation. Also from these views the forward velocities across the truncal valve can be measured with continuous wave Doppler to reveal any stenosis. This velocity should always be confirmed

with the stand-alone Doppler probe from the suprasternal and the high right and left subclavicular positions since these positions commonly yield higher velocities than interrogations from the apex.

Relationship of the Truncal Valve with the Atrioventricular Valves and with the Ventricles

There is always fibrous continuity between the truncal valve and the mitral valve. Discontinuity between the truncal and tricuspid valves is the norm due to the usual presence of a muscular ventriculoinfundibular fold (Fig. 25-4A).

As mentioned previously, in the majority of instances, the truncal valve overrides both ventricles in a balanced form; this has been seen in 16.5% to 80% of cases reported (2,4,8,9,20) (Fig. 25-3A). A right predominant truncus with overriding mostly over the right ventricle has been seen slightly less frequently, in 10.6% to 66.5% of cases (2,4,8,9,20) (Fig. 25-3B). Origin of the truncus exclusively from the right ventricle was reported by Bharati et al. (4) in 14.2% of their specimens and in 3% of the cases reported by Crupi et al. (8). Left predominance is much less frequent and has been observed in 2.8% to 16% of reported cases (2,4,8,9) (Fig. 25-3C).

The relationship between the truncal and atrioventricular valves can be examined echocardiographically from the parasternal long-axis view both in standard projection and tilted towards the right ventricular inflow, from the apical long-axis and from the four-chamber apical and subcostal views tilting the transducer superiorly towards the truncal valve. Simultaneously, from these same views, the relationship of the truncus with the ventricles and the degree and type of predominance can be ascertained.

Type of Truncus Arteriosus

In 1949, Collet and Edwards (2) proposed a classification of truncus arteriosus based on the site of origin of the pulmonary arteries, and it is still the one most commonly used today. It established four types of truncus arteriosus: Type I, in which a short pulmonary arterial trunk emerges from the truncus and divides into right and left pulmonary branches (Fig. 25-2A) (Echos. 25-4, 25-5; see color plate 90 following p. 364); Type II, in which there is no common pulmonary trunk, rather the right and left branches emerge separately but close to each other from the posterior wall of the truncus (Fig. 25-2B) (Echos. 25-6, 25-7; see color plate 91 following p. 364); Type III, in which there is also no common pulmonary trunk and both branches emerge from the truncus separately from either side of the truncus arteriosus (Fig. 25-2C); and Type IV, in which there are no pulmonary arteries and which should be considered a type of pulmonary atresia with ventricular communication rather

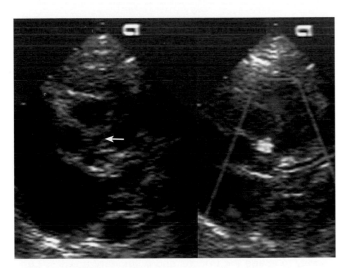

ECHO. 25-3. Short-axis view of a quadricuspid truncal valve. The *arrow* points to the regurgitant orifice in the middle of the valve. **Right:** Cross-section of the regurgitant jet occupying the orifice.

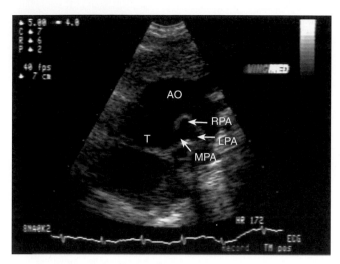

ECHO. 25-4. Suprasternal long-axis view of type I truncus with the origin of the common pulmonary trunk and its branches *(arrows)*. *MPA,* main pulmonary artery; *RPA,* right pulmonary artery; *LPA,* left pulmonary artery; *T,* truncus; *AO,* ascending aorta.

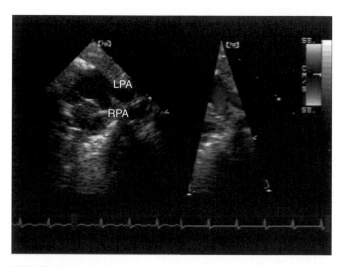

ECHO. 25-6. Left: Left subclavicular view of type II truncus with the origin of the right and left pulmonary arteries directly from the truncus without a common pulmonary trunk. **Right:** Color Doppler map of the flow from the truncus into the branch pulmonary arteries. *LPA,* left pulmonary artery; *RPA,* right pulmonary artery.

than a type of truncus arteriosus (8,31,43) (Fig. 25-2D) (Echo. 25-8; see color plate 92 following p. 364).

In Type I truncus, the short common pulmonary trunk usually emerges from the left lateral wall of the truncus or slightly posterolaterally (Fig. 25-2A) (Echo. 25-4). Occasionally, it can also have an anterolateral (42) or directly posterior (44) origin. Ordinarily, the truncus is larger than the pulmonary trunk, but in rare instances, the pulmonary has been reported as being larger than the truncus, almost always in association with interruption of the aortic arch (20). In Type III, anomalies of the origin of the pulmonary

arteries, such as crossed arteries, have been reported (45,46).

The type of truncus is determined echocardiographically by imaging the origin of the pulmonary arteries. The parasternal short-axis view aimed above the plane of the truncal valve and the high short-axis view (47) are particularly helpful to demonstrate the presence or absence of a common pulmonary trunk and the origin of the pulmonary branches (Echos. 25-5, 25-6). The parasternal long-axis views may also reveal the origin of the pulmo-

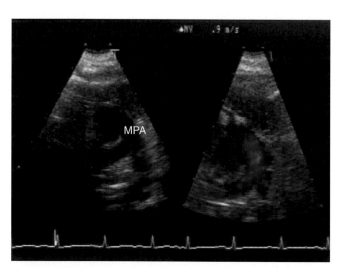

ECHO. 25-5. Left: Parasternal short-axis view of type I truncus showing the origin of the main pulmonary trunk and branches. **Right:** Color Doppler flow map demonstrating the flow from the truncus to the pulmonary arteries. A coronary artery is seen emerging from the truncus anteriorly. *MPA,* main pulmonary artery.

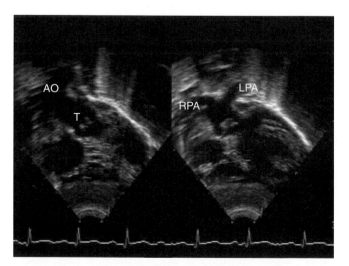

ECHO. 25-7. Subcostal view with the transducer aimed superiorly to image the truncus and pulmonary arteries. **Left:** View of the common truncus with the transverse aortic arch distally. **Right:** Origin of the branch pulmonary arteries directly from the truncus. *T,* truncus; *AO,* aorta; *RPA,* right pulmonary artery; *LPA,* left pulmonary artery.

nary arteries, particularly if they are posterior on the truncal wall. These views are also important to establish the differentiation between tetralogy of Fallot with pulmonary atresia, double-outlet right ventricle tetralogy type, and truncus arteriosus. The suprasternal and the subcostal oblique views can also aid in demonstrating the origin of the pulmonary arteries and establishing the type of truncus present (Echos. 25-4, 25-7). From the suprasternal notch long-axis view, the entire truncus can be seen, including the transverse arch and descending aorta, so interruption of the arch can be ruled out from this approach (Echo. 25-4). The suprasternal short-axis view usually demonstrates the right and left pulmonary branches and the presence of a common trunk. Doppler interrogation from these views using color flow mapping as well as spectral recording of velocities can help confirm the origin and branching of the pulmonary arteries and demonstrate any stenosis at these sites (Echos. 25-5, 25-6).

Origin and Distribution of the Coronary Arteries

There is a wide variety of patterns of origin and distribution of the coronary arteries in truncus arteriosus (4,5,8,9,36,48,49). The coronary ostia can have any location around the circumference of the truncal valve, with a slight predominance for the left coronary to originate from the left anterior area of the truncal annulus and for the right coronary to originate from the right anterior area

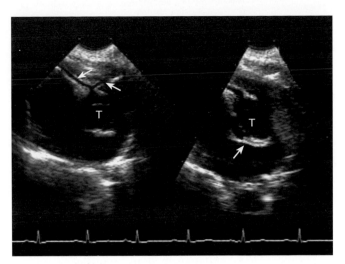

ECHO. 25-9. Parasternal short-axis view of the truncal root demonstrating the origins of coronary arteries. **Left:** The origin and proximal course of the right coronary artery is seen. The *arrows* point to the right coronary artery and a conal branch coursing anteriorly. **Right:** The right coronary artery is seen anteriorly. The *arrow* points to the origin and proximal left coronary artery coursing behind the truncus. *T,* truncus.

(36). However, coronaries originating from the posterior area of the annulus have been observed (36). The incidence of a single coronary varies between 4% and 19% of cases (4,5,8,9,36,48,49). It is surgically important to determine if there are major branches coursing in front of the anterosuperior wall of the right ventricle, which may occur in up to 13% of cases (36).

Echocardiographically, the origin and proximal distribution of the coronary arteries can be best established from a low parasternal short-axis view aiming towards the truncal valve superiorly. From this position, coronary ostia can be seen originating around any point along the circumference of the truncal annulus (Echo. 25-9). The proximal courses of the arteries should be followed if possible, particularly to determine if a major branch is crossing in front of the right ventricular outflow tract.

Associated Anomalies

Anomalies that have been described in association with truncus arteriosus include patent foramen ovale, ostium secundum atrial septal defects, patent ductus arteriosus not associated with interruption of the aortic arch, tricuspid insufficiency, tricuspid stenosis, tricuspid atresia, straddling tricuspid valve, mitral valve stenosis, mitral atresia, complete atrioventricular septal defects, multiple ventricular septal defects, absence of a pulmonary artery branch, right aortic arch, interruption of the aortic arch, hypoplasia of the aortic arch, coarctation of the aorta, double aortic arch, aberrant origin of the subclavian arteries, partial or total anomalous pulmonary venous drain-

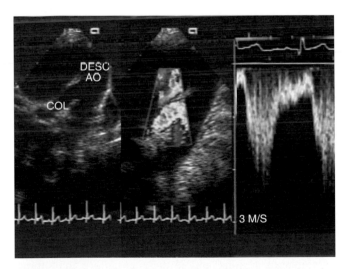

ECHO. 25-8. **Left:** Suprasternal long-axis view demonstrating the truncus and descending aorta. A large systemic-to-pulmonary collateral vessel is seen emerging from the underside of the transverse arch supplying the pulmonary circulation. This is an example of type IV truncus, which should instead be considered a form of pulmonary atresia with ventricular communication. **Middle:** The color Doppler flow map demonstrates the flow into the collateral vessel. **Right:** Spectral Doppler recording of the flow into the collateral vessel. It is exclusively left to right. *DESC AO,* descending aorta; *COL,* collateral vessel.

age, absence of the superior or inferior vena cava with azygous continuation, and left superior vena cava draining to the coronary sinus (2,4,9,20,31,37,42,50–52).

INTRAOPERATIVE AND POSTOPERATIVE EVALUATION

Pre-bypass the objectives would be to assess ventricular function and to attempt to confirm the type of truncus, size of the pulmonary branches, and coronary artery patterns. Ventricular function and size are best established through a transgastric transverse view (see Fig. 4-27A). Withdrawing the transducer to a four-chamber view reveals the ventricular septal defect, the atrioventricular valves, and the truncal override (see Fig. 4-28A,B). Anteflexion and further slight withdrawal of the transducer reveals the number, shape, location, and function of the cusps from a short axis of the truncal valve (see Fig. 4-29B,C). From this view, the coronary ostia are also seen and their proximal distribution can be followed with slight retroflexion and anteflexion of the transducer. The atrial septum should be examined from the transverse views for any atrial communication, which should be closed at surgery. The longitudinal views are used primarily to study the outflow tracts of both ventricles and the relationship of the truncus to them (see Fig. 4-29E,F). Regurgitation and/or stenosis of the truncal valve can be evaluated from these views. Depending on their location, the site and type of origin of the pulmonary arteries may be seen as well, although the transverse view, with the endoscope withdrawn to the base of the heart, affords a better evaluation of the branch pulmonary arteries (see Fig. 4-31A,B).

The post-bypass evaluation depends on the type of surgery performed. In most centers, a complete repair is performed initially without previous palliation, although occasionally prior banding of the common pulmonary trunk or of each individual pulmonary branch has been performed with mixed results. Complete surgical repair varies depending on the anatomic and functional characteristics of the truncus: correction of simple truncus arteriosus, correction of truncus with truncal valve replacement, and correction of truncus with interruption of the aortic arch (53).

Correction of simple truncus arteriosus consists of closing the ventricular septal defect leaving the truncus connected to the left ventricle and placing an extracardiac valved conduit from the right ventricle to the pulmonary artery (53). An important point according to Castaneda et al. (53) is to leave a potential atrial communication, especially in infants with large right-to-left shunts and Pao_2 of less than 0.40 Torr. They consider that this maneuver, which would allow a right-to-left shunt, reduces the physiopathologic consequences of poor right ventricular function during the early postoperative period following a complete repair and permits normal left ventricular output.

In the presence of significant stenosis or insufficiency of the truncal valve, it may have to be replaced at the time of surgery. Mild or moderate stenosis is acceptable; however, in severe stenosis, a valve commissurotomy is usually performed (53). Truncal valve insufficiency is more likely to require valve replacement since its presence increases mortality (53,54). When the truncal valve insufficiency is severe, the valve can be replaced with an aortic homograft between the left ventricle and the truncus, utilizing the anterior mitral leaflet to close the ventricular septal defect. A second homograft is then implanted between the right ventricle and the pulmonary arterial trunk or branches (55).

Repair of truncus arteriosus associated with aortic arch interruption involves placement of a homograft gusset between the ascending and descending aorta in order to reconstruct the arch. The right ventricle-to-pulmonary artery connection is established via implantation of an extracardiac conduit, and the ventricular septal defect is closed, similar to the repair of simple truncus arteriosus (53).

The post-bypass transesophageal study should start with a global assessment of ventricular size and function via a transgastric short-axis view (see Fig. 4-27A). This can be supplemented by evaluation of diastolic ventricular function from the inflow velocities of the ventricles recorded from the four-chamber transverse views and with examination of segmental wall motion from four- and two-chamber transverse and longitudinal views. The transverse four-chamber views (see Fig. 4-28A,B) allow detection of any significant residual shunting across the ventricular and atrial septa, evaluation of atrioventricular valve regurgitation, and the presence of truncal valve regurgitation. The longitudinal views reveal the reconstructed right ventricular outflow tract with the conduit. Although the conduit is sometimes difficult to see due to its unusual position in the chest, it is recommended that an attempt be made to record forward velocities across the length of the conduit with pulsed wave Doppler and to establish the presence and degree of regurgitation of the conduit valve, which can serve as a baseline for the late postoperative follow-up.

The long-term postoperative follow-up is primarily directed at the function of the right ventricular conduit and of the truncal valve, assuming no significant residual shunts or atrioventricular valve regurgitation. The truncal valve can degenerate with time, particularly if there are myxomatous lesions and if there are more than three leaflets. This evaluation should be carried out transthoracically from the standard parasternal long- and short-axis views and the apical and subcostal four-chamber and long-axis views. Recording of Doppler velocities across the valve as well as of the regurgitant jet, if any, should be performed to establish severity of the stenosis and/or insufficiency. The conduit between the right ventricle and the pulmonary artery(ies) is more difficult to evaluate; however, it should be searched for from the parasternal long- and short-axis views and the infraclavicular area as well as from the subcostal and suprasternal positions. The forward velocities across the conduit should be recorded with either the standard imaging probes or with the stand-alone nonimaging Doppler transducer if the conduit itself cannot be imaged, in order to confirm any significant stenosis. Regurgitation of the conduit valve should also be evaluated carefully. Besides direct recording of the regurgitant jet signals, the size of the right ventricular cavity and wall and the motion of the septum can serve as indirect measures of the functional status of the conduit.

REFERENCES

1. Lev M, Saphir O. Truncus arteriosus communis persistens. *J Pediatr* 1942;20:74–88.
2. Collet RW, Edwards JE. Persistent truncus arteriosus: a classification according to anatomic types. *Surg Clin North Am* 1949;29:1245–1270.
3. Van Praagh R, Van Praagh S. The anatomy of common aorticopulmonary trunk (truncus arteriosus communis) and its embryologic implications. A study of 57 necropsy cases. *Am J Cardiol* 1965;16:406–425.
4. Bharati S, McAllister HA, Rosenquist GC, Miller RA, Tatooles CJ, Lev M. The surgical anatomy of truncus arteriosus communis. *J Thorac Cardiovasc Surg* 1974;67:501–510.
5. Calder L, Van Praagh R, Van Praagh S, et al. Truncus arteriosus communis. Clinical, angiocardiographic, and pathologic findings in 100 patients. *Am Heart J* 1976;92:23–38.
6. Thiene G, Bortolotti U, Gallucci V, Terribile V, Pellegrino PA. Anatomical study of truncus arteriosus communis with embryological and surgical considerations. *Br Heart J* 1976;38:1109–1123.
7. Edwards JE. Persistent truncus arteriosus: a comment. *Am Heart J* 1976;92:1–2.
8. Crupi G, Macartney FJ, Anderson RH. Persistent truncus arteriosus. A study of 66 autopsy cases with special reference to definition and morphogenesis. *Am J Cardiol* 1977;40:569–578.
9. Butto F, Lucas RV Jr, Edwards JE. Persistent truncus arteriosus: pathologic anatomy in 54 cases. *Pediatr Cardiol* 1986;7:95–101.
10. Wilson J. A description of a very unusual malformation of the human heart. *Philos Trans R Soc Lond Biol Sci* 1798;18.346.
11. Buchanan A. Malformation of the heart. Undivided truncus arteriosus. Heart otherwise double. *Trans Pathol Soc Lond* 1864;15:89–91.
12. Beaver DC. Persistent truncus arteriosus and congenital absence of one kidney with other developmental defects. *Arch Pathol* 1993;15:51–54.
13. Davison G. A case of congenital heart disease with single arterial trunk. *J Anat* 1935;69:423–426.
14. Tynan MJ, Becker AE, Macartney FJ, Quero Jimenez M, Shinebourne EA, Anderson RH. Nomenclature and classification of congenital heart disease. *Br Heart J* 1979;41:544–553.
15. Kidd BSL. Persistent truncus arteriosus. In: Keith JD, Rowe RD, Vlad P, eds. *Heart disease in infancy and childhood.* 3rd ed. New York: Macmillan, 1978:457–469.
16. Hoffman JIE, Christianson R. Congenital heart disease in a cohort of 19,502 births with long-term follow-up. *Am J Cardiol* 1978;42:641–647.
17. Fyler DC. Report of the New England regional infant cardiac program. *Pediatrics* 1980;65:376–461.
18. Rowe RD, Freedom RM, Mehrizi A, Bloom KR. Truncus arteriosus. In: Rowe RD, Freedom RM, Mehrizi A, Bloom KR, eds. *The neonate with congenital heart disease.* 2nd ed. Philadelphia: WB Saunders, 1981:529–544.
19. Fyler DC. Truncus arteriosus. In: Fyler DC, ed. *Nadas pediatric cardiology.* Philadelphia: Hanley & Belfus, 1992:675–695.
20. Perez Martinez VM. Tronco arterial comun. In: Sanchez PA, ed. *Cardiologia pediatrica. Clinica y cirugia. Tomo I.* Barcelona: Salvat Editores SA, 1986:352–364.
21. De la Cruz MV, Sanchez Gomez C, Arteaga M, Arguello C. Experimental study of the development of the truncus and the conus in the chick embryo. *J Anat* 1977;123:661–686.
22. De la Cruz MV, Cayre R. Desarrollo embriologico del corazon y las grandes arterias. In: Sanchez PA, ed. *Cardiologia pediatrica. Clinica y cirugia. Tomo I.* Barcelona: Salvat Editores SA, 1986:10–18.
23. De la Cruz MV, Munoz Armas S, Castellanos L. *Development of the chick heart.* Baltimore: The Johns Hopkins Press, 1971.
24. Netter FH, Van Mierop LHS. Embryology. In: Netter FH, Yonkman FF, eds. *Heart.* Summit, NJ: CIBA Publications Department, 1969:111–130 *(The Ciba collection of medical illustrations, vol. 5).*
25. Kirby ML, Gale TF, Stewart DE. Neural crest cells contribute to aorticopulmonary septation. *Science* 1983;220:1059–1061.
26. Goor DA, Dische R, Lillehei CW. The Conotruncus. I. Its normal inversion and conus absorption. *Circulation* 1972;46:374–384.
27. Van Mierop LHS. Pathology and pathogenesis of the common cardiac malformations. *Cardiovasc Clin* 1970;2:27–59.
28. Van Mierop LHS, Patterson DF, Schnarr WR. Pathogenesis of persistent truncus arteriosus in light of observations made in a dog embryo with the anomaly. *Am J Cardiol* 1978;41:755–762.
29. Nishibatake M, Kirby ML, Van Mierop LHS. Pathogenesis of persistent truncus arteriosus and dextroposed aorta in the chick embryo after neural crest ablation. *Circulation* 1987;75:255–264.
30. Becker AE, Anderson RH. Single outlet of the heart. In: Becker AE, Anderson RH, eds. *Pathology of congenital heart disease. Postgraduate pathology series.* London: Butterworths, 1981:309–318.
31. Mair DD, Edwards WD, Fuster V, Seward FB, Danielson GK. Truncus arteriosus and aortopulmonary window. In: Anderson RH, Macartney FJ, Shinebourne EA, Tynan M, eds. *Paediatric cardiology. Vol. 2.* Edinburgh: Churchill Livingstone, 1987:913–929.
32. Bartelings MM, Gittenberger-de Groot AC. Morphogenetic considerations on congenital malformations of the outflow tract. Part 1: common arterial trunk and tetralogy of Fallot. *Int J Cardiol* 1991;32:213–230.
33. Carr I, Bharati A, Kusnoor VS, Lev M. Truncus arteriosus communis with intact ventricular septum. *Br Heart J* 1979;42:97–102.
34. Rosenquist GC, Bharati S, McAllister HA, Lev M. Truncus arteriosus communis: truncal valve anomalies associated with small conal or truncal septal defects. *Am J Cardiol* 1976;37:410–412.
35. Soto B, Pacifico AD. Truncus arteriosus. In: Soto B, Pacifico AD, eds. *Angiocardiography in congenital heart malformations.* Mount Kisco, NY: Futura Publishing, 1990:433–447.
36. De la Cruz MV, Cayre R, Angelini P, Noriega-Ramos N, Sadowinski S. Coronary arteries in truncus arteriosus. *Am J Cardiol* 1990;66:1482–1486.
37. Suzuki A, Ho SY, Anderson RH, Deanfield JE. Coronary arterial and sinusal anatomy in hearts with a common arterial trunk. *Ann Thorac Surg* 1989;48:792–797.
38. Becker AE, Becker MJ, Edwards JE. Pathology of the semilunar valve in persistent truncus arteriosus. *J Thorac Cardiovasc Surg* 1971;62:16–26.
39. Gelband H, Van Meter S, Gersony WM. Truncal valve abnormalities in infants with persistent truncus arteriosus. A clinicopathologic study. *Circulation* 1972;45:397–403.
40. Ledbetter MK, Tandon R, Titus JL, Edwards JE. Stenotic semilunar valve in persistent truncus arteriosus. *Chest* 1976;69:182–187.
41. Patel RG, Freedom RM, Bloom KR, Rowe RD. Truncal or aortic valve stenosis in functionally single arterial trunk. A clinical, hemodynamic and pathologic study of six cases. *Am J Cardiol* 1978;42:800–809.
42. Kirklin JW, Barrat-Boyes BG. Truncus arteriosus. In: Kirklin JW, Barrat-Boyes BG, eds. *Cardiac surgery. Morphology, diagnostic criteria, natural history, techniques, results, and indications. Vol. II.* 2nd ed. New York: Churchill Livingstone, 1993:1131–1151.
43. Sotomora RF, Edwards JE. Anatomic identification of so-called absent pulmonary artery. *Circulation* 1978;57:624–633.
44. Angelini P, Verdugo AL, Illera JP, Leachman RD. Truncus arteriosus communis. Unusual case associated with transposition. *Circulation* 1977;56:1107–1110.
45. Wolf WJ, Casta AS, Nichols M. Anomalous origin and malposition of the pulmonary arteries (crisscross pulmonary arteries) associated with complex congenital heart disease. *Pediatr Cardiol* 1986;6:287–291.

46. Diaz GF, Marquez A, Martinez VP, Marino B, Ruiz C. Truncus arteriosus comunis con interrupcion del arco aortico. Aspectos morfologicos y consideraciones quirurgicas. Estudio Cooperativo Internacional. *Rev Col Cardiol* 1994;6:251–257.

47. Rice MJ, Seward JB, Hagler DJ, Mair DD, Tajik AJ. Definitive diagnosis of truncus arteriosus by two-dimensional echocardiography. *Mayo Clin Proc* 1982;57:476–481.

48. Shrivastava S, Edwards JE. Coronary arterial origin in persistent truncus arteriosus. *Circulation* 1977;55:551–554.

49. Anderson KR, McGoon DC, Lie JT. Surgical significance of the coronary arterial anatomy in truncus arteriosus communis. *Am J Cardiol* 1978;41:76–81.

50. Daskalopoulos DA, Edwards WD, Driscoll DJ, Schaff HV, Danielson GK. Fatal pulmonary artery banding in truncus arteriosus with anomalous origin of circumflex coronary artery from right pulmonary artery. *Am J Cardiol* 1983;52:1363–1364.

51. Areias JC, Lopez JM. Common arterial trunk associated with absence of one atrioventricular connexion. *Int J Cardiol* 1987;17: 329–332.

52. Ceballos R, Soto B, Kirklin JW, Bargeron LM Jr. Truncus arteriosus. An anatomical-angiographic study. *Br Heart J* 1983;49:589–599.

53. Castaneda AR, Jonas RA, Mayer JE, Hanley FL. Truncus arteriosus. In: Castaneda AR, Jonas RA, Mayer JE, Hanley FL, eds. *Cardiac surgery of the neonate and infant.* Philadelphia: WB Saunders, 1994:281–293.

54. Hanley FL, Heinemann MK, Jonas RA, et al. Repair of truncus arteriosus in the neonate. *J Thorac Cardiovasc Surg* 1993;105: 1047–1056.

55. Elkins RC, Steinberg JB, Razook JD, Ward KE, Overholt ED, Thompson WM Jr. Correction of truncus arteriosus with truncal valvar stenosis or insufficiency using two homografts. *Ann Thorac Surg* 1990;50:728–733.

CHAPTER 26

Aortopulmonary Window

Lilliam M. Valdes-Cruz and Raul O. Cayre

Aortopulmonary window, aortopulmonary fenestration, or aortopulmonary septal defect is a rare malformation characterized by a communication between the ascending aorta and the pulmonary artery (1–9). It is differentiated from truncus arteriosus communis in that there are two clearly separated semilunar valve annuli (10). Consequently, it should not be termed "truncus arteriosus type B" or "truncus arteriosus without interventricular communication" (11) or "truncus arteriosus type V" (12).

It was first reported by Elliotson in 1830 (13). Its incidence varies between 0.15% and 0.20% of all cases with congenital cardiac anomalies (14,15).

EMBRYOLOGIC CONSIDERATIONS

The morphogenesis of aortopulmonary window involves the abnormal development of the aortopulmonary septum (15,16), which originates from cells in the neural crest (17) and divides the aortic sac into the ascending portion of the aorta and pulmonary arterial trunk (see Fig. 1-14C). The truncal and conal septa develop normally, so usually there is no ventricular communication and the semilunar valves are separate (18,19) (see Fig. 1-14A,B). Kutsche and Van Mierop (15) consider that there are three different types of aortopulmonary window, each with a different morphogenetic mechanism. The first type (15) is more or less round in shape and located in the proximal portion of the aortopulmonary septum, close to the valve leaflets (Figs. 26-1A, 26-2A). These authors suggest that it occurs due to failure of fusion between the aortopulmonary and the truncal septa. We consider this type to be secondary to a defect in the aortopulmonary septum at this level, rather than a failure of fusion with the truncal septum, since the defect in the vast majority of cases is not adjacent to the semilunar valve leaflets and there is a portion of aortopulmonary septum of variable length between the lower border of the defect and the level of the semilunar valve leaflets. In the second type of defect (15), the aortopulmonary septum has more than one spiral turn and the defect is formed by malalignment between the proximal and distal portions of the aortopulmonary septum (Figs. 26-1B, 26-2B). The third type (15) is usually a large defect lacking posterior or distal borders (Figs. 26-1C, 26-2C) and is due to a total absence of the aortopulmonary septum. There is a fourth type of aortopulmonary window with two defects of the aortopulmonary septum, described by Baronofsky et al. (3), which is extremely rare; its formation is also due to an abnormal development of the aortopulmonary septum (Figs. 26-1D, 26-2D).

ANATOMIC AND ECHOCARDIOGRAPHIC CONSIDERATIONS

As in all congenital cardiac malformations, the echocardiographic study should determine the visceroatrial situs and the systemic and pulmonary venous drainage sites. In addition, and specific to this defect, the following should be established: (a) type of aortopulmonary window; (b) associated anomalies; and (c) intra- and postoperative evaluation.

Type of Aortopulmonary Window

As mentioned above, there are four types of aortopulmonary window described (3,4,11,15,19–21). In the first type of Kustche and Van Mierop (15), also called "proximal defect" (19), the window is located between the left wall of the ascending aorta and the right wall of the pulmonary artery and there is a variable amount of tissue present between the lower border of the defect and the plane of the semilunar valve leaflets (Fig. 26-2A). Rarely, there can be a defect that extends proximally and is adjacent to the semilunar valves (22). The

459

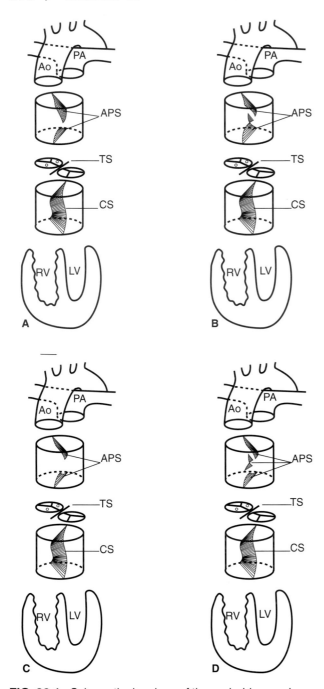

aorta and the anterior wall of the right pulmonary branch (21). The third type is one characterized by an almost complete absence of the aortopulmonary septum and has also been called "total defect" (20). In these cases, there is a remnant of aortopulmonary septum and the defect extends up to the bifurcation of the pulmonary artery (Fig. 26-2C). The presence of a double communication between the ascending aorta and the pulmonary artery (3) is very rare and would be the fourth type of aortopulmonary defect. In this case, the two defects are separated by a portion of aortopulmonary septum (Fig. 26-2D).

The echocardiographic views that reveal the presence of an aortopulmonary window are the parasternal long-axis view aiming laterally and superiorly to image both outflow tracts and great vessels, the parasternal short-

FIG. 26-1. Schematic drawings of the probable morphogenesis of the various anatomic types of aortopulmonary window. **A:** Defect proximal to the semilunar valves. **B:** Defect distal to the semilunar valves. **C:** Total defect. **D:** Double aorticopulmonary defect. *CS,* conal septum; *TS,* truncal septum; *APS,* aortopulmonary septum; *RV,* right ventricle; *LV,* left ventricle; *Ao,* aorta; *PA,* pulmonary artery.

second type of window, or distal aortopulmonary defect (19), consists of a communication between the level of the semilunar valve leaflets and the origin of the right pulmonary artery (15,19–21) (Fig. 26-2B). A variant of this type has been described in which the defect is located between the posterior wall of the ascending

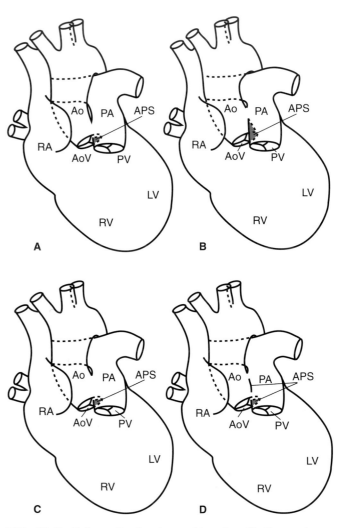

FIG. 26-2. Schematic drawings of hearts with the various anatomic types of aortopulmonary window. **A:** Defect proximal to the semilunar valves. **B:** Defect distal to the semilunar valves. **C:** Total defect. **D:** Double aortopulmonary defect. *APS,* aortopulmonary septum; *AoV,* aortic valve; *PV,* pulmonic valve; *RA,* right atrium; *RV,* right ventricle; *LV,* left ventricle; *Ao,* aorta; *PA,* pulmonary artery.

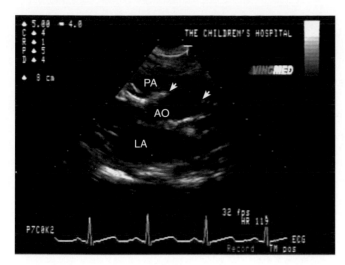

ECHO. 26-1. Parasternal long-axis view showing the presence of an aortopulmonary window (arrows). PA, pulmonary artery; AO, aorta; LA, left atrium.

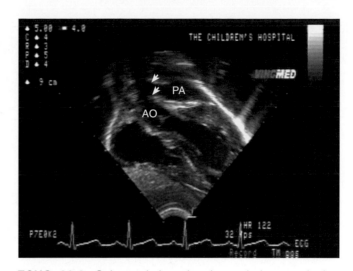

ECHO. 26-3. Subcostal view aimed superiorly towards the great arteries. The arrows point to the aortopulmonary window. AO, aorta; PA, pulmonary artery.

axis view, the subcostal coronal view, and the suprasternal long-axis view (Echos. 26-1–26-4; see color plate 93 following p. 364). From the parasternal long-axis view, tilting the transducer as described, two separate semilunar valves can be seen, and, depending on its location, the defect can also be appreciated (Echo. 26-1). The parasternal short-axis view has been shown to be very useful to demonstrate aortopulmonary windows (23,24). At the level of the valve leaflets, two separate annuli can be clearly identified, thereby differentiating it from truncus arteriosus communis, which only has one semilunar valve (Echo. 26-2). Tilting the transducer cephalically or moving it to a high paraster-

nal position reveals the presence of the window and allows differentiation from anomalous origin of the right pulmonary artery from the ascending aorta (25). The subcostal coronal view with cephalic inclination of the transducer towards the outflow tracts of the ventricles and the suprasternal long-axis view also permit demonstration of these defects (Echos. 26-3, 26-4).

Due to the thinness of the walls of the great arteries, there is commonly an echo dropout between them that should not be confused with an aortopulmonary window (Echo. 26-3; see color plate 94 following p.

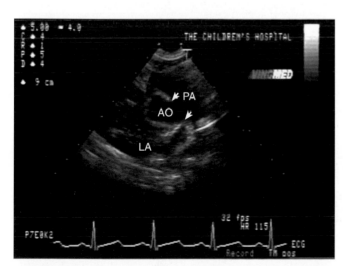

ECHO. 26-2. Parasternal short-axis view imaging the aortopulmonary window (arrows). PA, pulmonary artery; AO, aorta; LA, left atrium.

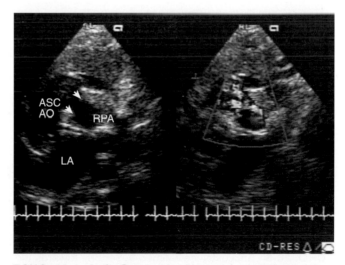

ECHO. 26-4. Left: Suprasternal long-axis view demonstrating the aortopulmonary window (arrows). Right: Color Doppler flow map of the shunting across the communication. ASC AO, ascending aorta; RPA, right pulmonary artery; LA, left atrium.

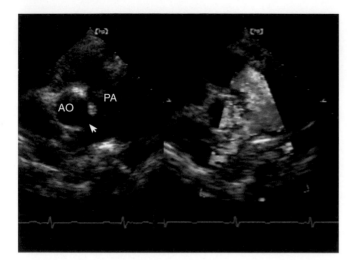

ECHO. 26-5. Parasternal short-axis view in a normal heart demonstrating a false echo dropout *(arrow)*, which should not be confused with a true aortopulmonary window. *AO,* aorta; *PA,* pulmonary artery.

364). Color Doppler flow mapping helps in the differential diagnosis since in the presence of a true window there is high-velocity aliased flows, either totally from left to right or commonly bidirectional (Echo. 26-6; see color plate 95 following p. 364). In addition, there is reversal of flow in the descending aorta during diastole due to run-off similar to that seen in aortic regurgitation or patent ductus arteriosus (26,27) (Echo. 26-7; see color plate 96 following p. 364). Spectral Doppler velocities and a color M-mode trace would help clarify the timing of shunting across the defect.

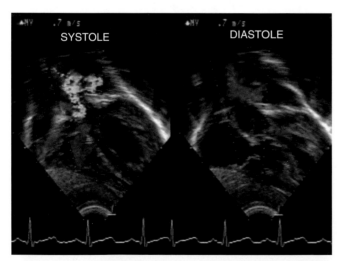

ECHO. 26-6. Subcostal view aimed superiorly towards the outflow tracts in the presence of an aortopulmonary window. The systolic frame demonstrates high-velocity aortic outflow and aliased shunting into the pulmonary artery through the window. The diastolic frame shows the lower velocity retrograde flow into the pulmonary artery.

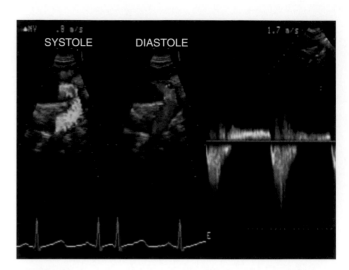

ECHO. 26-7. Color Doppler map of the flow in the descending aorta in the presence of an aortopulmonary window. Note the reversal of flow in the descending aorta during diastole due to the run-off into the pulmonary circulation. The spectral Doppler velocity recording demonstrates the slightly disturbed forward systolic flow and the reversed diastolic flow.

Associated Anomalies

Usually, aortopulmonary window presents as an isolated malformation. In the largest series published in the literature, the most common associated defect was a patent ductus arteriosus, present in 12% of cases (4). Others are ventricular septal defect with and without pulmonic stenosis, tetralogy of Fallot, double-outlet right ventricle, atrial septal defect, partial anomalous pulmonary venous drainage, subaortic stenosis, bicuspid aortic valve, coarctation of the aorta, interrupted aortic arch, right aortic arch, right pulmonary artery originating from the aorta, pulmonary arterial hypoplasia, anomalous origin of the left coronary artery from the pulmonary artery, and arteriovenous pulmonary fistula.

INTRAOPERATIVE AND POSTOPERATIVE EVALUATION

The pre-bypass intraoperative study should begin with an assessment of ventricular function, best done from the transgastric, transverse view of the short axis of the ventricles. This can be supplemented with other transverse and longitudinal views for specific segmental wall motion analysis and evaluation of diastolic function from the ventricular inflow velocities. The best projections to evaluate the aortopulmonary defect, its location, and its relationship to the semilunar valve leaflets are the longitudinal views (see Fig. 4-29E), where both outflow tracts and great arteries are seen side by side, and the basal transverse views (28) (see Fig. 4-31A,B).

Post-bypass the same sequence should be followed with

initial evaluation of the ventricular function followed by visualization of the site of surgery for any residual shunts. The surgical closure of these defects is accomplished either with a patch of pericardium or Dacron in the medium and large defects or with a simple suture closure in the small ones (29,30). In cases with associated anomalies, those should be studied specifically from the appropriate views.

REFERENCES

1. Dadds JH, Hoyle C. Congenital aortic septal defect. *Br Heart J* 1949;11:390–397.
2. Gibson S, Potts WJ, Langewisch WH. Aortic-pulmonary communication due to localized congenital defect of aortic septum. *Pediatrics* 1950;6:357–360.
3. Baronofsky ID, Gordon AJ, Grishman A, Steinfeld L, Kreel I. Aorticopulmonary septal defect. Diagnosis and report of case successfully treated. *Am J Cardiol* 1960;5:273–276.
4. Neufeld HN, Lester RG, Adams P Jr, Anderson RC, Lillehei CW, Edwards JE. Aorticopulmonary septal defect. *Am J Cardiol* 1962;9:12–25.
5. Morrow AG, Greenfield LJ, Braunwald E. Congenital aortopulmonary septal defect. Clinical and hemodynamic findings, surgical technique, and results of operative correction. *Circulation* 1962;25:463–476.
6. Bosher LH Jr, Moore McCue C. Diagnosis and surgical treatment of aortopulmonary fenestration. *Circulation* 1962;25:456–462.
7. Blieden LC, Moller JH. Aorticopulmonary septal defect. An experience with 17 patients. *Br Heart J* 1974;36:630–635.
8. Richardson JV, Doty DB, Rossi NP, Ehrenhaft J. The spectrum of anomalies of aortopulmonary septation. *J Thorac Cardiovasc Surg* 1979;78:21–27.
9. Lau KC, Calcaterra G, Miller GAH, et al. Aorto-pulmonary window. *J Cardiovasc Surg* 1982;23:21–27.
10. Crupi G, Macartney FJ, Anderson RH. Persistent truncus arteriosus. A study of 66 autopsy cases with special reference to definition and morphogenesis. *Am J Cardiol* 1977;40:569–578.
11. Van Praagh R, Van Praagh S. The anatomy of common aorticopulmonary trunk (truncus arteriosus communis) and its embryologic implications. A study of 57 necropsy cases. *Am J Cardiol* 1965;16:406–425.
12. Collet RW, Edwards JE. Persistent truncus arteriosus: a classification according to anatomic types. *Surg Clin North Am* 1949;29:1245–1270.
13. Elliotson J. Case of malformation of the pulmonary artery and aorta. *Lancet* 1830-31;1:247–248.
14. Rowe RD. Aortopulmonary septal defect. In: Keith JD, Rowe RD, Vlad P, eds. *Heart disease in infancy and childhood.* 3rd ed. New York: Macmillan, 1978:452–456.
15. Kutsche LM, Van Mierop LHS. Anatomy and pathogenesis of aorticopulmonary septal defect. *Am J Cardiol* 1987;59:443–447.
16. Cucci CE, Doyle EF, Lewis EW Jr. Absence of a primary division of the pulmonary trunk. An ontogenic theory. *Circulation* 1964;29:124–131.
17. Kirby ML, Gale TF, Stewart DE. Neural crest cells contribute to aorticopulmonary septation. *Science* 1983;220:1059–1061.
18. Goor DA, Lillehei CW. Aorticopulmonary window. In: Goor DA, Lillehei CW, eds. *Congenital malformations of the heart. Embryology, anatomy and operative considerations.* New York: Grune and Stratton, 1975:164–168.
19. Roca Llop J, Lozano Sainz C. Ventana aortopulmonar. In: Sanchez PA, ed. *Cardiologia pediatrica. Clinica y cirugia. Tomo I.* Barcelona: Salvat Editores SA, 1986:340–345.
20. Mori K, Ando M, Takao A, Ishikawa S, Imai Y. Distal type of aortopulmonary window. Report of 4 cases. *Br Heart J* 1978;40:681–689.
21. Crawford FA Jr, Watson DG, Joransen JA. Tetralogy of Fallot with coexisting type II aortopulmonary window. *Ann Thorac Surg* 1981;31:78–81.
22. Mair DD, Edwards WD, Fuster V, Seward JB, Danielson GK. Truncus arteriosus and aortopulmonary window. In: Anderson RH, Macartney FJ, Shinebourne EA, Tynan M, eds. *Paediatric Cardiology. Vol. II.* Edinburgh: Churchill Livingstone, 1987:913–929.
23. Rice MJ, Seward JB, Hagler DJ, Mair DD, Tajik AJ. Visualization of aortopulmonary window by two-dimensional echocardiography. *Mayo Clin Proc* 1982;57:482–487.
24. Smallhorn JF, Anderson RH, Macartney FJ. Two dimensional echocardiographic assessment of communications between ascending aorta and pulmonary trunk or individual pulmonary arteries. *Br Heart J* 1982;47:563–572.
25. King DH, Huhta JC, Gutgesell HP, Ott DA. Two dimensional echocardiographic diagnosis of anomalous origin of the right pulmonary artery from the aorta: differentiation from aortopulmonary window. *J Am Coll Cardiol* 1984;4:351–355.
26. Alboliras ET, Chin AJ, Barber G, Helton JG, Pigott JD. Detection of aortopulmonary window by pulsed and color Doppler echocardiography. *Am Heart J* 1988;115:900–902.
27. Balaji S, Burch M, Sullivan ID. Accuracy of cross-sectional echocardiography in diagnosis of aortopulmonary window. *Am J Cardiol* 1991;67:650–653.
28. Seward JB, Khandheria BK, Edwards WD, Oh JK, Freeman WK, Tajik AJ. Biplanar transesophageal echocardiography: anatomic correlations, image orientation and clinical applications. *Mayo Clin Proc* 1990;65:1193–1213.
29. Kirklin JW, Barrat-Boyes BG. Aortopulmonary window. In: Kirklin JW, Barrat-Boyes BG, eds. *Cardiac surgery. Morphology diagnostic criteria, natural history, techniques, results, and indications. Vol. II.* 2nd ed. New York: Churchill Livingstone, 1993:1153–1157.
30. Castaneda AR, Jonas RA, Mayer JE, Hanley FL. Aortopulmonary window. In: Castaneda AR, Jonas RA, Mayer JE, Hanley FL, eds. *Cardiac surgery of the neonate and infant.* Philadelphia: WB Saunders, 1994:295–300.

CHAPTER 27

Anatomically Corrected Malposition of the Great Arteries

Lilliam M. Valdes-Cruz and Raul O. Cayre

Anatomically corrected malposition of the great arteries is a rare congenital cardiac malformation characterized by atrioventricular concordance and ventriculoarterial concordance but an anomalous spatial relationship of the great vessels (1). The first anatomical description was reported by Theremin in 1895 (2), and the denomination of "anatomically corrected malposition" of the great arteries was suggested by Van Praagh et al. (3) instead of the so called "anatomically corrected transposition of the great arteries" (4,5). Its overall incidence is about 0.4% of all congenital cardiac malformations (6).

EMBRYOLOGIC CONSIDERATIONS

This defect was considered an embryological impossibility by Van Mierop and Wiglesworth (7), and this thought was initially shared by Van Praagh (8). However, various reports in the literature have served to confirm its existence (1,5,6,8–13).

In anatomically corrected malposition of the great arteries, the morphologic right atrium is connected to a morphologic right ventricle and the morphologic left atrium to a morphologic left ventricle; therefore, there is atrioventricular concordance (Fig. 27-1). It is most frequently found in situs solitus (Fig. 27-1A), although there have been descriptions in situs inversus (6,12) (Fig. 27-1B). The aorta emerges from the anatomic left ventricle and the pulmonary artery from the anatomic right ventricle; consequently, there is also ventriculoarterial concordance. However, the spatial position of the great arteries is abnormal. The aorta is typically anterior and to the left (L aorta) with respect to the pulmonary artery in cases of situs solitus (Fig. 27-1A) and anterior and to the right (D aorta) in situs inversus (Fig. 27-1B). The great vessels can also be side by side, with the aorta to the left in situs solitus

(L aorta) (Fig. 27-2A) or to the right in situs inversus (D aorta) (12) (Fig. 27-2B). Hearts with visceroatrial heterotaxy and those with atrioventricular univentricular connection are not included in this chapter.

In analyzing the probable morphogenesis of this lesion, the following should be considered: (a) visceroatrial situs; (b) bulboventricular looping; (c) conal septation; (d) truncal septation; and (e) aortopulmonary septation.

Visceroatrial Situs and Bulboventricular Looping

Since there is atrioventricular concordance, the bulboventricular looping is similar to that of the normal heart—that is, D looping in situs solitus (morphologic right ventricle to the right) or L looping in situs inversus (morphologic right ventricle to the left) (Figs. 27-1, 27-2).

Conal Septation

In cases of anatomically corrected malposition of the great arteries in situs solitus, the conal septum develops abnormally so that there is a sinistrodorsal conal crest and a dextroventral conal crest (Fig. 27-3A). The conal septum that is formed when these fuse has an abnormal direction from left to right and from posterior to anterior (see Fig. 26-3A), which results in the division of the conus into an anteromedial and a posterolateral conus (14).

In cases of side-by-side great arteries with L aorta, there is a dorsal or posterior conal crest and a ventral or anterior conal crest, which will give rise to a conal septum that has an anteroposterior direction, perpendicular to the frontal plane, which divides the conus into a lateral and a medial one (14,15) (Fig. 27-3B). The conus that will

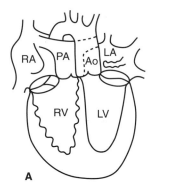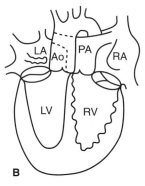

FIG. 27-1. Schematic drawings of hearts with anatomically corrected malposition of the great arteries with anterior aorta and posterior pulmonary artery. See text for details. **A:** Situs solitus. **B:** Situs inversus. *RA,* right atrium; *LA,* left atrium; *RV,* right ventricle; *LV,* left ventricle; *Ao,* aorta; *PA,* pulmonary artery.

be incorporated into the left ventricle in the late post loop stage is the medial one (14).

Truncal Septation

In cases with an anterior and leftward aorta, the truncal swellings appearing in the proximal end of the truncus are in a sinistrosuperior and a dextroinferior position similar to that in the normal heart (see Figs. 1-12B and 1-14B). As a result, the truncal septum has an orientation also similar to that in the normal heart—that is, from left to right and from posterior to anterior (Fig. 27-3A). These truncal swellings also give rise to the right and left posterior aortic cusps and the right and left anterior pulmonary cusps. The left intercalated truncal swelling forms the anterior aortic cusp and the right intercalated swelling the posterior pulmonary cusp.

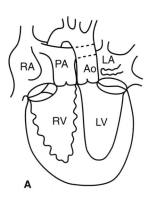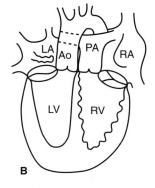

FIG. 27-2. Schematic drawings of hearts with anatomically corrected malposition of the great arteries with side-by-side great vessels. See text for details. **A:** Situs solitus. **B:** Situs inversus. *RA,* right atrium; *LA,* left atrium; *RV,* right ventricle; *LV,* left ventricle; *Ao,* aorta; *PA,* pulmonary artery.

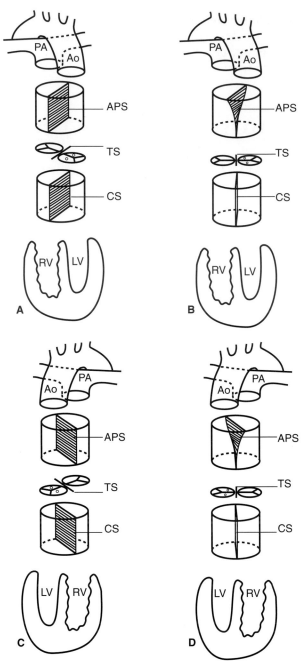

FIG. 27-3. Schematic representation of the probable morphogenesis of the various types of anatomically corrected malposition of the great arteries. **A:** Situs solitus with anterior and leftward aorta. **B:** Situs solitus with side-by-side great arteries and leftward aorta. **C:** Situs inversus with anterior and rightward aorta. **D:** Situs inversus with side-by-side great arteries and rightward aorta. *RV,* right ventricle; *LV,* left ventricle; *CS,* conal septum; *TS,* truncal septum; *APS,* aortopulmonary septum; *Ao,* aorta; *PA,* pulmonary artery.

Truncal swellings located superiorly and inferiorly would cause a truncal septum with an anteroposterior direction and side-by-side great arteries with leftward aorta (Fig. 27-3B). These swellings would also give rise to left anterior and posterior aortic cusps and the right anterior and posterior pulmonary cusps (Fig. 27-3B). The left aortic cusp would originate from the left intercalated truncal swelling and the right pulmonary cusp from the right intercalated truncal swelling.

Aortopulmonary Septation

The aortopulmonary septum develops abnormally in this defect. At the distal end of the truncus, the aortopulmonary septum has a left to right and posterior to anterior direction (14,15) (Fig. 27-3A,B). If the aorta is anterior and to the left, the aortopulmonary septum is straight rather than spiral (Fig. 27-3A), so the aorta that is anterior and leftward cephalically will connect to the anteromedial infundibulum of the anatomic left ventricle located on the left. The pulmonary artery located in a posterior and rightward position in its cephalic end will connect to the posterolateral infundibulum of the anatomic right ventricle located to the right.

With side-by-side great arteries and L aorta (Fig. 27-3B), the aortopulmonary septum would be directed from left to right and posterior to anterior at its cephalic end (14,15), but would adopt a semispiral rather than straight orientation, so that caudally it would have an anteroposterior direction. This results in the aorta having an anterior and leftward position cephalically, but assuming a leftward position as it connects to the medial infundibulum of the morphologic left ventricle located to the left. The pulmonary artery cephalically is located posteriorly and to the right, and connects with the lateral infundibulum of the anatomic right ventricle located to the right.

Hearts in situs inversus would be in mirror image to those in situs solitus (Fig. 27-3C,D).

ANATOMIC AND ECHOCARDIOGRAPHIC CONSIDERATIONS

This malformation has received several denominations in the literature, many of which are confusing: concordant atrioventricular relation and concordant ventriculoarterial relation with L position of the aorta (1), anatomically corrected transposition (4,5), aortic levoposition without ventricular inversion (6), transposition with bulbus inversion for hearts in situs solitus (16), transposition with sinoatrial inversion and ventricular inversion for hearts in situs inversus (16), isolated bulbar inversion in corrected transposition (17), L malposed great arteries with situs solitus, and concordant atrioventricular connection (18). Some authors have used the term anatomically corrected malposition of the great arteries in the presence of atrioventricular concordance, as well as atrioventricular discordance (8,11,12,19).

Even if at first glance it would appear simplistic, it is important to clarify the differences among complete

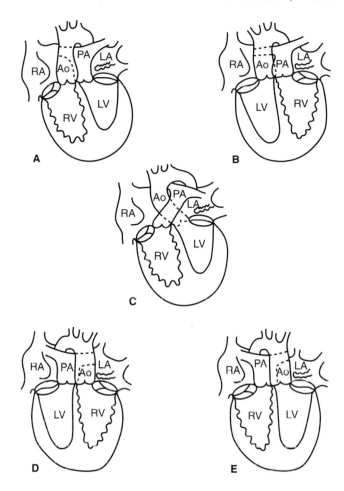

FIG. 27-4. Schematic drawings of hearts in situs solitus with various types of atrioventricular and ventriculoarterial connections. See text for details. **A:** Atrioventricular concordance and ventriculoarterial discordance (classic complete transposition of the great arteries). **B:** Atrioventricular discordance and ventriculoarterial concordance (isolated ventricular inversion). **C:** Atrioventricular concordance, ventriculoarterial concordance and normally related great arteries (normal heart). **D:** Atrioventricular discordance and ventriculoarterial discordance (congenitally corrected transposition of the great arteries). **E:** Atrioventricular concordance, ventriculoarterial concordance with malposition of the great arteries (anatomically corrected malposition). *RA,* right atrium; *LA,* left atrium; *RV,* right ventricle; *LV,* left ventricle; *Ao,* aorta; *PA,* pulmonary artery.

transposition of the great arteries, isolated ventricular inversion, congenitally corrected transposition of the great arteries, and anatomically corrected malposition of the great arteries (Fig. 27-4).

In complete transposition of the great arteries there is atrioventricular concordance with ventriculoarterial discordance; therefore, the physiology is that of transposition since the circulations are in parallel (Fig. 27-4A).

In isolated ventricular inversion there is atrioventricular discordance with ventriculoarterial concordance; therefore, the physiology is similar to that of complete transposition with parallel circulations (Fig. 27-4B).

In normal heart there is atrioventricular concordance and ventriculoarterial concordance; therefore, the circulations are in series, and the physiology is normal (Fig. 27-4C).

In congenitally corrected transposition of the great arteries there is atrioventricular discordance and ventriculoarterial discordance; therefore, the circulations are in series, and the physiology is normal (Fig. 27-4D). The clinical presentation will depend on the associated malformations.

In anatomically corrected malposition of the great arteries there is atrioventricular concordance and ventriculoarterial concordance, so the circulations are in series and the physiology is normal (Fig. 27-4E). As in corrected transposition, the clinical findings will depend on the associated anomalies.

The echocardiographic study in anatomically corrected malposition should include (a) visceroatrial situs and atrioventricular concordance; (b) ventriculoarterial concordance and infundibular morphology; (c) spatial relationship of the great vessels; (d) origin and distribution of the coronary arteries; (e) associated anomalies; and (f) intra- and postoperative evaluation.

Visceroatrial Situs and Atrioventricular Concordance

The details of establishing visceroatrial situs and atrioventricular concordance by echocardiography are covered in detail in Chapters 4 and 8.

In anatomically corrected malposition, there is atrioventricular concordance, which can occur in situs solitus or situs inversus (Fig. 27-1). The atrial morphology, the atrioventricular valves, the ventricular inlet, and trabecular portions are all similar to those found in the normal heart. The visceroatrial situs can be best examined from the subcostal abdominal short- and long-axis views, which allow the identification of the inferior vena cava and aorta and the drainage of the vena cava into the anatomic right atrium. The atrial appendages, which identify the atria anatomically, are best seen from the parasternal short-axis view (for the left) and from the long-axis parasternal view tilting the transducer towards the right ventricular inflow (for the right). The four-chamber views from the apex and subcostal windows are the best suited for demonstrating the anatomical characteristics of both atrioventricular valves and ventricles. The atrioventricular septum is present so the tricuspid valve is inserted lower than the mitral valve. The parasternal and subcostal short-axis views at ventricular level permit identification of the two papillary muscles, one anterolateral and one posteromedial, in the anatomic left ventricle and the moderator band in the anatomic right ventricle. Flow through these structures can be seen using color Doppler flow mapping and is similar to that in the normal heart.

Ventriculoarterial Concordance and Infundibular Morphology

The ventriculoarterial connection is concordant, but the spatial relation of the great arteries is abnormal and they arise from abnormal infundibula (1,6,18,20) (Fig. 27-3). Usually, in this malformation, the aorta occupies an anterior and leftward position relative to the pulmonary artery (1,5,6,9,11,13,18,20,21) (Figs. 27-1A, 27-3A), or it can be side by side in L position (9,10,12) (Figs. 27-2A, 27-3B). In the majority of cases, there are bilateral muscular infundibula causing discontinuity between the aortic and mitral valves and between the pulmonary and the tricuspid valves. Occasionally, however, there can be only a subaortic muscular infundibulum (11,13) or even absence of both muscular infundibula with aortic-mitral and pulmonary-tricuspid continuities (22).

In almost all instances, there is a malalignment between the infundibular and the trabecular muscular septa (6,18,20). The infundibular septum is commonly dextroposed (6,20), which allows the existence of a subaortic ventricular septal defect with overriding of the aorta over the interventricular septum. More rarely, the infundibular septum is levoposed, and there is a subpulmonary ventricular defect with overriding of the pulmonary artery. This malalignment between the infundibular and trabecular muscular septa can be considered part of the spectrum that comprises double-outlet right ventricle with anterior and leftward aorta when it overrides the septum more than 50% over the right ventricle (see Fig. 23-13A), anatomically corrected malposition of the great arteries (see Fig. 23-13B), and double-outlet left ventricle with anterior, leftward aorta when the pulmonary artery overrides the septum more than 50% over the left ventricle (6,23) (see Fig. 23-13C).

Echocardiographically, the apex and subcostal four-chamber views sweeping the transducer from posterior to anterior permit visualization of the ventriculoarterial concordance, the malalignment between the infundibular and interventricular septa, the ventricular defect, which is almost always present, and the degree of overriding of the aorta or pulmonary artery. These views along with the parasternal long- and short-axis views aiming from apex to base also demonstrate whether there is continuity between the semilunar and atrioventricular valves.

Doppler color flow mapping demonstrates the flows across the atrioventricular valves, the direction of shunting through the ventricular defect, and its physiologic relationship to either semilunar valve.

Spatial Relationship of the Great Vessels

In situs solitus, the aorta will usually have a position that is anterior and to the left of the pulmonary artery (Figs. 27-1A, 27-3A) or directly to the left in side-by-side relationship (Figs. 27-2A, 27-3B). In situs inversus, the aorta will be anterior and rightward (Figs. 27-1B, 27-3C) or directly to the right when the great vessels are side by side (Figs. 27-2B, 27-3D).

Anatomically corrected malposition of the great arteries with leftward aorta in a side-by-side relationship to the pulmonary artery can considered part of the spectrum that comprises double-outlet right and left ventricles with side-by-side great arteries and leftward aorta (see Fig. 23-12).

The echocardiographic demonstration of the great artery relationship is best accomplished through a parasternal short-axis view. When the aorta is anterior and to the left, it should be differentiated from corrected transposition of the great arteries, which has the same aortic to pulmonary orientation, but in the presence of atrioventricular discordance.

Origin and Distribution of the Coronary Arteries

In the majority of cases, the right-sided coronary artery emerges from the posterior right aortic cusp but branches into an anterior descending and a right coronary artery (Fig. 27-5A), whereas the circumflex coronary artery emerges from the posterior left aortic cusp and courses along the left atrioventricular sulcus (6,11,18,20,24). This pattern suggests the presence of ventricular inversion (6,11,18,24), thereby making the conclusive determination of atrioventricular concordance even more critical.

The coronary origin and distribution can also be similar to that of the normal heart since there is atrioventricular concordance. Namely, the left-sided coronary artery emerges from the left posterior aortic cusp and gives rise to the anterior descending and the circumflex (Fig. 27-5B); the right-sided coronary artery emerges from the posterior right aortic cusp and courses along the right atrioventricular sulcus (11,24).

There have been cases described with single coronary artery emerging from the right posterior cusp and dividing into a right, an anterior descending, and circumflex coronary arteries (12,24) (Fig. 27-5C). A single coronary artery has also been seen to emerge from the left posterior cusp of the aorta and cross between both great arteries before dividing into a right, an anterior descending, and circumflex coronary arteries (24) (Fig. 27-5D). A single coronary can also emerge from the left posterior aortic cusp and follow a trajectory in front of the aorta before dividing into right, anterior descending, and circumflex coronary arteries (24) (Fig. 27-5E).

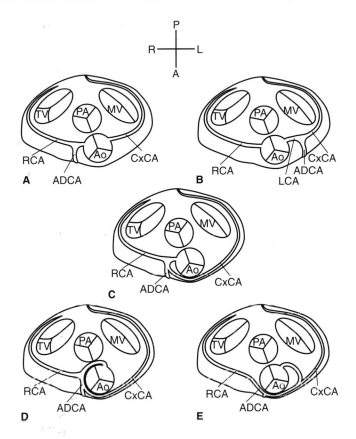

FIG. 27-5. A–E: Schematic representation of the various patterns of coronary arterial origin and distribution in anatomically corrected malposition of the great arteries. See text for details. *TV*, tricuspid valve; *MV*, mitral valve; *Ao*, aorta; *PA*, pulmonary artery; *RCA*, right coronary artery; *LCA*, left coronary artery; *ADCA*, anterior descending coronary artery; *CxCA*, circumflex coronary artery; *A*, anterior; *P*, posterior; *R*, right; *L*, left.

Echocardiographic demonstration of the origin and proximal course of the coronaries is best accomplished from the parasternal short-axis view. Once the origins are established, the transducer may have to be placed slightly lower or higher on the chest to follow the distribution of the branches.

ASSOCIATED ANOMALIES

The most common associated anomaly, almost always present, is a ventricular septal defect due to malalignment of the infundibular and interventricular septa, which can be subaortic or subpulmonary. Cases with muscular, subtricuspid (perimembranous), and doubly committed ventricular septal defects have also been described in the literature (1,21). The malalignment between the infundibular and ventricular septa can also cause obstruction of the outflow tracts, either subpulmonary, when there is dextroposition of the infundibular septum (1,6,20), or subaortic, when there is levoposition (11,20).

Other anomalies that have been seen with anatomically corrected malposition are isolated pulmonic valve stenosis (22), or associated with subvalve stenosis (1,5, 6,10,13), fibromuscular subaortic stenosis (21), ostium secundum atrial septal defect (5,6,9,12), juxtaposition of the left atrial appendage (1,6,9,10,13,21), right aortic arch (13), hypoplasia or atresia of the tricuspid valve associated with hypoplastic right ventricle (23), and coarctation of the aorta (21).

INTRAOPERATIVE AND POSTOPERATIVE EVALUATION

The intraoperative evaluation of this lesion is directed at the evaluation of associated anomalies.

The pre-bypass study should begin with assessment of the size and function of the ventricles, best performed from the transgastric short-axis view (see Fig. 4-27A,B). The four-chamber view obtained by withdrawing the transducer behind the heart (see Fig. 4-28A) will demonstrate the ventricular defect, the relationship to the semilunar valve, and the degree of override. The atrioventricular valve anatomy and function can also be determined from this position. Anteflexion of the transducer permits visualization of the coronary arterial origin and proximal distribution (see Fig. 4-29B,C). The atrial septal views reveal the presence of atrial shunting, which requires closure (see Fig. 4-30). The longitudinal views from the transgastric position with anteflexion (see Fig. 4-27D,E) reveal the outflows of both ventricles and permit the best alignment of the Doppler continuous wave sampling line to record the velocities and establish the presence and severity of any stenosis. The retrocardiac longitudinal views demonstrate the atrioventricular valves from different orthogonal cuts and the outflow tracts of both ventricles, although not with a favorable position for Doppler velocity interrogation (see Figs. 4-28C and 4-29E). From these views, however, the relationship of the great vessels to the ventricles and the continuity between the atrioventricular and semilunar valves can be appreciated.

The post-bypass study should also begin with the assessment of ventricular size and function from the transgastric position. The rest of the examination should address the possible presence of residual shunting at ventricular and/or atrial levels and of outflow tract obstruction.

In the presence of hypoplasia of the right ventricle, a univentricular repair of the Fontan type may be required (23), and an extracardiac conduit may need to be implanted if the subpulmonary obstruction cannot be relieved primarily (23).

The late postoperative follow-up should address the type of repair performed. Specifically, outflow tract obstructions may recur and should be evaluated periodically from the parasternal long-axis view of the outflow tract, the short-axis view, and the apical and subcostal coronal views. The examination of Fontan type of repairs should include evaluation of the systemic ventricular function and of the Fontan connection. The extracardiac conduits require serial evaluation of the forward gradients, ideally obtained at the proximal and distal anastomotic sites and at the valve itself in addition to assessment of regurgitation. There are no standard views for conduit evaluation, so this should be attempted from all possible windows, including recording of velocities with the stand-alone Doppler probe from high parasternal and subclavicular positions to assure detection of any significant stenosis or regurgitation.

REFERENCES

1. Kirklin JW, Pacifico AD, Bargeron LM Jr, Soto B. Cardiac repair in anatomically corrected malposition of the great arteries. *Circulation* 1973;48:153–159.
2. Theremin E. *Etudes sur les affections congenitales du coeur.* Paris: Asselin et Houzeau, 1895:83–84.
3. Van Praagh R, Perez-Trevino C, Lopez-Cuellar M, et al. Transposition of the great arteries with posterior aorta, anterior pulmonary artery, subpulmonary conus and fibrous continuity between aortic and atrioventricular valves. *Am J Cardiol* 1971;28:621–631.
4. Harris JS, Farber S. Transposition of the great cardiac vessels with special reference to the phylogenetic theory of Spitzer. *Arch Pathol* 1939;28:427–502.
5. Van Praagh R, Van Praagh S. Anatomically corrected transposition of the great arteries. *Br Heart J* 1967;29:112–119.
6. Otero Coto E, Quero Jimenez M, Cabrera A, Deverall PB, Caffarena JM. Aortic levopositions without ventricular inversion. *Eur J Cardiol* 1978;8:523–541.
7. Van Mierop LHS, Wiglesworth FW. Pathogenesis of transposition complexes. III. True transposition of the great vessels. *Am J Cardiol* 1963;12:233–239.
8. Van Praagh R. The story of anatomically corrected malposition of the great arteries [Editorial]. *Chest* 1976;69:2–4.
9. Freedom RM, Harrington DP. Anatomically corrected malposition of the great arteries. Report of two cases, one with congenital asplenia; frequent association with juxtaposition of atrial appendages. *Br Heart J* 1974;36:207–215.
10. Freedom RM, Harrington DP, White RI. The differential diagnosis of levo-transposed or malposed aorta. *Circulation* 1974;50:1040–1046.
11. Van Praagh R, Durnin RE, Jockin H, Wagner HR, Korns M, Garabedian H, Ando M, Calder AL. Anatomically corrected malposition of the great arteries (S,D,L). *Circulation* 1975;51:20–31.
12. Anderson RH, Becker AE, Losekoot TG, Gerlis LM. Anatomically corrected malposition of the great arteries. *Br Heart J* 1975;37:993–1013.
13. Bream PR, Elliot LP, Bargeron LM Jr. Plain film findings of anatomically corrected malposition: its association with juxtaposition of the atrial appendages and right aortic arch. *Radiology* 1978;126:589–595.
14. De la Cruz MV, Arteaga M, Quero-Jimenez M. Conexiones y relaciones ventriculo-arteriales. Clasificacion anatomica y embriogenesis. *Rev Lat Cardiol* 1981;2:66–75.
15. Anselmi G, Munoz OH, Espino Vela J, Arguello C. Side by side great arteries. Embryologic considerations. In: Mendes Oteo F, ed. *Side by side great arteries.* Caracas, Venezuela: Instituto Venezolano de Cardiologia, 1984:2–21.

16. Anderson RC, Lillehei WC, Lester RG. Corrected transposition of the great vessels of the heart. *Pediatrics* 1957;20:626–646.

17. Raghib G, Anderson RC, Edwards JE. Isolated bulbar inversion in corrected transposition. *Am J Cardiol* 1966;17:407–410.

18. Otero Coto E, Castaneda AR, Caffarena JM, Deverall PB, Cabrera A, Quero Jimenez M. L-malposed great arteries with situs solitus and concordant atrioventricular connection. *J Cardiovasc Surg* 1982;23:277–286.

19. Zakheim R, Mattioli L, Vaseenon T, Edwards W. Anatomically corrected malposition of the great arteries. *Chest* 1976;69:101–104.

20. Otero Coto E, Caffarena JM, Gomez-Ullate JM, Such Martinez M. Anatomically corrected malposition. Surgical repair. *J Cardiovasc Surg* 1980;21:367–370.

21. Colli AM, De Leval M, Somerville J. Anatomically corrected malposition of the great arteries: diagnostic difficulties and surgical repair of associated lesions. *Am J Cardiol* 1985;55:1367–1372.

22. Loya YS, Desai AG, Sharma S. Anatomically corrected malposition: a rare case with bilateral absence of a complete subarterial muscular infundibulum. *Int J Cardiol* 1991;30:131–134.

23. Kirklin JW, Barrat-Boyes BG. Anatomically corrected malposition of the great arteries. In: Kirklin JW, Barrat-Boyes BG, eds. *Cardiac surgery. Morphology, diagnostic criteria, natural history, techniques, results, and indications. Vol. 2.* 2nd ed. New York: Churchill Livingstone, 1993:1581–1584.

24. Neufeld HN, Schneeweiss A. Anatomically corrected malposition. In: Neufeld HN, Schneeweiss A, eds. *Coronary artery disease in infants and children.* Philadelphia: Lea & Febiger, 1983:94–96.

PART X

Anomalies of the Aortic Arches

CHAPTER 28

Coarctation of the Aorta

Lilliam M. Valdes-Cruz and Raul O. Cayre

Coarctation of the aorta is characterized by a narrowing of the aorta in the region adjacent to the union of the ductus arteriosus and the descending aorta. The first description of this malformation was by Johann F. Meckel (1714–74), who presented his case at the Royal Academy of Berlin in 1750, and it was published in the *Memoirs of the Academy* in 1768 (1). The first publication of a case was by J. B. Morgagni in 1760 (2). M. Paris in 1791 (3) described the typical pathological findings, and the first attempt at classification of the various types of coarctation was by L. M. Bonnet in 1903 (4). The incidence of coarctation of the aorta varies between 5.3% and 7.5% of all congenital cardiac anomalies (5–9).

EMBRYOLOGIC CONSIDERATIONS

The different segments of the thoracic aorta have different embryological origins (Fig. 28-1). The ascending aorta originates from the aortic sac. The aortic arch arises from the fourth left aortic arch; it has two segments—the transverse arch and the isthmus. The proximal portion of the transverse arch is that part of the aortic arch between the origin of the innominate artery and the left common carotid artery; the distal portion of the transverse arch is between the origin of the left common carotid and the left subclavian arteries. The aortic isthmus is that portion of the aortic arch between the origin of the left subclavian and the ductus arteriosus. The proximal transverse arch is considered hypoplastic if its external diameter is equal to or less than 60% of the diameter of the ascending aorta; the distal transverse arch is termed ''hypoplastic'' if its diameter is equal to or less than 50% of the ascending aorta; the isthmus is hypoplastic if it is equal to or less than 40% of the ascending aortic diameter (10).

The morphogenetic process giving rise to coarctation of the aorta continues to be controversial today. Reynaud in 1828 (11) was the first to establish a relationship between the closure and disappearance of the ductus arteriosus and aortic coarctation. This theory, in which the process of ductal obliteration is extended into the aorta, was supported by Craigie (12) and, as discussed in Bonet (13), by Hamernik in 1844 in *Prager Vierteljahr*. In 1855, Skoda (14) suggested two theories: one proposed that ductal tissue extended into the aortic wall, which became narrowed through the same process responsible for ductal closure; and the second one suggested that the aortic segment obliterated during fetal life due to some anomaly of the aortic wall proper. The extension of ductal tissue into the aorta was later confirmed by various authors (15–19); however, this theory alone cannot explain all cases of coarctation of the aorta.

Skoda's theory of ductal extension into the aortic wall was not substantiated by Clagett et al. (20) in histologic studies. These authors postulated that the embryologic origin of coarctation was related to the development of the aortic isthmus and the cephalic migration of the left subclavian artery (7th intersegmental artery) during early development. According to their theory, an abnormal degree of differential growth would result in a relatively excessive amount of aortic tissue, which would be redundant and protrude curtain-like inside the lumen of the aorta. Based on this same theory, Moffatt (21) considered coarctation to be due to an infolding of the wall of the left subclavian artery caused by its cephalic migration. Krediet (22) hypothesized that, during the process of migration of the left subclavian artery, proximal aortic tissue became incorporated into the subclavian artery, leaving a gap that would need to be filled by distal aortic tissue. If there was not sufficient aortic tissue to fill the gap, it would be filled by ductal tissue, resulting in a ring of ductal tissue surrounding the ostium of the aortic isthmus causing isthmic stenosis. Finally, Rosenberg (23) suggested that an abnormal development of the junction between the distal end of the 4th left aortic arch (isthmus), the distal end of the 6th left arch (ductus arteriosus), and the descending aorta would result in failure of reabsorp-

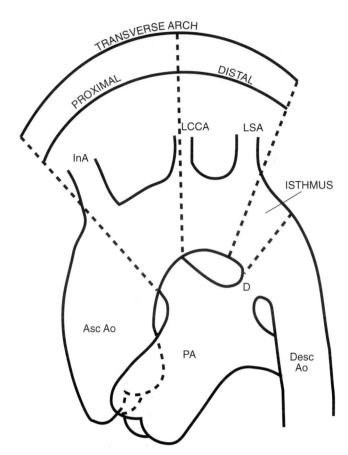

FIG. 28-1. Schematic drawing indicating the various segments of the aorta as well as the proximal and distal portions of the transverse aortic arch. *Asc Ao,* ascending aorta; *Desc Ao,* descending aorta; *D,* ductus arteriosus; *PA,* pulmonary artery; *InA,* innominate artery; *LCCA,* left common carotid artery; *LSA,* left subclavian artery.

tion of ductal tissue into the superior wall of the aorta, thereby causing a coarctation.

A theory based on hemodynamics during fetal life playing an important role in the morphogenesis of coarctation has been proposed recently (10,24–27).

ANATOMIC AND ECHOCARDIOGRAPHIC CONSIDERATIONS

The echocardiographic study of coarctation should include the site of the coarctation, the presence of tubular isthmic hypoplasia, the patency of the ductus arteriosus, and associated anomalies.

Various classifications and nomenclatures of coarctation of the aorta have been proposed based on the site of narrowing and the patency of the ductus (4,20,23,25,28–30). The first classification proposed by Bonnet (4) considered two types of coarctation of the aorta, one seen in the newborn and termed ''infantile type,'' and one seen in the adult and termed ''adult type.'' In his ''infantile type,'' the ''coarctation'' was proximal to the ductus and

characterized by diffuse narrowing of the isthmus with usual ductal patency (Fig. 28-2A). In his adult type of coarctation, the narrowing was at or distal to the site of insertion of the ductus, which was usually closed (Fig. 28-2B). However, it is presently accepted that his original description of the so-called ''infantile type'' of coarctation is actually tubular hypoplasia of the isthmus (31), which may or may not be associated with a discrete coarctation of the aorta (16,19,32) from which it has to be differentiated (31–33). Calling tubular hypoplasia of the transverse aorta a ''preductal coarctation'' (34) seems incorrect.

Tubular isthmic hypoplasia is characterized by long uniform narrowing of the aortic isthmus that has a histologically normal medial layer (31) (Fig. 28-2A). *Coarctation of the aorta,* on the other hand, is an abrupt narrowing of the aorta at, distal to, or proximal to the site of insertion

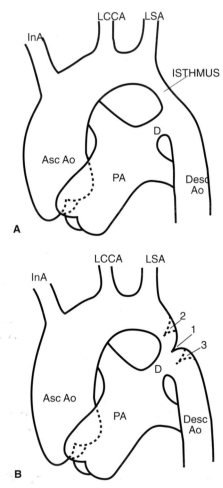

FIG. 28-2. Schematic drawing demonstrating hypoplasia of the aortic isthmus and the different anatomic locations of coarctation of the aorta. **A:** Isthmic hypoplasia. **B:** Coarctation of the aorta. *1,* ductal coarctation; *2,* preductal coarctation; *3,* postductal coarctation; *Asc Ao,* ascending aorta; *Desc Ao,* descending aorta; *D,* ductus arteriosus; *PA,* pulmonary artery; *InA,* innominate artery; *LCCA,* left common carotid artery; *LSA,* left subclavian artery.

of the ductus arteriosus (35) (Fig. 28-2B). Van Praagh et al. (36) consider that coarctation of the aorta is not preductal, postductal, or juxtaductal, but rather simply ductal.

The site of the coarctation is marked externally by a concavity or infolding that includes the entire aorta except for its inferior wall, into which the ductus inserts. Internally in the lumen, there is a sharply localized curtain-like infolding corresponding to the site of the external concavity, which includes the anterior, superior, and posterior walls of the aorta (31,35) opposite the ductus (Fig. 28-2B). Histologically, this curtain-like structure is characterized by a thickening of the media. In adolescents and adults, additional histologic changes are found, including thickening of the intima and an increase in the medial elastic lamina. These histologic changes transform the curtain-like infolding into a diaphragm-like membrane at the site of the coarctation (35). The wall immediately distal to the stricture usually has a localized lesion that protrudes from the intima and that consists of fibrosis and intimal thickening; this has been called a ''jet lesion'' (35).

Collateral circulation, which can develop to bridge the site of obstruction, was first noted by Meckel in 1827 (37) and Reynaud in 1828 (11) and later reviewed by King (33), Blackford (38), Abbott (39), and Edwards (40). Its development has been related to the position of the coarctation relative to the ductus arteriosus. If the coarctation is located distal to the ductus, ductal blood cannot flow into the descending aorta resulting in development of collaterals during fetal life allowing blood to flow to the lower body even after ductal closure postnatally. If the coarctation is proximal to the ductus, the blood from it can flow freely to the lower body so no collateral circulation develops during fetal life; as a consequence, the obstruction due to the coarctation becomes critical after the ductus closes postnatally (31).

The echocardiographic views used to assess the aortic

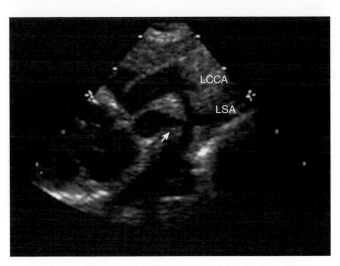

ECHO. 28-2. Suprasternal long-axis view of the aorta demonstrating hypoplasia of the distal transverse arch and isthmus and a paraductal coarctation. The *arrow* points to the ductus arteriosus, the distal limit of the isthmus. Note the increased distance between the left common carotid and the left subclavian arteries, an indirect sign of the presence of coarctation of the aorta. *LCCA*, left common carotid artery; *LSA*, left subclavian artery.

arch are the suprasternal long-axis and the high right and left parasternal views (41–46). In the suprasternal long-axis view, the entire aortic arch can be seen as well as the junction of the ductus and descending aorta (Echos. 28-1, 28-2); therefore, the presence of generalized aortic hypoplasia, or isthmic hypoplasia with or without an associated discrete coarctation, can be established (10,47). It is important to make measurements of the different aortic segments since there is normally a progressive decrease in aortic vessel size, particularly in the neonate and infant. The site(s) of narrowing can also be seen from the high parasternal views, which demonstrate the union of the ductus to the descending aorta (Echo. 28-3; see color plate 97 following p. 364). Echocardiographically the coarctation appears as an echodense shelf of tissue on the superior wall of the aorta obstructing its lumen. It is important to note that in neonates it is common to see a small shelf at the site of the ductal junction without obstruction which should not be confused with a coarctation (Echo. 28-4; see color plate 98 following p. 364).

Sometimes it is difficult to obtain a clear view of the entire aortic arch and isthmus from the suprasternal approach. In newborns particularly, the subcostal abdominal long-axis view can be useful. It should start with a short-axis abdominal view of the aorta and inferior vena cava followed by rotation of the transducer 90 degrees counterclockwise to achieve a longitudinal view of the descending aorta. Aiming the transducer superiorly, the descending aorta is followed into the thoracic descending portion, the aortic arch and the ascending aorta. The short-axis and longitudinal subcostal views of the descending aorta

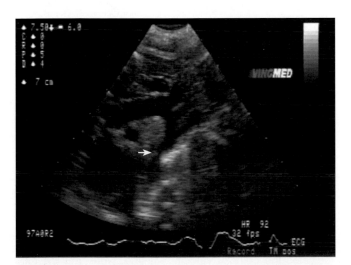

ECHO. 28-1. Suprasternal long-axis view of the aorta demonstrating the presence of a coarctation *(arrow).*

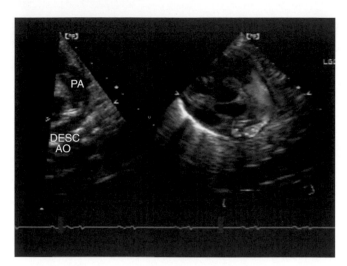

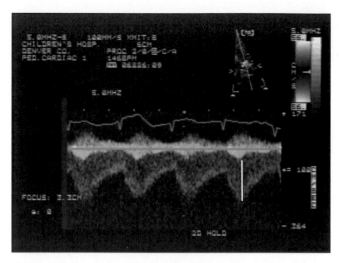

ECHO. 28-3. High parasternal short-axis view demonstrating the pulmonary artery, patent ductus arteriosus, and adjacent coarctation of the aorta. Note the normal forward flow in the main pulmonary artery. The pulmonary flow aliases at the site of the coarctation and supplies the descending aorta through a patent ductus arteriosus. *PA,* pulmonary artery; *DESC AO,* descending aorta.

ECHO. 28-5. Spectral Doppler velocity typical of severe coarctation of the aorta where the high velocity persists through diastole. If the proximal velocity exceeds 1 m/s, it should be subtracted from the maximal velocity to avoid overestimation of the trans-coarctation gradient. See text for details.

are also useful to demonstrate a reduced pulsatility, which is typical of coarctation.

Color Doppler flow mapping is helpful in confirming the diagnosis of coarctation since two-dimensional echocardiography sometimes cannot establish its presence conclusively. Color Doppler demonstrates the site of flow acceleration, the aliasing proximal and distal to the narrowed site (48) and the presence and direction of shunting

across a patent ductus arteriosus (Echo. 28-3). The color image also aids in the placement of the continuous wave sampling line to measure the velocity across the coarctation which can be used to estimate the gradient (49). The velocity proximal to the coarctation should always be measured with pulsed wave Doppler and, if greater than 1 m/s, it should be subtracted from the maximal velocity to avoid overestimation of the severity of the trans-coarctation gradient (Echo. 28-5).In these cases the appropriate modification of the Bernoulli equation would be gradient $= 4(V_2^2 - V_1^2)$.

The characteristics of the spectral Doppler curve re-

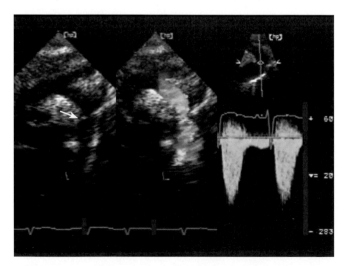

ECHO. 28-4. Left: Suprasternal long-axis view of the aorta in a neonate. There is a shelf at the site of the ductal junction *(arrow)* with slight narrowing at that site. **Middle:** Color Doppler flow map through the descending aorta. There is slight narrowing of the color flow and aliasing at the site of the shelf. **Right:** Spectral Doppler velocity recording through the descending aorta demonstrating low velocity, without the typical diastolic high-velocity flow.

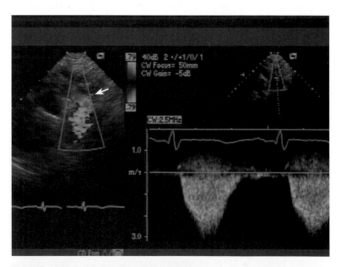

ECHO. 28-6. Color Doppler flow map and spectral velocity recording across a mild coarctation of the aorta. The *arrow* indicates the point of velocity aliasing. Note that the high velocity is recorded only in systole, without high-velocity diastolic flows.

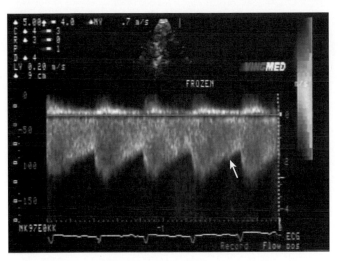

ECHO. 28-7. Spectral Doppler velocity across a severe coarctation of the aorta. The *arrow* points to the persistent high-velocity flow in diastole, indicating a persistent gradient.

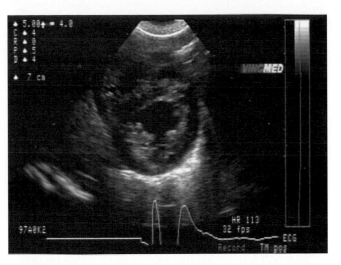

ECHO. 28-9. Parasternal short-axis view of the left ventricle demonstrating a reduced distance between the two papillary muscles, considered an indirect sign of the presence of coarctation.

corded across the coarctation site can be related to the hemodynamic consequences associated with the different degrees of severity of obstruction. In mild obstruction, the high velocity is only seen in systole (Echo. 28-6; see color plate 99 following p. 364); with increasing severity, the gradient is maintained during diastole as well, causing the typical Doppler pattern associated with coarctation where high velocities persist throughout the cardiac cycle (Echos. 28-5, 28-7). The Doppler velocities should be confirmed with a stand alone continuous wave probe which is considered more sensitive than the imaging/Doppler probes and

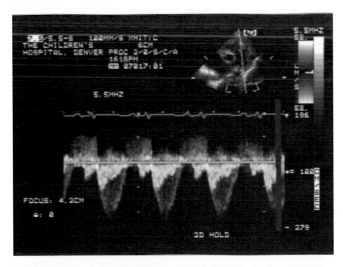

ECHO. 28-8. Spectral Doppler recording through a coarctation of the aorta with an associated patent ductus arteriosus. Note the double spectral signal. The more intense, lower velocity originates from the flow proximal to the coarctation site. The less intense, higher velocity represents the velocity across the coarctation. The maximal velocity recorded is 2.2 m/s and could be underestimated by the presence of a patent ductus arteriosus. See text for details.

which can also be easily placed in a variety of anatomical positions. In the presence of a patent ductus arteriosus the velocities recorded across the coarctation can be erroneously low since the pressure distal to the coarctation is maintained by ductal flow (50,51) (Echos. 28-3, 28-8). In many instances, the true severity of the coarctation cannot be determined until the ductus closes.

Distal displacement of the left subclavian artery has been used as an indirect echocardiographic sign of coarctation of the aorta when the distance between the left subclavian and the left common carotid arteries is 1.5 times greater than the distance between the left common carotid and the innominate arteries (52) (Echo. 28-2). Another sign suggestive of coarctation is a reduced distance between the papillary muscles of the left ventricle seen from the parasternal short-axis view compared to normals (53) (Echo. 28-9).

The so-called subclinical coarctation (54), pseudocoarctation (55), kinking (56), or buckling of the aorta (57) is an anomaly characterized by a deformity and mild narrowing of the aortic isthmus with variable degrees of proximal dilatation and tortuosity. It is different from coarctation in that there is no luminal obstruction, the gradient is either mild or nonexistent and there are no collaterals. The echocardiogram demonstrates the tortuosity of the aorta at the isthmus usually manifested by an inability to obtain a complete view of the arch and descending aorta from the same echocardiographic plane. The color Doppler flow pattern is usually somewhat disturbed, but no high-velocity or typical coarctation spectral pattern can be recorded.

Associated Anomalies

Isolated coarctation is seen in 18% to 22.5% of cases (7,30,32). The most frequently associated cardiac malformations are a patent ductus arteriosus and a bicuspid aortic valve. The ductus has been found to be patent in 64% to 95.5% of cases in various series (7,16,30,32,34,58,59). The finding of associated bicuspid aortic valve in 25.1% of cases was reported by Abbott in 1928 (39). Later reports find an even higher incidence between 25.1% and 46% (29,34,58–60) (Echo. 28-10).

Ventricular septal defects associated with coarctation are seen in 26% to 65% of cases (7,16,19,30,32,44,58–60). In 80% of cases in Anderson's pathologic series (61), the defect was of a specific perimembranous type, which extended into all parts of the ventricular septum adjacent to the central fibrous body with overriding of the aortic valve. Other types of ventricular septal defects seen are perimembranous with posterior deviation of the outlet septum and left ventricular outflow tract obstruction and outlet muscular defect (61). Atrioventricular septal defects have a variable incidence between 2% and 10% of cases (19,44,58,62).

A wide spectrum of anomalies of the mitral valve is seen frequently in association with coarctation and include mitral valve hypoplasia (59), stenosis (7,16,32,34,44), double orifice (34), arcade (34), and atresia (58,59). The parachute deformity of the mitral valve can be found in association with coarctation by itself or as part of the syndrome described by Shone et al. (63) characterized by a supravalvular mitral ring, parachute mitral valve, subaortic stenosis, and coarctation of the aorta (see Fig. 13-3).

Other anomalies found with coarctation can be atrial septal defect, patent foramen ovale, atrioventricular univentricular connection, complete transposition of the great arteries, corrected transposition of the great arteries, double outlet right ventricle, truncus arteriosus, hypoplastic left ventricle, subaortic stenosis, aortic stenosis, unicuspid aortic valve, aortic atresia, Ebstein anomaly, straddling tricus-

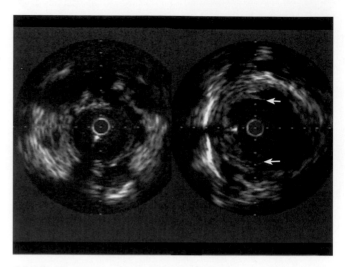

ECHO. 28-11. Intravascular ultrasound in coarctation of the aorta. **Left:** Site of coarctation prior to balloon dilatation. The site measures approximately 2 mm. **Right:** Site of coarctation after balloon dilatation. The *arrows* point to the intimal tears or flaps commonly noticed after the angioplasty.

pid valve, total or partial anomalous venous drainage, and left superior vena cava draining into the coronary sinus.

INTRAOPERATIVE AND POSTOPERATIVE EVALUATION

The intraoperative echocardiographic study in coarctation of the aorta is not routinely performed in our center except if it is in association with an intracardiac malformation requiring repair. These are covered in their specific chapters. However, other centers use transesophageal echocardiography to visualize coarctations in older children and adults (64–66).

Recently an increasing number of centers are using balloon angioplasty to relieve coarctation either primarily or if there is recurrent coarctation after surgery. In these instances, the use of intravascular ultrasound to examine the internal aortic wall has been useful both pre and post angioplasty (Echo. 28-11). In a recent study by Sohn et al. (67), intimal tears or flaps were seen in all cases of native and most cases of recoarctations immediately post balloon angioplasty with intravascular ultrasound, most of which were not seen by angiography. At follow-up, however, no patient has developed aneurysms and approximately half demonstrated a diminution in size or actual resolution of the tears. Further follow-up will be required using intravascular ultrasound before the final long-term results of this procedure are known.

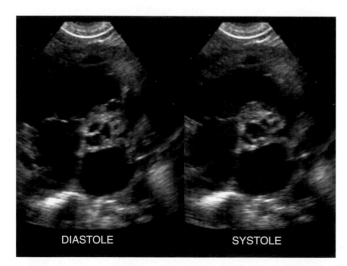

ECHO. 28-10. Parasternal short-axis view of a bicuspid aortic valve in association with coarctation of the aorta. Note there is an anterior and a posterior cusp. The raphe is in the anterior cusp.

REFERENCES

1. Jarcho S. Historical milestones. Coarctation of the aorta (Meckel, 1750; Paris, 1791). *Am J Cardiol* 1961;7:844–852.

2. Morgagni JB. De sedibus et causis morborum [Article 6]. *Epist* 1760;18.

3. Paris M. Retrecissement considerable de l'aorte pectorale observe a l'Hotel Dieu de Paris. *J Chir Desault* 1791;2:107–110.

4. Bonnet LM. Sur la lesion dite stenose congenitale de l'aorte, dans la region de l'isthme. *Rev Med* 1903;23:108–126,255–265,335–353,418–438,481–502.

5. Mitchell SC, Korones SB, Berendes HW. Congenital heart disease in 56,109 births. *Circulation* 1971;43:323–332.

6. Hoffman JIE, Christianson R. Congenital heart disease in a cohort of 19,502 births with long-term follow-up. *Am J Cardiol* 1978;42:641–647.

7. Fyler DC, Buckley LP, Hellebrand WE, Cohn HE. Report of the New England regional infant cardiac program. *Pediatrics* 1980;65:375–461.

8. Samanek M, Slavik Z, Zborilova B, Hrobonova V, Voriskova M, Skovranek J. Prevalence, treatment, and outcome of heart disease in live-born children: a prospective analysis of 91,823 live-born children. *Pediatr Cardiol* 1989;10:205–211.

9. Hoffman JIE. Incidence of congenital heart disease: I. Postnatal incidence. *Pediatr Cardiol* 1995;16:103–113.

10. Moulaert AJ, Bruins CC, Oppenheimer-Derkker A. Anomalies of the aortic arch and ventricular septal defects. *Circulation* 1976;53:1011–1015.

11. Reynaud A. Observation d'une obliteration presque complete de l'aorte, suivie de quelques reflexions, et precedee de l'indication des faits analogues, consignes dans les auteurs. *J Hebdomadaire Med* 1828;1:161–175.

12. Craigie D. Instance of obliteration of the aorta beyond the arch, illustrated by similar cases and observations. *Edinburgh Med Surg J* 1841;56:427–462.

13. Hamernik J. *Prager vierteljahr*, 1844. Cited by Bonnet LM. Sur la lesion dite stenose congenitale de l'aorte dans la region de l'isthme. *Rev Med* 1903;23:108–126,255–265,335–353,418–438,481–502.

14. Skoda J. Protokoll der Sections-Sitzung fur Physiologie und Pathologie. *Wochenblatt Ztschr Gesellsch Aerztez Wien* 1855;1:720.

15. Wielenga G, Dankmeijer J. Coarctation of the aorta. *J Pathol Bacteriol* 1968;95:265–274.

16. Ho SY, Anderson RH. Coarctation, tubular hypoplasia, and the ductus arteriosus. Histological study of 35 specimens. *Br Heart J* 1979;41:268–274.

17. Oppenheimer-Dekker A, Moene RJ, Moulaert AJ, Gittenberger-De Groot AC. Teratogenetic considerations regarding aortic arch anomalies associated with cardiovascular malformations. In: Pexieder T, ed. *Mechanisms of cardiac morphogenesis and teratogenesis. Perspectives in cardiovascular research. Vol. 5.* New York: Raven Press, 1981:485–500.

18. Elzenga NJ, Gittenberger-De Groot AC. Localized coarctation of the aorta. An age-dependent spectrum. *Br Heart J* 1983;49:317–323.

19. Elzenga NJ, Gittenberger-De Groot AC, Oppenheimer-Dekker A. Coarctation and other obstructive aortic arch anomalies: their relationship to the ductus arteriosus. *Int J Cardiol* 1986;13:289–308.

20. Clagett OT, Kirklin JW, Edwards JE. Anatomic variations and pathologic changes in coarctation of the aorta. A study of 124 cases. *Surg Gynecol Obstet* 1954;98:103–114.

21. Moffat DB. Pre- and post-natal changes in the left subclavian artery and their possible relationship to coarctation of the aorta. *Acta Anat* 1960;43:346–357.

22. Krediet P. An hypothesis of the development of coarctation in man. *Acta Morphol Neerl Scand* 1965;6:207–212.

23. Rosenberg HS. Coarctation of the aorta: morphology and pathogenetic considerations. In: Rosenberg HS, Bolande RP, eds. *Perspectives in pediatric pathology. Vol. 1.* Chicago: Year Book Medical Publisher, 1973:339–368.

24. Hutchins GM. Coarctation of the aorta explained as a branch-point of the ductus arteriosus. *Am J Pathol* 1971;63:203–209.

25. Rudolph AM, Heymann MA, Spitznas U. Hemodynamics considerations in the development of narrowing of the aorta. *Am J Cardiol* 1972;30:514–525.

26. Shinebourne EA, Elseed AM. Relation between fetal flow patterns, coarctation of the aorta, and pulmonary blood flow. *Br Heart J* 1974;36:492–498.

27. Hoffman JIE, Heymann MA, Rudolph AM. Coarctation of the aorta:

28. Evans W. Congenital stenosis (coarctation), atresia, and interruption of the aortic arch (a study of twenty-eight cases). *Q J Med* 1933;2:1–31.

29. Reifenstein GH, Levine SA, Gross RE. Coarctation of the aorta. A review of 104 autopsied cases of the "adult type," 2 years of age or older. *Am Heart J* 1947;33:146–168.

30. Keith JD. Coarctation of the aorta. In: Keith JD, Rowe RD, Vlad P, eds. *Heart disease in infancy and childhood.* 3rd ed. New York: Macmillan, 1978:736–760.

31. Edwards JE, Carey LS, Neufeld HN, Lester RG. Coarctation of the aorta. In: Edwards JE, Carey LS, Neufeld HN, Lester RG, eds. *Congenital heart disease. Correlation of pathologic anatomy and angiocardiography. Vol. II.* Philadelphia: WB Saunders, 1965:677–704.

32. Sinha SN, Kardatzke ML, Cole RB, Muster AJ, Wessel HU, Paul MH. Coarctation of the aorta in infancy. *Circulation* 1969;40:385–398.

33. King JT, Stenosis of the isthmus (coarctation) of the aorta and its diagnosis during life. Report of four cases. *Arch Intern Med* 1926;38:69–95.

34. Bharati S, Lev M. The surgical anatomy of the heart in tubular hypoplasia of the transverse aorta (preductal coarctation). *J Thorac Cardiovasc Surg* 1986;91:79–85.

35. Edwards JE, Christensen NA, Clagett OT, McDonald JR. Pathologic considerations in coarctation of the aorta. *Proc Staff Meet Mayo Clinic* 1948;23:324–332.

36. Van Praagh R, O'Connor B, Chacko KA. The pathologic anatomy of aortic coarctation. In: Crupi G, Parenzan L, Anderson RH, eds. *Perspectives in pediatric cardiology. Vol. 2. Pediatric cardiac surgery Part 1.* Mount Kisco, NY: Futura Publishing, 1989:261–263.

37. Meckel A. Verschliessung der aorta am vierten brustwirbel. *Arch Anat Physiol* 1827;345–354. Cited by Edwards JE, Clagett OT, Drake RC, Christensen NA. The collateral circulation in coarctation of the aorta. *Proc Staff Mayo Clinic* 1948;23.333–339.

38. Blackford LM. Coarctation of the aorta. *Arch Intern Med* 1928;41:702–735.

39. Abbott ME. Coarctation of the aorta of the adult type. II. A statistical study and historical retrospect of 200 recorded cases, with autopsy, of stenosis or obliteration of the descending arch in subjects above the age of two years. *Am Heart J* 1928;3:392–421,574–618.

40. Edwards JE, Clagett OT, Drake RL, Christensen NA. The collateral circulation in coarctation of the aorta. *Proc Staff Meet Mayo Clinic* 1948;23:333–339.

41. Sahn DJ, Allen HD, McDonald G, Goldberg SJ. Real-time cross-sectional echocardiographic diagnosis of coarctation of the aorta. A prospective study of echocardiographic-angiographic correlations. *Circulation* 1977;56:762–769.

42. Snider AR, Silverman NH. Suprasternal notch echocardiography: a two-dimensional technique for evaluating congenital heart disease. *Circulation* 1981;63:165–173.

43. Duncan WJ, Ninomiya K, Cook DH, Rowe RD. Noninvasive diagnosis of neonatal coarctation and associated anomalies using two-dimensional echocardiography. *Am Heart J* 1983;106:63–69.

44. Smallhorn JF, Huhta JC, Adams PA, Anderson RH, Wilkinson JL, Macartney FJ. Cross-sectional echocardiographic assessment of coarctation in the sick neonate and infant. *Br Heart J* 1983;50:349–361.

45. Huhta JC, Gutgesell HP, Latson LA, Huffines FD. Two-dimensional echocardiographic assessment of the aorta in infants and children with congenital heart disease. *Circulation* 1984;70:417–424.

46. Nihoyannopoulos P, Karas S, Sapsford RN, Hallidie-Smith K, Foale R. Accuracy of two-dimensional echocardiography in the diagnosis of aortic arch obstruction. *J Am Coll Cardiol* 1987;10:1072–1077.

47. Morrow WR, Huhta JC, Murphy DJ, McNamara DG. Quantitative morphology of the aortic arch in neonatal coarctation. *J Am Coll Cardiol* 1986;8:616–620.

48. Simpson IA, Sahn DJ, Valdes-Cruz LM, Chung KJ, Sherman FS, Swensson RE. Color Doppler flow mapping in patients with coarctation of the aorta: new observations and improved evaluation with color flow diameter and proximal acceleration as predictor of severity. *Circulation* 1988;77:736–744.

49. Carvalho JS, Redington AN, Shinebourne EA, Rigby ML. Continuous wave Doppler echocardiography and coarctation of the aorta: gradients and flow patterns in the assessment of severity. *Br Heart J* 1990;64:133–137.

50. Marx GR, Allen HD. Accuracy and pitfalls of Doppler evaluation of the pressure gradient in aortic coarctation. *J Am Coll Cardiol* 1986;7:1379–1385.

51. Wilson N, Sutherland GR, Gibbs JL, Dickinson DF, Keeton BR. Limitations of Doppler ultrasound in the diagnosis of neonatal coarctation of the aorta. *Int J Cardiol* 1989;23:87–89.

52. Kantoch M, Pieroni D, Roland JMA, Gingell RL. Association of distal displacement of the left subclavian artery and coarctation of the aorta. *Pediatr Cardiol* 1992;14:164–169.

53. Goldberg SJ, Gerlis LM, Ho SY, Butler Penilla M. Location of the left papillary muscles in juxtaductal aortic coarctation. *Am J Cardiol* 1995;75:746–750.

54. Souders CR, Pearson CM, Adams HD. An aortic deformity simulating mediastinal tumor: a subclinical form of coarctation. *Dis Chest* 1951;20:35–45.

55. Dotter CT, Steinberg I. Angiocardiography in congenital heart disease. *Am J Med* 1952;12:219–237.

56. Di Guglielmo L, Guttadauro M. Kinking of aorta: report of two cases. *Acta Radiol* 1955;44:121–128.

57. Stevens GM. Buckling of aortic arch (pseudocoarctation, kinking): a roentgenographic entity. *Radiology* 1958;70:67–73.

58. Becker AE, Becker MJ, Edwards JE. Anomalies associated with coarctation of aorta. Particular reference to infancy. *Circulation* 1970;41:1067–1075.

59. Rosenquist GC. Congenital mitral valve disease associated with coarctation of the aorta. A spectrum that includes parachute deformity of the mitral valve. *Circulation* 1974;49:985–993.

60. Pellegrino A, Deverall PB, Anderson RH, et al. Aortic coarctation in the first three months of life. An anatomopathological study with respect to treatment. *J Thorac Cardiovasc Surg* 1985;89:121–127.

61. Anderson RH, Lenox CC, Zuberbuhler JR. Morphology of ventricular septal defect associated with coarctation of aorta. *Br Heart J* 1983;50:176–181.

62. Kirklin JW, Barrat-Boyes BG. Coarctation of the aorta and interrupted aortic arch. In: Kirklin JW, Barrat-Boyes BG, eds. *Cardiac surgery. Morphology, diagnostic criteria, natural history, techniques, results, and indications. Vol. 2.* 2nd ed. New York: Churchill Livingstone, 1993:1263–1325.

63. Shone JD, Sellers RD, Anderson RC, Adams P Jr, Lillehei CW, Edwards JE. The developmental complex of "parachute mitral valve," supravalvular ring of left atrium, subaortic stenosis, and coarctation of the aorta. *Am J Cardiol* 1963;11:714–725.

64. Cyran SE, Kimball TR, Meyer RA, et al. Efficacy of intraoperative transesophageal echocardiography in children with congenital heart disease. *Am J Cardiol* 1989;63:594–598.

65. Stumper OFW, Elzenga NJ, Hess J, Sutherland GR. Transesophageal echocardiography in children with congenital heart disease: an initial experience. *J Am Coll Cardiol* 1990;16:433–441.

66. Ryan K, Sanyal RS, Pinheiro L, Nanda NC. Assessment of aortic coarctation and collateral circulation by biplane transesophageal echocardiography. *Echocardiography* 1992;9:277–285.

67. Sohn S, Rothman A, Shiota T, et al. Acute and follow-up intravascular ultrasound findings after balloon dilation of coarctation of the aorta. *Circulation* 1994;90:340–347.

CHAPTER 29

Complete Interruption of the Aortic Arch

Lilliam M. Valdes-Cruz and Raul O. Cayre

Complete interruption of the aortic arch is a rare malformation characterized by a complete absence of anatomic continuity between two segments of the aortic arch. Raphael J. Steidele (1) described the first case of this malformation in 1778, which was an interruption between the left subclavian and the ductus arteriosus. In 1818, Seidel (2) reported a case with interruption between the left common carotid and the left subclavian artery. The first case of interruption between the innominate and the left common carotid arteries was published by Weisman and Kesten in 1948 (3). These three types of complete interruption are the types A, B and C of the Celoria and Patton classification (4) (Fig. 29-1). The classification was later expanded by Freedom et al. (5) and Oppenheimer-Dekker et al. (6). Some authors call this malformation Steidele's complex (7,8). Its incidence varies between 1% and 1.3% of all congenital cardiac anomalies (9–12) and is found in 1.4% of all autopsies of children with congenital heart disease (13).

When there is an imperforate segment of the aortic arch represented by a fibrous ligament, this is called atresia of that particular segment (14–16) (Fig. 29-2). This should be differentiated from complete interruption, in which there is no fibrous ligament between the segments.

EMBRYOLOGIC CONSIDERATIONS

The morphogenetic processes that can result in the different types of aortic arch interruption are intimately related with the embryologic development of the aortic arches (see Fig. 1-16). The influence of blood flow in the development or involution of the aortic arch was mentioned by Congdon (17) and by Congdon and Wang (18) and later endorsed by many other authors (5,6,13, 14,16,19–23); however, this mechanism alone cannot explain all cases of interrupted arch, particularly those without associated cardiac malformations, which could cause reduced blood flow in the ascending aorta (24,25).

Type A complete interruption (Fig. 29-1A) is caused by a regression or atrophy of the segment of arch between the ductus arteriosus and the left subclavian artery (left dorsal aorta), after the seventh week of embryonic life (4,7,13,26). Type B (Fig. 29-1B) is produced as a result of failure of formation of the 4th left aortic arch, before the seventh week of gestation, which will determine that the left subclavian artery will not have its cephalic ascent and will remain connected with the descending aorta (4,7,13,26). Various mechanisms have been suggested in the formation of Type C interruption (Fig. 29-1C). Celoria and Patton have proposed two possible ones: (a) partial or complete failure in the formation of the 3rd and 4th left aortic arches with persistence of the dorsal aortic segment between these two arches as the left common carotid artery and (b) failure of connection between the outgrowth of the aortic sac and the 3rd and 4th aortic arches with fusion of these two arches to form the left common carotid artery (4). Van Praagh et al. (13) consider that this type of arch interruption is caused by an involution of the left distal portion of the aortic sac; this would cause an involution of the 4th left aortic arch and of the ventral origin of the 3rd left aortic arch with persistence of the left dorsal aorta between the 3rd and 4th arches, which normally involutes.

ANATOMIC AND ECHOCARDIOGRAPHIC CONSIDERATIONS

The echocardiographic study of complete interruption of the aortic arch should include the following: (a) morphology of the different types of interruption; (b) patent ductus arteriosus; (c) ventricular septal defect; (d) subaortic stenosis; (e) associated anomalies; and (f) intra- and postoperative evaluation.

Morphology of the Different Types of Interruption

The classification proposed by Celoria and Patton (4) divides the different types of interruption according to

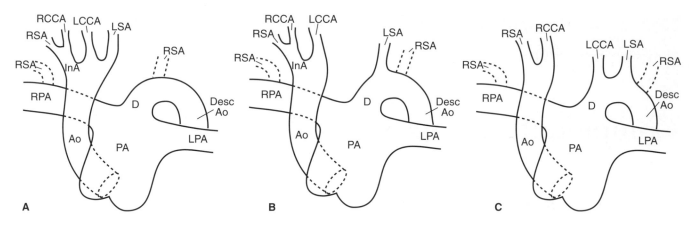

FIG. 29-1. Schematic drawings of the various anatomic types of complete interruption of the aortic arch according to the classification of Celoria and Patton (4) and the subtypes based on the anomalous origin of the right subclavian artery either from the right pulmonary artery or from the descending aorta. **A:** Complete interruption type A. **B:** Complete interruption type B. **C:** Complete interruption type C. *Ao,* aorta; *PA,* pulmonary artery; *D,* ductus arteriosus; *Desc Ao,* descending aorta; *RPA,* right pulmonary artery; *LPA,* left pulmonary artery; *InA,* innominate artery; *RCCA,* right common carotid artery; *LCCA,* left common carotid artery; *RSA,* right subclavian artery; *LSA,* left subclavian artery.

the site. Type A (Fig. 29-1A) is seen in 30% to 44% of cases (5,7,11,13,26). The ascending aorta is continuous with a portion of the aortic arch from which the brachiocephalic trunk and the left common carotid and the left subclavian arteries originate. The interruption is located between the left subclavian and the ductus arteriosus (Echo. 29-1; see color plate 100 following p. 364). Type B (Fig. 29-1B) is the most common form found in 50%

to 67% of series (5,7,11,13,26). The interruption is found between the left common carotid and the left subclavian artery, which originates from the descending aorta (Echo. 29-2). Type C (Fig. 29-1C) is rarely seen, having an incidence of 3% to 5% of cases (11,13,26). The interruption occurs between the innominate artery and the left common carotid artery (Echo. 29-3). In all types of interruption (A, B, or C), there are two subtypes based on the site of origin of the right subclavian artery: subtype 1, when it branches from the descending aorta (5,6), and subtype 2, when it originates from the right pulmonary artery (6) (Fig. 29-1).

In all types of interruption, there is a complete disconti-

FIG. 29-2. Schematic drawing of atresia of the aortic isthmus. Note the presence of a fibrous ligament between the distal portion of the transverse aortic arch and the descending aorta. *Ao,* aorta; *PA,* pulmonary artery; *D,* ductus arteriosus; *Desc Ao,* descending aorta; *InA,* innominate artery; *LCCA,* left common carotid artery; *LSA,* left subclavian artery.

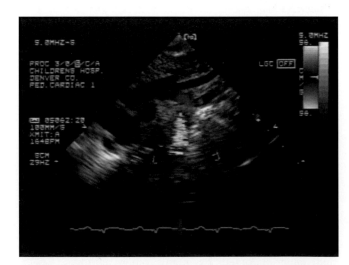

ECHO. 29-1. Suprasternal long-axis view of type A interruption of the aortic arch (between the left subclavian artery and the ductus arteriosus). The aliased flow seen in the descending aorta originates from the pulmonary artery through a patent ductus arteriosus.

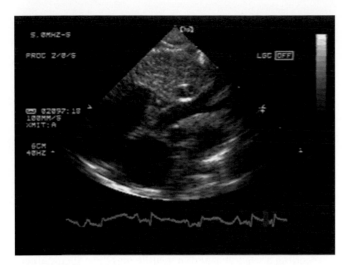

ECHO. 29-2. Suprasternal long-axis view of type B interruption of the aortic arch (between the left common carotid and left subclavian arteries).

nuity between the two segments of the aortic arch, and, contrary to atresia of an aortic segment, there is no fibrous ligament in between (Figs. 29-1, 29-2). The ascending aorta is smaller than the pulmonary artery, which is usually dilated. The descending aorta is almost always on the left, but there are isolated cases that have been described with a right descending aorta (27–31). There is a high association with DiGeorge syndrome, particularly in cases of a right descending aorta (31). Very rarely there can be aortic arch interruption with persistence of the 5th aortic arch (32–34). This arch normally involutes early in gestation in the human; however, when it persists, it allows continuity between the ascending and descending aorta and can be mistaken for a normal aortic arch.

The suprasternal long-axis and high right parasternal views are the classic ones to evaluate the aortic arch and identify the presence and site of interruption (35,36). Inability to demonstrate continuity between the ascending and descending aorta with an almost straight leftward-cephalic orientation of the transverse arch is highly suggestive of interruption (Echos. 29-1–29-3). A marked difference in size between the ascending aorta and pulmonary artery is also an indirect sign of aortic interruption (35). Structures and landmarks that should be specifically identified are the origin of the brachiocephalic trunk, of the left common carotid, and of the left subclavian artery. The right subclavian artery should be searched for and its origin localized also from these suprasternal views. Color Doppler flow mapping is of great utility in defining the discontinuity in the flow between the ascending and descending aorta (Echo. 29-1).

Patent Ductus Arteriosus

Presence of a patent ductus is almost the rule in this malformation (5,7,11,13,15,26). The clinical course de-

pends on the permeability of the ductus, which connects the pulmonary artery with the descending aorta (Fig. 29-1). This was called the "pulmonary-ductus-descending aorta trunk" by Evans (37).

The ductus is located on the same side as the descending aorta. In cases of anomalous origin of the right subclavian artery from the right pulmonary artery, there are bilateral ducti—one on the left between the descending aorta and the pulmonary trunk and one on the right between the right subclavian and the right pulmonary arteries (6,38). Extremely rarely the ductus is not patent, and the flow between the ascending and descending aorta is through collaterals (24,25,39,40).

The echocardiographic demonstration of the ductus arteriosus and the flow through it is accomplished from the same views as those used for the arch, and from the parasternal short-axis position (Echo. 29-1). Assessment of ductal permeability is important in the immediate neonatal period while patients are awaiting surgical repair on prostaglandin E1 infusion.

Ventricular Septal Defect

There is almost always a ventricular septal defect present (5,7,9,11,13,15,26,27,41). The frequent association of aortic arch interruption, patent ductus arteriosus, and ventricular septal defect led to the consideration of these as a trilogy (42).

In the majority of cases, the septal defect is of the infundibular type due to malalignment between the interventricular septum and the infundibular or outlet septum, which is displaced posteriorly and leftward, so that it comes to be located inside the left ventricular outflow

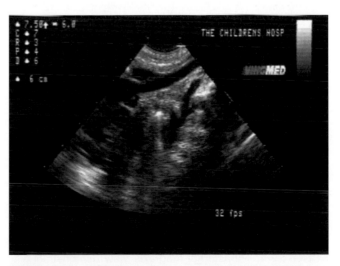

ECHO. 29-3. Suprasternal long-axis view of type C interruption of the aortic arch (between the innominate and the left common carotid arteries).

tract (5,13–15,27,41,43,44) (Echo. 29-4). Seen from the right, the defect is perimembranous, is located between the limbs of the septomarginal trabecula, and usually has outlet extensions towards the pulmonary valve (43,44). Less commonly it has trabecular or inlet extensions (44), or there is a totally muscular ring, thereby being a muscular outlet defect (43,44), muscular trabecular (5,41,45), or muscular inlet (41). On occasion, the defect can be subarterially doubly committed, in which case there is hypoplasia or absence of the outlet septum with fibrous continuity between the aortic valve and the pulmonary valve, which both form the roof of the defect (5,44). Multiple ventricular septal defects have also been described (41).

Echocardiographically, the ventricular septal defects can be studied from the same views as those described in detail in Chapter 10.

Subaortic Stenosis

The leftward and posterior displacement of the infundibular septum in cases of aortic interruption with malalignment ventricular septal defect results in various degrees of obstruction of the left ventricular outflow tract (5,7,13–16,26,27,41,44,45). The infundibular or outlet septum is then located within the left ventricular outflow tract and inserts in the anterolateral wall or in an anterolateral muscular band within the left ventricle (16,44). This anterolateral muscular band, which is found in 40% of normal hearts (46), can either worsen the obstruction caused by the infundibular displacement or be the primary cause of it in instances where the infundibular displacement is minimal (44). The other contributing factor in the

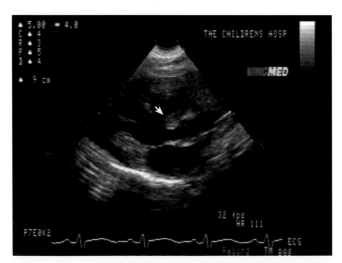

ECHO. 29-4. Parasternal long-axis view demonstrating a ventricular septal defect and posterior displacement of the infundibular septum *(arrow)* causing obstruction of the left ventricular outflow tract.

subaortic obstruction may be hypertrophy of the anterolateral wall of the left ventricle (44).

The echocardiographic views that best display the infundibular septal displacement and the obstruction of the outflow tract of the left ventricle are the parasternal long- and short-axis views, the apical outflow and long-axis views, and subcostal long- and short-axis views (Echo. 29-4). Due to the presence of an unrestrictive ventricular septal defect, Doppler cannot be used to estimate the degree of left ventricular outflow tract obstruction preoperatively, which would become manifest only after surgical closure of the defect. For this reason, various measurements have been used to predict obstruction. The ratio between the diameter of the left ventricular outflow tract averaged in systole and diastole and the diameter of the descending aorta averaged in systole and diastole obtained from the subcostal abdominal short-axis view at the level of the diaphragm has been shown to be lower than normal in infants with potential obstruction (47). More recently, Geva et al. (48) reported that a cross-sectional area of the left ventricular outflow tract of 0.7 cm^2/m^2 obtained from the parasternal or subcostal short-axis view in early systole was predictive of the development of subaortic obstruction postoperatively.

Associated Anomalies

Besides patent ductus arteriosus and ventricular septal defect, other reported anomalies have been bicuspid aortic valve (3,7,11,13,26,27,44,49), patent foramen ovale or ostium secundum atrial septal defect (3,7,9,11,13,36, 41,49,50), truncus arteriosus (5,6,11,13,19,26,35,36,41), complete transposition of the great arteries (5,6,9, 11,13,41,50–52), aortopulmonary window usually with intact ventricular septum (6,9,11,12,36,41,50,52,53), double outlet right ventricle (11,35,41,50,52), atrioventricular univentricular connection (9,11,52), left ventricular hypoplasia (9,41,49,52), atrioventricular septal defect (5,52), aortic valve stenosis (9,11), persistent left superior vena cava (13,41,50), total anomalous pulmonary venous drainage (11,52), congenitally corrected transposition of the great arteries (6), tricuspid atresia (6), straddling tricuspid valve (6), pulmonic valve stenosis (54), bicuspid pulmonic valve (49), and anomalous origin of the right pulmonary artery from the descending aorta (53,55).

INTRAOPERATIVE AND POSTOPERATIVE EVALUATION

The preoperative study through the transesophageal approach would not be of great utility in defining the type of interruption since the aortic arch may not be clearly visualized from this approach. It is used primarily to evaluate ventricular function and associated anomalies, most commonly the ventricular septal defect and the presence of left ventricular outflow tract obstruction. This is best accomplished starting from the transgastric short-axis view for global ventricular function (see Fig. 4-27A,B). Withdrawing the transducer to a four-chamber transverse view allows examination of the ventricular septum in its inlet, perimembranous, and trabecular portions (see Fig. 4-28A). It also permits study of the left ventricular outflow tract and aortic valve (see Fig. 4-29A). The longitudinal views complement the examination of the left ventricular outflow tract and also demonstrate the outlet extension of the ventricular septal defect (see Fig. 4-29E,F).

The postoperative study should also begin with evaluation of the ventricular function globally from the transgastric views and more segmentally from the transverse and longitudinal retrocardiac views. Residual ventricular septal defects can be seen with the help of color Doppler flow mapping from the same views as pre-bypass. The most important contribution of the postoperative study is the assessment of the left ventricular outflow tract. In this setting, after septal defect closure, obstructions become evident both anatomically as well as with Doppler velocity interrogation. The transverse four-chamber view (see Fig. 4-28A) serves as an initial general examination of the outflow tract. The longitudinal view (see Fig. 4-29E) permits a better analysis of the entire length of the left ventricular outflow although the angle for velocity interrogation is not favorable. For accurate recording of Doppler velocities, the best view is the transgastric longitudinal view of the outflow tracts (see Fig. 4-27E). In the late postoperative studies, it is not unusual to detect some tortuosity of the descending aorta at the site of the previous repair. Associated with it, there can be mild flow acceleration detected by color and/or spectral Doppler,

which is usually of no clinical significance (Echo. 29-5; see color plate 101 following p. 364).

REFERENCES

1. Steidele RJ. Sammlg. Verschiedener in der chirurgish praktik. *Lehrschule Germachten Beobb* 1777;2:114–116.
2. Seidel JF. *Index muse: anatomici kiliensis, quem praefatus est illustris D. (Joannes Leonardus) Fischer. Vol. XIV.* Kiliae: C. F. Mohr, 1818.
3. Weisman D, Kesten HD. Absence of transverse aortic arch with defects of cardiac septums. Report of a case simulating acute abdominal disease in a newborn infant. *Am J Dis Child* 1948;76:326–330.
4. Celoria GC, Patton RB. Congenital absence of the aortic arch. *Am Heart J* 1959;58:407–413.
5. Freedom RM, Bain HH, Esplugas E, Dische R, Rowe RD. Ventricular septal defect in interruption of aortic arch. *Am J Cardiol* 1977;39:572–582.
6. Oppenheimer-Dekker A, Gittenberger-de Groot AC, Roozendaal H. The ductus arteriosus and associated cardiac anomalies in interruption of the aortic arch. *Pediatr Cardiol* 1982;2:185–193.
7. Lie JT. The malformation complex of the absence of the arch of the aorta-Steidele's complex. *Am Heart J* 1967;73:615–625.
8. Takashina T, Ishikura Y, Yamane K, et al. The congenital cardiovascular anomalies of the interruption of the aorta-Steidele's complex. *Am Heart J* 1972;83:93–99.
9. Collins-Nakai RL, Dick M, Parisi-Buckley L, Fyler DC, Castaneda AR. Interrupted aortic arch in infancy. *J Pediatr* 1976;88:959–962.
10. Fyler DC, Buckley LP, Hellenbrand WE, Cohn HE. Report of the New England regional infant cardiac program. *Pediatrics* 1980;65:375–461.
11. Reardon MJ, Hallman GL, Cooley DA. Interrupted aortic arch: brief review and summary of eighteen-year experience. *Texas Heart Inst J* 1984;11:250–259.
12. Braunlin E, Peoples WM, Freedom RM, Fyler DC, Goldblatt A, Edwards JE. Interruption of the aortic arch with aorticopulmonary septal defect. An anatomic review. *Pediatr Cardiol* 1982;3:329–335.
13. Van Praagh R, Bernhard WF, Rosenthal A, Parisi LF, Fyler DC. Interrupted aortic arch: surgical treatment. *Am J Cardiol* 1971;27:200–211.
14. Moulaert AJ, Bruins CC, Oppenheimer-Dekker A. Anomalies of the aortic arch and ventricular septal defects. *Circulation* 1976;53:1011–1015.
15. Becker AE, Anderson RH. Malformations of the aortic arch. In: Becker AE, Anderson RH, eds. *Pathology of congenital heart disease.* London: Butterworths, 1981.321–338.
16. Moene RJ, Oppenheimer-Dekker A, Moulaert AJ, Wenink ACG, Gittenberger-de Groot AC, Roozendaal H. The concurrence of dimensional aortic arch anomalies and abnormal left ventricular muscle bundles. *Pediatr Cardiol* 1982;2:107–114.
17. Congdon ED. Transformation of the aortic-arch system during the development of the human embryo. *Contrib Embryol Carnegie Inst Washington* 1922;14:47–110.
18. Congdon ED, Wang HW. The mechanical processes concerned in the formation of the differing types of aortic arches of the chick and the pig and in the divergent early development of the pulmonary arches. *Am J Anat* 1926;37:499–520.
19. Steiner P, Finegold MJ. Truncus arteriosus with atresia of the aortic arch. *Arch Pathol* 1965;79:518–523.
20. Jaffe OC. The development of the arterial outflow tract in the chick embryo heart. *Anat Rec* 1967;158:35–42.
21. Rudolph AM, Heymann MA, Spitznas U. Hemodynamic considerations in the development of narrowing of the aorta. *Am J Cardiol* 1972;30:514–525.
22. Shinebourne EA, Elseed AM. Relation between fetal flow patterns, coarctation of the aorta, and pulmonary blood flow. *Br Heart J* 1974;36:492–498.
23. Moore GW, Hutchins GM. Association of interrupted aortic arch with malformations producing reduced blood flow to the fourth aortic arches. *Am J Cardiol* 1978;42:467–472.

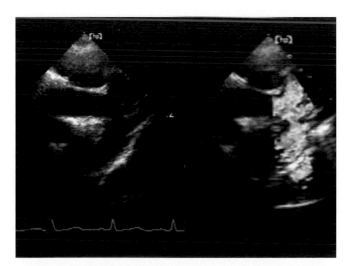

ECHO. 29-5. Suprasternal long-axis view of repaired interruption of the aortic arch. **Left:** Anatomic view demonstrating an apparently unobstructed arch. **Right:** Color Doppler flow map of the area of repair with aliasing of velocities indicating mild flow disturbance. This is usually of no clinical significance.

24. Pillsbury RC, Lower RR, Shumway NE. Atresia of the aortic arch. *Circulation* 1964;30:749–754.

25. Dische MR, Tsai M, Baltaxe HA. Solitary interruption of the aortic arch of the aorta. Clinicopathologic review of eight cases. *Am J Cardiol* 1975;35:271–277.

26. Roberts WC, Morrow AG, Braunwald E. Complete interruption of the aortic arch. *Circulation* 1962;26:39–59.

27. Becu LM, Tauxe WN, DuShane JW, Edwards JE. A complex of congenital cardiac anomalies: ventricular septal defect, biventricular origin of the pulmonary trunk, and subaortic stenosis. *Am Heart J* 1955;50:901–911.

28. Kleinerman J, Yang W, Hackel DB, Kaufman N. Absence of transverse aortic arch. *Arch Pathol* 1958;65:490–498.

29. Garcia OL, Hernandez FA, Tamer D, Poole C, Gelband H, Castellanos AW. Congenital bilateral subclavian steal. Ductus-dependent symptoms in interrupted aortic arch associated with ventricular septal defect. *Am J Cardiol* 1979;44:101–104.

30. Pierpont MEM, Zollikofer CL, Moller JH, Edwards JE. Interruption of the aortic arch with right descending aorta. A rare condition and a cause of bronchial compression. *Pediatr Cardiol* 1982;2:153–159.

31. Moerman P, Dumolin M, Lauweryns J, Van Der Hauwaert LG. Interrupted right aortic arch in DiGeorge syndrome. *Br Heart J* 1987;58:274–278.

32. Konishi T, Lizima T, Onai K, Kobayashi G, Kawabe M, Anzai T. Persistent fifth aortic arch complicated by coarctation of the aorta and aneurysm of left subclavian artery. *J Jpn Assoc Thorac Surg* 1981;29:1243–1248.

33. Da Costa AG, Iwahashi ER, Atik E, Rati MAN, Ebaid M. Persistence of hypoplastic and recoarcted fifth aortic arch associated with type A aortic arch interruption: surgical and balloon angioplasty results in an infant. *Pediatr Cardiol* 1992;13:104–106.

34. Juri R, Alday LE, De Rossi R. Interrupted fourth aortic arch with persistent fifth aortic arch and aortic coarctation-treatment with balloon angioplasty combined with surgery. *Cardiol Young* 1994;4:304–306.

35. Smallhorn JF, Anderson RH, Macartney FJ. Cross-sectional echocardiographic recognition of interruption of aortic arch between left carotid and subclavian arteries. *Br Heart J* 1982;48:229–235.

36. Riggs TW, Berry TE, Aziz KU, Paul MH. Two-dimensional echocardiographic features or interruption of the aortic arch. *Am J Cardiol* 1982;50:1385–1390.

37. Evans W. Congenital stenosis (coarctation), atresia, and interruption of the aortic arch (a study of twenty-eight cases). *J Med* 1933;2:1–31.

38. Barger JD, Creasman RW, Edwards JE. Bilateral ductus arteriosus associated with interruption of the aortic arch. *Am J Clin Pathol* 1954;24:441–444.

39. Milo S, Massini C, Goor DA. Isolated atresia of the aortic arch in

40. Sharratt GP, Carson P, Sanderson JM. Complete interruption of aortic arch, without persistent ductus arteriosus, in an adult. *Br Heart J* 1975;37:221–224.

41. Ho SY, Wilcox BR, Anderson RH, Lincoln JCR. Interrupted aortic arch—anatomical features of surgical significance. *Thorac Cardiovasc Surg* 1983;31:199–205.

42. Everts-Suarez EA, Carson CP. The triad of congenital absence of aortic arch (isthmus aortae), patent ductus arteriosus and interventricular septal defect—a trilogy. *Ann Surg* 1959;150:153–159.

43. Anderson RH, Lenox CC, Zuberbuhler JR. Morphology of ventricular septal defect associated with coarctation of aorta. *Br Heart J* 1983;50:176–181.

44. Al-Marsafawy HMF, Ho SY, Redington AN, Anderson RH. The relationship of the outlet septum to the aortic outflow tract in hearts with interruption of the aortic arch. *J Thorac Cardiovasc Surg* 1995;109:1225–1236.

45. Moene RJ, Oppenheimer-Dekker A, Wenink ACG. Relation between aortic arch hypoplasia of variable severity and central muscular ventricular septal defects: emphasis on associated left ventricular abnormalities. *Am J Cardiol* 1981;48:111–116.

46. Moulaert AJ, Oppenheimer-Dekker A. Anterolateral muscle bundle of the left ventricle, bulboventricular flange and subaortic stenosis. *Am J Cardiol* 1976;37:78–81.

47. Bove EL, Minich LL, Pridjian AK, et al. The management of severe subaortic stenosis, ventricular septal defect, and aortic arch obstruction in the neonate. *J Thorac Cardiovasc Surg* 1993;105:289–296.

48. Geva T, Hornberger LK, Sanders SP, Jonas RA, Ott DA, Colan SD. Echocardiographic predictors of left ventricular outflow tract obstruction after repair of interrupted aortic arch. *J Am Coll Cardiol* 1993;22:1953–1960.

49. Devloo-Blancquaert A, Titus JL, Edwards JE, Vallaeys JHJ, De Gezelle HRM, Coppens M. Interruption of the aortic arch and hypoplastic left heart syndrome. *Pediatr Cardiol* 1995;16:304–308.

50. Mehrizi A, Morrish HF. Interruption of the aortic arch. *Bull Johns Hopkins Hosp* 1962;111:127–142.

51. Bowers DE, Schiebler GL, Krovetz LJ. Interruption of the aortic arch with complete transposition of the great vessels. Hemodynamic and angiocardiographic data of a case diagnosed during life. *Am J Cardiol* 1965;16:442–448.

52. Esplugas E. Interruption of the aortic arch—anatomical, clinical and angiocardiographic observations. In: Godman M, Marquis RM, eds. *Paediatric cardiology. Vol. 2. Heart disease in the newborn.* Edinburgh: Churchill Livingstone, 1979:187–195.

53. Alva-Espinosa C, Jimenez-Arteaga S, Diaz-Diaz E, et al. Diagnosis of Berry syndrome in an infant by two-dimensional and color Doppler echocardiography. *Pediatr Cardiol* 1995;16:42–44.

54. Matsushita T, Nakajima T, Kishimoto H. Interruption of aortic arch associated with pulmonary valve stenosis. *Int J Cardiol* 1995;49:86–88.

55. Jew EW, Gross P. Aortic origin of the right pulmonary artery and absence of the transverse aortic arch. *Arch Pathol* 1952;53:191–194.

CHAPTER 30

Patent Ductus Arteriosus

Lilliam M. Valdes-Cruz and Raul O. Cayre

Patent ductus arteriosus is a congenital cardiac anomaly resulting from persistence of the ductus arteriosus, a vascular structure that in the fetus connects the pulmonary artery and the descending aorta. The first description of the ductus arteriosus was by Galen (A.D. 129–200), who described in the fetus a "small, third vessel" (ductus arteriosus) connecting the "venous artery" (pulmonary artery) with the "arteria magna" (aorta) (1,2). In addition, Galen mentioned that, after birth, all parts of the body grow, but that the ductus arteriosus not only does not grow but becomes progressively thinner and in the course of time wastes entirely away and dries up (1,2). The first mention of the term ductus arteriosus appeared in a book by Arantius, *De humano foetu libellus*, published in 1595 (3). In 1628, Harvey (4) mentioned that when the heart contracts in the embryo, blood is continually propelled through the arterial canal (ductus arteriosus) from the right ventricle to the aorta. The term "ductus of Botal" is improper because that author described the persistence of a foramen ovale as a large ductus; through a series of misinterpretations and incorrect translations, this was confused with the ductus arteriosus (5). Rokitansky (6,7) was the first to consider a patent ductus arteriosus as an isolated congenital malformation; Peacock (8) described cases of patent ductus arteriosus associated with complex congenital anomalies.

The incidence of an isolated patent ductus arteriosus varies between 4.7% and 12% of all cases of congenital heart disease (9–12) and reaches 17.8% to 20% in patients living at elevations over 9,900 feet (13). In premature infants, the incidence of a patent ductus is even higher. In infants weighing less than 1,750 g, the overall incidence of a hemodynamically significant ductus is 20.2%; in those weighing between 1,500 and 1,750 g, the incidence is 7%, and it is up to 42% in those weighing less than 1,000 g (14).

EMBRYOLOGIC CONSIDERATIONS

The ductus arteriosus is intimately related to the development of the aortic arches. Its presence in the fetus represents persistence of the distal portion of the left sixth aortic arch (see Fig. 1-16). Persistence of the distal portion of the right sixth aortic arch results in a right-sided ductus, whereas persistence of the distal portion of both the right and left sixth aortic arches gives rise to bilateral ducti.

Persistence of a ductus arteriosus as an isolated congenital anomaly results when it fails to close after birth. Functional ductal closure occurs from 10 to 15 hours after birth (15,16), and anatomic closure occurs in the second to third week of life (17). By 1 year of age, closure has occurred in 98.8% of children (18).

The processes by which the initial ductal closure takes place are not completely known. As mentioned by Langer in 1857, the ductus is similar to a muscular artery but differs histologically from the pulmonary artery and the aorta in having fewer elastic fibers and more muscular tissue (19). Generally, it is considered that the wall of the ductus comprises a thin adventitial layer in which are found vasa vasorum and nerve fibers, a media characterized by the presence of smooth-muscle fibers arranged spirally and few thin elastic fibers, and an intima made up of a thin layer of smooth endothelial cells, muscle fibers, and collagen; the intima is separated from the media by an internal elastic lamina (20–24). The primary mechanism of the functional closure of the ductus is the contraction of the spiral muscular fibers within its walls, caused by the increase in Pa_{O2} occurring immediately after birth (25–32). The response of the muscular fibers of the ductal wall is greater later in gestation, with a weak response in premature infants (27–32). The fact that the muscular layer of the ductus extends slightly into the wall of the pulmonary artery and the elastic tissue into the aortic wall could explain why ductal closure starts at the pulmonary end (33).

Prostaglandins, products of the metabolism of arachidonic acid, are potent vasoactive agents that keep the ductus open during fetal life (31,32,34–42). Prostaglandin E_2 (PGE_2) is the most potent for maintaining ductal permeability (32,40,43,44). The actual site of production of PGE$_2$ is not known. It has been postulated that PGE$_2$ may be produced locally within the ductal wall to act on the smooth-muscle fibers (32,41,42), and also in the placenta (32). Diminution in the levels of PGE$_2$ after placental extraction and inactivation in the lungs have also been mentioned as possible mechanisms contributing to the initial ductal constriction after birth (32).

The reason why infants recovering from respiratory distress syndrome have a greater incidence of patent ductus than those without respiratory distress is not known. Factors may include less cholinergic innervation of the ductus and/or diminution of the ductal response to oxygen (45).

In addition to functional closure, an active morphologic process contributes to anatomic closure. This is characterized by fragmentation of the internal elastic membrane, proliferation of the intima with formation of cushions that protrude into the ductal lumen, medial proliferation, and formation of mucoid lakes in the intima and internal third of the media, resulting in a hyaline mass that totally occludes the ductal lumen (22–24). In general, the process of ductal closure is complete by the first year of life (17,18,21), which explains why certain authors believe that patency after 1 year of age should be considered persistence of the ductus arteriosus (18,21,23).

The patent ductus arteriosus seen in infants with rubella syndrome differs histologically from the normal ductus, so it is considered that persistence in these cases is caused by an abnormal ductal wall. The wall is thinner, the internal elastic lamina is absent or poorly developed, intimal proliferation is completely absent, and there is moderate replacement of muscular and elastic tissue by collagen tissue (21,46).

ANATOMIC AND ECHOCARDIOGRAPHIC CONSIDERATIONS

The echocardiographic study of patent ductus arteriosus should determine (a) morphologic characteristics, location, and size of the ductus; (b) characteristics of the flow across the ductus; and (c) the types of associated anomalies. Echocardiographic study includes intraoperative and postoperative evaluation.

Morphologic Characteristics, Location, and Size of the Ductus

The ductus arteriosus is a vascular channel that originates from the posterosuperior aspect of the pulmonary arterial trunk at the level of the bifurcation or from the left pulmonary branch immediately after the bifurcation. It is directed posteriorly and slightly to the left toward the anterolateral wall of the aorta, which it joins at the junction of the aortic isthmus with the descending aorta.

It is distal and opposite to the site of drainage of the left subclavian artery (Fig. 30-1). In newborns, the ductus assumes a position that is more closely parallel to the aortic arch and forms a more acute angle with the aortic isthmus (47).

The ductus is almost always located on the left side in the presence of a left aortic arch (Fig. 30-1). Rarely, the ductus is on the left in the presence of a right aortic arch, in which case the ductus connects the left innominate artery or the left subclavian artery with the left pulmonary artery (48,49). The ductus is less commonly located on the right in the presence of a left aortic arch, between the right innominate artery or the right subclavian artery and the right pulmonary artery (48,50). Rarely, the ductus is found between the superior portion of the descending aorta and the right pulmonary artery in the presence of a right aortic arch (48,49). The presence of bilateral ducti with left aortic arch, right aortic arch, or double aortic arch has also been reported (48,51–53).

The size and length of the ductus are variable; it can be long and narrow, long and tortuous, or short and wide. Usually, it is equal to or larger in size than the descending aorta, and its length can range from a few millimeters to up to 1.8 cm (3). The shape of the ductus also varies. It can be cylindrical, having the same width throughout its length; hourglass-shaped, with a medial constriction; funnel-shaped, with the aortic end wider than the pulmonary end; or it can be aneurysmal. In this latter case, the

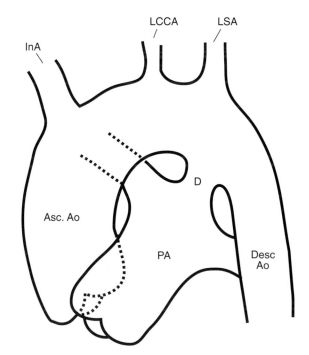

FIG. 30-1. Schematic drawing demonstrating the anatomic location of the ductus arteriosus. *Asc Ao*, ascending aorta; *Desc Ao*, descending aorta; *D*, ductus arteriosus; *PA*, pulmonary artery; *InA*, innominate artery; *LCCA*, left common carotid artery; *LSA*, left subclavian artery.

aortic end is always open, and the pulmonary end can be either open or closed (54–60). In infants under 2 months of age, the ductal aneurysm is fusiform in 83%, saccular in 5%, and dissecting in 12% of cases (60). Complications have been reported in 30% of cases, including compression of adjacent structures, rupture, embolism, and infection (54,57,59,60). Spontaneous resolution of a ductal aneurysm following localized thrombus formation and later fibrosis has been reported (59,60).

The echocardiographic views that allow study of the ductus are the parasternal and subcostal short-axis, the left or right high parasternal or subclavicular, and the suprasternal long- and short-axis views (61–66) (Echo. 30-1; see color plate 102 following p. 364. The best are the suprasternal long-axis and the high left or right parasternal views, with the transducer tilted toward the left or right, depending on which side the ductus is located. The left ductus is seen between the aortic arch and left pulmonary artery (Echo. 30-2; see color plate 103 following p. 364). These same views demonstrate the length, width, and shape of the ductus as well as any aneurysmal dilatation that may be present. Measurement of the ductal diameter by echocardiography has become important in recent years to assess the possibility for transcatheter closure with an umbrella device or a coil (67–70) (Echo. 30-3). These views are also useful for detection of residual shunts. In 41% of patients, a residual shunt can be seen immediately after coil embolization, and in 5%, a residual shunt can be appreciated up to 20 months after the procedure (70).

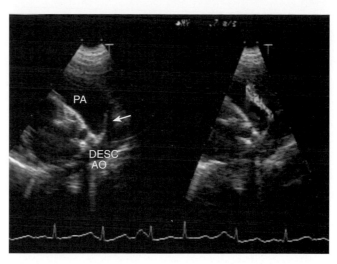

ECHO. 30-2. Left: High left sagittal view of the pulmonary artery and ductus arteriosus (*arrow*). Right: Color Doppler flow map of the left-to-right shunt across the patent ductus arteriosus. *PA*, pulmonary artery; *DESC AO*, descending aorta.

Characteristics of Flow across the Ductus

With normal pulmonary arterial pressure, the higher systemic pressure causes a continuous left-to-right shunt across the ductus. This can be confirmed from the parasternal short-axis, left subclavicular, and suprasternal views with spectral and color Doppler flow mapping (Echo. 30-4). Usually, the flow is seen along the outer or convex wall of the main pulmonary trunk, and it can reach the pulmonary valve. If the pulmonary trunk is dilated, there can be swirling of flow within the pulmonary artery, which is seen as flow away from the transducer (blue) along the inner curvature of the pulmonary

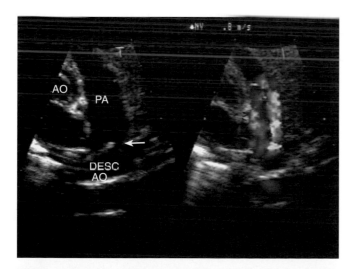

ECHO. 30-1. Parasternal short-axis view in the presence of a patent ductus arteriosus. Left: Anatomic image of the ductus (*arrow*) connecting the pulmonary artery and descending aorta. Right: Color Doppler flow map of a left-to-right shunt across a patent ductus arteriosus. Note the trace pulmonary insufficiency caused by the ductal jet striking the pulmonic valve. *AO*, aorta; *PA*, pulmonary artery; *DESC AO*, descending aorta.

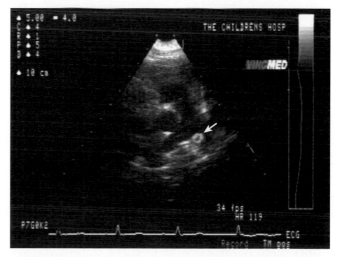

ECHO. 30-3. Parasternal short-axis view of the pulmonary artery showing a coil used to close a patent ductus arteriosus (*arrow*).

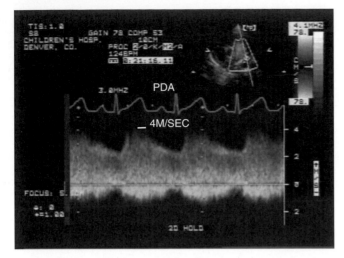

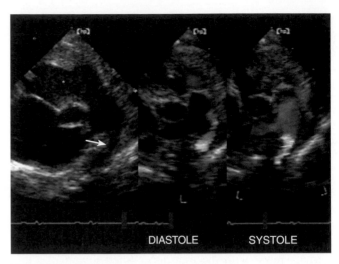

ECHO. 30-4. Spectral Doppler recording of a high-velocity flow across a restrictive ductus arteriosus in the presence of normal pulmonary artery pressures. The flow is continuous in the left-to-right direction because of the higher systemic pressure throughout the cardiac cycle. The velocity peaks at end-systole. *PDA,* patent ductus arteriosus.

ECHO. 30-6. Parasternal short-axis view of a ductus arteriosus in the presence of pulmonary hypertension. **Left:** Anatomic view of the large ductus (*arrow*). Note the dilated pulmonary artery. **Middle:** Color Doppler flow map of the left-to-right shunt across the ductus during diastole. **Right:** Color Doppler flow map of the right-to-left shunt across the ductus in systole.

artery. In the presence of pulmonary valve insufficiency, ductal flow can be seen crossing the valve into the right ventricular outflow tract. As a result of the runoff of flow into the pulmonary circulation, diastolic runoff can be recorded within the descending aorta (Echo. 30-5). If the pulmonary arterial resistance is high, approaching systemic levels, the shunt across the ductus is bidirectional, from right to left during systole and from left to right during diastole (Echos. 30-6, 30-7; see color plate 104 following p. 364). If the pulmonary arterial pressure is higher than the systemic pressure, the shunting can be

exclusively from right to left (reverse ductal shunting) (Echo. 30-8; see color plate 105 following p. 364). The residual shunt seen after device or coil embolization is usually very small, from left to right, and localized at the level of the ductal entrance into the left pulmonary artery.

Spectral Doppler offers a more detailed picture of ductal shunting. Various patterns of flow are seen, depending on the position of the sample volume and level of pulmonary arterial pressure.

With a large ductus and normal pulmonary resistance, the spectral Doppler varies according to the location of

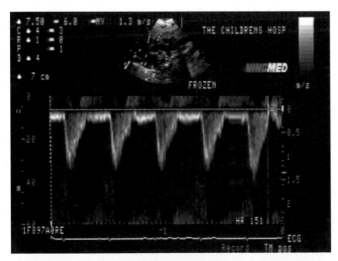

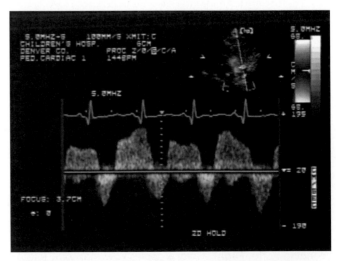

ECHO. 30-5. Spectral Doppler recording of the flow in the descending aorta in the presence of a ductus arteriosus. Note the low-velocity flow during diastole, reflecting the runoff into the pulmonary circulation.

ECHO. 30-7. Spectral Doppler recording of flow across a ductus arteriosus in the presence of elevated pulmonary arterial pressures. Note the left-to-right shunt in diastole and the right-to-left flow in systole. Both velocities are low.

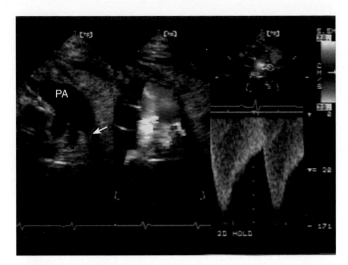

ECHO. 30-8. Patent ductus arteriosus in severe pulmonary hypertension. **Left:** *Arrow* points to the ductus. Note the very dilated main pulmonary artery. **Middle:** Color Doppler map of the flow in the main and proximal pulmonary arterial branches and in the ductus arteriosus. The ductal shunt is from right to left. **Right:** Spectral Doppler recording of the flow across the ductus. Note the continuous right-to-left flow persisting throughout the cardiac cycle. *PA*, pulmonary artery.

the sample volume. If it is inside the ductus or in the pulmonary end, the flow is continuous and of high velocity, peaking at end-systole (71) (Echo. 30-4). If the sample volume is above the pulmonic valve, spectral Doppler tracings demonstrate disturbed, low-velocity systolic flow away from the transducer, representing right ventricular outflow across the pulmonic valve, followed by high-velocity diastolic flow toward the transducer that begins in late systole and continues through diastole. If the sample volume is located in the descending aorta, antegrade systolic flow and retrograde diastolic flow are recorded (Echo. 30-5).

In the presence of a ductus and elevated pulmonary resistance, the spectral Doppler recording within the ductus itself or at its pulmonary arterial end is continuous and of low velocity, peaking in late systole (71) (Echo. 30-7). With higher pulmonary pressures, the diastolic left-to-right flow is abbreviated, and a right-to-left systolic flow starts in late diastole (Echo. 30-8).

Associated Anomalies

A patent ductus arteriosus can be found in isolation or associated with other congenital cardiac anomalies. In some of these latter instances, a patent ductus can be life-saving, and so they are called duct-dependent lesions. Duct-dependent lesions can be grouped as follows: (a) malformations in which the only source of pulmonary blood flow is the ductus, such as pulmonary atresia with

intact ventricular septum, tetralogy of Fallot with pulmonary atresia without systemic-to-pulmonary collaterals, and critical pulmonic valve stenosis of the newborn; (b) malformations in which the systemic flow depends on the permeability of the ductus, such as aortic atresia, hypoplastic left-heart syndrome, interrupted aortic arch, and severe aortic coarctation; and (c) malformations in which the ductus allows a mixture of parallel pulmonary and systemic circulations, such as complete transposition of the great arteries. In all of these instances, patency of the ductus must be maintained through the use of PGE_2. The diagnosis and monitoring of ductal patency before and during PGE_2 infusion have become essential in the management of these patients.

INTRAOPERATIVE AND POSTOPERATIVE EVALUATION

Intraoperative study of the ductus arteriosus is not routinely performed in our center.

Monitoring of residual shunting with transthoracic echocardiography after transcatheter closure of the ductus with a device or coil is routine and has been discussed above.

REFERENCES

1. Galen. De usu partium corporis humani. In: *Opera omnia*, Liber XV, Cap VI. Reprint of edition edited by Kuhn CG. *Claudii Galeni opera omnia. Medicorum Graecorum opera quae exstant.* Leipzig, Germany. Georg Olms Verlagsbuchhandlung Hildesheim, 1822, 1964:241–246.
2. Galen. *On the usefulness of the parts of the body*, Vol 2. Translated from the Greek with an introduction and commentary by Margaret Tallmadge May. Ithaca, NY: Cornell University Press, 1968:670–671.
3. Arantius GC. *De humano foetu libellus 1595.* Cited by Noback GJ, Rehman I. The ductus arteriosus in the human fetus and newborn infant. *Anat Rec* 1941;81:505–527.
4. Harvey W. *Exercitatio anatomica de motu cordis et sanguinis in animalibus.* Francofurti sumptibus Guglielmi Fitzeri 1628. An English translation with annotations by Chauncey D. Leake, 5th ed. Springfield, IL: Charles C Thomas Publisher, 1970:53–60.
5. Franklin KJ. Ductus venosus (Arantii) and ductus arteriosus (Botalli). *Bull Hist Med* 1941;9:580–584.
6. Rokitansky C. *Handbuch der speciellen pathologischen anatomie II Band.* Wien: Braunmuller and Seidel, 1844:387–388. Cited by Marquis RM. The continuous murmur of persistence of the ductus arteriosus—a historical review. *Eur Heart J* 1980;1:465–478.
7. Rokitansky C. *Ueber einige der Wichstigsten Krankheiten der arterien.* Wien: Aus der Kaiserlich-Koniglichen Hof-und Staatsdruckeral, 1852:54–55. Cited by Marquis RM. The continuous murmur of persistence of the ductus arteriosus—a historical review. *Eur Heart J* 1980;1:465–478.
8. Peacock TB. *Malformations of the human heart. With original cases.* Reprint of the edition published in 1858 by J Churchill, London. Boston: Mildford House, 1973.
9. Anderson RC. Causative factors underlying congenital heart malformations. I. Patent ductus arteriosus. *Pediatrics* 1954;14:143–152.
10. Fyler DC, Buckley LP, Hellebrand WE, Cohn HE. Report of the

New England Regional Infant Cardiac Program. *Pediatrics* 1980; 65[Suppl]:375–461.

11. Samanek M, Slavik Z, Zborilova B, Hrobonova V, Voriskova M, Skovranek J. Prevalence, treatment, and outcome of heart disease in live-born children: a prospective analysis of 91,823 live-born children. *Pediatr Cardiol* 1989;10:205–211.

12. Hoffman JIE. Incidence of congenital heart disease: I. Postnatal incidence. *Pediatr Cardiol* 1995;16:103–113.

13. Alzamora-Castro V, Battilana G, Abugattas R, Sialer S. Patent ductus arteriosus and high altitude. *Am J Cardiol* 1960;5:761–763.

14. Nadas AS. Mannheimer Lecture. XVIIIth Annual General Meeting of the Association of European Paediatric Cardiologists, Milan, May 12–15, 1981. *Pediatr Cardiol* 1982;3:71–76.

15. Moss AJ, Emmanouilides G, Duffe ER Jr. Closure of the ductus arteriosus in the newborn infant. *Pediatrics* 1963;32:25–30.

16. Rudolph AM, Scarpelli EM, Golinko RJ, Gootman NL. Hemodynamic basis for clinical manifestations of patent ductus arteriosus. *Am Heart J* 1964;68:447–458.

17. Mitchell SC. The ductus arteriosus in the neonatal period. *J Pediatr* 1957;51:12–17.

18. Christie A. Normal closing time of the foramen ovale and the ductus arteriosus. *Am J Dis Child* 1930;40:323–326.

19. Langer C. Zur anatomie der fotalen kaeislaufsorgane. *Z. Gesell Aertze* 1857;13:328. Cited by Cassels DE. Histology. In: Cassels DE, ed. *The ductus arteriosus.* Springfield, IL: Charles C Thomas Publisher, 1973:37–50.

20. Jager BV, Wollenman OJ Jr. An anatomical study of the closure of the ductus arteriosus. *Am J Pathol* 1942;18:595–613.

21. Cassels DE. *The ductus arteriosus.* Springfield, IL: Charles C Thomas Publisher, 1973.

22. Gittenberger-de Groot AC. Persistent ductus arteriosus: most probably a primary congenital malformation. *Br Heart J* 1977;39:610–618.

23. Ho SY, Anderson RH. Anatomical closure of the ductus arteriosus: a study in 35 specimens. *J Anat* 1979;128:829–836.

24. Gittenberger-de Groot AC, Van Ertbruggen I, Moulaert AJMG, Harinck E. The ductus arteriosus in the preterm infant: histologic and clinical observations. *J Pediatr* 1980;96:88–93.

25. Kennedy JA, Clark SL. Observations on the physiological reactions of the ductus arteriosus. *Am J Physiol* 1942;136:140–147.

26. Moss AJ, Emmanouilides GC, Adams FH, Chuang K. Response of ductus arteriosus and pulmonary and systemic arterial pressure to changes in oxygen environment in newborn infants. *Pediatrics* 1964;33:937–944.

27. McMurphy DM, Heymann MA, Rudolph AM, Melmon KL. Developmental changes in constriction of the ductus arteriosus: responses to oxygen and vasoactive agents in the isolated ductus arteriosus of the fetal lamb. *Pediatr Res* 1972;6:231–238.

28. Oberhansli-Weiss I, Heymann MA, Rudolph AM, Melmon KL. The pattern and mechanisms of response to oxygen by the ductus arteriosus and umbilical artery. *Pediatr Res* 1972;6:693–700.

29. Noel S, Cassin S. Maturation of contractile response of ductus arteriosus to oxygen and drugs. *Am J Physiol* 1976;231:240–243.

30. Clyman RI, Mauray F, Wong L, Heymann MA, Rudolph AM. The developmental response of the ductus arteriosus to oxygen. *Biol Neonate* 1978;34:177–181.

31. Clyman RI, Mauray F, Rudolph AM, Heymann MA. Age-dependent sensitivity of the lamb ductus arteriosus to indomethacin and prostaglandins. *J Pediatr* 1980;96:94–98.

32. Clyman RI, Heymann MA. Pharmacology of the ductus arteriosus. *Pediatr Clin North Am* 1981;28:77–93.

33. Neal WA, Mullet MD. Patent ductus arteriosus in premature infants: a review of current management. *Pediatr Cardiol* 1982;3:59–63.

34. Coceani F, Olley PM, Bodach E. Lamb ductus arteriosus: effects of prostaglandin synthesis inhibitors on the muscle tone and the response to prostaglandin E₂. *Prostaglandins* 1975;9:299–308.

35. Sharpe GL, Larsson KS. Studies on closure of the ductus arteriosus. X. *In vivo* effects of prostaglandin. *Prostaglandins* 1975;9:703–719.

36. Sharpe GL, Larsson KS, Thalme B. Studies on closure of the ductus arteriosus. XII. *In utero* effect of indomethacin and sodium salicylate in rats and rabbits. *Prostaglandins* 1975;9:585–596.

37. Heymann MA, Rudolph AM. Effects of acetylsalicylic acid on the ductus arteriosus and circulation in fetal lambs in utero. *Circ Res* 1976;38:418–422.

38. Friedman WF, Hirschklau MJ, Printz MP, Pitlick PT, Kirkpatrick SE. Pharmacologic closure of patent ductus arteriosus in the premature infant. *N Engl J Med* 1976;295:526–529.

39. Heymann MA, Rudolph AM, Silverman NH. Closure of the ductus arteriosus in premature infants by inhibition of prostaglandin synthesis. *N Engl J Med* 1976;295:530–533.

40. Clyman RI, Brett C, Mauray F. Circulating prostaglandin E₂ concentrations and incidence of patent ductus arteriosus in preterm infants with respiratory distress syndrome. *Pediatrics* 1980;66:725–729.

41. Coceani F, Olley PM. Role of prostaglandins, prostacyclin, and thromboxanes in the control of prenatal patency and postnatal closure of the ductus arteriosus. *Semin Perinatol* 1980;4:109–113.

42. Clyman RI. Ontogeny of the ductus arteriosus response to prostaglandins and inhibitors of their synthesis. *Semin Perinatol* 1980;4:115–124.

43. Coceani F, Bodach E, White E, Bishai I, Olley PM. Prostaglandin I₂ is less relaxant than prostaglandin E₂ on the lamb ductus arteriosus. *Prostaglandins* 1978;15:551–556.

44. Clyman RI, Mauray F, Roman C, Rudolph AM. PGE₂ is a more potent vasodilator of the lamb ductus arteriosus than is either PGI₂ or 6 keto PGF₁α. *Prostaglandins* 1978;16:259–264.

45. Neal WA, Bessinger FB Jr, Hunt CE, Lucas RV Jr. Patent ductus arteriosus complicating respiratory distress syndrome. *J Pediatr* 1975;86:127–131.

46. Swan C. A study of three infants dying from congenital defects following maternal rubella in the early stages of pregnancy. *J Pathol* 1944;56:289–295.

47. Mancini AJ. A study of the angle formed by the ductus arteriosus with the descending thoracic aorta. *Anat Rec* 1951;109:535–539.

48. Stewart JR, Kincaid OW, Edwards JE. *An atlas of vascular rings and related malformations of the aortic arch system.* Springfield, IL: Charles C Thomas Publisher, 1964.

49. Knight L, Edwards JE. Right aortic arch. Types and associated cardiac anomalies. *Circulation* 1974;50:1047–1051.

50. Heinrich WD, Perez Tamayo R. Left aortic arch and right descending aorta. Case report. *Am J Roentgenol* 1956;76:762–766.

51. Kelsey JR Jr, Gilmore CE, Edwards JE. Bilateral ductus arteriosus representing persistence of each sixth aortic arch. Report of a case in which there were associated isolated dextrocardia and ventricular septal defects. *Arch Pathol* 1953;55:154–161.

52. Barger JD, Bregman EH, Edwards JE. Bilateral ductus arteriosus with right aortic arch and right-sided descending aorta. Report of case. *Am J Roentgenol* 1956;76:758–761.

53. Freedom RM, Moes CAF, Pelech A, et al. Bilateral ductus arteriosus (or remnant): an analysis of 27 patients. *Am J Cardiol* 1984;53:884–891.

54. Falcone MW, Perloff JK, Roberts WC. Aneurysm of the nonpatent ductus arteriosus. *Am J Cardiol* 1972;29:422–426.

55. Heikkinen ES, Simila S, Laitinen J, Larmi T. Infantile aneurysm of the ductus arteriosus. Diagnosis, incidence, pathogenesis, and prognosis. *Acta Paediatr Scand* 1974;63:241–248.

56. Rutishauser M, Ronen G, Wyler F. Aneurysm of the nonpatent ductus arteriosus in the newborn. *Acta Paediatr Scand* 1977;66:649–651.

57. Fripp RR, Whitman V, Waldhausen JA, Boal DK. Ductus arteriosus aneurysm presenting as pulmonary artery obstruction: diagnosis and management. *J Am Coll Cardiol* 1985;6:234–236.

58. Jesseph JM, Mahony L, Girod DA, Brown JW. Ductus arteriosus aneurysm in infancy. *Ann Thorac Surg* 1985;40:620–622.

59. Malone PS, Cooper SG, Elliot M, Kiely EM, Spitz L. Aneurysm of the ductus arteriosus. *Arch Dis Child* 1989;64:1386–1388.

60. Lund JT, Hansen D, Brocks V, Jensen MB, Jacobsen JR. Aneurysm of the ductus arteriosus in the neonate: three case reports with a review of the literature. *Pediatr Cardiol* 1992;13:222–226.

61. Sahn DJ, Allen HD. Real-time cross-sectional echocardiographic imaging and measurement of the patent ductus arteriosus in infants and children. *Circulation* 1978;58:343–354.

62. Allen HD, Goldberg SJ, Valdes-Cruz LM, Sahn DJ. Use of echocardiography in newborns with patent ductus arteriosus: a review. *Pediatr Cardiol* 1982;3:65–70.

63. Smallhorn JF, Huhta JC, Anderson RH, Macartney FJ. Suprasternal

cross-sectional echocardiography in assessment of patent ductus arteriosus. *Br Heart J* 1982;48:321–330.

64. Huhta JC, Cohen M, Gutgesell HP. Patency of the ductus arteriosus in normal neonates: two-dimensional echocardiography versus Doppler assessment. *J Am Coll Cardiol* 1984;4:561–564.

65. Rigby ML, Pickering D, Wilkinson A. Cross sectional echocardiography in determining persistent patency of the ductus arteriosus in preterm infants. *Arch Dis Child* 1984;59:341–345.

66. Vick GW III, Huhta JC, Gutgesell HP. Assessment of the ductus arteriosus in preterm infants utilizing suprasternal two-dimensional/Doppler echocardiography. *J Am Coll Cardiol* 1985;5:973–977.

67. Gray DT, Fyler DC, Walker AM, Weinstein MC, Chalmers TC. Clinical outcomes and costs of transcatheter as compared with surgical closure of patent ductus arteriosus. *N Engl J Med* 1993;329:1517–1523.

68. Lloyd TR, Fedderly R, Mendelsohn AM, Sandhu SK, Beekman RH III. Transcatheter occlusion of patent ductus arteriosus with Gianturco coils. *Circulation* 1993;88:1412–1420.

69. Moore JW, George L, Kirkpatrick SE, et al. Percutaneous closure of the small patent ductus arteriosus using occluding spring coils. *J Am Coll Cardiol* 1994;23:759–765.

70. Shim D, Fedderly RT, Beekman RH III, et al. Follow-up of coil occlusion of patent ductus arteriosus. *J Am Coll Cardiol* 1996;28:207–211.

71. Hatle L, Angelsen B. Pulsed and continuous wave Doppler in diagnosis and assessment of various heart lesions. In Hatle L, Angelsen B, eds. *Doppler ultrasound in cardiology. physical principles and clinical applications*, 2nd ed. Philadelphia: Lea & Febiger, 1985:97–292.

CHAPTER 31

Vascular Rings and Pulmonary Sling

Lilliam M. Valdes-Cruz and Raul O. Cayre

There is a small group of abnormalities of the aortic arches that cause compression of the trachea and/or esophagus. These are the vascular rings and the pulmonary sling, or anomalous origin of the left pulmonary artery from the right pulmonary artery.

VASCULAR RINGS

Vascular rings comprise a group of vascular anomalies resulting from an abnormal development of the aortic arches, in which a partial or complete vascular ring causes compression of the trachea and/or esophagus. The first description of a vascular ring was that of Hommel in 1737, of a double aortic arch (1). The term vascular ring was first used by Gross in 1945 (2). The incidence of vascular rings varies between 0.8% and 1.3% of all cases of congenital heart disease (3–5).

EMBRYOLOGIC CONSIDERATIONS

The morphogenesis of vascular rings is intimately related to the development of the aortic arches (see Fig. 1-16). As the pharyngeal arches appear in a cephalocaudal sequence, along the lateral walls of the pharyngeal gut, the aortic sac contributes a right and a left arterial branch, which connect with the right and left dorsal aortas, respectively. This results in six pairs of arteries, called the aortic arches (6,7) (see Fig. 1-16A). As a consequence of the process of cephalization, the aortic arches undergo a series of transformations (see Fig. 1-16B). The first aortic arch is the first one to disappear, and it persists only as a portion of the maxillary arteries. The second aortic arch also disappears, giving rise to a portion of the stapedial arteries. The third aortic arch contributes to the development of the carotid arteries. The proximal portion becomes the common carotid arteries, and the distal portions, along with the segments of the right and left dorsal

aortas located between the first and second arches, give rise to the internal carotid arteries. The portion of the right and left dorsal aortas located between the third and fourth arches disappears. The transformations of the fourth aortic arch are different on each side. The proximal end of the right fourth arch and an elongation of the right portion of the aortic sac give rise to the right brachiocephalic or innominate artery. The distal portion of the right fourth arch develops into the proximal portion of the right subclavian artery. The distal portion of the right subclavian artery arises from the proximal segment of the caudal portion of the right dorsal aorta and from the seventh right intersegmentary artery. The distal segment of the caudal portion of the right dorsal aorta disappears. On the left side, the fourth arch becomes the transverse arch. The ascending aorta arises from the aortic sac and the descending aorta from the left dorsal aorta. The fifth aortic arch is inconstant, never well developed, and transitory. The sixth arch, in addition to connecting with the right and left dorsal aortas, also connects with the primitive right and left pulmonary arteries, which originate from the pulmonary capillary plexus. The proximal portion of the right sixth aortic arch gives rise to the proximal right pulmonary artery; the distal portion of the right sixth arch disappears. The proximal portion of the left sixth aortic arch gives rise to the left proximal pulmonary artery, and the distal portion of the sixth arch becomes the ductus arteriosus. The pulmonary trunk arises from the aortic sac. The left subclavian artery emerges from the left seventh intersegmentary artery.

Vascular rings are caused either by persistence of a segment of the aortic arches that normally disappears or by regression of a segment that normally remains patent (8–10). The probable morphogenesis of the various types of vascular rings, as proposed by Edwards (8,9), is based on variations of a hypothetical case of double aortic arch and bilateral ductus arteriosus.

Double aortic arch would be caused by normal development of the left fourth aortic arch and normal persistence of the caudal portion of the left dorsal aorta, which gives rise to a left aortic arch, along with abnormal persistence of the caudal portion of the right dorsal aorta, which would result in a right aortic arch (8–11) (Fig. 31-1A).

In cases of vascular ring with left aortic arch and aberrant right subclavian artery, there is normal development of the left fourth aortic arch and caudal portion of the left dorsal aorta. In addition, there is regression of the distal portion of the right fourth aortic arch, which normally gives rise to the proximal right subclavian artery, and a normal regression of the caudal portion of the right dorsal aorta. The right subclavian artery originates from an intersegmentary artery as a fourth branch of the left aortic arch (8–10) (Fig. 31-1B).

Regression of the left fourth aortic arch with persistence of the right fourth aortic arch, regression of a portion of the right dorsal aorta, and persistence of a portion of the

left dorsal aorta results in a right aortic arch with a left superior descending aorta (8–10). Persistence of a left ductus arteriosus or a left ductal ligament completes the vascular ring (Fig. 31-1C).

In cases of a right aortic arch with left retroesophageal ductus arteriosus, there is regression of the left fourth aortic arch and caudal portion of the left dorsal aorta with persistence of the fourth right aortic arch and right dorsal aorta. The left ductus arteriosus connects the left pulmonary artery with the right descending aorta through a remnant of the left dorsal aorta (8–10). The left ductus may or may not be patent; in the latter case, there is a left ductal ligament between the left pulmonary artery and descending aorta (Fig. 31-1D). When an aberrant left subclavian artery is present, this arises as the last branch of the superior descending aorta, and a left ductus or ductal ligament joins the left pulmonary branch with the left subclavian artery (Fig. 31-1E). This type of vascular ring

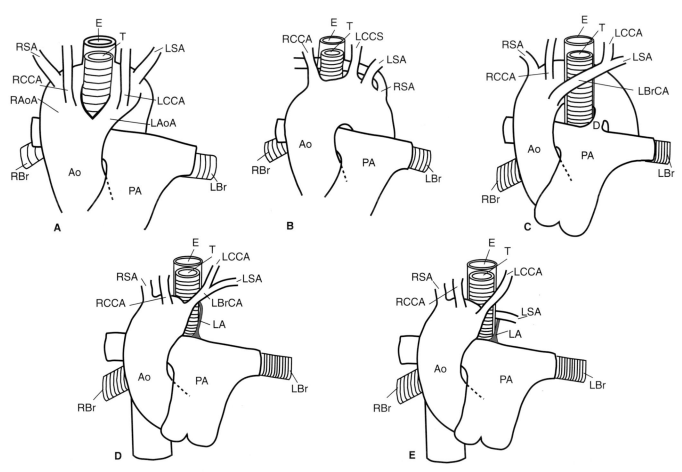

FIG. 31-1. Schematic drawings showing the most common types of vascular rings. **A:** Double aortic arch. **B:** Left aortic arch and aberrant right subclavian artery. **C:** Right aortic arch and left ductus arteriosus or ductal ligament. **D:** Right aortic arch and retroesophageal ductus arteriosus or ductal ligament. **E:** Right aortic arch, aberrant left subclavian artery, and left ductus arteriosus or ductal ligament. *Ao,* aorta; *PA,* pulmonary artery; *D,* ductus arteriosus; *LA,* ligamentum arteriosum; *RAoA,* right aortic arch; *LAoA,* left aortic arch; *RCCA,* right common carotid artery; *LCCA,* left common carotid artery; *RSA,* right subclavian artery; *LSA,* left subclavian artery; *LBrCA,* left brachiocephalic artery; *RBr,* right bronchus; *LBr,* left bronchus; *T,* trachea; *E,* esophagus.

is the result of regression of the left fourth aortic arch between the left carotid artery and left subclavian artery (8–10).

ANATOMIC AND ECHOCARDIOGRAPHIC CONSIDERATIONS

The echocardiographic study of vascular rings should examine (a) the anatomic characteristics of the various types of vascular rings and (b) any associated anomalies.

Anatomic Characteristics of Various Types of Vascular Rings

Double aortic arch (Fig. 31-1A) is the most common type of vascular ring, with an incidence of 33% to 73% of all cases of vascular rings (12–23). There are two patent aortic arches in 40% to 58% of cases and one atretic arch in 42% to 60% of reported cases (20,22,23). The ascending aorta is normally located, and it divides in front of the trachea into a right and a left arch. The right aortic arch is higher than the left, crosses above the right main bronchus, borders the right lateral wall of the trachea and the right lateral and posterior walls of the esophagus, and becomes continuous with the descending aorta, fused with the left aortic arch. At the point of union of the right arch with the descending aorta, there is frequently a small aortic diverticulum, which represents the posterior remnant of the left aortic arch (24). This diverticulum, also seen in cases of atresia of one of the arches, is called the diverticulum of Kommerell. The left aortic arch is inferior to the right arch; it crosses in front of the trachea and above the left main bronchus, borders the left lateral walls of the trachea and esophagus, and joins the right aortic arch posteriorly to become continuous with the descending aorta. The aorta descends on the left or slightly to the right of its usual position. The right aortic arch gives rise to the right common carotid artery and the right subclavian artery; the left arch gives rise to the left common carotid artery and the left subclavian artery. Usually, there is a ductus arteriosus or ductal ligament between the left pulmonary branch and left aortic arch (8,11,13,14,20,25–27). Edwards (8,24) classifies this type of double aortic arch with left descending aorta and left ductus arteriosus or ductal ligament as group I aortic arch anomalies. He also considers that there could exist a hypothetical case of double aortic arch with right descending aorta and a ductus or ductal ligament between the right pulmonary artery and the right aortic arch; he considers these as group II (8,24). Rarely, both arches are of the same size. More commonly, in 64% to 81% of reviewed cases, the right arch was larger than the left (12,13,16,18,20,22). In the remaining 19% to 36% of reported cases, the left arch was larger than the right (12,13,16,18,20,22).

Left aortic arch with aberrant right subclavian artery and a left ductus arteriosus or ligamentum arteriosum (Fig. 31-1B) is seen in 11% to 19% of all cases of vascular rings (13,14,20,22,23). The first case of aberrant subclavian artery was reported by Hunauld in 1735 (28). The term *disphagia lusoria* was utilized by Bayford in 1794 (29) to describe the symptoms of this type of vascular anomaly. The ascending aorta and left aortic arch are in their normal positions. An aberrant right subclavian artery arises either as a fourth branch of the aortic arch, beyond the origin of the left subclavian artery, or from the superior part of the descending aorta and courses toward the right, with a retroesophageal trajectory. An incomplete vascular ring is formed between the right common carotid artery and left aortic arch, which cross in front of the trachea, and the aberrant right subclavian artery, which courses behind the esophagus to cause dysphagia (dysphagia lusoria) rather than actual tracheoesophageal obstruction (8–10,15).

Right aortic arch and left ductus arteriosus or ductal ligament (Fig. 31-1C) is seen in 3% to 18% of all cases of vascular rings (3,12,20,22,23) and in 5.5% of all cases of right aortic arch (30). The ascending aorta is normally positioned and is continuous with a right aortic arch, which crosses above the right main bronchus, borders the right lateral wall of the trachea and esophagus, and follows a retroesophageal course to join a left and superior descending aorta. The presence of a left ductus arteriosus or ductal ligament completes the vascular ring.

Right aortic arch and retroesophageal ductus arteriosus (Fig. 31-1D) is seen in 11% of all cases of vascular rings (21). The ascending aorta is found in its normal position and is continuous with a right arch, which crosses above the right main bronchus, borders the right lateral wall of the trachea and esophagus, and joins the right descending aorta. A left ductus arteriosus or ductal ligament borders the left lateral wall of the trachea and esophagus and, after following a retroesophageal course, connects with either the right aortic arch or with the superior part of the right descending aorta beyond the origin of the right subclavian artery, thus forming a complete vascular ring.

Right aortic arch, aberrant left subclavian artery, and left ductus or ductal ligament (Fig. 31-1E) is the second most common type of vascular ring, comprising 22% to 48% of all cases (17,18,20–23). The ascending aorta is normal and continuous with the right aortic arch, which crosses above the right main bronchus and borders the right lateral walls of the trachea and esophagus to join the right descending aorta. The aberrant left subclavian artery emerges from the right aortic arch or from the superior part of the right descending aorta, beyond the origin of the right subclavian artery, and is directed to the left, coursing behind the esophagus. The vascular ring is completed by the presence of a left ductus arteriosus or ductal ligament between the left pulmonary artery and the aberrant left subclavian artery.

Left aortic arch with retroesophageal segment, right ductus arteriosus, and right descending aorta was described as a single case by Edwards in 1948 (31) and is very rare. The ascending aorta was continuous with a left aortic arch, which crossed above the left main bronchus, bordered the lateral left walls of the trachea and esophagus, and was directed toward the right, coursing behind the esophagus to join a right descending aorta. A ductal ligament connecting the right pulmonary artery with the descending aorta beyond the origin of the right subclavian artery completed the ring.

The echocardiographic study of vascular rings is approached from the suprasternal notch long- and short-axis views, the parasternal short-axis view, and the subcostal long-axis view (16,17,27,32–35). It is important to determine the presence of a left- or right-sided aortic arch or of a double arch. The suprasternal long-axis view and the high parasternal long-axis view allow visualization of the ascending aorta, a left arch, and the descending aorta. Inability to image the arch from this view usually suggests the presence of a right aortic arch, which can be brought into view by rotating the transducer counterclockwise approximately 30 degrees and aiming it to the patient's right. In cases of double aortic arch, the standard suprasternal long-axis view images the left-sided arch, and a rotation similar to that for a right aortic arch would demonstrate the right-sided arch (Echos. 31-1–31-3; see color plates 106 and 107 following p. 364). Also, sweeping the transducer anteriorly to posteriorly in a standard suprasternal long-axis position is useful to demonstrate the two arches (16). The subcostal long-axis view shows the double arch when the transducer is angled superiorly toward the two outflow tracts, where the ascending aorta

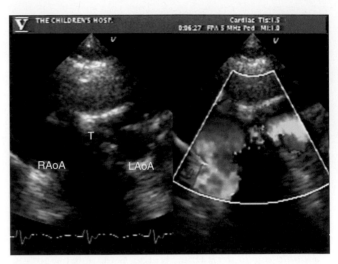

ECHO. 31-2. Suprasternal short-axis view demonstrating the two arches bifurcating from the aorta. *RAoA,* right aortic arch; *LAoA,* left aortic arch; *T,* trachea.

can be seen bifurcating into a right and a left arch (27). Visualization of position of the aorta relative to the echogenic, air-filled trachea from the parasternal short-axis or high parasternal view (32) or relative to the esophagus during ingestion of fluids from the suprasternal view (33) has been utilized to determine arch sidedness. In cases of right aortic arch with retroesophageal course and a left descending aorta, the image of the aortic arch can be confused with that of a normal left-sided arch; therefore, visualization of the first brachiocephalic vessel coursing toward the left and superiorly would indicate that the aortic arch is right-sided (34) (Echo. 31-4).

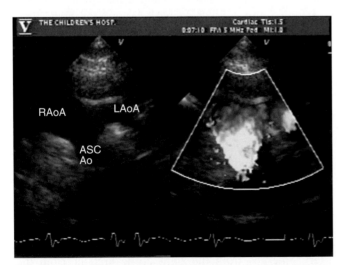

ECHO. 31-1. Short-axis suprasternal view aimed anteriorly demonstrating a double aortic arch. A segment of the ascending aorta is seen with the two arches emerging from it. The right arch is larger than the left. *ASC AO,* ascending aorta; *RAOA,* right aortic arch; *LAOA,* left aortic arch.

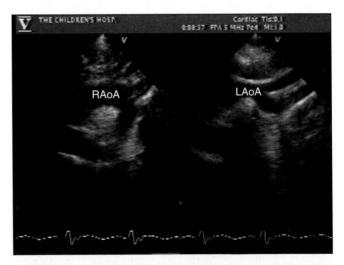

ECHO. 31-3. Suprasternal long-axis view demonstrating the length of the two aortic arches. **Left:** Right aortic arch seen by rotating the transducer toward the right. **Right:** Left aortic arch imaged from a standard transducer position. *RAoA,* right aortic arch; *LAoA,* left aortic arch.

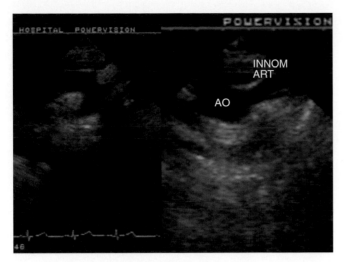

ECHO. 31-4. Suprasternal view of a right aortic arch. **Left:** Long-axis view obtained by rotating the transducer 30 degrees counterclockwise and aiming toward the patient's right. **Right:** Suprasternal short-axis view demonstrating the first brachiocephalic vessel coursing toward the left and superiorly. *INNOM ART,* innominate artery; *AO,* aorta.

Associated Anomalies

Double aortic arch has been associated with ventricular septal defect (14,20), coarctation of the aorta (16,20), aortic atresia (16), tetralogy of Fallot (14), and partial atrioventricular septal defect (13).

Right aortic arch, aberrant left subclavian artery, and left ductus or ductal ligament has been seen in association with ventricular septal defect (20).

Right aortic arch and left ductus arteriosus or ductal ligament has been seen with ventricular septal defect (13), partial atrioventricular septal defect (13), and tetralogy of Fallot (30).

Left aortic arch with aberrant right subclavian artery and left ductus or ductal ligament has been found with valvular pulmonic stenosis (13).

Left aortic arch with retroesophageal course and a right descending aorta has been seen with tetralogy of Fallot (36), coarctation of the aorta (36), ventricular septal defect (36), atrial septal defect (36), valvular pulmonic stenosis (36), double-outlet right ventricle (36), aberrant right subclavian artery (36), and absence of the left pulmonary artery branch (37).

PULMONARY SLING

Pulmonary sling or anomalous left pulmonary artery is a rare malformation of the aortic arches in which the left pulmonary artery originates from the right pulmonary artery. The first case of this type of malformation was reported by Glaevecke and Doehle in 1897 (38). Contro et al. in 1958 called it vascular sling (39). The incidence of pulmonary sling varies between 3% and 6% of all anomalies of the aortic arches (14,15,19,20,23).

EMBRYOLOGIC CONSIDERATIONS

The proximal portions of the right and left pulmonary arteries originate from the right and left sixth aortic arches, respectively. The distal portions are formed from the primitive right and left pulmonary arteries, which originate from the pulmonary capillary plexus (see Fig. 1-16B).

The embryologic origin of pulmonary sling is not clearly known. It has been postulated that it can be the result of absence of development of the left sixth aortic arch, which normally gives rise to the proximal portion of the left pulmonary artery. The vascular supply to the left lung would be accomplished through an anomalous vessel originating from the sixth right aortic arch (40,41). For this reason, some consider that an anomalous left pulmonary branch is not truly a left pulmonary artery but a collateral vessel or an aberrant branch of the right pulmonary artery (10,15).

ANATOMIC AND ECHOCARDIOGRAPHIC CONSIDERATIONS

The echocardiographic study of pulmonary sling should consider the (a) the anatomic characteristics of the malformation and (b) any associated anomalies.

Anatomic Characteristics of the Malformation

In pulmonary sling, the main pulmonary trunk is normally located and continuous with the right pulmonary artery; the left pulmonary artery has an anomalous origin (Fig. 31-2). The left pulmonary artery emerges from the posterior wall of the right pulmonary artery, crosses above the right main bronchus, and is directed to the left, crossing between the trachea and esophagus to reach the left hilum in the usual manner. Gikonyo et al. (42) reported a case of partial pulmonary sling in which the left upper lobe was supplied by an accessory left pulmonary artery emerging from the main pulmonary trunk but the rest of the left lung was supplied by the anomalous left pulmonary artery originating from the right pulmonary artery.

The echocardiographic study of pulmonary sling can be accomplished from the subcostal long- and short-axis views and the parasternal short-axis view (43,44) (Echos. 31-5, 31-6; see color plate 108 following p. 364). Absence of the normal bifurcation of the main pulmonary trunk with absence of the left branch is characteristic of this anomaly. Further, the presence of an echo-free zone in the posterior wall of the right pulmonary artery is sugges-

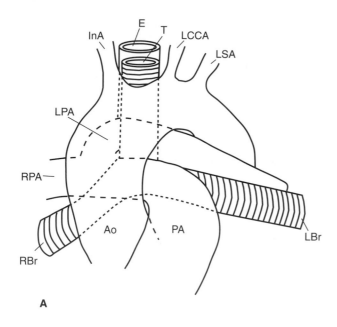

A

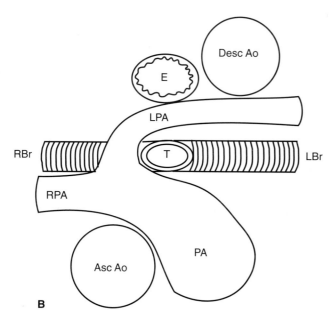

B

FIG. 31-2. Schematic drawings of pulmonary artery sling. **A:** Origin of the left pulmonary artery from the right pulmonary artery. **B:** Relationship of the left pulmonary artery to the trachea and esophagus. *Ao*, aorta; *Asc Ao*, ascending aorta; *Desc Ao*, descending aorta; *PA*, pulmonary artery; *RPA*, right pulmonary artery; *LPA*, left pulmonary artery; *InA*, innominate artery; *LCCA*, left common carotid artery; *LSA*, left subclavian artery; *RBr*, right bronchus; *LBr*, left bronchus; *T*, trachea; *E*, esophagus.

tive of anomalous origin of the left pulmonary branch. Color Doppler flow mapping is of great utility to demonstrate flow from the right to the left pulmonary artery (Echo. 31-6). In cases in which the echogenic, air-filled trachea can be demonstrated, it is found to the left of the site of anomalous origin of the left branch from the right pulmonary artery (Echos. 31-5, 31-6). Echocardiographic

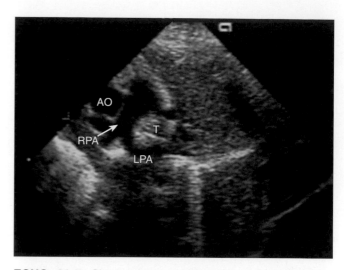

ECHO. 31-5. Short-axis view of the pulmonary arteries in anomalous origin of the left pulmonary artery from the right pulmonary artery (pulmonary sling). The air-filled trachea is seen to the left of the left pulmonary artery. *Arrow* points to the right pulmonary artery. *AO*, aorta; *RPA*, right pulmonary artery; *LPA*, left pulmonary artery; *T*, trachea.

pitfalls in the diagnosis of pulmonary sling include the presence of a large branch of the right pulmonary artery supplying the right upper lobe, simulating a pulmonary sling. A ductus arteriosus or left atrial appendage can also simulate a normally positioned left pulmonary artery (43).

Associated Anomalies

Anomalies that have been found in association with pulmonary sling are patent ductus arteriosus (14,15,19,

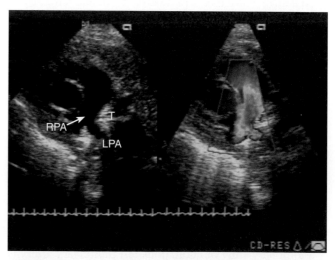

ECHO. 31-6. Short-axis view of a pulmonary sling (same patient as in Echo. 31-5). **Left:** Anatomic image of anomalous origin of the left pulmonary artery from the right pulmonary artery. **Right:** Color Doppler map of the flow in the pulmonary arteries. *RPA*, right pulmonary artery; *LPA*, left pulmonary artery.

20,41,45–47), ventricular septal defect (14,15,19,40, 42,46,48–51), valvular pulmonic stenosis (40,46), quadricuspid pulmonic valve (42), patent foramen ovale (51), atrial septal defect (15,41,42,45,47), partial atrioventricular septal defect (45), bicuspid aortic valve (47), complete transposition of the great arteries (19), tricuspid atresia (19), tetralogy of Fallot (41,45,50), pulmonary atresia (42), truncus arteriosus (42,43), scimitar syndrome (19), left superior vena cava draining into the coronary sinus (19,39,42,45–47), left superior vena cava draining into the left atrium with absence of the coronary sinus (42), aberrant right subclavian artery (19), and atrioventricular univentricular connection with anterior and rightward aorta and posterior and leftward pulmonary artery (39).

REFERENCES

1. Hommel L. Commercium litterarium Norimbergae, 1737:161. Cited by Ekstrom G, Sandblom P. Double aortic arch. Acta Chir Scand 1951–52;102:183–202.
2. Gross RE. Surgical relief for tracheal obstruction from a vascular ring. N Engl J Med 1945;233:586–590.
3. Fontana RS, Edwards JE. Vascular-ring malformations of the aortic arch system: age at death and distribution according to sex of patients in the pathologic material of the Mayo Clinic. In: Fontana RS, Edwards JE, eds. Congenital cardiac disease: a review of 357 cases studied pathologically. Philadelphia: WB Saunders, 1962: 124–125.
4. Fyler DC, Buckley LP, Hellenbrand WE, Cohn HE. Report of the New England Regional Infant Cardiac Program. Pediatrics 1980; 65[Suppl]:375–461.
5. Park SC, Zuberbuhler FR. Vascular ring and pulmonary sling. In: Anderson RH, Macartney FJ, Shinebourne EA, Tynan M. Paediatric cardiology, Vol 2. Edinburgh: Churchill Livingstone, 1987: 1123–1136.
6. Congdon ED. Transformation of the aortic arch system during development of the human embryo. Contrib Embryol 1922;14:47–110.
7. Barry A. Aortic arch derivatives in the human adult. Anat Rec 1951; 111:221–238.
8. Edwards JE. Anomalies of the derivatives of the aortic arch system. Med Clin North Am 1948;32:925–949.
9. Edwards JE. Malformations of the aortic arch system manifested as "vascular rings." Lab Invest 1953;2:56–75.
10. Steward JR, Kincaid OW, Edwards JE. An atlas of vascular rings and related malformations of the aortic arch system. Springfield, IL: Charles C Thomas Publisher, 1964.
11. Ekstrom G, Sandblom P. Double aortic arch. Acta Chir Scand 1951–52;102:183–202.
12. Gross RE, Neuhauser EBD. Compression of the trachea or esophagus by vascular anomalies. Surgical therapy in 40 cases. Pediatrics 1951;7:69–83.
13. Eklof O, Ekstrom G, Eriksson BO, et al. Arterial anomalies causing compression of the trachea and/or the esophagus. A report of 30 symptomatic cases. Acta Paediatr Scand 1971;60:81–89.
14. Binet JP, Langlois J. Aortic arch anomalies in children and infants. J Thorac Cardiovasc Surg 1977;73:248–252.
15. Idriss FS, Nikaidoh H, DeLeon SY, Koopot R. Surgery for vascular anomalies causing obstruction of the trachea and esophagus. In: Tucker BL, Lindesmith GG, eds. First clinical conference on congenital heart disease. New York: Grune & Stratton, 1979:125–156.
16. Murdison KA, Andrews BAA, Chin AJ. Ultrasonographic display of complex vascular rings. J Am Coll Cardiol 1990;15:1645–1653.
17. Lillehei CW, Colan S. Echocardiography in the preoperative evaluation of vascular rings. J Pediatr Surg 1992;27:1118–1121.
18. Chun K, Colombani PM, Dudgeon DL, Haller JA Jr. Diagnosis and management of congenital vascular rings: a 22-year experience. Ann Thorac Surg 1992;53:597–603.
19. Backer CL. Vascular rings, slings, and tracheal rings. Mayo Clin Surg 1993;68:1131–1133.
20. Van Son JAM, Julsrud PR, Hagler DJ, et al. Surgical treatment of vascular rings: the Mayo Clinic experience. Mayo Clin Surg 1993; 68:1056–1063.
21. Kirklin JW, Barrat-Boyes BG. Vascular ring and sling. In: Kirklin JW, Barrat-Boyes BG, eds. Cardiac surgery. Morphology, diagnostic criteria, natural history, techniques, results, and indications, Vol 2, 2nd ed. New York: Churchill Livingstone, 1993:1365–1382.
22. Roberts CS, Biemann Othersen H Jr, Sade RM, Smith CD III, Tagge EP, Crawford FA. Tracheoesophageal compression from aortic arch anomalies: analysis of 30 operatively treated children. J Pediatr Surg 1994;29:334–338.
23. Van Son JAM, Julsrud PR, Hagler DJ, et al. Imaging strategies for vascular rings. Ann Thorac Surg 1994;57:604–610.
24. Edwards JE. "Vascular rings" related to anomalies of the aortic arches. Mod Concepts Cardiovasc Dis 1948;17:19–20.
25. Gordon S. Double aortic arch. J Pediatr 1947;30:428–437.
26. Shaw DL. An aorta with a double arch. JAMA 1897;28:538–540.
27. Sahn DJ, Valdes-Cruz LM, Ovitt TW, et al. Two-dimensional echocardiography and intravenous digital video subtraction angiography for diagnosis and evaluation of double aortic arch. Am J Cardiol 1982;50:342–346.
28. Hunauld. Examen de quelques parties d'un singe. Hist Acad Roy Sci 1735;2:516–523. Cited by Steward JR, Kincaid OW, Edwards JE. An atlas of vascular rings and related malformations of the aortic arch system. Springfield, IL: Charles C Thomas Publisher, 1964.
29. Bayford D. An account of a singular case of obstructed deglutition. Med Soc London Mem 1794;2:275–286. Cited by Steward JR, Kincaid OW, Edwards JE. An atlas of vascular rings and related malformations of the aortic arch system. Springfield, IL: Charles C Thomas Publisher, 1964.
30. Schneeweiss A, Blieden L, Shem-Tov A, Deutsch V, Neufeld HN. Retroesophageal right aortic arch. Pediatr Cardiol 1984;5:191–196.
31. Edwards JE. Retro-esophageal segment of the left aortic arch, right ligamentum arteriosum and right descending aorta causing a congenital vascular ring about the trachea and esophagus. Proc Staff Meet Mayo Clin 1948;23:108–116.
32. Shrivastava S, Berry JM, Einzig S, Bass JL. Parasternal cross-sectional echocardiographic determination of aortic arch sidedness: a new approach. Am J Cardiol 1985;55:1236–1238.
33. Huhta JC. Aortic arch. In: Huhta JC, ed. Pediatric imaging/Doppler ultrasound of the chest: extracardiac diagnosis. Philadelphia: Lea & Febiger, 1986:59–75.
34. Kveselis DA, Snider AR, Dick M II, Rocchini AP. Echocardiographic diagnosis of right aortic arch with a retroesophageal segment and left descending aorta. Am J Cardiol 1986;57:1198–1199.
35. Enderlein MA, Silverman NH, Stanger P, Heymann MA. Usefulness of suprasternal notch echocardiography for diagnosis of double aortic arch. Am J Cardiol 1986;57:359–360.
36. Arisan Ergin M, Jayaram N, LaCorte M. Left aortic arch and right descending aorta: diagnostic and therapeutic implications of a rare type of vascular ring. Ann Thorac Surg 1981;31:82–85.
37. Whitman G, Stephenson LW, Weinberg P. Vascular ring: left cervical aortic arch, right descending aorta, and right ligamentum arteriosum. J Thorac Cardiovasc Surg 1982;83:311–315.
38. Glaevecke, Doehle. Ueber eine seltene angeborene anomalie del pulmonalarterie. Munchen Med Wochenschr 1887;44:950. Cited by Steward JR, Kincaid OW, Edwards JE. An atlas of vascular rings and related malformations of the aortic arch system. Springfield, IL: Charles C Thomas Publisher, 1964.
39. Contro S, Miller RA, White H, Potts WJ. Bronchial obstruction due to pulmonary artery anomalies. I. Vascular sling. Circulation 1958; 17:418–423.
40. Jue KL, Raghib G, Amplatz K, Adams P Jr, Edwards JE. Anomalous origin of the left pulmonary artery from the right pulmonary artery. Report of two cases and review of the literature. Am J Roentgenol 1965;95:598–610.
41. Bamman JL, Ward BH, Woodrum DE. Aberrant left pulmonary artery. Clinical and embryologic factors. Chest 1977;72:67–71.

42. Gikonyo BM, Jue KL, Edwards JE. Pulmonary vascular sling: report of seven cases and review of the literature. *Pediatr Cardiol* 1989; 10:81–89.

43. Yeager SB, Chin AJ, Sanders SP. Two-dimensional echocardiographic diagnosis of pulmonary artery sling in infancy. *J Am Coll Cardiol* 1986;7:625–629.

44. Gnanapragasam JP, Houston AB, Jamieson MPG. Pulmonary artery sling: definitive diagnosis by colour Doppler flow mapping avoiding cardiac catheterisation. *Br Heart J* 1990;63:251–252.

45. Jacobson JH II, Morgan BC, Andersen DH, Humphreys GH II. Aberrant left pulmonary artery. A correctable cause of respiratory obstruction. *J Thorac Cardiovasc Surg* 1960;39:602–612.

46. Lubbers WJ, Tegelaers WHH, Losekoot TG, Becker AE. Aberrant origin of left pulmonary artery (vascular sling). Report of the clinical and anatomic features in three patients. *Eur J Cardiol* 1975;2: 477–483.

47. Sade RM, Rosenthal A, Fellows K, Castaneda AR. Pulmonary artery sling. *J Thorac Cardiovasc Surg* 1975;69:333–346.

48. Lenox CC, Crisler C, Zuberbuhler JR, et al. Anomalous left pulmonary artery. Successful management. *J Thorac Cardiovasc Surg* 1979;77:748–752.

49. Backer CL, Ilbawi MN, Idriss FS, DeLeon SY. Vascular anomalies causing tracheoesophageal compression. Review of experience in children. *J Thorac Cardiovasc Surg* 1989;97:725–731.

50. Murdison KA, Weinberg PM. Tetralogy of Fallot with severe pulmonary valvar stenosis and pulmonary vascular sling (anomalous origin of the left pulmonary artery from the right pulmonary artery). *Pediatr Cardiol* 1991;12:189–191.

51. Ziemer G, Heinemann M, Kaulitz R, Freihorst J, Seidenberg J, Wilken M. Pulmonary artery sling with tracheal stenosis: primary one-stage repair in infancy. *Ann Thorac Surg* 1992;54:971–973.

CHAPTER 32

Anomalies of the Systemic Venous Connection

Lilliam M. Valdes-Cruz and Raul O. Cayre

Anomalies of the systemic venous connections can be observed in hearts with situs solitus, situs inversus, and situs ambiguus. Occurrence of these anomalies with normal (situs solitus) or inverted (situs inversus) atrial arrangement is uncommon, with an incidence of 3.6% (1). They comprise a series of venous malformations, including (a) anomalies of connection of the right superior vena cava, (b) persistence of the left superior vena cava, (c) anomalies of connection of the inferior vena cava, (d) anomalies of the hepatic veins, and (e) anomalies of the coronary sinus.

Anomalies of systemic venous connection associated with visceral heterotaxy are discussed in Chapter 8.

EMBRYOLOGIC CONSIDERATIONS

The right and left common cardinal veins receive the anterior and posterior cardinal veins and drain laterally and cephalically into the sinus venosus. The intercardinal anastomosis permits blood flow between the right and left anterior cardinal veins (see Figs. 1-9–1-11).

The right common cardinal vein and the caudal end of the proximal portion of the right anterior cardinal vein give rise to the superior vena cava. The cephalic end of the proximal portion of the anterior right cardinal vein gives rise to the right brachiocephalic vein, and the intercardinal anastomosis persists as the innominate vein and left brachiocephalic vein (see Fig. 1-9C).

The transverse and proximal portions of the left horn of the sinus venosus give rise to the coronary sinus. The distal portion of the left horn of the sinus venosus and the left common cardinal vein become obliterated, giving rise to the ligament of Marshall. The caudal portion of the left anterior cardinal vein becomes the oblique vein, and the cephalic portion persists as the highest intercostal vein (see Fig. 1-9C).

The vitelline veins or right and left omphalomesenteric veins, before draining into the caudal and medial portions of the sinus venosus, give rise to an anastomotic vascular network at the level of the septum transversum, called the hepatic sinusoids. The proximal portions of the vitelline veins, which connect the hepatic sinusoids with the sinus venosus, are called the right and left hepatocardiac channels (see Fig. 1-10A). The hepatic veins originate from the hepatic sinusoids, and the suprahepatic portion of the inferior vena cava originates from the right hepatocardiac channel (see Fig. 1-10B,C).

Obliteration of the right common cardinal vein, along with obliteration of the proximal portion of the right anterior cardinal vein, will result in the absence of a right superior vena cava. As a consequence, the right brachiocephalic vein will drain into a persistent left superior vena cava via an innominate vein (2).

A connection of the right superior vena cava with the left atrium will be the result of malposition of the right horn of the sinus venosus, which would be found in the cephalic portion of the sinus venosus but displaced toward the left. This causes the right superior vena cava to drain directly into the left atrium (3).

Failure of obliteration of the distal portion of the left horn of the sinus venosus and of the left common cardinal vein, along with persistence of the caudal portion of the left anterior cardinal vein, will result in persistence of a left superior vena cava that drains into the coronary sinus. Failure of development of the sino-atrial fold, which separates the transverse portion and the left horn of the sinus venosus from the left atrium, causes failure of development of the coronary sinus. The persistent left superior vena cava would then drain directly into the left atrium (4).

In the rare case described by Effler et al. (5), with situs solitus, absence of the right inferior vena cava, and presence of a left inferior vena cava in continuation with the azygous venous system, the embryologic explanation might be a failure of development of the right inferior vena cava and development of a left venous system (2). In this case, there would also have been obliteration of the right hepatocardiac channel and drainage of the hepatic veins directly into the right atrium. In instances in which the inferior vena cava drains directly into the left atrium, there would have been obliteration of the right and persistence of the left hepatocardiac channel.

The morphogenetic mechanism causing direct connection of the hepatic veins with the atria or coronary sinus is not completely understood. An anomalous persistence of hepatocardiac channels has been postulated (2).

The embryologic origin of stenosis or atresia of the coronary sinus ostium is not known. It has been proposed that there could be abnormal persistence of the portion of the right valve of the sinus venosus, which would finally give rise to the thebesian valve (6).

ANATOMIC AND ECHOCARDIOGRAPHIC CONSIDERATIONS

The echocardiographic study of anomalies of the systemic venous connection should determine (a) the type of anomalous venous connection and (b) the presence of any associated anomalies, and should include intraoperative and postoperative evaluation.

Type of Anomalous Venous Connection

The various types of anomalous systemic venous connection that can be seen in normal or inverted atrial arrangement (situs solitus or situs inversus, respectively) include anomalies of the right superior vena cava, persistence of the left superior vena cava, and anomalies of the inferior vena cava, hepatic veins, and coronary sinus.

Anomalies of the right superior vena cava comprise absence of the right superior vena cava and direct connection of the right superior vena cava to the left atrium (Fig. 32-1A,B).

Absence of the right superior vena cava with persistence of a left superior vena cava was originally described in 1862 (7) (Fig. 32-1A). The incidence of this malformation in hearts with situs solitus is very low, approximately 0.1% (8). In these cases, the right superior vena cava is totally absent. The right brachiocephalic vein drains through the innominate vein into a persistent left superior vena cava, which usually connects with the coronary sinus, although it can also connect directly with the left atrium if unroofing of the coronary sinus is present (9) (Fig. 32-1A). Rarely, an atretic right superior vena cava can be represented by a fibrous cord (10,11).

Connection of the right superior vena cava to the left atrium is also very rare in hearts with situs solitus (3,12–17). The right superior vena cava is normally situated; however, within the pericardial sac, it is directed toward the left, draining into the roof of the left atrium (Fig.

32-1B). The inferior vena cava drains normally into the right atrium, and no persistent left superior vena cava is seen in the majority of cases (12,14–17). Gueron et al. (13) published a case with an inferior vena cava draining into the left atrium. A case of dilated and tortuous right superior vena cava has been reported by Braudo et al. (12). The interatrial septum can be intact (12,14,17) or can have a patent foramen ovale or an atrial septal defect (13,15,16). A connection of the right superior vena cava with both atria has been reported by Shapiro et al. (18) and by Bharati and Lev (19).

Persistent left superior vena cava is the most commonly observed anomaly of the systemic veins seen in hearts with situs solitus or situs inversus (Fig. 32-1A, C–E). Its incidence varies between 2% and 3% (8,20).

A persistent left superior vena cava draining into a coronary sinus is the most common (Fig. 32-1C). The left superior vena cava receives the left brachiocephalic vein, descends in front of the aortic arch and left pulmonary artery, and is continuous with a dilated coronary sinus, through which it drains into the right atrium. Between 45% and 50% of cases have a venous connection between the two cavae through the innominate vein (1,2). The right superior vena cava and the inferior vena cava drain normally into the right atrium, except in the rare cases of absence or atresia of the right superior vena cava (7–11) (Fig. 32-1A).

A persistent left superior vena cava draining directly into the left atrium (Fig. 32-1D) also descends in front of the aortic arch and left pulmonary artery and drains into the roof of the left atrium between the left upper pulmonary vein and left atrial appendage; the coronary sinus is absent (4,9,21,22). The right superior vena cava and the inferior vena cava drain normally into the right atrium, and the innominate vein is usually present. As a rule, there is a defect in the lower portion of the interatrial septum of the coronary sinus type or an unroofed coronary sinus; however, two cases with an intact interatrial septum have been reported (23,24).

A persistent left superior vena cava draining into the left pulmonary veins is extremely rare (Fig. 32-1E). The first description was reported by Wilson in 1798 (25). McCotter (26) described a case in which the left superior vena cava was connected with the left upper pulmonary vein, which drained into the left atrium at a higher than normal position; the lower left and the right pulmonary veins drained normally (Fig. 32-1E). After reading these two reports, the possibility of these cases actually being partial anomalous drainage of the upper left pulmonary vein into a persistent left superior vena cava cannot be ruled out.

Anomalies of the inferior vena cava in the presence of situs solitus or situs inversus are exceptional and include absence of the suprahepatic segment and drainage into the left atrium (Fig. 32-1F–H).

Absence of the suprahepatic segment and continuation

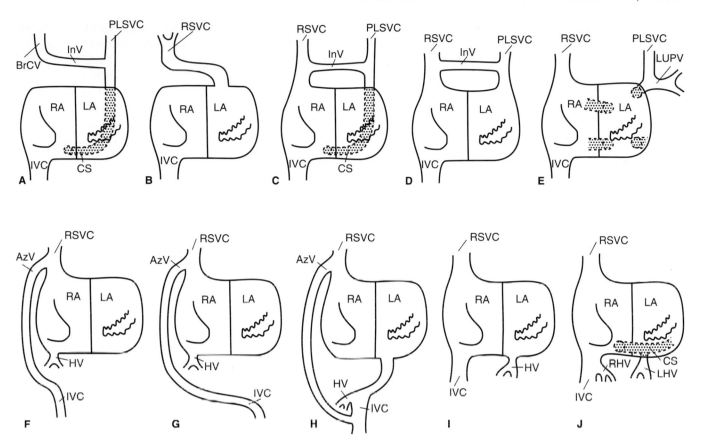

FIG. 32-1. Schematic drawings of the various types of anomalies of the systemic venous connection in hearts with situs solitus. **A:** Absence of the right superior vena cava. **B:** Anomalous connection of the right superior vena cava to the left atrium. **C:** Persistent left superior vena cava draining into the coronary sinus. **D:** Persistent left superior vena cava draining into the left atrium. **E:** Persistent left superior vena cava draining into the left upper pulmonary vein. **F:** Absence of the suprahepatic segment of the inferior vena cava with azygous continuation. **G:** Absence of the suprahepatic segment of the inferior vena cava with leftward thoracic and abdominal segments of the inferior vena cava and azygous continuation. **H:** Inferior vena cava draining into the left atrium. **I:** Total anomalous connection of the hepatic veins to the left atrium. **J:** Partial anomalous connection of the left hepatic vein with the coronary sinus. *BrCV,* brachiocephalic vein; *InV,* innominate vein; *PLSVC,* persistent left superior vena cava; *IVC,* inferior vena cava; *RSVC,* right superior vena cava; *LUPV,* left upper pulmonary vein; *AzV,* azygous vein; *HV,* hepatic veins; *RHV,* right hepatic vein; *LHV,* left hepatic vein; *CS,* coronary sinus; *RA,* right atrium; *LA,* left atrium.

with the azygous venous system (Fig. 32-1F) is seen in the majority of cases of bilateral left-sidedness syndrome and is extremely rare in the presence of situs solitus (1), having an incidence well under 0.3% (27). The suprahepatic portion of the inferior vena cava is absent and there is continuation with the azygous vein, which drains into the superior vena cava. The hepatic veins drain normally into the right atrium. Effler et al. (5) reported a case in which the abdominal and thoracic portions of the inferior vena cava were found on the left side of the spine; at the level of the seventh thoracic vertebra, the vena cava took a rightward direction and became continuous with the azygous vein, which drained into the superior vena cava. The suprahepatic portion of the inferior vena cava was absent, and the hepatic veins drained directly into the right atrium (Fig. 32-1G).

Connection of the inferior vena cava to the left atrium has been rarely reported in the presence of situs solitus (28–31). These authors describe an inferior vena cava that is positioned normally below the diaphragm, but above the diaphragm it is directed toward the left and drains into the left atrium (Fig. 32-1H). The hepatic veins drain into the inferior vena cava, and in all cases a dilated azygous vein drains into the right superior vena cava, which connects normally to the right atrium. The interatrial septum was intact in all cases described. Gueron et al. reported one case of total systemic venous connection with the left atrium, where the right superior vena cava, the inferior vena cava, and the coronary sinus drained into the left atrium and an atrial septal defect was present (13).

Anomalies of the hepatic veins are also very rare in the

presence of situs solitus or situs inversus (Fig. 32-1I,J). In the case reported by Yee (32), there was total anomalous connection of the hepatic veins with the left atrium (Fig. 32-1I). Partial anomalous connection of the left hepatic vein to the coronary sinus was published by Nabarro in 1903 (33) (Fig. 32-1J).

Anomalies of the coronary sinus include atresia of the coronary sinus ostium, connection of the coronary sinus to the inferior vena cava, hypoplasia of the coronary sinus, and unroofed coronary sinus syndrome. The latter is discussed in Chapter 9.

In atresia of the coronary sinus ostium, the coronary sinus is present, but atresia of the ostium into the right atrium results in retrograde drainage of the coronary venous blood into a persistent left superior vena cava. The latter drains either into the right superior vena cava via an innominate vein (34), into the innominate vein only (35), or directly into the left atrium (35).

Connection of the coronary sinus to the inferior vena cava immediately before drainage of the inferior vena cava into the right atrium was reported by Basu in 1932 (36). In this case, a persistent left superior vena cava was connected to the coronary sinus.

Hypoplasia of the coronary sinus usually occurs with coronary veins draining directly into the atrial chambers (35).

The echocardiographic study of anomalies of the right superior vena cava is accomplished by using the subcostal coronal and sagittal (long- and short-axis) views and the suprasternal views. Color Doppler flow mapping demonstrates flow of the right brachiocephalic vein via the innominate vein into the coronary sinus or left atrium in the absence of a right superior vena cava (Echo. 32-1).

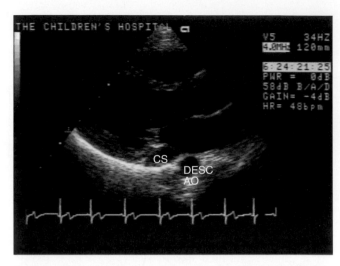

ECHO. 32-2. Parasternal long-axis view demonstrating a dilated coronary sinus. Note the position of the descending aorta, which should not be confused with the coronary sinus. *CS*, coronary sinus; *DESC AO*, descending aorta.

A right superior vena cava draining into the left atrium would also be seen on color Doppler mapping.

A persistent left superior vena cava draining into the coronary sinus is usually suspected when a dilated coronary sinus is seen posterior to the aortic root in the parasternal long-axis view (Echo. 32-2). This can be confirmed from the parasternal and suprasternal notch short-axis views with angulation of the transducer toward the left (Echo. 32-3). Color Doppler would demonstrate flow directed away from the transducer along the left side of

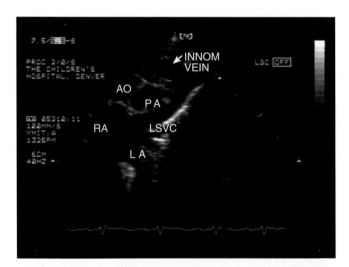

ECHO. 32-1. Suprasternal short-axis view with the transducer aimed to the left to image a persistent left superior vena cava draining into the right atrium. The innominate vein connects to the left superior vena cava. *AO*, aorta; *PA*, pulmonary artery; *INNOM VEIN*, innominate vein; *LSVC*, left superior vena cava; *LA*, left atrium.

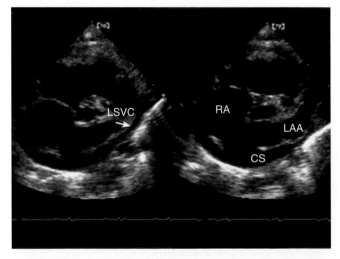

ECHO. 32-3. Parasternal short-axis view of a persistent left superior vena cava draining into the coronary sinus. **Left:** The left superior vena cava courses below the left atrium and drains into the coronary sinus posteriorly. **Right:** The coronary sinus is dilated. The left atrial appendage can be seen from this view and should not be mistaken for a left superior vena cava. *LSVC*, left superior vena cava; *RA*, right atrium; *CS*, coronary sinus; *LAA*, left atrial appendage.

the left atrium. A left superior vena cava draining directly into the roof of the left atrium is seen from the parasternal long- and short-axis views by aiming the transducer superiorly and toward the left, and also from the suprasternal short-axis view by angling the transducer toward the left, as described above for drainage into the coronary sinus. Color Doppler is of considerable help in demonstrating this drainage site (Echo. 32-4; see color plate 109 following p. 364). The short-axis suprasternal view is useful to demonstrate bilateral superior venae cavae and their drainage sites (Echo. 32-5).

Anomalous connections of the inferior vena cava and hepatic veins are best seen from the abdominal and the subcostal views. Cases with azygous or hemiazygous continuation of the inferior vena cava can be documented through the abdominal short-axis view. An azygous vein is seen to the right and posteriorly, and a hemiazygous vein to the left and posterior to the descending aorta (1) (see Echo. 8-10). The drainage of these veins, either into the right superior vena cava or into a persistent left superior vena cava, is appreciated from the suprasternal long- and short-axis views and from the subcostal short-axis view (see Echo. 8-11). Anatomic demonstration can be greatly enhanced with the use of color Doppler flow mapping to document the direction of flow and site of drainage.

Associated Anomalies

Cardiac malformations that have been reported in association with systemic venous anomalies include atrial

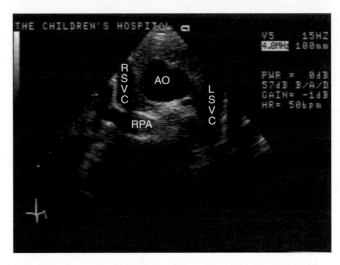

ECHO. 32-5. Suprasternal short-axis view demonstrating the presence of bilateral superior venae cavae. *AO*, aorta; *RSVC*, right superior vena cava; *LSVC*, left superior vena cava; *RPA*, right pulmonary artery.

septal defects, ventricular septal defects, patent ductus arteriosus, patent foramen ovale, tetralogy of Fallot, atrioventricular univentricular connection, pulmonary atresia with ventricular septal defect, pulmonic stenosis, double-outlet right ventricle, atrioventricular septal defect, bicuspid pulmonic valve, coarctation of the aorta, subaortic stenosis, aortic atresia, tricuspid stenosis, ventriculoarterial discordance, interrupted aortic arch, truncus arteriosus, partial anomalous pulmonary venous drainage, and pulmonary arteriovenous fistulas (1,4,8–11,13,15–17,19, 21,26–28,31,32)

INTRAOPERATIVE AND POSTOPERATIVE EVALUATION

In general, transesophageal echocardiography is not particularly helpful in the diagnosis of systemic venous anomalies in children. The proximal portions of the superior and inferior venae cavae can be visualized from the longitudinal view of the atria, so that anomalies at these sites would be demonstrated (37) (see Fig. 4-30D). Persistence of the left superior vena cava draining into the coronary sinus can be seen from the longitudinal inflow view of the left ventricle (the two-chamber equivalent view) by counterclockwise and leftward rotation of the transducer (37,38) (see Fig. 4-28C). Dilatation of the coronary sinus can be appreciated from the transverse four-chamber view with retroflexion of the transducer to image the diaphragmatic wall of the heart (see Fig. 4-28A). The postoperative evaluation is primarily directed toward follow-up of the repaired associated anomalies. Nonetheless, anatomic and Doppler examination of the sites of the systemic venous repair can be accomplished transthoracically.

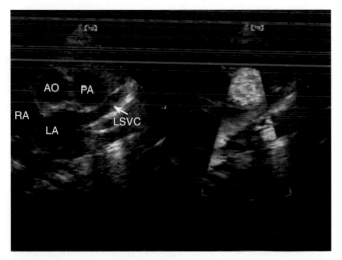

ECHO. 32-4. Suprasternal short-axis view with the transducer tilted to the left to demonstrate the persistence of a left superior vena cava draining into the roof of the left atrium. **Left:** Anatomic image of the connection between the left superior vena cava (*arrow*) and the left atrium. The left-sided pulmonary veins are also seen in this view connecting normally to the left atrium. **Right:** Color Doppler image of the flow of the left superior vena cava into the left atrium. The flow within the pulmonary artery is also seen in this frame. *AO*, aorta; *PA*, pulmonary artery; *RA*, right atrium; *LA*, left atrium; *LSVC*, left superior vena cava.

REFERENCES

1. Huhta JC, Smallhorn JF, Macartney FJ, Anderson RH, De Leval M. Cross-sectional echocardiographic diagnosis of systemic venous return. *Br Heart J* 1982;48:388–403.
2. Goor DA, Lillehei CW. Anomalous systemic venous connections. In: Goor DA, Lillehei CW, eds. *Congenital malformations of the heart.* New York: Grune & Stratton, 1975:398–413.
3. Kirsch WM, Carlsson E, Hartmann AF. A case of anomalous drainage of the superior vena cava into the left atrium. *J Thorac Cardiovasc Surg* 1961;41:550–556.
4. Raghib G, Ruttenberg HD, Anderson RC, Amplatz K, Adams P, Edwards JE. Termination of left superior vena cava in left atrium, atrial septal defect, and absence of coronary sinus. A developmental complex. *Circulation* 1965;31:906–918.
5. Effler DB, Greer AE, Sifers EC. Anomaly of the vena cava inferior. Report of fatality after ligation. *JAMA* 1951;146:1321–1322.
6. Lucas RV Jr, Krabill KA. Abnormal systemic venous connections. In: Emmanouilides GC, Riemenschneider TA, Allen HD, Gutgesell HP, eds. *Moss and Adams heart disease in infants, children, and adolescents. Including the fetus and young adult,* Vol I, 5th ed. Baltimore: Williams & Wilkins, 1995:874–902.
7. Halbertsma MJ. Vena cava superior sinistra. *Nederl Tijdschr Geneesk* 1862;6:610. Cited by Karnegis JN, Wang Y, Winchell P, Edwards JE. Pesistent left superior vena cava, fibrous remnant of the right superior vena cava and ventricular septal defect. *Am J Cardiol* 1964;14:573–577.
8. Lenox CC, Zuberbuhler JR, Park SC, et al. Absent right superior vena cava with persistent left superior vena cava: implications and management. *Am J Cardiol* 1980;45:117–122.
9. Choi JY, Anderson RH, Macartney FJ. Absent right superior caval vein (vena cava) with normal atrial arrangement. *Br Heart J* 1987;57:474–478.
10. Karnegis JN, Wang Y, Winchell P, Edwards JE. Persistent left superior vena cava, fibrous remnant of the right superior vena cava and ventricular septal defect. *Am J Cardiol* 1964;14:573–577.
11. Miller GAH, Ongley PA, Rastelli GC, Kirklin JW. Surgical correction of total anomalous systemic venous connection: report of case. *Mayo Clin Proc* 1965;40:532–538.
12. Braudo M, Beanlands DS, Trusler G. Anomalous drainage of the right superior vena cava into the left atrium. *Can Med Assoc J* 1968;99:715–719.
13. Gueron M, Hirsh M, Borman J. Total anomalous systemic venous drainage into the left atrium. Report of a case of successful surgical correction. *J Thorac Cardiovasc Surg* 1969;58:570–574.
14. Park HM, Smith ET, Silberstein EB. Isolated right superior vena cava draining into left atrium diagnosed by radionuclide angiocardiography. *J Nucl Med* 1973;14:240–242.
15. Vazquez-Perez J, Frontera-Izquierdo P. Anomalous drainage of the right superior vena cava into the left atrium as an isolated anomaly. Rare case report. *Am Heart J* 1979;97:89–91.
16. Alpert BS, Rao PS, Moore V, Covitz W. Surgical correction of anomalous right superior vena cava to the left atrium. *J Thorac Cardiovasc Surg* 1981;82:301–305.
17. Park HM, Summerer MH, Preuss K, Armstrong WF, Mahomed Y, Hamilton DJ. Anomalous drainage of the right superior vena cava into the left atrium. *J Am Coll Cardiol* 1983;2:358–362.
18. Shapiro EP, Al-Sadir J, Campbell NPS, Thilenius OG, Anagnostopoulos CE, Hays P. Drainage of right superior vena cava into both atria. Review of the literature and description of a case presenting with polycythemia and paradoxical embolization. *Circulation* 1981;63:712–717.
19. Bharati S, Lev M. Direct entry of the right superior vena cava into the left atrium with aneurysmal dilatation and stenosis at its entry into the right atrium with stenosis of the pulmonary veins: a rare case. *Pediatr Cardiol* 1984;5:123–126.
20. Soto B, Pacifico AD. Anomalies of the systemic venous return. In: Soto B, Pacifico AD, eds. *Angiocardiography in congenital heart malformations.* Mount Kisco, NY: Futura Publishing, 1990:105–119.
21. LePere RH, Kohler CM, Klinger P, Lowry JK. Intrathoracic venous anomalies. *J Thorac Cardiovasc Surg* 1965;49:599–614.
22. Blank E, Zuberbuhler JR. Left to right shunt through a left atrial left superior superior vena cava. *Am J Roentgenol* 1968;103:87–92.
23. Davis WH, Jordaan FR, Snyman HW. Persistent left superior vena cava draining into the left atrium as an isolated anomaly. *Am Heart J* 1959;57:616–622.
24. Hurwitt ES, Escher DJW, Citrin LI. Surgical correction of cyanosis due to entrance of left superior vena cava into left auricle. *Surgery* 1955;38:88–93.
25. Wilson J. A description of a very unusual formation of the human heart. *Phil Trans R Soc London* 1798;88:346–356.
26. McCotter RE. Three cases of the persistence of the left superior vena cava. *Anat Rec* 1915–1916;10:371–383.
27. Anderson RC, Adams P, Burke B. Anomalous inferior vena cava with azygous continuation (infrahepatic interruption of the inferior vena cava). Report of 15 new cases. *J Pediatr* 1961;59:370–383.
28. Gardner DL, Cole L. Long survival with inferior vena cava draining into left atrium. *Br Heart J* 1955;17:93–97.
29. Meadows WR, Bergstrand I, Sharp JT. Isolated anomalous connection of a great vein to the left atrium; the syndrome of cyanosis and clubbing, "normal heart," and left ventricular hypertrophy on electrocardiogram. *Circulation* 1961;24:669–676.
30. Venables AW. Isolated drainage of the inferior vena cava to the left atrium. *Br Heart J* 1963;25:545–548.
31. Black H, Smith GT, Goodale WT. Anomalous inferior vena cava draining into the left atrium associated with intact interatrial septum and multiple pulmonary arteriovenous fistulae. *Circulation* 1964;29:258–267.
32. Yee KF. Anomalous termination of a hepatic vein in the left atrium. *Arch Pathol* 1968;85:219–223.
33. Nabarro D. Two hearts showing peculiarities of the great veins. *J Anat Physiol* 1903;37:382. Cited by Mantini E, Grondin CM, Lillehei CW, Edwards JE. Congenital anomalies involving the coronary sinus. *Circulation* 1966;33:317–327.
34. Harris WG. A case of bilateral superior venae cavae with a closed coronary sinus. *Thorax* 1960;15:172–173.
35. Mantini E, Grondin CM, Lillehei CW, Edwards JE. Congenital anomalies involving the coronary sinus. *Circulation* 1966;33:317–327.
36. Basu BN. Persistent "left superior vena cava," "left duct of Cuvier" and "left horn of the sinus venosus." *J Anat* 1932;66:268–270.
37. Seward JB, Khandheria BK, Edwards WD, Oh JK, Freeman WK, Tajik AJ. Biplanar transesophageal echocardiography: anatomic correlations, image orientation, and clinical applications. *Mayo Clin Proc* 1990;65:1193–1213.
38. Nanda NC, Pinheiro L, Sanyal R, Jain H, Van TB, Rosenthal S. Transesophageal echocardiographic examination of left-sided superior vena cava and azygous and hemiazygos veins. *Echocardiography* 1991;8:731–740.

CHAPTER 33

Anomalies of the Pulmonary Venous System

Lilliam M. Valdes-Cruz and Raul O. Cayre

Anomalies of the pulmonary venous system comprise a group of malformations that include (a) anomalous pulmonary venous connection, (b) atresia of the common pulmonary vein, and (c) stenosis of the pulmonary veins. In this chapter, we consider cases presenting with situs solitus or with mirror-image atrial arrangement (situs inversus). Cases associated with visceral heterotaxies are discussed in Chapter 8.

ANOMALOUS PULMONARY VENOUS CONNECTION

The failure of anatomic and physiologic union of one or all pulmonary veins with the left atrium has been given various denominations, such as anomalies of the pulmonary veins (1–6), congenital anomalies of the pulmonary veins (7), transposition of the pulmonary veins (8,9), drainage of the pulmonary veins into the right side of the heart (10–12), abnormal disposition of the pulmonary veins (13,14), anomalous pulmonary veins (15,16), anomalous pulmonary return (17), anomalies of the pulmonary venous return (18), anomalous pulmonary venous return (19–23), anomalous pulmonary venous drainage (24–31), and anomalous pulmonary venous connection (32–47). The existence of a physiologically anomalous pulmonary venous drainage in the presence of normal pulmonary venous connection, as occurs in hearts with atrial septal defects, has led to use of the term anomalous pulmonary venous connection, proposed by Edwards (32), to refer to the lack of union of some or all pulmonary veins with the left atrium.

The first classification of this anomaly was proposed in 1942 by Brody (10), who recognized two types: total, in which all pulmonary veins connect with the right atrium or a systemic venous tributary of the right atrium, and incomplete, in which some of the pulmonary veins connect with the right atrium or a systemic venous tributary of the right atrium. This was later called partial type

(6,17,20,23,28,32,38,39). Becker and Anderson (48,49) categorize these malformations as anomalies of unilateral connection when only one lung, either left or right, drains anomalously; these can be partial, in which only one part of the lung is involved, or complete, in which the entire lung is involved. There can also be two variants of the bilateral type: partial, in which only one part of both lungs drains anomalously, or complete, in which the entire venous drainage of both lungs is abnormal.

In this chapter, we use the more conventional terminology of total anomalous pulmonary venous connection when all pulmonary veins drain into the right atrium or a tributary vein of the right atrium, and partial anomalous pulmonary venous connection when some of the pulmonary veins drain into the right atrium or a tributary vein of the right atrium.

EMBRYOLOGIC CONSIDERATIONS

The lung buds, which originate from a subdivision of the respiratory diverticulum, are surrounded by a vascular plexus called the splanchnic plexus (50–54). Later, the splanchnic plexus establishes connections with the cardinal venous system and with the umbilicovitelline venous system and gives rise to the pulmonary venous plexus, within which the pulmonary veins develop, thereby serving as the drainage of the pulmonary venous flow (50–54). Simultaneously, an endothelial sprout grows from the superior wall of the left atrium toward the pulmonary vascular plexus, giving rise to the common pulmonary vein. This acquires a lumen and connects with the pulmonary venous plexus, which bifurcates into right and left pulmonary veins; these then subdivide further into two additional branches (55). When the common pulmonary vein connects with the pulmonary venous plexus, the latter loses its connection with the splanchnic plexus and therefore with the cardinal and umbilicovitelline veins. The common pulmonary vein and later the pulmonary veins themselves become incorporated into the posterior wall of the left atrium, with the result that four pulmonary veins drain directly into it (18,32).

Failure of complete connection of the common pulmonary vein with the pulmonary venous plexus results in persistence of one or more of the connections between the pulmonary venous plexus and the system of cardinal veins and umbilicovitelline veins, giving rise to a total anomalous pulmonary venous connection to the right atrium or to one of its tributary veins (18,32,54,56–58). Partial connection of the common pulmonary vein with the pulmonary venous plexus gives rise to a partial anomalous pulmonary venous connection to the right atrium or to one of its venous tributaries (18,32,54,56).

Total Anomalous Pulmonary Venous Connection

In total anomalous pulmonary venous connection, there is no communication between the left atrium and pulmonary veins, which drain via a common collector directly into the right atrium or into one of the veins that drain into the right atrium. The first case of this malformation was reported in 1798 by Wilson (59) in a 7-day-old infant with additional cardiac anomalies (cor biloculare). The first report of an isolated case was published by Friedlowsky in 1868 (60).

The real incidence of total anomalous pulmonary venous connection is difficult to establish because most publications include these cases with the visceral heterotaxies. Nonetheless, an incidence of 2.6% of all congenital cardiac anomalies has been reported for isolated total anomalous pulmonary venous connection (61).

ANATOMIC AND ECHOCARDIOGRAPHIC CONSIDERATIONS

The echocardiographic study of total anomalous pulmonary venous connection should establish, in addition to the visceroatrial situs, the following: (a) type of pulmonary venous connection, (b) presence of pulmonary venous obstruction, (c) size of the cardiac cavities, and (d) presence of associated anomalies. The intraoperative and postoperative evaluation of all pulmonary venous anomalies is discussed at the end of the chapter.

Type of Pulmonary Venous Connection

The classification most commonly used is that proposed by Darling et al. (11), who recognized four types according to the anatomic level where the connection is established: type I (supracardiac), type II (cardiac), type III (infracardiac), and type IV (mixed, in which connections are established into two or more levels).

Type I, supracardiac type, is seen in 43% to 58% of

cases of total anomalous pulmonary venous connection (5,10,11,16,25,31,33). Connections can be established to the left innominate vein, right superior vena cava, or azygous vein (Fig. 33-1A–C).

Connection to the left innominate vein is the most common variety and is seen in 50% to 85% of all cases (5,10,11,16,25,31,33) (Fig. 33-1A). The anatomic characteristics are similar in most cases. The right pulmonary veins course behind the left atrium and join a common collector, which also receives the left pulmonary veins and ascends vertically on the left side of the mediastinum. This collector, also called the vertical vein (6), ascends in front of the left pulmonary artery, left main bronchus, and aortic arch and connects with a dilated left innominate vein, which drains normally into the superior vena cava. Occasionally, the vertical vein can course between the left pulmonary artery and left main bronchus, resulting in obstruction of the pulmonary venous drainage at that site (37).

Connection to the right superior vena cava, the second most common variety, is seen in 15% to 40% of all supracardiac cases (5,10,11,25,31,33) (Fig. 33-1B). In this type of connection, the four pulmonary veins also join a common collector behind the left atrium; this ascends on the right side, courses in front of the right pulmonary hilum, and usually drains into the posterior wall of the superior vena cava (11).

Connection to the azygous vein is rare, occurring in 1% to 10% of cases. In these instances, the common collector drains into the azygous vein (17,31,33,62,63) (Fig. 33-1C).

Type II, cardiac type, is found in 23% to 43% of all cases of total anomalous pulmonary venous connection (5,6,10,11,16,17,25,31,33). The connection can be to the coronary sinus or directly to the right atrium (Fig. 33-1D–F).

Connection to the coronary sinus is the most common variety, being found in 48% to 72% of cases of the cardiac type (5,6,10,11,16,17,25,31,33). The common collector drains directly into the coronary sinus at the level of the atrioventricular sulcus (Fig. 33-1D).

Connection directly to the right atrium is seen in 38% to 52% of all cases of the cardiac type of connection (5,6,10,11,16,17,25,31,33). Two variants can be seen: the common venous collector can drain into the posterosuperior wall of the right atrium (Fig. 33-1E), or the four pulmonary veins can drain separately into the posterior wall of the right atrium (Fig. 33-1F).

Type III, infracardiac or infradiaphragmatic type, is seen in 10% to 23% of all cases of total anomalous pulmonary venous connection (5,6,10,11,16,17,25,31,33). In these cases, the four pulmonary veins form a common collector behind the left atrium. It is located in front and slightly to the left of the esophagus and courses downward, crosses the diaphragm at the level of the esophageal hiatus, and establishes a connection with a systemic vein

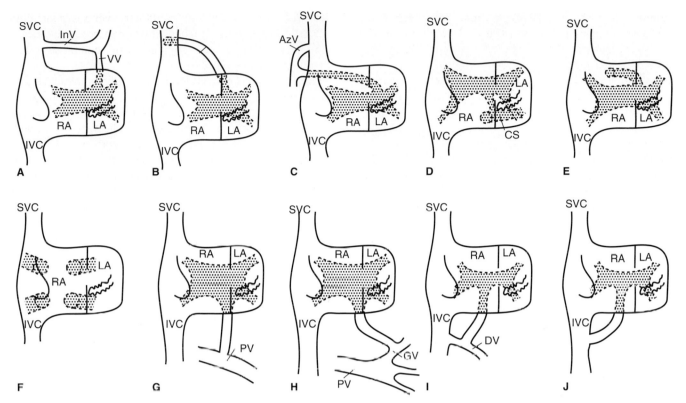

FIG. 33-1. Schematic drawings of the various types of total anomalous pulmonary venous connection in hearts with situs solitus. **A:** To the innominate vein. **B:** To the right superior vena cava. **C:** To the azygous vein. **D:** To the coronary sinus. **E:** To the right atrium through a common collector. **F:** To the right atrium through four separate connections. **G:** To the portal vein. **H:** To the gastric vein. **I:** To the ductus venosus. **J:** To the inferior vena cava. *RA*, right atrium; *LA*, left atrium; *SVC*, superior vena cava; *IVC*, inferior vena cava; *InV*, innominate vein; *VV*, vertical vein; *AzV*, azygous vein; *CS*, coronary sinus; *PV*, portal vein; *GV*, gastric vein; *DV*, ductus venosus.

(Fig. 33-1G–J). In the majority of cases, there is only one systemic venous connection, but there can also be several venous channels (6). In most instances, the anomalous connection is established with the portal vein (Fig. 33-1G) or one of its tributaries, usually the gastric vein (Fig. 33-1H). Less commonly, the connection can be established with the ductus venosus (5,6,11,25,31,33,62,64) (Fig. 33-1I) or with the inferior vena cava (5,10,31,33,62) (Fig. 33-1J). Isolated cases of anomalous connection to a hepatic vein have been reported (31,33,62).

In *type IV, mixed type,* the pulmonary veins drain into two or more of the sites described above. The incidence of this type varies between 2% and 15% of all cases of total anomalous pulmonary venous connection (10,11, 17,25,31,33).

Two-dimensional echocardiography has been of great utility in the noninvasive diagnosis of the various types of total anomalous pulmonary venous connection (41,43). Inability to visualize pulmonary veins draining into the left atrium from the suprasternal short-axis view, apical four-chamber view, and/or subcostal four-chamber view should alert the operator of the possibility of anomalous pulmonary venous connection. Further, dilation of the

cavities of the right side of the heart and flat to paradoxical septal motion are characteristic of the volume overload of the right side seen in total anomalous pulmonary venous connection.

In the supracardiac type, the suprasternal views demonstrate the common collector located below the right pulmonary artery (Echo. 33-1); with counterclockwise and slightly leftward rotation of the transducer, the vertical vein can be seen coursing upward into a dilated left innominate vein, which eventually drains into the right superior vena cava (Echo. 33-2; see color plate 110 following p. 364). Color and spectral Doppler can be very useful in confirming the flows within these structures (Echo. 33-2). Venous flow toward the transducer (red) would differentiate a vertical vein from a persistent left superior vena cava, in which the flow would be directed away from the transducer (blue). The long-axis suprasternal view permits visualization of the connection of the common collector to the vertical vein and/or directly to the superior vena cava or azygous vein. Color Doppler is particularly useful to rule out mixed sites of connection (Echo. 33-3; see color plates 111 and 112 following p. 364). From the apical and subcostal views, the common

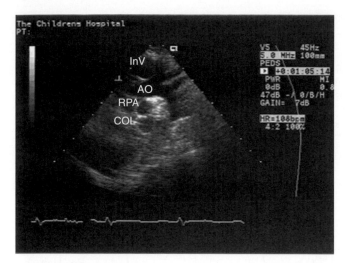

ECHO. 33-1. Suprasternal long-axis view showing the common venous collector located below the right pulmonary artery in total anomalous pulmonary venous connection to a vertical vein. *AO*, aorta; *RPA*, right pulmonary artery; *COL*, common venous collector; *InV;* innominate vein.

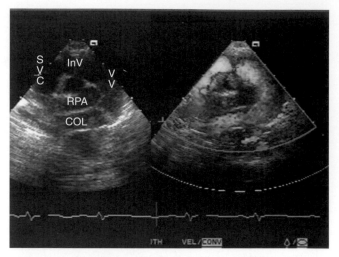

ECHO. 33-2. Suprasternal view of total anomalous venous connection to a vertical vein. The common venous collector is seen connecting with the vertical vein, which in turn joins a dilated innominate vein and the right superior vena cava. Anatomic image **(left)** and color Doppler image **(right)** of the drainage of the common venous collector into the vertical vein, innominate vein, and superior vena cava. *SVC*, superior vena cava; *InV*, innominate vein; *VV*, vertical vein; *RPA*, right pulmonary artery; *COL*, common venous collector.

collector can also be seen behind the left atrium (Echo. 33-4A). The connection of the vertical vein to the superior vena cava can be demonstrated with cranial angulation of the transducer and slight rotation toward the right (Echo. 33-4B; see color plate 113 following p. 364). Connection to the azygous vein may be more difficult to visualize but is usually seen from the subcostal view, with the transducer angled cranially.

Connection to the coronary sinus can be evaluated from the parasternal long-axis view, apical four-chamber view. and subcostal four-chamber view (Echos. 33-5, 33-6; see color plate 114 following p. 364). From these views, the coronary sinus appears dilated, and the common collector can be seen entering it posteriorly. Color Doppler flow mapping aids in the identification of the increased flow

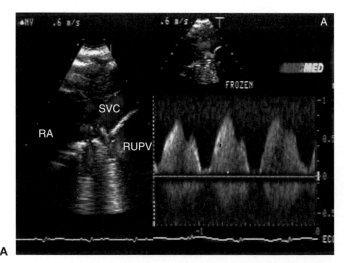

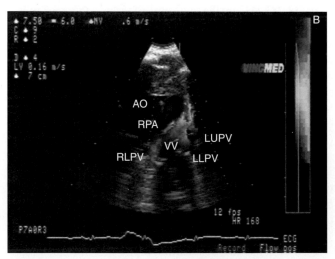

ECHO. 33-3. Color Doppler and spectral Doppler recordings in a case of total anomalous pulmonary venous connection, mixed type. **A:** Right subclavicular view **(left)** demonstrating the connection of the right upper pulmonary vein to the superior vena cava directly, and the spectral Doppler recording **(right)** of the velocities at the site of connection of the pulmonary vein to the superior vena cava. **B:** Color Doppler flow image identifying the three remaining pulmonary veins draining into a vertical vein. *RA*, right atrium; *SVC*, superior vena cava; *RUPV*, right upper pulmonary vein; *AO*, aorta; *RPA*, right pulmonary artery; *RLPV*, right lower pulmonary vein; *LUPV*, left upper pulmonary vein; *LLPV*, left lower pulmonary vein; *VV,* vertical vein.

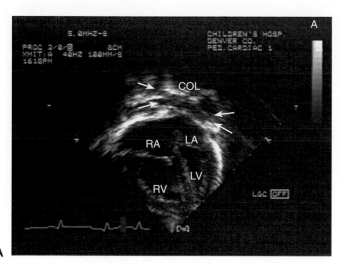

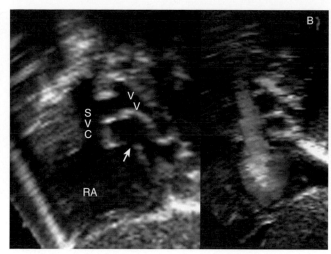

ECHO. 33-4. Images from a case with total anomalous pulmonary venous connection to a vertical vein. **A:** Apical four-chamber view demonstrating the common venous collector situated behind the left atrium. The *arrows* point to the four pulmonary veins entering the collector. Note that the cavities of the left side of the heart are small. **B:** Anatomic image **(left)** and color Doppler image **(right)** from the subcostal sagittal position of the connection of the vertical vein to the right superior vena cava through an innominate vein. *RA*, right atrium; *LA*, left atrium; *RV*, right ventricle; *LV*, left ventricle; *COL*, common venous collector; *SVC*, superior vena cava; *VV*, vertical vein.

into the coronary sinus as well as the flow from the pulmonary veins into the common collector. Connections directly into the posterior wall of the right atrium can also be demonstrated from these views, and the direction and velocity of flow confirmed with color and spectral Doppler (Echo. 33-7; see color plate 115 following p. 364).

The common collector in the infradiaphragmatic type of connection can also be identified from the parasternal (Echo. 33-8), apical, subcostal, and suprasternal short-axis views, behind the left atrium and below the right pulmonary artery. The collector, however, is directed downward toward the diaphragm, and flow toward the liver can be seen on color Doppler flow mapping (Echo. 33-9; see color plate 116 following p. 364). From the subcostal abdominal short-axis view, immediately below the diaphragm, a vascular structure can be seen to the left of the inferior vena cava and in front and to the right of the aorta; this is the descending vertical vein (42,65,66) (Echo. 33-10; see color plate 117 following p. 364). The

ECHO. 33-5. Images from a case with total anomalous pulmonary venous connection to the coronary sinus. Apical four-chamber view **(left)** of the dilated coronary sinus opening into the right atrium (*arrow*). Color Doppler image **(right)** of the flow from the coronary sinus into the right atrium. *RA*, right atrium; *RV*, right ventricle; *LV*, left ventricle; *CS*, coronary sinus.

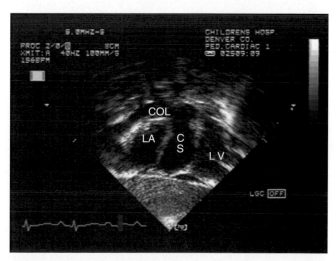

ECHO. 33-6. Subcostal view of the common venous collector connecting to a dilated coronary sinus. *LA*, left atrium; *COL*, common venous collector; *CS*, coronary sinus; *LV*, left ventricle.

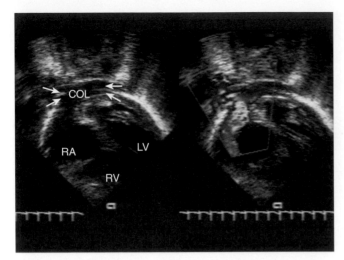

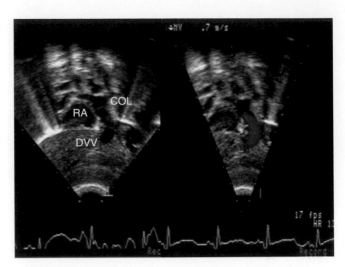

ECHO. 33-7. Subcostal view of total anomalous venous connection directly to the right atrium. **Left:** Anatomic image demonstrating the four pulmonary veins (*arrows*) connecting to a common venous collector, which in turn connects to the right atrium. **Right:** Color Doppler image of the flow from the collector into the right atrium. *COL*, common venous collector; *RA*, right atrium; *RV*, right ventricle; *LV*, left ventricle.

ECHO. 33-9. Images from a case with total anomalous venous connection, infradiaphragmatic type. **Left:** Anatomic image of the pulmonary veins joining a common collector, which connects to a descending vertical vein directed toward the liver. **Right:** Color Doppler image of the flow in the descending vertical vein. *RA*, right atrium; *COL*, common venous collector; *DVV*, descending vertical vein.

subcostal abdominal long-axis view also demonstrates the presence of the descending vertical vein, in front of the descending aorta. Both subcostal abdominal views permit identification of the site of connection into the portal vein or its tributaries, the ductus venosus, or the inferior vena cava. The venous return into the right atrium via the

inferior vena cava or one of its tributaries can be appreciated from the parasternal right ventricular inflow view (Echo. 33-11; see color plate 118 following p. 364).

Presence of Pulmonary Venous Obstruction

Obstructions to the pulmonary venous drainage can occur in all types of total anomalous connection. Obstructions can be seen at the junction of the pulmonary veins to the common collector, throughout the length of the

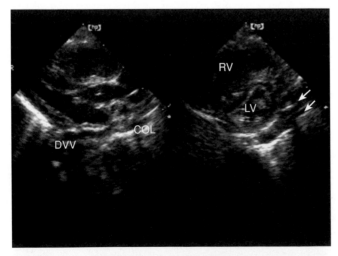

ECHO. 33-8. Parasternal views of total anomalous pulmonary venous connection, infradiaphragmatic type. **Left:** Long-axis view demonstrates the common venous collector and descending vertical vein. **Right:** Short-axis view of the ventricle shows the pulmonary veins connecting to a common venous collector behind the left ventricle (*arrows*). Note that the left ventricle is considerably smaller than the right ventricle. *COL*, common venous collector; *DVV*, descending vertical vein; *RV*, right ventricle; *LV*, left ventricle.

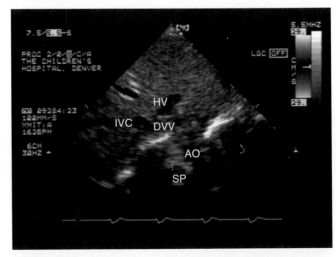

ECHO. 33-10. Abdominal short-axis view of total anomalous pulmonary venous connection, infradiaphragmatic type, showing the descending vertical vein in cross section. *HV*, hepatic vein; *IVC*, inferior vena cava; *DVV*, descending vertical vein; *AO*, aorta; *SP*, spine.

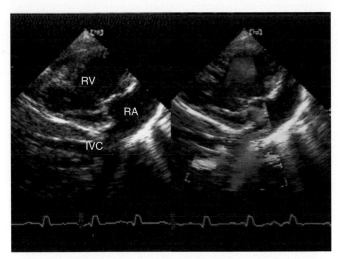

ECHO. 33-11. Parasternal long-axis view with the transducer tilted toward the right ventricular inflow in total anomalous pulmonary venous connection, infradiaphragmatic type. **Left:** The view demonstrates the connection of the inferior vena cava and the returning venous channel to the right atrium. **Right:** The color Doppler image illustrates the flow of the pulmonary venous channel at the inferior vena caval-right atrial-hepatic junction. *RV,* right ventricle; *RA,* right atrium; *IVC,* inferior vena cava.

collector, or at the site of the anomalous connection of the collector (Echo. 33-12). The mechanisms that produce obstruction include intrinsic anomalies of the venous walls, with hypertrophy of the media and adventitia and proliferation of the intima (21,45). In some cases of anomalous connection to the innominate vein, an obstruction can be caused by extrinsic compression when the common collector ascends behind the left pulmonary artery and in front of the left main bronchus (37,45). In the cardiac type of anomalous connection into the coronary sinus, obstructions can be seen at the drainage site of the common collector into the coronary sinus (67,68) or into the right atrium.

The majority of infradiaphragmatic anomalous connections are obstructive (14,34,46,64). Obstruction can result from compression of the descending vertical vein at the diaphragmatic hiatus, from increased resistance of the hepatic sinusoids when the connection is to the portal vein or its tributaries, or from constriction of the ductus venosus.

Color Doppler flow mapping permits demonstration of the presence of obstructions by color aliasing at the site(s) resulting from the increased flow velocity. This can be confirmed with spectral Doppler.

Size of the Cardiac Cavities

The right atrium and ventricle are dilated and hypertrophied in all cases of total anomalous pulmonary venous connection. The pulmonary artery is also dilated. The

left atrium is usually small and sometimes it is virtually reduced to the left atrial appendage because the venous portion of the atrium is absent. The left ventricular cavity is smaller than normal, and its size is further reduced by bulging of the interventricular septum to the left as a result of the volume overload of the right ventricle. The size of the left ventricle measured by echocardiography has been helpful in predicting the surgical outcome of this lesion (69). Patients with a ratio of the thickness of the left ventricular posterior wall in diastole to the left ventricular cavity dimension in diastole (*LVPWd/LVEDD*) of more than 0.86 and a left ventricular end-diastolic dimension of less than 38 mm/m^2 have been found to have higher perioperative mortality (69).

The echocardiographic views that permit assessment of the size of the ventricular cavities are the parasternal long- and short-axis views, the four-chamber apical and subcostal views, and the subcostal short-axis view (Echos. 33-4, 33-8). The M-mode traces derived from the parasternal short- or long-axis views are utilized to measure the actual wall and cavity sizes for comparison with normal values.

Associated Anomalies

In almost all cases of total anomalous pulmonary venous connection, an interatrial communication or patent foramen ovale is present. Exceptions have been the case reported by Hastreiter et al. (35) with patent ductus arteriosus and closed foramen ovale and the case reported by Delisle et al. (63) with intact interatrial septum and multiple ventricular septal defects. Other reported associated

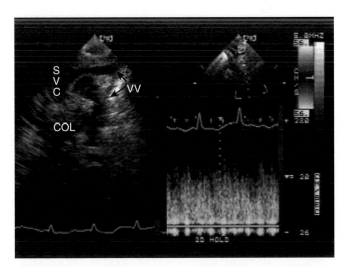

ECHO. 33-12. Images from a case with total anomalous pulmonary venous connection to a vertical vein with obstruction within the vertical vein (*arrows*). Note the high-velocity, disturbed flow recorded with the spectral Doppler. *SVC,* superior vena cava; *VV,* vertical vein; *COL,* common venous collector.

anomalies in cases without visceral heterotaxy have been patent ductus arteriosus, ventricular septal defect, complete transposition of the great arteries, congenitally corrected transposition, pulmonary atresia with ventricular septal defect, interruption of the aortic arch and ventricular septal defect, tetralogy of Fallot, and double-outlet right ventricle (29,31,43,67,70).

Partial Anomalous Pulmonary Venous Connection

In partial anomalous pulmonary venous connection, one or several of the pulmonary veins drain into the right atrium or into one of the venous tributaries of the right atrium. In 1739, Winslow (71) published the first case of anomalous connection of the right upper pulmonary vein into the superior vena cava. The incidence of partial anomalous venous connection in patients with congenital heart disease varies between 0.4% and 0.7% (10,15, 39,72), and it represents 14% of all pulmonary venous anomalies (6).

ANATOMIC AND ECHOCARDIOGRAPHIC CONSIDERATIONS

The echocardiographic study of partial anomalous pulmonary venous connection should determine (a) the type of connection and (b) the presence of associated anomalies.

Type of Partial Anomalous Pulmonary Venous Connection

Anomalous connections of the right-sided pulmonary veins are much more common than those of the left-sided veins. The anomalous connections can be to the right atrium, superior vena cava, or inferior vena cava.

Partial connections into the right atrium are found in 26% to 47% of cases (10,39). These include a number of variants (Fig. 33-2A–C). The right upper pulmonary vein can drain into the posterior wall of the right atrium (Fig. 33-2A), both right-sided veins can drain into the right atrium (Fig. 33-2B), or both right-sided veins and the left

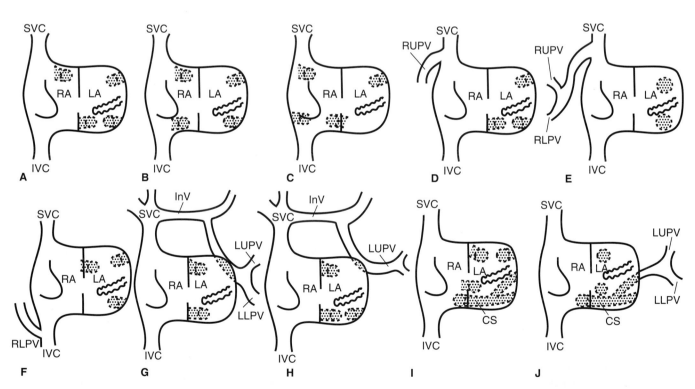

FIG. 33-2. Schematic drawings of the various types of partial anomalous pulmonary venous connections in hearts with situs solitus. **A:** Right upper pulmonary vein to the right atrium. **B:** Right pulmonary veins to the right atrium. **C:** Right pulmonary veins and left lower pulmonary vein to the right atrium. **D:** Right upper pulmonary vein to the superior vena cava. **E:** Right pulmonary veins to the superior vena cava. **F:** Right lower pulmonary vein to the inferior vena cava. **G:** Left pulmonary veins to the innominate vein. **H:** Left upper pulmonary vein to the innominate vein. **I:** Left lower pulmonary vein to the coronary sinus. **J:** Left pulmonary veins to the coronary sinus. *RA*, right atrium; *LA*, left atrium; *SVC*, superior vena cava; *IVC*, inferior vena cava; *RUPV*, right upper pulmonary vein; *RLPV*, right lower pulmonary vein; *InV*, innominate vein; *LUPV*, left upper pulmonary vein; *LLPV*, left lower pulmonary vein; *CS*, coronary sinus.

lower pulmonary vein can drain anomalously directly into the right atrium (Fig. 33-2C).

In 34% of cases of partial anomalous pulmonary venous connection, one or both right-sided veins are connected to the superior vena cava (Fig. 33-2D,E).

Connection of the right pulmonary veins to the suprahepatic portion of the inferior vena cava is seen in only 3% of cases of partial anomalous pulmonary venous connection (10) (Fig. 33-2F). This type of connection is hardly ever found as an isolated lesion; rather, it is associated with pulmonary anomalies such as abnormal lobulation and bronchial distribution, hypoplasia of the pulmonary artery, partial anomalous pulmonary flow from the systemic circulation, and dextroposition of the heart (26,73–77). The term "scimitar syndrome" (76) was proposed by Neill et al. to refer to the radiologic appearance of the pulmonary venous drainage into the inferior vena cava.

Anomalous connections of the left-sided pulmonary veins are much rarer and have been reported in 2% to 4% of all cases of partial anomalous pulmonary venous connection (10,78). These can be to the innominate vein, coronary sinus, or inferior vena cava (Fig. 33-2G–J).

Connection to the innominate vein can be complete, with both left-sided pulmonary veins connected anomalously (Fig. 33-2G), or only the left upper pulmonary vein can be thus connected (10,23,40,78–80) (Fig. 33-2H).

Connection of one lower left pulmonary vein (Fig. 33-2I) or both left-sided veins (Fig. 33-2J) to the coronary sinus is extremely rare (10,23,78). Only one case of connection of the left-sided pulmonary veins to the inferior vena cava has been reported in the literature (81).

The same views as those described for the identification of total anomalous pulmonary venous connection can be used for partial types. These include the suprasternal short- and long-axis views and the apical and subcostal four-chamber views. The spectral Doppler signal of the pulmonary venous flow in scimitar syndrome differs from normal in that it has one systolic-diastolic phase that includes late systole and early diastole and lacks the venous flow reversal (reverse "a" wave) normally associated with atrial contraction (82).

Associated Anomalies

Between 3% and 15% of atrial communications of the ostium secundum type are associated with partial anomalous pulmonary venous connection (39,83,84). Between 80% and 95% of atrial septal defects of the superior vena caval type are associated with a partial anomalous pulmonary venous connection, either directly to the superior vena cava or to the point where the superior vena cava connects to the right atrium (85–89). Associated atrial septal defects were found in 30% of cases of anomalous left-sided pulmonary venous connection reported by Van Meter et al. (23) and in one of the cases reported by

Neirotti et al. (40). Other associated anomalies include patent ductus arteriosus, patent foramen ovale, ventricular septal defect, tetralogy of Fallot, pulmonary atresia, pulmonic stenosis, aortic stenosis, coarctation of the aorta, and mitral insufficiency (10,23,40).

ATRESIA OF THE COMMON PULMONARY VEIN

In 1962, Lucas et al. (58) used the term atresia of the common pulmonary vein to indicate an extremely rare anomaly characterized by absence of connection of the pulmonary veins to the heart or a systemic vein. The case of atresia of the common pulmonary vein, previously published by Edwards et al. (57), had a total anomalous connection of the pulmonary veins to the superior vena cava. The incidence of atresia of the common pulmonary vein was 0.3% of necropsy cases of congenital heart disease (90).

EMBRYOLOGIC CONSIDERATIONS

A morphogenetic mechanism that has been suggested to explain this malformation includes a normal connection of the common pulmonary vein to the pulmonary venous plexus and later obliteration of the connection between the common pulmonary vein and left atrium. This would occur after the primitive connections between the splanchnic plexus and the cardinal and umbilicovitelline venous systems had disappeared (34,57,58).

ANATOMIC AND ECHOCARDIOGRAPHIC CONSIDERATIONS

The anatomic characteristics of this malformation include normal development of the four pulmonary veins, which converge to form a common pulmonary venous collector located behind the left atrium. Between the common collector and the posterior wall of the left atrium is a fibrous cord, which represents the atretic portion of the common pulmonary vein. A fibrous cord between the common venous collector and the right atrium and a fibrous cord between the common collector and the left brachiocephalic vein have both been reported (90). There is no connection of the pulmonary veins or common collector to the heart or systemic veins that would allow pulmonary venous outflow. Lucas et al. (58) hypothesized that one possible path of pulmonary venous outflow would be provided by anastomoses between the bronchopulmonary veins and the systemic veins. These same authors mention that in one of their three published cases, a dilated right bronchial vein originated from the right pulmonary hilum and coursed toward the esophagus, where it established connections with dilated esophageal venous channels; they assume that the bronchial vein represented the only exit for pulmonary venous flow (58). Nakib et al. (6) reported a case of atresia of the common pulmonary vein in which a series of small venous channels originating from the inferior wall of the common collector descended to fuse with the esophageal wall, and another case in which the veins from each lung separately established a connection with the paratracheal venous plexus via capillary-like channels. In all cases, a patent foramen ovale or atrial communication and a patent ductus arteriosus were present.

We have not studied any case with atresia of the common pulmonary vein, nor have we found a published report of the echocardiographic findings in this lesion.

STENOSIS OF THE PULMONARY VEINS

In this anomaly, the pulmonary veins connect normally to the left atrium; however, one or more of the veins are stenosed, either along a segment or at the point where they connect to the left atrium. In 1951, Reye (91) published the first case of this malformation. Its incidence is 0.1% of all cases of congenital heart disease (61).

EMBRYOLOGIC CONSIDERATIONS

The imperfect development of one or more individual pulmonary veins has been suggested as the mechanism that would result in stenosis of the pulmonary veins (54). Edwards (92) considers that the stenosis is caused by an abnormal incorporation of the common pulmonary vein into the left atrium.

ANATOMIC AND ECHOCARDIOGRAPHIC CONSIDERATIONS

The echocardiographic study of pulmonary vein stenosis should determine (a) the location and type of stenosis and (b) the presence of associated anomalies.

Location and Type of Stenosis

Three types of stenosis have been reported. In the first, the length of the stenosis is variable and the stenotic segment can extend into the lung parenchyma. This has been called hypoplasia of the pulmonary veins (6). The second type is characterized by the presence of a fibrous diaphragm in the extrapulmonary portion of the pulmonary veins (93). The third type, in which stenosis is found at the point of connection of one or several veins to the left atrium, has been called localized pulmonary

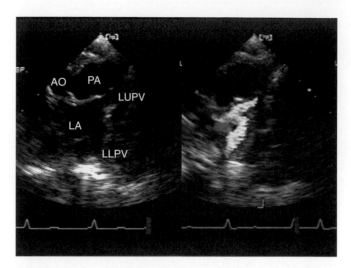

ECHO. 33-13. Suprasternal short-axis view demonstrating stenosis of the left-sided pulmonary veins. **Left:** The anatomic image suggests narrowing at the junction of the left pulmonary veins to the left atrium. **Right:** The color Doppler image demonstrates aliasing of the velocities at the sites of obstruction. *AO*, aorta; *PA*, pulmonary artery; *LUPV*, left upper pulmonary vein; *LLPV*, left lower pulmonary vein; *LA*, left atrium.

vein stenosis (6) (Echo. 33-13; see color plate 119 following p. 364).

The suprasternal long- and short-axis views as well as the apical and subcostal four-chamber views would allow determination of the size of the individual pulmonary veins. Spectral and color flow mapping would document the higher velocities at the sites(s) of drainage of the stenotic vein(s) (Echo. 33-13). The flow pattern on Doppler is unusual in that it is continuous, without the normal variations seen during the cardiac cycle (94).

Associated Anomalies

Approximately 50% of cases of pulmonary vein stenosis are associated with cardiac malformations (95), which include patent foramen ovale, atrial septal defect, ventricular septal defect, and absence of the right pulmonary artery (6,95,96).

INTRAOPERATIVE AND POSTOPERATIVE EVALUATION

The intraoperative transesophageal examination of total anomalous pulmonary venous connection is somewhat difficult because of the proximity of the structures to the endoscope, positioned in the esophagus. Nonetheless, because the common venous collector is posterior to the left atrium, it is seen as a structure separated from the left atrium by a wall. The best view to appreciate its presence and location is the four-chamber transverse view, with the endoscope positioned behind the left atrium (see Fig. 4-28A). Flow within the confluence may not be well recorded because it is of low velocity and the incident angle for color or spectral Doppler may not be favorable. Rotating the transducer toward the right and left may demonstrate one or more pulmonary veins draining into the collector, thereby confirming the diagnosis. Because the majority of cases involve supracardiac connection to the right superior vena cava directly, via a vertical vein or an azygous vein, the views demonstrating the superior vena cava would be helpful in demonstrating flow disturbance resulting from the anomalous drainage. These would be the longitudinal atrial/caval view (see Fig. 4-30D) and the transverse horizontal view at the level of the great vessels, where the superior vena cava would be seen in cross section to the right of the ascending aorta (see Fig. 4-31A). The cardiac type of connection into the coronary sinus can be appreciated from the transverse four-chamber view, with retroflexion of the transducer to visualize the coronary sinus, which would be enlarged and characterized by a high-velocity flow within (see Fig. 4-28A). In the infradiaphragmatic type of connection, the collector would be present behind the left atrium and immediately in front of the esophagus, but flow emerging from it would be directed downward. This might be detected by advancing the endoscope farther and following the flow within the collector by means of color Doppler mapping; the flow would appear to be away from the transducer (blue). In all these cases, there would also be the characteristically dilated right-sided cardiac structures, with the smaller left-sided chambers seen from the transverse four-chamber view.

Partial anomalous pulmonary venous connection of right pulmonary veins to the right superior vena cava can be seen from the same views as described above for visualizing the right superior vena cava. These views would also show dilation of the right-sided structures with flat to paradoxical septal motion, although not as severe as that seen in total anomalous return.

The late postoperative transthoracic study in these cases would emphasize visualization and Doppler interrogation of the pulmonary venous flow at the site of the surgical anastomosis of the common collector to the left atrium. Rarely, stenosis at this level may develop postoperatively. Interrogation of the velocity of all four pulmonary veins with spectral and color Doppler flow mapping would be necessary to confirm normal flow patterns and velocities. This would be conducted from the same views as described previously in this chapter—namely, the suprasternal short-axis view and the apical and subcostal four-chamber views.

The atrial septum should be examined from the subcostal four-chamber view for the presence of residual defects. Lastly, the right-sided cardiac structures become normal in size and the left-sided chambers enlarge after surgical repair of these anomalies. This should be evaluated serially along with assessment of the systolic and diastolic ventricular function.

REFERENCES

1. Schroder R. Uber anomalien der pulmonalvenen, zugleich ein beitrag zum cor biloculare. *Virchows Archiv Pathol Anat Physiol Klin Med* 1911;205:122–138.
2. MacCready PB. Anomalies of the pulmonary veins. *Bull Johns Hopkins Hosp* 1918;29:271–275.
3. Cords E. Ein fall von teilweiser erhaltung der V. cava sup. sin. zusammen mit einer anomalie der Vv. pulmonales. *Anat Anz* 1921;54:491–495.
4. Abbott ME. Congenital cardiac disease. In: Osler W, ed. *Modern medicine. Its theory and practice. I. Original contributions by American and foreign authors*, Vol 4, 3rd ed. Philadelphia: Lea & Febiger, 1927:612–812.
5. Parsons HG, Purdy A, Jessup B. Anomalies of the pulmonary veins and their surgical significance. Report of three cases of total anomalous pulmonary venous return. *Pediatrics* 1952;9:152–166.
6. Nakib A, Moller JH, Kanjuh VI, Edwards JE. Anomalies of the pulmonary veins. *Am J Cardiol* 1967;20:77–90.
7. Gander G. Un cas d'anomalie congénitale des veines pulmonaires. *Ann d'Anat Pathol* 1937;14:225–229.
8. Nagel A. Eine transposition aller lungenvenen in den rechten vorhof. *Virchows Archiv Pathol Anat Physiol Klin Med* 1936;297:343–350.
9. Muller WH Jr. The surgical treatment of transposition of the pulmonary veins. *Ann Surg* 1951;134:683–693.
10. Brody H. Drainage of the pulmonary veins into the right side of the heart. *Arch Pathol* 1942;33:221–240.
11. Darling RC, Rothney WB, Craig JM. Total pulmonary venous drainage into the right side of the heart. *Lab Invest* 1957;6:44–64.
12. Bahnson HT, Spencer FC, Neill CA. Surgical treatment of thirty-five cases of drainage of pulmonary veins to the right side of the heart. *J Thorac Surg* 1958;36:777–802.
13. Butler H. Abnormal disposition of the pulmonary veins. *J Anat* 1952;86:485–486.
14. Butler H. An abnormal disposition of the pulmonary veins. *Thorax* 1952;7:249–254.
15. Hughes CW, Rumore PC. Anomalous pulmonary veins. *Arch Pathol* 1944;37:364–366.
16. Smith JC. Anomalous pulmonary veins. *Am Heart J* 1951;41:561–568.
17. Gott VL, Lester RG, Lillehei CW, Varco RL. Total anomalous pulmonary return. An analysis of thirty cases. *Circulation* 1956;13:543–552.
18. Neill CA. Development of the pulmonary veins. With reference to the embryology of anomalies of pulmonary venous return. *Pediatrics* 1956;18:880–887.
19. Harris GBC, Neuhauser EBD, Giedion A. Total anomalous pulmonary venous return below the diaphragm. The roentgen appearances in three patients diagnosed during life. *Am J Roentgenol* 1960;84:436–441.
20. Blake HA, Hall RJ, Manion WC. Anomalous pulmonary venous return. *Circulation* 1965;32:406–414.
21. Haworth SG. Total anomalous pulmonary venous return. Prenatal damage to pulmonary vascular bed and extrapulmonary veins. *Br Heart J* 1982;48:513–524.
22. Fyler DC. Total anomalous pulmonary venous return. In: Fyler DC, ed. *Nadas' pediatric cardiology*. Philadelphia: Hanley & Belfus, 1992:683–691.
23. Van Meter C Jr, LeBlanc JG, Culpepper WS III, Ochsner JL. Partial anomalous pulmonary venous return. *Circulation* 1990;82[Suppl IV]:IV-195–IV-198.
24. Snellen HA, Albers FH. The clinical diagnosis of anomalous pulmonary venous drainage. *Circulation* 1952;6:801–816.
25. Keith JD, Rowe RD, Vlad P, O'Hanley JH. Complete anomalous pulmonary venous drainage. *Am J Med* 1954;16:23–38.
26. Frye RL, Marshall HW, Kincaid OW, Burchell HB. Anomalous pulmonary venous drainage of the right lung into the inferior vena cava. *Br Heart J* 1962;24:696–702.

27. Cooley DA, Balas PE. Total anomalous pulmonary venous drainage into inferior vena cava: report of successful surgical correction. *Surgery* 1962;51:798–804.

28. Snellen HA, Van Ingen HC, Hoefsmit ECM. Patterns of anomalous pulmonary venous drainage. *Circulation* 1968;38:45–63.

29. Steeg CN, Ellis K, Gersony WM. Total anomalous pulmonary venous drainage with ventricular septal defect. *Am Heart J* 1973;86:341–346.

30. Skovranek J, Tuma S, Urbancova D, Samanek M. Range-gated pulsed Doppler echocardiographic diagnosis of supracardiac total anomalous pulmonary venous drainage. *Circulation* 1980;61:841–847.

31. Bharati S, Lev M. Total anomalous pulmonary venous drainage. In: Bharati S, Lev M, eds. *The pathology of congenital heart disease. A personal experience with more than 6,300 congenitally malformed hearts.* Mt. Kisco, NY: Futura Publishing, 1996:609–626.

32. Edwards JE. Pathologic and developmental considerations in anomalous pulmonary venous connection. *Proc Staff Meet Mayo Clin* 1953;28:441–452.

33. Burroughs JT, Edwards JE. Total anomalous pulmonary venous connection. *Am Heart J* 1960;59:913–931.

34. Lucas RV Jr, Adams P Jr, Anderson RC, Varco RL, Edwards JE, Lester RG. Total anomalous pulmonary venous connection to the portal venous system: a cause of pulmonary venous obstruction. *Am J Roentgenol* 1961;86:561–575.

35. Hastreiter AR, Paul MH, Molthan ME, Miller RA. Total anomalous pulmonary venous connection with severe pulmonary venous obstruction. A clinical entity. *Circulation* 1962;25:916–928.

36. Fontana RS, Edwards JE. Total anomalous pulmonary venous connection: age at death and distribution according to sex of patients in the pathologic material of the Mayo Clinic. In: Fontana RS, Edwards JE, eds. *Congenital cardiac disease. A review of 357 cases studied pathologically.* Philadelphia: WB Saunders, 1962:133–137.

37. Elliott LP, Edwards JE. The problem of pulmonary venous obstruction in total anomalous pulmonary venous connection to the left innominate vein [Editorial]. *Circulation* 1962;25:913–915.

38. Edwards JE, Carey LS, Neufeld HN, Lester RG. Partial anomalous pulmonary venous connection. In: Edwards JE, Carey LS, Neufeld HN, Lester RG, eds. *Congenital heart disease. Correlation of pathologic anatomy and angiocardiography,* Vol I. Philadelphia: WB Saunders, 1965:225–234.

39. Kalke BR, Carlson RG, Ferlic RM, Sellers RD, Lillehei CW. Partial anomalous pulmonary venous connections. *Am J Cardiol* 1967;20:91–101.

40. Neirotti R, Gonzalez-Lavin L, Ross DN. Anomalous pulmonary venous connexions of left lung associated with valvular heart disease. Report of two cases. *Br Heart J* 1972;34:969–973.

41. Smallhorn JF, Sutherland GR, Tommasini G, Hunter S, Anderson RH, Macartney FJ. Assessment of total anomalous pulmonary venous connection by two-dimensional echocardiography. *Br Heart J* 1981;46:613–623.

42. Snider AR, Silverman NH, Turley K, Ebert PA. Evaluation of infradiaphragmatic total anomalous pulmonary venous connection with two-dimensional echocardiography. *Circulation* 1982;66:1129–1132.

43. Huhta JC, Gutgesell HP, Nihill MR. Cross sectional echocardiographic diagnosis of total anomalous pulmonary venous connection. *Br Heart J* 1985;53:525–534.

44. Smallhorn JF, Freedom RM. Pulsed Doppler echocardiography in the preoperative evaluation of total anomalous pulmonary venous connection. *J Am Coll Cardiol* 1986;8:1413–1420.

45. Lucas RV Jr, Lock JE, Tandon R, Edwards JE. Gross and histologic anatomy of total anomalous pulmonary venous connections. *Am J Cardiol* 1988;62:292–300.

46. Wang JK, Lue HC, Wu MH, Young ML, Wu FF, Wu JM. Obstructed total anomalous pulmonary venous connection. *Pediatr Cardiol* 1993;14:28–32.

47. Lee ML, Wang JK, Wu MH, Chu SH, Lue HC. Unusual form of total anomalous pulmonary venous connection with double drainage. *Pediatr Cardiol* 1995;16:301–303.

48. Becker AE, Anderson RH. Anomalies of the pulmonary veins. In: Becker AE, Anderson RH, eds. *Pathology of congenital heart disease.* London: Butterworth-Heineman, 1981:53–61.

49. Becker AE, Anderson RH. Anomalous pulmonary venous return. In: Becker AE, Anderson RH, eds. *Cardiac pathology. An integrated text and colour atlas.* New York: Raven Press, 1982:10.11–10.13.

50. Brown AJ. The development of the pulmonary vein in the domestic cat. *Anat Rec* 1913;7:299–330.

51. Buell CE Jr. Origin of the pulmonary vessels in the chick. *Contrib Embryol* 1922;14:11–28.

52. Auer J. The development of the human pulmonary vein and its major variations. *Anat Rec* 1948;101:581–594.

53. Butler H. Some derivatives of the foregut venous plexus of the albino rat, with reference to man. *J Anat* 1952;86:95–109.

54. Lucas RV Jr, Anderson RC, Amplatz K, Adams P Jr, Edwards JE. Congenital causes of pulmonary venous obstruction. *Pediatr Clin North Am* 1963;10:781–836.

55. Arey LB. The heart and circulation changes. In: Arey LB, ed. *Developmental anatomy. A textbook and laboratory manual of embryology,* 7th ed. Philadelphia: WB Saunders, 1966:375–395.

56. Van Mierop LHS. Pathology and pathogenesis of the common cardiac malformations. *Cardiovasc Clin* 1970;2:27–59.

57. Edwards JE, DuShane JW, Alcott DL, Burchell HB. Thoracic venous anomalies. III. Atresia of the common pulmonary vein, the pulmonary vein draining wholly into the superior vena cava (case 3). IV. Stenosis of the common pulmonary vein (cor triatriatum) (case 4). *Arch Pathol* 1951;51:446–460.

58. Lucas RV Jr, Woolfrey BF, Anderson RC, Lester RG, Edwards JE. Atresia of the common pulmonary vein. *Pediatrics* 1962;29:729–739.

59. Wilson J. A description of a very unusual formation of the human heart. *Phil Trans R Soc London* 1798;88:346. Cited by Burroughs JT, Edwards JE. Total anomalous pulmonary venous connection. *Am Heart J* 1960;59:913–931.

60. Friedlowsky A. Einen fall von fehlen des atrium sinistrum. *Vrtljs f prakt Heilk* 1868;98:45.

61. Fyler DC, Buckley LP, Hellenbrand WE, Cohn HE. Total anomalous pulmonary venous return. Report of the New England Regional Infant Cardiac Program. *Pediatrics* 1980;65:375–461.

62. Edwards JE, Carey LS, Neufeld HN, Lester RG. Total anomalous pulmonary venous connection. In: Edwards JE, Carey LS, Neufeld HN, Lester RG, eds. *Congenital heart disease. Correlation of pathologic anatomy and angiocardiography,* Vol I. Philadelphia: WB Saunders, 1965:268–288.

63. Delisle G, Ando M, Calder AL, et al. Total anomalous pulmonary venous connection: report of 93 autopsied cases with emphasis on diagnostic and surgical considerations. *Am Heart J* 1976;91:99–122.

64. Edwards JE, DuShane JW. Thoracic venous anomalies. I. Vascular connection of the left atrium and the left innominate vein (levoatriocardinal vein) associated with mitral atresia and premature closure of the foramen ovale (case 1). II. Pulmonary veins draining wholly into the ductus venosus (case 2). *Arch Pathol* 1950;49:517–537.

65. Cooper MJ, Teitel DF, Silverman NH, Enderlein MA. Study of the infradiaphragmatic total anomalous pulmonary venous connection with cross-sectional and pulsed Doppler echocardiography. *Circulation* 1984;70:412–416.

66. Del Torso S, Goh TH, Venables AW. Echocardiographic findings in the liver in total anomalous pulmonary venous connection. *Am J Cardiol* 1986;57:374–375.

67. Whight CM, Barrat-Boyes BG, Calder AL, Neutze JM, Brandt PWT. Total anomalous pulmonary venous connection. Long-term results following repair in infancy. *J Thorac Cardiovasc Surg* 1978;75:52–63.

68. Arciniegas E, Henry JG, Green EW. Stenosis of the coronary sinus ostium. An unusual site of obstruction in total anomalous pulmonary venous drainage. *J Thorac Cardiovasc Surg* 1980;79:303–305.

69. Rodriguez AM, Marin D, Cayre RO, et al. Total anomalous pulmonary venous return: prognostic value of left ventricular size for surgical outcome. An echocardiographic study. *J Am Soc Echocardiogr* 1994;7:S21(abst).

70. Kirklin JW, Barrat-Boyes BG. Total anomalous pulmonary venous connection. In: Kirklin JW, Barrat-Boyes BG, eds. *Cardiac surgery. Morphology, diagnostic criteria, natural history, techniques, results, and indications,* Vol 1, 2nd ed. New York: Churchill Livingstone, 1993:645–673.

71. Winslow. *Mem Acad Roy Sci* 1739:113. Cited by Brody H. Drainage

of the pulmonary veins into the right side of the heart. *Arch Pathol* 1942;33:221–240.

72. Healey JE Jr. An anatomic survey of anomalous pulmonary veins: their clinical significance. *J Thorac Surg* 1952;23:433–444.

73. Dotter CT, Hardisty NM, Steinberg I. Anomalous right pulmonary vein entering the inferior vena cava: two cases diagnosed during life by angiocardiography and cardiac catheterization. *Am J Med Sci* 1949;218:31–36.

74. McKusick VA, Cooley RN. Drainage of right pulmonary vein into inferior vena cava. Report of a case, with a radiologic analysis of the principal types of anomalous venous return from the lung. *N Engl J Med* 1955;252:291–301.

75. Halasz NA, Halloran KH, Liebow AA. Bronchial and arterial anomalies with drainage of the right lung into the inferior vena cava. *Circulation* 1956;14:826–846.

76. Neill CA, Ferencz C, Sabiston DC, Sheldon H. The familial occurrence of hypoplastic right lung with systemic arterial supply and venous drainage: "scimitar syndrome." *Bull Johns Hopkins Hosp* 1960;107:1–21.

77. Kiely B, Filler J, Stone S, Doyle EF. Syndrome of anomalous venous drainage of the right lung to the inferior vena cava. A review of 67 reported cases and three new cases in children. *Am J Cardiol* 1967;20:102–116.

78. Bauer A, Korfer R, Bircks W. Left-to-right shunt at atrial level due to anomalous venous connection of left lung. Report of seven cases. *J Thorac Cardiovasc Surg* 1982;84:626–630.

79. Dean JC, Fox GW. A left pulmonary vein emptying into the left innominate. *Wis Med J* 1928;27:120–122.

80. Jack R, Lee H. An anomaly of the left pulmonary vein. *Anat Rec* 1928;39:359–363.

81. D'Cruz IA, Arcilla RA. Anomalous venous drainage of the left lung into the inferior vena cava. *Am Heart J* 1964;67:539–544.

82. Salazar J. Scimitar syndrome: five cases examined with two-dimensional and Doppler echocardiography. *Pediatr Cardiol* 1995;16:283–286.

83. Beerman LB, Zuberbuhler FR. Atrial septal defect. In: Anderson RH, Macartney FJ, Shinebourne EA, Tynan M. *Pediatric cardiology*, Vol 1. Edinburgh: Churchill Livingstone, 1987:541–562.

84. Gotsman MS, Astley R, Parsons CG. Partial anomalous pulmonary venous drainage in association with atrial septal defect. *Br Heart J* 1965;27:566–571.

85. Swan HJC, Kirklin JW, Becu LM, Wood EH. Anomalous connection of right pulmonary veins to superior vena cava with interatrial communications: hemodynamic data in eight cases. *Circulation* 1957;16:54–66.

86. Lewis FJ. High defects of the atrial septum. *J Thorac Cardiovasc Surg* 1958;36:1–11.

87. Cooley DA, Ellis PR, Bellizi ME. Atrial septal defects of the sinus venosus type: surgical considerations. *Dis Chest* 1961;39:185–192.

88. Davia JE, Cheitlin MD, Bedynek JL. Sinus venosus atrial septal defect: analysis of fifty cases. *Am Heart J* 1973;85:177–185.

89. Ettedgui JA, Siewers RD, Anderson RH, Park SC, Pahl E, Zuberbuhler JR. Diagnostic echocardiographic features of the sinus venosus defect. *Br Heart J* 1990;64:329–331.

90. Deshpande JR, Kinare SG. Atresia of the common pulmonary vein. *Int J Cardiol* 1991;30:221–226.

91. Reye RDK. Congenital stenosis of the pulmonary veins in their extrapulmonary course. *Med J Aust* 1951;1:801–802.

92. Edwards JE. Congenital stenosis of pulmonary veins. Pathologic and developmental considerations. *Lab Invest* 1960;9:46–66.

93. Binet JP, Bouchard F, Langlois J, Chetochine F, Conso JF, Pottemain M. Unilateral congenital stenosis of the pulmonary veins. *J Thorac Cardiovasc Surg* 1972;63:397–402.

94. Smallhorn JF, Pauperio H, Benson L, Freedom RM, Rowe RD. Pulsed Doppler assessment of pulmonary vein obstruction. *Am Heart J* 1985;110:483–486.

95. Sade RM, Freed MD, Matthews EC, Castaneda AR. Stenosis of individual pulmonary veins. Review of the literature and report of a surgical case. *J Thorac Cardiovasc Surg* 1974;67:953.

96. Bini RM, Cleveland DC, Ceballos R, Bargeron LM Jr, Pacifico AD, Kirklin JW. Congenital pulmonary vein stenosis. *Am J Cardiol* 1984;54:369–375.

PART XII

Anomalies of the Coronary Arteries

CHAPTER 34

Congenital Anomalies of the Coronary Arteries

Lilliam M. Valdes-Cruz and Raul O. Cayre

The congenital anomalies of the coronary arteries include coronary fistulae, anomalous origin of one or both coronary arteries from the pulmonary artery, and congenital aneurysms. The anomalies of origin and distribution of the coronary arteries associated with the various congenital cardiac malformations, as well as the ventriculocoronary communications seen in pulmonary atresia with intact ventricular septum and with hypoplastic left heart syndrome, are discussed in their corresponding chapters.

CORONARY FISTULAE

Coronary fistulae are rare malformations characterized by an anomalous connection of a coronary artery with a cardiac chamber or major thoracic vessel. The first description of a communication between the coronary arteries and the right ventricle was mentioned by Vieussens (1) in a letter addressed to Monsieur Boudin, Premier Medicin de Monseigneur le Dauphin et Conseiller d'Etat, dated July 9, 1705 and published in 1706. The incidence of this type of malformation is one in 50,000 of all congenital heart disease (2,3) and comprises 43% of all major congenital anomalies of the coronary arteries (4).

EMBRYOLOGIC CONSIDERATIONS

In the early stages of cardiac development, the ventricular walls are nourished initially by imbibition of the circulating blood (5) and later by intramyocardial sinusoids that originate from the intertrabecular spaces (6–9). In the fifth week of development, two endothelial vascular networks appear in the subepicardial space at the level of the atrioventricular and interventricular sulci (10–12) (see Fig. 1-15). These subepicardial vascular networks initially establish contact with the intramyocardial sinusoids. Later, when they come in contact with the wall of the truncus arteriosus either through coronary buds (10–13)

or through the development of small channels in its wall (14–16), the connection with the intramyocardial sinusoids is lost. The subepicardial endothelial vascular networks give rise to the trunk and branches of the coronary arteries.

The presence of a fistula between one or both coronaries and a cardiac chamber is due to an abnormal persistence of the connection between the subepicardial vascular network and the intertrabecular spaces or intramyocardial sinusoids (3,17–20). In cases where there is a fistula between a coronary artery and the pulmonary artery, the coronary sinus or a systemic vein, the fistula is due to an abnormal connection between the subepicardial network and the pulmonary artery, the coronary sinus or the tributary vein.

ANATOMIC AND ECHOCARDIOGRAPHIC CONSIDERATIONS

The echocardiographic study of coronary fistulae should establish the following: (a) the anatomic characteristics of the fistula, the coronary artery from which it originates and the site of drainage; and (b) associated anomalies.

Anatomic Characteristics of the Fistula, the Coronary Artery from Which It Originates, and the Site of Drainage

In the presence of coronary fistulae, there is a communication between the coronary system at high pressure and a cardiac chamber or vessel at a constant or intermittent low pressure. Of the 241 cases of coronary fistula reviewed by us in the literature, 98.8% (238/241) had normal origin of both coronary arteries from the aorta. A single coronary artery was found in two cases (0.8%) and an anomalous origin of the right coronary artery from the

527

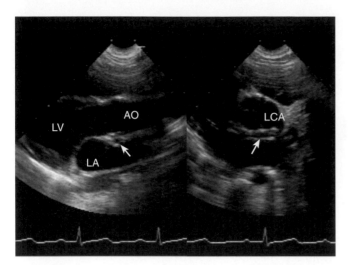

ECHO. 34-1. Left: Cross-section of dilated fistula between the left coronary artery and the right atrium *(arrow)*. **Right:** Long axis of the left coronary artery to right atrial fistula *(arrow)*. *AO,* aorta; *LV,* left ventricle; *LA,* left atrium.

pulmonary artery in one case (0.4%) (2,3,17–19,21–40). The fistula can originate from the proximal portion of the coronary artery or a branch, from the mid portion of the vessel, or from its terminal end. The artery or arteries involved are tortuous and dilated, and 19% to 36% of cases have aneurysmal dilatation in the region of the fistula (2,3). The wall of the coronary artery has medial thickening, an increase in the amount of elastic fibers between the muscular fibers, and mild intimal thickening in the region close to the entrance of the fistula (18). Generally, the fistula has only one drainage site, but occasionally there can be two or more. It can form an angiomatous network with multiple vessels having one or more drainage points.

Of the 241 cases reviewed, the right coronary artery was involved in 105 (44%) (2,3,17–19,21,22,24,28–31,33–39); the left coronary artery in 131 (54%) (2,3,17–19,23,26–40); both coronary arteries in three instances (1.2%) (3,33,38); and a single coronary artery in two cases (0.8%) (25,39). The most frequent site of drainage of the fistula was the right ventricle in 89 cases (37%), either at the apex, the outflow tract, or the inflow (2,3,17–19,25,28–39). The fistula was to the main pulmonary artery in 77 cases (32%) (2,3,17–19,23,29,30,33–36,38,40); the right atrium in 39 cases (16%) (2,3,19,22,29,31,33–36,38); the coronary sinus in 12 cases (5%) (3,21,24,30,34–36); the left ventricle in 12 cases (5%) (2,17,19,38); the left atrium in six cases (2.6%) (2,3,30,33,36); the superior vena cava in two cases (0.8%) (27,30); the bronchial veins in two cases (0.8%) (2); a persistent left superior vena cava draining into the coronary sinus in one case (0.4%) (26); and the right pulmonary artery in one case (0.4%) (2).

When there is a fistula into the right atrium, the right ventricle, the pulmonary artery, the coronary sinus, or a systemic vein, there is a left-to-right or systemic to pulmonary shunt. When the fistula is established to the left atrium or left ventricle, there is a coronary-systemic arterial shunt. The fistula causes disturbance to the coronary flow, which can result in myocardial ischemia, heart failure, or myocardial infarction. There can also be bacterial endocarditis, coronary arteriosclerosis, thrombosis, or rupture of the aneurysmal dilatation in the region of the fistula with sudden death. Only two cases of spontaneous closure have been reported in the literature (35,41).

Two-dimensional echocardiography with color Doppler flow mapping has been shown to be of utility in demonstrating coronary fistulae (35,42). The views from which the location, trajectory, and site of entry of the fistulae can be studied are the parasternal long- and short-axis views, the apical four- and two-chamber views, and the subcostal four-chamber and short-axis views. Visualization of a dilated proximal coronary artery or of a dilated branch and of another coronary artery of normal size, particularly in the presence of a continuous murmur, should raise the suspicion of a coronary fistula (Echo. 34-1). With adequate angulation of the transducer, the trajectory and site of drainage of the fistula can be demonstrated. The chamber or vessel into which the fistula drains is dilated. Color Doppler flow mapping is useful in showing disturbed continuous flow within the fistulous coronary artery and the vessel receiving its drainage or a jet if the fistula ends within a chamber (Echo. 34-2; see color plate 120 following p. 364). Spectral Doppler records continuous flow with late systolic and early diastolic accentuation. In cases where the coronary fistula drains into the pulmonary artery, the presence of two coronary arteries emerging normally from the aorta would allow differentiation from anomalous origin of the coronary artery from the pulmonary; however, these can be difficult

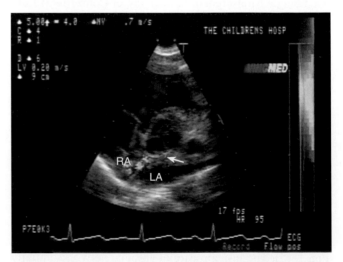

ECHO. 34-2. Short axis of the aorta demonstrating the color Doppler flow image of the fistulous drainage of a left coronary artery into the right atrium *(arrow)*. *RA,* right atrium; *LA,* left atrium.

to determine conclusively, so aortography with or without selective coronary arteriography may be required. Retrograde diastolic flow may be seen in the descending aorta if the shunt is large.

Associated Anomalies

Coronary fistulae have been reported in association with ventricular septal defects (2), patent ductus arteriosus (2,3,31,35), valve pulmonic stenosis (2,25), atrial septal defect (25), prolapse of the mitral valve (2), tricuspid regurgitation (2), mitral regurgitation (2,3), double outlet right ventricle and valve pulmonic stenosis (2), valve aortic stenosis (2), and left superior vena cava draining into the coronary sinus (26).

ANOMALOUS ORIGIN OF A CORONARY ARTERY FROM THE PULMONARY ARTERY

Anomalous origin of a coronary artery from the pulmonary artery is a rare abnormality of the coronary arteries that occurs in 0.25% to 0.50% of all congenital heart disease (20,43). It comprises 57% of all major coronary arterial malformations (4). The first description of a case of anomalous origin of a right coronary artery from the pulmonary artery was reported by Brooks in 1886 (44). The first case of anomalous origin of a left coronary artery was reported by Abbott in 1908 (45). Tow in 1931 (46) published the first case of origin of both coronary arteries from a common trunk that emerged from the left pulmonary artery in a patient with truncus arteriosus. In 1934, Grayzel (47) reported a case with both coronary arteries originating separately from the main pulmonary arterial trunk.

EMBRYOLOGIC CONSIDERATIONS

Anomalous origin of one or both coronary arteries from the pulmonary artery would be the result of an abnormal connection of the subepicardial vascular network with the region of the wall of the truncus arteriosus that will give rise to the pulmonary artery. Normally it would establish connection with the region giving origin to the aorta.

ANATOMIC AND ECHOCARDIOGRAPHIC CONSIDERATIONS

The echocardiographic study of anomalous origin of one or both coronary arteries from the pulmonary artery should include the following: (a) identification of the anomalous coronary artery and the site of origin; and (b) associated anomalies.

Identification of the Anomalous Coronary Artery and the Site of Origin

The left coronary artery, is the one most commonly seen arising from the pulmonary artery, comprising 92% of all cases reviewed by us in the literature (4,28,34,48–57). A case of anomalous origin of a left coronary artery from the left pulmonary artery in the presence of truncus arteriosus has been reported by Hallman (28).

The left coronary artery emerges from the left posterior sinus of Valsalva of the pulmonary artery and its size can be normal or hypoplastic. The right coronary artery emerges normally from the right anterior aortic sinus and is generally dilated. The presence of collaterals between the right and left coronary arteries results in blood flow from the right coronary artery, which is under systemic pressure, to the left coronary arterial system and retrogradely into the pulmonary artery. The presence or absence of these collaterals serves as the basis of a clinical classification of anomalous origin of the coronary from the pulmonary artery, infantile type, in which there are no or very few collaterals and adult type in which the collateral circulation is well developed (56). Patients with few collaterals present with greater degrees of myocardial ischemia and/or infarction and therefore with more severe mitral regurgitation. The mitral valve apparatus can show signs of dysplasia, probably secondary in origin, and the left ventricle is dilated and histologically has evidence of chronic ischemia with interstitial fibrosis and endocardial thickening (56).

Origin of a right coronary artery from the pulmonary artery is much rarer (43,58–62). It has been seen in 6% of all reported cases of anomalous coronary origin from

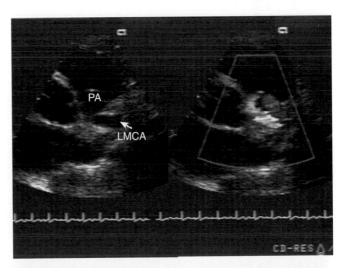

ECHO. 34-3. Parasternal short-axis view demonstrating anomalous origin of the left coronary artery from the pulmonary artery. **Left:** Anatomic image indicating the anomalous coronary artery (arrow). **Right:** Color Doppler image of the flow of the left coronary artery into the pulmonary artery. *PA,* pulmonary artery; *LMCA,* left main coronary artery.

the pulmonary artery (4,28,34,48–62). Usually patients have few symptoms. The incidence of anomalous origin of both coronary arteries separately (4,47,48,63) or through a common trunk (46,64) from the pulmonary artery comprises only 2% of all cases of anomalous coronary arterial origin from the pulmonary artery (4,28,34,48–64).

Anomalous origin of the left anterior descending coronary artery from the pulmonary artery has been reported in two cases (65,66). Two additional cases have also been reported of anomalous origin of the circumflex branch from the pulmonary artery (67,68).

The echocardiographic demonstration of anomalous origin of one or both coronaries from the pulmonary is best accomplished from the parasternal long- and short-axis views, the subcostal short-axis view, and the high left subclavicular view (Echo. 34-3; see color plate 121 following p. 364). A dilated and dysfunctional left ventricle is common, and this can be evaluated from the parasternal long- and short-axis view, the apical four-chamber, two-chamber, and long-axis views. The presence and severity of the mitral regurgitation can also be evaluated from these multiple views. The parasternal short-axis view demonstrates absence of a connection between the involved coronary artery and the aorta, although it is not uncommon to record the appearance of a connection giving the false impression of normal origin; this by itself should not be interpreted as the presence of a normally arising coronary artery. Spectral and color Doppler mapping of the flow within the pulmonary artery is extremely helpful to characterize the drainage of an anomalous coronary artery. The flow is continuous, of low velocity, and directed towards the transducer (red) on the color map (Echos. 34-3, 34-4).

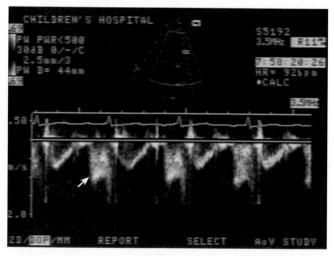

ECHO. 34-4. Spectral Doppler tracing of the velocity recorded at the site of drainage of the flow from an anomalous left coronary artery into the pulmonary artery *(arrow).*

Associated Anomalies

Anomalous origin of one or both coronary arteries from the pulmonary artery has been seen in association with ventricular septal defect (51,54,56,59), patent ductus arteriosus (48,51,56), patent foramen ovale (48,53), atrial septal defect (51,53,56), valve pulmonic stenosis (54), coarctation of the aorta (48,56), bicuspid aortic valve (64), bicuspid pulmonic valve (56), aortopulmonary window (59), tricuspid atresia (47), and truncus arteriosus (28,46).

CONGENITAL ANEURYSM OF THE CORONARY ARTERIES

Aneurysms of the coronary arteries can have various origins such as micotic, arteriosclerotic, traumatic, and syphilitic or be associated with periarteritis nodosa, necrotizing arteritis, coronary arteriovenous fistulae, and mucocutaneous lymph node syndrome (Kawasaki's disease), or be congenital (69–75). Isolated congenital aneurysms are extremely rare, and their actual incidence is not known. The first reported case of a coronary aneurysm, of micotic origin, was by Bougon in 1812 (76). In the review by Scott in 1948 (77), the first report of a presumably congenital aneurysm is attributed to Peste in 1843.

EMBRYOLOGIC CONSIDERATIONS

The morphogenetic mechanism causing congenital aneurysms of the coronary arteries is not known. Forbus in 1930 (78) suggested that the origin could be similar to that of cerebral artery aneurysms, namely an incomplete development of the vessel wall with thinning of the elastic and muscular layers at the site of bifurcation of the arteries.

ANATOMIC AND ECHOCARDIOGRAPHIC CONSIDERATIONS

The echocardiographic study of congenital aneurysms of the coronary arteries should include the following: (a) characteristics and location of the aneurysm(s); and (b) associated anomalies.

Characteristics and Location of the Aneurysm(s)

Congenital aneurysms of the coronary arteries are usually single. They can be found in any one of the coronary arteries or in both simultaneously. Most frequently, they are located at the site of bifurcation of the coronary arteries, particularly at the origin of the anterior descending coronary artery. Their size can be variable, from a few millimeters to several centimeters (79–84). Histologically, there are areas of thinning of the arterial wall with irregular deposits of hyaline and plaques of calcified material (83). Rupture or thrombosis are common complications.

The echocardiographic views that best demonstrate coronary aneurysms are the parasternal short-axis and the apical and subcostal outflow views. Differentiation between congenital and acquired aneurysm is not possible echocardiographically so the clinical presentation is essential in the diagnosis. Aneurysms in the proximal right or left coronary arteries, at the bifurcation of the left main coronary artery, and in the proximal portions of the left anterior descending and the circumflex arteries are easily seen by two-dimensional echocardiography, classically from the parasternal short-axis view. The transducer may need to be positioned slightly higher or lower on the chest wall to demonstrate greater lengths of the coronary branches. The posterior descending coronary artery can be evaluated coursing along the posterior septum from the parasternal view.

Associated Anomalies

Congenital aneurysms of the coronary arteries usually present as isolated lesions, without associated cardiac anomalies. There has been one case reported by Kalke and Edwards (73) with a bicuspid aortic valve.

INTRAOPERATIVE AND POSTOPERATIVE EVALUATION

Intraoperative transesophageal study has been shown to be very useful in the localization and surgical treatment of coronary fistulae in the pediatric population (39). The

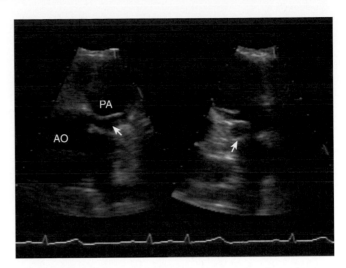

ECHO. 34-6. **Left:** Parasternal short-axis view demonstrating a dilated tunnel used to redirect an anomalous left coronary from the pulmonary artery into the aorta *(arrow).* **Right:** Cross-section of the tunnel *(arrow).* Note the dilatation of the tunnel appreciated in both views. *AO,* aorta; *PA,* pulmonary artery.

transverse four-chamber view (see Fig. 4-28A) with the adjunctive use of color Doppler flow mapping shows the dilated coronary artery with continuous, disturbed flow within its lumen and at the site of drainage into a cardiac chamber. Stevenson et al. (39) reported the utility of observing the disappearance of the fistulous flow and/or of additional fistulous drainage sites during surgical treatment of this lesion using transesophageal color Doppler flow mapping.

More recently, coronary fistulae have been closed with transcatheter delivery of coils, thereby avoiding open heart surgery. The coils can usually be seen on echocardiography and any residual flow assessed with transthoracic

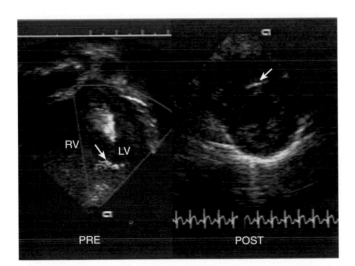

ECHO. 34-5. Images from a case of coronary fistulae. **Left:** Apical view of a coronary fistula draining into the right ventricle *(arrow).* **Right:** Short-axis view demonstrating the coil used to close the fistulous connection *(arrow). RV,* right ventricle; *LV,* left ventricle.

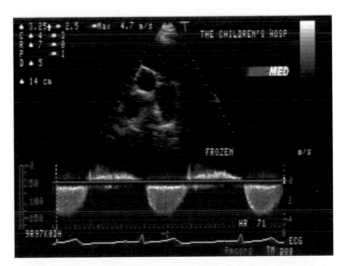

ECHO. 34-7. Spectral Doppler recording of the flows across the pulmonic valve in the same patient as in Echo. 34-6. The tunnel has caused pulmonary stenosis and regurgitation.

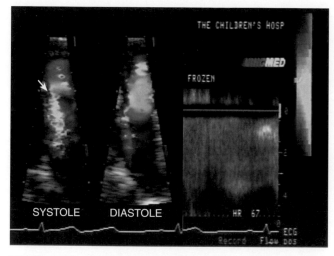

ECHO. 34-8. Color Doppler and spectral velocity recording of a fistula between the left coronary artery and the pulmonary artery (arrow) after tunnel repair of anomalous origin of the left coronary artery from the pulmonary artery. Images were obtained from the same patient as in Echos. 34-6 and 34-7. The recordings demonstrate continuous, high-velocity flow from the left coronary artery to the pulmonary artery.

imaging (Echo. 34-5; see color plate 122 following p. 364).

Anomalous origin of a coronary artery from the pulmonary artery can be seen from the longitudinal view at the level of the outflow tracts (see Fig. 4-29E) and from the transverse view at basal level (see Fig. 4-31A), where the greater length of the main pulmonary artery can be recorded. Color Doppler flow mapping aids in the demonstration of the anomalous flow draining into the pulmonary trunk. The left ventricular size and function, as well as the wall motion abnormalities commonly present in this lesion, can be evaluated from the transgastric short-axis view (see Fig. 4-27A) as well as from the retrocardiac transverse four-chamber view and the longitudinal two-chamber equivalent view (see Fig. 4-28).

Postoperatively, the site of repair of the anomalous left coronary should be assessed carefully for signs of obstruction. This can be accomplished best through the parasternal short-axis view (Echos. 34-6–34-8; see color plate 123 following p. 364).

REFERENCES

1. Vieussens R. *Nouvelles decouvertes sur le coeur.* Paris, 1706. Cited by Wearn JT, Mettier SR, Klumpp TG, Zschiesche LJ. The nature of the vascular communications between the coronary arteries and the chambers of the heart. *Am Heart J* 1933;9:143–164.
2. Urrutia CO, Falaschi G, Ott DA, Cooley DA. Surgical management of 56 patients with congenital coronary artery fistulas. *Ann Thorac Surg* 1983;35:300–307.
3. Chen Y, Belboul A, Roberts D. The surgical management of congenital coronary artery fistula. *Coron Artery Dis* 1994;5:995–1000.
4. Ogden JA. Congenital anomalies of the coronary arteries. *Am J Cardiol* 1970;25:474–479.
5. Dbaly J, Ostadal B, Rychter Z. Development of the coronary arteries in rat embryos. *Acta Anat* 1968;71:209–222.
6. Licata RH. A continuation study of the development of the blood supply of the human heart. Part II: the deep or intramural circulation. *Anat Rec* 1956;124:326(abst).
7. Manasek FJ. The ultrastructure of embryonic myocardial blood vessels. *Dev Biol* 1971;26:42–54.
8. Rychter Z, Ostadal B. Fate of "sinusoidal" intertrabecular spaces of chick embryo heart wall after the origination of coronary bed. *Folia Morphol* 1971;19:31–44.
9. Rychter Z, Rychterova V. Angio- and myoarchitecture of the heart wall under normal and experimentally changed morphogenesis. In: Pexieder T, ed. *Perspectives in cardiovascular research. Mechanisms of cardiac morphogenesis and teratogenesis.* New York: Raven Press, 1981:431–452.
10. Ogden J. The origin of the coronary arteries. *Circulation* 1968; 38[Suppl VI]:150.
11. Sissman N. Developmental landmarks in cardiac morphogenesis: comparative chronology. *Am J Cardiol* 1970;25:141–148.
12. Hirakow R. Development of the cardiac blood vessels in staged human embryos. *Acta Anat* 1983;115:220–230.
13. Conte G, Pellegrini A. On the development of the coronary arteries in human embryos, stages 14–19. *Anat Embryol* 1984;169:209–215.
14. Bogers AJJC, Gittenberger-de Groot AC, Dubbeldam JA, Huysmans HA. The inadequacy of existing theories on development of the proximal coronary arteries and their connections with the arterial trunks. *Int J Cardiol* 1988;20:117–122.
15. Gittenberger-de Groot AC, Bogers AJJC, Poelmann RE, Peault BM, Huysmans HA. Development of the coronary arterial orifices. *Ann NY Acad Sci* 1990;588:377–379.
16. Waldo K, Kirby ML. A new perspective on the development of the coronary arteries in the chick embryo. *Ann NY Acad Sci* 1990;588: 459–460.
17. Gasul BM, Arcilla RA, Fell EH, Lynfield J, Bicoff JP, Luan LL. Congenital coronary arteriovenous fistula. Clinical, phonocardiographic, angiocardiographic and hemodynamic studies in five patients. *Pediatrics* 1960;25:531–560.
18. Neufeld HN, Lester RG, Adams P Jr, Anderson RC, Lillehei CW, Edwards JE. Congenital communication of a coronary artery with a cardiac chamber or the pulmonary trunk ("coronary artery fistula"). *Circulation* 1961;24:171–179.
19. McNamara JJ, Gross RE. Congenital coronary artery fistula. *Surgery* 1969;65:59–69.
20. Vlodaver Z, Neufeld HN, Edwards JE. Anomalous communication of a coronary artery with a cardiac chamber or major thoracic vessel. In: Vlodaver Z, Neufeld HN, Edwards JE, eds. *Coronary arterial variations in the normal heart and in congenital heart disease.* New York: Academic Press, 1975:43–77.
21. Halpert B. Arteriovenous communication between the right coronary artery and the coronary sinus. *Heart* 1929–31;15:129–133.
22. Edwards JE, Gladding TC, Weir AB. Congenital communication between the right coronary artery and the right atrium. *J Thorac Surg* 1958;35:662–673.
23. Amplatz K, Aguirre J, Lillehei CW. Coronary arteriovenous fistula into main pulmonary artery. Preoperative diagnosis by selective aortography. *JAMA* 1960;172:1384–1386.
24. Yenel F. Coronary arteriovenous communication. Report of a case and review of the literature. *N Engl J Med* 1961;265:577–580.
25. Anselmi G, Munoz S, Blanco P, Carbonell L, Puigbo JJ. Anomalous coronary artery connecting with the right ventricle associated with pulmonary stenosis and atrial septal defect. *Am Heart J* 1961;62: 406–414.
26. Stansel HC Jr, Fenn JE. Coronary arteriovenous fistula between the left coronary artery and persistent left superior vena cava complicated by bacterial endocarditis. *Ann Surg* 1964;160:292–296.
27. Gensini GG, Palacio A, Buonanno C. Fistula from circumflex coronary artery to superior vena cava. *Circulation* 1966;33:297–301.
28. Hallman GL, Cooley DA, Singer DB. Congenital anomalies of the coronary arteries: anatomy, pathology, and surgical treatment. *Surgery* 1966;59:133–144.
29. Sakakibara S, Yokoyama M, Takao A, Nogi M, Gomi H. Coronary arteriovenous fistula. Nine operated cases. *Am Heart J* 1966;72: 307–314.

30. Effler DB, Sheldom WC, Turner JJ, Groves LK. Coronary arteriovenous fistulas: diagnosis and surgical management. Report of fifteen cases. *Surgery* 1967;61:41–50.

31. Taber RE, Gale HH, Lam CR. Coronary artery–right heart fistulas. *J Thorac Cardiovasc Surg* 1967;53:84–92.

32. Daniel TM, Graham TP, Sabiston DC. Coronary artery–right ventricular fistula with congestive heart failure: surgical correction in neonatal period. *Surgery* 1970;67:985–994.

33. Oldham HN Jr, Ebert PA, Young WG, Sabiston DC Jr. Surgical management of congenital coronary artery fistula. *Ann Thorac Surg* 1971;12:503–513.

34. Levin DC, Fellows KE, Abrams HL. Hemodynamically significant primary anomalies of the coronary arteries. Angiocardiographic aspects. *Circulation* 1978;58:25–34.

35. Liberthson RR, Sagar K, Berboken JP, Weintraub RM, Levine FH. Congenital coronary arteriovenous fistula. Report of 13 patients, review of the literature and delineation of management. *Circulation* 1979;59:849–854.

36. Lowe JE, Oldham HN Jr, Sabiston DC Jr. Surgical management of congenital coronary artery fistulas. *Ann Surg* 1981;194:373–380.

37. Ludomirsky A, Danford DA, Glasow PF, Blumenschein SD, Murphy DJ Jr, Huhta JC. Evaluation of coronary artery fistula by color-flow Doppler echocardiography. *Echocardiography* 1987;4:383–386.

38. Karagoz HY, Zorlutuna YI, Babacan KM, et al. Congenital coronary artery fistulas. Diagnostic and surgical considerations. *Jpn Heart J* 1989;30:685–694.

39. Stevenson JG, Sorensen GK, Stamm SJ, McCloskey JP, Hall DG, Rittenhouse EA. Intraoperative transesophageal echocardiography of coronary artery fistulas. *Ann Thorac Surg* 1994;57:1217–1221.

40. Achtel RA, Zaret BL, Iben AB, Hurley EJ. Surgical correction of congenital left coronary artery–main pulmonary artery fistula in association with anomalous right coronary artery. *J Thorac Cardiovasc Surg* 1975;70:46–51.

41. Griffiths SP, Ellis K, Hordof AJ. Spontaneous complete closure of a congenital coronary artery fistula. *J Am Coll Cardiol* 1983;2:1169–1173.

42. Velvis H, Schmidt KG, Silverman NH, Turley K. Diagnosis of coronary artery fistula by two dimensional echocardiography, pulsed Doppler ultrasound and color flow imaging. *J Am Coll Cardiol* 1989;14:968–976.

43. Tyler DC, Buckley LP, Hellenbrand WE, Cohn HE. Report of the New England Regional Infant Cardiac Program. *Pediatrics* 1980;65[Suppl]:375–461.

44. Brooks H St J. Two cases of an abnormal coronary artery of the heart arising from the pulmonary artery: with some remarks upon the effect of this anomaly in producing cirsoid dilatation of the vessels. *J Anat Physiol* 1886;20:26. Cited by Edwards JE. Anomalous coronary arteries with special reference to arteriovenous-like communications. *Circulation* 1958;17:1001–1006.

45. Abbott ME. Anomalous origin from the pulmonary arteries. In: Osler W, ed. *"Osler" modern medicine. Its theories and practice.* Vol. 4. Philadelphia: Lea & Febiger, 1908:420. Cited by Vlodaver Z, Neufeld HN, Edwards JE. Anomalous origin of the coronary arteries from the pulmonary trunk. In: Vlodaver Z, Neufeld HN, Edwards JE, eds. *Coronary arterial variations in the normal heart and in congenital heart disease.* New York: Academic Press, 1975:78–108.

46. Tow A. Cor biloculare with truncus arteriosus and endocarditis. *Am J Dis Child* 1931;42:1413–1416.

47. Grayzel DM, Tennant R. Congenital atresia of the tricuspid orifice and anomalous origins of the coronary arteries from the pulmonary artery. *Am J Pathol* 1934;10:791–794.

48. Alexander RW, Griffith GC. Anomalies of the coronary arteries and their clinical significance. *Circulation* 1956;14:800–805.

49. Nadas AS, Gamboa R, Hugenholtz PG. Anomalous left coronary artery originating from the pulmonary artery. Report of two surgically treated cases with a proposal of hemodynamic and therapeutic classification. *Circulation* 1964;29:167–175.

50. Lundquist C, Amplatz K. Anomalous origin of the left coronary artery from the pulmonary artery. *Am J Roentgenol* 1965;95:611–620.

51. Sabiston DC Jr, Orme SK. Congenital origin of the left coronary artery from the pulmonary artery. *J Thorac Cardiovasc Surg* 1968;9:543–552.

52. Cazzaniga M, Herraiz Sarachaga I, Cayre R, et al. Origen anomalo de la arteria coronaria izquierda. Presentacion de cinco casos. *An Esp Pediatr* 1983;18:1–10.

53. Midgley FM, Watson DC Jr, Scott LP, et al. Repair of anomalous origin of the left coronary artery in the infant and small child. *J Am Coll Cardiol* 1984;4:1231–1234.

54. Cottrill CM, Davis D, McMillen M, O'Connor WN, Noonan JA, Todd EP. Anomalous left coronary artery from the pulmonary artery: significance of associated intracardiac defects. *J Am Coll Cardiol* 1985;6:237–242.

55. Bunton R, Jonas RA, Lang P, Rein AJJT, Castaneda AR. Anomalous origin of left coronary artery from pulmonary artery. Ligation versus establishment of a two coronary artery system. *J Thorac Cardiovasc Surg* 1987;93:103–108.

56. Smith A, Arnold R, Anderson RH, et al. Anomalous origin of the left coronary artery from the pulmonary trunk. Anatomic findings in relation to pathophysiology and surgial repair. *J Thorac Cardiovasc Surg* 1989;98:16–24.

57. Kesler KA, Pennington DG, Nouri S, et al. Left subclavian–left coronary artery anastomosis for anomalous origin of the left coronary artery. Long-term follow-up. *J Thorac Cardiovasc Surg* 1989;98:25–29.

58. Jordan RA, Dry TJ, Edwards JE. Anomalous origin of right coronary artery from the pulmonary trunk. *Proc Staff Meet Mayo Clin* 1950;25:673–678.

59. Burroughs JT, Schmutzer KJ, Linder F, Neuhaus G. Anomalous origin of the right coronary artery with aortico-pulmonary window and ventricular septal defect. Report of a case with complete operative correction. *J Cardiovasc Surg* 1962;3:142–148.

60. Wald S, Stonecipher K, Baldwin BJ, Nutter DO. Anomalous origin of the right coronary artery from the pulmonary artery. *Am J Cardiol* 1971;27:677–681.

61. Tingelstad JB, Lower RR, Eldredge WJ. Anomalous origin of the right coronary artery from the main pulmonary artery. *Am J Cardiol* 1972;30:670–673.

62. Bregman D, Brennan FJ, Singer A, et al. Anomalous origin of the right coronary artery from the pulmonary artery. *J Thorac Cardiovasc Surg* 1976;72:626–630.

63. Blake HA, Manion WC, Mattingly TW, Baroldi G. Coronary artery anomalies. *Circulation* 1964;30:927–940.

64. Goldblatt E, Adams APS, Ross IK, Savage JP, Morris LL. Single-trunk anomalous origin of both coronary arteries from the pulmonary artery. Diagnosis and surgical management. *J Thorac Cardiovasc Surg* 1984;87:59–65.

65. Schwartz RP, Robicsek F. An unusual anomaly of the coronary system: origin of the anterior (descending) interventricular artery from the pulmonary trunk. *J Pediatr* 197;78:123–126.

66. Probst P, Pachinger O, Koller H, Nierderberger M, Kaindl F. Origin of anterior descending branch of left coronary artery from pulmonary trunk. *Br Heart J* 1976;38:523–525.

67. Honey M, Lincoln JCR, Osborne MP, DeBono DP. Coarctation of aorta with right aortic arch. Report of surgical correction in two cases: one with associated anomalous origin of left circumflex coronary artery from the right pulmonary artery. *Br Heart J* 1975;37:937–945.

68. Ott DA, Cooley DA, Pinsky WW, Mullins CE. Anomalous origin of circumflex coronary artery from right pulmonary artery. Report of a rare anomaly. *J Thorac Cardiovasc Surg* 1978;76:190–194.

69. Packard M, Wechsler HF. Aneurysm of the coronary arteries. *Arch Intern Med* 1929;43:1–14.

70. Harris PN. Aneurysmal dilatation of the cardiac coronary arteries. Review of the literature and report of a case. *Am J Cardiol* 1937;13:89–98.

71. Scott DH. Aneurysm of the coronary arteries. *Am Heart J* 1948;36:403–421.

72. Crocker DW, Sobin S, Thomas WC. Aneurysms of the coronary arteries. Report of three cases in infants and review of the literature. *Am J Pathol* 1957;33:819–843.

73. Kalke B, Edwards JE. Localized aneurysms of the coronary arteries. *Angiology* 1968;19:460–470.

74. Kawasaki T, Kosaki F, Okawa S, Shigematsu I, Yanagawa H. A new infantile acute febrile mucocutaneous lymph node syndrome (MLNS) prevailing in Japan. *Pediatrics* 1974;54:271–276.

75. Ludomirsky A, O'Laughlin MP, Reul GJ, Mullins CE. Congenital aneurysm of the right coronary artery with fistulous connection to the right atrium. *Am Heart J* 1990;119:672–675.

76. Bougon. *Biblioth Med* 1812;37:183. Cited by Packard M, Weschler HF. Aneurysm of the coronary arteries. *Arch Intern Med* 1929;43: 1–14.

77. Peste. *Arch Gen Med* 1843;2:472. Cited by Scott DH. Aneurysm of the coronary arteries. *Am Heart J* 1948;36:403–421.

78. Forbus WD. On the origin of miliary aneurysms of the superficial cerebral arteries. *Bull Johns Hopkins Hosp* 1930;47:239–284.

79. Sherkat A, Kavanagh-Gray D, Edworthy J. Localized aneurysms of the coronary arteries. *Radiology* 1967;89:24–26.

80. Sayegh S, Adad W, Macleod CA. Multiple aneurysms of the coronary arteries. *Am Heart J* 1968;76:252–258.

81. Ghahramani A, Iyengar R, Cunha D, Jude J, Sommer L. Myocardial infarction due to congenital coronary arterial aneurysm (with successful saphenous vein bypass graft). *Am J Cardiol* 1972;29:863–867.

82. Dawson JE Jr, Ellison RG. Isolated aneurysm of the anterior descending coronary artery. Surgical treatment. *Am J Cardiol* 1972;29:868–871.

83. Vlodaver Z, Neufeld HN, Edwards JE. Congenital aneurysm of a coronary artery. In: Vlodaver Z, Neufeld HN, Edwards JE, eds. *Coronary arterial variations in the normal heart and in congenital heart disease.* New York: Academic Press, 1975:38–42.

84. Seabra-Gomes R, Sommerville J, Ross DN, Emanuel R, Parker DJ, Wong M. Congenital coronary artery aneurysms. *Br Heart J* 1974;36:329–335.

PART **XIII**

Miscellaneous

CHAPTER 35

Echocardiographic Evaluation of Pulmonary Hypertension

D. Dunbar Ivy

Echocardiography is the most useful noninvasive tool to evaluate the presence, etiology, and severity of pulmonary hypertension (1,2). Echocardiography allows differentiation between primary and secondary pulmonary hypertension and aids in diagnosing the cardiac lesions responsible for pulmonary hypertensive states, in many cases obviating the need for cardiac catheterization prior to surgical repair. This chapter describes a general diagnostic approach to the diagnosis and evaluation of pulmonary hypertension by echocardiography. The M-mode, two-dimensional, and Doppler findings will be presented in detail. Furthermore, the newer technique of intravascular ultrasound will be discussed in the evaluation of pulmonary hypertension.

Normally, pulmonary vascular resistance is high *in utero* and falls rapidly following birth, reaching adult levels by several months of age (3,4). However, in patients with certain congenital cardiac lesions, such as a large ventricular septal defect or hypoplastic left heart syndrome, pulmonary vascular resistance does not fall to normal levels after birth and may increase with age. For most congenital cardiac lesions, early surgical repair effectively prevents progression of pulmonary vascular disease, but in some instances pulmonary hypertension may continue and even worsen despite early surgical repair (5,6).

Pulmonary hypertension may have primary or secondary etiologies. Primary or unexplained pulmonary hypertension is defined by the exclusion of all other causes. In contrast, secondary pulmonary hypertension is associated with a known etiology, such as congenital heart disease.

Many congenital cardiac lesions cause pulmonary hypertension (Table 35-1). In patients with increased pulmonary blood flow due to left-to-right shunting, such as a large ventricular septal defect, patent ductus arteriosus or atrioventricular septal defects, pulmonary vascular resis-

tance is higher than normal at birth and may fall, resulting in worsening congestive heart failure. Usually, if these defects are repaired prior to 2 years of age, pulmonary vascular resistance will return to normal over time. However, in some instances, irreversible pulmonary hypertension may occur prior to 2 years of age, thereby preventing surgical repair (7). Likewise, if the defect is unnoticed until right-to-left shunting occurs, Eisenmenger's syndrome develops with irreversible pulmonary vascular disease. The age at which these lesions cause irreversible pulmonary vascular disease varies; therefore, each patient must be individually evaluated for the presence and severity of pulmonary hypertension to determine the timing of surgical repair. Generally, patients with large ventricular septal defect or patent ductus arteriosus do not develop irreversible pulmonary vascular changes before 2 years of age (8–10). Contrary to patients with large ventricular septal defects, less than 20% of patients with large atrial septal defects will develop inoperable pulmonary vascular disease if not repaired by the third decade of life (11). Patients with atrioventricular septal defect may develop irreversible pulmonary vascular disease earlier than patients with other left-to-right shunt lesions, especially if associated with Down's syndrome. The combination of high pressure and high flow appears to be a more potent stimulus for the development of pulmonary hypertension than a lesion associated with high flow alone.

Patients with cyanotic congenital cardiac lesions may also develop pulmonary hypertension. In fact, one of the lesions with the most rapid development of irreversible pulmonary hypertension is complete transposition of the great arteries with ventricular septal defect (12,13). Hypoxia with the presence of left-to-right shunting also appears to be a potent stimulus for the development of pulmonary vascular disease. Other cyanotic lesions with associated pulmonary hypertension include truncus arteri-

TABLE 35-1. Congenital cardiac lesions associated with pulmonary hypertension

Increased pulmonary blood flow
  Acyanotic
    Ventricular septal defect
    Atrial septal defect
    Atrioventricular septal defect
    Patent ductus arteriosus
    Aortico-pulmonary window
  Cyanotic
    Complete transposition of the great arteries with VSD
    Truncus arteriosus
    Univentricular heart (high-flow)
Cyanotic heart disease
  Complete transposition of the great arteries
  Tetralogy of Fallot (pulmonary atresia/VSD)
Increased pulmonary venous pressure
  Coarctation of the aorta (left ventricular diastolic dysfunction)
  Hypoplastic left heart syndrome
  Shone complex
  Mitral stenosis
  Supravalvar mitral ring
  Cor triatriatum
  Pulmonary vein stenosis
  Pulmonary veno-occlusive disease
  Total anomalous pulmonary venous return
Anomalies of the pulmonary artery or pulmonary vein
  Origin of a pulmonary artery from the aorta
  Unilateral "absence" of a pulmonary artery
  Scimitar syndrome
Palliative shunting operations
  Waterston anastomosis
  Potts anastomosis
  Blalock-Taussig anastomosis

osus, tetralogy of Fallot (pulmonary atresia), and univentricular atrioventricular connection with high pulmonary blood flow.

Lesions causing increased pulmonary venous pressure, such as hypoplastic left heart syndrome, mitral stenosis, pulmonary vein stenosis, cor triatriatum, total anomalous pulmonary venous return, or left ventricular diastolic dysfunction as seen in coarctation of the aorta, also develop pulmonary hypertension. Generally, pulmonary hypertension due to increased pulmonary venous pressure from congenital heart disease will reverse upon repair of the lesion; however, this is not universal, as some patients with congenital mitral stenosis (14,15) or total anomalous pulmonary venous return (16,17) may develop progressive pulmonary venous occlusion and pulmonary hypertension.

Pulmonary hypertension may also be seen in lesions with anomalies of the pulmonary arteries or pulmonary veins. Origin of one pulmonary artery from the aorta and unilateral "absence" of a pulmonary artery (pulmonary artery attached to the aorta by a thread-like remnant of the ductus arteriosus) are examples (18,19). Infantile scimitar syndrome, with pulmonary venous return of the right pulmonary veins to the inferior vena cava, may also be asso-

ciated with severe pulmonary hypertension secondary to abnormal shunting, pulmonary vein stenosis, a reduced pulmonary vascular bed, or associated lesions (20).

Finally, some palliative shunting operations, designed to increase pulmonary blood flow, occasionally lead to the development of pulmonary hypertension. Whereas only 10% of patients with a Blalock-Taussig shunt (subclavian artery to pulmonary artery) will develop early onset pulmonary vascular disease (21), as many as 30% of patients with a Waterston (ascending aorta to right pulmonary artery) or Potts (descending aorta to left pulmonary artery) anastomosis will develop pulmonary hypertension.

For many patients, the decision to perform corrective cardiac surgery requires a combination of diagnostic approaches. Rabinovitch et al. (22) recommend a three-pronged approach to children with pulmonary hypertension and congenital heart disease. Cardiac catheterization (23), lung biopsy (24–26), and quantitative pulmonary wedge angiograms (27,28) are utilized to determine surgical risk. In patients with an uncertain severity of pulmonary hypertension by echocardiography, this combined approach to the assessment of the presence, severity, and reactivity of pulmonary hypertension is necessary to determine the operability and survivability following cardiac surgery.

M-MODE ECHOCARDIOGRAPHY

The early echocardiographic evaluation of pulmonary hypertension was performed using M-mode echocardiography, which included observation of abnormalities of pulmonic valve motion and later evolved into measurement of right ventricular time intervals.

Initial studies of the pattern of pulmonic valve motion in patients with pulmonary hypertension revealed the absence of the "a" wave after atrial contraction, a negative e-f slope, suggesting loss of the normal posterior valve motion in diastole, and the presence of mid-systolic notching or fluttering (29). Further studies showed that the degree of "a" wave dips correlated with the degree of pulmonary hypertension (30). In a study by Nanda et al. (30), patients with more severe grades of pulmonary hypertension had absence of "a" dips, whereas patients with less severe pulmonary hypertension had small "a" dips. Contrast M-mode allowed for further differentiation between patients with normal pulmonary artery pressure and those with pulmonary hypertension, and provided an explanation for the early closure of the pulmonic valve in pulmonary hypertension (31). In these studies, contrast M-mode revealed that patients with early closure of the pulmonic valve showed abnormal retrograde flow of contrast in mid to late systole. Other studies using M-mode and Doppler ultrasound showed an early systolic flow velocity peak in the pulmonary artery of patients with pulmonary hypertension, the timing of which correlated with mean pulmonary artery pressure. Patients with normal pulmonary artery pressure had a higher midsystolic pulmonary flow velocity than patients with pulmonary hypertension (65.4 ± 140 cm/s versus 342 ± 85 cm/s) (32,33). Interestingly, the study of a patient with Eisenmenger's syndrome showed a reopening of the pulmonary valve in late systole (34). Although these techniques were fairly specific, further studies showed that these abnormalities of pulmonic valve motion were not adequately sensitive for determination of the presence of pulmonary hypertension (35–37). For example, in the study by Acquatella et al. (37), there was no correlation between the pulmonary valve ''a'' wave amplitude and hemodynamic assessment.

Hirschfeld et al. (38) found a more quantitative correlation of pulmonary artery pressure and pulmonary vascular resistance with M-mode measurement of right ventricular systolic and diastolic time intervals than by evaluation of the pattern of pulmonic valve motion. Increased pulmonary artery diastolic pressure, mean pulmonary artery pressure, and pulmonary vascular resistance result in an increase in the ratio of right ventricular preejection period (PEP) to right ventricular ejection time (ET) by causing an increase in the PEP and no change or a decrease in the ET. This study also demonstrated that the ratio PEP/ET is uninfluenced by heart rate and age, whereas either of these measurements alone may be influenced by both age and heart rate. In children with congenital heart disease, a PEP/ET ratio under 0.30 was 97% specific for pulmonary vascular resistance less than 3 Wood units, whereas all patients with pulmonary vascular resistance over 5 units had a ratio of PEP/ET greater than 0.40 (38). Other studies have also evaluated the use of right ventricular systolic and diastolic time intervals in evaluation of pulmonary hypertension (39–42).

Although most studies have shown a linear relationship between pulmonary artery pressure and the ratio of PEP/ET, the utility of right ventricular time intervals may be limited by many variables (41), including heart rate, contractility, interventricular conduction disturbances, and the ability to obtain adequate measurements in patients with obesity or lung disease. In children with ventricular septal defect, Silverman et al. (41) found no relationship between mean pulmonary artery pressure or pulmonary vascular resistance and the ratio of PEP/ET. Furthermore, because of the scatter of the measurements, application of the PEP/ET ratio for a particular patient may be limited. Boyd et al. (43) found that right heart failure, right bundle branch block, or elevated right atrial pressure altered systolic time intervals such that there was no correlation between these intervals and the level of pulmonary pressure. Using the Burstin method for estimation of peak pulmonary artery pressure, incorporating the period of isovolumetric diastole between pulmonary valve closure and tricuspid valve opening, Stevenson et al. (44) found a close correlation between predicted and actual peak pulmonary artery pressure ($r = 0.86$). All patients with a peak systolic pulmonary artery pressure less than 40 mmHg at catheterization had a predicted pressure less than 40 mmHg by echocardiography. However, less accuracy was found using M-mode measurements with heart rates above 155 beats/min (44).

M-mode and Doppler studies of isovolumetric contraction time intervals of the right ventricle and isovolumetric relaxation time intervals of the left ventricle correlate well with measurements of pulmonary artery pressure and may alleviate some of the difficulties associated with measurements in patients with elevated heart rates. One study has shown a relationship between the isovolumetric contraction time of the right ventricle and measurement of pulmonary artery pressure (45). Burstin et al. (46) initially studied the isovolumetric contraction time between closure of the tricuspid valve and opening of the pulmonary valve in relation to pulmonary hypertension in patients with congenital heart disease. The nomogram designed by Burstin was used by Hatle (47) in comparing pulmonary artery pressure at catheterization and the right ventricular isovolumetric contraction time. In this study, the nomogram used by Burstin took into account the heart rate, but assumed that right atrial pressure was normal. At high heart rates, an isovolumetric contraction time greater than 100 ms suggests the presence of pulmonary hypertension, but accurate measurement of the isovolumetric contraction time may be difficult at heart rates greater than 150 beats per minute. At lower heart rates, an increase in isovolumetric contraction time of greater than 25 ms is suggestive of pulmonary hypertension. Bourlon et al. (48) studied systolic and diastolic time intervals to assess pulmonary artery pressure in patients with complete transposition of the great arteries. The ratio of the isovolumetric relaxation time of the left ventricle (IRT) to the left ventricular ejection time (LVET) correlated best with systolic pulmonary artery pressure. Patients with a negative IRT/LVET ratio had a pulmonary artery systolic pressure lower than 35 mmHg (48) and a mean pulmonary artery pressure less than 25 mmHg.

TWO-DIMENSIONAL ECHOCARDIOGRAPHY

Two-dimensional echocardiography may provide clues to the severity and sequelae of pulmonary hypertension. An enlarged right atrium, hypertrophied and dilated right ventricle (49), and enlarged main pulmonary artery segment may be seen with pulmonary hypertension (Echo. 35-1). Right ventricular pressure overload may also cause flattening or bulging of the interventricular septum into the left ventricular cavity, leading to left ventricular diastolic abnormalities or changes in isovolumetric relaxation of the left ventricle (Echo. 35-2). Prolapse of the pulmonary valve may predict pulmonary hypertension with the ratio of pulmonary artery to systemic artery pres-

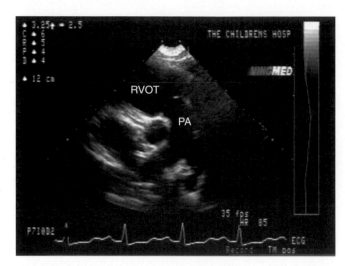

ECHO. 35-1. Parasternal short-axis view demonstrating a dilated right ventricle and main pulmonary artery in the presence of pulmonary hypertension. *RVOT,* right ventricular outflow tract; *PA,* pulmonary artery.

sure ratio greater than 0.5; however, the sensitivity and specificity of this finding is unknown (50).

Changes in the shape of the interventricular septum may provide semiquantitative information about the severity of pulmonary hypertension. In a study by King et al. (51), the degree of curvature of the interventricular septum provided a marker of right ventricular systolic hypertension. An increase in the septal radius curvature greater than two times normal had good correlation with near systemic right ventricular systolic pressure. Few studies have been performed to quantitate the relationship between flattening of the interventricular septum and the degree of pulmonary hypertension (52–55), but generally it is thought that right ventricular hypertension is present if systolic flattening of the interventricular septum is present (Echo. 35-2).

Contrast echocardiography allows demonstration of the direction of intracardiac shunting and thus estimation of relative intracardiac pressures and pulmonary vascular resistance. For example, contrast echocardiography may provide detection of right-to-left shunting in patent ductus arteriosus (56), or across a patent foramen ovale in response to hypoxia in a patient with primary pulmonary hypertension (see Echo. 9-2).

DOPPLER ECHOCARDIOGRAPHY

The addition of pulsed Doppler velocimetry has added further information to the evaluation of pulmonary hypertension by echocardiography. With pulmonary hypertension, the peak flow velocity is unchanged, whereas the acceleration time is decreased with an increase in acceleration rate and preejection time. Thus, the peak velocity is reached earlier in systole with a decrease in flow during mid systole in comparison with patients with normal pulmonary artery pressure (57). Thus, many authors have described notching or a ''W'' pattern of the pulmonary artery flow pattern in patients with pulmonary hypertension (Echo. 35-3).

Several authors have examined the relationship of the Doppler flow pattern to pulmonary artery pressure and/or pulmonary vascular resistance (57–68) (Table 35-2). In general, the acceleration time and the ratio of the acceleration time to ET have been used to estimate the presence and degree of pulmonary hypertension.

Kitabatake et al. (57) initially described that patients with pulmonary artery hypertension had shorter pulmonary flow acceleration times on Doppler spectral traces.

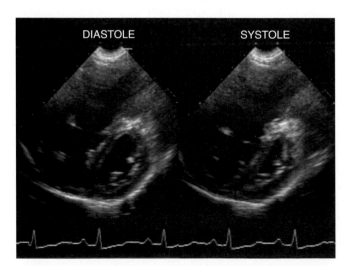

ECHO. 35-2. Parasternal short-axis view of a dilated right ventricle compressing the left ventricle. Note the posterior bulging of the interventricular septum in systole.

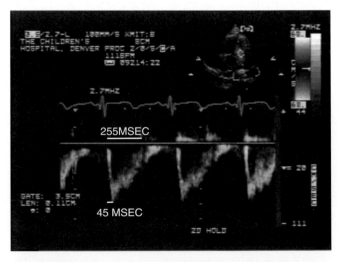

ECHO. 35-3. Spectral Doppler velocity waveform of the pulmonary artery in pulmonary hypertension. Note the rapid acceleration time and the notching of the systolic curve due to decreased flow in mid systole.

TABLE 35-2. Pulmonary artery systolic time intervals in pulmonary hypertension

Reference	Hemodynamic variable	AT	ET	PEP	AT/ET	PEP/ET	PEP/AT	Population
Kitabatake et al. (57)	m/PAP <20 mmHg	137 ± 24 ms[a]	304 ± 38 ms	N/A	0.45 ± 0.05	N/A	N/A	Adults
	m/PAP >20 mmHg	97 ± 20 ms	284 ± 37 ms	N/A	0.34 ± 0.05	N/A	N/A	
Dabestani et al. (58)	m/PAP <20 mmHg	134 ± 20 ms[a]	302 ± 38 ms	96 ± 20 ms	N/A	N/A	N/A	Adults
	m/PAP >20 mmHg	88 ± 25 ms	278 ± 51 ms	93 ± 15 ms	N/A	N/A	N/A	
Kosturakis et al. (60)	s/PAP <30 mmHg	150 ± 30 ms[a]	343 ± 42 ms	88 ± 3 ms	0.44 ± 0.05	0.26 ± 0.35	N/A	Children w/CHD
	s/PAP <30 mmHg	82 ± 30 ms	289 ± 56 ms	80 ± 2 ms	0.31 ± 0.08	0.32 ± 0.13	N/A	
Isobe et al. (62)	m/PAP ≤19 mmHg	144 ± 16 ms[a]	317 ± 33 ms	99 ± 21 ms	0.45 ± 0.05[a]	0.35 ± 0.09[a]	0.70 ± 0.17	Adults
	m/PAP ≥20 mmHg	79 ± 16 ms	N/A	N/A	0.30 ± 0.06	0.45 ± 0.11	1.50 ± 0.35	
Martin-Duran et al. (59)	m/PAP <20 mmHg	143 ± 30 ms[a]	N/A	N/A	0.44 ± 0.06[a]	0.28 ± 0.08[a]	N/A	Mixed
	m/PAP >20 mmHg	75 ± 20 ms	N/A	N/A	0.25 ± 0.05	0.39 ± 0.10	N/A	
Friedman et al. (63)	Control	125 ± 12 ms[a]	318 ± 18 ms[a]	N/A	0.40 ± 0.03	N/A	N/A	Children
	PPH	66 ± 18 ms	207 ± 38 ms	N/A	0.34 ± 0.10	N/A	N/A	

[a] p < 0.05.
Systolic time intervals of patients with pulmonary hypertension according to various published series. m, mean; s, systolic; PPH, primary pulmonary hypertension; CHD, congenital heart disease; AT, acceleration time; ET, ejection time; PEP, preejection period; N/A, not studied.

In this study, patients with mean pulmonary artery pressure less than 20 mmHg had an acceleration time of 137 ± 24 ms, whereas patients with mean pulmonary artery pressure greater than 20 mmHg had an acceleration time of 97 ± 20 ms. Both the acceleration time and the ratio of acceleration time to ET had a high negative correlation with mean pulmonary artery pressure ($r = -0.90$). Likewise, Dabestani et al. (58) found that patients with mean pulmonary artery pressure less than 20 mmHg had an acceleration time of 134 ± 20 ms, whereas patients with mean pulmonary artery pressure greater than 20 mmHg had an acceleration time of 88 ± 25 ms. In patients with an acceleration time less than 120 ms, there was a negative correlation between acceleration time and mean pulmonary artery pressure (58). Kosturakis et al. (60) performed similar studies and found that acceleration time and the ratio of acceleration time to ET correlated better than measurement of the PEP, right ventricular ET, or the ratio of preejection time to ET in patients with pulmonary hypertension and congenital heart disease. In contrast, Isobe et al. (62) found that the best correlation between mean pulmonary artery pressure and Doppler time intervals was with the ratio of right ventricular preejection time to acceleration time with a sensitivity of 93% and specificity of 97% using a ratio of 1.1. Finally, Hatle and Angelsen (69) showed that patients without pulmonary hypertension had the combination of Doppler measured right ventricular preejection time/ET under 0.34 and right ventricular acceleration time/ET over 0.36.

The measurement of right ventricular time intervals may be affected by many of the same factors as the M-mode time intervals. Heart rate, ventricular function, right ventricular preload and afterload, the presence of bundle branch block, cardiac output, right atrial pressure, and Doppler sampling site all may affect measurement of Doppler time intervals. Most investigators place the spectral Doppler sample volume guided by two-dimensional imaging within the central distal main pulmonary artery at a visual intercept angle near 0 in order to minimize errors from sampling sites and angle dependence of Doppler. It is generally thought that Doppler time intervals correlate better with pulmonary artery pressure and are easier to obtain than the intervals derived by M-mode echocardiography. However, the variability of the measurement of the Doppler time intervals in a particular patient makes the use of Doppler time intervals less than optimal in the evaluation of pulmonary hypertension (41,64–66).

Another method of estimating pulmonary artery pressure involves calculation of right ventricular systolic pressure by Doppler techniques. In the absence of subvalve, valve, or supravalve pulmonary stenosis, right ventricular systolic pressure is equal to pulmonary artery systolic pressure.

The Bernoulli equation relates the velocity of blood flow between two adjacent structures to the pressure drop between them:

$$P_1 - P_2 = \frac{1}{2}\rho(V_2^2 - V_1^2) + \rho\int_1^2 \frac{dV}{dt}ds + R(V)$$

where P_1 = pressure proximal to the obstruction; P_2 = pressure distal to the obstruction; V_1 = velocity proximal to the obstruction; V_2 = velocity in the jet distal to the obstruction; ρ = mass density of blood; dV = change in velocity that occurs over the time period dt; ds = distance over which the decrease in pressure occurs; R = viscous resistance in the vessel; V = velocity of blood flow. For most intracardiac blood flow phenomena, the formula has been simplified to:

$$P = 4V^2$$

where P is the pressure gradient in mmHg between the structures and V is the maximal velocity of blood flow between them in meters per second (m/s). As such, in order to estimate the right ventricular systolic pressure there must be either tricuspid valve insufficiency or a ventricular septal defect. Pulmonary artery systolic pressure may be directly estimated in the presence of a systemic to pulmonary artery communication as well.

Both patients with normal pulmonary artery pressure and those with pulmonary hypertension frequently have some degree of tricuspid regurgitation detectable by spectral and color Doppler (69). Measurement of the velocity of tricuspid regurgitation should be performed from several views (apical four-chamber, parasternal short-axis) until the highest velocity is obtained. Frequently continuous wave Doppler is utilized guided by the color Doppler image (Echo. 35-4; see color plate 124 following p. 364). As the modified Bernoulli equation estimates, the pressure gradient between the right atrium and the right ventricle,

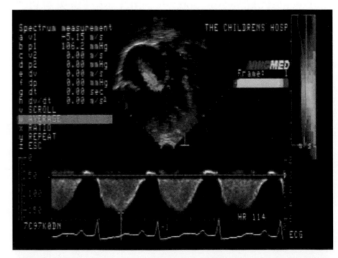

ECHO. 35-4. Spectral Doppler velocity traces from a tricuspid regurgitant jet. Note the high velocity and the slow acceleration seen in pulmonary hypertension.

right atrial pressure must be added to the result of the Bernoulli calculation to determine right ventricular systolic pressure (70–73). Thus the equation for estimation of right ventricular systolic pressure from the tricuspid regurgitant jet velocity is:

$$RVSP = 4V^2 + RA_m$$

where RVSP = right ventricular systolic pressure, V = the maximal tricuspid regurgitation jet velocity, and RA_m = right atrial mean pressure. Direct measurement of right atrial pressure with a central venous catheter is the preferred method; however, this is usually not available. Right atrial pressure may be difficult to calculate by physical examination and echocardiographic findings, so it is usually assumed to be 5 mmHg in normal patients and 10 to 15 mmHg in patients with moderate to severe pulmonary hypertension or right heart failure. Berger et al. (73) have derived a formula to estimate pulmonary systolic pressure without estimation of right atrial pressure:

$$PASP = 4V^2 \times 1.23 \text{ mmHg}$$

where PASP = pulmonary artery systolic pressure, and V = maximal tricuspid regurgitation jet velocity.

Pulmonary artery systolic pressure may also be estimated in the presence of an interventricular communication (74–77) (see Echo. 10-17). This method is valid only in the absence of right and left ventricular outflow tract obstruction and may be calculated by the equation:

$$RVSP = SBP - 4V^2$$

where RVSP = right ventricular systolic pressure, SBP = simultaneous systemic systolic blood pressure determined by sphygmomanometry (assumed to be equal to the systolic left ventricular pressure), and V = maximal velocity across the ventricular septal defect (left ventricular to right ventricular systolic pressure gradient). The main pitfall of this technique is the possibility of overestimating right ventricular peak systolic pressure if the highest peak velocity is not obtained across the interventricular communication. Perimembranous ventricular septal defects are best interrogated from the parasternal and subcostal long-axis windows, whereas muscular defects are best interrogated from the parasternal or subcostal short-axis views. The apical views are useful also if the Doppler sampling line can be aligned with the direction of flow. Another drawback of this approach is that the systemic systolic pressure by sphygmomanometry may overestimate the left ventricular pressure. Finally, errors may occur in the estimation of right ventricular systolic pressure secondary to the time lag between right ventricular peak pressure and left ventricular peak pressure. As echocardiography measures the peak instantaneous pressure gradient, and cardiac catheterization measurements are routinely performed between the two peaks of the pressure

curves, it is possible to have no difference in peak-to-peak pressure measured at catheterization and have a gradient detected by echocardiography. One author noted a 25 mmHg gradient by Doppler in a patient without any peak-to-peak pressure gradient measured at catheterization (75).

Pulmonary artery systolic pressure may be estimated directly in patients with systemic to pulmonary artery communications (78). In a series of 25 patients with patent ductus arteriosus, pulsed wave Doppler distinguished between those with pulmonary hypertension and those with normal pulmonary artery pressure (see Echos. 30-4–30-8). Although there was good correlation between abbreviated ductal flow and increased pulmonary artery pressure, there was no linear correlation between duration of diastolic flow and pulmonary artery pressure. The authors concluded that patients with pandiastolic ductal flows do not have pulmonary hypertension, which would preclude ductal closure (78).

Pulmonary artery diastolic pressure may also be estimated using the modified Bernoulli equation to measure the end diastolic pressure gradient between the pulmonary artery and the right ventricle (79). This is usually accomplished by measuring the velocity at the "shoulder" of the pulmonary regurgitant Doppler curve (Echo. 35-5; see color plate 125 following p. 364). The incidence of pulmonary regurgitation is greater in patients with pulmonary hypertension than in those with normal pulmonary artery pressure (80). Furthermore, Yock et al. (70) noted an incidence of pulmonary valve regurgitation in 40% of normal patients. Masuyama et al. (79) found that the Doppler-determined pressure gradient at end-diastole correlated with catheter measurement of the pressure gradient between the pulmonary artery and the right ventricle at end-diastole ($r = 0.94$) and with pulmonary artery end-

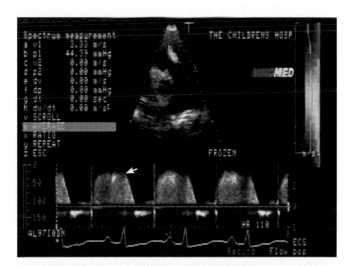

ECHO. 35-5. Spectral Doppler recording of a pulmonary insufficiency curve. The velocity at the "shoulder" of the waveform is high *(arrow)*, indicating the presence of elevated pulmonary end-diastolic pressures.

diastolic pressure ($r = 0.92$). In addition, pulmonary regurgitant flow velocity was higher as pulmonary artery pressure increased (79). Difficulties of this technique relate to the Doppler incident angle, and to the hemodynamic state of the patient. In the presence of severe pulmonary regurgitation and possibly severe right heart failure, the end-diastolic pressure gradient across the pulmonary valve will be affected since an elevated right ventricular end-diastolic pressure will result in lower end-diastolic Doppler velocities.

Clinically, measurement of tricuspid valve regurgitation and pulmonic valve regurgitation are more useful in the routine evaluation of patients with pulmonary hypertension. Measurement of pulmonary artery pressure by use of the modified Bernoulli equation has several advantages over estimation by Doppler time intervals. The Bernoulli equation utilizes blood flow velocity, which is directly related to intracardiac pressure differences. Furthermore, measurement of this velocity is not affected by many of the variables that affect Doppler systolic time intervals, such as heart rate, contractility, and conduction disturbances. However, care must be taken to measure the peak velocity accurately in order to estimate the pressure difference without errors. One study found estimation of pulmonary artery pressure by measurement of peak tricuspid regurgitation velocity superior to other Doppler techniques (67).

INTRAVASCULAR ULTRASOUND

Classically, evaluation of the pulmonary vasculature has depended on several diagnostic tools: echocardiography, hemodynamic evaluation by cardiac catheterization, wedge angiography, and lung biopsy. Each of these techniques has inherent limitations. Recently, intravascular ultrasound has been used to study the appearance of the pulmonary arterial tree in order to determine both structural and functional changes in pulmonary hypertension (81–86).

The use of intravascular ultrasound to evaluate structural changes in pulmonary hypertension is exciting as this technique provides the opportunity to image the distal pulmonary vasculature directly during cardiac catheterization. Pulmonary hypertension causes a progression of structural changes within the lung. The initial stage involves increased muscularity of small distal pulmonary arteries and arterioles with distal extension of smooth muscle. Intimal proliferation is rarely seen during the first year in congenital heart defects causing pulmonary hypertension. Medial hypertrophy also precedes the initial lesions of plexogenic arteriopathy.

Heath and Edwards (26) classified the pulmonary vascular changes by light microscopy in patients with pulmonary hypertension. Six grades of pulmonary vascular changes were described: Grade I—medial hypertrophy;

Grade II—intimal hyperplasia; Grade III—vessel lumen mostly occluded by intimal hyperplasia; Grade IV—arterial dilatation; Grades V and VI—angiomatoid formation and fibrinoid necrosis (26). This classification is limited by the lack of severe changes in patients under two years of age (88) and the lack of homogeneity in the distribution of lesions throughout the lung (89). Reid, Hislop, and Haworth (90–92) found that abnormal extension of muscle into peripheral pulmonary arteries that are normally nonmuscular was more reliable than the Heath-Edwards changes. Rabinovitch et al. (24) formulated a quantitative classification of hypertensive vascular changes. The stages in their schema are as follows: Grade A—extension of muscle into peripheral arteries that are usually nonmuscular; Grade B—medial muscle of small intraacinar arteries thicker than usual; and Grade C—reduced number of intraacinar arteries.

Although the clinical utility of direct intravascular evaluation of pulmonary arteries remains to be determined, several authors have shown a good correlation between intravascular ultrasound measurements and pulmonary artery pressure or lung histological changes. Berger et al. (82) showed that pulsatility of the pulmonary artery was related to vessel size. Ishii et al. (84) found that intravascular images correlated with lung biopsy findings in vitro, and that normal patients had only one layer visible by intravascular imaging, whereas all patients with pulmonary hypertension had three visible layers. Changes observed with intravascular ultrasound imaging correlated well with the histopathologic grade in this in vitro study (84).

We performed IVUS, pulmonary wedge angiography,

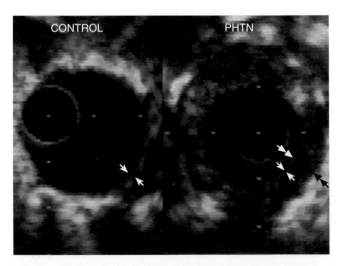

ECHO. 35-6. Intravascular ultrasound image of a patient with normal pulmonary artery pressures **(left)** and one with pulmonary hypertension **(right)**. Note that the normal patient has only one visible middle layer *(arrows)*, which is not hypertrophied. The patient with pulmonary hypertension has two visible layers: the inner *(single arrows)* and middle *(double arrows)* layers.

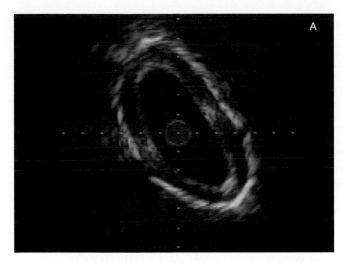
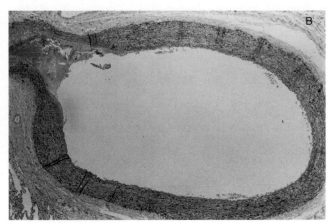

ECHO. 35-7. Intravascular ultrasound **(A)** and histologic cut **(B)** from the lungs of a patient with Eisenmenger's syndrome and suprasystemic pulmonary arterial pressures. Note the similarity between the two images. The inner and middle layers are both severely hypertrophied.

and assessed vasoreactivity to inhaled nitric oxide and oxygen in 8 patients with normal pulmonary artery pressure and in 15 patients with pulmonary hypertension undergoing cardiac catheterization (81). IVUS study revealed abnormalities of elastic pulmonary arteries in children with pulmonary artery hypertension compared to controls. Patients with pulmonary hypertension had a thicker media (0.32 ± 0.17 versus 0.15 ± 0.01 mm, p < 0.05), percent wall thickness (29 ± 3 versus 16 ± 2%, p < 0.05), and diminished pulsatility (p < 0.05) than controls. The intima was not visualized in any control patient, but was seen in 9 out of 15 patients with pulmonary hypertension. Patients without pulmonary hypertension had two visible layers, while patients with pulmonary hypertension had two to three visible layers (Echos. 35-6, 35-7). In children with pulmonary hypertension baseline mean pulmonary artery pressure correlated with intimal thickness, number of layers visualized, percent wall thickness, and thickness of the media.

Pulmonary artery wedge angiography correlated with baseline mean pulmonary artery pressure and pulmonary vascular resistance as well as with IVUS findings of wall thickness and intimal thickness. The inner layer was not visualized in any patient who had grade 1 wedge angiograms nor in 86% of patients with grade 2 wedge angiograms. All patients with grade 4 and 80% of patients with grade 3 wedge angiograms had a visible intima. However, vasoreactivity to inhaled nitric oxide and oxygen did not correlate with structural assessment of the pulmonary vasculature by intravascular imaging or wedge angiography.

Intravascular imaging of small pulmonary arteries allows for direct visualization of structural changes in elastic pulmonary arteries in children with pulmonary hypertension and may complement current techniques utilized in the evaluation of children with pulmonary hypertension.

In summary, echocardiography provides an important diagnostic tool in the evaluation of patients with pulmonary hypertension. Both the etiology and severity of pulmonary hypertension may readily be determined by echocardiography. Future studies using transthoracic and intravascular imaging should decrease the need for more invasive techniques in the evaluation of patients with pulmonary hypertension.

REFERENCES

1. Zellers T, Gutgesell HP. Noninvasive estimation of pulmonary artery pressure. *J Pediatr* 1989;114:735–741.
2. Robinson PJ, Macartney FJ, Wyse RK. Non-invasive diagnosis of pulmonary hypertension. *Int J Cardiol* 1986;11:253–259.
3. Rudolph AM. The changes in the circulation after birth. Their importance in congenital heart disease. *Circulation* 1970;41:343–359.
4. Rudolph AM, Auld PAM, Golinko RJ. Pulmonary vascular adjustments in the neonatal period. *Pediatrics* 1961;28:28–34.
5. Wagenvoort CA. Lung biopsies and pulmonary vascular disease. In: Weir EK, Reeves JT, eds. *Pulmonary hypertension.* Mt. Kisco, NY: Futura Publishing, 1984:393–437.
6. Rabinovitch M, Keane JF, Norwood WI, Castaneda AR. Vascular structure in lung tissue obtained at biopsy correlated with pulmonary hemodynamic findings after repair of congenital heart defects. *Circulation* 1984;69:655–667.
7. Alt B, Shikes RH. Pulmonary hypertension in congenital heart disease: irreversible vascular changes in young infants. *Pediatr Pathol* 1983;1:423–434.
8. Hallidie-Smith KA, Hollman A, Cleland WP, Bentall HH, Goodwin JF. Effects of surgical closure of ventricular septal defects upon pulmonary vascular disease. *Br Heart J* 1969;31:246–260.
9. Friedli B, Kidd BSL, Mustard WT, Keith JD. Ventricular septal defect with increased pulmonary vascular resistance. *Am J Cardiol* 1974;33:403–409.
10. Reid JM, Stevenson JG, Coleman EN, et al. Moderate to severe pulmonary hypertension accompanying patent ductus arteriosus. *Br Heart J* 1964;26:600–605.
11. Besterman E. Atrial septal defect with pulmonary hypertension. *Br Heart J* 1961;23:587–598.
12. Reid LD. Structure and function in pulmonary hypertension; new perceptions. *Chest* 1986;89:279–288.
13. Viles PH, Ongley PA, Titus JL. The spectrum of pulmonary vascu-

lar disease in transposition of the great arteries. *Circulation* 1969; 40:31–41.

14. Scott WC, Miller DC, Haverich A, et al. Operative risks of mitral replacement: discriminant analysis of 1,329 procedures. *Circulation* 1985;72[Suppl II]:II-108–II-119.

15. John S, Bashi VV, Jairaj PS, et al. Closed mitral valvotomy: early results and long-term follow-up of 3,724 consecutive patients. *Circulation* 1983;68:891–896.

16. Katz NM, Kirklin JW, Pacifico AD. Concepts and practices in surgery for total anomalous pulmonary venous connection. *Ann Thorac Surg* 1978;25:479–487.

17. Fleming WH, Clark EB, Dooley KJ, et al. Late complications following surgical repair of total anomalous pulmonary venous return below the diaphragm. *Ann Thorac Surg* 1979;27:435–439.

18. Nakamura Y, Yasui H, Kado H, Yonenga K, Shiokawa Y, Tokunaga S. Anamolous origin of the right pulmonary artery from the ascendng aorta. *Ann Thorac Surg* 1991;52:1285–1291.

19. Pool PE, Vogel JHK, Blount SG. Congenital unilateral absence of a pulmonary artery: the importance of flow in pulmonary hypertension. *Am J Cardiol* 1962;10:706–732.

20. Dupuis C, Charaf LAC, Breviere GM, Abou P. "Infantile" form of the scimitar syndrome with pulmonary hypertension. *Am J Cardiol* 1993;71:1326–1330.

21. Paul MH, Miller RA, Potts WJ. Long-term results of aortic-pulmonary anastomosis for tetralogy of Fallot: analysis of the first 100 cases eleven to thirteen years after operation. *Circulation* 1961; 23:525–533.

22. Rabinovitch M. Problems of pulmonary hypertension in children with congenital cardiac defects. *Chest* 1988;93[Suppl]:119S–126S.

23. Ivy DD, Wolfe RR, Abman SH. Congenital heart disease. In: Peacock AJ, ed. *The pulmonary circulation: a handbook for clinicians.* London: Chapman & Hall Medical, 1996.

24. Rabinovitch M, Haworth SG, Castaneda AR. Lung biopsy in congenital heart disease: a morphometric approach to pulmonary vascular disease. *Circulation* 1978;58:1107–1122.

25. Rabinovitch M, Castaneda AR, Reid L. Lung biopsy with frozen section as a diagnostic aid in patients with congenital heart defects. *Am J Cardiol* 1981;47:77–84.

26. Heath D, Edwards JE. The pathology of hypertensive pulmonary vascular disease. *Circulation* 1958;18:533–547.

27. Rabinovitch M, Keane JF, Fellows KE, Castaneda AR, Reid L. Quantitative analysis of the pulmonary wedge angiogram in congenital heart defects. Correlation with hemodynamic data and morphometric findings in lung biopsy tissue. *Circulation* 1981;63:152–164.

28. Nihill MR, McNamara DG. Magnification pulmonary wedge angiography in the evaluation of children with congenital heart disease and pulmonary hypertension. *Circulation* 1978;58:1094–1106.

29. Weyman AE, Dillon JC, Feigenbaum H, Chang S. Echocardiographic patterns of pulmonary valve motion with pulmonary hypertension. *Am J Cardiol* 1974;50:905–910.

30. Nanda NC, Gramiak R, Robinson TI, Shah PM. Echocardiographic evaluation of pulmonary hypertension. *Circulation* 1974;50:575–581.

31. Meltzer RS, Valk NK, ten Cate F, Visser CA, Roelandt J. Contrast echocardiography in pulmonary hypertension: observations explaining the early closure of the pulmonic valve. *Am Heart J* 1983; 106:1394–1398.

32. Zeiher AM, Bonzel T, Wollschlager H, Hohnloser S, Hust MH, Just H. Noninvasive evaluation of pulmonary hypertension by quantitative contrast M-mode echocardiography. *Am Heart J* 1986;111: 297–306.

33. Turkevich D, Groves BM, Micco A, Trapp JA, Reeves JT. Early partial systolic closure of the pulmonic valve relates to severity of pulmonary hypertension. *Am Heart J* 1988;115:409–418.

34. Haugland H, Vik-Mo H. Echocardiographic characteristics of pulmonary and aortic valve motion in the Eisenmenger's syndrome from ventricular septal defect. *Am J Cardiol* 1984;54:927–929.

35. Lew W, Karliner JS. Assessment of pulmonary valve echogram in normal subjects and in patients with pulmonary arterial hypertension. *Br Heart J* 1979;42:147–161.

36. Marin-Garcia J, Moller JH, Mirvis DM. The pulmonic valve echogram in the assessment of pulmonary hypertension in children. *Pediatr Cardiol* 1983;4:209–214.

37. Acquatella H, Schiller NB, Sharpe DN, Chatterjee K. Lack of correlation between echocardiographic pulmonary valve morphology and simultaneous pulmonary arterial pressure. *Am J Cardiol* 1979;43: 946–950.

38. Hirschfeld S, Meyer R, Schwartz DC, Korfhagen J, Kaplan S. The echocardiographic assessment of pulmonary artery pressure and pulmonary vascular resistance. *Circulation* 1975;52:642–650.

39. Gutgesell HP. Echocardiographic estimation of pulmonary artery pressure in transposition of the great arteries. *Circulation* 1978;57: 1151–1153.

40. Spooner EW, Perry BL, Stern AM, Sigmann JM. Estimation of pulmonary/systemic resistance ratios from echocardiographic systolic time intervals in young patients with congenital or acquired heart disease. *Am J Cardiol* 1978;42:810–816.

41. Silverman NH, Snider AR, Rudolph AM. Evaluation of pulmonary hypertension by M-mode echocardiography in children with ventricular septal defect. *Circulation* 1980;61:1125–1132.

42. Oberhansli I, Branden G, Girod M, Friedli B. Estimation of pulmonary artery pressure by ultrasound. A study comparing simultaneously recorded pulmonary valve echogram and pulmonary arterial pressures. *Pediatr Cardiol* 1982;2:123–130.

43. Boyd MJ, Williams IP, Turton CWG, Brooks N, Leech G, Millard FJC. Echocardiographic method for the estimation of pulmonary artery pressure in chronic lung disease. *Thorax* 1980;35:914–919.

44. Stevenson JG, Kawabori I, Guntheroth WG. Noninvasive estimation of peak pulmonary artery pressure by M-mode echocardiography. *J Am Coll Cardiol* 1984;4:1021–1027.

45. Johnson GL, Meyer RA, Korfhagen J, Schwartz DC, Kaplan S. Echocardiographic assessment of pulmonary arterial pressure in children with complete right bundle branch block. *Am J Cardiol* 1978;41:1264–1269.

46. Burstin L. Determination of pressure in the pulmonary artery by external graphic recordings. *Br Heart J* 1967;29:396–404.

47. Hatle L, Angelsen BA, Tromsdal A. Non-invasive estimation of pulmonary artery systolic pressure with Doppler ultrasound. *Br Heart J* 1981;45:157–165.

48. Bourlon F, Fouron JC, Battle-Diaz J, Ducharme G, Davignon A. Relation between isovolumic relaxation period of left ventricle and pulmonary artery pressure in d-transposition of the great arteries. *Br Heart J* 1980;43:226–231.

49. Shah A, Schwartz H, Class RN. Unusual echocardiographic findings in primary pulmonary hypertension. *Arch Intern Med* 1983;143: 820–822.

50. Robinson PJ, Wyse RK, Macartney FJ. Significance of pulmonary valve prolapse: a cross-sectional echocardiographic study. *Br Heart J* 1984;52:266–271.

51. King ME, Braun H, Goldblatt A, Liberthson R, Weymann AE. Interventricular septal configuration as a predictor of right ventricular systolic hypertension in children: a cross-sectional echocardiographic study. *Circulation* 1983;68:68–75.

52. Shimada R, Takeshita A, Nakamura M. Noninvasive assessment of right ventricular systolic pressure in atrial septal defect: analysis of the end-systolic configuration of the ventricular septum by two-dimensional echocardiography. *Am J Cardiol* 1984;53:1117–1123.

53. Akaishi M, Nakamura Y. Noninvasive assessment of right ventricular systolic pressure in atrial septal defect [Letter]. *Am J Cardiol* 1984;54:1170.

54. Trowitzsch E, Ostrejz M, Evers D, Engert J, Brode P. Echocardiographic proof of pulmonary hypertension with irreversible increased resistance in the pulmonary circulation as a complication after placement of a ventriculo-atrial shunt for internal hydrocephalus. *Eur J Pediatr Surg* 1992;2:361–364.

55. Forker AD, Wilson CS, Weaver WF. Illustrative echocardiogram. Eisenmenger's syndrome, pulmonary valvular insufficiency, and paradoxic septal motion. *Chest* 1974;65:202–203.

56. Dick C, Asinger RW. Contrast echocardiographic detection of a right-to-left shunting patent ductus arteriosus. *J Am Soc Echocardiogr* 1989;2:198–201.

57. Kitabatake A, Inoue M, Asao M, et al. Noninvasive evaluation of pulmonary hypertension by a pulsed Doppler technique. *Circulation* 1983;68:302–309.

58. Dabestani A, Mahan G, Gardin JM, et al. Evaluation of pulmonary artery pressure and resistance by pulsed Doppler echocardiography. *Am J Cardiol* 1987;59:662–668.

59. Martin-Duran R, Larman M, Trugeda A, et al. Comparison of Doppler-determined elevated pulmonary arterial pressure with pressure measured at cardiac catheterization. Am J Cardiol 1986;57: 859–863.

60. Kosturakis D, Goldberg SJ, Allen HD, Loeber C. Doppler echocardiographic prediction of pulmonary arterial hypertension in congenital heart disease. Am J Cardiol 1984;53:1110–1115.

61. Matsuda M, Sekiguchi T, Sugishita Y, Kuwako K, Iida K, Ito I. Reliability of non-invasive estimates of pulmonary hypertension by pulsed Doppler echocardiography. Br Heart J 1986;56:158–164.

62. Isobe M, Yazaki Y, Takaku F, et al. Prediction of pulmonary arterial pressure in adults by pulsed Doppler echocardiography. Am J Cardiol 1986;57:316–321.

63. Friedman DM, Bierman FZ, Barst R. Gated pulsed Doppler evaluation of idiopathic pulmonary artery hypertension in children. Am J Cardiol 1986;58:369–370.

64. Serwer GA, Cougle AG, Eckerd JM, Armstrong BE. Factors affecting the use of the Doppler-determined time from flow onset to maximal pulmonary artery velocity for measurement of pulmonary artery pressure in children. Am J Cardiol 1986;58:352–356.

65. Panidis IP, Ross J, Mintz GS. Effect of sampling site on assessment of pulmonary artery blood flow by Doppler echocardiography. Am J Cardiol 1986;58:1145–1147.

66. Mallery JA, Gardin JM, King SW, Ey S, Henry WL. Effects of heart rate and pulmonary artery pressure on Doppler pulmonary artery acceleration time in experimental acute pulmonary hypertension. Chest 1991;100:470–473.

67. Chan KL, Currie PJ, Seward JB, Hagler DJ, Mair DD, Tajik AJ. Comparison of three Doppler ultrasound methods in the prediction of pulmonary artery pressure. J Am Coll Cardiol 1987;9:549–554.

68. Hatle L, Angelsen B. Doppler ultrasound in cardiology. 2nd ed. Philadelphia: Lea & Febiger, 1985.

69. Maciel DC, Simpson IA, Valdes-Cruz LM, et al. Color flow mapping studies of physiologic pulmonary and tricuspid regurgitation: evidence for true regurgitation as opposed to a valve closing volume. J Am Soc Echocardiogr 1991;4:589–597.

70. Yock PG, Popp RL. Noninvasive estimation of right ventricular systolic pressure by Doppler ultrasound in patients with tricuspid incompetence. Circulation 1984;70:657–662.

71. Currie PJ, Seward JB, Chan KL, et al. Continuous wave Doppler determination of right ventricular pressure: a simultaneous Doppler-catheterization study in 127 patients. J Am Coll Cardiol 1985;6: 750–756.

72. Homer HP, Takenn BL, Posma JL, Lie KI. Noninvasive measurement of right ventricular systolic pressure by combined color coded and continuous-wave Doppler ultrasound. Am J Cardiol 1988;61: 668–671.

73. Berger M, Haimowitz A, Van Tosh A, Berdoff RL, Goldberg E. Quantitative assessment of pulmonary hypertension in patients with tricuspid regurgitation using continuous wave Doppler ultrasound. J Am Coll Cardiol 1985;6:359–365.

74. Hatle L, Rokseth R. Noninvasive diagnosis and assessment of ventricular septal defect by Doppler ultrasound. Acta Med Scand 1981; 645[Suppl]:47–56.

75. Murphy DJ, Ludomirsky A, Huhta JC. Continuous-wave Doppler in children with ventricular septal defect: noninvasive estimation of interventricular pressure gradient. Am J Cardiol 1986;57:428–432.

76. Marx GR, Allen HD, Goldberg SJ. Doppler echocardiographic estimation of systolic pulmonary artery pressure in pediatric patients with interventricular communications. J Am Coll Cardiol 1985;6: 1132–1137.

77. Silbert DR, Brunson SC, Schiff R. Determination of right ventricular pressure in the presence of a ventricular septal defect using continuous wave Doppler ultrasound. J Am Coll Cardiol 1986;8: 379–384.

78. Stevenson JG, Kawabori I, Guntheroth WG. Noninvasive detection of pulmonary hypertension in patent ductus arteriosus by pulsed Doppler echocardiography. Circulation 1979;60:355–359.

79. Masuyama T, Kodama K, Kitabatake A, Sato H, Nanto S, Inoue M. Continuous-wave Doppler echocardiographic detection of pulmonary regurgitation and its application to noninvasive estimation of pulmonary artery pressure. Circulation 1986;74:484–492.

80. Waggoner AD, Quinones MA, Young JB, et al. Pulsed Doppler echocardiographic detection of right-sided valve regurgitation. Experimental results and clinical significance. Am J Cardiol 1981;47: 279–286.

81. Ivy D, Neish S, Knudson O, et al. Intravascular ultrasonic characteristics and vasoreactivity of the pulmonary vasculature in children with pulmonary hypertension. Am J Cardiol 1998;81;740–748.

82. Berger RMF, Cromme-Dijkhuis AH, Van Vliet AM, Hess J. Evaluation of the pulmonary vasculature and dynamics with intravascular ultrasound imaging in children and infants. Pediatr Res 1995;38: 36–41.

83. Ricou F, Nicod PH, Moser KM, Peterson KL. Catheter-based intravascular ultrasound imaging of chronic thromboembolic pulmonary disease. Am J Cardiol 1991;67:749–752.

84. Ishii M, Kato H, Kawano T, et al. Evaluation of pulmonary artery histopathologic findings in congenital heart disease: an in vitro study using intravascular ultrasound imaging. J Am Coll Cardiol 1995; 26:272–276.

85. Kravitz KD, Scharf GR, Chandrasekaran K. In vivo diagnosis of pulmonary atherosclerosis. Role of intravascular ultrasound. Chest 1994;106:632–634.

86. Scott PJ, Essop AR, Al-Ashab W, Deaner A, Parsons J, Williams G. Imaging of pulmonary vascular disease by intravascular ultrasound. Int J Card Imaging 1993;9:179–184.

87. Porter TR, Taylor DO, Fields J, et al. Direct in-vivo evaluation of pulmonary arterial pathology in chronic congestive heart failure with catheter-based intravascular ultrasound imaging. Am J Cardiol 1993;71:754–757.

88. Wagenvoort CA, Nauta J, Van der Schaar PJ, Weeda HWH, Wagenvoort N. The pulmonary vasculature in complete transposition of the great vessels, judged from lung biopsies. Circulation 1968;38: 746–754.

89. Heath D, Helmholz HF, Burchell HB, DuShane JW, Kirklin JW, Edwards JE. Relation between structural changes in the small pulmonary arteries and the immediate reversibility of pulmonary hypertension following closure of ventricular and atrial septal defects. Circulation 1958;18:1167–1174.

90. Haworth SG. Pulmonary vascular disease in different types of congenital heart disease: implications for interpretation of lung biopsy findings in early childhood. Br Heart J 1984;52:557–571.

91. Hislop A, Haworth SG, Shinebourne EA, Reid L. Quantitative structural analysis of pulmonary vessels in isolated ventricular septal defects in infancy. Br Heart J 1975;37:1014–1021.

92. Haworth SG, Reid L. A morphometric study of regional variation in lung structure in infants with pulmonary hypertension and congenital heart defect. A justification of lung biopsy. Br Heart J 1978; 40:825–831.

Subject Index

Page numbers followed by *f* refer to figures, page numbers followed by *e* refer to echocardiograms, and page numbers followed by *t* refer to tables.